Brief Contents

Unit 1
How Nurses Think 1

Chapter 1	Evolution of Nursing Thought & Action 3
Chapter 2	Clinical Judgment 7
Chapter 3	The Steps of the Nursing Process 12
Chapter 4	Evidence-Based Practice: Theory & Research 25
Chapter 5	Ethics & Values 31

Unit 2
Factors Affecting Health 39

Chapter 6	Life Span: Infancy Through Middle Adulthood 41
Chapter 7	Life Span: Older Adults 53
Chapter 8	Experiencing Wellness: Health & Illness 59
Chapter 9	Stress & Adaptation 79
Chapter 10	Psychosocial Health & Illness 89
Chapter 11	Promoting Family Health 101
Chapter 12	Caring in Multicultural Healthcare Environments 108
Chapter 13	Spirituality 118
Chapter 14	Experiencing Loss 126

Unit 3
Essential Nursing Interventions 139

Chapter 15	Communication & Therapeutic Relationships 141
Chapter 16	Patient Education 149
Chapter 17	Interprofessional Partnerships: Documenting & Reporting 156
Chapter 18	Measuring Vital Signs 172
Chapter 19	Health Assessment 198
Chapter 20	Promoting Asepsis & Preventing Infection 302
Chapter 21	Promoting Safety 331
Chapter 22	Facilitating Hygiene 345
Chapter 23	Administering Medications 391

Unit 4
Supporting Physiological Functioning 477

Chapter 24	Nutrition 479
Chapter 25	Urinary Elimination 516
Chapter 26	Bowel Elimination 559
Chapter 27	Sensation, Perception, & Response 595
Chapter 28	Pain 605
Chapter 29	Physical Activity & Immobility 616
Chapter 30	Sexual Health 638
Chapter 31	Sleep & Rest 650
Chapter 32	Skin Integrity & Wound Healing 658
Chapter 33	Oxygenation 705
Chapter 34	Circulation & Perfusion 758
Chapter 35	Hydration & Homeostasis 767
Chapter 36	Caring for the Surgical Patient 810

Unit 5
Nursing Functions 835

Chapter 37	Community & Home Health Nursing 837
Chapter 38	Informatics 846
Chapter 39	Legal Accountability 851
Chapter 40	Leading & Managing 859

Credits 864

Index 866

DAVIS ADVANTAGE for

Wilkinson's FUNDAMENTALS OF NURSING

Thinking, Doing, and Caring

FIFTH EDITION

Volume Two

Leslie S. Treas, PhD, RN, CPNP-PC, NNP-BC

Karen L. Barnett, DNP, RN

Mable H. Smith, PhD, JD, MN, NEA-BC

F.A. DAVIS
Philadelphia

F. A. Davis Company
1915 Arch Street
Philadelphia, PA 19103
www.fadavis.com

Copyright © 2024 by F. A. Davis Company

Copyright © 2024 by F. A. Davis Company. All rights reserved. This book is protected by copyright. No part of it may be reproduced, stored in a retrieval system, or transmitted in any form or by any means, electronic, mechanical, photocopying, recording, or otherwise, without written permission from the publisher.

Printed in China

Last digit indicates print number: 10 9 8 7 6 5 4 3 2 1

Senior Acquisitions Editor: Jacalyn Sharp
Senior Content Project Manager: Amy Romano
Design and Illustrations Manager: Carolyn O'Brien

ISBN: 978-1-7196-4798-4

As new scientific information becomes available through basic and clinical research, recommended treatments and drug therapies undergo changes. The author(s) and publisher have done everything possible to make this book accurate, up to date, and in accord with accepted standards at the time of publication. The author(s), editors, and publisher are not responsible for errors or omissions or for consequences from application of the book, and make no warranty, expressed or implied, in regard to the contents of the book. Any practice described in this book should be applied by the reader in accordance with professional standards of care used in regard to the unique circumstances that may apply in each situation. The reader is advised always to check product information (package inserts) for changes and new information regarding dose and contraindications before administering any drug. Caution is especially urged when using new or infrequently ordered drugs.

Library of Congress Cataloging-in-Publication Data

Names: Treas, Leslie S., author. | Barnett, Karen L., author. | Smith, Mable H., author. | Wilkinson, Judith M., 1946- Davis advantage for fundamentals of nursing.
Title: Davis advantage for Wilkinson's fundamentals of nursing: theory, concepts, and applications / Leslie S. Treas, Karen L. Barnett, Mable H. Smith.
Other titles: Advantage for Wilkinson's fundamentals of nursing
Description: Fifth edition. | Philadelphia, PA: F.A. Davis Company, [2024] | Preceded by Davis advantage for fundamentals of nursing / Judith M. Wilkinson, Leslie S. Treas, Karen L. Barnett, Mable H. Smith. Fourth edition. [2020]. | Includes bibliographical references and index.
Identifiers: LCCN 2023015270 (print) | LCCN 2023015271 (ebook) | ISBN 9781719647977 (v. 1 ; hardcover) | ISBN 9781719647984 (v. 2 ; paperback) | ISBN 9781719650540 (ebook)
Subjects: MESH: Nursing Process | Nursing Care | Nursing Theory
Classification: LCC RT49 (print) | LCC RT49 (ebook) | NLM WY 100.1 | DDC 610.73—dc23/eng/20230516
LC record available at https://lccn.loc.gov/2023015270
LC ebook record available at https://lccn.loc.gov/2023015271

Authorization to photocopy items for internal or personal use, or the internal or personal use of specific clients, is granted by F. A. Davis Company for users registered with the Copyright Clearance Center (CCC) Transactional Reporting Service, provided that the fee of $.25 per copy is paid directly to CCC, 222 Rosewood Drive, Danvers, MA 01923. For those organizations that have been granted a photocopy license by CCC, a separate system of payment has been arranged. The fee code for users of the Transactional Reporting Service is: 978-1-7196-4798-4/23 0 + $.25.

Preface

We chose our book title carefully. We have used the words *theory, concepts, application, thinking, doing,* and *caring* because we believe that excellent nursing requires an equal mix of knowledge, thought, and action. Nurses use all of these to express caring. It is knowledge and its application—not just the tasks nurses do—that delineate the various levels of nursing. Even so, skillful performance of tasks is essential to full attainment of the nursing role.

We present our material in two volumes to enable students to focus on material suitable for use in specific venues. Volume 2 is a compact, easy-to-carry reference to use in the skills lab and in clinical experiences. This volume contains practical, step-by-step information for safely performing nursing actions and interacting with real patients. Rationales for each action explain the why behind the what to help you practice nursing based on concepts rather than cookbook-style action. Volume 2 offers practice-based forms, assessment questionnaires, and other clinical tips, but it is not limited to skills and procedures. It includes both thinking and doing, the same as Volume 1; however, the emphasis is unique in each volume. Volume 2 works seamlessly with Volume 1, the skills videos, and Davis Advantage to provide a user-friendly learning experience that will surely stimulate new enthusiasm for learning. For example, throughout Volume 2, students are offered a family case study, known as Caring for the Williams Family, through which they apply our full-spectrum model of nursing to learn about the nursing role, the healthcare system, and the real-world application of the content in Volume 1.

Other features in each chapter of this volume include critical-thinking activities (Critical Thinking and Clinical Judgment), step-by-step procedures, Clinical Insights (with rationales), assessment guidelines and tools, a summary of the main points covered in Volume 1, and a knowledge map of the concepts discussed in the chapter. These features will be useful during each student's clinical day. In addition, Thinking About the Procedures exercises to tie the procedures to the skills videos are available on the Davis's Nursing Skills Videos Web site on www.fadavis.com.

Volume 2 (as well as Volume 1) will appeal to nontraditional students of the technological generation, encourage independent learning, promote critical thinking, support a variety of learning styles, and assure students that it is possible to achieve excellent nursing despite today's challenges.

We hope you will read the other introductory material in the front of Volume 1. It explains the philosophical underpinnings for this text and describes in more detail how to use the various pieces of this highly integrated learning package, which is flexible enough to accommodate a variety of teaching styles and curriculums.

Contents

Unit 1
How Nurses Think   1

CHAPTER 1
Evolution of Nursing Thought & Action   3
Caring for the Williams Family   3
Clinical Reasoning   4
    Critical Thinking and Clinical Judgment   4
Knowledge Map   6

CHAPTER 2
Clinical Judgment   7
Caring for the Williams Family   7
Clinical Reasoning   8
    Applying the Full-Spectrum Nursing Model   8
    Critical Thinking and Clinical Judgment   9
Knowledge Map   11

CHAPTER 3
The Steps of the Nursing Process   12
Caring for the Williams Family   12
Assessment Guidelines and Tools   13
    Evaluation Checklist   15
    Functional Ability Assessment   17
    Applying the Full-Spectrum Nursing Model   19
    Critical Thinking & Clinical Judgment   20
Knowledge Map   24

CHAPTER 4
Evidence-Based Practice: Theory & Research   25
Caring for the Williams Family   25
Clinical Reasoning   26
    Applying the Full-Spectrum Nursing Model   26
    Critical Thinking and Clinical Judgment   26
Knowledge Map   30

CHAPTER 5
Ethics & Values   31
Caring for the Williams Family   31
Practical Knowledge: Clinical Application   32
Clinical Insights   32
Clinical Insight 5-1: Using the MORAL Model for Ethical Decision Making   32
Clinical Insight 5-2: Guidelines for Advocacy   33
Clinical Reasoning   33
    Applying the Full-Spectrum Nursing Model   33
    Critical Thinking and Clinical Judgment   34
Knowledge Map   38

Unit 2
Factors Affecting Health   39

CHAPTER 6
Life Span: Infancy Through Middle Adulthood   41
Caring for the Williams Family   41

vii

viii   CONTENTS

Practical Knowledge: Clinical Application   42
Procedures   42
Procedure 6-1: Assessing for Abuse   43
Assessment Guidelines & Tools   48
    Fetal Development   48
    Apgar Scoring   50
Clinical Reasoning   50
    Applying the Full-Spectrum Nursing Model   50
    Critical Thinking and Clinical Judgment   50
Knowledge Map   52

CHAPTER 7
Life Span: Older Adults   53

Caring for the Williams Family   53
Practical Knowledge: Clinical Application   54
Assessment Guidelines and Tools   54
    Assessment for All Older Adults   54
Clinical Reasoning   55
    Applying the Full-Spectrum Nursing Model   55
    Critical Thinking and Clinical Judgment   56
Knowledge Map   58

CHAPTER 8
Experiencing Wellness: Health & Illness   59

Caring for the Williams Family   59
Procedures   60
Procedure 8-1: Admitting a Patient to a Nursing Unit   60
Procedure 8-2: Transferring a Patient to Another Unit in the Agency   63
Procedure 8-3: Transferring a Patient to a Long-Term Care Facility   64
Procedure 8-4: Discharging a Patient From the Healthcare Facility   66
Clinical Insights   69
Clinical Insight 8-1: Preparing the Room for an Admission   69
Forms   70
    Discharge Assessment/Instructions   70
Assessment Guidelines and Tools   72
    Health Promotion: Physical Fitness Assessment   72
    Lifestyle and Risk Assessment   73
Clinical Reasoning   75
    Applying the Full-Spectrum Nursing Model   75
    Critical Thinking and Clinical Judgment   76
Knowledge Map   78

CHAPTER 9
Stress & Adaptation   79

Caring for the Williams Family   79
Practical Knowledge: Clinical Application   80
Clinical Insights   80
Clinical Insight 9-1: Dealing With Angry Patients   80
Clinical Insight 9-2: Crisis Intervention Guidelines   81
Assessment Guidelines and Tools   82
    The Holmes-Rahe Social Readjustment Scale   82
    Assessing for Stress: Questions to Ask   83
Clinical Reasoning   84
    Applying the Full-Spectrum Nursing Model   84
    Critical Thinking and Clinical Judgment   85
Knowledge Map   88

CHAPTER 10
Psychosocial Health & Illness   89

Caring for the Williams Family   89
Practical Knowledge: Clinical Application   90
Clinical Insights   90
Clinical Insight 10-1: Assessing Self-Concept   90
Clinical Insight 10-2: Performing a Self-Esteem Inventory   91
Clinical Insight 10-3: Identifying Depressed Patients Who Should Be Referred for Evaluation   92
Assessment Guidelines and Tools   93
    Anxiety Assessment Guide   93
    Depression Assessment Guide: Patient Health Questionnaire (PHQ-9)   94
    Differentiating Depression and Dementia   95
Clinical Reasoning   95
    Applying the Full-Spectrum Nursing Model   95
    Critical Thinking and Clinical Judgment   96
Knowledge Map   100

CHAPTER 11
Promoting Family Health   101

Caring for the Williams Family   101
Practical Knowledge: Clinical Application   102
Clinical Insights   102
Clinical Insight 11-1: Conducting a Family Assessment   102

Assessment Guidelines and Tools 103
  Assessing Family Developmental Tasks 103
Clinical Reasoning 104
  Applying the Full-Spectrum Nursing Model 104
  Critical Thinking and Clinical Judgment 105
Knowledge Map 107

CHAPTER 12
Caring in Multicultural Healthcare Environments 108

Caring for the Williams Family 108
Practical Knowledge: Clinical Application 109
Clinical Insights 109
Clinical Insight 12-1: Understanding Biological Variations 109
Clinical Insight 12-2: Communicating With Clients Who Speak a Different Language 110
Assessment Guidelines and Tools 111
  Obtaining Minimum Cultural Information 111
  Cultural Assessment Using the Transcultural Assessment Model 112
Clinical Reasoning 113
  Applying the Full-Spectrum Nursing Model 113
  Critical Thinking and Clinical Judgment 114
Knowledge Map 117

CHAPTER 13
Spirituality 118

Caring for the Williams Family 118
Practical Knowledge: Clinical Application 119
Clinical Insights 119
Clinical Insight 13-1: Types of Prayers 119
Clinical Insight 13-2: Praying With Clients 120
Assessment Guidelines and Tools 121
  The HOPE Approach to Spiritual Assessment: Examples of Questions 121
  SPIRIT Assessment 122
Clinical Reasoning 123
  Applying the Full-Spectrum Nursing Model 123
  Critical Thinking and Clinical Judgment 123
Knowledge Map 125

CHAPTER 14
Experiencing Loss 126

Caring for the Williams Family 126
Practical Knowledge: Clinical Application 127
Clinical Insights 127
Clinical Insight 14-1: Communicating With People Who Are Grieving 127
Clinical Insight 14-2: Helping Families of Dying Patients 127
Clinical Insight 14-3: Caring for the Dying Person: Meeting Physiological Needs 128
Clinical Insight 14-4: Caring for the Dying Person: Meeting Psychological Needs 130
Clinical Insight 14-5: Providing Postmortem Care 130
Assessment Guidelines and Tools 132
  Assessing Grief and Loss 132
Clinical Reasoning 134
  Applying the Full-Spectrum Nursing Model 134
  Critical Thinking and Clinical Judgment 134
Knowledge Map 138

Unit 3
Essential Nursing Interventions 139

CHAPTER 15
Communication & Therapeutic Relationships 141

Caring for the Williams Family 141
Practical Knowledge: Clinical Application 142
Clinical Insights 142
Clinical Insight 15-1: Collaborative Professional Communication 142
Clinical Insight 15-2: Communicating With SBARQ* 143
Clinical Insight 15-3: Communicating With Clients From Another Culture 144
Assessment Guidelines and Tools 144
  Communication 144
Clinical Reasoning 145
  Applying the Full-Spectrum Nursing Model 145
  Critical Thinking and Clinical Judgment 146
Knowledge Map 148

CHAPTER 16

Patient Education 149

Caring for the Williams Family 149

Practical Knowledge: Clinical Application 150

Assessment Guidelines and Tools 150
Learning Assessment 150

Clinical Reasoning 151
Applying the Full-Spectrum Nursing Model 151
Critical Thinking and Clinical Judgment 152

Knowledge Map 155

CHAPTER 17

Interprofessional Partnerships: Documenting & Reporting 156

Caring for the Williams Family 156

Practical Knowledge: Clinical Application 157

Clinical Insights 157

Clinical Insight 17-1: Giving Oral Reports 157

Clinical Insight 17-2: Receiving Telephone and Verbal Prescriptions 159

Clinical Insight 17-3: Guidelines for Documentation 159

Clinical Insight 17-4: Guidelines for Paper Health Records 163

Tables 163
Abbreviations Commonly Used in Healthcare 163

Documentation Forms 166
Adult Admission History Electronic Screen 166
Nursing Assessment Flowsheets are Comprehensive Charting Documents 167

Clinical Reasoning 168
Applying the Full-Spectrum Nursing Model 168
Critical Thinking and Clinical Judgment 168

Knowledge Map 171

CHAPTER 18

Measuring Vital Signs 172

Caring for the Williams Family 172

Practical Knowledge: Clinical Application 173

Procedures 173

Procedure 18-1: Assessing Body Temperature 173
Procedure 18-1A: Taking an Axillary Temperature 174
Procedure 18-1B: Taking an Oral Temperature 175
Procedure 18-1C: Taking a Rectal Temperature 175
Procedure 18-1D: Taking a Temporal Artery Temperature 176
Procedure 18-1E: Taking a Tympanic membrane Temperature 177
Procedure 18-1F: Taking a Skin Temperature Using a Chemical Strip Thermometer 178

Procedure 18-2: Assessing peripheral Pulses 179
Procedure 18-2A: Assessing the Radial Pulse 180
Procedure 18-2B: Assessing the Brachial Pulse 180
Procedure 18-2C: Assessing the Carotid Pulse 181
Procedure 18-2D: Assessing the Dorsalis Pedis Pulse 181
Procedure 18-2E: Assessing the Femoral Pulse 182
Procedure 18-2F: Assessing the Posterior Tibial Pulse 182
Procedure 18-2G: Assessing the Popliteal Pulse 182
Procedure 18-2H: Assessing the Temporal Pulse 183

Procedure 18-3: Assessing the Apical Pulse 184

Procedure 18-4: Assessing for an Apical-Radial Pulse Deficit 186

Procedure 18-5: Assessing Respirations 187

Procedure 18-6: Measuring Blood Pressure 189

Clinical Insights 193

Clinical Insight 18-1: Choosing a Blood Pressure Cuff Size 193

Clinical Insight 18-2: Taking an Accurate Blood Pressure 193

Clinical Insight 18-3: Teaching Your Patient About Hypertension 194

Clinical Reasoning 194
Applying the Full-Spectrum Nursing Model 194
Critical Thinking and Clinical Judgment 195

Knowledge Map 197

CHAPTER 19

Health Assessment 198

Caring for the Williams Family 198

Practical Knowledge: Clinical Application 199

Procedures 199

Procedure 19-1: Performing the General Survey 200
Procedure 19-2: Assessing the Skin 206
Procedure 19-3: Assessing the Hair 215
Procedure 19-4: Assessing the Nails 216
Procedure 19-5: Assessing the Head and Face 218
Procedure 19-6: Assessing the Eyes 220
Procedure 19-7: Assessing the Ears and Hearing 227
Procedure 19-8: Assessing the Nose and Sinuses 232
Procedure 19-9: Assessing the Mouth and Oropharynx 234
Procedure 19-10: Assessing the Neck 238
Procedure 19-11: Assessing the Breasts and Axillae 240
Procedure 19-12: Assessing the Chest and Lungs 244

Procedure 19-13: Assessing the Heart and Vascular System   250

Procedure 19-14: Assessing the Abdomen   257

Procedure 19-15: Assessing the Musculoskeletal System   263

Procedure 19-16: Assessing the Sensory-Neurological System   272

Procedure 19-17: Assessing the Male Genitourinary System   285

Procedure 19-18: Assessing the Female Genitourinary System   290

Procedure 19-19: Assessing the Anus and Rectum   294

Procedure 19-20: Brief Bedside Assessment   295

Clinical Insights   297

Clinical Insight 19-1: Performing Percussion   297

Clinical Insight 19-2: Performing Auscultation   298

Clinical Insight 19-3: Assisting With a Speculum Examination   298

Knowledge Map   301

CHAPTER 20

Promoting Asepsis & Preventing Infection   302

Caring for the Williams Family   302

Practical Knowledge: Clinical Application   303

Procedures   303

Procedure 20-1: Hand Hygiene   303
  Procedure 20-1A: Using Soap and Water   303
  Procedure 20-1B: Using Alcohol-Based Handrubs   304

Procedure 20-2: Donning Personal Protective Equipment (PPE)   305

Procedure 20-3: Removing Personal Protective Equipment (PPE)   307

Procedure 20-4: Surgical Hand Washing: Traditional Method   309

Procedure 20-5: Surgical Hand Washing: Brushless System   311

Procedure 20-6: Sterile Gown and Gloves (Closed Method)   314

Procedure 20-7: Sterile Gloves (Open Method)   316

Procedure 20-8: Sterile Fields   318
  Procedure 20-8A: Setting Up a Sterile Field   318
  Procedure 20-8B: Adding Supplies to a Sterile Field   319
  Procedure 20-8C: Adding Sterile Solutions to a Sterile Field   320

Clinical Insights   321

Clinical Insight 20-1: Guidelines for Hand Hygiene   321

Clinical Insight 20-2: Providing a Clean Patient Environment   322

Clinical Insight 20-3: Following CDC Standard Precautions   323

Clinical Insight 20-4: Following Transmission-Based Precautions   325

Diagnostic Testing   327

Common Tests for Evaluating the Presence of or Risk for Infection   327

Clinical Reasoning   327

Applying the Full-Spectrum Nursing Model   327
Critical Thinking and Clinical Judgment   328

Knowledge Map   330

CHAPTER 21

Promoting Safety   331

Caring for the Williams Family   331

Practical Knowledge: Clinical Application   332

Procedures   332

Procedure 21-1: Using Bed and Chair Monitoring Devices   332

Procedure 21-2: Using Restraints   334

Clinical Insights   338

Clinical Insight 21-1: Choking Rescue Maneuver   338

Clinical Insight 21-2: Preventing Needlestick Injury   338

Clinical Insight 21-3: What You Should Know About Using Restraints   339

Assessment Guidelines and Tools   340

Clinical Reasoning   341

Applying the Full-Spectrum Nursing Model   341
Critical Thinking and Clinical Judgment   342

Knowledge Map   344

CHAPTER 22

Facilitating Hygiene   345

Caring for the Williams Family   345

Practical Knowledge: Clinical Application   346

Procedures   346

Procedure 22-1: Bathing: Providing a Complete Bed Bath Using a Prepackaged Bathing Product   346

Procedure 22-2: Bathing: Using a Basin and Water   351

Procedure 22-3: Providing Perineal Care   352

Procedure 22-4: Providing Foot Care   355

Procedure 22-5: Brushing and Flossing the Teeth   358

Procedure 22-6: Providing Denture Care   361

Procedure 22-7: Providing Oral Care for an Unconscious Patient   363

Procedure 22-8: Shampooing the Hair   366
  Procedure 22-8A: Shampooing the Hair for a Patient on Bedrest Using Rinse-Free Shampoo   366
  Procedure 22-8B: Shampooing the Hair Using Rinse-Free Shampoo Cap   367
  Procedure 22-8C: Shampooing the Hair Using a Basin and Water   367
Procedure 22-9: Providing Beard and Mustache Care   369
Procedure 22-10: Shaving a Patient   370
Procedure 22-11: Removing and Caring for Contact Lenses   372
Procedure 22-12: Caring for Artificial Eyes   374
Procedure 22-13: Caring for Hearing Aids   375
Procedure 22-14: Making an Unoccupied Bed   377
Procedure 22-15: Making an Occupied Bed   380
Clinical Insight   383
Clinical Insight 22-1: Assisting With a Shower or Tub Bath   383
Assessment Guidelines and Tools   384
  Guidelines for Assessing Hygiene   384
Clinical Reasoning   386
  Applying the Full-Spectrum Nursing Model   386
  Critical Thinking and Clinical Judgment   386
Knowledge Map   390

CHAPTER 23

Administering Medications   391

Caring for the Williams Family   391
Practical Knowledge: Clinical Application   392
Procedures   392
Medication Guidelines: Steps to Follow for All Medications (Regardless of Type or Route)   392
Procedure 23-1: Administering Oral Medications   396
  Procedure 23-1A: Administering Medication Through an Enteral Tube   398
Procedure 23-2: Administering Ophthalmic Medication   400
  Procedure 23-2A: Irrigating the Eyes   402
Procedure 23-3: Administering Otic Medication   403
Procedure 23-4: Administering Nasal Medication   405
Procedure 23-5: Administering Vaginal Medication   407
Procedure 23-6: Inserting a Rectal Suppository   409
  Procedure 23-6A: Inserting a Macy Catheter   411
Procedure 23-7: Applying Medication to Skin   412
  Procedure 23-7A: Applying Topical Lotion, Cream, and Ointment   413
  Procedure 23-7B: Applying Topical Aerosol Spray   413
  Procedure 23-7C: Applying Prescribed Powder   413
  Procedure 23-7D: Applying Transdermal Medication   413
Procedure 23-8: Administering Metered-Dose Inhaler (MDI) Medication   415
Procedure 23-9: Preparing, Drawing Up, and Mixing Medication   417
  Procedure 23-9A: Drawing Up Medication From Ampules   418
  Procedure 23-9B: Drawing Up Medication From Vials   419
  Procedure 23-9C: Mixing Medication From Two Vials   421
  Procedure 23-9D: Mixing Medications From One Ampule and One Vial   423
  Procedure 23-9E: Using a Prefilled Cartridge and Single-Dose Vial—For Intravenous Administration   424
Procedure 23-10: Recapping Needles Using a One-Handed Technique   426
  Procedure 23-10A: Recapping Contaminated Needles   427
  Procedure 23-10B: Recapping Sterile Needles   427
Procedure 23-11: Administering Intradermal Medication   428
Procedure 23-12: Administering Subcutaneous Medication   431
Procedure 23-13: Locating Intramuscular Injection Sites   434
  Procedure 23-13A: Locating the Ventrogluteal Site   434
  Procedure 23-13B: Locating the Deltoid Site   435
  Procedure 23-13C: Locating the Vastus Lateralis Site   435
  Procedure 23-13D: Locating the Rectus Femoris Site   436
Procedure 23-14: Administering an Intramuscular Injection   437
  Procedure 23-14A: Intramuscular Injection: Traditional Method   437
  Procedure 23-14B: Intramuscular Injection: Z-Track Method   438
Procedure 23-15: Adding Medications to Intravenous Fluids   440
Procedure 23-16: Administering IV Push Medication   441
  Procedure 23-16A: Administering IV Push Medications Through a Primary IV Line   442
  Procedure 23-16B: Administering IV Push Medications Through an Intermittent Device (IV Lock) When No Extension Tubing Is attached to the Venous Access Device   443
  Procedure 23-16C: Administering IV Push Medications Through an intermittent Device With IV Extension Tubing   444
Procedure 23-17: Administering medication by Intermittent Infusion   446
  Procedure 23-17A: Using a Piggyback Administration Set With a Gravity Infusion   446
  Procedure 23-17B: Using a Piggyback Administration Set With an Infusion Pump   447
  Procedure 23-17C: Using a Volume-Control Administration Set   448

CONTENTS xiii

Procedure 23-18: Administering Medication Through a Central Venous Access Device (CVAD) 450

Practical Knowledge: Clinical Application 453

Clinical Insights 453

Clinical Insight 23-1: Taking Action After a Medication Error 453

Clinical Insight 23-2: Using Prefilled Unit-Dose Systems 454

Clinical Insight 23-3: Reconstituting Medication 455

Clinical Insight 23-4: Measuring Dosage When Changing Needles 456

Clinical Insight 23-5: Mixing Two Kinds of Insulin in One Syringe 457

Clinical Insight 23-6: Administering Anticoagulant Medication Subcutaneously 458

Tables: Abbreviations 459

Common Medication-Related Abbreviations 459
Table Institute for Safe Medication Practices (ISMP) List of Error-Prone Abbreviations, Symbols, and Dose Designations 460

Measuring and Calculating Dosage 466

Medication Measurement Systems 466
Calculating Dosages 467

Clinical Reasoning 469

Applying the Full-Spectrum Nursing Model 469
Critical Thinking & Clinical Judgment 470

Knowledge Map 475

Unit 4
Supporting Physiological Functioning 477

CHAPTER 24
Nutrition 479

Caring for the Williams Family 479

Practical Knowledge: Clinical Application 480

Procedures 480

Procedure 24-1: Checking Fingerstick (capillary) Blood Glucose Levels 480

Procedure 24-2: Inserting Nasogastric and Nasoenteric Tubes 483

Procedure 24-3: Administering Feedings Through Gastric and Enteric Tubes 488

Procedure 24-3A: Administering Feedings Through Gastric and Enteric Tubes using a Closed System: Infusion Pump 489

Procedure 24-3B: Administering Feedings Through Gastric and Enteric Tubes using an Open System: Syringe 490

Procedure 24-4: Removing a Nasogastric or Nasoenteric Tube 493

Procedure 24-5: Administering Parenteral Nutrition 494

Procedure 24-6: Administering Lipids 498

Clinical Insights 500

Clinical Insight 24-1: Measurements to Evaluate Body Composition 500

Clinical Insight 24-2: Assisting patients With Meals 502

Clinical Insight 24-3: Monitoring Patients Receiving Enteral Nutrition 503

Clinical Insight 24-4: Monitoring and Maintenance Interventions for Patients Receiving Parenteral Nutrition 504

Assessment Guidelines and Tools 505

Screening for Nutrition Problems 505
Subjective Global Assessment 505
Nutrition Screening Initiative (NSI) for Older Adults: Indications of Impaired Nutrition Status 505
Mini-Nutritional Assessment 506
Focused Assessment 506
Focused Nutrition Assessment 506

Diagnostic Testing 510

Tests Reflecting Nutrition Status: Norms 510

Clinical Reasoning 510

Applying the Full-Spectrum Nursing Model 510
Critical Thinking and Clinical Judgment 511

Knowledge Map 515

CHAPTER 25
Urinary Elimination 516

Caring for the Williams Family 516

Practical Knowledge: Clinical Application 517

Procedures 517

Procedure 25-1: Measuring Postvoid Residual Urine Volume With a Portable Bladder Scanner 517

Procedure 25-2: Obtaining a Urine Specimen for Testing 519

Procedure 25-2A: Collecting a Clean-Catch Urine Specimen 520
Procedure 25-2B: Obtaining a Sterile Urine Specimen From a Catheter 521
Procedure 25-2C: Collecting a 24-Hour Urine Specimen 521

Procedure 25-3: Inserting an Intermittent Urinary Catheter (Straight Catheter) 523

Procedure 25-4: Inserting an Indwelling Urinary Catheter 529

Procedure 25-5: Applying an External (Condom) Urinary Catheter 535

Procedure 25-6: Removing an Indwelling Catheter 537

Procedure 25-7: Irrigating the Bladder or Catheter 540
   Procedure 25-7A: Intermittent Bladder or Catheter Irrigation 540
   Procedure 25-7B: Continuous Bladder Irrigation 542

Clinical Insight 544

Clinical Insight 25-1: Teaching Clients About Clean, Intermittent Self-Catheterization 544

Assessment Guidelines and Tools 545
   Urinary Elimination History Questions 545
   Guidelines for Physical Assessment for Urinary Elimination 546

Diagnostic Testing 547
   Urinalysis 547
   Blood Studies: BUN and Creatinine 548
   Studies of the Urinary System 549
   Nursing Care Plan 551

Clinical Reasoning 555
   Applying the Full-Spectrum Nursing Model 555
   Critical Thinking and Clinical Judgment 556

Knowledge Map 558

CHAPTER 26

Bowel Elimination 559

Caring for the Williams Family 559

Practical Knowledge: Clinical Application 560

Procedures 560

Procedure 26-1: Testing Stool for Occult Blood 560

Procedure 26-2: Placing and Removing a Bedpan 562
   Procedure 26-2A: Placing a Bedpan 563
   Procedure 26-2B: Removing a Bedpan 564

Procedure 26-3: Administering an Enema 565
   Procedure 26-3A: Administering a Cleansing Enema 566
   Procedure 26-3B: Administering a Prepackaged Enema 567
   Procedure 26-3C: Administering an Oil-Retention Enema 568
   Procedure 26-3D: Administering a Return-Flow Enema 568

Procedure 26-4: Removing Stool Digitally 569

Procedure 26-5: Inserting a Rectal Tube 571

Procedure 26-6: Changing an Ostomy Appliance 573

Procedure 26-7: Irrigating a Colostomy 577

Procedure 26-8: Placing Fecal Drainage Devices 579
   Procedure 26-8A: Applying an External Fecal Collection System 580
   Procedure 26-8B: Inserting an Indwelling Fecal Drainage Device 581

Clinical Insights 583

Clinical Insight 26-1: Caring for a Patient With an Indwelling Fecal Drainage Device 583

Clinical Insight 26-2: Guidelines for Ostomy Care 584

Assessment Guidelines and Tools 585
   Bowel Elimination 585

Diagnostic Testing 586
   Direct Visualization Studies of the Gastrointestinal Tract 586
   Indirect Visualization Studies of the Gastrointestinal Tract 587
   Nursing Care Plan 589

Clinical Reasoning 591
   Applying the Full-Spectrum Nursing Model 591
   Critical Thinking and Clinical Judgment 592

Knowledge Map 594

CHAPTER 27

Sensation, Perception, & Response 595

Caring for the Williams Family 595

Practical Knowledge: Clinical Application 596

Procedures 596

Procedure 30-1: Performing Otic Irrigation 596

Clinical Insights 598

Clinical Insight 30-1: Communicating With Clients Who Are Visually Impaired 598

Clinical Insight 30-2: Communicating With Clients Who Are Hearing Impaired 598

Assessment Guidelines and Tools 599
   Hearing Screening in Older Adults 599
   Other Sensory Assessment Tools 599
   Nursing History: Overall Sensory–Perceptual Status 599
   Bedside Assessment of Sensory Function 601

Clinical Reasoning 601
   Applying the Full-Spectrum Nursing Model 601
   Critical Thinking & Clinical Judgment 602

Knowledge Map 604

CHAPTER 28

Pain 605

Caring for the Williams Family 605

Practical Knowledge Knowing How 606

Procedure 606

Procedure 28-1: Setting Up and managing Patient-Controlled Analgesia by Pump 606

Clinical Insight   609
Clinical Insight 28-1: Caring for the Patient With an Epidural Catheter   609
Assessment Guidelines and Tools   610
  Pain Assessment   610
  Pain Relief Diary   611
  Richmond Agitation–Sedation Scale   612
  Opioid Risk Tool—Revised (ORT-R)   612
Clinical Reasoning   613
  Applying the Full-Spectrum Nursing Model   613
  Critical Thinking and Clinical Judgment   613
Knowledge Map   615

CHAPTER 29
Physical Activity & Immobility   616

Caring for the Williams Family   616
Practical Knowledge: Clinical Application   617
Procedures   617
Procedure 29-1: Moving and Turning Patients in Bed   617
  Procedure 29-1A: Moving a Patient Up in Bed   618
  Procedure 29-1B: Turning a Patient in Bed   619
  Procedure 29-1C: Logrolling a Patient   620
Procedure 29-2: Transferring Patients   622
  Procedure 29-2A: Transferring a Patient From Bed to Stretcher   622
  Procedure 29-2B: Dangling a Patient at the Side of the Bed   623
  Procedure 29-2C: Transferring a Patient From Bed to Chair   624
Procedure 29-3: Assisting With Ambulation   625
  Procedure 29-3A: Assisting With Ambulation (One Nurse)   626
  Procedure 29-3B: Assisting With Ambulation (Two Nurses)   627
Clinical Insights   628
Clinical Insight 29-1: Applying Principles of Body Mechanics   628
Clinical Insight 29-2: Performing Passive Range-of-Motion Exercises   629
Clinical Insight 29-3: Assisting With Physical Conditioning Exercises to Prepare for Ambulation   629
Clinical Insight 29-4: Teaching Patients to use Walking Aids   630
Assessment Guidelines and Tools   632
  Assessing Activity and Exercise   632
Clinical Reasoning   634
  Applying the Full-Spectrum Nursing Model   634
  Critical Thinking and Clinical Judgment   635
Knowledge Map   637

CHAPTER 30
Sexual Health   638

Caring for the Williams Family   638
Practical Knowledge: Clinical Application   639
Clinical Insights   639
Clinical Insight 30-1: Providing Care After Sexual Assault   639
Clinical Insight 30-2: Guidelines for Taking a Sexual History   640
Clinical Insight 30-3: Teaching your Patient to Use a Condom   641
Tables   642
  Methods of Contraception   642
Assessment Guidelines and Tools   644
  Guidelines and Questions for Taking a Sexual History   644
Clinical Reasoning   645
  Applying the Full-Spectrum Nursing Model   645
  Critical Thinking and Clinical Judgment   646
Knowledge Map   649

CHAPTER 31
Sleep & Rest   650

Caring for the Williams Family   650
Practical Knowledge: Clinical Application   652
Assessment Guidelines and Tools   652
  Questions for a Sleep History   652
  Sleep Log   653
Clinical Reasoning   653
  Applying the Full-Spectrum Nursing Model   653
  Critical Thinking and Clinical Judgment   654
Knowledge Map   657

CHAPTER 32
Skin Integrity & Wound Healing   658

Caring for the Williams Family   658
Practical Knowledge: Clinical Application   659
Procedures   659
Procedure 32-1: Obtaining a Wound Culture by Swab   659
Procedure 32-2: Performing a Sterile Wound Irrigation   662

CONTENTS

Procedure 32-3: Taping a Dressing 665
Procedure 32-4: Removing and Applying Dry Dressings 666
Procedure 32-5: Removing and Applying Wet-to-Damp Dressings 668
Procedure 32-6: Applying a Negative Pressure Wound Therapy (NPWT) Device 671
   Procedure 32-6A: Open-Pore Reticulated Polyurethane Foam Therapy (i.e., Vacuum-Assisted Closure [VAC]) 672
   Procedure 32-6B: Gauze Dressing Application (i.e., Chariker–Jeter Method) 674
Procedure 32-7: Applying and Removing a Transparent Film Dressing 676
Procedure 32-8: Applying a Hydrating Dressing (Hydrocolloid or Hydrogel) 678
Procedure 32-9: Placing Skin Closures 680
Procedure 32-10: Applying Binders 682
Procedure 32-11: Applying Bandages 684
Procedure 32-12: Removing Sutures and Staples 688
   Procedure 32-12A: Removing Sutures 688
   Procedure 32-12B: Removing Staples 689
Procedure 32-13: Shortening a Wound Drain 690
Procedure 32-14: Emptying a Closed-Wound Drainage System 691

Clinical Insights 693
Clinical Insight 32-1: Applying Local Heat Therapy 693
Clinical Insight 32-2: Applying Local Cold Therapy 694

Assessment Guidelines and Tools 694
   History Questions for Skin and Wound Assessment 694
   Physical Examination: Wound Assessment 695
   Braden Scale for Predicting Pressure Sore Risk 696
   Norton Pressure Sore Risk Assessment Scale 697
   PUSH Tool for Evaluation of Pressure Ulcers 698

Diagnostic Testing 700
   Tests for Assessing Wounds 700

Clinical Reasoning 701
   Applying the Full-Spectrum Nursing Model 701
   Critical Thinking and Clinical Judgment 701

Knowledge Map 704

CHAPTER 33

Oxygenation 705

Caring for the Williams Family 705
Practical Knowledge: Clinical Application 706
Procedures 706
Procedure 33-1: Collecting a Sputum Specimen 706
   Procedure 33-1A: Collecting an Expectorated Sputum Specimen 707
   Procedure 33-1B: Collecting a Suctioned Sputum Specimen 708
Procedure 33-2: Monitoring Pulse Oximetry (Arterial Oxygen Saturation) 709
Procedure 33-3: Performing Percussion, Vibration, and Postural Drainage 712
Procedure 33-4: Administering Oxygen 714
Procedure 33-5: Performing Tracheostomy Care Using Modified Sterile Technique 719
   Procedure 33-5A: Performing Tracheostomy Care Using Sterile Technique 721
Procedure 33-6: Performing Tracheostomy or Endotracheal Suctioning (Open System) 726
Procedure 33-7: Performing Tracheostomy or Endotracheal Suctioning (Inline Closed System) 729
Procedure 33-8: Performing Orotracheal and Nasotracheal Suctioning (Open System) 730
Procedure 33-9: Performing Upper Airway Suctioning 734
Procedure 33-10: Caring for Patients Requiring Mechanical Ventilation 737
Procedure 33-11: Setting Up Disposable Chest Drainage Systems 740
Procedure 33-12: Inserting an Oropharyngeal Airway 744
Procedure 33-13: Inserting a Nasopharyngeal Airway 746

Clinical Insights 748
Clinical Insight 33-1: Tips for Obtaining Accurate Pulse Oximetry Readings 748
Clinical Insight 33-2: Guidelines for Preventing Aspiration 748
Clinical Insight 33-3: Oxygen Therapy Safety Precautions 749
Clinical Insight 33-4: Caring for Patients With Endotracheal Airways 749
Clinical Insight 33-5: Managing Chest Tubes 750

Assessment Guidelines and Tools 751
   Oxygenation 751

Diagnostic Testing 752
   Lung Volumes and Capacities 752
   Tests Related to Oxygenation 753
   Reading a Tuberculin Skin Test Result 754

Clinical Reasoning 754
   Applying the Full-Spectrum Nursing Model 754
   Critical Thinking and Clinical Judgment 755

Knowledge Map 757

Assessment Guidelines and Tools   103
  Assessing Family Developmental Tasks   103
Clinical Reasoning   104
  Applying the Full-Spectrum Nursing Model   104
  Critical Thinking and Clinical Judgment   105
Knowledge Map   107

CHAPTER 12
Caring in Multicultural Healthcare Environments   108

Caring for the Williams Family   108
Practical Knowledge: Clinical Application   109
Clinical Insights   109
Clinical Insight 12-1: Understanding Biological Variations   109
Clinical Insight 12-2: Communicating With Clients Who Speak a Different Language   110
Assessment Guidelines and Tools   111
  Obtaining Minimum Cultural Information   111
  Cultural Assessment Using the Transcultural Assessment Model   112
Clinical Reasoning   113
  Applying the Full-Spectrum Nursing Model   113
  Critical Thinking and Clinical Judgment   114
Knowledge Map   117

CHAPTER 13
Spirituality   118

Caring for the Williams Family   118
Practical Knowledge: Clinical Application   119
Clinical Insights   119
Clinical Insight 13-1: Types of Prayers   119
Clinical Insight 13-2: Praying With Clients   120
Assessment Guidelines and Tools   121
  The HOPE Approach to Spiritual Assessment: Examples of Questions   121
  SPIRIT Assessment   122
Clinical Reasoning   123
  Applying the Full-Spectrum Nursing Model   123
  Critical Thinking and Clinical Judgment   123
Knowledge Map   125

CHAPTER 14
Experiencing Loss   126

Caring for the Williams Family   126
Practical Knowledge: Clinical Application   127
Clinical Insights   127
Clinical Insight 14-1: Communicating With People Who Are Grieving   127
Clinical Insight 14-2: Helping Families of Dying Patients   127
Clinical Insight 14-3: Caring for the Dying Person: Meeting Physiological Needs   128
Clinical Insight 14-4: Caring for the Dying Person: Meeting Psychological Needs   130
Clinical Insight 14-5: Providing Postmortem Care   130
Assessment Guidelines and Tools   132
  Assessing Grief and Loss   132
Clinical Reasoning   134
  Applying the Full-Spectrum Nursing Model   134
  Critical Thinking and Clinical Judgment   134
Knowledge Map   138

Unit 3
Essential Nursing Interventions   139

CHAPTER 15
Communication & Therapeutic Relationships   141

Caring for the Williams Family   141
Practical Knowledge: Clinical Application   142
Clinical Insights   142
Clinical Insight 15-1: Collaborative Professional Communication   142
Clinical Insight 15-2: Communicating With SBARQ*   143
Clinical Insight 15-3: Communicating With Clients From Another Culture   144
Assessment Guidelines and Tools   144
  Communication   144
Clinical Reasoning   145
  Applying the Full-Spectrum Nursing Model   145
  Critical Thinking and Clinical Judgment   146
Knowledge Map   148

CHAPTER 16

Patient Education 149

Caring for the Williams Family 149

Practical Knowledge: Clinical Application 150

Assessment Guidelines and Tools 150
  Learning Assessment 150

Clinical Reasoning 151
  Applying the Full-Spectrum Nursing Model 151
  Critical Thinking and Clinical Judgment 152

Knowledge Map 155

CHAPTER 17

Interprofessional Partnerships: Documenting & Reporting 156

Caring for the Williams Family 156

Practical Knowledge: Clinical Application 157

Clinical Insights 157

Clinical Insight 17-1: Giving Oral Reports 157

Clinical Insight 17-2: Receiving Telephone and Verbal Prescriptions 159

Clinical Insight 17-3: Guidelines for Documentation 159

Clinical Insight 17-4: Guidelines for Paper Health Records 163

Tables 163
  Abbreviations Commonly Used in Healthcare 163

Documentation Forms 166
  Adult Admission History Electronic Screen 166
  Nursing Assessment Flowsheets are Comprehensive Charting Documents 167

Clinical Reasoning 168
  Applying the Full-Spectrum Nursing Model 168
  Critical Thinking and Clinical Judgment 168

Knowledge Map 171

CHAPTER 18

Measuring Vital Signs 172

Caring for the Williams Family 172

Practical Knowledge: Clinical Application 173

Procedures 173

Procedure 18-1: Assessing Body Temperature 173
  Procedure 18-1A: Taking an Axillary Temperature 174
  Procedure 18-1B: Taking an Oral Temperature 175
  Procedure 18-1C: Taking a Rectal Temperature 175
  Procedure 18-1D: Taking a Temporal Artery Temperature 176
  Procedure 18-1E: Taking a Tympanic membrane Temperature 177
  Procedure 18-1F: Taking a Skin Temperature Using a Chemical Strip Thermometer 178

Procedure 18-2: Assessing peripheral Pulses 179
  Procedure 18-2A: Assessing the Radial Pulse 180
  Procedure 18-2B: Assessing the Brachial Pulse 180
  Procedure 18-2C: Assessing the Carotid Pulse 181
  Procedure 18-2D: Assessing the Dorsalis Pedis Pulse 181
  Procedure 18-2E: Assessing the Femoral Pulse 182
  Procedure 18-2F: Assessing the Posterior Tibial Pulse 182
  Procedure 18-2G: Assessing the Popliteal Pulse 182
  Procedure 18-2H: Assessing the Temporal Pulse 183

Procedure 18-3: Assessing the Apical Pulse 184

Procedure 18-4: Assessing for an Apical-Radial Pulse Deficit 186

Procedure 18-5: Assessing Respirations 187

Procedure 18-6: Measuring Blood Pressure 189

Clinical Insights 193

Clinical Insight 18-1: Choosing a Blood Pressure Cuff Size 193

Clinical Insight 18-2: Taking an Accurate Blood Pressure 193

Clinical Insight 18-3: Teaching Your Patient About Hypertension 194

Clinical Reasoning 194
  Applying the Full-Spectrum Nursing Model 194
  Critical Thinking and Clinical Judgment 195

Knowledge Map 197

CHAPTER 19

Health Assessment 198

Caring for the Williams Family 198

Practical Knowledge: Clinical Application 199

Procedures 199

Procedure 19-1: Performing the General Survey 200

Procedure 19-2: Assessing the Skin 206

Procedure 19-3: Assessing the Hair 215

Procedure 19-4: Assessing the Nails 216

Procedure 19-5: Assessing the Head and Face 218

Procedure 19-6: Assessing the Eyes 220

Procedure 19-7: Assessing the Ears and Hearing 227

Procedure 19-8: Assessing the Nose and Sinuses 232

Procedure 19-9: Assessing the Mouth and Oropharynx 234

Procedure 19-10: Assessing the Neck 238

Procedure 19-11: Assessing the Breasts and Axillae 240

Procedure 19-12: Assessing the Chest and Lungs 244

Procedure 19-13: Assessing the Heart and Vascular System   250

Procedure 19-14: Assessing the Abdomen   257

Procedure 19-15: Assessing the Musculoskeletal System   263

Procedure 19-16: Assessing the Sensory-Neurological System   272

Procedure 19-17: Assessing the Male Genitourinary System   285

Procedure 19-18: Assessing the Female Genitourinary System   290

Procedure 19-19: Assessing the Anus and Rectum   294

Procedure 19-20: Brief Bedside Assessment   295

Clinical Insights   297

Clinical Insight 19-1: Performing Percussion   297

Clinical Insight 19-2: Performing Auscultation   298

Clinical Insight 19-3: Assisting With a Speculum Examination   298

Knowledge Map   301

CHAPTER 20

Promoting Asepsis & Preventing Infection   302

Caring for the Williams Family   302

Practical Knowledge: Clinical Application   303

Procedures   303

Procedure 20-1: Hand Hygiene   303
  Procedure 20-1A: Using Soap and Water   303
  Procedure 20-1B: Using Alcohol-Based Handrubs   304

Procedure 20-2: Donning Personal Protective Equipment (PPE)   305

Procedure 20-3: Removing Personal Protective Equipment (PPE)   307

Procedure 20-4: Surgical Hand Washing: Traditional Method   309

Procedure 20-5: Surgical Hand Washing: Brushless System   311

Procedure 20-6: Sterile Gown and Gloves (Closed Method)   314

Procedure 20-7: Sterile Gloves (Open Method)   316

Procedure 20-8: Sterile Fields   318
  Procedure 20-8A: Setting Up a Sterile Field   318
  Procedure 20-8B: Adding Supplies to a Sterile Field   319
  Procedure 20-8C: Adding Sterile Solutions to a Sterile Field   320

Clinical Insights   321

Clinical Insight 20-1: Guidelines for Hand Hygiene   321

Clinical Insight 20-2: Providing a Clean Patient Environment   322

Clinical Insight 20-3: Following CDC Standard Precautions   323

Clinical Insight 20-4: Following Transmission-Based Precautions   325

Diagnostic Testing   327

Common Tests for Evaluating the Presence of or Risk for Infection   327

Clinical Reasoning   327

  Applying the Full-Spectrum Nursing Model   327
  Critical Thinking and Clinical Judgment   328

Knowledge Map   330

CHAPTER 21

Promoting Safety   331

Caring for the Williams Family   331

Practical Knowledge: Clinical Application   332

Procedures   332

Procedure 21-1: Using Bed and Chair Monitoring Devices   332

Procedure 21-2: Using Restraints   334

Clinical Insights   338

Clinical Insight 21-1: Choking Rescue Maneuver   338

Clinical Insight 21-2: Preventing Needlestick Injury   338

Clinical Insight 21-3: What You Should Know About Using Restraints   339

Assessment Guidelines and Tools   340

Clinical Reasoning   341

  Applying the Full-Spectrum Nursing Model   341
  Critical Thinking and Clinical Judgment   342

Knowledge Map   344

CHAPTER 22

Facilitating Hygiene   345

Caring for the Williams Family   345

Practical Knowledge: Clinical Application   346

Procedures   346

Procedure 22-1: Bathing: Providing a Complete Bed Bath Using a Prepackaged Bathing Product   346

Procedure 22-2: Bathing: Using a Basin and Water   351

Procedure 22-3: Providing Perineal Care   352

Procedure 22-4: Providing Foot Care   355

Procedure 22-5: Brushing and Flossing the Teeth   358

Procedure 22-6: Providing Denture Care   361

Procedure 22-7: Providing Oral Care for an Unconscious Patient   363

Procedure 22-8: Shampooing the Hair 366
  Procedure 22-8A: Shampooing the Hair for a Patient on Bedrest Using Rinse-Free Shampoo 366
  Procedure 22-8B: Shampooing the Hair Using Rinse-Free Shampoo Cap 367
  Procedure 22-8C: Shampooing the Hair Using a Basin and Water 367
Procedure 22-9: Providing Beard and Mustache Care 369
Procedure 22-10: Shaving a Patient 370
Procedure 22-11: Removing and Caring for Contact Lenses 372
Procedure 22-12: Caring for Artificial Eyes 374
Procedure 22-13: Caring for Hearing Aids 375
Procedure 22-14: Making an Unoccupied Bed 377
Procedure 22-15: Making an Occupied Bed 380

Clinical Insight 383
Clinical Insight 22-1: Assisting With a Shower or Tub Bath 383

Assessment Guidelines and Tools 384
  Guidelines for Assessing Hygiene 384

Clinical Reasoning 386
  Applying the Full-Spectrum Nursing Model 386
  Critical Thinking and Clinical Judgment 386

Knowledge Map 390

CHAPTER 23

Administering Medications 391

Caring for the Williams Family 391
Practical Knowledge: Clinical Application 392
Procedures 392
Medication Guidelines: Steps to Follow for All Medications (Regardless of Type or Route) 392
Procedure 23-1: Administering Oral Medications 396
  Procedure 23-1A: Administering Medication Through an Enteral Tube 398
Procedure 23-2: Administering Ophthalmic Medication 400
  Procedure 23-2A: Irrigating the Eyes 402
Procedure 23-3: Administering Otic Medication 403
Procedure 23-4: Administering Nasal Medication 405
Procedure 23-5: Administering Vaginal Medication 407
Procedure 23-6: Inserting a Rectal Suppository 409
  Procedure 23-6A: Inserting a Macy Catheter 411
Procedure 23-7: Applying Medication to Skin 412
  Procedure 23-7A: Applying Topical Lotion, Cream, and Ointment 413
  Procedure 23-7B: Applying Topical Aerosol Spray 413
  Procedure 23-7C: Applying Prescribed Powder 413
  Procedure 23-7D: Applying Transdermal Medication 413
Procedure 23-8: Administering Metered-Dose Inhaler (MDI) Medication 415

Procedure 23-9: Preparing, Drawing Up, and Mixing Medication 417
  Procedure 23-9A: Drawing Up Medication From Ampules 418
  Procedure 23-9B: Drawing Up Medication From Vials 419
  Procedure 23-9C: Mixing Medication From Two Vials 421
  Procedure 23-9D: Mixing Medications From One Ampule and One Vial 423
  Procedure 23-9E: Using a Prefilled Cartridge and Single-Dose Vial—For Intravenous Administration 424
Procedure 23-10: Recapping Needles Using a One-Handed Technique 426
  Procedure 23-10A: Recapping Contaminated Needles 427
  Procedure 23-10B: Recapping Sterile Needles 427
Procedure 23-11: Administering Intradermal Medication 428
Procedure 23-12: Administering Subcutaneous Medication 431
Procedure 23-13: Locating Intramuscular Injection Sites 434
  Procedure 23-13A: Locating the Ventrogluteal Site 434
  Procedure 23-13B: Locating the Deltoid Site 435
  Procedure 23-13C: Locating the Vastus Lateralis Site 435
  Procedure 23-13D: Locating the Rectus Femoris Site 436
Procedure 23-14: Administering an Intramuscular Injection 437
  Procedure 23-14A: Intramuscular Injection: Traditional Method 437
  Procedure 23-14B: Intramuscular Injection: Z-Track Method 438
Procedure 23-15: Adding Medications to Intravenous Fluids 440
Procedure 23-16: Administering IV Push Medication 441
  Procedure 23-16A: Administering IV Push Medications Through a Primary IV Line 442
  Procedure 23-16B: Administering IV Push Medications Through an Intermittent Device (IV Lock) When No Extension Tubing Is attached to the Venous Access Device 443
  Procedure 23-16C: Administering IV Push Medications Through an intermittent Device With IV Extension Tubing 444
Procedure 23-17: Administering medication by Intermittent Infusion 446
  Procedure 23-17A: Using a Piggyback Administration Set With a Gravity Infusion 446
  Procedure 23-17B: Using a Piggyback Administration Set With an Infusion Pump 447
  Procedure 23-17C: Using a Volume-Control Administration Set 448

Procedure 23-18: Administering Medication Through a Central Venous Access Device (CVAD)   450

Practical Knowledge: Clinical Application   453

Clinical Insights   453

Clinical Insight 23-1: Taking Action After a Medication Error   453

Clinical Insight 23-2: Using Prefilled Unit-Dose Systems   454

Clinical Insight 23-3: Reconstituting Medication   455

Clinical Insight 23-4: Measuring Dosage When Changing Needles   456

Clinical Insight 23-5: Mixing Two Kinds of Insulin in One Syringe   457

Clinical Insight 23-6: Administering Anticoagulant Medication Subcutaneously   458

Tables: Abbreviations   459
  Common Medication-Related Abbreviations   459
  Table Institute for Safe Medication Practices (ISMP) List of Error-Prone Abbreviations, Symbols, and Dose Designations   460

Measuring and Calculating Dosage   466
  Medication Measurement Systems   466
  Calculating Dosages   467

Clinical Reasoning   469
  Applying the Full-Spectrum Nursing Model   469
  Critical Thinking & Clinical Judgment   470

Knowledge Map   475

Unit 4
Supporting Physiological Functioning   477

CHAPTER 24
Nutrition   479

Caring for the Williams Family   479

Practical Knowledge: Clinical Application   480

Procedures   480

Procedure 24-1: Checking Fingerstick (capillary) Blood Glucose Levels   480

Procedure 24-2: Inserting Nasogastric and Nasoenteric Tubes   483

Procedure 24-3: Administering Feedings Through Gastric and Enteric Tubes   488
  Procedure 24-3A: Administering Feedings Through Gastric and Enteric Tubes using a Closed System: Infusion Pump   489
  Procedure 24-3B: Administering Feedings Through Gastric and Enteric Tubes using an Open System: Syringe   490

Procedure 24-4: Removing a Nasogastric or Nasoenteric Tube   493

Procedure 24-5: Administering Parenteral Nutrition   494

Procedure 24-6: Administering Lipids   498

Clinical Insights   500

Clinical Insight 24-1: Measurements to Evaluate Body Composition   500

Clinical Insight 24-2: Assisting patients With Meals   502

Clinical Insight 24-3: Monitoring Patients Receiving Enteral Nutrition   503

Clinical Insight 24-4: Monitoring and Maintenance Interventions for Patients Receiving Parenteral Nutrition   504

Assessment Guidelines and Tools   505
  Screening for Nutrition Problems   505
  Subjective Global Assessment   505
  Nutrition Screening Initiative (NSI) for Older Adults: Indications of Impaired Nutrition Status   505
  Mini-Nutritional Assessment   506
  Focused Assessment   506
  Focused Nutrition Assessment   506

Diagnostic Testing   510
  Tests Reflecting Nutrition Status: Norms   510

Clinical Reasoning   510
  Applying the Full-Spectrum Nursing Model   510
  Critical Thinking and Clinical Judgment   511

Knowledge Map   515

CHAPTER 25
Urinary Elimination   516

Caring for the Williams Family   516

Practical Knowledge: Clinical Application   517

Procedures   517

Procedure 25-1: Measuring Postvoid Residual Urine Volume With a Portable Bladder Scanner   517

Procedure 25-2: Obtaining a Urine Specimen for Testing   519
  Procedure 25-2A: Collecting a Clean-Catch Urine Specimen   520
  Procedure 25-2B: Obtaining a Sterile Urine Specimen From a Catheter   521
  Procedure 25-2C: Collecting a 24-Hour Urine Specimen   521

Procedure 25-3: Inserting an Intermittent Urinary Catheter (Straight Catheter)   523

Procedure 25-4: Inserting an Indwelling Urinary Catheter   529

Procedure 25-5: Applying an External (Condom) Urinary Catheter 535
Procedure 25-6: Removing an Indwelling Catheter 537
Procedure 25-7: Irrigating the Bladder or Catheter 540
  Procedure 25-7A: Intermittent Bladder or Catheter Irrigation 540
  Procedure 25-7B: Continuous Bladder Irrigation 542

Clinical Insight 544
Clinical Insight 25-1: Teaching Clients About Clean, Intermittent Self-Catheterization 544

Assessment Guidelines and Tools 545
  Urinary Elimination History Questions 545
  Guidelines for Physical Assessment for Urinary Elimination 546

Diagnostic Testing 547
  Urinalysis 547
  Blood Studies: BUN and Creatinine 548
  Studies of the Urinary System 549
  Nursing Care Plan 551

Clinical Reasoning 555
  Applying the Full-Spectrum Nursing Model 555
  Critical Thinking and Clinical Judgment 556

Knowledge Map 558

CHAPTER 26

Bowel Elimination 559

Caring for the Williams Family 559

Practical Knowledge: Clinical Application 560

Procedures 560

Procedure 26-1: Testing Stool for Occult Blood 560
Procedure 26-2: Placing and Removing a Bedpan 562
  Procedure 26-2A: Placing a Bedpan 563
  Procedure 26-2B: Removing a Bedpan 564
Procedure 26-3: Administering an Enema 565
  Procedure 26-3A: Administering a Cleansing Enema 566
  Procedure 26-3B: Administering a Prepackaged Enema 567
  Procedure 26-3C: Administering an Oil-Retention Enema 568
  Procedure 26-3D: Administering a Return-Flow Enema 568
Procedure 26-4: Removing Stool Digitally 569
Procedure 26-5: Inserting a Rectal Tube 571
Procedure 26-6: Changing an Ostomy Appliance 573
Procedure 26-7: Irrigating a Colostomy 577
Procedure 26-8: Placing Fecal Drainage Devices 579
  Procedure 26-8A: Applying an External Fecal Collection System 580
  Procedure 26-8B: Inserting an Indwelling Fecal Drainage Device 581

Clinical Insights 583
Clinical Insight 26-1: Caring for a Patient With an Indwelling Fecal Drainage Device 583
Clinical Insight 26-2: Guidelines for Ostomy Care 584

Assessment Guidelines and Tools 585
  Bowel Elimination 585

Diagnostic Testing 586
  Direct Visualization Studies of the Gastrointestinal Tract 586
  Indirect Visualization Studies of the Gastrointestinal Tract 587
  Nursing Care Plan 589

Clinical Reasoning 591
  Applying the Full-Spectrum Nursing Model 591
  Critical Thinking and Clinical Judgment 592

Knowledge Map 594

CHAPTER 27

Sensation, Perception, & Response 595

Caring for the Williams Family 595

Practical Knowledge: Clinical Application 596

Procedures 596

Procedure 30-1: Performing Otic Irrigation 596

Clinical Insights 598
Clinical Insight 30-1: Communicating With Clients Who Are Visually Impaired 598
Clinical Insight 30-2: Communicating With Clients Who Are Hearing Impaired 598

Assessment Guidelines and Tools 599
  Hearing Screening in Older Adults 599
  Other Sensory Assessment Tools 599
  Nursing History: Overall Sensory–Perceptual Status 599
  Bedside Assessment of Sensory Function 601

Clinical Reasoning 601
  Applying the Full-Spectrum Nursing Model 601
  Critical Thinking & Clinical Judgment 602

Knowledge Map 604

CHAPTER 28

Pain 605

Caring for the Williams Family 605

Practical Knowledge Knowing How 606

Procedure 606

Procedure 28-1: Setting Up and managing Patient-Controlled Analgesia by Pump 606

Clinical Insight 609

Clinical Insight 28-1: Caring for the Patient With an Epidural Catheter 609

Assessment Guidelines and Tools 610
  Pain Assessment 610
  Pain Relief Diary 611
  Richmond Agitation–Sedation Scale 612
  Opioid Risk Tool—Revised (ORT-R) 612

Clinical Reasoning 613
  Applying the Full-Spectrum Nursing Model 613
  Critical Thinking and Clinical Judgment 613

Knowledge Map 615

CHAPTER 29
Physical Activity & Immobility 616

Caring for the Williams Family 616

Practical Knowledge: Clinical Application 617

Procedures 617

Procedure 29-1: Moving and Turning Patients in Bed 617
  Procedure 29-1A: Moving a Patient Up in Bed 618
  Procedure 29-1B: Turning a Patient in Bed 619
  Procedure 29-1C: Logrolling a Patient 620

Procedure 29-2: Transferring Patients 622
  Procedure 29-2A: Transferring a Patient From Bed to Stretcher 622
  Procedure 29-2B: Dangling a Patient at the Side of the Bed 623
  Procedure 29-2C: Transferring a Patient From Bed to Chair 624

Procedure 29-3: Assisting With Ambulation 625
  Procedure 29-3A: Assisting With Ambulation (One Nurse) 626
  Procedure 29-3B: Assisting With Ambulation (Two Nurses) 627

Clinical Insights 628

Clinical Insight 29-1: Applying Principles of Body Mechanics 628

Clinical Insight 29-2: Performing Passive Range-of-Motion Exercises 629

Clinical Insight 29-3: Assisting With Physical Conditioning Exercises to Prepare for Ambulation 629

Clinical Insight 29-4: Teaching Patients to use Walking Aids 630

Assessment Guidelines and Tools 632
  Assessing Activity and Exercise 632

Clinical Reasoning 634
  Applying the Full-Spectrum Nursing Model 634
  Critical Thinking and Clinical Judgment 635

Knowledge Map 637

CHAPTER 30
Sexual Health 638

Caring for the Williams Family 638

Practical Knowledge: Clinical Application 639

Clinical Insights 639

Clinical Insight 30-1: Providing Care After Sexual Assault 639

Clinical Insight 30-2: Guidelines for Taking a Sexual History 640

Clinical Insight 30-3: Teaching your Patient to Use a Condom 641

Tables 642
  Methods of Contraception 642

Assessment Guidelines and Tools 644
  Guidelines and Questions for Taking a Sexual History 644

Clinical Reasoning 645
  Applying the Full-Spectrum Nursing Model 645
  Critical Thinking and Clinical Judgment 646

Knowledge Map 649

CHAPTER 31
Sleep & Rest 650

Caring for the Williams Family 650

Practical Knowledge: Clinical Application 652

Assessment Guidelines and Tools 652
  Questions for a Sleep History 652
  Sleep Log 653

Clinical Reasoning 653
  Applying the Full-Spectrum Nursing Model 653
  Critical Thinking and Clinical Judgment 654

Knowledge Map 657

CHAPTER 32
Skin Integrity & Wound Healing 658

Caring for the Williams Family 658

Practical Knowledge: Clinical Application 659

Procedures 659

Procedure 32-1: Obtaining a Wound Culture by Swab 659

Procedure 32-2: Performing a Sterile Wound Irrigation 662

Procedure 32-3: Taping a Dressing 665
Procedure 32-4: Removing and Applying Dry Dressings 666
Procedure 32-5: Removing and Applying Wet-to-Damp Dressings 668
Procedure 32-6: Applying a Negative Pressure Wound Therapy (NPWT) Device 671
  Procedure 32-6A: Open-Pore Reticulated Polyurethane Foam Therapy (i.e., Vacuum-Assisted Closure [VAC]) 672
  Procedure 32-6B: Gauze Dressing Application (i.e., Chariker–Jeter Method) 674
Procedure 32-7: Applying and Removing a Transparent Film Dressing 676
Procedure 32-8: Applying a Hydrating Dressing (Hydrocolloid or Hydrogel) 678
Procedure 32-9: Placing Skin Closures 680
Procedure 32-10: Applying Binders 682
Procedure 32-11: Applying Bandages 684
Procedure 32-12: Removing Sutures and Staples 688
  Procedure 32-12A: Removing Sutures 688
  Procedure 32-12B: Removing Staples 689
Procedure 32-13: Shortening a Wound Drain 690
Procedure 32-14: Emptying a Closed-Wound Drainage System 691

Clinical Insights 693
Clinical Insight 32-1: Applying Local Heat Therapy 693
Clinical Insight 32-2: Applying Local Cold Therapy 694
Assessment Guidelines and Tools 694
  History Questions for Skin and Wound Assessment 694
  Physical Examination: Wound Assessment 695
  Braden Scale for Predicting Pressure Sore Risk 696
  Norton Pressure Sore Risk Assessment Scale 697
  PUSH Tool for Evaluation of Pressure Ulcers 698
Diagnostic Testing 700
  Tests for Assessing Wounds 700
Clinical Reasoning 701
  Applying the Full-Spectrum Nursing Model 701
  Critical Thinking and Clinical Judgment 701
Knowledge Map 704

CHAPTER 33

Oxygenation 705

Caring for the Williams Family 705
Practical Knowledge: Clinical Application 706
Procedures 706
Procedure 33-1: Collecting a Sputum Specimen 706
  Procedure 33-1A: Collecting an Expectorated Sputum Specimen 707
  Procedure 33-1B: Collecting a Suctioned Sputum Specimen 708
Procedure 33-2: Monitoring Pulse Oximetry (Arterial Oxygen Saturation) 709
Procedure 33-3: Performing Percussion, Vibration, and Postural Drainage 712
Procedure 33-4: Administering Oxygen 714
Procedure 33-5: Performing Tracheostomy Care Using Modified Sterile Technique 719
  Procedure 33-5A: Performing Tracheostomy Care Using Sterile Technique 721
Procedure 33-6: Performing Tracheostomy or Endotracheal Suctioning (Open System) 726
Procedure 33-7: Performing Tracheostomy or Endotracheal Suctioning (Inline Closed System) 729
Procedure 33-8: Performing Orotracheal and Nasotracheal Suctioning (Open System) 730
Procedure 33-9: Performing Upper Airway Suctioning 734
Procedure 33-10: Caring for Patients Requiring Mechanical Ventilation 737
Procedure 33-11: Setting Up Disposable Chest Drainage Systems 740
Procedure 33-12: Inserting an Oropharyngeal Airway 744
Procedure 33-13: Inserting a Nasopharyngeal Airway 746

Clinical Insights 748
Clinical Insight 33-1: Tips for Obtaining Accurate Pulse Oximetry Readings 748
Clinical Insight 33-2: Guidelines for Preventing Aspiration 748
Clinical Insight 33-3: Oxygen Therapy Safety Precautions 749
Clinical Insight 33-4: Caring for Patients With Endotracheal Airways 749
Clinical Insight 33-5: Managing Chest Tubes 750
Assessment Guidelines and Tools 751
  Oxygenation 751
Diagnostic Testing 752
  Lung Volumes and Capacities 752
  Tests Related to Oxygenation 753
  Reading a Tuberculin Skin Test Result 754
Clinical Reasoning 754
  Applying the Full-Spectrum Nursing Model 754
  Critical Thinking and Clinical Judgment 755
Knowledge Map 757

Knowledge Map

CRITICAL-THINKING SKILLS
- Contextual awareness
- Considering alternatives
- Using credible sources
- Reflecting skeptically
- Analyzing assumptions

CRITICAL-THINKING ATTITUDES
- Independent thinking
- Intellectual curiosity
- Intellectual humility
- Intellectual empathy
- Intellectual courage
- Intellectual perseverance
- Fair-mindedness

Critical thinking

Nursing knowledge

Nursing process

Theoretical: Knowing WHY

Practical: Knowing HOW

- Assessing
- Diagnosing
- Planning outcomes
- Planning interventions
- Implementing
- Evaluating

CHAPTER 3

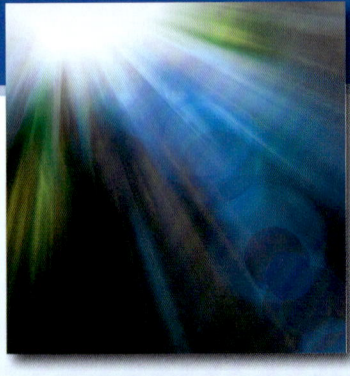

The Steps of the Nursing Process

STUDENT RESOURCES

The questions and exercises in Volume 2 allow you to practice the kind of thinking you will use as a full-spectrum nurse. Critical-thinking questions usually have more than one correct answer, so we do not provide "correct" answers for these features. It is more important to develop your nursing judgment than to just cover content. You will learn by discussing the questions with your peers. If you are still unsure, see the Davis Advantage chapter resources for suggested responses.

 To explore learning resources for this chapter,

 Go to www.DavisAdvantage.com and find:

Answers and Suggested Responses for all questions in this chapter
Concept Map
Knowledge Map
References and Bibliography

Key Concepts

Assessment
Nursing diagnosis
Planning outcomes
Planning interventions
Implementation
Evaluation

Related Concepts

See the Concept Map on Davis Advantage.

Caring for the Williams Family

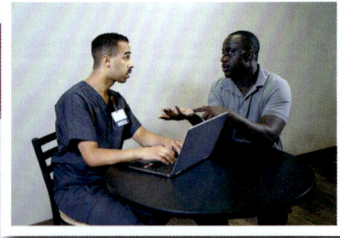

Review the scenario of Stanley Williams in the front of this book. As the clinic nurse, you have written the following nursing diagnostic statement: Overweight related to inappropriate food choices and serving size as evidenced by body mass index (BMI) of 30.7.

A. Write at least two short-term and two long-term goals for Mr. Williams based on this diagnostic statement. Remember that your goals must be realistic, and consider Mr. Williams' other health problems.

B. Based on the outcomes (goals) you wrote, identify four possible interventions to address the diagnosis and outcomes.

C. Review the interventions and identify two that would be most appropriate for Mr. Williams given all the information you have about his health status.

D. Write a nursing prescription for each of the two interventions you identified earlier.

E. How will you evaluate whether Mr. Williams has met his goal?

ASSESSMENT GUIDELINES AND TOOLS

FOLLOW-UP CARE

When to call the doctor; symptom management (pain, nausea); plan for meeting outcomes not met during hospitalization:

Call your primary physician to find out if an insurance referral form is needed for follow-up appointments.
After discharge, you need to call for an appointment to see physician.
Clinic/Physician   Phone #   Date   Time
_____   _____   _____   _____   or ____days ____weeks ____months
_____   _____   _____   _____   or ____days ____weeks ____months
_____   _____   _____   _____   or ____days ____weeks ____months

Plans for follow-up Labs/Tests/Treatments
Date   Time   Test/Treatment   Location   Ordered by

PERSONAL CARE

Bathing: ❏ No restrictions ❏ Other:

Treatment/Therapy/Wound or Skin Care/ Supplies Needed   2-Day Supply Sent Home ?   ❏ Yes

ACTIVITY/REHAB

❏ No restrictions   ❏ Do not climb stairs   ❏ Drive_____   ❏ Return to Work _____
❏ Do not lift   ❏ May lift up to ____ lbs   ❏ Weight Bearing ____ #   ❏ Other

DIET

❏ No restrictions   ❏ Other:

Food/Drug Interactions: ❏ Coumadin   ❏ MAO Inhibitors   ❏ Other:

MEDICAL EQUIPMENT

❏ 2nd pair of TED hose given

COMMUNITY RESOURCES

Referral Resource	Agency	Phone #	
Home IV Therapy			Transportation Arrangements for discharge: ___
Home Health			
Home Oxygen			Education/Community Resources:_____
Home PT/OT/Speech			
Ask-A-Nurse		816-932-0000	

Preprinted Discharge Instruction Sheet given to patient   ❏ NA ❏ Yes
List Instruction Sheets:

I understand these instructions and agree with this plan of care _____
                                                                  Patient/SO Signature

MULTIDISCIPLINARY DISCHARGE INSTRUCTIONS
Shawnee Mission Medical Center
9100 W. 74th Street
Shawnee Mission, Kansas 66204

Form # 60869 Revised: 4/01 PILOT Page 1 of 2

Source: Courtesy of Shawnee Mission Health System, Shawnee Mission, KS

Elements for review		Client A	Client B	Client C	Client D
Activity/Task Level of client stability	Describe activity/task: Score the client's level of stability: **Client condition:** 0 – Is chronic/stable/predictable 1 – Has minimal potential for change 2 – Has moderate potential for change 3 – Has unstable/acute/strong potential for change				
Level of NAP competence	Score the NAP competence in completing delegated nursing care activities in the defined client population: **NAP is:** 0 – Expert in activities to be delegated, in defined population 1 – Experienced in activities to be delegated, in defined population 2 – Experienced in activities but not in defined population 3 – Novice in performing activities and in defined population				
Level of licensed nurse competence	Score the licensed nurse's competence in relation to both knowledge of providing nursing care to a defined population and competence in implementation of the delegation process: 0 – Expert in the knowledge of nursing needs/activities of defined client population *and* expert in the delegation process 1 – Either expert in knowledge of needs/activities of defined client population and competent in delegation *or* experienced in the needs/activities of defined client population and expert in the delegation process 2 – Experienced in knowledge of needs/activities of defined client population *and* competent in the delegation process 3 – Either experienced in knowledge of needs/activities of defined client population *or* competent in the delegation process 4 – Novice in knowledge of defined population *and* novice in delegation				
Potential for harm	Score the potential level of risk the nursing care activity has for the client *(risk is probability of [the client] suffering harm)*: 0 – None 1 – Low 2 – Medium 3 – High				
Frequency	Score based on how often the NAP has performed the specific nursing care activity: 0 – Performed at least daily 1 – Performed at least weekly 2 – Performed at least monthly 3 – Performed less than monthly 4 – Never performed				
Level of decision making	Score the decision-making needed, related to the specific nursing care activity, client (both cognitive and physical status) and client situation: 0 – Does not require decision making 1 – Minimal level of decision making 2 – Moderate level of decision making 3 – High level of decision making				
Ability for self care	Score the client's level of assistance needed for self-care activities: 0 – No assistance 1 – Limited assistance 2 – Extensive assistance 3 – Total care or constant attendance				
	Total Score				

Scoring: A low score on the grid suggests that an activity can be safely delegated. For example if a client's stability is ranked 3 (unstable) and the level of NAP competence is also 3 (novice in the activity), then you probably should *not* delegate to that NAP. Each agency should establish a policy regarding the individual and/or total scores to be considered acceptable for delegating.

Source: Used by permission from the National Council of State Boards of Nursing (NCSBN), Chicago, IL (1997). Retrieved February 1, 2008, from the NCSBN web site (www.ncsbn.org)

Evaluation Checklist

Instructions: Check the appropriate response and follow the associated instructions

Assessment Review

1. Were the assessment data complete and accurate?
   ___ YES. No action.
   ___ NO. Reassess client. Record the new data. Change care plan as indicated

2. Have all data been validated, as needed?
   ___ YES. No action.
   ___ NO. Validate with client (by interview and physical examination), significant others, or other professionals. Record validation (or failure to validate). Change care plan as indicated.

3. Have new data become available that require changes in the plan (e.g., a different problem etiology, new goals/ outcomes, new medical orders)?
   ___ NO. No action.
   ___ YES. Record the new data in the progress notes; redefine problem, goals, nursing orders, as needed.

4. Has the patient's condition changed?
   ___ NO. No action.
   ___ YES. Record data about present health status. Change care plan as indicated.

→ *Move to a review of the diagnosis step.* ←

Diagnosis Review

1. Is the diagnosis relevant and related to the data?
   ___ YES. No action.
   ___ NO. Revise the diagnosis.

2. Is the diagnosis well supported by the data?
   ___ YES. No action.
   ___ NO. Collect more data. Support or revise diagnosis.

3. Has the problem status changed (actual, potential, possible)?
   ___ NO. No action.
   ___ YES. Restate the problem.

4. Is the diagnosis stated clearly?
   ___ YES. No action.
   ___ NO. Revise the diagnostic statement.

5. Does the etiology correctly reflect the factors contributing to the problem?
   ___ YES. No action.
   ___ NO. Revise the etiology.

6. Is the problem one that can be treated primarily by nursing actions?
   ___ YES. No action.
   ___ NO. Label as collaborative and consult appropriate health professional.

7. Is the diagnosis specific and individualized to the patient?
   ___ YES. No action.
   ___ NO. Revise diagnosis. Revise outcomes and nursing orders as suggested by the new nursing diagnosis.

8. Does the problem (diagnosis) still exist?
   ___ YES. No action.
   ___ NO. Delete diagnosis and related outcomes and nursing orders.

→ *Proceed to a review of client goals.* ←

Planning Review: Outcomes

1. Have nursing diagnoses been added or revised?
   ___ NO. No action.
   ___ YES. Write new outcomes.

2. Are the outcomes realistic in terms of patient abilities and agency resources?
   ___ YES. No action.
   ___ NO. Revise outcomes.

3. Was sufficient time allowed for outcome achievement?
   ___ YES. No action.
   ___ NO. Revise time frame.

4. Do the outcomes address all aspects of the client's problem?
   ___ YES. No action.
   ___ NO. Write additional outcomes.

Evaluation Checklist *(continued)*

5. Do the expected outcomes, as written, demonstrate resolution of the problem specified in the nursing diagnosis?
   ___ YES. No action.   ___ NO. Revise outcomes.
6. Have client priorities changed, or has the focus of care changed?
   ___ NO. No action.   ___ YES. Revise outcomes.
7. Is the client in agreement with the goals?
   ___ YES. No action.   ___ NO. Get client input. Write outcomes valued by the client.

→ Proceed to a review of nursing orders. ←

Planning Review: Nursing Orders

1. Have nursing diagnoses or outcomes been added or revised in previous review steps?
   ___ NO. No action.   ___ YES. Write new nursing orders.
2. Are the nursing orders clearly related to the stated patient outcomes?
   ___ YES. No action.   ___ NO. Revise or develop new nursing orders.
3. Is the rationale sufficient to justify the use of the nursing order?
   ___ YES. No action.   ___ NO. Revise or develop new nursing orders.
4. Are the nursing orders unclear or vague, so that other staff may have had questions about how to implement them?
   ___ NO. No action.   ___ YES. Revise nursing orders. Add details to make more specific or individualized to the patient.
5. Do the nursing orders include instructions for timing of the activities?
   ___ YES. No action.   ___ NO. Revise nursing orders: add times, schedules.
6. Was an order clearly and obviously ineffective?
   ___ NO. No action.   ___ YES. Delete it.
7. Are the orders realistic in terms of staff and other resources?
   ___ YES. No action.   ___ NO. Revise orders or obtain resources.
8. Have new resources become available that might enable you to change the goals or nursing orders?
   ___ NO. No action.   ___ YES. Write new goals or nursing orders reflecting the new capabilities.
9. Do the nursing orders address all aspects of the client's health goals?
   ___ YES. No action.   ___ NO. Add new nursing orders.

→ Proceed to a review of implementation step ←

Implementation Review

1. Did the nurse [or NAP] get client input at each step in developing and implementing the plan?
   ___ YES. No action.   ___ NO. Obtain client input, revise plan and implementation as needed. [Coach NAP or role model, as needed.]
2. Were the nursing interventions acceptable to the patient?
   ___ YES. No action.   ___ NO. Consult patient; change nursing orders or implementation approach.
3. Did the nurse [NAP] prepare the patient for implementation of the nursing order (e.g., explain what the patient should expect or do)?
   ___ YES. No action.   ___ NO. Continue same plan, but prepare patient before implementing. Reevaluate.
4. Did the nurse [NAP] have adequate knowledge and skills to perform techniques and procedures correctly?
   ___ YES. No action.   ___ NO. Continue same plan. Have someone else implement or help the nurse [or NAP] to acquire the needed knowledge or skills. If neither of these is possible, delete nursing order.

(continued)

5. Did client or family comply with the therapeutic regimen? Were self-care activities performed correctly?
   __ YES. No action.
   __ NO. Reassess motivation, knowledge, and resources. Add outcomes and nursing orders aimed at teaching, motivating, and supporting, patient in carrying out the regimen. Set time for reevaluation.

6. Did other staff members follow the nursing orders?
   __ YES. No action.
   __ NO. Implement the omitted nursing orders or ensure that others will do so. Set time for reevaluation. Find out why order was not carried out.

7. Was the plan of care implemented in a manner that communicated caring?
   __ YES. No action.
   __ NO. This is a problem that must be addressed by personal and staff development.

After making the necessary revisions to the care plan, implement the new plan and begin the nursing cycle again.

Source: Wilkinson, J. (2011). *Nursing process and critical thinking* (5th ed.). Upper Saddle River, NJ: Prentice Hall, pp. 325–327.

Functional Ability Assessment

The Joint Commission (2020) requires an initial functional ability assessment "based on the patient's condition." These three functional assessment tools are commonly used:

The Karnofsky Performance scale (Karnofsky & Burchenal, 1949). This tool is used primarily in palliative care settings to assess functional abilities at the end of life. To see the scale,

Go to http://www.npcrc.org/files/news/karnofsky_performance_scale.pdf

The Katz Index of ADL scale (1963). This instrument is one of the best for assessing independent performance in very basic areas. It assigns 1 point for independence in each of the following areas: bathing, dressing, toileting, transfer, continence, and feeding. Nurses often use the data to plan staffing and appropriate placement of patients. The accompanying Focused Assessment box addresses functions similar to those assessed by the Katz scale. To see the Katz scale,

Go to the ConsultGeri Web site at https://hign.org/sites/default/files/2020-06/Try_This_General_Assessment_2.pdf

Lawton Instrumental Activities of Daily Living (IADL) scale (1969). This easy-to-use tool is particularly helpful in assessing a person's ability to independently perform the more sophisticated tasks of everyday life, such as shopping. Identifying early functional decline is important for discharge planning. The Lawton scale is especially useful for older adults, who may begin to have functional decline within 48 hours of hospital admission (Graf, 2008; Lawton & Brody, 1969).

Patient Assessment Tool—Lawton Instrumental Activities of Daily Living.

Date: _____   Name: _____

Please check the box that most applies for each activity:

Activity	Needs no help (2 pts. each)	Needs some help (1 pt. each)	Unable to do at all (0 pts. each)
1. Using the telephone	___	___	___
2. Getting to places beyond walking distance	___	___	___
3. Grocery shopping	___	___	___
4. Preparing meals	___	___	___
5. Doing housework or handyman work	___	___	___
6. Doing laundry	___	___	___
7. Taking medications	___	___	___
8. Managing money	___	___	___

Total score: ___ =   (___ x 2 =) ___ +   (___ x 1 =) ___ +   0

A patient is awarded 2 points for each area in which he/she can function totally without help, 1 point in those areas that they need some help, and 0 points for those activities that somebody else must do completely for them. The maximum score is 16, minimum score is 0.

Like other evaluations, the IADL scale provides a baseline of data that can be compared with the results of future evaluations. (Note that some activities may be gender specific. Omit these items if the patient does not usually perform those tasks.)

Permission obtained from M. Powell Lawton, Ph.D., Philadelphia Geriatric Center, Philadelphia, PA. May be used freely for patient assessment. Formatted and posted May 25, 1996, to www.acsu.buffalo.edu/~drstall/assessmenttools.html by Robert S. Stall, M.D.

Special Needs Assessment: Questions for Assessing Independence in Activities of Daily Living

Focused Assessment

Mobility
Does the client require devices (e.g., cane, crutches, walker, wheelchair) for support?

Transfer
Can the client get in and out of bed and in and out of a chair without assistance?

If not, how much help does the client need?

Is the client completely confined to bed?

Bathing
Can the client perform a sponge bath, tub bath, or shower bath with no help?

If not, specifically what assistance does the client need?

Dressing
Can the client get all necessary clothing from drawers and closets and get completely dressed without help?

If not, specifically what assistance does the client need?

Feeding
Can the client feed themselves without assistance?

If not, specifically what assistance does the client need (e.g., help with cutting meat, tube feeding)?

Toileting
Can the client go to the bathroom, use the toilet, clean themselves, and rearrange clothing without help?

If a night bedpan or commode is used, can the client empty and clean it independently?

If the client needs help with these activities, specifically what does it include?

Continence
Does the client independently control urination and bowel movements?

If not, how often is the client incontinent of bladder or bowel?

Does the client require an indwelling urinary catheter?

CHAPTER 2　Clinical Judgment　　11

Knowledge Map

CRITICAL-THINKING SKILLS
- Contextual awareness
- Considering alternatives
- Using credible sources
- Reflecting skeptically
- Analyzing assumptions

CRITICAL-THINKING ATTITUDES
- Independent thinking
- Intellectual curiosity
- Intellectual humility
- Intellectual empathy
- Intellectual courage
- Intellectual perseverance
- Fair-mindedness

Critical thinking

Nursing knowledge

Nursing process

Theoretical: Knowing WHY

Practical: Knowing HOW

- Assessing
- Diagnosing
- Planning outcomes
- Planning interventions
- Implementing
- Evaluating

CHAPTER 3

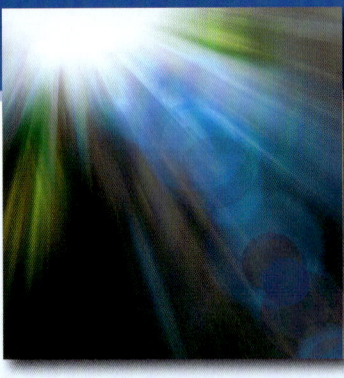

The Steps of the Nursing Process

STUDENT RESOURCES

The questions and exercises in Volume 2 allow you to practice the kind of thinking you will use as a full-spectrum nurse. Critical-thinking questions usually have more than one correct answer, so we do not provide "correct" answers for these features. It is more important to develop your nursing judgment than to just cover content. You will learn by discussing the questions with your peers. If you are still unsure, see the Davis Advantage chapter resources for suggested responses.

 To explore learning resources for this chapter,

 Go to www.DavisAdvantage.com and find:

Answers and Suggested Responses for all questions in this chapter
Concept Map
Knowledge Map
References and Bibliography

Key Concepts

Assessment
Nursing diagnosis
Planning outcomes
Planning interventions
Implementation
Evaluation

Related Concepts

See the Concept Map on Davis Advantage.

Caring for the Williams Family

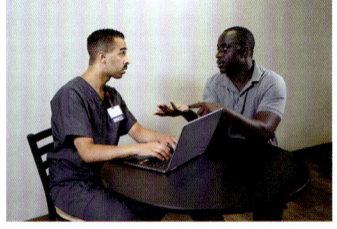

Review the scenario of Stanley Williams in the front of this book. As the clinic nurse, you have written the following nursing diagnostic statement: Overweight related to inappropriate food choices and serving size as evidenced by body mass index (BMI) of 30.7.

A. Write at least two short-term and two long-term goals for Mr. Williams based on this diagnostic statement. Remember that your goals must be realistic, and consider Mr. Williams' other health problems.

B. Based on the outcomes (goals) you wrote, identify four possible interventions to address the diagnosis and outcomes.

C. Review the interventions and identify two that would be most appropriate for Mr. Williams given all the information you have about his health status.

D. Write a nursing prescription for each of the two interventions you identified earlier.

E. How will you evaluate whether Mr. Williams has met his goal?

12

ASSESSMENT GUIDELINES AND TOOLS

FOLLOW-UP CARE	When to call the doctor; symptom management (pain, nausea); plan for meeting outcomes not met during hospitalization: Call your primary physician to find out if an insurance referral form is needed for follow-up appointments. After discharge, you need to call for an appointment to see physician. Clinic/Physician Phone # Date Time _____ _____ _____ _____ or _____ days _____ weeks _____ months _____ _____ _____ _____ or _____ days _____ weeks _____ months _____ _____ _____ _____ or _____ days _____ weeks _____ months Plans for follow-up Labs/Tests/Treatments Date Time Test/Treatment Location Ordered by
PERSONAL CARE	**Bathing:** ❏ No restrictions ❏ Other: **Treatment/Therapy/Wound or Skin Care/ Supplies Needed** 2-Day Supply Sent Home ? ❏ Yes
ACTIVITY/ REHAB	❏ No restrictions ❏ Do not climb stairs ❏ Drive _____ ❏ Return to Work _____ ❏ Do not lift ❏ May lift up to _____ lbs ❏ Weight Bearing _____ # ❏ Other
DIET	❏ No restrictions ❏ Other: Food/Drug Interactions: ❏ Coumadin ❏ MAO Inhibitors ❏ Other:
MEDICAL EQUIPMENT	❏ 2nd pair of TED hose given
COMMUNITY RESOURCES	**Referral Resource** **Agency** **Phone #** Transportation Arrangements for discharge: ___ Home IV Therapy _____ _____ Home Health _____ _____ Home Oxygen _____ _____ Education/Community Resources: _____ Home PT/OT/Speech _____ _____ Ask-A-Nurse _____ 816-932-0000

Preprinted Discharge Instruction Sheet given to patient   ❏ NA   ❏ Yes
List Instruction Sheets:

I understand these instructions and agree with this plan of care _____
                                                            Patient/SO Signature

MULTIDISCIPLINARY DISCHARGE INSTRUCTIONS
Shawnee Mission Medical Center
9100 W. 74th Street
Shawnee Mission, Kansas 66204

Form # 60869 Revised: 4/01 PILOT Page 1 of 2

Source: Courtesy of Shawnee Mission Health System, Shawnee Mission, KS

Elements for review		Client A	Client B	Client C	Client D
Activity/Task Level of client stability	Describe activity/task: Score the client's level of stability: **Client condition:** 0 – Is chronic/stable/predictable 1 – Has minimal potential for change 2 – Has moderate potential for change 3 – Has unstable/acute/strong potential for change				
Level of NAP competence	Score the NAP competence in completing delegated nursing care activities in the defined client population: **NAP is:** 0 – Expert in activities to be delegated, in defined population 1 – Experienced in activities to be delegated, in defined population 2 – Experienced in activities but not in defined population 3 – Novice in performing activities and in defined population				
Level of licensed nurse competence	Score the licensed nurse's competence in relation to both knowledge of providing nursing care to a defined population and competence in implementation of the delegation process: 0 – Expert in the knowledge of nursing needs/activities of defined client population *and* expert in the delegation process 1 – Either expert in knowledge of needs/activities of defined client population and competent in delegation *or* experienced in the needs/activities of defined client population and expert in the delegation process 2 – Experienced in knowledge of needs/activities of defined client population *and* competent in the delegation process 3 – Either experienced in knowledge of needs/activities of defined client population *or* competent in the delegation process 4 – Novice in knowledge of defined population *and* novice in delegation				
Potential for harm	Score the potential level of risk the nursing care activity has for the client *(risk is probability of [the client] suffering harm):* 0 – None 1 – Low 2 – Medium 3 – High				
Frequency	Score based on how often the NAP has performed the specific nursing care activity: 0 – Performed at least daily 1 – Performed at least weekly 2 – Performed at least monthly 3 – Performed less than monthly 4 – Never performed				
Level of decision making	Score the decision-making needed, related to the specific nursing care activity, client (both cognitive and physical status) and client situation: 0 – Does not require decision making 1 – Minimal level of decision making 2 – Moderate level of decision making 3 – High level of decision making				
Ability for self care	Score the client's level of assistance needed for self-care activities: 0 – No assistance 1 – Limited assistance 2 – Extensive assistance 3 – Total care or constant attendance				
	Total Score				

Scoring: A low score on the grid suggests that an activity can be safely delegated. For example if a client's stability is ranked 3 (unstable) and the level of NAP competence is also 3 (novice in the activity), then you probably should *not* delegate to that NAP. Each agency should establish a policy regarding the individual and/or total scores to be considered acceptable for delegating.

Source: Used by permission from the National Council of State Boards of Nursing (NCSBN), Chicago, IL (1997). Retrieved February 1, 2008, from the NCSBN web site (www.ncsbn.org)

Evaluation Checklist

Instructions: Check the appropriate response and follow the associated instructions

Assessment Review

1. Were the assessment data complete and accurate?
   - ___ YES. No action.
   - ___ NO. Reassess client. Record the new data. Change care plan as indicated

2. Have all data been validated, as needed?
   - ___ YES. No action.
   - ___ NO. Validate with client (by interview and physical examination), significant others, or other professionals. Record validation (or failure to validate). Change care plan as indicated.

3. Have new data become available that require changes in the plan (e.g., a different problem etiology, new goals/ outcomes, new medical orders)?
   - ___ NO. No action.
   - ___ YES. Record the new data in the progress notes; redefine problem, goals, nursing orders, as needed.

4. Has the patient's condition changed?
   - ___ NO. No action.
   - ___ YES. Record data about present health status. Change care plan as indicated.

→ *Move to a review of the diagnosis step.* ←

Diagnosis Review

1. Is the diagnosis relevant and related to the data?
   - ___ YES. No action.
   - ___ NO. Revise the diagnosis.

2. Is the diagnosis well supported by the data?
   - ___ YES. No action.
   - ___ NO. Collect more data. Support or revise diagnosis.

3. Has the problem status changed (actual, potential, possible)?
   - ___ NO. No action.
   - ___ YES. Restate the problem.

4. Is the diagnosis stated clearly?
   - ___ YES. No action.
   - ___ NO. Revise the diagnostic statement.

5. Does the etiology correctly reflect the factors contributing to the problem?
   - ___ YES. No action.
   - ___ NO. Revise the etiology.

6. Is the problem one that can be treated primarily by nursing actions?
   - ___ YES. No action.
   - ___ NO. Label as collaborative and consult appropriate health professional.

7. Is the diagnosis specific and individualized to the patient?
   - ___ YES. No action.
   - ___ NO. Revise diagnosis. Revise outcomes and nursing orders as suggested by the new nursing diagnosis.

8. Does the problem (diagnosis) still exist?
   - ___ YES. No action.
   - ___ NO. Delete diagnosis and related outcomes and nursing orders.

→ *Proceed to a review of client goals.* ←

Planning Review: Outcomes

1. Have nursing diagnoses been added or revised?
   - ___ NO. No action.
   - ___ YES. Write new outcomes.

2. Are the outcomes realistic in terms of patient abilities and agency resources?
   - ___ YES. No action.
   - ___ NO. Revise outcomes.

3. Was sufficient time allowed for outcome achievement?
   - ___ YES. No action.
   - ___ NO. Revise time frame.

4. Do the outcomes address all aspects of the client's problem?
   - ___ YES. No action.
   - ___ NO. Write additional outcomes.

Evaluation Checklist *(continued)*

5. Do the expected outcomes, as written, demonstrate resolution of the problem specified in the nursing diagnosis?
   __ YES. No action.   __ NO. Revise outcomes.
6. Have client priorities changed, or has the focus of care changed?
   __ NO. No action.   __ YES. Revise outcomes.
7. Is the client in agreement with the goals?
   __ YES. No action.   __ NO. Get client input. Write outcomes valued by the client.

→ *Proceed to a review of nursing orders.* ←

Planning Review: Nursing Orders

1. Have nursing diagnoses or outcomes been added or revised in previous review steps?
   __ NO. No action.   __ YES. Write new nursing orders.
2. Are the nursing orders clearly related to the stated patient outcomes?
   __ YES. No action.   __ NO. Revise or develop new nursing orders.
3. Is the rationale sufficient to justify the use of the nursing order?
   __ YES. No action.   __ NO. Revise or develop new nursing orders.
4. Are the nursing orders unclear or vague, so that other staff may have had questions about how to implement them?
   __ NO. No action.   __ YES. Revise nursing orders. Add details to make more specific or individualized to the patient.
5. Do the nursing orders include instructions for timing of the activities?
   __ YES. No action.   __ NO. Revise nursing orders: add times, schedules.
6. Was an order clearly and obviously ineffective?
   __ NO. No action.   __ YES. Delete it.
7. Are the orders realistic in terms of staff and other resources?
   __ YES. No action.   __ NO. Revise orders or obtain resources.
8. Have new resources become available that might enable you to change the goals or nursing orders?
   __ NO. No action.   __ YES. Write new goals or nursing orders reflecting the new capabilities.
9. Do the nursing orders address all aspects of the client's health goals?
   __ YES. No action.   __ NO. Add new nursing orders.

→ *Proceed to a review of implementation step* ←

Implementation Review

1. Did the nurse [or NAP] get client input at each step in developing and implementing the plan?
   __ YES. No action.   __ NO. Obtain client input, revise plan and implementation as needed. [Coach NAP or role model, as needed.]
2. Were the nursing interventions acceptable to the patient?
   __ YES. No action.   __ NO. Consult patient; change nursing orders or implementation approach.
3. Did the nurse [NAP] prepare the patient for implementation of the nursing order (e.g., explain what the patient should expect or do)?
   __ YES. No action.   __ NO. Continue same plan, but prepare patient before implementing. Reevaluate.
4. Did the nurse [NAP] have adequate knowledge and skills to perform techniques and procedures correctly?
   __ YES. No action.   __ NO. Continue same plan. Have someone else implement or help the nurse [or NAP] to acquire the needed knowledge or skills. If neither of these is possible, delete nursing order.

(continued)

5. Did client or family comply with the therapeutic regimen? Were self-care activities performed correctly?
   ___ YES. No action.
   ___ NO. Reassess motivation, knowledge, and resources. Add outcomes and nursing orders aimed at teaching, motivating, and supporting, patient in carrying out the regimen. Set time for reevaluation.

6. Did other staff members follow the nursing orders?
   ___ YES. No action.
   ___ NO. Implement the omitted nursing orders or ensure that others will do so. Set time for reevaluation. Find out why order was not carried out.

7. Was the plan of care implemented in a manner that communicated caring?
   ___ YES. No action.
   ___ NO. This is a problem that must be addressed by personal and staff development.

After making the necessary revisions to the care plan, implement the new plan and begin the nursing cycle again.

Source: Wilkinson, J. (2011). *Nursing process and critical thinking* (5th ed.). Upper Saddle River, NJ: Prentice Hall, pp. 325–327.

Functional Ability Assessment

The Joint Commission (2020) requires an initial functional ability assessment "based on the patient's condition." These three functional assessment tools are commonly used:

- **The Karnofsky Performance scale** (Karnofsky & Burchenal, 1949). This tool is used primarily in palliative care settings to assess functional abilities at the end of life. To see the scale,

  Go to http://www.npcrc.org/files/news/karnofsky_performance_scale.pdf

- **The Katz Index of ADL scale** (1963). This instrument is one of the best for assessing independent performance in very basic areas. It assigns 1 point for independence in each of the following areas: bathing, dressing, toileting, transfer, continence, and feeding. Nurses often use the data to plan staffing and appropriate placement of patients. The accompanying Focused Assessment box addresses functions similar to those assessed by the Katz scale. To see the Katz scale,

  Go to the ConsultGeri Web site at **https://hign.org/sites/default/files/2020-06/Try_This_General_Assessment_2.pdf**

- **Lawton Instrumental Activities of Daily Living (IADL) scale** (1969). This easy-to-use tool is particularly helpful in assessing a person's ability to independently perform the more sophisticated tasks of everyday life, such as shopping. Identifying early functional decline is important for discharge planning. The Lawton scale is especially useful for older adults, who may begin to have functional decline within 48 hours of hospital admission (Graf, 2008; Lawton & Brody, 1969).
- Patient Assessment Tool—Lawton Instrumental Activities of Daily Living.

Date: _____   Name: _____

Please check the box that most applies for each activity:

Activity	Needs no help (2 pts. each)	Needs some help (1 pt. each)	Unable to do at all (0 pts. each)
1. Using the telephone	___	___	___
2. Getting to places beyond walking distance	___	___	___
3. Grocery shopping	___	___	___
4. Preparing meals	___	___	___
5. Doing housework or handyman work	___	___	___
6. Doing laundry	___	___	___
7. Taking medications	___	___	___
8. Managing money	___	___	___

Total score: ___ =   (___ x 2 =) ___ +   (___ x 1 =) ___ +   0

A patient is awarded 2 points for each area in which he/she can function totally without help, 1 point in those areas that they need some help, and 0 points for those activities that somebody else must do completely for them. The maximum score is 16, minimum score is 0.

Like other evaluations, the IADL scale provides a baseline of data that can be compared with the results of future evaluations. (Note that some activities may be gender specific. Omit these items if the patient does not usually perform those tasks.)

Permission obtained from M. Powell Lawton, Ph.D., Philadelphia Geriatric Center, Philadelphia, PA. May be used freely for patient assessment. Formatted and posted May 25, 1996, to www.acsu.buffalo.edu/~drstall/assessmenttools.html by Robert S. Stall, M.D.

Special Needs Assessment: Questions for Assessing Independence in Activities of Daily Living

Focused Assessment

Mobility
Does the client require devices (e.g., cane, crutches, walker, wheelchair) for support?

Transfer
Can the client get in and out of bed and in and out of a chair without assistance?

If not, how much help does the client need?

Is the client completely confined to bed?

Bathing
Can the client perform a sponge bath, tub bath, or shower bath with no help?

If not, specifically what assistance does the client need?

Dressing
Can the client get all necessary clothing from drawers and closets and get completely dressed without help?

If not, specifically what assistance does the client need?

Feeding
Can the client feed themselves without assistance?

If not, specifically what assistance does the client need (e.g., help with cutting meat, tube feeding)?

Toileting
Can the client go to the bathroom, use the toilet, clean themselves, and rearrange clothing without help?

If a night bedpan or commode is used, can the client empty and clean it independently?

If the client needs help with these activities, specifically what does it include?

Continence
Does the client independently control urination and bowel movements?

If not, how often is the client incontinent of bladder or bowel?

Does the client require an indwelling urinary catheter?

Applying the Full-Spectrum Nursing Model

PATIENT SITUATION

You have now admitted Todd from the ED. Refer to the Meet Your Patient scenario for the data you need to answer the following questions. According to the ED report, Todd's admitting medical diagnosis is chronic renal failure. He is married, 58 years old, and employed, and he has a long-standing history of type 2 diabetes mellitus (DM). During the past 3 days, he reports that he has developed swelling and decreased sensation in his legs and difficulty walking, which he describes as "slight loss of mobility." You have many questions concerning Todd's immediate and long-term needs, which include the following:

His medication regimen	What laboratory tests have been completed
His compliance with his diabetes treatment plan	How severe his renal dysfunction has become
The extent to which his family is involved	His safety needs

After you obtain necessary data, you need to organize and analyze them to form some initial impressions about what they mean. Here are examples:

- Admitting diagnosis is chronic renal failure; anticipate a problem with fluid balance.

- Decreased sensation in lower extremities; patient may have problems with mobility and safety.

- Diabetes: Todd is at risk for impaired skin and tissue integrity.

- Diabetes and renal failure require complex treatment regimens and self-care: Is Todd managing his therapy effectively? If not, is it because he is not motivated to do so?

When Todd and his family arrive on your unit, you begin gathering comprehensive data. From that, you then make a list of Todd's health problems in order of priority.

THINKING

1. *Theoretical Knowledge:* What theoretical knowledge will you need to identify the collaborative problems and nursing diagnoses for Todd?

2. *Critical Thinking (Inquiry Based on Credible Sources):*
   a. What resources would you use to find out more about the pathophysiology of renal failure? How do you know the source is credible?

   b. When you are making your assessments of Todd, who is your best source of data? Why?

DOING

3. *Nursing Process (Diagnosis/Analyzing Cues):*
   a. Write one collaborative problem for Todd. If you do not know the potential complications of chronic renal failure, look them up in a medical-surgical or pathophysiology textbook. Explain why you would not use a nursing diagnosis to describe the problem.

   b. After further assessment, you observe that Todd's skin is intact and without redness or lesions. Write a nursing diagnosis (problem and etiology) to describe your concerns about his skin.

   c. Based on Maslow's hierarchy of needs, which problem has the highest priority?

CARING

4. *Ethical Knowledge:* The scenario does not provide enough information for you to identify the ethical dimensions of Todd's care. However, based on what you already know about him, speculate about some things that might create ethical questions for you.

PATIENT SITUATION

5. *Patient Preferences:* Think critically about the patient's preferences and concerns. Suppose that Todd's main concern is not the same as the high-priority problem you identified. Speculate about some other concerns he might have. What other things might he want to have resolved that could—for him—be more important than his chronic renal failure? Aside from his physical condition, what life concerns do you think Todd might have right now?

Critical Thinking & Clinical Judgment

1. Recall the definition of subjective data. Make a list of patients from whom you might not be able to get subjective data or who might give unreliable data. One example is a baby who cannot talk yet. How many others can you think of?

2. What are some factors that might make it difficult, but not impossible, for a patient to provide you with subjective data? One example is when the person is severely anxious.

3. For each of the factors in question 2, state what you could do to facilitate collection of reliable subjective data from that person.

4. The following are excerpts from criteria in the American Nurses Association (ANA) (2021) professional practice. Standard 1. For each criterion, write an example of what would constitute evidence (proof) that the standard is being followed in a healthcare agency. (The first one is done for you.)

    a. "Collects data . . . in a systematic and ongoing process."
    I would look in the care plan for nursing orders that call for some kind of assessment on a scheduled basis. For example, an order might read, "Temperature q4hr" or "Check dressing for drainage once per shift." I would also look at the nursing notes, especially for flow sheets (e.g., vital sign flow sheets, input and output records, neurological checks) to see whether assessment findings were recorded at regular intervals. I would look for nursing diagnoses or other conclusions they have charted in the nurses' notes (e.g., stating that the medication has effectively relieved pain). Other evidence would be to observe the nurses doing systematic and ongoing data collection. I would also perform my physical assessment in a systematic way, using the same order (unless otherwise indicated).

    b. "Engages the healthcare consumer and other interprofessional team members in holistic, culturally sensitive data collection."

    c. "Prioritizes data collection based on the healthcare consumer's immediate condition, or the anticipated needs . . ."

    d. "Uses evidence-based assessment techniques, instruments, tools, available data, information, and knowledge relevant to the situation to identify patterns and variances."

    e. "Documents relevant data accurately and in a manner accessible to the interprofessional team."

5. You have a homebound client with diabetes who has the beginning of a pressure injury. You have been treating the client for impaired skin integrity related to decreased circulation and mobility. However, the client's skin continues to break down.

    a. Your client has diabetes mellitus type 2. What type of problem is that (medical, nursing, or collaborative)?

    b. What is the client's nursing diagnosis?

c. The client has impaired skin integrity. The break in the body's first line of defense (intact skin) increases the risk for infection. Write a problem statement reflecting that risk nursing diagnosis.

6. Merle Quinn is visiting a family planning clinic where she has just been informed that she is 6 weeks pregnant. She looks worried and makes the following statements: "This is a shock. I've just started a new business, and I need to work 7 days a week to make it go. . . . I don't know if I'm ready to be a mother. . . ." Her husband agrees: "I just don't see how we can afford this. We don't even have any insurance now."

"Still," Mrs. Quinn says, "I don't see how I could deal with having an abortion. My parents would be devastated. I'm sure they'd never speak to me again." Her husband says, "Not to speak of the fact that the Church forbids it. It would be a sin."

A week later, Mrs. Quinn calls the clinic in tears. She says she has not been able to eat or sleep and that she doesn't know what to do about her pregnancy. "I don't want this baby, but I can't bring myself to have an abortion." You diagnose her with decisional conflict related to unexpected or unwanted pregnancy and possibly assume that she believes that abortion is her only alternative, as evidenced by statements of indecision, tearfulness, and inability to sleep. You make an appointment to see Mr. and Mrs. Quinn that same day. Imagine that you are writing the care plan for the Quinns.

a. Analyze your assumptions. What values and beliefs do you have that may influence the goals you write for the Quinns? Specifically, how could your values affect the goals you write?

b. Develop a short-term goal to address the problem clause of this nursing diagnosis. The goal should be one you expect the Quinns to be able to achieve during their appointment that same day.

c. You also write a goal: "By the end of this visit, clients will verbalize and demonstrate decreased anxiety and stress." Which part of the nursing diagnosis does this goal address?

d. The NOC standardized outcomes linked to the diagnosis of decisional conflict are the following (definitions are given):

Decision Making: Ability to choose between two or more alternatives

Information Processing: Ability to acquire, organize, and use information

Participation: Health Care Decisions: Personal involvement in selecting and evaluating healthcare options

Which of those outcomes is most important for the Quinns to achieve *today*? Why?

e. Now imagine that you have written the following individualized goals/outcomes for today's visit with the Quinns:
By the end of this visit, clients will:

1. Verbalize and demonstrate decreased anxiety and stress.

2. Verbalize awareness that they have options for coping with whatever decision they make about the pregnancy.

3. Discuss with the nurse options for continuing or terminating the pregnancy.

4. Verbalize intent to discuss their feelings with family (i.e., their parents).

5. Verbalize intent to discuss feelings with a member of the clergy.

6. Decide whether to continue the pregnancy.

- Why is outcome 2 so important?

- What would you have had to assume to write outcome 4?

- What would you have had to assume to write outcome 5?

- Which of the outcomes is/are probably *not* appropriate for today's visit? Why?

7. You are working a 12-hour shift (7 p.m. to 7 a.m.) on a medical unit at a local hospital. You will be caring for six adult patients. Make a list of the theoretical and practical knowledge you need about the patients to begin organizing your work for the shift. You may not yet have enough experience to make a complete list, but speculate about the kinds of information you think you might need. For example, to organize your work, you will need to know whether you have a UAP or an LVN/LPN to assist you or whether you are providing total care for the patients.

8. Alma Newport, who is 80 years old, has diabetes, severe arthritis, and mild dementia secondary to Alzheimer disease. She lives alone. She refuses to consider an assisted living facility or nursing home, although her primary provider and children, who live out of town, believe it would be safer for her to do so. On more than one occasion, she has forgotten to turn off a stove burner while cooking, burning the contents of the pan and smoking up the house.

    A home health nurse visits Mrs. Newport once a week. The physician wants Mrs. Newport to check and record her blood sugar levels before each meal. When the nurse asks, she says her blood sugar level is "OK" and shows the nurse the record she has kept, on which she has recorded many extremely low readings (e.g., 17, 20, 80, 24, 17 mg/dL). When the nurse checks Mrs. Newport's blood sugar, she obtains a reading of 210 mg/dL. After calibrating the glucose meter, the nurse writes the following care plan:

    Nursing Diagnosis:

    Deficient knowledge related to cognitive deficits secondary to dementia.

    Desired Outcomes:

    Mrs. Newport will demonstrate correct method for checking her blood sugar by next visit.

    Mrs. Newport will obtain correct readings.

    Nursing Orders:

    Teach correct method of fingerstick and checking blood glucose.

    Evaluate patient's technique at each visit.

    Over the next few weeks, the home health nurse checks Mrs. Newport's log and fingerstick method at each visit. The logs continue to show low readings, and Mrs. Newport remains unable to perform a fingerstick blood glucose test correctly despite repeated demonstrations.

    a. Evaluate Mrs. Newport's progress. Has she met, partially met, or not met the desired outcome?

    b. What possible reasons may account for your evaluation of Mrs. Newport's outcome status?

       Hints:

       1. Use your theoretical knowledge and personal experience with physical changes that occur with aging.

       2. Use the data you have about Mrs. Newport.

       3. Use your practical knowledge about nursing diagnoses.

9. A UAP is helping a patient with a shower when their pager goes off. After ensuring the patient's safety, the UAP goes into the hallway and answers the page. You observe that the UAP is still wearing gloves. How would you handle this situation?

What Are the Main Points in This Chapter?

- Assessment is a systematic, ongoing process of collecting, categorizing, and recording holistic data about client health status.
- Nursing assessments focus on client responses to illness and stressors rather than on identifying disease processes.
- Validating data helps to ensure that they are accurate, complete, and factual and you should involve patients in verifying and prioritizing their problems.
- Nursing diagnosis is the unique obligation of the professional nurse; it cannot be delegated.
- An accurate nursing diagnosis is the foundation for the plan of care because it directs the choice of client-centered goals and nursing interventions.
- Collaborative problems are potential physiological complications of diseases, treatments, or diagnostic studies that nurses monitor and help to prevent but that cannot be treated primarily by independent nursing interventions.
- A diagnostic statement consists basically of "problem + etiology"; however, a variety of formats is needed to describe client health status.
- In general, the problem side of the diagnostic statement directs the choice of goals; the etiology directs the choice of nursing interventions.
- During the planning outcomes phase, you will derive goals/expected outcomes from identified nursing diagnoses.
- Goals/expected outcomes (1) suggest nursing interventions, (2) serve as criteria for use in the evaluation step of the nursing process, and (3) provide motivation for patients and nurses.
- To ensure continuity of care, you should begin discharge planning with the initial patient assessment.
- A holistic, individualized patient care plan contains information needed to address (1) basic needs and ADLs, (2) medical and collaborative therapies, (3) nursing diagnoses and collaborative problems, and (4) special teaching and/or discharge needs.
- Standardized approaches to care planning include institutional policies and procedures, protocols, unit standards of care, standardized care plans, critical pathways, and integrated plans of care (IPOCs).
- Computer-assisted care planning helps ensure that the nurse considers a variety of interventions and does not overlook common and important interventions; it reduces the time spent on paperwork.
- Nursing-sensitive goals (expected outcomes, predicted outcomes, desired outcomes) describe the changes in patient health status that are intended to result from and can be influenced by nursing interventions.
- For every nursing diagnosis, you must state one "essential" goal—one that, if achieved, would demonstrate problem resolution or improvement.
- Goals should be concrete, specific, and observable; they should be valued by the patient/family; and they should not conflict with the medical treatment plan.
- Nursing interventions are treatments that nurses perform (1) in response to nursing diagnoses and (2) for the purpose of achieving client outcomes.
- Nursing interventions are performed for the purpose of assessing health status, preventing and treating disease/illness, and promoting health.
- The RN is responsible for choosing interventions and writing nursing orders; however, the RN can delegate actual performance of some interventions to UAPs and LPN/LVNs.
- Nursing orders, written on the nursing care plan, consist of the detailed instructions for performing nursing interventions.
- Implementation is the nursing process phase in which you perform or delegate the nursing activities that were planned in preceding steps.
- Delegation is the transfer of responsibility for an action while retaining the accountability for the outcome—this implies that you must supervise those to whom you delegate care.
- The final activity in the implementation step is documentation of the care provided. Documenting client responses is actually a part of the evaluation phase; however, you will document both at the same time, often in the same note.
- Evaluation is the final step of the nursing process. It is a planned, ongoing, systematic activity in which you use predetermined standards and criteria to make judgments about (1) patient progress toward health goals; (2) the effectiveness of the nursing care plan; and (3) the overall quality of care on a unit, in an organization, or in a geographical area.
- Quality improvement programs are specially designed to promote excellence in nursing. They include structure, process, and outcomes evaluation.

Knowledge Map

ASSESSMENT
- Nursing
  - Health
  - Environment
  - Client
    - Response to illness
    - Understanding of illness
- Collect and Validate Data
  - Subjective
  - Objective
- Document Data
  - Graphic flowsheet
  - Medication administration record
  - Discharge summary
- Organize Data
  - Nursing framework
  - Non-nursing framework

DIAGNOSING
- Problem or Diagnostic Label
  - Actual, risk, possible, syndrome, wellness
- Etiology (Related to Clause)
- Defining Characteristics
- Diagnostic Reasoning
  - Clustering cues
  - Analyzing & interpreting data
  - Identifying problem etiology
  - Drawing conclusions and making inferences
  - Verifying the problem
  - Prioritizing problems
  - Identifying types of nursing diagnoses

PLANNING
- Types
  - Formal/informal
  - Initial
  - Ongoing
  - Discharge planning
- Comprehensive Care Plans
  - Standardized
  - Individualized
  - Discharge or teaching
  - Computerized
- Standardized Language
  - NANDA
  - NOC
  - CCC
  - Omaha
  - Nursing framework
  - Non-nursing framework

INTERVENTIONS
- Achieve Client Goals and Outcomes
- Address Etiology of Nursing Diagnosis
- Based on Theory and Evidence Based Practice
- Nursing Orders
  - Date
  - Action verbs
  - Nursing behavior
  - Time/limits
  - Signature

IMPLEMENTATION
- Do or Delegate
- Promote Patient Participation
- Promote Patient Adherence
- Coordinate Care
- Delegate tasks using '5-Rights of Delegation'

EVALUATION
- Patient Progress Measured:
  - Based on goals and outcomes
  - Based on standards & criteria
- Final Step:
  - Revising the care plan

CHAPTER 4

Evidence-Based Practice: Theory & Research

STUDENT RESOURCES

The questions and exercises in this book allow you to practice the kind of thinking you will use as a full-spectrum nurse. Critical-thinking questions usually have more than one right answer, so we do not provide "correct" answers for these features. Try to answer these questions yourself. It is more important to develop your nursing judgment than to just cover content. You will learn more by discussing the questions with your peers. If you are still unsure, see the Davis Advantage chapter resources for suggested responses.

To explore learning resources for this chapter,

Go to www.DavisAdvantage.com and find:

Answers and Suggested Responses for all questions in this chapter
Concept Map
Knowledge Map
References and Bibliography

Key Concepts

Evidence-based practice
Nursing research
Nursing theory
Theory

Related Concepts

See the Concept Map on Davis Advantage.

Caring for the Williams Family

Stanley Williams arrives at the clinic for a follow-up visit. As you may recall, he has been diagnosed with hypertension. At a previous visit, you wrote this nursing diagnosis: Obesity related to inappropriate food choices and serving size, as evidenced by a body mass index (BMI) of 30.7. Today you have gathered the following intake data:

Blood pressure: 174/96 mm Hg
Heart rate: 88 beats/min
Respiratory rate: 18 breaths/min
Temperature: 98.5°F
Weight: 233 lb

A. What observations can you make about today's data in comparison with those of his initial visit?

B. As part of the treatment plan for Mr. Williams, you have been asked to educate him about a diet to assist with weight loss and hypertension management. How would you determine the most appropriate diet to include in your treatment plan?

C. Several sources recommend the DASH (Dietary Approaches to Stop Hypertension) eating plan. Go online and search for "Dietary Approaches to Stop Hypertension." Is there sufficient research to support incorporating this information into Mr. Williams' treatment plan? If so, describe the research and summarize the DASH eating plan.

CLINICAL REASONING
Applying the Full-Spectrum Nursing Model

PATIENT SITUATION

You are caring for a 90-year-old patient in a long-term care facility. He is completely dependent for performing activities of daily living (ADLs). In addition, he has been unresponsive, cannot swallow safely, and has been receiving fluids and nutrition through a feeding tube for many months. His adult grandson has recently discovered a living will in which the patient had stated that he does not wish to be kept alive by "artificial means, including being tube fed." The grandson, John, insists that the patient's wishes be honored, but the patient's son (Mr. Lee) threatens a lawsuit if the caregivers discontinue the feedings. They argue loudly, and Mr. Lee yells to his son, "You just want him gone because you're in a hurry to get his money!"

THINKING

1. *Theoretical Knowledge:* What facts are important to know to decide whether to stop the feedings?

2. *Critical Thinking (Analyzing Cues):* Without thinking too much, what is your first thought about what is causing the disagreement between Mr. Lee and his son, John? Examine your assumption. How certain are you that it is valid? What else might be going on in their lives to cause father and son to disagree on this issue?

DOING

3. *Clinical Judgment (Assessment/Recognizing Cues):* To provide some information about the patient that might be helpful in restoring peace between Mr. Lee and John, what patient assessments should you make?

CARING

4. *Ethical Knowledge:* State one ethical issue involved in this case—or one moral problem that the case would present for you if you were involved in it.

▶ Go to **Davis Advantage, Resources, Chapter 4, Applying the Full-Spectrum Nursing Model—Suggested Responses**.

Critical Thinking and Clinical Judgment

1. Recall the scenario about Mr. Khatri (Meet Your Patient) in Volume 1. Imagine you are the home health nurse providing care to a frail older man in his home. Mr. Khatri is visibly upset and is grabbing at the belt around his waist as he sits in the chair. He is crying out to his deceased mother to come and take him to her. Using any nursing theory you wish, or your own idea, describe each of the four concepts of a theory as they apply in this scenario:

    a. Patient (Who is the patient? How do you know?)

    b. Nurse (Who is the nurse? What is she doing that is "nursing"?)

    c. Health (Is the patient healthy? What is the patient's state of health?)

    d. Environment (Where is the nurse–patient encounter occurring?)

2. Recall Maslow's hierarchy of needs. Give one example of a specific nursing intervention a nurse could do to meet each of those needs. If you think the nurse cannot address a need, explain why.

   a. Physiological

   b. Safety and security (mental and physical protection)

   c. Love and belonging

   d. Self-esteem (achievement, reputation)

   e. Cognitive needs (knowledge, self-awareness)

   f. Aesthetic needs (beauty, balance, form)

   g. Self-actualization (personal growth, fulfillment)

   h. Transcendence (helping others to self-actualize)

3. You are an emergency department nurse taking care of a 4-year-old child who has had a bike accident. The child has an open abrasion and a few cuts that will require some minor care. However, he is frightened and crying.

   a. Using Nightingale's theory, what interventions might you use?

   b. Using Watson's theory, what might you do?

   c. Using Henderson's theory, what would be the focus of your interventions?

   d. Choose one of the following theories: Neuman, Orem, or Rogers. Describe how that theory would direct you in this case.

4. You are working the night shift, and while making your 2 a.m. rounds, you are surprised as you look into the room of 22-year-old Angela Kindred and see her mother sitting at her bedside and sobbing. Visits are not encouraged at that time of night, and you did not know Mrs. Kindred was on the unit. Even though Angela's leukemia is terminal, you understood from the nurse on the day shift that the family, as well as Angela, had accepted the inevitable outcome.

   a. Explain how you can demonstrate caring to this mother who will soon lose her beloved daughter.

   b. Look at Watson's (1988) 10 caring processes, repeated as follows from the textbook. How can you use them to demonstrate caring to this mother and daughter? Be specific in your answers.

Watson's 10 Caring Processes

1. Forming a humanistic–altruistic system of values
2. Instilling faith and hope
3. Cultivating sensitivity to self and others
4. Forming helping and trusting relationships
5. Conveying and accepting the expression of positive and negative feelings
6. Systematic use of the scientific problem-solving method that involves caring process
7. Promoting transpersonal teaching–learning
8. Providing for supportive, protective, and corrective mental, physical, sociocultural, and spiritual environment
9. Assisting with gratification of human needs
10. Sensitivity to existential–phenomenological forces

5. You are a nurse in an urgent care clinic taking care of a 3-year-old with wounds from a dog bite. The child is frightened, even though his mother is sitting in the treatment room with him. You ask the mother to hold the child while he is being treated and restrain him, if necessary.

    In reflecting on this intervention afterward, you decide to find the best evidence for your intervention to be certain that you will want to use it in similar situations in the future. Write a PICOT question to guide your literature search. Write each part, then write the full statement.

    P—
    I—
    C—
    O—
    T—
    Full statement of the question:

6. Read analytically an article in a research journal. Answer the following questions about the article:

    a. What is the article about as a whole? Answer using one sentence.

    b. What are the author's main conclusions?

    c. Do you think these conclusions are true? If not, why not?

    d. Is this article of any significance in nursing? That is, how could it be used to improve patient care or nursing education?

7. For each of the following concepts, use critical thinking to describe how or why it is important to nursing, patient care, or nursing theory and research. Note that these are *not* to be merely definitions.

Nursing theory	Nursing research
The science of human caring	Institutional review board
From novice to expert	Informed consent
Culturally competent care	Research utilization
Evidence-based practice	Analytical reading

What Are the Main Points in This Chapter?

- The four components of a nursing theory are person, nurse, environment, and health.
- A theory is developed by recognizing a need or by having an idea for an improvement, using research to determine whether the idea is effective, and then using the research process to define a theory.
- Theories help nurses (1) find meaning in their experiences of nursing; (2) organize their thinking around pertinent ideas; and (3) develop new, evidence-based ideas and insights into the work they do.
- Nurses use theories as an evidence-based framework for their nursing practice.
- Three leaders in nursing caring theories are Dr. Jean Watson, Dr. Patricia Benner, and Dr. Madeleine Leininger.
- Nursing research is a systematic, objective process of analyzing phenomena of importance in nursing.
- Quantitative research may be generalized to populations similar to the sample studied, presuming the sample represents the greater group. Influencing factors are controlled and the data are analyzed using suitable statistical methods.
- Qualitative research is conducted to gain understanding of a phenomenon or concept, or explain behavior, perceptions, or ideas. This type of research commonly examines the lived experience of a person or group of people by interview and observation of a small number of participants.
- The research process is a systematic way of organizing, preparing, and presenting research.

- Research participants (people in a research study) are protected from harm by specific laws and regulations.
- The two main responsibilities of the institutional review board are (1) to protect the research participants from harm and (2) to ensure that the research is of value.
- Components of informed consent include the following:
  - Right to not be harmed
  - Right to full disclosure
  - Right to self-determination (right to say no)
  - Rights of privacy and confidentiality
- Evidence-based nursing requires evaluating scientific research based on sound methodology and statical procedures to find the best evidence and then applying it in practice.
- The process of finding best evidence consists of identifying a clinical nursing problem, formulating a searchable question, searching the literature, evaluating the quality of the research, and integrating the research into practice.
- The PICOT format is a structure used to formulate a searchable clinical question. The parts of a PICOT question are **p**atient problem, **i**ntervention, **c**omparison intervention, **o**utcome, and **t**ime.

Knowledge Map

Theorists:
- Henderson: Basic needs
- Peplau: Interpersonal relationships
- Nightingale: Environment
- Watson, Benner, Leininger: Caring

NURSING THEORY — contributes to → **EVIDENCE-BASED PRACTICE** ← contributes to — **NURSING RESEARCH**

Evidence-Based Practice stimulates/contributes to Nursing Theory.

Nursing Theory:
- Inductive and deductive reasoning
- assists in:
  - Finding meaning
  - Organizing thoughts
  - Developing evidence-based ideas
- includes:
  - Phenomena
  - Assumptions
  - Concepts
  - Definitions
  - Statements
  → Person, Environment, Health, Nursing

Nursing Research employs **SCIENTIFIC METHOD**:
- QUANTITATIVE
- QUALITATIVE

Quantitative:
- ID problem
- Clarify purpose
- Review literature
- Develop framework
- Formulate hypothesis
- Define variables
- Select sample
- Conduct pilot
- Analyze data
- Interpret findings
- Share findings

CHAPTER 5

Ethics & Values

STUDENT RESOURCES

The questions and exercises in this book allow you to practice the kind of thinking you will use as a full-spectrum nurse. Critical-thinking questions usually have more than one right answer, so we do not provide "correct" answers for these features. Try to answer these questions yourself. It is more important to develop your nursing judgment than to just cover content. You will learn more by discussing the questions with your peers. If you are still unsure, see the Davis Advantage chapter resources for suggested responses.

To explore learning resources for this chapter,

Go to www.DavisAdvantage.com and find:

Answers and Suggested Responses for all questions in this chapter
Concept Map
Knowledge Map
References and Bibliography

Key Concepts

Morals
Nursing ethics
Values

Related Concepts

See the Concept Map on Davis Advantage.

Example Client Conditions

Moral distress
Whistleblowing

Caring for the Williams Family

Charlene Williams, Stanley Williams' mother, has hypertension. She is forgetful about taking her medicines. Since her husband died, she has had periods of depression. When asked about her medicines, she often replies, "It doesn't really matter since my husband died. If I die, what difference will it make?"

Charlene was scheduled to have lunch with friends but did not arrive. When her friends called the house, they got no answer. At the end of lunch, one of Charlene's friends decided to call Stanley to inform him of her concerns about his mother. Stanley found his mother unresponsive on the kitchen floor. He called 911, and she was brought to the hospital by ambulance. At the hospital, the emergency department (ED) physician tells Stanley that his mother has had a massive stroke (brain attack) brought on by uncontrolled hypertension. He

(Continued)

31

Caring for the Williams Family (continued)

asks Stanley whether Charlene has an advance directive. She does not. The physician asks Stanley to consider what level of care to offer his mother. He tells Stanley that comprehensive treatment would include intubation, mechanical ventilation, and tube feeding support. The physician thinks it is unlikely that she will have significant recovery from this stroke.

Stanley tells you, "I want everything done for my mother. I lost my father this year, and I'm not going to lose her, too." Nadine, Stanley's wife, reminds you that Charlene has been depressed since her husband died and has expressed a desire to die. Because Stanley and Nadine are not in agreement about the course of action, no decision is communicated. Charlene's condition continues to deteriorate, and the ED physician feels he must intubate her, place her on a ventilator, and admit her to the ICU according to hospital protocol.

A. You are aware of Charlene's statements and her poor compliance with treatment. What, if any, concerns do you have about this course of action?

B. Charlene's condition continues to decline. Stanley is informed that the "only thing keeping your mother alive is the ventilator and IV medicines." Do you consider this heroic treatment?

C. How would you approach Stanley to speak with him about how he is feeling?

D. Stanley and Nadine have asked to meet with the team providing care to Charlene. They announce that they would like all the "heroic measures to end." They request that Charlene be allowed to die. Could you participate in this care? With what actions would you be comfortable? With what actions would you be uncomfortable?

Practical Knowledge clinical application

Practical knowledge in nursing ethics primarily involves communication and problem-solving skills. We have included one model of ethical decision making as well as guidelines for patient advocacy for your quick reference in clinical situations.

CLINICAL INSIGHTS

Clinical Insight 5-1 ▸ Using the MORAL Model for Ethical Decision Making

- **M—Massage the dilemma.** Identify and define the issues in the dilemma. Consider the options of all the major players in the dilemma and their value systems. This includes patients, family members, nurses, physicians, religious representatives, and other interdisciplinary healthcare members. Identify the information gaps.
- **O—Outline the options.** Examine all the options, including those that are less realistic and conflicting. This stage is only for considering options and not for making final decisions.
- **R—Resolve the dilemma.** Review issues and options, applying principles of ethics to each option. Decide the best option based on the views of all those concerned in the dilemma.
- **A—Act by applying the chosen option.** This step is usually the most difficult because it requires actual implementation, whereas the previous steps allow for only dialogue and discussion.
- **L—Look back and evaluate.** Reflect on the entire process and evaluate all steps, including the implementation. No process is complete without thorough evaluation. Ensure that those involved can follow through on the final option. If not, a second decision may be required, and the process must begin again at the first step.

Practice Resources
Badruddin, S. (2016); Yoder-Wise, P. (2019).

Clinical Insight 5-2 ➤ Guidelines for Advocacy

The following principles will help you to function effectively as an advocate.

- **Keep the ethical principle of patient autonomy in mind.**
- **Know and document the facts** of the case.
- **Know the arguments** of those who oppose the patient. Use role playing to develop a strategy for responding to the arguments.
- **Have a sound base of support for your actions.** Be familiar with any policies or laws that apply.
- **Form a coalition of allies,** if you can. Get consultation. Communicate, inform, and clarify their collaborative roles.
- **Intervene high enough in the hierarchy** to get the job done. If the difficulty is with a provider or an organizational policy, merely going to the charge nurse will not be enough. You will need to communicate with nurse administrators or other agency administrators.
- **Demonstrate to the system** how it is defeating its own goals (e.g., for patient care).
- **Avoid getting into a power struggle** if possible (use the preceding steps first). If you must, decide how far you need to go and whether you are willing to go that far. You will need to enlist people with more power in the system than you have (e.g., family members, providers, administrators).
- **Be aware of client vulnerability.** When possible, avoid confrontation. If there is risk for the client (as in a power contest), be sure the client is aware of his risks and possible gains; then let him choose how far to take the situation.
- **Have alternative actions.** Assess risks realistically. Weigh them against potential gains.

CLINICAL REASONING
Applying the Full-Spectrum Nursing Model
PATIENT SITUATION

Read the following summary of the Kithari and Kirschner article:

Kothari, S., & Kirschner, K. (2006). Abandoning the golden rule: The problem with "putting ourselves in the patient's place." *Topics in Stroke Rehabilitation, 13*(4), 68–73.

A large body of evidence documents the difficulties healthcare professionals have in predicting what their patient believes or wishes. These difficulties extend from these predictions:

- Very specific patient wishes, such as for life-sustaining therapies
- More global assessments of patients' lives as a whole (e.g., their quality of life)

One explanation for this phenomenon is that healthcare professionals, either consciously or unconsciously, adopt "golden rule thinking." This refers to our attempts to understand another person's situation by imagining what we would believe or want under similar circumstances—in other words, putting ourselves in the patient's place.

Although golden rule thinking would seem to be a promising strategy, studies show that it results in inaccurate presumptions of a patient's wishes or beliefs. These presumptions, in turn, have significant clinical and ethical implications. That is, they cause healthcare professionals and families to make decisions for the patient that are, in reality, *not* what the patient would want. The thinking goes like this:

I should put myself in the patient's place.   Therefore, the patient probably wants X.

If I were the patient, I would want X.   Because the patient probably wants X, we will do X.

This thinking process can have different results: (1) The patient really does want X, so you have met his needs. (2) The patient really wanted Y, so you did not meet his needs.

THINKING

1. *Theoretical Knowledge:* What is the golden rule, or what does it say?

2. *Critical Thinking (Inquiry):* What is one thing that could be done ahead of time to prevent the need for golden rule thinking? Explain why that would work.

DOING

3. *Nursing Process (Assessment):* If the patient's wishes are unknown, instead of thinking what *you* would want, how could you get an idea of what the patient might want?

CARING

4. *Self-Knowledge:* What is your earliest memory of being taught the golden rule?

5. *Ethical Knowledge:* Which ethical principle does the golden rule seem to try to follow: autonomy, nonmaleficence/beneficence, fidelity, veracity, or justice?

Critical Thinking and Clinical Judgment

1. Some examples of ethical issues you may encounter are end-of-life issues, abortion or other reproductive issues, breaches of patient confidentiality, and incompetent or illegal practices of colleagues. Think about a time when you have witnessed an ethical challenge in the clinical area.

    a. Describe the situation.

    b. How well equipped did you feel to handle the situation?

    c. What guided your thoughts and actions?

2. At the beginning of this chapter in Volume 1, Alan (Meet Your Patients), a teenager, had been injured in a soccer game. Without a blood transfusion, he may die, but because his family is of the Jehovah's Witnesses faith, Alan's parents have refused to grant permission for his transfusion. Considering each of the abilities required for ethical agency, state whether you think these people have the abilities in the following lettered list: Alan, Alan's parents, the physician/surgeon, the nurse. Explain your thinking. An ethical agent must be able to do the following:

    a. Perceive the difference between good and evil, right and wrong.

    Alan   Physician/surgeon

    Parents   Nurse

    b. Understand abstract ethical principles.

    Alan   Physician/surgeon

    Parents   Nurse

    c. Reason and apply ethical principles to make decisions, weigh alternatives, and plan ways to achieve goals.

    Alan   Physician/surgeon

    Parents   Nurse

    d. Decide and choose freely.

        Alan   Physician/surgeon

        Parents   Nurse

    e. Act according to his choice; this assumes both the power and the capability to act.

        Alan   Physician/surgeon

        Parents   Nurse

3. Consider Alan's situation again. Analyze the situation (a) using a deontological framework and ethical principles and then (b) using a utilitarian framework. Focus on this question: Is it ethical to try hard to influence the parents to consent to allow a blood transfusion?

    a. Deontology

    b. Utilitarianism

    c. Did you reach a different conclusion depending on the framework you selected?

4. You are a busy nurse with a caseload of eight patients. One patient, Lily, is the mother of the hospital administrator. She had surgery 3 days ago and is progressing nicely, but she is very demanding and requires a great deal of assistance to be repositioned in bed and to move from bed to chair. She has frequent visitors, including children and young grandchildren. In the next room is a patient with a history of drug abuse who had emergency surgery this morning. She speaks little English and seems very anxious. She has nausea and pain and needs a transfusion of a unit of packed red blood cells this evening. Her boyfriend is at the desk requesting to bring her 3-year-old daughter to the unit so that she may see her mother. The visiting policy says that children must be at least 12 years old to visit the unit. Consider what aspects of justice apply to this situation and how it might be most equitably handled. Focus on the principle of justice.

5. An example of the feminist ethical approach arises in deciding whether to allocate federal healthcare resources to younger people (e.g., education, day care, free immunizations) or to older adults (e.g., prescription drug insurance, long-term care). Feminist reasoning would be as follows:

    a. In the United States, older women outnumber older men.

    b. Older women tend to be poorer and are more likely to be alone than are men.

    c. Therefore, if healthcare for older adults were to be rationed, it would negatively affect women more than it would men.

    d. Thus, more healthcare resources should be allocated to older adults, especially women.

        1. Analyze this decision using a deontological framework. Explain your reasoning, as was done above.

        2. Analyze this decision using a consequentialist framework. Explain your reasoning.

6. Deception can take various forms, from intentional lying to nondisclosure of information or partial disclosure of information. Think about your duty to tell the truth. Is there ever a time when being completely honest is not the best nursing intervention? Do you consider withholding information the same as lying?

7. Review the following scenario. Examine your self-knowledge, and work through the steps of the values clarification process (choosing, prizing, and acting). A 40-year-old couple with no other children learn that their unborn child has Down syndrome. The couple need to make a difficult decision because the mother is 18 weeks pregnant.

   a. How would you feel about this couple if they chose to have this child and insisted on doing everything possible to keep the baby alive even if it is born with severe handicaps?

   b. Do you think that your professional relationship with this couple would change if they chose to terminate the pregnancy?

   c. How can you help the couple clarify their values?

      (1) List alternatives.

      (2) Examine the possible consequences of the alternative choices.

      (3) Choose freely.

      (4) Feel good about the choice that has been made.

      (5) Affirm the choice to others.

      (6) Act on the choice.

      (7) Act with a consistent pattern.

What Are the Main Points in This Chapter?

- Ethics is a formal process for deciding right and wrong conduct in situations where issues of values and morals arise.
- *Nursing ethics* refers to ethical questions that arise out of nursing practice.
- Morals are learned and internalized throughout the life span. Carol Gilligan proposed that moral development and reasoning are different among men and women.
- Ethical agency is the ability to make ethical choices and to be responsible for one's ethical actions. In practice, nurses sometimes make moral decisions that they are not able to carry out.
- Moral distress is the inability to carry out moral decisions.
- Whistleblowing occurs when a person identifies in the workplace an incompetent, unethical, or illegal situation or actions of others and then appeals to someone who may have the power to stop it.
- Nursing ethics problems arise from technological advances, the needs of a multicultural population, cost containment efforts in healthcare, the nature of nursing work, and the nature of the nursing profession.
- Nurses have complex obligations and multiple complex relationships within healthcare organizations (e.g., with employers, providers, patients, families, and other nurses).
- Ethical decisions are affected by a person's developmental stage, values, ethical frameworks and principles, and professional guidelines.
- Attitudes are mental dispositions or feelings toward a person, object, or idea.
- A belief is something that one accepts as true.
- A value is a belief that you have about the worth of something; a value is highly prized and expressed through behaviors, feelings, and decisions.
- Values are transmitted through social interaction.
- Value neutrality means that we attempt to understand our own values regarding an issue and to know when to put them aside, if necessary, to become nonjudgmental.
- Values clarification is the process of becoming conscious of and naming one's values. Nurses can assist clients with values clarification.
- Six important ethical principles are autonomy, nonmaleficence, beneficence, fidelity, veracity, and justice.

- Consequentialist theories are ethical theories in which the rightness or wrongness of an action depends on the consequences of the act rather than on the nature of the act itself.
- The principle of utility states that a "good" act is one that produces the greatest good for the greatest number of people.
- Deontological theories consider an action to be right or wrong independent of its consequences.
- Feminist ethics asserts that focusing on deontological principles distracts one from dealing with larger social issues and that objectivity is impossible.
- Ethics of care directs attention to a patient's specific situation viewed within the context of his or her life narrative. It emphasizes feelings but not at the expense of some conventional ethical principles, such as autonomy, nonmaleficence, or beneficence.
- Nurses can obtain ethical guidance from professional codes of ethics, standards of practice, and the American Hospital Association's *Patient Care Partnership*.
- The principle of autonomy underlies informed consent—clients' right to decide for themselves whether they will agree to a proposed procedure or treatment.
- Specific ethical issues the nurse is likely to encounter may involve abortion, allocation of resources, issues of confidentiality, end-of-life issues (e.g., advance directives, DNAR/AND prescriptions, life-sustaining treatments, informed consent, organ transplantation), and reproductive technologies.
- Not all moral problems are dilemmas. A dilemma is a particular kind of moral problem. It is a painful situation in which a choice must be made between two equally undesirable actions. There is no clearly right or wrong option.
- One method of working through an ethical problem is to perform assessment and diagnosis, as in the nursing process; then use the mnemonic MORAL: **m**assage the dilemma, **o**utline the options, **r**esolve the dilemma, **a**ct by applying the chosen option, and **l**ook back and evaluate.
- A good compromise preserves the integrity of all parties when there is disagreement among them in a moral situation.
- Nurses should be patient advocates because (1) their professional role requires it, (2) they have special knowledge that the patient does not have, (3) they have a special relationship with patients, and (4) one aspect of the nursing role is to defend patient's autonomous decisions.
- The nurse's role as an advocate is to inform, support, and communicate.

Knowledge Map

Age, maturity level, environmental stimuli *influence* →

STAGES OF MORAL DEVELOPMENT
- Piaget
- Kohlberg
- Gilligan

MORALS — Broad consideration of right and wrong

NURSING ETHICS

ETHICS — Formal process for making moral decisions

Moral decisions ---- used in making ---- **Bioethics**

FACTORS AFFECTING MORAL DECISIONS
- Values
- Beliefs
- Attitudes
- Moral principles
  - Autonomy, fidelity
  - Nonmaleficence
  - Beneficence, veracity
- Moral frameworks
- Professional guidelines

NURSING ETHICS — Ethical questions that involve nursing actions

RELATED CONCEPTS
- Ethical agency
- Moral distress
- Moral outrage
- Whistle-blowing

To maintain ethical practice:
- Clarify own values
- Assist client with value clarification
- Be familiar with ethical decision-making models
- Understand concepts of compromise
- Understand obligation in ethical decisions

Factors contributing to ethical problems:
- Societal factors
- Nature of nursing work
- Nature of nursing profession

UNIT 2

Factors Affecting Health

6 **Life Span: Infancy Through Middle Adulthood**

7 **Life Span: Older Adults**

8 **Experiencing Wellness: Health & Illness**

9 **Stress & Adaptation**

10 **Psychosocial Health & Illness**

11 **Promoting Family Health**

12 **Caring in Multicultural Healthcare Environments**

13 **Spirituality**

14 **Experiencing Loss**

CHAPTER 6

Life Span: Infancy Through Middle Adulthood

STUDENT RESOURCES

The questions and exercises in this section allow you to practice the kind of thinking you will use as a full-spectrum nurse. Critical-thinking questions usually have more than one right answer, so we do not provide "correct" answers for these features. It is more important to develop your nursing judgment than to just cover content. You will learn more by discussing the questions with your peers. If you are still unsure, see the Davis Advantage chapter resources for suggested responses.

To explore learning resources for this chapter,

Go to www.DavisAdvantage.com and find:

Answers and Suggested Responses for all questions in this chapter
Concept Map
Knowledge Map
References and Bibliography

Key Concepts

Growth
Development
Stages

Related Concepts

See the Concept Map on Davis Advantage.

Caring for the Williams Family

Review the scenario of Stanley Williams in the front of this book. Answer the following questions based on that scenario:

A. Evaluate Mr. Williams' physical health status in comparison with what is expected for someone in his age group.

B. Mr. Williams and his wife are raising their 3-year-old granddaughter. What effect might this have on Mr. Williams' ability to accomplish his developmental tasks?

PracticalKnowledge clinical application

One important aspect of developmental care across the life span is to identify abuse and intervene for patients who are being abused.

PROCEDURES

You will find information on elder abuse in Chapter 10; however, the following procedure can be used for patients of all ages.

Keep in mind that if there is an injury, it's possible that it was inflicted. The following flow chart and Procedure 6-1 will aid you in identifying cases of abuse.

Possible Abuse Flow Chart

```
                              Start
                                │
                                ▼
              Has there been a delay in seeking treatment for injuries
                                and/or illness?
                ┌───────────────┴───────────────┐
                ▼                               ▼
               NO                              YES
                │                               │
                ▼                               │
        Are injuries consistent with history? ──► NO
                │                               │
                ▼                               │
               YES                              │
                │                               │
                ▼                               │
        Is there a history of frequent injuries ──► YES
                and/or illness?                 │
                │                               │
                ▼                               │
               NO                               │
                │                               │
                ▼                               │
        Is behavior appropriate for the patient's ──► NO
                developmental level?            │
                │                               │
                ▼                               ▼
               YES                              │
                │                               │
                ▼                               ▼
        Low risk of abuse               High risk of abuse
```

Procedure 6-1 ■ Assessing for Abuse

▶ For steps to follow in *all* procedures, refer to the Universal Steps for All Procedures found on the inside back cover of this text.

Preprocedure Assessments

- If you suspect sexual abuse, request that a forensic nurse or sexual assault nurse examiner (SANE) be present.
  A forensic nurse and a SANE are specially trained to identify findings that indicate abuse, to support the patient, and to handle the evidence to ensure validity in a court of law.
- Assess for abuse routinely in older or vulnerable adults and women of childbearing age and any time a child, dependent person, or spouse has an injury.

Even in the absence of a strong base of evidence to support screening, The Joint Commission requires that all patients be screened for abuse and domestic violence.

Delegation

Key Point: *Assessment is a nursing responsibility and cannot be delegated.*

▶ When performing the procedure, always identify your patient, according to agency policy, by using two identifiers, and be attentive to standard precautions, hand hygiene, patient safety and privacy, body mechanics, and documentation.

▶ Privacy and confidentiality are extremely important for this procedure.

Procedure Steps

Obtain a Focused Health History.

1. **Interview the patient and family members or caregivers separately.** In case of more than one caregiver, separate them for the interview.
   A person experiencing abuse may be afraid to talk in the presence of the abuser. Victims have often been intimidated and will usually support the abuser's version of events. If two adults accompany a child, it may be that one of them is abusing both the partner and the child. To help rule that out, separate the caregivers to be certain that they tell the same story.

2. **Approach the subject in a nonthreatening and caring manner.** For example, you might say, "The law requires us to ask about certain injuries. We are not accusing you of anything. I know you care about your child/parent/spouse and want to do everything possible for their health."

3. **Consider the patient's developmental and cognitive level** in assessing whether the story of how the injury occurred is consistent with the injuries.
   The patient must be developmentally capable of performing an activity in the situation where the injury occurred. For example, an infant is not likely to have opened a medication bottle and taken the pills; if a child cannot yet walk, it is not likely that they reached up to pull a hot pan off the stove.

4. **Observe the patient's behavior.** Is it inconsistent with the patient's developmental level?
   In the presence of the abuser, it is common for the victim of abuse to appear passive and withdrawn and avoid eye contact. The victim may exhibit anxiety or fear, may look to the parent or caregiver before answering questions, may be overly compliant, or may let the abuser answer the questions.

5. **Ask about the injury or incident.** Ask detailed questions about how and when the injury occurred or the illness began: "When did this injury happen or when did you first begin to feel ill?" "How did you get this injury?" "What happened to you?" "What have you been doing to treat your symptoms since you first became ill?"
   A delay in treatment of 12 to 18 hours may indicate abuse. If the details of the history of an injury change during the interview, the likelihood of abuse increases.

6. **Ask about past injuries or incidents:** "Have you ever had similar injuries?" "Have you ever required emergency care in the past?"
   Abusive behavior typically occurs repeatedly. If an injury is caused by abuse, the patient is most likely to have experienced abuse in the past and will have evidence of old injuries.

7. **Ask about the patient's usual diet:** "What do you usually eat for breakfast? Lunch? Dinner? What kind of snacks do you have during the day?"
   Neglect and/or abuse may be in the form of an inadequate or inappropriate diet.

Assess for Sexual Abuse.

8. **Ask directly whether the patient has been touched** inappropriately or forced to have sexual relations.
   Whenever possible, question the patient directly so that your question will not be misunderstood.

9. **Ask whether the patient has genitourinary symptoms:** "Have you had any burning or itching when you urinate? How about any vaginal discharge?"
   In a child, genitourinary symptoms may indicate sexual abuse or neglect.

10. **Does the child display knowledge or interest in sexual acts** inappropriate to their age or even seductive behavior?

11. **Does the child appear to avoid another person** or display unusual behavior—either very aggressive or very passive?

12. **Does the victim display destructive behaviors,** such as alcohol or drug abuse, self-mutilation, or suicide attempts?

13. **Is the victim pregnant,** particularly if no intimate relationship is known or the victim is very young?

(continued on next page)

UNIT 2 Factors Affecting Health

Procedure 6-1 ■ Assessing for Abuse (continued)

Assess for Psychological Abuse.

14. **Ask parents or caregivers,** "Are there family members or friends who help you with problems?"
    Isolation is a risk factor for abuse. Parents or caregivers may not have the support they need.

15. **Ask the patient, "Whom do you talk to** when you are having problems?"
    An abuser will try to isolate the victim from family and friends over time. Ask questions to determine what the relationship is between the victim and family and friends.

16. **Ask, "Tell me how you feel about yourself."**
    An abuser demeans and degrades the victim so that the victim has low self-worth and feels that the "punishment" is deserved; conversely, the victim may desire the attention of the abuser, even if it is in the form of abuse.

17. **Observe if the child acts fearful,** shies away from touch, or appears to be afraid to go home.

18. **Ask, "Who manages the family finances,** and how are decisions made regarding spending?" (for adults)
    An abuser frequently controls all the finances and restricts the resources of the victim. Abusers typically seek control of victims by fostering dependency and powerlessness.

Perform a Focused Physical Assessment.

19. **If sexual abuse is suspected** from the interview, have a forensic nurse or SANE present, if possible.
    For any sexual examination, always have a witness in the room to protect the patient and the examiner.

20. **Assess the current injury,** and look for evidence of previous injuries. Look for the following cues:
    a. Bruises that form an outline of a hand, cord loop, buckle, or belt
        *Injuries of different ages and multiple injuries may show a pattern of abuse. Be careful to assess the bruise accurately. Some home treatments may cause what looks like bruising. For example, **moxibustion** (includes such actions as firmly rubbing a warm spoon down the affected area) is used in some Asian cultures.*
    b. Injuries that are inconsistent with the history of the injuries or are of varying stages (e.g., bruises of different colors, cuts in varying stages of healing)
    c. Obvious nonaccidental burns, such as burns to both feet and lower legs from immersion in hot water
        One method of abuse is to immerse the victim's hands or feet in scalding water. The resulting injury has a well-defined border and usually appears on both extremities.
    d. Circular burns, possibly from cigarettes
        Burns at several locations on the body are signs of abuse.
    e. Bite marks
    f. Oral ecchymosis (injury from forced oral sex)
        Forced oral sex will cause injuries to the mouth.
    g. Bruising at the crease above the eyelids, tense fontanel if the victim is an infant, hyphema, subconjunctival hemorrhage or retinal bleeding, detached retina, ruptured tympanic membrane

    KEY POINT: *Injuries to the head are common in abuse. Abusive head trauma (AHT, previously referred to as shaken-baby syndrome) is one of the most common and most serious injuries in young children.*

    h. Bleeding or bruising of genitalia, poor sphincter tone, encopresis (poor bowel control), and bruises on inner thighs
    i. Positive culture result for sexually transmitted infection (STI) or positive pregnancy test result
        An STI, particularly in a child, can indicate sexual abuse.
    j. Bruises on wrists and ankles from being restrained
        Abused individuals may be tied or locked in a closet or other small space.
    k. Refer to the figure for typical features of injuries that may be nonaccidental:
        Injuries to both sides of the body
        Injuries to soft tissues
        Injuries in the "triangle of safety": ears, side of face, neck, and top of the shoulders
        Accidental injuries in the triangle of safety are unusual. Accidental injuries are usually over bony prominences. One suspicious pattern is the "swimsuit zone" on the trunk, breast, abdomen, genitalia, and buttocks. ▼

Black eyes, especially bilateral
Soft tissues of cheeks
Intra-oral injuries
Forearm raised to protect self
Chest and abdomen
Groin or genital injury
Inner aspects of thighs
Soles of feet

Ears – especially pinch marks involving both sides of the ear
The "triangle of safety"
Inner aspects of arms
Back and side of trunk, except directly over the bony spine

21. **Assess whether the injuries are consistent with the history.**
    If the injuries are not consistent with the history, you must assume abuse.

22. **Observe for signs of neglect:**
    - Malnutrition, such as a distended abdomen, or weight markedly below ideal body weight
    - Excess body weight for height and age
    - Poor hygiene, including oral hygiene
    - Ingrown nails
    - Untreated sores or pressure sores or other medical conditions
    - Matted hair
    - Dehydration
    - Confusion
    - Clothing that is inappropriate for the weather, such as heavy, full-length pants and long-sleeved shirts on hot days
    - Long periods a young child or a frail older adult is left alone without care or supervision

    Signs of neglect occur because of long-term starvation or underfeeding, poor personal care, untreated sores or injuries, and inadequate fluid intake. Neglect can also result in childhood obesity because of poor-quality food, erratic eating patterns, and poor supervision of the diet.

After the Examination.

23. **If the forensic nurse or primary care provider determines** that abuse has occurred, follow legal procedures to ensure that all evidence is secured. If possible, have a forensic nurse and social worker work with the patient.
    In situations where a violation of the law has occurred, strict procedures are essential to ensure that your findings can be used in a court of law and to protect yourself against legal liability.

24. **Provide referrals, if appropriate,** for the abused person, partner, family member, or caregiver to obtain assistance in escaping the abusive situation and/or stopping the abuse.
    Resources are available to assist the abused individual and to assist the parent or caregiver to stop the abuse. Be aware of local and national resources.

25. **Report concerns regarding abuse,** according to agency and state guidelines.
    Key Point: *Suspected child and elder abuse must be reported to the appropriate agency, according to federal and state laws. Spousal abuse may be mandatory to report, depending on state law. The Joint Commission has mandated that all cases of possible abuse or neglect be immediately reported in the hospital.*

26. **Treat physical injuries,** or refer to the primary care provider for medical care, as needed.
    Detection and prevention of abuse require the collaborative efforts of the healthcare team.

? What if . . .

- **My patient is a child? Are there any special assessments I should make or actions I should take?**

Follow steps 1 through 6, with these modifications:

Note: *The interview is important in ruling out sexual abuse in children. Physical findings are often absent, even when the perpetrator admits to penetration of the child's genitalia. Most expert interviewers do not interview children younger than age 3 years.*

a. To assess for sexual abuse, ask whether the patient has been touched inappropriately:
   - *Child older than age 2 years:* Ask about being touched in the "private parts."
   - *Older child:* Ask, "Sometimes people you know may touch or kiss you in a way that you feel is strange or wrong. Has this ever happened to you?"
   - *Adolescent:* Ask, "Sometimes people touch you in ways you feel are wrong. This can be frightening, and it is wrong for people to do that to you. Has this ever happened to you?"

b. Ask the parent or caregiver:
   - "Has the child started wetting the bed or soiling himself?"
   - "Does the child have fears that seem unreasonable?"

   Abuse may result in regression to former behaviors. Symptoms of sexual abuse in children may be general and nonspecific, such as sleep disturbances, bed-wetting, or excessive fears.

   - "Has the child been masturbating or sexually acting out with other children?"

   A child who is sexually abused may exhibit inappropriate sexual behavior.

   - "Has the child ever run away? If they leave, do they go somewhere safe?" "Is the child/adolescent sexually active?"

   An abused child may have feelings of low self-worth and may demonstrate risk-taking behaviors, such as running away to places that are unsafe.

c. To assess for psychological abuse, ask the parent or caregiver:
   - "Was the child a result of a planned pregnancy? What were the pregnancy, birth, and postpartum period like?"

   Risk factors for abuse include an unplanned pregnancy, complications during pregnancy, stressors (e.g., moving, illness, loss of job, divorce), a difficult pregnancy or birth, and lengthy stay in the neonatal intensive care unit.

   - "How would you describe the child now?"

   An abusive parent may describe the child as a "problem child" who is always doing something wrong. The opposite is sometimes seen, when the child is described as "perfect."

   - "How does the child's behavior compare with that of others in the family?"

   Determine whether the parent sees the child differently from his siblings. This is a risk factor for abuse.

   - "Has the child had physical or emotional problems in the past?"

   A history of physical or emotional problems may indicate abuse.

   - "What are your expectations of the child's behavior [e.g., school performance, following instructions]?"

   The expectations of parents or caregivers who are more likely to abuse a child may be that the child will "always be a problem" or will be a "perfect" son or daughter.

   - "What form of discipline works best with the child?"

(continued on next page)

Procedure 6-1 ■ Assessing for Abuse (continued)

Determine whether the parents or caregivers use physical or emotional punishment that may be abusive or disproportionate for the act or situation.

- "Do you have any history of depression, anxiety, difficulty coping with situations or everyday life, or other history of mental health problems?"
  Mental health disorders interfere with a person's ability to perceive others and situations in a realistic and appropriate way. When coping is compromised, the risk for abuse escalates.

d. Perform a physical assessment. Signs of physical abuse and neglect in children include the following:
- Bruises on head, face, ears, buttocks, and lower back that are inconsistent with the history of the injury and are at varying stages of healing (different colors)
- Hemorrhage of the eye, detached retina, ruptured ear drum
  Bruising may occur in different patterns. One pattern is the "swimsuit zone" on the trunk, breast, abdomen, genitalia, and buttocks. Children often have accidental bruises over bony areas, but usually not on the abdomen. Injuries to the head are common in abuse. AHT syndrome may cause detached retina(s), hemorrhages, and subdural hematomas.

- Assess for abdominal pain and other nonspecific complaints.
  Abdominal pain may be a symptom of sexual abuse in children. Signs of sexual abuse may be general and nonspecific in children.

? What if...

■ **My patient is an older adult? Are there any special assessments I should make or actions I should take?**

a. Ask the patient's caregiver:
- "Describe the patient's personal support network. Who visits the patient? How often does the patient have visitors?"
  As in spousal abuse, people who victimize older people often isolate the person from any support network.
- "Who is the patient's primary healthcare provider?"
  Multiple healthcare providers, or lack of a provider, can be an indication of abuse. The caregiver may bring the patient to a different physician with each injury or illness to avoid discovery.
- "Has the patient ever received the wrong dose of medication?"
  Getting the wrong medication or dosage of medication (especially oversedation) may indicate abuse or inability to provide safe care.
- "Who manages the patient's finances?"
  Financial abuse is a fairly common form of abuse in this population. Determine who has control of the older person's finances and makes the decisions regarding spending.

b. Ask the patient:
- "Do you feel safe in your home?"
  The patient who is being abused does not feel safe. Keep in mind that abandonment is a form of abuse.
- "Tell me about your usual day." "Are you able to take care of yourself?" "Who helps you shower and dress?" or "Do you require help with showering or dressing?" "Who is responsible for grocery shopping and cooking in your home?" "How do you get to your appointments or other places you want or need to go?"
  To determine the patient's usual level of self-care

c. Observe for signs of self-neglect.

? What if...

■ **You feel that you are, or the patient is, in immediate danger?**

If the patient's safety or your safety is at risk, immediate intervention is required. You may need to secure the area (e.g., by closing the door), notify the in-house security officer, and then call the police.

Evaluation
- Determine whether abuse may have occurred.
- Ensure that appropriate agencies have been notified of the possible abuse.
- Evaluate whether it is safe to let the patient leave the facility.

Patient Teaching
- Inform the patient, parent, partner, and/or caregiver of local resources for prevention or intervention in situations of child, spousal, or elder abuse.
- Inform the patient that abuse is suspected. Ask for their perceptions of the situation.
- Emphasize to the patient that her safety is the primary concern.

Home Care
- If potential abuse is identified in the home, follow agency and state legal guidelines.
- If the patient's safety is at risk, immediate intervention is required. You may need to notify the police or call an ambulance. Be sure to carry a fully charged cell phone with you.
- If you believe that you are at risk for harm (common in abusive situations), leave the setting before notifying the police.

Documentation
- Follow legal requirements for documenting possible abuse, including disposition of potential evidence.

- If possible, take pictures of the injuries by using a digital camera, and include them in the charting. Place a ruler or other common object next to the injury for reference by a third-party viewer.

Photos must be saved and stored in-house because of the requirement to protect confidentiality.

Chart all findings factually—do not add any interpretations. For example:

Do Chart:

A 4-year-old boy admitted with second-degree burns to both feet, extending to midpoint of shins. Father says, "I put him in the bathtub and didn't realize how hot the water was."

Do Not Chart:

A 4-year-old boy admitted with immersion burns to both feet, extending to midpoint of shins, as found in abuse.

Practice Resources

Carson, 2018; Dudas et al., 2019

ASSESSMENT GUIDELINES & TOOLS

Fetal Development	
STAGE	**DESCRIPTION**
Week 4 End of first lunar month	Length: ¼ in. (0.6 cm) Appearance: Curled upon itself with head touching tail. Signs of formation of arm and leg buds. Liver formed. Heart present. Begins to pulsate about the 14th to 24th day. Primitive blood cells present. Beginnings of brain present.
Weeks 6–8 Second lunar month	Length: 1 in. (2.5 cm) Weight: 1/30 oz (1 g) Chambers of heart develop. Rapid brain development occurring. Primitive limbs present. Fingers and toes begin to form. Face develops. Eyes, ears, nose appear. Palate and upper lip forming. Gastrointestinal tract developing. Part of intestine still in umbilical cord. Urogenital systems forming. Head disproportionately large due to rapid brain development. Organogenesis completed.
Weeks 9–12 Third lunar month	Length: 3 in. (7.5 cm) Weight: 1 oz (28 g) Growth and maturation of structures continues. Head disproportionately large. Brain shows structural features. Eyelids fused. Nail beds form on fingers and toes. Bile present in intestines. Spontaneous movements present. Ossification centers in bones begin to appear. Enamel-forming cells and dentin forming. Kidney secretion by 10th week. Bone marrow begins to form blood cells. Distinguishing sexual traits evident. Respiratory-like movements (reflex activity) present. Intestines retracted from umbilical cord into abdomen. Palate completed fused. Neck well defined.
Weeks 13–16 Fourth lunar month	Length: 6 to 7 in. (15.2 to 17.7 cm) Weight: 4 oz (112 g) Fetus active. Mother may experience quickening. Skeleton calcified and visible on x-ray film. Downy lanugo on head. Placenta distinct. Blood vessels visible beneath transparent skin. Heart actually circulating blood through fetal body. Increasing amount of respiratory movements can be detected by sonogram. Enzymes ptyalin and pepsin being secreted. Fetal thyroid gland begins functioning by the 14th week. Total body blood volume: Less than 100 mL. Amount of amniotic fluid present: 150 to 280 mL.

Fetal Development—cont'd

STAGE	DESCRIPTION
Weeks 17–20 Fifth lunar month	Length: 10 in. (25.4 cm) Weight: 8 to 10 oz (224 to 280 g) Fetal heart sounds evident with stethoscope. Scalp hair visible. Lanugo present, especially on shoulders. Skin less transparent. Eyebrows present. Vernix caseosa present. Fingernails and toenails apparent. Some fat deposits present.
Weeks 21–24 Sixth lunar month	Length: 12 in. (30.5 cm) Weight: 1½ lb (672 g) Skin wrinkled, pink, translucent. Increasing amounts of vernix caseosa present. Eyebrows and eyelashes well defined. External ear soft, flat, shapeless. Lanugo covering entire body. Some breathing effort evident.
Weeks 25–28 Seventh lunar month	Length: 15 in. (37.5 cm) Weight: 2½ lb (1120 g) Skin red, wrinkled, covered with vernix caseosa. Looks like a "little old man." Membranes disappear from eyes. Eyelids open. Scalp hair well developed. Fingernails and toenails present. Subcutaneous fat present. Testes at internal inguinal ring or below.
Weeks 29–32 Eighth lunar month	Length: 15 to 17 in. (37.5 to 42.5 cm) Weight: 3½ to 4 lb (1568 to 1792 g) Skin pink and smooth. Areola of breast visible but flat. Testicles begin descent down inguinal canal (may be in scrotal sac), or Labia majora small and separated, clitoris prominent. Hair fine and wooly. One or two creases evident on anterior portion of soles. Deposits of subcutaneous fat present. Can be conditioned to respond to sounds outside of mother's body.
Weeks 33–36 Ninth lunar month	Length: 19 in. (47.5 cm) Weight: 5 to 6 lb (2240 to 2688 g) Increased fat deposits give body and limbs a more rounded appearance. Skin thicker, whiter. Lanugo disappearing. Sole creases involve anterior two thirds of foot. Breast tissue develops beneath nipples.
Weeks 37–40 Tenth lunar month	Length: 20 in. (50 cm) Weight: 7 to 7½ lb (3136 to 3360 g) After 38 weeks, considered full term. Body plump. Lanugo gone from face. Vernix caseosa disappearing, present in varying amounts. Testes in scrotum (male). Labia majora meet in midline and cover labia minora and clitoris (female). Ear well defined. Erect from head. Uniform color to eyes (a slate hue). Acquires antibodies from mother.

Source: Polan, E., & Taylor, D. (2019). *Journey Across the Life Span: Human Development and Health Promotion,* 6th ed. Philadelphia: F.A. Davis.

Apgar Scoring			
CATEGORY	0	1	2
Breathing effort	Not breathing	Respirations slow (<30 breaths/min) or irregular	Infant cries well
Heart rate (by stethoscope)	None	<100 beats/min	>100 beats/min
Muscle tone	Loose and floppy	Some muscle tone, weak flexion	Active motion, full flexion
Grimace response or reflex irritability (response to stimulation such as mild pinch)	No reaction	Grimace	Grimace and cough, sneeze, or vigorous cry
Skin color	Pale blue	Pink with blue extremities	Entire body is pink

Source: Medline Plus, U.S. National Library of Medicine, National Institutes of Health. Retrieved from http://www.nlm.nih.gov/medlineplus/ency/article/003402.htm.

CLINICAL REASONING
Applying the Full-Spectrum Nursing Model

PATIENT SITUATION

Lani Ettinger is a 30-year-old woman, married, with three school-age children. She has just had a mastectomy (removal of a breast) after a positive biopsy result for cancer. There were no complications during surgery; the cancer was removed at an early stage, and she is expected to recover completely. As you are helping her prepare to leave the hospital, she begins crying.

THINKING

1. *Theoretical Knowledge:* What are Havighurst's developmental tasks of young adulthood?

2. *Critical Thinking (Contextual Awareness):* Which of those developmental tasks is/are most likely to be affected by Lani's mastectomy and her emotional reaction to it?

DOING

3. *Nursing Process (Assessment/ Recognizing Cues):* When you see Lani crying, what do you need to do?

CARING

4. *Self-Knowledge:* Suppose Lani tells you, "My husband has gone to get the car, but when he was here, he didn't want to hug me or kiss me. I asked him if he still loves me, and he didn't say anything. He was crying when he left." What would your feelings be about the husband? You do not need to speculate on exactly what his actions meant; just imagine what your initial feelings would be.

Critical Thinking and Clinical Judgment

1. Now that you have an understanding of the stages of growth and development, let us return to the three pediatric patients you met in Meet Your Patients, in Volume 1. All three children have been diagnosed with pneumonia. You have introduced yourself to Tamika's grandmother and Miguel's mother and have spoken by phone to Carrie's mother. Each is asking you how this hospitalization will affect their child or grandchild.

   - Tamika, a 3-year-old, lives with her grandparents. Her grandmother is present only during the afternoon visiting hours because she has to care for her husband, who suffers from numerous health problems.

- Miguel, a 2-month-old, lives with his mother. Since his admission yesterday, his mother has stayed at his bedside and provided most of her son's care. Miguel's mother is 17 years old and is very concerned about her son's condition.
- Carrie, a 13-year-old, lives with her parents. Both parents are able to visit only during the evening visiting hours after they leave work.

   a. Based on Erikson's stages of development, compare the developmental stages of Tamika, Miguel, and Carrie.

   b. How will nursing care differ for each child?

   c. Analyze each caregiver's developmental stage, and discuss the impact it may have on health teaching.

   d. Would it be a good idea to have the children's caregivers meet for a group teaching session to provide information about pneumonia? Explain.

2. For each of the following concepts, use critical thinking to describe how or why it is important to nursing, patient care, or growth and development. Note these are *not* to be merely definitions.

Ego defense mechanisms

Cognitive development

Psychosocial development

Fetal development

Infant development

Reflexes

Toddler development

Preschooler development

School-age development

Puberty

Adolescent development

Young adult development

Middle adult development

What Are the Main Points in This Chapter?

- Growth and development occur across the life span in a predictable pattern.
- Developmental theories help nurses identify what to expect behaviorally, cognitively, socially, and morally from patients at various ages.
- Fetal growth begins at the time of conception and continues for 10 lunar months until birth.
- Critical adaptations at birth include the establishment of respirations and independent circulation, thermoregulation, and the production of urine.
- Between birth and 1 year, infants develop a sense of trust when the caregiver provides the child with love, warmth, and food.
- The toddler period (1 to 3 years) is the time when the child explores the environment and attempts to become autonomous.
- In the preschool period (4 to 5 years) children are able to separate from their parents, communicate needs through language, and control bodily functions.
- The school-age child (6 to 12 years) begins to develop relationships outside the home. This leads to increasing confidence and independence.
- In the adolescent period (12 to 18 years) children establish their own identities and begin to make decisions that will affect their future.
- The young adult (20 to 40 years) leaves home and begins to function as an independent person.
- Middle adulthood (40 to 65 years) is a time when people balance aspirations with reality. It is often a time when the needs of their children diminish, whereas the needs of their aging parents increase.
- Growth and developmental differences result in each age group's having specific health problems requiring specific assessment techniques. Data from these assessments are used to plan and provide care and anticipatory guidance that are developmentally appropriate.
- Abuse of both children and adults is common. Assess all patients for signs of abuse.

Knowledge Map

UNIT 2 Factors Affecting Health

GROWTH: Physical changes that occur over time

DEVELOPMENT: Process of adapting to one's environment over time

DEVELOPMENT THROUGH THE LIFE SPAN

NATURE Versus NURTURE

Nurses use theoretical knowledge of development to plan and implement age-appropriate care.

PRINCIPLES OF GROWTH AND DEVELOPMENT
- Predictable pattern still unique to each individual
- Growth: Cephalocaudal pattern
- Development: Proximodistal pattern
- Development of simple skills separate and independent; then integrated into complex skills
- Each body system grows at its own rate
- Body system functions differentiate over time

THEORIES OF DEVELOPMENT

HAVIGHURST: DEVELOPMENTAL TASK:
Six life stages with associated tasks

FREUD: PSYCHOANALYTIC:
Four forces: Id, ego, superego, and unconscious mind

PIAGET: COGNITIVE DEVELOPMENT:
Adaptation; assimilation; accommodation

ERIKSON: PSYCHOSOCIAL DEVELOPMENT:
Eight stages of development throughout the lifespan

KOHLBERG: MORAL DEVELOPMENT:
Age-related moral reasoning: Progressively higher reasoning

FOWLER: SPIRITUAL DEVELOPMENT:
Age-related development of faith

CHAPTER 7

Life Span: Older Adults

STUDENT RESOURCES

The questions and exercises in this book allow you to practice the kind of thinking you will use as a full-spectrum nurse. Critical-thinking questions usually have more than one right answer, so we do not provide "correct" answers for these features. It is more important to develop your nursing judgment than to just cover content. You will learn more by discussing the questions with your peers. If you are still unsure, see the Davis Advantage chapter resources for suggested responses.

To explore learning resources for this chapter,

Go to www.DavisAdvantage.com and find:

Answers and Suggested Responses for all questions in this chapter
Concept Map
Knowledge Map
References and Bibliography

Key Concepts

Developmental changes
Functional status
Older adulthood

Related Concepts

See the Concept Map on Davis Advantage.

Example Client Conditions

Dementia
Elder abuse
Frail elderly

Caring for the Williams Family

Stanley Williams' father, Tyrone Williams, is 80 years old and has multiple health problems. He has hypertension and heart disease. Although he had surgery for prostate cancer many years ago, the cancer has now metastasized. Because health was declining rapidly, Stanley and Nadine moved Tyrone and his wife, Charlene, into their home last year. Both Stanley and Nadine work outside the home, so the elderly Charlene cares for her husband as best she can during the day. Stanley is too weak to get out of bed without help, and his wife is not strong enough to support him. She cooks for him, but he eats only a few bites, then pushes the plate away. Stanley telephones today to say, "We can't take care of him safely at home any longer. Can you tell me how to get him admitted to a hospital or a nursing home?"

(Continued)

Caring for the Williams Family (continued)

A. What other ideas do you have for helping the Williams family to care or to find care for Tyrone other than placing him in a hospital or nursing home?

B. Stanley's first concern seems to be about getting help for his father. What do you think his next concern will be?

C. What actual data do you have about Tyrone's nutrition status?

D. What else do you need to know to fully assess Tyrone's nutrition status? If you do not know the answer to this, you will find some information in the Assessment sections of this chapter in Volume 1. For more complete information, refer to Screening for Nutrition Problems and Focused Nutrition Assessment in Chapter 24, Volume 2. Also

➤ Go to **Assessment** in Chapter 24 of Volume 1.

E. Would you consider Tyrone to be a frail elderly person? Why or why not?

Practical Knowledge
clinical application

ASSESSMENT GUIDELINES AND TOOLS

Assessments for All Older Adults

Focused Assessment

- **Vital signs**—Be aware that the normal ranges for VS are slightly different for older adults (see Chapter 18). For example, the average body temperature is lower.
- **Height measurement**—Compare with previous height (as a screen for osteoporosis). Especially important past age 65.
- **Weight and body mass index (BMI)**, calculated.
- **Lipid panel screening**—Total cholesterol, triglycerides, high-density lipoprotein (HDL), low-density lipoprotein (LDL), and ratios.
- **Blood glucose screening.**
- **Annual clinical breast examination**—For female patients aged 50 to 74 years (U.S. Preventive Services Task Force, January 2016).
- **Breast self-awareness**—Patients should know how their breasts normally look and feel and report any breast changes to a healthcare provider right away. Breast self-examination is an option for patients throughout their life span.
- **Biannual mammogram or thermography**—For female patients aged 55 and older. Screening should continue as long as a patient is in good health and is expected to live 10 more years or longer.

   The American Cancer Society (ACS) (2022) recommends that women with average risk of breast cancer should undergo regular screening mammography starting at age 45 years. Female patients aged 45 to 54 years should be screened annually, and patients 55 years and older should transition to biennial screening or have the opportunity to continue screening annually.

- **Cervical cancer screening (Pap test)**—Female patients over age 65 who have had regular cervical cancer testing in the past 10 years with normal results should not be tested for cervical cancer. Once testing is stopped, it should not be started again. Patients with a history of a serious cervical precancer should continue to be tested for at least 20 years after that diagnosis, even if testing goes beyond age 65.
  - A patient who has had her uterus and cervix removed (a total hysterectomy) for reasons not related to cervical cancer and who has no history of cervical cancer or serious precancer should not be tested (ACS, 2022).
- **Colon cancer screening**—The USPSTF (May 2019) recommends screening for colorectal cancer using fecal occult blood testing, sigmoidoscopy, or colonoscopy in adults, beginning at age 50 years and continuing to age 75 years. Intervals for recommended screening strategies include the following:
  - **Annual screening with high-sensitivity fecal occult blood testing.**
  - **Sigmoidoscopy**—Every 5 years, with high-sensitivity fecal occult blood testing every 3 years.
  - **Screening colonoscopy**—Every 10 years.

Focused Assessment

Assessments for All Older Adults—cont'd

➤ **Screening CT** *colonographies,* or "virtual colonoscopies," are particularly safe for older adults as a noninvasive test that requires no sedation or anesthesia. The American Cancer Society considers CT colonography as a first-line colon-cancer screening to be as effective as the traditional colonoscopy. The USPSTF (May 2019) recommends the decision to screen older adults aged 76 to 85 years should be an individual one, taking into account the patient's overall health and screening history.

➤ **Digital rectal examination (for male patients)** may be done to detect an enlarged prostate. Enlargement can indicate either benign prostatic hypertrophy or prostate cancer. Before deciding whether to be screened, patients should discuss with their clinician the potential benefits and harms of screening and incorporate their values and preferences in the decision.

➤ **Serum prostate-specific antigen (PSA)** level (for male patients) is a more sensitive indicator than the digital rectal examination. Some guidelines encourage yearly screening for men over age 50; some caution against routine screening; others make decisions on an individual basis. The USPSTF recommends that patients ages 55 to 69 years discuss the potential benefits and harms of PSA screening for prostate cancer with their healthcare provider, but recommends against PSA screening for patients ages 70 years and older (USPSTF, 2018a).

➤ **Eye examination**—Every 2 years if there are no problems; otherwise annually, particularly if the older adult has chronic conditions such as hypertension, cardiovascular disease, or diabetes.

➤ **Bone-density scan**—Recommended for all female patients ages 65 years and older as a routine screening for osteoporosis. For patients at increased risk for osteoporotic fractures (postmenopausal, tobacco smoking, history of fragility fractures, low body weight), screening should begin at age 60 years (USPSTF, 2018b). The test is also recommended for male patients older than age 70.

CLINICAL REASONING
Applying the Full-Spectrum Nursing Model

PATIENT SITUATION

Alvin Bell, 82 years old, was just discharged from the hospital after a myocardial infarction (heart attack). On your first home visit to supervise the medication regimen, you notice that the house looks as though it has not been cleaned in weeks. Piled on every flat surface, including the floor, is what appears to be months' accumulations of newspapers, magazines, and other clutter. Dishes are piled in the sink, apparently from before the hospitalization. There is hardly any food in the cupboard. When you weigh Alvin, you see that there is a 3 lb weight loss in the 3 days since discharge. The client admits to not eating well: "I'm not hungry, and it's too much trouble." As you talk with Alvin, you learn that his wife died of cancer 7 months ago. Alvin says, "I don't know what to do without her. I hate living alone. I don't have much reason for going on." Alvin is alert and oriented but talks and moves very slowly.

THINKING

1. *Theoretical Knowledge:*

    a. What do you know about depression in older adults? Do you have enough knowledge of that topic to be able to assess whether Alvin is depressed? If not, what resources would you use to find out? (List specific resources. That is, give the URL; don't just say "the Internet." Give the name or author of the book, not just "my psych-nursing book.")

    b. You will also need to know whether it is normal for appetite to decrease in older adults, and what their caloric needs are compared with the needs of other age groups. Where can you go to find this information?

2. *Critical Thinking (Considering Alternatives):*

   a. As you survey Alvin's overall situation, what is your first impulse to improve the situation? What questions come to you?

   b. What community services might be helpful for Alvin?

   c. How would you handle referrals? Would you leave a list of telephone numbers? Would you call the agencies yourself? Explain your thinking.

DOING

3. *Practical Knowledge:* In your physical examination of Alvin, you find no old or recent bruises or other injuries. However, because of the depression and weight loss, you wonder about neglect or financial abuse. What questions could you ask to find out?

CARING

4. *Self-Knowledge:* Think of one patient you have cared for who has something in common with Mr. Bell. Describe the way(s) in which they are alike.

Critical Thinking and Clinical Judgment

1. Margaret O'Malley, age 67, tells you that even though she has new reading glasses, she still cannot see as well as she would like to for reading or sewing. She says, "My eyes often feel dry and scratchy. I wonder if something is wrong."

   a. What would you advise her to do that might improve her reading ability?

   b. What age-related change do you think may be causing Mrs. O'Malley's eyes to feel dry and scratchy?

2. Tony King, age 78, is having difficulty controlling his diabetes. Because he leads a sedentary life, his physician has advised him to take daily walks to help regulate his blood sugar. Mr. King says, "Doc, I can't do that. With the arthritis in my back and hips, every step is agony. I walk just enough to take care of myself, get to the store, come here, and do whatever I have to. I'm already taking a lot of drugs for the pain; I can't take more when I walk." What kind of program could the physician recommend to Mr. King?

3. For each of the following concepts, use critical thinking to describe how or why it is important to nursing, patient care, or growth and development. Note that these are *not* to be merely definitions.

   a. Gender disparities in life expectancy

   b. Age distribution in the population (population pyramid)

   c. Aging in place

What Are the Main Points In This Chapter?

- The number of older adults (ages 65 and older) in the United States has risen significantly because of increasing life expectancy.
- Older adulthood is a time of transition. Most health problems of older adults are chronic in nature and often affect ability to live independently.
- Most older adults live independently.
- Aging can be examined from a life expectancy, percentage of total population, or life-span perspective.
- Aging in place means that as they age, persons live in their own age-friendly residences and receive supportive services for their changing needs rather than move to another location or alternative type of housing.
- Retirement communities are planned and built specifically to provide elder-friendly dwellings and environments for independent living and allow older adults to "downsize" their dwelling.
- Continuing care retirement communities (CCRC) offer a wide range of living accommodations, including residential living, assisted living, skilled nursing care, rehabilitation, and dementia care on a large campuslike setting.
- Assisted-living facilities (ALFs) are congregate residential settings that provide or coordinate personal services, 24-hour supervision and assistance, activities, and health-related services.
- Nursing care facilities, or nursing homes, provide skilled and unskilled nursing care for older adults and adults with disabilities.
- The stages of older adulthood are referred to as the *young-old* (ages 65 to 74), *middle-old* (ages 75 to 84), and *oldest-old* (ages 85 and older).
- The fastest-growing segment of older adults is the oldest-old, some of whom are the frail elderly and *centenarians* (people over 100 years old).
- Older adults learn new material more slowly. However, there is no loss of intelligence as a person ages.
- Disengagement theory and activity theory attempt to explain the psychosocial development of older adults.
- **Dementia,** a loss of cognitive ability, is not a normal result of aging. It is important to differentiate dementia from depression, acute confusion, or delirium that may be precipitated by dehydration, infection, or a medication side effect or overdose. Alzheimer disease is the primary form of dementia.
- Developmental differences result in each age group's having specific health problems requiring specific assessment techniques. Data from these assessments are used to plan and provide care and anticipatory guidance that are developmentally appropriate.
- Older adults should have an annual physical examination, including a focused assessment of functional status.
- Frailty is a set of characteristics that describe a heightened state of vulnerability for developing adverse health outcomes.
- Abuse of adults is common. Assess all patients for signs of abuse.
- Suspicion of elder abuse must be reported to adult protection services and/or the authority designated by law in each state.

Knowledge Map

GROWTH: Physical changes that occur over time

DEVELOPMENT: Process of adapting to one's environment over time

DEVELOPMENT THROUGH THE LIFE SPAN

STAGES OF OLDER ADULTHOOD
Young-old: Ages 65 to 74
Middle-old: Ages 75 to 84
Oldest-old: Age 85+
Centenarians
Frail elderly

Nurses use theoretical knowledge of development to plan and implement age-appropriate care.

THEORIES OF AGING
Wear-and-tear theory
Genetic theories
Cellular malfunction
Autoimmune reaction

ASSESSMENTS
- Annual physical exam
- Recommended screening (e.g., colon cancer, mammogram)
- Functional status
- Depression
- Cognitive status (e.g., dementia)

POTENTIAL PROBLEMS
Dementia
Elder abuse
Frailty
Adult failure to thrive
Risk for delayed development

CHAPTER 8

Experiencing Wellness: Health & Illness

STUDENT RESOURCES

The questions and exercises in this book allow you to practice the kind of thinking you will use as a full-spectrum nurse. Critical-thinking questions usually have more than one right answer, so we do not provide "correct" answers for these features. It is more important to develop your nursing judgment than to just cover content. You will learn more by discussing the questions with your peers. If you are still unsure, see the Davis chapter resources for suggested responses.

To explore learning resources for this chapter,

Go to www.DavisAdvantage.com and find:

Answers and Suggested Responses for all questions in this chapter
Concept Map
Knowledge Map
References and Bibliography

Key Concepts

Health
Health experience
Health promotion
Health protection
Illness
Illness experience
Illness prevention
Wellness

Related Concepts

See the Concept Map on Davis Advantage.

Caring for the Williams Family

Stanley Williams has recently been diagnosed with hypertension, obesity, and degenerative joint disease (DJD). He is struggling with these diagnoses. He tells his wife, Nadine, "I feel so old now. These are the kinds of things my parents are dealing with." At a clinic visit, Stanley tells you, "It's hard to think of myself as sick. I've been depressed ever since Dr. Johnson told me about his findings. Now he's asked me to get some laboratory work. I'm afraid he may find even more problems." If you need help answering the following questions,

Go to **Chapter 8, Figure 8-1: The Health-Illness Continuum** and **Figure 8-2: Dunn's Health Grid** in Volume 1.

(Continued)

Caring for the Williams Family (continued)

A. Identify the disruptions that Stanley must deal with based on these diagnoses. Explain your reasons for choosing these disruptions.

B. How would you evaluate Stanley's health status?

C. What kinds of activities could you suggest to Stanley to improve his health status?

D. What stage of illness behavior is Stanley exhibiting regarding his recent medical diagnoses?
Practical Knowledge Clinical Application
Practical knowledge in this chapter means using the nursing process to apply what you have learned about how people experience health, wellness, and illness.

PROCEDURES

The procedures in this chapter will help you admit, transfer, and discharge patients in such a way that you can begin to establish trust at the first patient contact.

Procedure 8-1 ■ Admitting a Patient to a Nursing Unit

> For steps to follow in *all* procedures, refer to the Universal Steps for All Procedures on the inside back cover.

Equipment

- Identifying armband (if this has not been supplied by the admissions department)
- Patient's chart, including provider prescriptions and nursing admission record
- Thermometer, blood pressure cuff, and stethoscope
- Scales for height and weight
- Gown
- Admission pack (e.g., water pitcher, soap, comb, toothbrush, mouthwash, and facial tissues)
- Nursing care plan or clinical pathway, if one has already been made
- Hospital brochures, Patient Care Partnership, and other forms
- Admission assessment form

Delegation

A registered nurse is responsible for managing medical orders and assessing the patient's need for nursing care in all settings, although this may vary in some specifics according to hospital policy, the law, and regulations. Most other admission activities can be delegated to unlicensed assistive personnel (UAP) if the patient is stable.

Preprocedure Assessments

- Assess for signs of emotional and/or physical distress.
- Assess ability to ambulate and/or move.
- Assess ability to communicate and understand what is occurring.

> When performing the procedure, always identify your patient according to agency policy, using two identifiers, and be attentive to standard precautions, hand hygiene, patient safety and privacy, body mechanics, and documentation.

Procedure Steps

1. **Ensure placement of patient labels** (e.g., on the chart, at the bedside, outside the door).

2. **Introduce yourself to the patient and family.** Explain who you are. Do not be afraid to tell a patient that you are a nursing student.
   Many patients are aware that students have more time to spend with them than doctors do. Talking to the patient and family reassures them and provides information about the patient's level of consciousness and awareness, social relationships, and so on.

3. **Assist the patient into a hospital gown.**
   If the patient is able to stand, assist them into a gown before weighing them to obtain the most accurate weight.

4. **Measure height and weight** while the patient stands on a floor scale, if possible. If they are unable to stand, transfer them into the bed and measure their weight using a bed scale.
   Weigh in the same manner each time to ensure accuracy.

5. **Assist the patient into the bed.**
   Get the patient comfortable before continuing the admission to prevent overtiring them.

6. **✚ Check the patient's identification band** to ensure the information, including allergies, is correct. Verify this information with the patient or family.

   Questioning the patient about allergies and verifying with the family will ensure that the information is accurate and documented on the wristband and the chart.

7. **Measure vital signs.**

   Measuring the vital signs before completing the rest of the admission ensures that you will be aware of the patient's status. If the vital signs are abnormal, further assess the patient's condition before continuing. Report your findings to the admitting care provider.

8. **Complete the nursing admission assessment,** including health history and physical assessment. Be sure to include the patient's expectations and concerns. For inpatients, this must be completed within 24 hours after admission. All patients should be screened on admission for risk for pressure injuries. (Chapter 19 contains a step-by-step approach to physical assessment.)

   An admission assessment is needed to identify problems and establish a baseline. The Joint Commission requires that each patient have an admission assessment performed by a registered nurse.

9. **Check that the list of the patient's current medications** (created in the admitting department) is complete and accurate. Usually the patient's own medications are sent home with the family, or they may be sent to pharmacy for storage.

   It is important to know what medications the patient has been taking. The pharmacy will identify medicines from home when necessary. When medications are ordered and given during the patient's stay, they are compared with those on the list so any discrepancies can be resolved.

10. **Orient the patient to the room.**

    These actions ensure that the patient and family will be able to call for assistance if needed and increase the patient's and family's level of comfort and ability to function in the hospital setting. Remember that one of the disruptions associated with illness is anxiety about the unknown. If you tell your patient what to expect, you help to minimize their anxiety.

    a. Make sure the patient knows how to use the bed, the call light, and any equipment that you expect them to use.
    b. Point out the location of personal care items.
    c. Show the patient the location of the restroom.
    d. If you will be measuring the patient's intake and output, tell the patient so during your orientation.

    If the patient is alert, they may be able to assist you with these measures.

11. **Explain hospital routines,** including use of side rails, mealtimes, and so on. Answer the patient's and family's questions.

    Hospitalization takes away control of basic decisions. Knowing the routines and available choices increases patient and family comfort.

12. **Verify with the patient all other admission data** on the chart for completeness and accuracy.

    Basic data, such as name, address, marital status, name of admitting care provider, admitting diagnosis, consent to treatment, and so on, will usually be obtained in the admitting office. However, you will need to be sure all the admitting information is complete; if it is not, then complete it.

13. **Ask the patient whether they have an advance directive** (e.g., power of attorney or living will). If so, place a copy in the hospital record. If not, explain the purpose of the document and give the patient a form to fill out if they wish to do so. (See Chapters 12 and 41, Volume 1, if you need more information about advance directives.)

    Advance directives enable patients to indicate their preferences about treatments and prolonging life.

14. **Advise the patient of his privacy rights under Health Insurance Portability and Accountability Act (HIPAA).** See that they have a written explanation of their privacy rights (see Chapter 41 as needed).

15. **Inventory the patient's belongings.** Encourage the family to take home valuable items and money. If that is not possible, arrange to have valuables placed in the hospital safe. Most agencies require money in excess of $5.00 to be sent home or to the cashier's office.

    Patient belongings, including valuables, are frequently lost during hospitalization. Documenting the disposition of everything ensures being able to return the belongings to the patient upon discharge.

16. **Complete or ensure that all admission orders (prescriptions)** have been completed (e.g., laboratory tests, medications, diet and fluid orders).

    Unless it is an unscheduled admission, diagnostic tests are usually completed on an outpatient basis before admission to the hospital. However, some prescriptions might need to be done immediately, whereas others can be delayed. Make sure the prescriptions are completed in the most appropriate time frame.

17. **Ensure patient comfort** (e.g., positioning, pain, water at bedside).

18. **✚ Make one last safety check** (i.e., call light within reach, bed in low position, side rails up as appropriate, equipment functioning properly).

19. **Before leaving, ask if you can do anything else** for the patient and family.

20. **Initiate the care plan or clinical pathway.**

    Identifying the patient's priority problems enables the nurse to develop the most appropriate nursing orders.

(continued on next page)

Procedure 8-1 ■ Admitting a Patient to a Nursing Unit (continued)

? What if...

- **The patient may be at risk for falls?**

  Perform fall risk assessment as appropriate to the patient and according to agency policy.

  Falls are common in inpatient facilities, especially among older adults. If a patient has risk factors for falls, risk reduction measures can be instituted.

- **The patient has special care needs?**

  When the patient has special needs, such as allergies, a nothing by mouth (NPO) prescription, or an "intake and output" prescription, post patient care reminders at the head of the bed or at the door to remind other care providers.

- **The patient needs a more in-depth assessment in some areas?**

  Perform special needs assessments as relevant to the care and condition of the patient (social situation, nutrition and hydration status, functional abilities, spiritual and cultural variables). If these are warranted, they must be completed within 24 hours after admission or before surgery.

  In-depth assessment of these topics is not a part of all admission assessments but should be done if the patient's condition warrants.

- **The patient has a learning disability?**

  If possible, preadmissions should be arranged for the patient and main caregiver. This allows more time to discuss issues of consent, alleviate anxiety, and set up links with a learning disability specialist or social worker.

  - Allow more time for the admission process, or the preadmission process if that has been arranged.
  - Use short sentences, with one idea at a time.
  - Include the caregiver in the admission process, but encourage the patient to participate as much as possible.
  - Document the main caregiver and contact numbers.
  - Expect the patient to be anxious.
  - Include special communication and personal needs in the plan of care.
  - Give the patient hospital information with pictures, such as those given to children, if appropriate for the patient's developmental level.

- **The patient is an older adult?**

  Ask all older adults if they have had any falls in the past year. If they report a fall, observe them as they stand up from a chair without using their arms, walk several paces, and return ("get up and go"). If they are steady, no further assessment is required. If there is unsteadiness or if the person reports more than one fall, further assessment is required.

  The incidence and severity of fall-related complications rise steadily after age 60. Fall rates in nursing homes and hospitals are almost three times the rate for those living at home.

- **The patient is a child?**

  Use a friendly approach.

  The first priority is to establish a trusting relationship with the child and parents to alleviate fears and anxiety. Children younger than 3 years may fear being separated from parents. Older children usually worry more about what is going to happen to them.

  - Explain the visiting and rooming-in policies to the parents.
  - Ask about the child's usual routine (e.g., toileting, bedtime rituals, favorite foods).
  - Speak to the child directly if she is old enough to understand.
  - Direct the family to the bathroom, playroom, television, and snack room, if those are available.
  - Encourage the parents to bring toys and other favorite items from home.

  It helps the child feel more comfortable in the unfamiliar surroundings.

Documentation

- Document all assessment findings on the admission database provided by the institution.
- Document an admission note and any teaching or other interventions in the nursing notes or flowsheet (according to agency policy).
- Recall that a discharge plan is created on admission. You will find forms for discharge assessment and teaching under Forms, after the Procedures in this chapter.

Practice Resources

The American Geriatrics Society (n.d.); The Joint Commission (2021, 2022); McKenzie, Lasater, Delander, et al. (2017).

Procedure 8-2 ■ Transferring a Patient to Another Unit in the Agency

➤ For steps to follow in all procedures, refer to the Universal Steps for All Procedures on the inside back cover.

Equipment
- Medical record or chart
- Care plan
- Patient's medications
- Supplies for any ongoing treatments
- Patient's belongings, clothes, and personal care articles
- Standardized handoff form, if available
- A utility cart, if belongings are numerous
- Wheelchair or transfer cart
- If patient must be transferred with equipment running (e.g., portable oxygen), obtain it ahead of time and set it up for the transfer

Delegation
If the patient's condition allows, you can delegate the physical transfer of the patient and have the UAP move the patient's belongings to the other room. However, as the nurse, you are responsible for obtaining and completing the necessary records, making the final assessment, and gathering and checking the medications. You must also give the handoff report to another nurse.

Preprocedure Assessments
- Make a final brief focused physical assessment.
- Assess the patient's mobility and ability to assist.
- Assess for emotional and/or physical distress (administer medications, as needed).
- Assess the patient's ability to communicate and understand what is occurring.

➤ When performing the procedure, always identify your patient according to agency policy, using two identifiers, and be attentive to standard precautions, hand hygiene, patient safety and privacy, body mechanics, and documentation.

Procedure Steps

1. **✚ Obtain the number of personnel needed** to make a safe transfer.
   For efficiency and patient and staff safety.

2. **✚ Gather the patient's medications and label them** correctly for the new room.
   This ensures availability of medications when the patient arrives at the new unit; helps prevent medication administration errors.

3. **Notify the receiving unit** of the time to expect the transfer. Also notify other departments (e.g., dietary, pharmacy, admitting), primary care provider, and family of the transfer.
   You need to schedule the transfer with the receiving nurse so they can plan their work and so you can arrange the transfer time to limit the number of interruptions during the handoff. Limiting interruptions minimizes the possibility of communication errors (e.g., forgetting information). Other departments must have the transfer data so that services such as meals and physical therapy treatments will not be interrupted. The primary care provider and family, of course, need to know where to find the patient.

4. **Gather the patient's personal belongings and supplies,** including treatment-related supplies and equipment (e.g., isolation supplies, clean dressings) and patient records. Place on a utility cart if necessary.
   Having the supplies and equipment ready to go makes the transfer more efficient for you and less stressful for the patient.

5. **Bring the wheelchair or transfer cart** to the bedside and assist the patient to the chair or cart. If you're using a wheelchair, the patient can hold the pan of supplies; if using a bed or cart, place supplies on the bed.

6. **Take the patient to the new room** and give the handoff report. Follow agency procedure for handoff reports. However, the method chosen should allow both the giver and the receiver of patient information the opportunity for questioning.
   a. If you need to review content of an oral handoff report, see Chapter 15. In general, the report should include name, age, sex, care providers, surgical procedures, medical diagnoses, medications, allergies, laboratory data, special equipment (e.g., oxygen, suction), the patient's current health status, and whether there are advance directives and resuscitation status. Identify the nursing diagnoses and priorities for nursing care.
   b. Consistently use a structured framework or memory aid to guide the handoff process and the oral report.
   The objective of a handoff is to provide accurate information about the patient. The information communicated must be accurate to ensure patient safety.
   c. ✚ Be sure to point out to the nurse if the patient is taking corticosteroids, anticoagulants, diabetes medications, antibiotics, or narcotic analgesics.
   These medications can have serious side effects and need careful monitoring.

(continued on next page)

Procedure 8-2 ■ Transferring a Patient to Another Unit in the Agency (continued)

Evaluation

With the receiving nurse, evaluate the patient's response to the move. The receiving nurse will take vital signs and make a preliminary admission assessment.

Documentation

- Just before moving, document as much information as you can, including the patient's status at that time.
- After handoff, document the information reported in the handoff, the name and title of the person who received the patient, and your report.
- Sign the note. Some agencies have a standardized form for the transfer note.

Example of Documentation

3/13/XX____1615.____Patient transferred to room 501 by stretcher, with both side rails up, with assistance of one. Temperature 104.8°F, pulse 100 beats/min, BP 138/88, respirations 20 breaths/min and shallow. Drowsy upon arrival. Responds to verbal stimuli with moaning. Last pain medication given at 15:15. Denies pain when asked. No urine noted since 12:00 pm; will encourage voiding by offering urinal every 2 hr. #22 IV in RAC and #18 IV in R hand flushed with 3 mL of normal saline; flushes without redness, edema, or induration. Receiving 3 L/min of oxygen during transfer. Placed on 3 L/min in room; will wean oxygen as tolerated. Handoff report given to Linda Hamm, RN. ————————Sarah Fields, RN

Practice Resources
Ernst, McComb, & Ley (2018); The Joint Commission (2021, 2022).

Procedure 8-3 ■ Transferring a Patient to a Long-Term Care Facility

➤ For steps to follow in *all* procedures, refer to the Universal Steps for All Procedures on the inside back cover.

Equipment
- Health record or chart
- Care plan
- Patient's medications
- Supplies for any ongoing treatments
- Patient's belongings, clothes, and personal care articles
- Standardized transfer form, if available
- A utility cart, if belongings are numerous
- Wheelchair or transfer cart

Delegation
If the patient's condition allows, you can delegate the physical transfer of the patient and have the UAP move the patient's supplies and belongings. However, as the nurse, you are responsible for obtaining and completing the necessary records, making the final assessment, and gathering and checking the medications. You must also give the handoff report to another nurse.

Preprocedure Assessments
- Make a final brief focused physical assessment.
- Assess the patient's mobility and ability to assist.
- Assess for emotional and/or physical distress (administer medications, as needed).
- Assess the patient's ability to communicate and understand what is occurring.

➤ When performing the procedure, always identify your patient according to agency policy, using two identifiers, and be attentive to standard precautions, hand hygiene, patient safety and privacy, body mechanics, and documentation.

Procedure Steps

1. **Notify the patient and family well in advance** of the upcoming transfer to another facility. Include information about the reasons the patient is being transferred as well as any alternatives to transfer.
   Allows them time to adjust emotionally and to make any necessary plans.

2. **Prepare the patient's records.** Send a copy of the patient's health record, including a copy of the comprehensive nursing assessment and a detailed nursing care plan, as well as prescriptions and cards for future appointments, to the receiving facility. The originals remain with the hospital.
   This ensures continuity of care, thus minimizing patient stress.

3. **Gather and pack the patient's personal items** and treatment supplies to send to the long-term care facility with the patient.
   Having the supplies and equipment ready to go makes the transfer more efficient for you.

4. ✚ Be certain the medications are labeled correctly.
   This ensures availability and correct administration of medications when the patient arrives at the new facility.

5. **Coordinate the transfer.** Determine which agency will arrange transportation for the patient.
   Notify the receiving facility of the time to expect the transfer and of any special equipment the patient will need (e.g., IV pole, portable oxygen); notify other hospital departments

(e.g., dietary, pharmacy, admitting), primary care provider, and family of the transfer.

You need to schedule the transfer with the receiving agency so they can plan their work and so you can arrange the transfer at a time that will limit the number of interruptions during the transfer. Other in-house departments must have the transfer data so that services such as meals and physical therapy treatments will be discontinued. The primary care provider and family, of course, need to know where to find the patient.

6. **Just before transfer, make your final quick assessment and sign off your charting** (usually there is a preprinted standardized discharge form for this purpose).

   It is important to complete documentation in a timely manner, but it is also important to provide the most recent assessment data to the long-term care facility.

7. **Take the patient off the unit** and out of the hospital after you are notified that transportation has arrived (or delegate this task). Alternatively, a transporter may come to your unit to get the patient. (Note: Some agencies ask you to remove the patient's identification band at time of transfer.)

   Keeping the patient on the unit for as long as practical helps to minimize anxiety and fatigue that may occur from a long wait in the hospital lobby.

8. **Give an oral report** to the nurse at the long-term care facility. You will usually give a telephone report unless a nurse comes to your hospital to accompany the patient. As appropriate for the care, treatment, and services provided, the report should include the following:
   a. The reason the patient is being transferred
   b. The patient's physical and psychosocial status
   c. A summary of care, treatment, and services provided and progress toward outcomes
   d. Referrals and community resources provided to the patient

   A report helps ensure continuity of care and provides a baseline for later changes in the patient's health status.

- **It is best to consistently use a structured framework** or memory aid to guide the handoff process and the oral report.

   The objective of a handoff report is to provide accurate information about the patient. The information communicated must be accurate to ensure patient safety.

- **Notify the long-term care agency** if the patient is colonized or infected with methicillin-resistant *Staphylococcus aureus* (MRSA) or other contagious microorganisms.

   The facility can arrange for and communicate any special isolation or care activities to their staff. MRSA is a serious problem for long-term care residents.

- **Be sure to point out to the nurse if the patient is taking** corticosteroids, anticoagulants, diabetes medications, antibiotics, or narcotic analgesics.

   These medications confer particularly high risk of adverse postdischarge drug events, and the long-term-care nurses will need to continue careful monitoring.

? What if...

- **The patient has IV lines and other equipment that cannot be turned off?**

   It is common to transfer patients with IV lines. Some wheelchairs are equipped with an IV pole, or you may need to hold the IV bag while taking the patient to the transporting vehicle. If so, always hold the bag well above the patient's chest and arm so that blood does not back up in the tubing. Also, you should notify the long-term care facility so they will have the necessary equipment in the transport vehicle. Portable oxygen and suction are also available for patients who must have them. Usually the receiving facility will bring these, but you need to coordinate that in advance.

- **When you are ready to transfer the patient, their condition worsens and they become unstable?**

   Perform interventions to stabilize the patient, call for help if needed, and notify the medical provider. Notify the transporter and the long-term care center of the change and postpone the transfer until further medical assessment is done.

Evaluation

The receiving nurse at the long-term care facility will evaluate the patient's response to the move.

Documentation

- Just before the transfer, document your final assessment and complete the agency's discharge summary.
- You will probably put your final nursing note on a transfer or discharge summary, as required by agency policy.

Practice Resources

Ernst et al. (2018); The Joint Commission (2021); Patton et al. (2017).

Procedure 8-4 ■ Discharging a Patient From the Healthcare Facility

➤ For steps to follow in *all* procedures, refer to the Universal Steps for All Procedures on the inside back cover.

Equipment
- Health record or chart
- Patient's medications
- Supplies for any ongoing treatments
- Patient's belongings, clothes, and personal care articles
- Standardized discharge form, if available, with instructions for patient
- A utility cart, if belongings are numerous
- Wheelchair

Delegation
If the patient's condition allows, you can delegate to the UAP such tasks as packing belongings, helping the patient dress, and taking the patient out of the facility. However, as the nurse, you are responsible for obtaining and completing the necessary records, making the final assessment, gathering and checking the medications, and coordinating care.

Preprocedure Assessments
- Make a final brief focused physical assessment.
- Assess the patient's mobility.
- Assess for emotional and/or physical distress.
- Assess the patient's ability to communicate and understand what is occurring.

➤ When performing the procedure, always identify your patient according to agency policy, using two identifiers, and be attentive to standard precautions, hand hygiene, patient safety and privacy, body mechanics, and documentation.

Procedure Steps

1. **Notify the patient and family** as much in advance of the discharge as possible. This is often done early in the hospital stay.
   Allows them time to adjust emotionally and to make any necessary plans.

A Day or Two Before Discharge (Steps 2 and 3)

2. **Make or confirm necessary arrangements.**
   a. Arrange for or help the family arrange for services (e.g., home healthcare, physical therapy, IV therapy, social worker) that will be needed at home.
      NOTE: To reimburse for home care, insurers require a physician's prescription for all services, and the patient must meet certain eligibility criteria.
   b. Confirm or arrange for equipment needed in the home (e.g., portable oxygen).
   c. Confirm or arrange for transportation.
   d. Make necessary referrals (e.g., medical specialists, physical therapists); book appointments, if necessary, and if in line with agency policy.
      Hospital stays are short, and many patients are still ill enough to require complex treatments and care by family members when they go home.

3. **Communicate and provide teaching** to the patient and caregivers.
   Patients who have a clear understanding of their after-hospital care (e.g., medications, follow-up visits) are 30% less likely to visit the emergency department or be readmitted than patients who lack this information (Roberts et al., 2019).
   a. Discuss the patient's diagnosis, care needs, and functional abilities with the family/caregiver.
   b. Train the patient and caregiver in the use of equipment. Arrange for follow-up evaluation at home to check that equipment is working and being used correctly and that further training is given if needed.
      In the stress of illness and the disruption of transition home, patients may not retain what they are taught in the hospital. Therapies will be ineffective if equipment is used incorrectly, so follow-up is essential to help avoid further illness and hospital readmission.
   c. Educate about medication use and side effects.
      Medication errors at home are a frequent cause of adverse events and readmissions to the hospital.
   d. Ask relatives or the caregiver to bring clothing for the patient to wear home, if needed.
      If this was an unplanned admission, the patient may have come in nightwear and a robe.

Day of Discharge (Steps 4 Through 16)

4. **Make and document final assessments.**
   a. Assess that the patient's condition remains as expected.
   b. Confirm that the patient has house keys, heating is turned on, and food is available.
   c. Follow up on diagnostic and laboratory test results.

5. **Bring a wheelchair or other transport** device to the bedside.

6. **Make final notifications.**
   a. Contact the family or guardian; confirm transportation.
   b. Notify community service agencies and home health nursing of the discharge, as needed.

7. **Gather prescriptions and instruction sheets,** including a list of current medications and appointment cards; give to the patient along with the discharge instructions at discharge. **Key Point:** Be certain that either the patient or caregiver can read the instructions. Inadequate literacy has been shown to be a risk factor for readmission.

8. **Gather and pack the patient's personal items** and treatment supplies.
   Having the supplies and equipment ready to go makes the transfer more efficient for you and less stressful for the patient and family.

9. ✚ **Prepare the patient's medications.** Be certain the medications are labeled correctly, pack them, and record which medications they are taking home.
   This ensures availability and correct administration of medications when the patient arrives home. It also provides a legal record that the patient left with the medications.

10. **Review discharge instructions** with patient and caregiver (and provide a written copy to take home):
    a. Medication instructions
    b. Symptom management and treatments
    c. Information about provider and location for the follow-up appointment(s)
    d. How to obtain further care, treatment, and services, as needed
    e. How and when to call the physician or primary care provider, including signs of a change in condition
    f. Emergency contact
    g. Diet restrictions
    h. Maintenance of hydration
    i. Activities of daily living, focusing on safety and mobility
    Teaching should occur throughout the hospital stay. However, it is important to reinforce with a last-minute summary and written instructions to take home. With the stress of illness and anticipation of discharge, patients may not retain what they are taught.

11. **Address any questions or concerns** of the patient and caregiver.
    This ensures the ability to safely transition to home.

12. **Give new prescriptions,** as well as reminder cards for outpatient appointments (e.g., with physicians, social services), to the patient.
    This ensures continuity of care, thus minimizing patient stress.

13. **Document your final nursing note and complete the discharge summary** (the patient often receives a copy of the summary). The patient needs a copy of (1) his instructions for care at home, which may be called a discharge plan; and (2) his discharge summary, a summary of the progress of his illness and treatment from admission through discharge. Some agencies combine these into one form.
    It is important to document the patient's condition at the time he leaves the unit. This provides a baseline for comparison if his condition should deteriorate after discharge.

14. **Accompany the patient off the unit** and out of the hospital (or delegate this task) when you are notified that transportation has arrived.
    Keeping the patient on the unit for as long as practical helps to minimize the anxiety and fatigue that may occur from a long wait in the hospital lobby while a family member brings a car to the door.

15. **Notify the admissions department** of the discharge. Depending on agency policy, notify the primary care or admitting physician.
    This will stop all scheduled services, such as meals, and notify the housekeeping department that the room needs to be cleaned.

16. **Ensure the patient's records are sent** to the medical records department.
    Whether paper or electronic, the chart is a legal document and remains permanently in storage in the medical records department.

? What if...

- ✚ Near the time of discharge, the patient's condition worsens and the patient becomes unstable?
  Perform interventions to stabilize the patient, call for help if needed, and notify the provider.
  Notify the family that discharge will be delayed.
  Communicate with other hospital departments and community agencies as necessary.

- ■ **The patient is an older adult?**
  Allow for more time to dress and leave the hospital.
  Allow for more time to communicate, teach, and answer questions.
  Obtain feedback to be certain the caregivers have heard and understood instructions.
  Consider having a geriatric nurse specialist make follow-up home visits.
  Hearing, visual, and mobility deficits become more common with advanced age.

- ✚ **The patient is taking "high-risk" drugs after discharge?**
  Medications with a high risk of adverse events include corticosteroids, anticoagulants, diabetes medications, antibiotics, antianxiety agents, sedatives, and narcotic analgesics.
  Provide teaching for patient, family, and other caregivers throughout the hospital stay. A day or two before discharge, review teaching with patient and family; evaluate their understanding. On discharge, summarize medication precautions and provide clear written instructions. Be sure the patient and family can read them.

(continued on next page)

Procedure 8-4 ■ Discharging a Patient From the Healthcare Facility (continued)

Evaluation

A few weeks after discharge, the facility will contact the patient to evaluate the quality and appropriateness of the discharge process. This may be done by making a home visit, telephoning, or sending a questionnaire. As a nurse, you may or may not be involved in this evaluation. The best evaluation of the multidisciplinary care will be whether the patient must be readmitted to the acute care facility.

Documentation

- For the health record, the primary provider will write a discharge progress note that contains the following information:
  Reason for hospitalization
  Significant findings during the stay, including significant changes in status since admission
  Procedures performed; care, treatment, and services provided during the stay
  Status of goals for the stay
  Condition at discharge

- Agency policy determines the format and content of nursing documentation. This is often a combination of a structured discharge form or checklist and a narrative progress note. Regardless of format, you should document the following information:
  - Your final assessment of the patient's health status
  - Information and teaching provided to the patient and caregivers
  - Referrals, medications
  - How patient left the unit (e.g., in wheelchair) and who accompanied him (e.g., spouse, name of staff member)

  The Joint Commission (2008) recommends standardized formats for documentation.

  To see examples of discharge summaries, see Forms, later in this chapter.

Practice Resources

Agency for Healthcare Research and Quality (2014a, 2014b); Alper et al. (2017); The Joint Commission (2022); Lim et al. (2016).

CLINICAL INSIGHTS

Clinical Insight 8-1 ➤ Preparing the Room for an Admission

Delegation
As a general rule, these tasks can be delegated to unlicensed assistive personnel (UAPs). The nurse is responsible for evaluating and supervising as well as for setting up special equipment (although the UAP may obtain it from storage).

Clean the Room
Agencies differ; however, it is common for the housekeeping department to clean the room and change the bed linens when a patient is discharged, so you should find the room ready for your preparations. The rest of these guidelines assume that fact.

Prepare the Bed
- Position the bed according to patient status. If the patient is ambulatory, put the bed in the lowest position and lock the wheels. If the patient will arrive on a stretcher, place the bed at stretcher height.
- If necessary, rearrange the furniture to allow easy access to the bed.
- Fold back the top linens to "open" the bed (see the figure).
- The patient may need to go to bed immediately, so it should be ready when they arrive.

Prepare Routine Supplies
- Most agencies have an admission pack containing lotion, tissues, water pitcher, and drinking cup. Open it and put it in the room.
- Place a hospital gown on the bed and nonslip footwear by the bedside. Patients may choose to wear their own sleep clothing, though.

Prepare Equipment
You will need the following:
- A stethoscope, thermometer, and blood pressure cuff in the room for taking vital signs
- A scale for measuring and weighing the patient
- If the patient is not ambulatory, a bedpan, urinal, and perhaps a bedside commode
- A clean-catch urine specimen container if laboratory work has not already been done

Set up and check special equipment (e.g., oxygen, suction, cardiac monitor, pulse oximeter, IV pump).

Prepare the Environment
Turn on the lights and adjust the room temperature. Open or close curtains, as needed.

FORMS

The forms in this section are copies that are put into the patient's permanent record in paper form. Many agencies have computer-based discharge processes, however.

Fishermen's HOSPITAL

Discharge Assessment/Instructions

Date of Discharge	Time of Discharge	Mode of Discharge ☐ Ambulatory ☐ Wheelchair ☐ Stretcher ☐ Ambulance	Accompanied by:
Belongings sent with patient/family ☐ Yes ☐ No		Personal Medications sent with patient family ☐ Yes ☐ No	
Temp	P	Discharge Destination	Transfer Information Sent
R	BP	☐ Home ☐ AMA ☐ Facility_____ ☐ Home Health	☐ Yes ☐ No

Special Instructions

Patient Assessment and Health Status

	Yes	No		Yes	No		Yes	No
Afebrile	☐	☐	Skin Intact	☐	☐	Hygiene	☐	☐
Able to live independently	☐	☐	Eating Well	☐	☐	Self-Care	☐	☐
Pain Controlled	☐	☐	Adequate Hydration	☐	☐	Assist	☐	☐
Oriented	☐	☐				Total Care	☐	☐
Appropriate Behavior	☐	☐				Adequate Elimination	☐	☐
Functions Independently	☐	☐						

Additional Comments:

Weight monitoring daily   Avoid all tobacco products

Instructions

Diet
☐ No Restrictions

Activity
☐ No Restrictions

Special Equipment/Treatment
☐ No Restrictions

Discharge Medications (Name, Amount, Special Instructions)
☐ No Meds   See Patient Education

Special Instructions/Discharge Summary
Call MD or go to the ER if symptoms worsen

☐ Pt or Caregiver given instructions about and counseled on potential for drug-food interactions

Physician Follow-up Appointment	Outpatient Visit
Referral ☐ None Required	

I have received all personal belongings.
I have received a copy and understand the above Instructions.
I have received a copy of the Patient Education form.

Patient Identification

Signature/Responsible Party

Physician/Nurse Signature   Date

0916065

CHAPTER 8 Experiencing Wellness: Health & Illness

Fishermen's HOSPITAL

3301 Overseas Highway, Marathon, FL 33050 • Ph 305-743-5533 • Fax 305-743-3962

Allergies/Reactions		No known drug allergies ☐		IN-PATIENT Circle Y to continue or N to not continue and sign below to authenticate order.		AT DISCHARGE Circle Y to continue at same dose or N to not continue or document any changes in dose.		
MEDICATION NAME (Include Herbal, OTC, Vitamins)	Dose / Route / Freq	Reason Taken	LAST DOSE DATE/TIME	\multicolumn{2}{c}{Continue on Admission}	\multicolumn{2}{c}{Continue at home on same dose}	Continue with the following changes:
Patient takes no medication ☐								
				Y	N	Y	N	
				Y	N	Y	N	
				Y	N	Y	N	
				Y	N	Y	N	
				Y	N	Y	N	
				Y	N	Y	N	
				Y	N	Y	N	
				Y	N	Y	N	
				Y	N	Y	N	
				Y	N	Y	N	
				Y	N	Y	N	
				Y	N	Y	N	
				Y	N	Y	N	

Source-of-Medication list *(check all used):*
___ Bottles/List
___ Patient/Family
___ Retail pharmacy_____
___ MD office records
___ Previous discharge medical record
___ Medication Administration Record from _____
___ Med Reconciliation Form

Meds:
___ Sent home with_____
___ Removed
    Sent to Pharmacy for approval

New medications prescribed for patient discharge:			
Meds	Dose / Route / Freq		Reason

ADMITTING NURSE SIGNATURE   DATE   DISCHARGE NURSE SIGNATURE   DATE

Patient Education Form

Page ___ of ___

FORM N-100, Rev. 12-07   White: Chart   Yellow: Patient

ASSESSMENT GUIDELINES AND TOOLS

Focused Assessment

Health Promotion: Physical Fitness Assessment

Cardiorespiratory Fitness

There are many modes of testing, such as field tests (walking or running), motor-driven treadmills, stationary bicycles, and step testing.

- **Field tests** for running are good for children. A 9-year-old child should be able to complete a 1-mile run in approximately 10 minutes, and a 17-year-old boy should be able to complete a 1-mile run in approximately 7.5 minutes (U.S. Department of health and Human Services, 2013).

- The **step test** is appropriate for most adults. Using a 12-inch bench, instruct the participant to step up and down at a rate of 24 steps per minute for 3 minutes. At the end of 3 minutes, the participant should check their heart rate. Stop testing immediately if the participant has any chest pain, shortness of breath, or lightheadedness. Results depend on age and sex and are available in the following charts.

Step Test Evaluation Charts

3-Minute Step Heart Rate Test (Male)

Physical condition	18–25 yr	26–35 yr	36–45 yr	46–55 yr	56–65 yr	66+ yr
Excellent	<79	<81	<83	<87	<86	<88
Good	79–89	81–89	83–96	87–97	86–97	88–96
Above average	90–99	90–99	97–103	98–105	98–103	97–103
Average	100–105	100–107	104–112	106–116	104–112	104–113
Below average	106–116	108–117	113–119	117–122	113–120	114–120
Poor	117–128	118–128	120–130	123–132	121–129	121–130
Very poor	>128	>128	>130	>132	>129	>130

3-Minute Step Heart Rate Test (Female)

Physical condition	18–25 yr	26–35 yr	36–45 yr	46–55 yr	56–65 yr	66+ yr
Excellent	<85	<88	<90	<94	<95	<90
Good	85–98	88–99	90–102	94–104	95–104	90–102
Above average	99–108	100–111	103–110	105–115	105–112	103–115
Average	109–117	112–119	111–118	116–120	113–118	116–122
Below average	118–126	120–126	119–128	121–129	119–128	123–128
Poor	114–140	114–138	129–140	130–135	129–139	129–134
Very poor	>140	>138	>140	>135	>139	>134

Muscular Fitness

- **Muscle strength** is recorded as weight pushed (or lifted) divided by body weight. For example, if a female participant weighing 150 pounds is able to lift 86 pounds, she will have a muscular strength score of 86 divided by 150, or 0.57.
  - Instruct the participant warm up and stretch before the test. Weight benches are ideal sites for testing upper-body and leg strength.
  - Compare the value obtained to normative standards or to previous personal scores to evaluate improvement.
- **Muscle endurance** is evaluated by the push-up or curl-up (crunch) test. Ask the participant to perform as many push-ups or curl-ups as possible without pausing.
  - The number of repetitions is the score. Once again, compare scores to norms or previous performance.

Flexibility

The **sit-and-reach test** evaluates low back and hip (trunk) flexion.

- Ask the participant to sit on a floor mat with legs fully extended and feet flat against a box. Have them extend arms and hands forward as far as possible and hold for a count of 3.
- Using a ruler, measure the distance in inches that the participant can reach beyond the proximal edge of the box. If the person cannot reach the edge, measure the distance of the fingertips from the edge, and report it as a negative number.
- Norms for trunk flexion vary among male and female individuals. The desired range for male participants is +1 to +5 inches; for female participants it is +2 to +6 inches (Murdaugh et al., 2018).

Focused Assessment

Lifestyle and Risk Assessment

The following is an example of an HRA.

Name _____ Age _____ Sex _____

Health View

In general, how would you say your present health is?

☐ Excellent ☐ Good ☐ Fair

☐ Very good ☐ Poor

General Practices

1. **Physical activity.** How many days each week do you get at least 30 minutes of physical activity, such as brisk walking, cycling, active gardening, active dance, swimming, jogging, or active sports?

2. **Strength exercises.** How many days each week do you do strength-building exercises, such as weightlifting or isometric exercises?

3. **Smoking status.** Indicate your present smoking status.

   ☐ Current smoker ☐ Ex-smoker

   ☐ Nonsmoker, never smoked regularly

   Environmental smoke. Do you live with or work with smokers and breathe secondhand smoke regularly?

   ☐ Yes ☐ No

4. **Alcohol.** How many drinks do you typically have on a day you drink? *One drink is a bottle or can of beer (12 oz), a glass of wine or wine cooler (3.5 oz), or a shot glass of liquor (1.5 oz).*

   ☐ Never drink.

   ☐ Have no more than one drink in a day.

   ☐ Have no more than two drinks in a day.

   ☐ Sometimes have three or four drinks in a day.

   ☐ Sometimes have five or more drinks in a day.

5. **Sleep.** How many hours of sleep do you usually get each night?

Eating Practices

6. **Breakfast.** How many days each week do you usually eat breakfast (more than just coffee and a roll)?

7. **Bread/grains.** How many servings of whole-grain breads and cereals do you eat daily? *One serving = 1 slice bread, ½ cup dry cereal, ½ cup cooked oatmeal or other whole-grain cereal or brown rice.*

8. **Fruits and vegetables.** How many servings of fruits and vegetables do you eat daily? *One serving = ½ cup fruit or vegetables.*

9. **High-fat and high-cholesterol foods.** How often do you eat foods high in saturated fat and cholesterol (e.g., steak, hamburger, hot dog, sausage, bacon, cheese, fried chicken, French fries, ice cream, cheesecake, or other desserts)?

   ☐ Daily

   ☐ 3 or more times a week

   ☐ Seldom or never

10. **Nuts/seeds.** How many servings of nuts do you usually eat each week? *One serving = 1 oz or a small handful, or 2 tablespoons of natural nut butter.*

11. **Legumes.** How many times a week do you eat legumes (peas, beans, lentils, garbanzos)? *One serving = ½ cup cooked.*

12. **Refined foods.** How often do you eat highly refined foods (soda pop, snack foods, chips, refined cereals, pastry, candy)?

    ☐ Daily

    ☐ 3 or more times a week

    ☐ Seldom or never

13. **Weight.** How many pounds have you gained since you were 21 to 24? (Enter 0 if you weigh the same, weigh less, or are younger than 21 years.)

14. **Water intake.** How many glasses (8 oz) of water do you typically drink each day? _____

Mental/Social Health

15. **Happiness.** How happy have you been during the past month?

    ☐ Very happy

    ☐ Pretty happy

    ☐ Not too happy

    ☐ Very unhappy

16. **Mood/feelings**

    (a) During the past month, have you often been bothered by feeling down, depressed, or hopeless?

    ☐ Yes ☐ No

    (b) During the past month, have you often been bothered by having little interest or pleasure in doing things?

    ☐ Yes ☐ No

    (c) Have your feelings in the past month caused you significant distress or impaired your ability to function socially or at work or school?

    ☐ Yes ☐ No

17. **Stress and coping.** How much of the time do you feel stressed out and unable to cope with life?

    ☐ Seldom or never

    ☐ Occasionally

    ☐ Much of the time

    ☐ Most of the time

Social Support

18. **Support.** Do you have family or friends you can get help from if needed?

    ☐ Yes ☐ No

19. **Social interaction.** Do you have frequent social contact with family or friends?

    ☐ Yes ☐ No

(Continued)

Lifestyle and Risk Assessment—cont'd

Community

20. **Community support.** Do you meet regularly with a faith community or other group that gives you support, comfort, meaning, and direction in your life?

    ☐ Yes   ☐ No

Safety

21. **Seat belts.** What percentage of the time do you wear seat belts when riding in a car? _____

22. **Smoke alarm.** Do you have a working smoke alarm on each floor of your home, including the area in which you sleep?

    ☐ Yes   ☐ No   ☐ Don't know for sure

23. **Helmet.** When biking or in-line skating do you always wear a helmet and protective gear?

    ☐ Yes   ☐ No

24. **Substance use and driving.** Do you ever drive soon after drinking alcohol or taking drugs or ride with someone who has been using illicit substances or alcohol?

    ☐ Yes   ☐ No

Safer Sex

25. **Practice safer sex.**

    (a) Are you in a monogamous relationship?

    ☐ Yes   ☐ No

    (b) Do you always use condoms, or abstain from sexual relations?

    ☐ Always   ☐ Don't always practice safer sex

Preventive Examinations

26. Do you keep current on recommended preventive examinations (see following list) and immunizations?

    ☐ Yes   ☐ No   ☐ Don't know for sure

Recommended Preventive Examinations

- Periodic checkup, including blood pressure, height and weight, and cholesterol check as recommended by your doctor
- Pap tests within the last year, for female individuals 21 years or older
- Mammogram within last 2 years, for female individuals 45 or older
- Colorectal cancer screening for all persons 45 or older
- Prostate examination, for men 50 or older
- Flu immunization, for everyone 6 months and older
- Pneumonia immunizations, for everyone 65 or older

Height _____

Weight _____

Blood pressure _____

Blood cholesterol _____ (mg/dL)

_____ **Scoring**

_____

Your score is the number of good health indicators you meet out of the 17 possible listed (below) in this assessment. The higher your score, the healthier your lifestyle. The average health lifestyle score is 9.4.

Health indicator	Guidelines for good health
1. Physical activity	Get 30 or more minutes of physical activity most days of the week.
2. Strength training	Do strength-building exercises at least twice per week.
3. Not smoking	Avoid all tobacco use and frequent exposure to secondhand smoke.
4. Alcohol use	Alcohol is not recommended, but if you drink alcohol, limit to 1 to 2 drinks in a day.
5. Adequate rest	Get adequate rest (at least 7 hours of sleep daily for best health).
6. Breakfast daily	Eat a nutritious breakfast daily for optimal physical and mental performance.
7. Whole grains	Choose whole-grain breads and cereals (at least 3 servings per day).
8. Fruits and vegetables	Eat at least 5 servings of fruits and vegetables daily.
9. Fat, cholesterol	Limit high-fat meats, whole milk, and butter. Vegetable oils are healthier than oils from animals.

Lifestyle and Risk Assessment—cont'd

Focused Assessment

Health indicator	Guidelines for good health
10. Nuts and legumes	Nuts such as almonds contain healthy fats and protect against heart disease. Legumes prevent carbohydrate cravings, prevent metabolic syndrome, provide protein and energy, protect against cancer, and are a source of calcium and other vitamins and minerals.
11. Healthy weight	Maintain a healthy weight by eating well and participating in regular, moderate-intensity physical activity.
12. Mental health	Develop effective coping skills and maintain a happy, hopeful outlook.
13. Social support	Maintain good social support and frequent contact with family and friends.
14. Community	Participate regularly in a faith community or other group that provides meaning, direction, and support in your life.
15. Safety	Be safety conscious; wear safety belts in the car and helmets when biking.
16. Safer sex	Remain in a monogamous relationship, or always use condoms, or abstain.
17. Regular examinations	Get regular examinations, including age- and sex-recommended preventive examinations.

Source: Adapted from Hall, D. R. (2004). *Lifestyle check assessment.* Nashville, TN: Vanderbilt University Health and Wellness.

CLINICAL REASONING
Applying the Full-Spectrum Nursing Model

PATIENT SITUATION

Recall Evelyn (Meet Your Patient, in Volume 1). She is 87 years old and has lived in a nursing home for the past 5 years. She has CHF, hypertension, diabetes, macular degeneration resulting in near blindness, a severe hearing deficit, urinary incontinence, and immobility resulting from a hip fracture. Despite these limitations, she keeps current in the lives of all her family members and friends. At the nursing home, staff members confide in Evelyn, and she knows about their children, their romances, and the gossip around the nursing home. Whenever there is an election, she makes sure that she gets to vote. She "reads" every audio book she can get her hands on.

Recently Evelyn was admitted to the hospital in severe CHF. When leaving the nursing home, she told her pastor, "I don't want to die yet. I'm having too much fun!" You notice that the papers from the nursing home do not contain an advance directive, and it was not mentioned in their report to you.

THINKING

1. *Critical Thinking (Considering Alternatives):*

    a. What are some possible reasons that no advance directive exists?

    b. Which of those seems most likely to you?

    c. How might you find out about the status of Evelyn's advance directive?

DOING

2. *Nursing Process (Diagnosis/Recognizing Cues):* On the care plan from the nursing home, there were two nursing diagnoses:

    a. Urgent urinary incontinence related to difficulty ambulating to bathroom

    b. Impaired skin integrity related to immobility and incontinence

    Which of these can you remove from the care plan for now? Explain your decision.

CARING

3. *Self-Knowledge:* The next day, despite aggressive treatment, Evelyn's condition worsens. She is not responding to verbal stimuli and her oxygen level is decreasing. There is discussion about putting her on a ventilator.

   a. What would you be feeling?

   b. If Evelyn has an advance directive that indicates "no ventilator," how would that change your feelings?

   c. If there is an advance directive that indicates "do everything possible to keep me alive," how would that change your feelings?

   Note: We are not asking you what you would do; rather, you should consider how you would feel.

Critical Thinking and Clinical Judgment

1. Describe your personal view of health.

2. Identify a person in your life, personally or professionally, who personifies health. What characteristics do you identify in this person that represent health? What factors do you think contribute to this person's health status?

3. Use the nursing process to develop a plan to improve your personal health.

4. What attributes, resources, or life experiences do you have to offer in your role as a nurse?

5. While you are working in a physician's office, a 70-year-old woman is referred to you for counseling regarding health protection activities. She is hypertensive and obese.

   a. How does her age affect your assessments and communication?

   b. What type of learning aids might be needed?

   c. What health screenings are appropriate for this patient?

6. The following is a group of clients who wish to enroll in a health promotion program.

   - Jennifer Kaska is 23 years old and was diagnosed with diabetes mellitus at the age of 12 years. She checks her blood sugar and administers insulin as needed. She runs 3 miles 3 days per week.

   - Maurice Rosenthal is 47 years old with no known illness. He is 6 feet tall and weighs 240 pounds. His body mass index (BMI) is 33 kg/m^2, indicating obesity. He takes no routine medication, only acetaminophen for occasional headaches.

   - Clara Fenton is 83 years old and has been diagnosed with hypertension, emphysema, and osteoporosis. She takes 10 prescription medications daily in addition to a multivitamin and an occasional laxative.

   Discuss the pros and cons of providing a group program that includes all three of these clients.

7. L. F. is a 50-year-old man with heart disease. He had coronary artery bypass surgery 1 month ago. He has stopped going to his prescribed cardiac rehabilitation program because of the distance he must travel to the rehabilitation center. Discuss at least two approaches for working with this client.

8. Cecelia Kent is 32 years old. She takes no medications and has annual physical examinations. She walks 4 to 5 miles 5 days per week and lifts light weights two or three times per week. She eats a low-fat, low-salt, low-sugar diet. She has never smoked and drinks only limited alcohol.

   a. She asks you to recommend further health promotion activities. How would you respond?

   b. How could you incorporate Cecelia into a health promotion class that includes Jennifer Kaska, Maurice Rosenthal, and Clara Fenton (from question 2)?

9. For each of the following concepts, use critical thinking to describe how or why it is important to nursing, patient care, or health promotion. Note that these are not to be merely definitions.

Health	Lifestyle
Wellness	Hardiness
Health promotion	Health screenings
Illness	Health education
Disruptions	Response to illness
Illness prevention	Health illness continuum

What Are the Main Points in This Chapter?

- Health is a complex phenomenon that involves physical, mental, and spiritual aspects. Having good health is an almost universal desire.
- Wellness is a way of life oriented toward optimal health and well-being.
- Health promotion refers to helping clients develop an optimal state of health.
- There are three levels of activities for health protection: primary, secondary, and tertiary prevention. Primary interventions are designed to prevent or slow the onset of disease. Secondary interventions are designed to detect illnesses in early stages. Tertiary interventions focus on stopping the disease from progressing and on rehabilitation.
- Life and wellness require nourishment. Nourishment comes in the form of food, exercise, sleep, relationships, meaningful work, the environment, and memories.
- The person with an illness rarely perceives the experience as a medical diagnosis. Instead, illness is usually described in terms of how it makes the person feel, such as pain, sadness, loss, fatigue, or being overwhelmed.
- People dealing with life-threatening illness have to figure out how to live and still be dying. Dealing with death is one of the most difficult experiences you will face as a nurse.
- Nurses deal with people who have been thrust into new life situations, situations they did not ask for and for which they were not prepared.
- Several factors influence a person's responses to disruptions. These factors include age; family patterns; culture; hardiness; support; access to healthcare resources; the stage and nature of the illness; and the intensity, duration, and multiplicity of the disruption.
- Chronic illnesses are a large and growing healthcare concern, especially among older adults.
- You can ease patients' disruptions experienced during admission, transfers, and discharge from a healthcare setting by discharge planning, communication, coordination, and teaching.
- As a nurse, you will need to cultivate a healing presence. Listening, being attentive, being willing to learn from those in your care, and recognizing and respecting others' ways of coping are behaviors associated with a healing presence.
- Most people experience health, illness, and wellness as an ever-changing continuum on which they move.
- Your healing presence may be the most memorable aspect of nursing care that you have to offer.
- Health promotion activities for all age groups include nutrition, exercise, safety concerns, changing unhealthy lifestyles, immunizations, and screenings.
- Health promotion activities may be conducted in acute care facilities, workplaces, local communities, or schools.
- A health promotion assessment involves obtaining a health history, physical examination, fitness assessment, lifestyle and risk appraisal, life stress review, assessment of healthcare beliefs, nutrition assessment, and screening activities.
- Health screening activities are designed to detect disease at an early stage so that treatment can begin before there is an opportunity for disease to spread or reduce the quality of life.
- Health screening activities vary based on developmental stage and identified risk factors.
- Nurses promote health through role models, counseling, health education, and providing and facilitating support.

Knowledge Map

EXPERIENCING WELLNESS, HEALTH & ILLNESS

WELLNESS
- A state of optimal health
- Well-being
- Integration of body, mind, and spirit
- Influenced by attitude and lifestyle choices

HEALTH
- Perfect body
- Absence of illness/disease
- Something one can buy
- Ideal state of physical and mental well-being
- Power of the soul to cope with varying body conditions

ILLNESS
- To some, a disease
- Response to a disruption in health
- A lived experience
- Unique to each individual
- Not a medical diagnosis

RN Role

FACTORS THAT INFLUENCE HEALTH
- Genetics; gender; age; developmental stage
- Nutrition
- Activity level
- Quantity/quality of sleep/rest
- Meaningful work
- Lifestyle choices
- Family relationships
- Culture
- Spirituality
- Environment
- Finances
- Hardiness

FACTORS THAT DISRUPT HEALTH
- Physical disease
- Injury
- Mental illness
- Pain
- Loss
- Impending death
- Competing demands
- The unknown
- Imbalance
- Isolation

LEVELS OF PREVENTION
- Primary
- Secondary
- Tertiary

STAGES OF ILLNESS BEHAVIOR
- Experiencing symptoms
- Sick role behavior
- Seeking professional care
- Dependence on others
- Recovery

HEALTH PROMOTION
- Physical Fitness Assessment
- Lifestyle and Role Appraisal
- Life Stress Review
- Health Beliefs
- Nutritional Assessment
- Health Screenings

INTERVENTIONS
- Role Modeling
- Counseling
- Health Education
- Support Lifestyle Change

NATURE OF ILLNESS
- Acute
- Chronic
  - Exacerbation
  - Remission

CHAPTER 9

Stress & Adaptation

STUDENT RESOURCES

The questions and exercises in this book allow you to practice the kind of thinking you will use as a full-spectrum nurse. Critical-thinking questions usually have more than one right answer, so we do not provide "correct" answers for these features. Try to answer these questions yourself. It is more important to develop your nursing judgment than to just cover content. You will learn more by discussing the questions with your peers. If you are still unsure, see the Davis Advantage chapter resources for suggested responses.

To explore learning resources for this chapter,

Go to www.DavisAdvantage.com and find:

Answers and Suggested Responses for all questions in this chapter
Concept Map
Knowledge Map
References and Bibliography

Key Concepts

Adaptation
Coping
Stress

Related Concepts

See the Concept Map on Davis Advantage.

Example Client Conditions

Panic
Post-traumatic stress disorder (PTSD)

Caring for the Williams Family

After having a comprehensive physical examination at the family health center, Nadine Williams has been scheduled to have a mammogram and laboratory screenings. When she arrives at the clinic for her mammogram, she tells you she is very nervous. "I have a good friend who just found out she has breast cancer. She's very depressed now. Do I really have to do this test?"

(Continued)

Caring for the Williams Family (continued)

A. What kind of stress is Nadine experiencing?

B. Three days later, the radiologist contacts Nadine requesting that she return to the family health center for additional films of the upper outer quadrant of the right breast. "There are some calcifications I want to check out," explains the radiologist.
- What factors might affect Nadine's adaptation to this stress?
- Evaluate what you know about Nadine's perception of her stress, her overall health status, her support system, and her coping methods. What more do you need to know about these topics to fully answer this question?

C. Later, Nadine calls the office frantically explaining that she is very upset about this recent event. She says, "Not knowing is killing me. I'm so nervous I can't stand it. I can't sleep. I can't eat." She asks how she can handle the stress until she comes in for the additional tests next week. What strategies would you recommend to help Nadine deal with the stress?

Practical Knowledge clinical application

CLINICAL INSIGHTS

Clinical Insight 9-1 ▶ Dealing With Angry Patients

- **Be aware of how you are responding to angry patients.** Are you relieving your own stress, or are you relieving the client's stress? If you respond angrily to relieve your own stress, you may provoke further anger in the patient and even escalate the situation to the point of aggression.
- **Remind yourself not to take anger personally;** remind family members and colleagues of this as well.
- **Recognize that anger and anxiety are normal feelings when facing adversity,** such as a life-threatening or debilitating illness. Do not discount feelings by saying, "Please don't be so angry" or "You shouldn't talk like that" or "Everything will be OK; don't worry."
- **Encourage the client and family to express feelings** verbally and appropriately.
- **Listen instead of defending.** If the patient says, "Everything about this place stinks!" keep the following in mind:
  Do not defend. Don't respond with a comment such as "We really are trying to do the best we can for you."
  Do encourage the person to express their feelings or give you more information: "You seem really angry; what's going on?" or "Maybe I can help. Tell me a little more about what stinks."
- **Do not take responsibility for the patient's anger.** It is not your fault, so don't apologize—unless you really *do* have something to apologize for.
- **Remain calm;** this reassures the patient and keeps the emotion from escalating.
- **Help the patient identify what is causing the anger** and try to meet those needs.
- ■ **Be alert to your own and the patient's safety needs.**

  Do not allow a patient to get between you and the door if the person seems to be violent.
  Do not wear a stethoscope around your neck, dangling jewelry, or anything a patient might use to hurt you.
  Do not go into a room alone with a patient who seems to have the potential for violence.
  Do not turn your back on an angry patient.
  Remain at least an arm's length away from an angry and potentially violent patient.
  Key Point: Be sure you know how to call for help from staff or security personnel if you think you or someone else is in danger.
  Key Point: If you believe the patient's anger may escalate to violence, your priority is your own safety and the safety of others in the area.
  Also refer to the NIC intervention Anger Control Assistance (Wagner, Butcher, Bulechek, et al., 2022).

Clinical Insight 9-2 ▶ Crisis Intervention Guidelines

Assess the Situation.
What is the nature of the patient's condition and the severity of the crisis?

Ensure Safety
- Call for help if you or the patient is in physical danger.
- Do not leave the patient unless you think you are in imminent danger.
- First ensure your own safety; then provide for the patient's safety.

Defuse the Situation
- Keep in mind that a person in crisis may not be in control of their actions.
- Try to calm the person verbally.
- Attempt physical restraint only as a last resort and only when there is enough help to do it safely for both the staff and the patient.

Decrease the Person's Anxiety
- Reassure the person that they are in a safe place and that you are concerned and want to help.
- Explain gently but firmly that you need the person's help and cooperation.
- Help the person to vent feelings of fear, guilt, and anger.
- Use physical contact very cautiously. The person in turmoil may interpret touch as aggression or a sexual approach.

Determine the Problem
- Find out what the patient believes to be the cause of the crisis.
- Remain calm, and do not pressure the patient to give reasons. Any tension on your part will create further panic in the patient.

Decide on the Type of Help Needed
- You may be able to calm the person enough for them to understand what just happened, or you may not. Evaluate your ability to calm the patient based on your assessment of their coping skills and resources.
- Put in place the help needed to restore the person to a minimal level of functioning. This may require long-term treatment. In that case, make the necessary referrals.

Return the Person to a Precrisis Level of Functioning
- *Crisis counseling.* The goal is to provide immediate relief, solve the most urgent problems, and give long-term counseling, if needed. Crisis centers often rely on telephone or online counseling ("hotlines").
- *Home visits.* If virtual counseling is not adequate or if observations of the home environment are needed, home visits may be necessary.

ASSESSMENT GUIDELINES AND TOOLS

Focused Assessment

The Holmes-Rahe Social Readjustment Scale

This is a way to check your stress level, measured in "life change units." Of course, it is not possible to score the exact intensity of stress. However, this will give you a general idea of your stress level and should provide some insight into the sources of your stress. The following are based on the number of life change units over a 1- to 2-year period:

Over 300 points (major amount of change): 80% chance of major illness

200–299 (moderate amount of change): 50% chance of major illness

150–199 (mild amount of change): 33% chance of major illness

0–149 (insignificant amount of change): Minimal chance of major illness

Of course, your personality and your ability to cope also determine the likelihood of your becoming ill.

Life event	Life change units	Life event	Life change units
Death of spouse	100	Son or daughter leaving home	29
Divorce	73	Trouble with in-laws	29
Marital separation	65	Outstanding personal achievement	28
Imprisonment	63	Spouse begins or stops work	26
Death of a close family member	63	Beginning or ending school	26
Personal injury or illness	53	Change in living conditions	25
Marriage	50	Revision of personal habits	24
Dismissal from work	47	Trouble with boss	23
Marital reconciliation	45	Change in work hours or conditions	20
Retirement	45	Change in residence	20
Change in health of family member	44	Change in schools	20
Pregnancy	40	Change in recreation	19
Sexual difficulties	39	Change in church activities	19
Gain of new family member	39	Change in social activities	18
Business readjustment	39	Minor mortgage or loan	17
Change in financial state	38	Change in sleeping habits	16
Change in number of arguments with spouse	35	Change in number of family reunions	15
Major mortgage	32	Change in eating habits	15
Foreclosure of mortgage or loan	30	Vacation	13
Change in responsibilities at work	29		

Source: Reprinted from Holmes, T., & Rahe, R. (1967). Social readjustment rating scale. *Journal of Psychosomatic Research, 11*(2), 213–218. doi:10.1016/0022-3999(67)90010-4. Reprinted with permission from Elsevier.

Focused Assessment

Assessing for Stress: Questions to Ask

1. **Assess stressors and risk factors.** Ask the client to complete a stress inventory, such as the preceding Holmes-Rahe Social Readjustment Scale. Then ask the client the following questions:
   - What is causing the most stress in your life?
   - On a scale of 1 to 10 (where 1 is "not much" and 10 is "extreme"), rate the stress you are experiencing in each of these areas: work or school, finances, community responsibilities, your health, health of a family member, family relationships, family responsibilities, relationships with friends.
   - How long have you been dealing with the stressful situation(s)?
   - Can you track the accumulation of stress in your life?
   - How long have you been under this stress?

   Note the client's developmental stage and determine whether he is functioning as expected for this stage. Review Chapter 9 if you need help to identify developmental milestones. To help you assess for stressors that can be predicted to occur in each stage, you might ask questions such as these:
   - What challenges do you face as a result of your life and your age?
   - Have you had recent life changes?
   - Do you anticipate any life changes?

   TO REVIEW DEVELOPMENTAL STAGE MILESTONES AND CHANGES,

   ➤ Go to **Chapters 5 and 6,** in Volume 1. Also see Chapter 9, **Box 9-1: Stressors Throughout the Life Span,** in Volume 1.

2. **Assess coping methods and adaptation.**
   - What coping strategies have you used previously? What was successful, and what was not successful?
   - Tell me about previous experiences you have had with stressful situations in your life.
   - What do you usually do to handle stressful situations? (If the client needs prompting, you can ask, "Do you cry, get angry, avoid people, talk to family or friends, do physical exercise, pray? Some people laugh or joke, others meditate, others try to control everything, and others just work hard, or look for a solution. What is your usual response?")
   - How well do these methods usually work for you?
   - What have you been doing to cope with the present situation?
   - How well is that working?
   - During the interview, you should also observe for the use of psychological defense mechanisms.

   TO REVIEW PSYCHOLOGICAL DEFENSE MECHANISMS,

   ➤ Go to Chapter 9, **Table 9-1: Psychological Defense Mechanisms,** in Volume 1.

   - If the patient has not exhibited any defense mechanisms, you could ask about the common ones. For example, "Do you ever cope with a situation by denying it exists or just by trying to put it out of your mind?"
   - Also ask the client about physiological changes and diseases caused by ongoing stress. Check the client's records for a history of somatoform disorders. Ask the client these questions:
     - What physical illnesses do you have? How long have you had them?
     - What, if any, physical changes have you noticed?
     - Do you have other physical conditions, such as hypertension, cardiac disease, diabetes, arthritis, joint pains, or cancer?

   TO REVIEW FINDINGS THAT MIGHT INDICATE MALADAPTATION TO STRESS,

   ➤ Go to Chapter 9, **Table 9-2: Organic Disorders Brought About by Failure of Adaptive Mechanisms,** in Volume 1.

3. **Assess physiological responses to stress.**

   The following are examples of questions you should ask:
   - What do you do to stay healthy?
   - Tell me about your health habits.
   - How often do you have a checkup?
   - What are your health concerns?

4. Assess emotional and behavioral responses to stress.

   Emotional Responses
   - Anger
   - Anxiety
   - Depression
   - Fear
   - Feelings of inadequacy
   - Low self-esteem
   - Irritability
   - Lack of motivation
   - Lethargy

   Behavioral Responses
   - Crying, emotional outbursts
   - Dependence
   - Poor job performance
   - Substance use and abuse
   - Sleeplessness (or sleeping too much)
   - Change in eating habits
   - Decrease in quality of job performance
   - Preoccupation or distraction
   - Listlessness

(Continued)

Focused Assessment

Assessing for Stress: Questions to Ask—cont'd

- Increased absenteeism
- Increased number of accidents
- Reduced interest in social situations or relationships
- Rebellion, acting out

Examples of Assessment Questions

- Do you use tobacco products?
- How much alcohol do you drink every day?
- What do you eat? What is your typical eating pattern?
- How much fluid do you drink daily?
- How many hours do you sleep at night? Do you feel rested when you wake up? Do you take naps?
- Do you often wake up very early in the morning and have difficulty getting back to sleep?
- What prescribed medications, vitamins, nonprescription medications, or dietary supplements do you take?
- What regular physical activity do you engage in?
- How much time do you spend at work versus at leisure and play?
- Do you constantly take work home with you? Or think about work almost all the time?
- How do you relax?
- Have you given up activities and relationships you previously enjoyed because you don't have enough time or are too tired?
- How do you express anger? What typically causes you frustration?
- Do you try to be perfect?
- Would you describe yourself as having the stress-filled lifestyle of a type A personality?
- How often do you find yourself feeling hopeless? Sad?

5. Assess cognitive responses to stress.
   - Difficulty concentrating
   - Poor judgment
   - Decrease in accuracy (e.g., in counting money)
   - Forgetfulness
   - Decreased problem-solving ability
   - Decreased attention to detail
   - Difficulty learning
   - Narrowing of focus
   - Preoccupation, distraction

6. Assess support systems.
   - Tell me about your home. Describe your living environment. (Make a home visit, if possible, or contact the case manager or social worker to arrange a home evaluation.)
   - Who are the persons who provide the most support for you? In what ways do they support you?
   - What support is available from family, friends, significant others, community agencies, and clergy that you may not have required until now?
   - Do you have or do you seek spiritual support?
   - How has your stress affected the family?
   - What are your financial resources? What are your financial obligations?

CLINICAL REASONING
Applying the Full-Spectrum Nursing Model

PATIENT SITUATION

Mrs. Williams, a 76-year-old woman, was admitted yesterday after suffering a stroke that paralyzed her right side. She has had diabetes and high blood pressure for many years. Since the stroke, she has been unable to speak clearly and becomes frustrated as she attempts to communicate her needs. Her daughter says Mrs. Williams is a proud, independent, and tidy woman who has been living alone since her husband's death last year. Until her stroke, she had been driving her car, cleaning the house, doing her grocery shopping, and maintaining her yard and garden. She wears eyeglasses for reading and driving and has a hearing aid, although she rarely uses it.

THINKING

1. *Theoretical Knowledge:*

   a. What stroke risk factors probably functioned as stressors for Mrs. Williams? (*Hint:* Look up stroke risk factors in a medical-surgical nursing or pathophysiology text or online.)

   b. What are common stressors for patients who must be hospitalized?

2. *Critical Thinking (Contextual Awareness):*

   a. Now that Mrs. Williams is in the hospital, what new stressors might she have?

DOING

3. *Practical Knowledge:* What might you advise Mrs. Williams' daughter to do to help her mother adapt more comfortably to the stressors in the hospital?

4. *Nursing Process (Nursing Diagnosis/Analyzing Cues):* Based on only the data in the scenario, write one or two nursing diagnoses for Mrs. Williams. Do not use potential diagnoses. Remember, the defining characteristics must be present in the scenario. State the data you would need to make diagnoses more descriptive.

CARING

5. *Self-Knowledge:* Imagine yourself in Mrs. Williams' situation.

   a. What is the one thing that would cause you the most stress? Why would that be the most stressful thing?

   b. What is the single most important thing you would want your nurse to do for you?

Critical Thinking and Clinical Judgment

1. Gloria and her husband, John (Meet Your Patient, in Volume 1), live in a residential community, and John commutes from there to work in a nearby city. Gloria runs an accounting business from their home. They have two teenage boys who are active in sports, church activities, Boy Scouts, and the school band. The boys need transportation to their various activities. Gloria and John teach Sunday school and are Boy Scout leaders. Gloria's mother needs knee replacement surgery and so cannot take care of Gloria's father, who is in the early stage of Alzheimer disease. In addition to her own home responsibilities, Gloria must go to her parents' house to prepare meals and to provide care for her parents during the day. Gloria's sister comes at 8:00 p.m. to sleep in the parents' home during the night.

   a. What resources may be available to help Gloria?

   b. What stress-reducing techniques can you suggest to help Gloria?

   c. What may reduce John's stress?

   d. On a scale of 1 to 10 (1 being low and 10 being high), what number will you give to Gloria's stress level?

2. Look again at Gloria and John's situation. Using the following list of defense mechanisms, create a possible scenario for each. That is, what might Gloria (or John) say and/or do if using one of the defense mechanisms in this situation? If you need to review psychological defense mechanisms,

   > Go to **Table 9-1,** in Volume 1.

   a. **Avoidance**—unconsciously staying away from events or situations that might open feelings of aggression or anxiety.

   b. **Conversion**—changing emotional conflict into physical symptoms that have no physical basis.

   c. **Denial**—transforming reality by refusing to acknowledge thoughts, feelings, desires, or impulses. This is an unconscious response; the person is *not* consciously lying.

d. **Displacement**—"Kicking the dog." Transferring emotions, ideas, or wishes from one original object or situation to a substitute inappropriate person or object that is perceived to be less powerful or less threatening.

e. **Reaction formation**—similar to compensation, except the person develops the exact opposite trait. The person is aware of their feelings but acts in ways opposite to what they are really feeling.

3. Maria is a nursing student. She works part-time to maintain health insurance coverage for herself and her children and to earn tuition money for school. She has to study after the children are in bed, so she gets little sleep herself. Her grades are low and do not reflect Maria's true knowledge level. Maria's nursing faculty suggests that she seek counseling for dealing with examination anxiety and learn about test-taking strategies. She realizes she may fail nursing school without this counseling, but she does not know how she will fit weekly sessions into her already full schedule.

   a. List Maria's stressors.

   b. *Self-knowledge:*

      - What life experiences do you have that may help you to understand Maria's situation?

      - How could these same life experiences interfere with your empathy for and understanding of Maria?

      - How much of Maria's story can you identify with as being part of your own experience now?

   c. Which interventions do you think would be most helpful to Maria: (1) helping her to change her perception of her stressors, or (2) the health promotion activities discussed in Volume 1? Explain your reasoning.

   d. Before deciding specifically how to help Maria, what data do you still need?

   e. Based on the information you have, what do you think Maria's two most important goals are?

   f. If you discover that Maria's most important goals are to (1) provide for her children and (2) succeed in nursing school, how might you use this information to help her?

4. *Self-knowledge:* In Volume 1, you listed your stressors. Let's assess further.

   a. What are your two (or three) *most* important goals? List them in order of importance.

   b. What support do you have that can help you to achieve each of these goals?

5. *Self-knowledge and theoretical knowledge:* Lead a partner through a visualization exercise; then reverse roles, and have your partner lead you through it.

   a. Before beginning, what were your thoughts and feelings about the exercise?

   b. After doing the visualization exercise, how did you feel? Did you feel more relaxed?

   c. How do you think your attitudes and perceptions before the exercise affected how you felt *after* the exercise?

6. For each of the following concepts, use critical thinking to describe how or why it is important to nursing, patient care, or stress and adaptation. Note that these are *not* to be merely definitions.

   Stress

   Developmental stressors

   Coping strategies

   Psychological defense mechanisms

   Inflammatory response

   Somatoform disorders

   Relaxation techniques for stress reduction

What Are the Main Points in This Chapter?

- Stress is a disturbance in normal homeostasis caused by internal or external stimuli called *stressors*.
- Adaptive coping techniques are those that offer healthy choices to the person and reduce the negative effects of stress.
- Approaches to coping include altering the stressor, adapting to the stressor, and avoiding the stressor.
- Whether the outcome of stress is positive (adaptation) or negative (disease) depends on the balance between the strength and duration of the stressors and the effectiveness of the person's coping methods.
- The three stages of Selye's general adaptation syndrome (GAS) are alarm, resistance, and exhaustion. Each stage in GAS produces different physical or psychological responses.
- In the alarm stage of GAS, responses are produced primarily by adrenal hormones, epinephrine, mineralocorticoids, and the sympathetic nervous system.
- The exhaustion stage can lead to stress-induced illness, burnout, or death.
- The two most common responses of local adaptation syndrome (LAS) are the reflex pain response and the inflammatory response.
- Examples of psychological responses are anxiety, fear, anger, and ego defense mechanisms.
- Psychological defense mechanisms are unconscious mental mechanisms that help decrease the inner tension associated with stressors; when overused, they are maladaptive.
- Unsuccessful adaptation can lead to crisis, organic disease (e.g., stomach ulcers), somatoform disorders (e.g., hypochondriasis), and psychological disorders (e.g., mental illness).
- Crisis exists when (1) an event in a person's life drastically changes his or her routine and is perceived as a threat to self, and (2) the person's usual coping methods are ineffective, resulting in high anxiety and reduced ability to function.
- Burnout occurs when nurses or other professionals cannot cope effectively with the demands of the workplace.
- You should assess for data about the patient's stressors, risk factors, coping and adaptation, support systems, and psychosocial and physiological responses to stress.
- Interventions for stress must be individualized to the patient. They include (1) health promotion activities for preventing and improving the ability to cope with stressors; (2) managing anxiety, fear, and anger; (3) stress management techniques that focus on discharging tension or producing relaxation; (4) techniques to alter perception (i.e., cognitive restructuring and positive self-talk); (5) identifying and using support systems; (6) reducing the stress of hospitalization; (7) providing spiritual support; (8) crisis intervention; (9) stress management in the workplace; and (10) making referrals.

Knowledge Map

COPING STRATEGIES
- Alter stressor
- Adapt to stressor
- Avoid stressor

TYPES OF STRESS
- Distress
- Eustress
- Internal
- External
- Developmental
- Situational
- Physiological
- Psychological

STRESS

INFLUENCING FACTORS
- Overall health
- Support system
- Perception of stressor
- Age
- Life experience
- Developmental level

POTENTIAL OUTCOME

increases

ADAPTATION

Responses — *When it fails* → **DISEASE**

PHYSIOLOGICAL RESPONSES
- Selye's GAS: Autonomic nervous system and endocrine system; alarm, resistance, recovery/exhaustion
- Local adaptation: Reflex pain and inflammatory response

PSYCHOLOGICAL DISORDERS
- Crisis
- Burnout
- Post-traumatic stress disorder

SPIRITUAL RESPONSES
- Prayer
- Meditation
- Religious affiliation

SOMATOFORM
- Hypochondriasis
- Somatization
- Pain disorders
- Malingering

PSYCHOLOGICAL RESPONSES
- Anxiety
- Fear
- Ego defense mechanisms
- Anger
- Depression

ORGANIC RESPONSES
- Heart disease
- Diabetes
- Irritable bowel syndrome
- Ulcers
- Autoimmune disorders

CHAPTER 10

Psychosocial Health & Illness

STUDENT RESOURCES

The questions and exercises in this book allow you to practice the kind of thinking you will use as a full-spectrum nurse. Critical-thinking questions usually have more than one right answer, so we do not provide "correct" answers for these features. Try to answer these questions yourself. It is more important to develop your nursing judgment than to just cover content. You will learn more by discussing the questions with your peers. If you are still unsure, see the Davis Advantage chapter resources for suggested responses.

To explore learning resources for this chapter,

Go to www.DavisAdvantage.com and find:

Answers and Suggested Responses for all questions in this chapter
Concept Map
Knowledge Map
References and Bibliography

Key Concepts

Anxiety
Depression
Psychosocial health
Self-concept

Related Concepts

See the Concept Map on Davis Advantage.

Caring for the Williams Family

Recall the case of Stanley Williams. Mr. Williams has been diagnosed with hypertension, obesity, and degenerative joint disease. At clinic visits he has made the following comments: "Every time I come in here, I get some new diagnosis. I guess it's amazing I'm not dead yet. I thought I had a lot more time left, but I'm not so sure anymore." When you ask him what his main concerns are, he tells you, "Just take a look at me! I'm a mess. Nothing is turning out the way I planned. I might as well just die now. It would save my family a lot of grief."

A. What information do you need in order to respond to Mr. Williams?

B. How should you respond to Mr. Williams?

C. What actions should you take?

D. What conclusions can you make about Mr. Williams' self-concept (body image, role performance, personal identity, and self-esteem)? What additional information do you need about his self-concept?

Practical Knowledge clinical application

This section provides guidelines and forms for assessing self-concept, self-esteem, anxiety, and depression, which are basic to psychosocial health and illness. In addition, you will find tables of selected standardized outcomes and interventions to consider when planning care for patients with problems related to anxiety and depression.

CLINICAL INSIGHTS

Clinical Insight 10-1 ▶ Assessing Self-Concept

Assessment category	Examples of assessment questions
Body image	■ When you look in the mirror, what do you see? ■ How do you think others see you? ■ How does your current ability to engage in work and leisure activities compare with how you would like to be?
Role performance	■ What are your three or four major roles (e.g., daughter, parent, student)? ■ How successful are you in each of these roles? ■ How important is it to you to be successful in each of these roles? ■ What is interfering with your ability to perform any of these roles? What can you do about it? ■ How did you see yourself before your illness/injury/loss? ■ How do you see yourself now?
Personal identity	■ How would you describe yourself to others? ■ What special abilities do you have? ■ How do you think others see you?
Self-esteem (also refer to the Assessment Box, Performing a Self-Esteem Inventory)	■ How do you feel about yourself? ■ What do you like about yourself? ■ To what extent do you feel you are in control of your life? ■ If you could change one thing about yourself, what would it be? ■ Where would you like to be 5 years from now? ■ How realistic are your expectations of yourself? ■ How do you see your illness/injury/loss in relation to yourself?

Clinical Insight 10-2 ▶ Performing a Self-Esteem Inventory

Place a check mark in the column that most closely describes the client's answer to each statement. Each check is worth the number of points listed.

	3 Often or a great deal	2 Sometimes	1 Seldom or occasionally	0 Never or not at all
1. I become angry or hurt when criticized.				
2. I am afraid to try new things.				
3. I feel stupid when I make a mistake.				
4. I have difficulty looking people in the eye.				
5. I have difficulty making small talk.				
6. I feel uncomfortable in the presence of strangers.				
7. I am embarrassed when people compliment me.				
8. I am dissatisfied with the way I look.				
9. I am afraid to express my opinions in a group.				
10. I prefer staying home alone rather than participating in group social situations.				
11. I have trouble accepting teasing.				
12. I feel guilty when I say no to people.				
13. I am afraid to make a commitment to a relationship for fear of rejection.				
14. I believe that most people are more competent than I am.				
15. I feel resentment toward people who are attractive and successful.				
16. I have trouble thinking of any positive aspects about my life.				
17. I feel inadequate in the presence of authority figures.				
18. I have trouble making decisions.				
19. I fear the disapproval of others.				
20. I feel tense, stressed out, or uptight.				

Problems with low self-esteem are indicated by items scored with a 3 or by a total score higher than 46.
Source: Townsend, M. C. (2018). *Psychiatric mental health nursing: Concepts of care in evidence-based practice* (9th ed.). Philadelphia: F. A. Davis.

Clinical Insight 10-3 ➤ Identifying Depressed Patients Who Should Be Referred for Evaluation

TWO YES/NO QUESTIONS

One way to identify depression that is more than simple, situational depression is to ask the following two questions. A yes answer merits a referral.
1. Over the past 2 weeks, have you felt down, depressed, or hopeless?
2. Over the past 2 weeks, have you felt little interest or pleasure in doing things?

SIGECAPS

Another method is to use the mnemonic SIGECAPS, a concise version of the *DSM-IV-TR* diagnostic criteria. Ask the patient whether they have experienced for 2 or more weeks:
- **S**leep increase/decrease
- **I**nterest in formerly compelling or pleasurable activities diminished
- **G**uilt, low self-esteem
- **E**nergy poor
- **C**oncentration poor
- **A**ppetite increase/decrease
- **P**sychomotor agitation or retardation
- **S**uicidal ideation

Both of the following require referral for evaluation and treatment:
- **Major depression** = depressed mood or interest *plus* 4 SIGECAPS for 2 or more weeks
- **Mild depression (mood disorder)** = depressed mood or interest *plus* 3 SIGECAPS most days for 2 or more years

Source: U.S. Preventive Services Task Force. (2016). Depression in adults: Screening. https://www.uspreventiveservicestaskforce.org/uspstf/recommendation/depression-in-adults-screening.

IN SAD CAGES

Some people prefer a mnemonic from an older source, IN SAD CAGES, which you would use in essentially the same way. Ask the patient whether they have experienced for 2 or more weeks:
- **I**nterest reduced
- **N**egative thoughts
- **S**leep disturbance
- **A**ppetite change
- **D**ecreased confidence or self-esteem
- **C**oncentration reduced
- **A**ffect blunt or flat
- **G**uilt
- **E**nergy reduced
- **S**uicidal ideation

The original reference does not include a suggested total that requires referral. However, you can assume that the more symptoms, the more severe the depression. We suggest the following:
- **IN** (reduced interest and negative thoughts or depressed mood) plus 4 of the other **SAD CAGES** requires referral.

Do not try to differentiate mild and major depression with this method.

Adapted from Leng, L. B. (2011). Overview of major depressive disorder. *The Singapore Family Physician, 37*(4), 18–21.

ASSESSMENT GUIDELINES AND TOOLS

Anxiety Assessment Guide

Rating scale: none = 0, mild = 1, moderate = 2, severe = 3, disabling (panic) = 4

Physiological Effects	Rating	Psychological Effects	Rating
Shortness of breath (dyspnea)	____	Depersonalization (unreal)	____
Choking sensation	____	Feeling "on edge"	____
Dry mouth	____	Poor concentration	____
Pounding heart, increased heart rate	____	Poor memory	____
Chest pain	____	Depressed mood	____
Increased sweating and clamminess	____	Loss of interest	____
Feeling faint, dizzy, unsteady	____	Restlessness	____
Nausea and abdominal upsets	____	Sense of panic	____
Numbness (pins and needles)	____	Worry, anticipation of the worst	____
Hot/cold flashes	____	Irritability	____
Trembling, shaking	____	Nightmares	____
Muscle tension and aches	____	Feeling of fear and foreboding	____
Exaggerated startle response	____	Excessive apprehension	____
Difficulties in falling asleep and staying asleep	____	Feeling lack of control	____

ASSESSING OVERALL SCORES

0–28	Mild anxiety
29–56	Moderate anxiety
57–84	Severe anxiety
85–112	Disabling anxiety

Creating a total score from this table can help you assess whether overall anxiety is mild, moderate, severe, or disabling. However, individual physiological or psychological symptoms that are rated as severe (3) or disabling (4) may be more important and relevant to your nursing assessment. For example, your patient's overall or total assessment may be 26 (in the mild range, 0–27), but they have rated "excessive apprehension" as 4 (disabling).

Focused Assessment

Depression Assessment Guide: Patient Health Questionnaire (PHQ-9)

This valid and reliable measure of depression was developed in 1999 by Pfizer, Inc. It can be self-administered (Kroenke, Spitzer, & Williams, 2001). It may be useful across cultures (Chen, Huang, Chang, et al., 2006).

Over the past 2 weeks, how often have you been bothered by any of the following problems? (Check or circle your answers.)

	Not at all	Several days	More than half the days	Nearly every day
1. Little interest or pleasure in doing things	0	1	2	3
2. Feeling down, depressed, or hopeless	0	1	2	3
3. Trouble falling or staying asleep, or sleeping too much	0	1	2	3
4. Feeling tired or having little energy	0	1	2	3
5. Poor appetite or overeating	0	1	2	3
6. Feeling bad about yourself—or that you are a failure or have let yourself or your family down	0	1	2	3
7. Trouble concentrating on things, such as reading the newspaper or watching television	0	1	2	3
8. Moving or speaking so slowly that other people could have noticed; or the opposite—being so fidgety or restless that you have been moving around a lot more than usual	0	1	2	3
9. Thoughts that you would be better off dead or of hurting yourself in some way	0	1	2	3

ADD COLUMNS ☐ + ☐ + ☐

TOTAL: ☐

10. If you checked off any problems, how difficult have these problems made it for you to do your work, take care of things at home, or get along with other people?

    Not difficult at all   _____
    Somewhat difficult   _____
    Very difficult   _____
    Extremely difficult   _____

(Healthcare professional: For interpretation of total, please refer to the accompanying score card. [Note to students: Interpretation requires training. You should report the patient's score to your instructor or your immediate supervising nurse.])

Source: Pfizer, Inc. http://www.phqscreeners.com.

Focused Assessment

Differentiating Depression and Dementia

Use this tool to help identify older adults who should be referred for further evaluation to determine whether symptoms are related to depression or dementia.

➤ To determine whether the patient should be referred to a mental health professional, refer to the Clinical Insight 10-3: Identifying Depressed Patients Who Should Be Referred for Evaluation.

➤ To determine whether the patient should be referred to a mental health professional, refer to Clinical Insight 10-3.

Key Point: *Confusion may be present in patients with depression as well as those who have dementia or delirium.*

Characteristic	Depression	Dementia
Cause/triggers	Loss (e.g., of spouse, of independence); stress	Physiological causes (e.g., Alzheimer disease, brain infarcts)
Onset	Acute or chronic; can be related to specific events	Chronic, gradual, and insidious
Course	Varies, depending on cause	Progressive, over a long period
Alertness	Usually reduced	Usually normal
Memory	Memory loss and forgetfulness	Recent and remote memory impaired; loss of recent memory is first sign; some loss of common knowledge
Thinking	Inability to concentrate	Difficulty with abstraction and word finding, especially nouns; difficulty with calculations; decreased judgment
Response to questions	Often says, "I don't know"	Answers inappropriately or with "near misses"
Language	Speaks slowly; slow to respond to verbal stimuli	Disoriented, rambling, incoherent; difficulty using nouns
Sleep	Difficulty falling asleep, early morning awakening, much day sleeping	Sleep fragmented; awakens often during night
Reversibility	Potential	Irreversible, progressive

Source: Adapted from Edwards, N. (2003). Differentiating the three D's: Delirium, dementia, and depression. *MedSurg Nursing: Official Journal of the Academy of Medical-Surgical Nurses, 12*(6), 347–357.

CLINICAL REASONING
Applying the Full-Spectrum Nursing Model
PATIENT SITUATION

Matthew has been admitted to the emergency department with extensive wounds to both forearms, including tendon and vascular damage, from a suicide attempt. Matthew seems very quiet, almost withdrawn, and answers most of your questions in monosyllables.

Matthew reports the following: He is the third child in a family of five. Matthew's middle-class parents are now retired, and his brothers and sisters are scattered across the country in large cities. Although Matthew claims his schooling years were unremarkable, he reminisces about several occasions when he was bullied and physically beaten by gangs of older adolescents.

Matthew further states that he graduated from Harvard Law School and became vice president of an influential law firm. Despite his apparent success in life, he has continued to question his self-worth since childhood. Plagued by worries and depression that have increased over the past few years, he says he wrote a note indicating that he now realizes what a failure he is and proceeded to slash both of his forearms with a sharp razor.

Matthew reports that he has not been eating much, feels tired all the time, and has no interest in going outside the house. He says, "I just don't feel like doing anything; I just want to sleep all the time."

THINKING

1. *Theoretical Knowledge:* Using just the information you have in the Patient Situation, use the SIGECAPS method outlined in Clinical Insight 10-3 to assess Matthew's level of depression. You will need to assume that he is reporting what he has experienced in the past 2 weeks (unless he is obviously referring to the past).

2. *Critical Thinking (Inquiry):* What items of the SIGECAPS cannot be completed with the information in the Patient Situation? What do you need to ask Matthew to complete them?

DOING

3. *Nursing Process (Implementation/Taking Action):* Based on your SIGECAPS data, what do you need to do right away (or be certain it was done in the emergency department)?

CARING

4. *Self-Knowledge:* What do you have in common with Matthew that might help you to empathize with him?

5. *Ethical Knowledge:* Try to put aside your own beliefs now, and answer the following questions from the perspective of (a) Matthew and (b) one of your nursing colleagues on the unit:

   a. Give one reason to support Matthew's claim that he has a right to commit suicide if his despair is too deep to bear.

   b. Give one reason to support a colleague's claim that Matthew does not have a right to commit suicide, no matter how he feels.

Critical Thinking and Clinical Judgment

1. Review the scenario about Karli (Meet Your Patient from Volume 1):

   You are caring for a 16-year-old patient named Karli who is suffering from fractures to both arms and several ribs as well as extensive first- and second-degree burns to 30% of her body after a motor vehicle accident. Karli was driving her parents' car home from her part-time job when she lost control of the car and crashed into a wall. The car exploded in flames. A passerby quickly reported the accident, and fast action by the emergency response team saved Karli's life.

   Karli is suffering from a moderate amount of shock and pain. She alternates among outbursts of anger, self-directed sarcasm, and despondence. She tells you that she cannot understand how the accident happened, that one moment she was adjusting the car radio, and the next moment she awoke in the hospital. Then suddenly she explodes. "It's not fair! I just took my eyes off the road for a second; that's all!" She bursts into tears. Picking at her bandages, she sobs, "No one will ever love me the way I'm going to look. My life is over. I hate myself!" You take her hand. "I used to be pretty," she says, "but now I'll look like a freak! What did I do to deserve this? I know plenty of kids who drive drunk or high all the time. I wasn't doing anything wrong!
   Why did this happen to me?"

   a. Now that you have completed Chapter 10 in Volume 1, make a list of the multiple physical, psychological, and social issues that you would need to consider in developing a comprehensive care plan for Karli.

   b. Compare your list with the one you made when you first began reading the chapter. How is it different? Or is it the same?

2. In the Meet Your Patient scenario, Karli perceives herself as unlovable "looking this way." Which of the following nursing activities do you think might be helpful in *exploring and changing her perception?* For those you *do not* choose, explain why.

   Role Enhancement
   - Help the patient distinguish ideal and actual self. Help her describe realistic roles and expectations tailored to specific health changes.
   - Compare realistic roles with previous and less functional roles.

   Conflict Mediation
   - Provide a quiet, private, neutral setting for mediation to take place.
   - Maintain your own neutrality in the process; do not "take sides."

   Promoting Family Integrity
   - Encourage and facilitate communication among family members.
   - Encourage family members to care for the patient as much as possible.

   Family Mobilization
   - Help the family to identify strengths they can use to support the patient.
   - Teach family members how to provide home care for the patient.
   - Help the family identify community resources and/or support groups.
   - With the patient's permission, keep the family informed about the patient's progress.

   Enhancing Socialization
   - Explore and reinforce the individual's established relationships.
   - Provide opportunities to rehearse relationship-building skills.
   - Investigate, assist, and promote any developing relationships with persons who have similar interests and goals.
   - Provide information and links to community activities that relate to the person's past, current, and future interests.
   - Promote access to education in social skills development.
   - Encourage the patient to communicate and engage in interpersonal relationship activities by providing ongoing positive feedback.
   - Organize small, cohesive group activities.
   - Provide or act as a role model where appropriate.

3. Mrs. King is being admitted into the orthopedics unit for a scheduled total knee replacement. Even though she appears to be in good health for a 72-year-old woman, you are concerned about her excessive weight, which can be described as moderate to severe obesity. You are troubled by how the obesity may negatively affect postsurgical recovery, wound healing, and mobility.

   a. What theoretical knowledge will you draw on to plan care to meet her biopsychosocial needs?

   b. What assumptions are you making? What stereotypes do you have that might affect your understanding of Mrs. King's situation?

   c. What do you think might be contributing to Mrs. King's obesity?

   d. What facts do you have to support those ideas?

   e. How could you find out for sure what is contributing to Mrs. King's obesity?

4. Day by day, you notice that your patient is eating less and complaining about constipation and tiredness. You carefully review their nutrition requirements against the food menu as well as check nursing records for bowel movements. You have exhausted your initial search for obvious reasons that your patient's appetite has changed. After sitting down next to your patient, you cannot help noticing how tired they look.

   a. What psychosocial problem do you suspect (low self-esteem, depression, anxiety, or disturbed personal identity)?

   b. What cues do you have to support your inference in (a)?

   c. Objective data in their chart indicate that the patient has been eating very little and that they have been having bowel movements only every 3 or 4 days—and even then only with a laxative or enema. What other symptom do you need to investigate further?

   d. How could you obtain more information about that symptom?

   e. Think of depressed people you have known or depressed patients you have cared for. What have you found to be difficult about dealing with them?

5. Edna Jackson is 42 years old. She has had a hysterectomy (removal of her uterus). Her surgery was uncomplicated, her overall health is good, and she is expected to make a full and rapid physical recovery. Her husband was not present when she was admitted and has not been in to see her since the surgery. He did not want her to have the surgery. He told Edna that he doesn't know whether he will want to have sex with her when she is no longer "a whole woman." He has had casual affairs during their marriage, which Edna has tolerated because she feels that difficulty is balanced by the many positive benefits of their relationship, which include a "good sex life."

   Edna has seven brothers and sisters, and she has five children of her own, ages 23, 21, 18, 6, and 4. She comes from a culture and a religion that value children and motherhood. She believes she is a good mother, although she must work full-time outside the home. Edna is an office manager—respected by her boss and by those who work for her. She has an internal locus of control and evaluates her job performance as "better than most people would do."

   a. Look at the context. What aspects of this situation may negatively affect Mrs. Jackson's recovery?

   b. Based on your answers in (a), what nursing diagnoses might be useful in describing the psychosocial aspects of Mrs. Jackson's health? (State both the problem and the etiology.)

   c. What strengths does Mrs. Jackson have that may help her to avoid and/or overcome those problems?

6. The following questions refer to earlier information about Matthew, a man admitted to the emergency department following a suicide attempt.

   a. After Matthew's tendon and vascular repair, he is admitted to your medical-surgical unit. What, broadly speaking, are your first two priorities for Matthew's care?

   b. Which of these nursing diagnoses—suicide risk or risk for self-harm—would you use, and why?

   c. Prioritize the following interventions for Matthew. Rank them (1 = highest rank, 4 = lowest rank). Explain your thinking.

   ____ Refer to a mental health professional for help with his depression.

   ____ Examine Matthew's belongings and the room for anything he might use to harm himself.

   ____ Encourage Matthew to tell you if he begins having thoughts of suicide.

   ____ Begin establishing a therapeutic relationship and gaining his trust.

   d. Evaluate your self-knowledge. To plan comprehensive care for Matthew, in what areas do you need to increase your theoretical and practical knowledge? How will you do that?

7. For each of the following concepts, use critical thinking to describe how or why it is important to nursing, patient care, or psychosocial health and illness. Note that these are *not* to be merely definitions.

Self-concept

Self-esteem

Body image

Biopsychosocial well-being

Anxiety

Defense mechanisms

Depression

Therapeutic relationships

Hopelessness

What Are the Main Points in This Chapter?

- Health and well-being are influenced by psychological, social, and spiritual development.
- Psychosocial theory provides a way to understand people as interactions of psychological and social events.
- Self-concept is one's overall view of oneself; it answers this question: "Who do you think you are?"
- Self-concept is developed throughout the life span and is influenced by multiple factors. Four dimensions contribute to self-concept: body image, role performance, personal identity, and self-esteem.
- Body image is a person's mental image of their physical self.
- Role performance consists of the actions a person takes and the behaviors they demonstrate in fulfilling a role, such as the role of a student.
- Personal identity is a person's view of oneself as a unique human being, different and separate from all others.
- Self-esteem evaluations arise from the differences between the ideal and the actual self.
- Communication skills are important because psychosocial information is personal and sometimes sensitive.
- When you formulate psychosocial diagnoses, it is difficult, but important, to determine what is cause and what is effect.
- Many of the NOC standardized psychosocial outcomes are found in the domains of psychosocial health and family health.
- Many of the NIC standardized psychosocial interventions are found in the behavioral and family domains.
- Anxiety is a common emotional response to a (usually unknown) stressor; it results from psychological conflicts, and it is accompanied by physical symptoms (e.g., trembling).
- Assessment should identify the presence, level, and cause of anxiety.
- Interventions for anxiety should help the patient become aware that they are anxious, identify the source of anxiety, and deal with the symptoms it produces.
- Depression is characterized by diminished interest or pleasure in previously enjoyed activities, sadness, emptiness, a flat or hollow feeling (absence of feeling), tearfulness, difficulty concentrating, feelings of worthlessness, and some physical symptoms (e.g., constipation).
- Assessment of depression includes a comprehensive history of mood, thoughts, behavior, and physical status.
- If you suspect severe depression, you should refer the patient to a mental health specialist; if there is a risk of suicide, referral should be immediate.
- In communicating with depressed persons, it is important to not be overly cheerful and to avoid phrases such as "cheer up."

Knowledge Map

PSYCHOSOCIAL HEALTH

ANXIETY
- Vague emotional response to threat to basic needs
- Intensity and duration determine whether anxiety is a normal response

DEPRESSION
- Sadness to major depression
- Withdrawal, flat affect

Factors influencing **SELF-CONCEPT**:
- GENDER
- SOCIO-ECONOMIC STATUS
- DEVELOPMENTAL LEVEL
- FAMILY AND PEER RELATIONS
- INTERNAL INFLUENCES

BODY IMAGE
- Mental image of physical self
- Involves cognition and sensory input
- Ideal versus perceived body image

ROLE PERFORMANCE
- Actions taken, behavior demonstrated
- Role strain
- Role conflict

PERSONAL IDENTITY
- View of self
- Constant
- Learned through socialization

SELF-ESTEEM
- How I like myself
- Expectations of myself versus true abilities
- Ideal versus actual self

ILLNESS influences body image, affects role performance, impairs personal identity, precipitates a crisis in self-esteem

CHAPTER 11

Promoting Family Health

STUDENT RESOURCES

The questions and exercises in this book allow you to practice the kind of thinking you will use as a full-spectrum nurse. Critical-thinking questions usually have more than one right answer, so we do not provide "correct" answers for these features. Try to answer these questions yourself. It is more important to develop your nursing judgment than to just cover content. You will learn more by discussing the questions with your peers. If you are still unsure, see the Davis Advantage chapter resources for suggested responses.

To explore learning resources for this chapter,

Go to www.DavisAdvantage.com and find:

Answers and Suggested Responses for all questions in this chapter
Concept Map
Knowledge Map
References and Bibliography

Key Concepts
Family
Family nursing

Related Concepts
See the Concept Map on Davis Advantage.

Example Client Conditions

Caring for the Williams Family

Kayla Robinson, 3 years old, is the eldest grandchild of Stanley and Nadine Williams. Until recently, Kayla lived with her mother, Jayden Robinson (Stanley and Nadine's daughter). Jayden had been diagnosed with schizophrenia at age 18 years. Initially she was functioning adequately on her medications; however, she has not been taking her medications, and her condition has been worsening for the past year. When Jayden became unable to care for Kayla, Stanley and Nadine assumed the child's care. Jayden rarely visits Kayla. Stanley and Nadine convinced Jayden to obtain residential care at a mental health facility. Stanley tells you at a clinic visit that he wishes his family were "normal."

(Continued)

Caring for the Williams Family (continued)

A. What do you need to clarify about Stanley's statement about his family?

B. What do *you* think Stanley means by a "normal" family?

C. How would you respond to Stanley's comments?

D. What effect might this new family structure have on Stanley's and Nadine's health?

E. How might you promote family functioning for the Williams family? What assessments should you make? What interventions should you consider?

F. What personal values or biases do you have that may affect your ability to care for the Williams family?

PracticalKnowledge clinical application

Material in this section will help you to assess and plan care for families.

CLINICAL INSIGHTS

Clinical Insight 11-1 ▸ Conducting a Family Assessment

In general, a family assessment should include the following:

Identifying data	Include such information as name, address, phone number, cultural/ethnic background, religious identification, social affiliation.
Family composition	For each member of the family, include gender identity, age, relationship, date and place of birth, occupation, and education.
Family history and developmental stage	This refers to the stages and developmental tasks in the Focused Assessment: Assessing Family Development Tasks.
Environmental data	Include a description of the home, neighborhood, larger community, family's social supports, and their transactions with the community.
Family structure	■ *Identify the structural type* (e.g., two parents, single parent). Also assess: 　■ *Communication patterns:* Functional and dysfunctional patterns, the way emotions are expressed, and contextual variables that affect communication 　■ *Power and role structures:* How are family decisions made? What are the roles of each member? Have there been changes in these? 　■ *Family values:* What are their values? What are their priorities? Are there value conflicts in the family?
Family functions	Assess the effectiveness of the family's: 　■ *Nurturing:* Are the members close? Are they separate or connected? 　■ *Socialization and child-rearing:* Who is [are] the socializing agent[s] for the children? What are their child-rearing practices? Are needs for play being met?
Health beliefs, values, and behaviors	■ How do they define health and illness? ■ What are their dietary, sleep, physical, and drug habits? ■ What are their dental and medical health practices, including physicals, eye examinations, immunizations, and exercise patterns? ■ Do they have access to health services?

Clinical Insight 11-1 ▸ Conducting a Family Assessment—cont'd

Family stressors and coping	■ What are their stressors (e.g., financial, family communication or relationships, neighbors, holidays, children's behavior)? ■ What successful coping strategies have they used? ■ What dysfunctional strategies are present?
Abuse and violence within the family	Because of the prevalence of abuse and knowing that families are likely to be ashamed to discuss it, you should assess every family member for any signs of abuse or neglect. For detailed guidelines, go to Procedure 6-1, Assessing for Abuse.

ASSESSMENT GUIDELINES AND TOOLS

Focused Assessment

Assessing Family Developmental Tasks

Stages and children's ages	Tasks
Beginning family No children	▸ Relinquishing the family of origin as the major emotional and economic resource ▸ Gaining a sense of autonomy and independence ▸ Making the relationship/marriage work; investment in spouse as the major emotional resource ▸ Finding a place in the kin network of each partner ▸ Exploring options for career development ▸ Deciding whether to have children
Childbearing family Ages newborn to 2 years	▸ Achieving pregnancy and birth ▸ Adjusting to life changes after birth and to the infant's needs ▸ Determining ways to meet all members' needs ▸ Renegotiating marriage ▸ Increasing contact with extended family
"No longer newlyweds" (with no children) No children; ages not applicable	▸ Establishing a sense of the permanence of the relationship ▸ Establishing long-term residency ▸ Being involved in the community/promoting the well-being of the community ▸ Focusing on or establishing professional careers
Family with preschool children Ages 3–5 years	▸ Adjusting to increased costs associated with family life ▸ Socializing the preschoolers ▸ Coping with loss of parental energy and privacy 3–5 years
Mature family (with no children) Ages not applicable	▸ Renegotiating relationship on basis of more maturity ▸ Adjusting to changing levels of responsibility in work and community ▸ If not done already, achieving financial security
Family with school-age children Ages 6–12 years	▸ Adjusting to the needs and demands of growing children ▸ Promoting joint decision making among parents and children ▸ Encouraging and supporting educational and school-related activities
Family with teenagers and young adults Ages 13–20 years	▸ Maintaining open communication among family members ▸ Reinforcing ethical and moral values ▸ For teens, balancing independence with parental rules

(Continued)

Focused Assessment

Assessing Family Developmental Tasks—cont'd

Stages and children's ages	Tasks	
Family launching young adults Ages 18–30 years	▸ Maintaining support to young adults as they leave the security of family ▸ Rediscovering marriage	
Postparental family Adults	▸ Preparing for retirement ▸ Adjusting to children's moving into new phases of adulthood, marriage or other relationship, and childbearing and to becoming a grandparent	
Middle-aged couple (with no children)	▸ Accepting that it may be too late to reconsider childbearing or child-rearing ▸ Reaching the peak of a career or realizing that the peak may not occur ▸ Planning for retirement	None
Aging family (also applies to family with no children)	▸ Adjusting to retirement and changes associated with aging ▸ Adjusting to the loss of a spouse and friendships	Adult *(or none)*

Source: Adapted from Denham, S., et al. (2016). *Family Focused Nursing Care.* Philadelphia, PA: F.A. Davis; Duvall, E. (1988). Family development's first forty years. *Family Relations, 37*(1), 127–134; Friedman, M., et al. (2003). *Family nursing: Research, theory, and practice* (5th ed.). Upper Saddle River, NJ: Prentice Hall; Kaakinen, J., et al. (Eds.). (2018). *Family health care nursing: Theory, practice and research* (6th ed.). Philadelphia, PA: F.A. Davis.

CLINICAL REASONING
Applying the Full-Spectrum Nursing Model

PATIENT SITUATION

Sandra Jackson, a 22-year-old single mother of an 18-month-old child, has type 1 diabetes mellitus. Her blood glucose levels have been unstable, primarily during times of stress and illness. Sandra lives with her mother, two younger sisters, and a brother. She has recently ended the relationship with her boyfriend. Sandra is trying to find a second job to meet the financial responsibilities of raising a child. She is showing physical signs of depression and distress (e.g., apathy, anorexia, excessive sleeping, and episodes of crying). During your home visit, Sandra says, "Something is really wrong with me. I can't snap out of this feeling of darkness. Life is too hard for me and is nothing but pain. I can't take it anymore and want it to be over." You believe she needs immediate mental health support.

THINKING

1. *Theoretical Knowledge:*

    a. What facts and principles do you already know about stress and depression?

    b. How does the emotional illness of one family member affect others living in the home and the family as a whole?

2. *Critical Thinking (Inquiry/Recognize Cues):*

    a. What factors in Sandra's life are possibly contributing to her feelings of hopelessness and thoughts of self-harm?

    b. Name at least three nursing diagnoses that would best suit Sandra's health needs.

DOING

3. *Practical Knowledge (Clinical Reasoning):* Based on the knowledge you have about stress and depression (see item 1 in this section), how would you educate the family on the best way to support Sandra?

4. *Nursing Process (Evaluation):* What measures would you identify to determine whether your nursing plan of care was effective?

CARING

5. *Self-Knowledge:*

    a. How comfortable would you be caring for a patient who is at risk for self-injury?

    b. What is one problem with Sandra and her family that was not described in the scenario that could possibly arise?

6. *Ethical Knowledge:* What ethical concerns might you have for a woman with a young child who is at risk for self-injury but has no financial resources to cover the expenses of mental healthcare?

Critical Thinking and Clinical Judgment

1. You are caring for a 58-year-old woman who was admitted for surgery of the foot. Today is the second day you have cared for the client. You notice that the family seems quiet and subdued. You ask the client whether something is wrong. She says that her 16-year-old niece ran away from home with her 19-year-old boyfriend.

    a. Name two things in this scenario that you, as a nurse, *cannot* change.

    b. Do the client and her family have a problem that you *can* help them with? How can you find out?

    c. Imagine you were your client (the aunt). What concerns would you have?

    d. Try to depict this situation by using systems theory. Draw circles for each system involved, and show where the systems interact.

    e. Use your self-knowledge. What biases or values do you have that might affect your thinking in this case, either positively or negatively?

2. You are caring for a 45-year-old man who was involved in a serious car accident. He suffered severe head trauma and, if he lives, probably will have serious deficits. He was admitted 24 hours ago and has not made significant improvements. The family is aware of his status and likely outcome.

    a. What are some concerns this family might have?

    b. Using structural–functional theory, describe how this family might be affected.

    c. How can you help this family?

3. You are caring for a 3-year-old child who has had a fall and is being discharged. As you are reviewing the discharge instructions, the child's mother reveals that she and the child spent last night in a hotel because of violence in the home. She tells you that her husband (the child's stepfather) drinks excessively and at times has become violent, hitting her but not the child. She did not call him when they went to the emergency room and is afraid to go home.

    a. What do you think might be the mother's main concerns?

    b. Do you think this is a common problem or an unusual problem?

c. What is the developmental stage of this family?

d. What theoretical knowledge do you need to help this family?

e. What kinds of help do you think are needed if she decides to escape from her husband?

f. How could you help her at this moment?

4. For each of the following concepts, use critical thinking to describe how or why it is important to nursing, client care, or the family. Note that these are *not* to be merely definitions.

Family relationships	Family as the unit of care
Blended families	Family health risk factors
Communication	The national economy
Systems theory	Health beliefs
Structural–functional theories	Family coping mechanisms
Developmental theory	Unexpected illness
Family interactional theory	

What Are the Main Points in This Chapter?

- *Family* is not limited to the traditional definition of a husband, a wife, and their children; defined more broadly, it is a group of individuals who provide physical, emotional, economic, and/or spiritual support while maintaining involvement in each other's lives.
- Families are structured in a variety of ways. Three examples are the grandparent family, blended families, and single-parent families.
- Family nursing views the family from three perspectives: as the context for care of an individual, as the unit of care, and as a system.
- Wellness of each member is critical to the health of the family unit.
- Under general systems theory, the family is viewed as a system in interaction with other systems (e.g., other families, groups, communities, and individuals).
- Under structural–functional theories, families are viewed as social systems with a focus on outcomes.
- Developmental theories focus on family stages: beginning family, childbearing family, family with preschool children, family with school-age children, family with teenagers and young adults, family launching young adults, postparental family, and aging family.
- Family interactional theory views the family as a unit of interacting personalities with a major emphasis on family roles.
- The family teaches health beliefs, values, and behaviors to its individual members.
- Assessment of family communication patterns consists of interviewing the family and the individual seeking care as well as astute observation by the nurse.
- How families cope with everyday life situations and hospitalization can influence the effectiveness of care rendered.
- Nurses can promote family wellness by addressing both individual and family concerns.
- The family can be a source of support or a source of difficulties for the ill person.

CHAPTER 11 Promoting Family Health 107

Knowledge Map

CHALLENGES TO HEALTH
- Poverty
- Disease
- Homelessness
- Violence
- HIV/AIDS
- Developmental changes

FAMILY RISK FACTORS
- Adapting to new roles
- Financial needs
- Adolescent's risk-taking behaviors
- Children leaving home
- Illness
- Sandwich generation

FAMILY STRUCTURES
- Single parent
- Without children
- Extended
- Single individuals
- Blended families
- Families with adopted and foster children

interrelated

occur in response to; and modify

FAMILY COPING PATTERNS — *affect* →

FAMILY THEORIES
- General systems theory
- Structural–functional theories
- Developmental theories
- Family interactional theory

guide thinking about

FAMILY COMMUNICATION PATTERNS — *influence and reflect* →

FAMILY HEALTH

HOLISTIC FAMILY NURSING

INDICATORS OF FAMILY HEALTH
- State of family well-being
- Sense of belonging and connectedness
- Shared responsibility
- Trust and respect
- Spending time together, sharing rituals and traditions
- Flexibility
- Commitment: working together to maintain the family
- Spiritual well-being
- Respect for privacy of individual members
- Positive, effective communication
- Ability to compromise and disagree
- Appreciation and affection for each other
- Responding to the needs and interests of all members
- Egalitarian distribution of power
- Health-promoting lifestyle of individual members

CHAPTER 12

Caring in Multicultural Healthcare Environments

STUDENT RESOURCES

The questions and exercises in this book allow you to practice the kind of thinking you will use as a full-spectrum nurse. Critical-thinking questions usually have more than one correct answer, so we do not provide "correct" answers" for these features. Try to answer these questions yourself. It is more important to develop your nursing judgment than to just cover content. You will learn by discussing the questions with your peers. If you are still unsure, see the Davis Advantage chapter resources for suggested responses.

To explore learning resources for this chapter,

Go to www.DavisAdvantage.com and find:

Answers and Suggested Responses for all questions in this chapter
Concept Map
Knowledge Map
References and Bibliography

Key Concepts

Cultural Competence
Culture

Related Concepts

See the Concept Map on Davis Advantage.

Caring for the Williams Family

Review the initial assessment of Stanley Williams just before Chapter 1.

A. How might the Williams family's cultural heritage affect their health beliefs?

B. What factors would you want to consider when performing a cultural assessment of the Williams family?

108

Practical Knowledge clinical application

Information in this section may be useful for assessing and communicating with clients of cultures different from your own.

CLINICAL INSIGHTS

Clinical Insight 12-1 ➤ Understanding Biological Variations

Racial categories tend to undermine the recognition of genetic similarity and diversity among individuals and human populations. You learned the following information in biology class:

- Genetics is the study of the function, effect, and heredity of a particular gene.
- Genes are units of heredity made up of DNA or RNA.
- Individuals have about 20,000 genes that carry information that determines their traits.
- Most people have the same genes with about 1% difference between people.
- A gene contains information for a specific trait or characteristic.
- DNA stores and transfers biological information for all the traits.
- Alleles are different forms of the same gene with small differences in their sequence of DNA bases. An individual has two alleles for each gene, inheriting one from each parent. Alleles determine the uniqueness of each person's physical features. For example, we all have the gene for eye color, but the allele determines the specific color.

A 2002 landmark study supports the trend toward ancestry composition rather than racial classifications. Researchers found that almost half (46.7%) of the 4,199 alleles present in the sample appeared in the seven represented regions: Africa, Europe, the Middle East, Central/South Asia, East Asia, Oceania, and America. They did not find a symbolic allele characteristic exclusive to a single group. Instead, researchers found that only 7.4% of alleles were exclusive to one region. Even then, only about 1% occurred in people in that region.

Thus, the concept of ancestry is preferred over that of race. While a client's racial background can help you understand and address social vulnerabilities and barriers to care, it should not be used to determine biological variations. Chou (2017) notes that ancestry provides a context of how a person's history unfolds based on the geographical origins of their ancestors. The identification of diseases based on regional descent (e.g., cystic fibrosis common in Northern European) can guide healthcare providers to be more inclusive in making diagnoses and prevent stereotyping based on race (e.g., sickle cell anemia associated with the African American population instead of individuals from sub-Saharan African).

Nurse's Role

Knowledge: As a nurse, you should understand genetics, genomic information, and ancestry. Since the 2003 Human Genome Project, genetic testing has grown tremendously. Healthcare providers use genetic testing to identify a patient's predisposition to certain diseases or disorders. Similarly, direct-to-consumer testing allows consumers to identify their risk for conditions such as diabetes, depression, and so on. Patients will rely on you to help them understand and reinforce genetics in screening and prevention initiatives.

Family Assessment: Conduct a three-generation family assessment that includes first, second, and third relatives' genetic risk factors. Collaborate with the provider to make a referral for potential high-risk genetic disorders.

Advocacy: Understanding the influence of genetics on a drug or disease can identify situations where advocacy is needed to promote treatment or genetic testing for patients.

Patient Education: Your patients may not understand genetics and its impact on disease risk and outcomes. A primary role of the nurse is to provide patient education on the basics of genetics.

Practice Resources

Chou (2017); Gannon (2016); Montgomery et al. (2017); National Human Genome Research Institute (updated 2020); Paz & Mitchel (2016); Rosenberg et al. (2002).

Clinical Insight 12-2 ➤ Communicating With Clients Who Speak a Different Language

When possible, use a qualified interpreter or a translator.
- A **translator** merely restates into the targeted language.
- An **interpreter** is specially trained to provide the meaning behind spoken words from one language to another. An interpreter can serve as a cultural broker by conveying the client's responses to questions and by providing general information about the client's culture (Centers for Disease Control and Prevention, 2018).

When using any type of interpreter do the following:
- Because of confidentiality issues, avoid asking a family member, especially a child or spouse, to act as an interpreter.
- Avoid using an interpreter who is socially or politically incompatible with the client.
- Be aware of gender and age differences and consider cultural norms.
- Have the interpreter spend some time alone with the patient.
- Ask the interpreter to interpret the words used by the healthcare provider as closely as possible, except where literal translation might be offensive or misunderstood. In such cases, an interpreter (compared with a translator) would provide the meaning of your words in terms acceptable to the client.
- Do not use metaphors ("happy as a clam") or medical jargon.
- Observe nonverbal communication (e.g., body language) when the client is listening and talking to the interpreter.
- Address your questions to the client, not the interpreter.
- Maintain eye contact with both the client and interpreter. Speak slowly and distinctly, facing the client; do not speak loudly.
- Ask one question at a time; allow time for interpretation and response from the client before asking another question.
- Use active rather than passive voice (e.g., say, "The doctor will see you tomorrow" rather than "You will be seen by the doctor tomorrow").
- Be aware that many clients can understand more words than they can express.
- Have health education materials translated into the client's language or have an interpreter audiotape or videotape instructions.

If there is no one available to interpret for you:
In addition to the preceding strategies, you should do the following (Munoz & Luckmann, 2005):
- Greet the client with respect. Greet the person formally, using Mr., Ms., and so forth, until given permission to do otherwise. People in some groups consider it disrespectful to use a person's first name.
- Identify the client's primary language and use any words that you are familiar with in their language to show that you are trying to communicate.
- Use the Internet or computer software to translate words into the client's native language.
- If appropriate, use a third language that both of you speak.
- Speak slowly and clearly, using simple sentences to talk about one question or need at a time.
- Use gestures to help convey meaning.
- Restate in different words, if needed.
- Use pictures or diagrams.
- Be aware that some clients may answer yes even if they don't understand what you have said.

Practice Resources

Munoz & Luckmann (2005); Centers for Disease Control and Prevention (2018).

ASSESSMENT GUIDELINES AND TOOLS

Focused Assessment

Obtaining Minimum Cultural Information

You should obtain at least this much cultural information from every client. For some, you may need a more in-depth assessment.

- Begin the interview with open-ended questions, such as the following:

    I would like to know more about your family.

    Who will be able to help you when you go home?

    What do you do to help keep yourself well?

- When you and the client are comfortable, be sure to ask a question such as "What concerns you the most about your illness and treatment?" This allows you to focus on the individual rather than just on their culture.

- You will not need to perform an in-depth cultural assessment on every patient, but you will need to recognize situations in which this is needed.

Language(s) spoken; proficiency in the language of the host country	▸ What language(s) do you speak? ▸ Are you comfortable speaking [English], or would you like to have an interpreter?
Length of time client has been here; where client was raised	▸ Where were you raised? ▸ How long have you lived here?
Ethnic affiliation and identity	▸ With what racial and ethnic group(s) do you identify? ▸ How closely do you identify with the values of those groups?
Usual religious practices	▸ What religion do you practice, if any? ▸ Are there any special beliefs, rituals, or practices you want us to be aware of?
Nonverbal communication style	▸ (You will need to observe the patient and draw on your theoretical knowledge of the patient's cultural group for this information.)
Family roles, primary decision maker	▸ Who is in your family? ▸ What is your role in your family? ▸ Who makes most of the decisions? ▸ How are decisions made in your family? ▸ Whom should I talk to for decisions about your healthcare?
Social support in the new country	▸ Do you have family and friends here? ▸ Whom can you go to when you need help? ▸ Where do you work? ▸ Will you need any help with your healthcare expenses?

Sources: Giger, J. (2016). *Transcultural nursing: Assessment and intervention* (7th ed.). St. Louis, MO: Elsevier; Spector, R. (2017). *Cultural diversity in health and illness* (9th ed.). Upper Saddle River, NJ: Pearson Education; Suzuki, L. A., & Ponterotto, J. G. (2007). *Handbook of multicultural assessment: Clinical, psychological, and educational applications* (3rd ed.). San Francisco, CA: Jossey-Bass.

Focused Assessment

Cultural Assessment Using the Transcultural Assessment Model

Assess information listed in the following categories.

Cultural Uniqueness
- Cultural and ethnic identification
- Place of birth
- Time in country

Communication
- Voice quality
- Pronunciation and enunciation
- Use of silence
- Use of nonverbal communication
- Touch
- Spoken language

Space
- Degree of comfort
- Distance in conversations
- Definition of space
- Body movement

Social Organization
- Normal state of health
- Marital status
- Number of children
- Parents living or deceased
- Friends
- Work
- Leisure

Time
- Orientation to time
- View of time
- Physiochemical reaction to time

Environmental Control
- Locus of control
- Value orientation
- Health and illness beliefs

Biological Variations
- Physical assessment (including body structure, skin color, skin discoloration, hair color and distribution, other visible physical characteristics, weight, height, laboratory variances)
- Susceptibility to illness
- Nutritional preferences
- Psychological characteristics

Other

In addition to the Giger categories, obtain information about the following:
- Educational experiences (formal and informal)
- Family patterns of healthcare
- Family role and function
- Healthcare beliefs and practices (folk and professional)
- Religious practices and beliefs
- Social networks
- Values orientation

Source: Adapted from Giger, J. (2016). *Transcultural nursing: Assessment and intervention* (7th ed.). St. Louis, MO: Elsevier.

CLINICAL REASONING
Applying the Full-Spectrum Nursing Model

PATIENT SITUATION

Mrs. Vasquez, a 70-year-old Mexican American woman, has diabetes mellitus and has come to the hospital because of a sore on her lower leg that will not heal. Mrs. Vasquez, a widow, cares for herself at home. She speaks only a little English and has some difficulty understanding your questions. After great effort on your part, you determine that she has missed her last appointment with her diabetes specialist because she has no transportation, so she has just been putting a dressing on the sore. Mrs. Vasquez tells you that she loves to see her grandchildren, who visit often, and that she enjoys cooking and eating Mexican food. She also says that she believes she is sick because she has displeased God. However, God is a source of comfort and assurance to her. She prays a lot and has rosary beads in her hand.

THINKING

1. *Theoretical Knowledge (Recall of Facts and Principles):* List six important culture specifics.

2. *Critical Thinking (Application of Knowledge):* Based on your theoretical knowledge, what are your expectations about communicating with Mrs. Vasquez?

3. *Critical Thinking (Compare and Contrast):* Compare your expectations to the actual data you have about her ability to communicate.

DOING

4. *Nursing Process (Assessment):* What are some pertinent cultural data that you should assess for Mrs. Vasquez?

5. *Nursing Process (Analysis/Diagnosis):* Which nursing diagnosis do you think would be best for planning Mrs. Vasquez's care? (Recall that the etiology should suggest your nursing interventions, and the diagnostic label should suggest the expected patient outcomes.) Explain your reasoning.

    - Noncompliance (with clinic appointments) related to lack of transportation
    - Skin integrity impairment related to self-treatment of ulcer
    - Noncompliance (with clinic appointments) related to beliefs about God and illness

CARING

6. *Self-Knowledge:* What areas of commonality do you have with Mrs. Vasquez around which you might form a caring relationship?

7. *Self-Knowledge:* Do you agree with Mrs. Vasquez that illness may be caused by displeasing God?

8. *Ethical Knowledge:* Suppose you do not agree with Mrs. Vasquez's assessment that she is ill because she has displeased God. Discuss whether you would explain to her that this is most likely not true and then teach her about the cause of diabetic ulcers.

Critical Thinking and Clinical Judgment

1. Mrs. Vasquez, a 70-year-old Mexican American woman, has diabetes mellitus and has come to the hospital because of a sore on her lower leg that will not heal. Review the details of Mrs. Vasquez's case in the preceding Full Spectrum Nursing Model situation.

   a. Identify Mrs. Vasquez's cultural data, and group it under the following culture specifics:

Communication	Social organization
Space	Environmental control
Time orientation	Biological variations

   b. You have learned that cultural data can have implications for nursing care. Answer each of the following:
   - What additional information should you assess for in this situation?
   - What biases do you have that affect your thinking in this situation?

2. An Asian woman comes to your clinic for assessment of her blood pressure. In casual conversation, she tells you that her oldest daughter is about to be married. She reveals that her daughter has some type of anemia for which she needs medication. She tells you that she has recently heard terrible stories about sickle cell anemia and is afraid that this is what her daughter has.

   a. What additional data do you need to collect to answer this client's questions?

   b. What assurances, if any, can you give this client about her daughter?

3. At times, nurses must care for clients who do not speak their language. This poses a challenge to nurses who strive to provide culturally competent care to all clients. Even with the assistance of interpreters, this can be difficult because of some barriers, such as differing dialects, street talk, and jargon. Keeping these facts in mind, answer the following questions:

   a. What options do you have when you encounter a person who cannot speak English?

   b. How do you communicate with such a client if no interpreter is available?

   c. What biases do you have about such a situation? Why?

4. Alma is of European descent; she is White. She is a Roman Catholic and believes abortion is wrong. She believes that it should be illegal to own a gun. She is a nursing student.

   Violetta's parents came to the United States from Europe. They were born in France. Before that, her great-grandparents lived in Africa. Violetta is Black. She is Roman Catholic, and she believes that abortion is wrong. She believes that it should be illegal to own a gun. She is a nursing student.

   Darcy is of European descent; she is White. She laughs at the idea of religion, saying, "Nobody's 'up there' looking out for me; and when you're dead, you're dead." Darcy is a gang member and always carries a gun in her purse or her pocket. She did not finish high school, and she has had two abortions.

   All of the women live in the United States. Which two women do you think share the most cultural commonalities? Explain your thinking.

5. Helen is a 52-year-old divorced woman. Her only child, Tamika, is incarcerated for prostitution and possession of narcotics. Helen is now raising her two grandchildren, Calvin, age 13 years, and Jevetta, age 2 years. Helen is a nursing assistant at the local hospital. It is hard for her to make ends meet because she has hypertension and diabetes, for which she takes several medications, including insulin, when she can afford them. Helen has not applied for medical assistance because she believes she should be able to take care of herself, but she does receive assistance for Jevetta's day-care costs. In addition to her grandchildren, Helen has a large group of friends, many of whom attend her church. She has little time to spend with her

friends since she took custody of the children. Jevetta has been admitted to the hospital for asthma. You are Jevetta's student nurse.

   a. Using your data collection skills, think of diagnostic labels that you could apply to Jevetta and to Helen as Jevetta's caregiver.

   b. What resources may be helpful to Helen?

6. Examine the following nursing diagnosis labels. For this set of labels, write an etiology that might be caused by cultural differences. The first one is completed for you as an example.

   - Body nutrition (excess), *related to patient's lack of knowledge about how to adapt preferred ethnic foods to prescribed low-fat diet.*

   - Health maintenance alterations

   - Role performance alteration

   - Anxiety

   - Powerlessness

   - Knowledge deficit

7. For the following set of labels, explain or give an example of how the nurse might misdiagnose or misperceive the data because of cultural differences. The first one is done for you.

   - Decisional conflict

The nurse might ask a woman to make some decision about her care. The woman may seem indecisive and unable to reach a conclusion. The reason might be that the husband is the decision maker in the family. When the husband arrives, the Decisional Conflict ("problem") may no longer exist.

   - Confusion

   - Socialization alteration

   - Nonadherence

   - Pain (acute or chronic)

8. For each of the following concepts, use critical thinking to describe how or why it is important to nursing, patient care, or cultural competence. Note that these are *not* to be merely definitions.

Culture	Cultural competence
Subculture	Transcultural nursing
Ethnicity	Giger and Davidhizar assessment model
Race	Biological variations among cultures
Religion	Prejudice and racism
Acculturation	Professional (e.g., nursing) subculture
Health and illness belief	Cultural sensitivity
Health and illness practice	Cultural awareness
Phenomena of culture	Culture universals
Ethnocentric	Culture specifics
Folk medicine	

What Are the Main Points in This Chapter?

- The cultural and ethnic composition of North America has changed dramatically over the past several decades, making it essential that nurses understand the healthcare beliefs and practices of diverse populations.
- Culture includes shared values, beliefs, norms, and practices that guide a particular group's thinking, decision making, and actions in a patterned way.
- Through acculturation, most ethnic and cultural groups modify some of their traditional cultural characteristics, values, beliefs, and practices.
- You should be familiar with the common characteristics of different cultural groups in your community.
- The U.S. Census Bureau (2022) has identified and divided the population into numerous racial categories:

    White
    Black or African American
    American Indian or Alaska Native
    Asian
    Native Hawaiian or Other Pacific Islander

- The Census Bureau (2020) categories for ethnicity (or "origin") are (1) Hispanic, Latino, or Spanish and (2) Not Hispanic, Latino, or Spanish.
- **Culture universals** (commonalities) are the values, beliefs, and practices that people from *all* cultures share. **Culture specifics** (diversities) are those values, beliefs, and practices that are unique to a culture.
- A **cultural archetype,** similar to a model, is an example of something that is recurrent and has its basis in facts. A **cultural stereotype** is a widely held but oversimplified and unsubstantiated belief that all people of a certain racial or ethnic group are alike in certain respects.
- Six organizing phenomena of culture that influence health include communication patterns, space, social organization, time, environmental control, and biological variations.
- Healthcare providers cannot understand the health beliefs and practices of diverse populations if they view them through the lens of the conventional (Western) culture of healthcare.
- Several "alternative" healing systems exist. Remedies have been passed down from generation to generation and include the use of herbs, customs, and rituals.
- An understanding of cultural concepts, theories, and models can help develop cultural competence.
- Ethnocentrism, stereotyping, prejudice, and racism are barriers to culturally competent care.
- When assessing a client and making nursing diagnoses, you must consider the client's cultural values, beliefs, and practices related to health and healthcare.
- Culturally competent care requires a nonjudgmental attitude, self-awareness, sensitivity, respect for differences, theoretical knowledge, and the desire to be culturally competent.

Knowledge Map

CHAPTER 12 Caring in Multicultural Healthcare Environments

CULTURAL SPECIFICS
- Time orientation
- Communication
- Space/boundaries
- Environment
- Biological variations
- Social organization

CULTURAL BELIEFS
- Religion
- Politics
- Philosophy
- Education
- Economy
- Technology

CULTURAL UNIVERSALS
- Values
- Beliefs
- Practices

affect → **HEALTH** ← *affects* — **HEALTHCARE SYSTEM**

- Complementary therapies
- Biomedical/professional
- Folk medicine
- Alternative medicine

are necessary for

consists of — **CULTURE**

- Learned
- Taught
- Shared
- Dynamic
- Complex
- Diverse

are

DOMINANT CULTURE

CULTURALLY COMPETENT HEALTHCARE

THEORISTS
- Purnell & Paulanka
- Leininger
- Campinha-Bacote

Minority groups — *are* — Fewer in number

SUBCULTURES
- Gender
- Ethnicity
- Race
- Religion
- Healthcare
- Nursing

VULNERABLE POPULATIONS
- Homeless
- Poor
- Mentally ill
- Disabled
- Age-related

BARRIERS
- Lack of knowledge
- Sexism
- Ethnocentrism
- Stereotyping
- Prejudice
- Racism

CHAPTER 13

Spirituality

STUDENT RESOURCES

The questions and exercises in this book allow you to practice the kind of thinking you will use as a full-spectrum nurse. Critical-thinking questions usually have more than one right answer, so we do not provide "correct" answers for these features. Try to answer these questions yourself. It is more important to develop your nursing judgment than to just cover content. You will learn more by discussing the questions with your peers. If you are still unsure, see the Davis Advantage chapter resources for suggested responses.

To explore learning resources for this chapter,

Go to www.DavisAdvantage.com and find:

Answers and Suggested Responses for all questions in this chapter
Concept Map
Knowledge Map
References and Bibliography

Key Concepts

Spirituality
Religion
Spiritual care

Related Concepts

See the Concept Map on Davis Advantage.

Caring for the Williams Family

Kayla Robinson is the 3-year-old granddaughter of Stanley and Charlene Williams. Stanley and Charlene are both practicing Muslims. Kayla's mother, Jayden, is the Williams' daughter. Jayden feels that religion is "a waste of time" and does not attend services at the local mosque. Kayla has had no formal religious experiences or attended any Islamic center.

A. At a clinic visit, Stanley asks you what you think about keeping religion away from a child. How would you respond?

B. Stanley explains his views on the situation: "I think she should have a strong religious foundation. She needs to understand the significance of our prayers. She has no connection to our prophet." Do you agree with this statement? Explain your views.

C. You realize that Stanley is concerned for Kayla and Jayden. How would you feel about this situation? What would you say to Stanley?

Practical Knowledge clinical application

In this section, you will find guidelines for performing focused spiritual assessments.

CLINICAL INSIGHTS

Clinical Insight 13-1 ▶ Types of Prayers

Prayer has a variety of purposes, expressions, and meanings to clients and their families, as well as to nurses themselves. For many people, prayer provides for periods of intimacy with the divine, reveals the presence and love of the divine, and serves as a powerful source of comfort and hope. For those who embrace the power and influence of prayer, it supports their spiritual journeys and may help them experience forgiveness, love, hope, trust, and meaning.

Intercession	Praying for the needs of others	*Christian prayer*
Faith	Belief that a problem will be resolved by God	*Christian prayer*
Consecration and dedication	Seeking direction from God on an issue or to make a decision	*Christian prayer*
Committal	To relieve oneself of burden (worry, fear) associated with trying to handle a problem	*Christian prayer*
Metta or compassion meditation	Prayer for well-being, peace, happiness, courage, patience, and other virtues	*Buddhist prayer*
Refuge	Identify three sources of refuge	*Buddhist prayer*
Healing	Elimination of hardship and for healing	*Prophet Muhammad; Islam prayer*
Thanks	Thanks rendered throughout all generations for lives, souls, and miracles	*Jewish prayer*
Healing	The Mi Sheberach is the prayer for physical cure as well as spiritual healing, asking for blessing, compassion, restoration, and strength	*Jewish prayer*
Peace	Prayer for peace among nations and they shall not learn war	*Jewish prayer*
Life	Prayer for a long life	*Native American prayer*
Learn from the earth	Prayer to learn positive life traits from the earth	*Native American prayer*

Adapted from these sources:
Beliefnet. (2020). *Essential prayers of world religions*. https://www.beliefnet.com/faiths/prayer/essential-prayers-of-world-religions.aspx.
Episcopal Church USA. (1979). *Book of common prayer*. Random House.
Johnson, K. (n.d.). Types of prayer. https://www.prayeronline.org.au/types-of-prayer.
Cheatham, D. (2008). *Kinds of prayer—A brief review*. https://evangelnorth.net/wp-content/uploads/2021/01/All-Manner-of-Prayers.pdf.
Jesuitresource.org. (n.d.). Prayer index. Xavier University Center for Mission and Identity. https://www.xavier.edu/jesuitresource/online-resources/prayer-index/index.
Jesuitresource.org. (n.d.). Buddhist prayers. Xavier University Center for Mission and Identity. https://www.xavier.edu/jesuitresource/online-resources/prayer-index/buddhist-prayers.
Pearls of Wisdom. (n.d.). Native American wisdom quotes. http://www.sapphyr.net/natam/.
Stanley, C. (2011). *Handle with prayer: Unwrap the source of God's strength for living*. David Cook.

Clinical Insight 13-2 ▸ Praying With Clients

Because there is a rich diversity in religious expression, keep the following guidelines in mind when you pray for or with clients:

- **Ask how the client prefers to address the divine.** Some people prefer the use of parental language in their prayers, for example, *Father God* or *Divine Mother*. Some use the word *Jehovah, Yahweh,* or *Allah*. Patients may address one or more of multiple Gods, each of whom has several names. Do not be afraid to seek direction from the client in these matters: Most people are honored to be able to explain their beliefs and practices to someone who is open to the experience.
- **Before the prayer begins, ask the client whether any rituals or religious items are necessary.** Some patients may want water to wash the mouth, nostrils, and hands before beginning prayer. Others may want to hold rosary beads or a set of beads called a mala. Others may have a prayer cloth or other item that needs to be accessible.
- **Always feel free to pray or not to pray.** Never feel that you are being forced to do or say something that makes you uncomfortable.
- **Do not be a compulsive "prayer" or a compulsive avoider of prayer.** Always make sure that the client (and/or family) is comfortable with prayer if they have not yet requested it.
- **Know that there are appropriate times and places for the offering of prayer.** Prayer at the bedside may be most appropriate, although it may make people uncomfortable in a crowded waiting room. Perhaps the statement "I will be praying for you and your family" might be more appropriate for some clients than actually praying aloud at that moment.
- **When a client asks for prayer, consider using this reply:** "I would be honored to offer prayer. What would you like me to *especially* address in the prayer?" Knowing what the client hopes for in prayer gives you an idea of the type of prayer the person is requesting.
- **When the client tells you what they want you to pray for, be sure to focus your prayer around the request.**
    - It is always good to summarize the results of previous conversations with the client and their needs in the course of your prayer. For example, imagine that a client with cancer who has been treated with chemotherapy now finds their blood counts are coming back to normal levels. The chemotherapy treatment seems successful at this point, but the client is afraid of a relapse and asks you to pray for the cancer to be cured.
    - Analyze the situation in terms of what has happened in the past, what is happening now, and what the client is requesting. This will help you organize your thoughts and then put them in the form of a prayer.
- **Perhaps you would want to take the client's hand in yours (if appropriate, based on your intuition and the nature of your nurse–client relationship) and compose a prayer in the following manner:** Dear [Lord], I give you thanks that [John] has done so well with his treatments. Please continue to help him be strong and open to your healing presence. We pray for his family, doctors, and nurses that all may be a part of [John's] continued healing and sense of comfort. I pray that the treatments that he is receiving, together with the prayers that we are offering, may all be effective in his care and in the treatment of his cancer. Watch over [John], and visit us all at this time with your healing presence. [Amen.]
- **When a terminally ill client requests a prayer for a cure, total healing, or a miracle, you may be challenged.** Knowing how to offer prayers that are "realistic" allows for the occurrence of miracles and healings of all types while also keeping in perspective the physical realities of the nature of disease and the reality of death.
- **If composing a prayer is difficult for you, you may want to ask the patient to identify scriptures that are meaningful to them or** whether they have examples of sacred writings from which you might be allowed to read. Perhaps the client has a favorite prayer or a text from an authoritative source that brings comfort and hope.
- **It is common for most prayers to include a request for divine help and direction for the client's healthcare team.** This expresses the reality that we are all working together for a common good and purpose and that we depend on each other (and a divine presence, in some cases) for our welfare and place in life.
- **Once the prayer is over, thank the client for asking you to participate.** In that way you can ask whether you can be of any further assistance.

ASSESSMENT GUIDELINES AND TOOLS

Focused Assessment—HOPE

The HOPE Approach to Spiritual Assessment: Examples of Questions

Mnemonic	Examples of questions
H—Sources of **hope**, meaning, comfort, strength, peace, love, and connection	What are your sources of internal support? What do you hold onto to get you through difficult times? For some people, religious or spiritual beliefs are a source of comfort in dealing with life's ups and downs. Is this true for you?
O—**Organized** religion	Do you belong to a religious or spiritual community? Does it help you? How important is this to you? What aspects of your religion are helpful to you?
P—**Personal** spirituality or **practices**	Do you believe in a higher power or divine being? What is your relationship with this power or being? Do you have personal spiritual beliefs that are not a part of organized religion? If so, what are they? What aspects of your spirituality are most helpful to you (e.g., meditation, prayer, reading scripture, listening to music, nature)?
E—**Effects** on medical care and end-of-life issues	Has your illness affected your relationship with the divine? Or your ability to do the things that usually help you spiritually? Are you concerned about conflicts between your beliefs and your healthcare treatment plan? Do you have any dietary restrictions or other practices I should know about in planning your care? Would you like to speak to a clinical chaplain (or community spiritual leader)?

Source: Based on Gowri, A., & Hight, E. (2001). Spirituality and medical practice: Using the HOPE questions as a practical tool for spiritual assessment. *American Family Physician, 63,* 36–41.

Focused Assessment—SPIRIT

SPIRIT Assessment

- Obtain information from the patient when possible.
- For an emergency admission or if the patient cannot give information, consult the next of kin or a designated power of attorney (DPOA) as soon as possible for information.

S—Spiritual/religious belief system

Religion, tradition, sect, or denominational affiliation

Text/writing(s) that provide a source of authority and codes for behavior

Name and phone number of supporting or affiliated church, synagogue, temple, or other place of worship

Past experience with a belief system (positive or negative)

Beliefs related to health, illness, healthcare, healthcare providers, Western medicine, adjuvant therapies, herbal or natural healing methods or techniques

Beliefs about suffering, terminal or chronic illness, advance directives, autopsy, organ donation

Stigmas related to illness, if applicable

P—Personal spirituality

Individual beliefs and practices of affiliation that the patient or family accepts and attempts to follow (may be directly or indirectly related to the aforementioned assessment areas)

Individual beliefs that may differ or even be contrary to affiliation beliefs

Whether spirituality is a part of personal experience of religion or a separate entity

Level of comfort discussing spirituality

Whether personal spirituality is viewed positively or negatively at the present time

I—Integration within a spiritual community

Name and title of religious or spiritual leader or authority figure(s)

Names and titles of religious groups that may need to be contacted: prayer group leader, prayer chain support person, shaman, medicine man or woman, men's or women's group within denomination

Role of patient or individual in any of the aforementioned groups

R—Ritualized practices and restrictions

Activities that patient's or family's faith encourages or forbids

Needs for modesty and covering of body parts or appendages

Any special beliefs or needs in relation to drawing blood or to laboratory tests or procedures

Dietary needs and restrictions: food preferences, preparation of foods, and location of food preparation areas

Gender-specific roles and responsibilities of care providers

Prayer needs and restrictions: Who delivers and offers such practices?

Articles or other materials needed for worship, devotion, or prayer (rosaries, prayer beads, prayer books, religious tracts, Bibles, crosses, prayer shawls or cloths)

I—Implications for medical care

Beliefs and practices that healthcare providers should remember while providing care

Specific medications that may not be administered and withheld, implications for pain control

Specific medical procedures or products that may not be administered (abortion, blood products)

Communication patterns and needs for effective care delivery: Who makes decisions? What is the role of parents or guardians when children or other vulnerable populations are the recipients of care? Does the guardian reflect the beliefs of the patient, if these are known?

T—Terminal events planning

Wishes for advance directives (cardiopulmonary resuscitation, intubation, ventilator assist, feeding tubes)

Wishes for transplantation or organ donation

Need for religious services (last rites, ministries of healing, baptism, initiation, confession, communion)

Clergy or ministry groups to be contacted and when

Ideas of an afterlife

Treatment of the body at the time of death

Funeral planning

Adapted from these sources:

Maugans, T. (1996). The SPIRITual History. *Archives of Family Medicine,* 5(1), 11–16.

Highfield, M. E. F. (2000). Providing spiritual care to patients with cancer. *Clinical Journal of Oncology Nursing,* 4(3), 115–120.

CLINICAL REASONING
Applying the Full-Spectrum Nursing Model

PATIENT SITUATION

Review the Meet Your Patient scenario to answer the questions about Charles Johnson, a 75-year-old divorced man with newly diagnosed cancer of the lung. He is unsure whether he wants to have the chemotherapy his provider recommends to try to increase his life span.

> Go to **Chapter 13, Meet Your Patient**, in Volume 1.

THINKING

1. *Theoretical Knowledge (Recall of Facts and Principles):* Define *forgiveness* and explain the benefits of forgiving self and others.

2. *Critical Thinking (Application of Knowledge):* Based on your theoretical knowledge about forgiveness, with whom might Mr. Johnson need to reconcile? Why do you think so?

DOING

3. *Practical Knowledge (HOPE Assessment):* Use the Focused Assessment: The HOPE Approach to Spiritual Assessment: Examples of Questions, and enter Mr. Johnson's data. Identify sections for which you need additional data.

CARING

4. *Self-Knowledge:* How is your religious background similar to or different from Mr. Johnson's?

5. *Self-Knowledge:* (a) How would you feel if Mr. Johnson said to you, "Church folk are all a bunch of hypocrites, if you ask me. I choose not to be a part of any of that"? (b) How would you respond?

6. *Ethical Knowledge:* Imagine that Mr. Johnson's sister comes to visit and leaves some religious pamphlets on a chair, where he will not see them before she leaves. What would you do?

Critical Thinking and Clinical Judgment

1. A 5-year-old boy was admitted to the hospital last night with a fever of 103°F (39.4°C). He was diagnosed with a serious infection that is easily treated with intravenous (IV) antibiotics. However, based on their religious beliefs, his parents do not want antibiotics administered to their son. They have called their religious practitioner to visit as soon as possible.

   a. What practical knowledge do you have that will give you some insight into this situation?

   b. What essential piece of knowledge do you need that is *not* given in this scenario?

   c. If the parents do not agree to accept IV antibiotics for their son, what can you do to (1) ensure that he receives treatment and (2) support their spiritual needs?

2. A woman is admitted to the emergency department and gives birth to a premature baby boy who is in severe respiratory distress. The woman is a devout Roman Catholic. What interventions could you use to ensure holistic spiritual care in this emergency situation?

3. Interview nurses in the area where you have your clinical experiences. Discuss the interviews with classmates.

    a. Ask them to describe spiritual problems their patients have had.

    b. Ask them to tell you of any spiritual interventions they have used with patients and how effective they believe them to be.

    c. Ask them how comfortable they are in using spiritual interventions, especially prayer.

4. For each of the following concepts, use critical thinking to describe how or why it is important to nursing, patient care, or spirituality. Note that these are *not* to be merely definitions.

    Spirituality and religion

    Nursing research in religion and healthcare

    Major religions and healthcare

    The nurse and spirituality

    Assessment of the spiritual domain of care

    Spiritual care nursing interventions

    Spiritual well-being

What Are the Main Points in This Chapter?

- Spirituality is a powerful force in the lives of many patients.
- Nursing has historical roots in religion and spirituality.
- Nurses work with other disciplines to provide spiritual care.
- Religion is a sort of "map" that outlines and integrates essential beliefs, values, and codes of conduct into a manner of living.
- Spirituality, like a journey, takes place over time and involves the accumulation of life experiences and understandings. It is the attempt to find meaning, value, and purpose in life.
- Religion and spirituality affect health and well-being; in turn, health and well-being affect a person's religion and spirituality.
- Research suggests that patients' beliefs in religion and spirituality are important to healthcare outcomes; however, it does not explain *how* or *why* this is so.
- The more you know about similarities in and differences among the world's major religions, the more you will be able to offer comprehensive, compassionate care to patients.
- People, even within the same religion, vary greatly in the degree to which they follow the rituals and practices of their own religion.
- Self-knowledge helps you to avoid abuses of spiritual care (e.g., imposing your religion on a patient).
- Barriers to spiritual care include (1) lack of awareness of spirituality in general and of your own spiritual belief system, (2) differences in spirituality between you (the nurse) and the patient, (3) fear that your spiritual knowledge is insufficient, and (4) fear of where spiritual discussions might lead.
- Nursing interventions related to spiritual care require you to be self-aware, fully present, supportive, empathetic, and nonjudgmental and to have a desire to benefit the patient.
- When a patient asks you to pray, you must determine whether they wish you to pray *for* or *with* him, and you should ask what they would like you to *especially* address in the prayer.
- A miracle does not necessarily involve the notion of a cure; miracles are more often events that proceed according to natural law but still have a powerful impact on the person's expectations.

CHAPTER 13 Spirituality 125

Knowledge Map

Illness leads to → **FAITH**
Illness leads to loss of → **HOPE**
Illness fosters struggles with → **LOVE**

STRUGGLES
- Doubt
- Guilt
- Anger
- Worthlessness

JOYS
- Awareness
- Self
- Gifts
- Talents

- Need to achieve, create
- Who am I?
- Why am I?

- Joy and heartbreak
- Conditional versus unconditional love
- Possibility of loss

FAITH — **HOPE** — **LOVE**

BELIEFS AND ESSENTIAL VALUES
- Rituals
- Sacraments
- Theology
- Eschatology
- Order
- Sin
- Salvation
- Higher self

RELIGION ↔ **SPIRITUALITY**

"THE JOURNEY"
- Experiences/beliefs
- Joy and pain = growth
- Finding meaning
- Possibilities for connection to the divine

- Judaism
- Christianity
- Christian Science
- Jehovah's Witness
- Mormon
- Islam, Baha'i
- Rastafarianism
- Buddhism
- Hinduism, Sikhism
- Native American

- Atheist
- Agnostic

Spirituality can be → Separate concepts → Combine as religion

HEALTH
- Longevity
- Health outcomes
- Disease process
- Motivation

affect

SPIRITUAL CARE
- Examine biases
- Be open
- Access resources

deter ←

- Lack of awareness of spirituality
- Spiritual differences
- Fears of addressing spiritual needs

CHAPTER 14

Experiencing Loss

STUDENT RESOURCES

The questions and exercises in Volume 2 allow you to practice the kind of thinking you will use as a full-spectrum nurse. Critical-thinking questions usually have more than one correct answer, so we do not provide "correct" answers for these features. Try to answer these questions yourself. It is more important to develop your nursing judgment than to just cover content. You will learn by discussing the questions with your peers. If you are still unsure, see the Davis Advantage chapter resources for suggested responses.

To explore learning resources for this chapter,

Go to www.DavisAdvantage.com and find:

Answers and Suggested Responses for all questions in this chapter
Concept Map
Knowledge Map
References and Bibliography

Key Concepts

Death and dying
End-of-life care
Grief
Loss

Related Concepts

See the Concept Map on Davis Advantage.

Caring for the Williams Family

At a clinic visit, Stanley Williams tells you that his father's health is declining rapidly. Mr. Williams tells you, "I thought he was doing okay. I knew he had surgery for his prostate, so I thought it was all over. Lately he's been having lots of low back and hip pain. So my mom begged him to go to the doctor, and he told him he has cancer all over." Mr. Williams shakes his head and looks away from you. You notice sadness in his eyes.

Mr. Williams tells you that his family has avoided discussions about serious illness and death. "It just never got discussed. The whole idea made my parents uncomfortable. When my father got sick the first time, he refused to discuss it. 'I'm going to get better. Don't even think about it,' he would say." Now Mr. Williams feels the need to discuss this situation with his parents but doesn't know how to bring up the topic. He asks for your advice.

Caring for the Williams Family (continued)

A. What would you think and feel when you see Stanley's sadness and when he asks for this advice?

B. What would you advise Mr. Williams?

C. What type of grief is Mr. Williams experiencing?

D. Examine the factors that affect grief. Apply these factors to Mr. Williams' situation. You will need to review the family history included in the introduction to the Williams family (in the front of this book) to fully answer this question. Indicate whether the information for any of the factors to be evaluated is insufficient.

Practical Knowledge
clinical application

In this section are guidelines for performing focused spiritual assessments.

CLINICAL INSIGHTS

Clinical Insight 14-1 ▶ Communicating With People Who Are Grieving

Perfect your listening skills. Listen for what is *not* said as well as what is said.

Be alert for and respond to nonverbal cues with appropriate touch and eye contact. A smile, a gentle touch, sitting with a patient, and eye contact all relay a message of genuine care and concern. You may not need to say very much at all.

Encourage and accept expressions of feelings.
- Receiving expressions of intense feelings (e.g., anger and guilt) may be painful for you. It may help to remember that it is therapeutic for people to express their feelings.
- You do not need to change the person's feelings or "make them better." As much as we would like to do this, it is not possible.
- You do need to validate the person's feelings (e.g., "It is normal to feel that way; it is okay").

Reassure the person that it is not wrong to feel anger, guilt, relief, or other feelings they may believe to be unacceptable. A dying patient might say, "I know it's awful, but I feel so angry with God for not curing this disease." Or a bereaved spouse might admit, "I shouldn't feel this way, but I'm relieved that it's finally over." Patients need to hear you say their feelings are not wrong or bad and that they are going through a normal process.

Increase your self-awareness. Become more conscious of your own attitudes and feelings regarding death and dying. *If you are comfortable with your perspective, you will be able to hear patients' expressions of anger, guilt, frustration, fear, and loneliness more comfortably.*

Continue to communicate with dying patients even if they are in a coma. Encourage family members to do so as well.
- Talk to the patient. Tell them what is going on around them, what care you are providing, and when you or others enter or are about to leave the room.
- Avoid discussing the dying person as though they were not present. *Research indicates that patients continue to hear even though they cannot respond, sometimes up to the moment of death.*

Practice Resources
Keeley (2017); Meichsner et al. (2020); Pfeifer & Head (2018); Saretta et al. (2022); Wynton (2019).

Clinical Insight 14-2 ▶ Helping Families of Dying Patients

- **View the family as your unit of care.** *Family members often rate communication with clinicians as one of their most important needs.*
- **Provide information, support, and a listening ear.** Include specific facts about the patient's condition and prognosis and whom to call about changes in condition.
- **Communicate medical updates daily.** *Information can relieve anxiety and is useful to the family when making decisions.*
- **Encourage family members to help with care if they are able.** Instruct and supervise as appropriate. If family members are not physically or emotionally able to provide care, accept that. *This helps meet their need to be useful, promotes family ties, and makes the patient more comfortable.*
- **Encourage family members to ask questions.** *They may hesitate to do so for various reasons (e.g., they may not want to interrupt busy care providers).*

(Continued)

Clinical Insight 14-2 ▶ Helping Families of Dying Patients—cont'd

- **Listen actively to the patient's and family's concerns.** Make eye contact; clarify when you do not understand. *This helps you avoid misinterpreting the family's concerns and needs.*
- **Help the family to understand the goals of care and solve problems when needed.**
- **Follow up with other healthcare team members promptly** if the family has questions that are outside your scope of practice.
- **Arrange for a formal interprofessional meeting with the family** soon after the patient's admission, if possible. Discussions should cover personal, cultural, and religious traditions (e.g., how prayers are to be conducted, how the body is to be handled after death).
- **Encourage the family to visit the hospital chapel and to speak with a chaplain** or with their own spiritual adviser.
- **Provide anticipatory guidance regarding the stages of loss and grief** so that they will know what to expect after their loved one dies.
- **Acknowledge the family's feelings** and the loss they are experiencing. *Many times family members begin the grieving process before the loved one dies.*
- **Help the family members explore past coping mechanisms;** reinforce successful past coping mechanisms.
- **Refer for ethics consultation** if decision making may become a problem.
- **Remind family members and significant others to take care of themselves.** *Watching a loved one die is a very difficult experience. A sensitive, caring nurse can make it a little easier.*
  - Many times they need "permission" to go to eat or to go home and rest.
- If the patient is near death and family and friends do not want to leave the patient's side, make them as comfortable as possible.
- Provide comfortable chairs, coffee, and snacks (according to organizational policy), and be alert for other needs they may have.
- **Teach the family what to expect regarding medications, treatments, and signs of approaching death.** *If family members know what is normal, they will be less likely to panic or fear the inevitable.*
- **As physical signs of death become apparent, keep the family informed.** You may say something like "Her blood pressure is becoming difficult to hear. That is one of the signs that she is closer to death." Help the family to understand what the patient is experiencing, because this may be very different from what they are seeing.
- **Reassure families of patients who become withdrawn near the time of death** that this does not mean the patient is rejecting them, but only that their body is conserving energy and that they have come to terms with dying and letting go of connections with life.
- **When approaching death is apparent, ask family members directly, "Do you want to be present while he is dying?"** Tell them what to expect, if they do not know.
- **When an expected death occurs, shift the focus of your care** to the family and those who were caregivers. *Death does not end the relationship; family and caregivers need support during bereavement.*

Practice Resources
Bloomer, M., et al. (2022); Flugelman, M. (2021); Hendson & Davies (2018); The Joint Commission (2014); Keely (2017); O'Sullivan et al. (2021).

Clinical Insight 14-3 ▶ Caring for the Dying Person: Meeting Physiological Needs

Active dying usually occurs over a period of 10 to 14 days (although it can take as little as 24 hours). The "final hours" refer to the last 4 to 48 hours of life, in which failure of body systems results in death.

- **Encourage the patient to be as independent as possible.** *This helps the patient to maintain a sense of control.*
- **Provide adequate pain control.** *This can be a major issue for patients and caregivers. In fact, dying patients are often more concerned about pain and loss of control than about dying itself. Pain is difficult to assess in semiconscious or unconscious patients. See Chapter 28 if you need more information about pain management.*
  - Dispel the myths about pain medication (e.g., addiction, overdose). Effective pain control medications exist and can be administered by various routes. Assure the patient and family that the focus is on pain control and not addiction to analgesics.
- Respect the patient's informed decision to refuse pain medications. For example, a patient may prefer to endure pain in order to be awake and alert when the family is at the bedside.
- Follow the prescribed pain protocols to ensure that pain is controlled.
- To ensure pain control, administer pain medication on a regular schedule instead of waiting until the patient asks (prn).
- Teach and perform nonpharmacological pain control measures when you judge these may be helpful (e.g., meditation, heat/cold therapies, massage, distraction, imagery, deep breathing, and herbal-scented lotions). It

Clinical Insight 14-3 ▶ Caring for the Dying Person: Meeting Physiological Needs—cont'd

may be soothing to play soft music, add "white noise," or turn off the television.
- Patients who are near death may moan or grunt as they breathe; this does not necessarily indicate pain. Be sure that families understand this. When accompanied by agitation and restlessness, these symptoms may indicate terminal delirium, which may require medications for control.

■ **Monitor the patient's energy level.** *Fatigue is a normal part of the dying process. Most dying patients sleep much of the time.*
- Perform hygiene and other care if the patient tires easily or lacks the energy for self-care (i.e., ADLs).
- Remove environmental stressors that interfere with sleep (e.g., noise, too much light, a room that is too hot or too cold).
- Identify psychosocial stressors (e.g., depression, anxiety, fear) that may keep the patient awake (see Clinical Insight 14-4).

■ **Maintain skin integrity.** *During the final hours of life, the goal changes from preserving skin integrity to providing comfort. Realize that during this time even excellent care may not prevent skin breakdown.*
- Turn the patient frequently unless contraindicated. Refer to the pain control interventions in the preceding list.
- Assess for increased diaphoresis and/or incontinence.
- Maintain adequate nutrition.

■ **If the patient is comatose or unconscious, provide special care for the eyes** so they do not become too dry. Many agencies use a form of artificial tears for this purpose.

■ **If the patient is not able to take fluids, wet the lips and mouth frequently with cool water** or with a prepared product to prevent dryness and cracking of lips and mucous membranes of the nose, mouth, and eyes. ✚ There is some evidence that glycerin swabs dry the mucous membranes and should not be used.

■ **Provide artificial hydration (unless the patient has an advance directive requesting no artificial hydration)** per nasogastric (NG) or IV route. *IV fluids can cause edema, nausea, and even pain in a patient who is actively dying. Dehydration is thought not to cause distress during the last hours and may even be protective (Emanuel et al., 2015; Mayo Clinic Staff, 2020).*

■ **Take the vital signs often, unless contraindicated;** observe for decreased level of consciousness and pallor.

■ **Assess and provide interventions for constipation, urinary retention, and incontinence.** *Constipation may be associated with decreased fluid intake, inactivity, weakness, hypercalcemia, hyperkalemia, and lack of privacy. It can contribute to pain, nausea, vomiting, and anorexia, so intervention is an important comfort measure. Incontinence may occur because of fatigue and loss of sphincter control. It can be distressing to patients and family members.*
- Administer laxatives, stool softeners, and lubricants for constipation.
- Catheterize the patient if they are unable to void and the bladder becomes distended.
- Use pads for incontinence, but change them frequently to prevent skin breakdown and, near the end, to promote comfort.
- Use a rectal tube if diarrhea is severe.

■ **Intervene for "death rattle"** if it occurs and if it is distressing to the family.
- Turn the patient on the side and elevate the head of the bed.
- Administer antispasmodic and anticholinergic medications if necessary.

■ **Provide medication for other symptoms,** such as nausea and breathlessness.

■ **Continue to speak to the patient as if they can hear.**

■ **Do not talk about the patient to others in their presence.** *The patient is usually able to hear even after they can no longer respond to sounds and other stimuli. Assume the unconscious patient hears everything.*

■ **Document changes in vital signs and level of consciousness.** Record intake and output, noting changes. Document the times of cardiac arrest and cessation of respirations.

Practice Resources

DerSarkissian (2020); Emanuel et al. (2015); The Joint Commission (2014); Mayo Clinic Staff (2020); National Institute on Aging (2017); Zhu et al. (2021).

Clinical Insight 14-4 ▶ Caring for the Dying Person: Meeting Psychological Needs

Patients experience many emotions at end of life, including anger, sadness, depression, fear, relief, loneliness, and grief. At this time, communication and support are most helpful. Discussing concerns and issues is a viable means of coping.

- **If there is an advance directive or living will, locate the documents.** Review the documents to be certain you understand the patient's wishes. If you have not already done so, notify all relevant health professionals of the existence of these documents.
- **Answer all questions honestly.**
- **Explain all care and treatments even if the patient is unconscious.** *They may still be able to hear.*
- **Realize that the patient may feel he is losing control.**
  - Help the person recognize what they do have control over.
  - Include the patient in care decisions as much as they are able.
- **Attend to social needs.** *Relationships are a priority at this time. Some patients may simply need to keep the bonds with family members and friends intact. For other patients, this may be a time to reestablish or mend relationships.*
  - Notify family members when the patient wishes to see them.
  - Allow the patient and family to discuss death at their own pace.
  - Offer to contact a chaplain or other spiritual leader if the patient chooses.
  - Pray with the patient if they request it and you are comfortable doing so.
- **Encourage the patient to express feelings.** Be prepared to accept a wide range of feelings, including anger, hopelessness, loneliness, and depression.
- **Early in the dying process, assess the sources of financial support** for the patient and family. *Finances may be a concern and may place an additional burden on the family, or the patient may feel they are a burden to care for.*
- **Be aware of sexual needs.** Provide realistic information about these issues. For example, suggest ways a couple can be close and affectionate at this time. Be aware that expressions of sexuality may change as a person becomes closer to death. *Some people may feel it is not right to have sexual feelings when the person they love is dying. Others may be afraid of harming the patient if they are sexually intimate.*
- **When the patient is very near death, focus on relieving symptoms** (e.g., pain, nausea) and emotional distress.
- **If the person can communicate, ask about immediate concerns:**
  - "Are you in pain?" "Are you comfortable?"
  - "What are you afraid of now?"
  - "What can we do to help you go peacefully?"
  - "Whom do you want in the room with you right now?"
- **If the patient asks, "Am I dying?" be honest and provide information that aligns with cultural beliefs and practices.**
- **If the patient cannot communicate, ask a significant other what the patient would want.** Ask the family member or person who is most likely to know.
- **When the patient is very near death, it may be helpful to say something like "Your family will be fine"** rather than "It is okay for you to go now." *Be aware that some people seem to wait to die until after a significant date (birthday, anniversary, and so on) has passed. Others wait for family to gather, whereas others wait until loved ones leave so they will not upset the family by dying in their presence.*

Practice Resources

Abramson (2022); DerSarkissian (2020); Emanuel et al. (2015); Galbadage et al. (2020); Mayo Clinic Staff (2020); National Institute on Aging (2017); Zhu (2021).

Clinical Insight 14-5 ▶ Providing Postmortem Care

Supporting the Family

- **At the moment of death, do not interrupt or intrude on the family.** Wait quietly and observe, or if they would feel more comfortable being alone with the patient, leave the room. Give them as much time as they need. When they move away from the body, or have expressed their last goodbyes, then it is time to assess the patient and report the lack of vital signs.
- **Immediately after death, express sympathy to the family.** This is very important. Make a simple statement, such as "I am sorry for your loss." Avoid statements that interpret the situation for the family, such as "It's God's will." Also avoid attempts to mitigate the family member's grief, such as "It will get better in time," or "You still have your son."
- **If the family wishes to be alone with the body,** straighten the bedcovers and make the patient look as natural as possible. Remove any tubes, IV lines, and so on, according to the institution's policy, and have the patient positioned in a way that appears comforting (e.g., bedcovers pulled up, hands at the side).
- **Be accepting of family members' behavior at this time,** no matter how strange it may seem to you. A family might want to take a picture, or the spouse may lie down beside the deceased person.

Clinical Insight 14-5 ▶ Providing Postmortem Care—cont'd

- **If no family members are present, identify the next of kin** and be sure the family is informed of the patient's death.
- **If family members arrive after the death, offer to take them to the bedside.**
- **If family members wish to be involved in postmortem care,** encourage them to do so. This can facilitate their grieving process.
- **Ask whether each family member wishes to spend time alone with the deceased person, and arrange for them to do so.** Never remove the body until the family is ready. Viewing the body is useful to many individuals.
- **Ask, "How can I help?" "What do you need?" "What would you like for me to do?"**
- **Locate personal effects and give them to the family/next of kin.** If you cannot remove a ring, wrap it with gauze, tape it in place, and tie the gauze to the wrist to prevent subsequent loss.

Legal Responsibilities

- **Notify the primary provider of the death.** Usually the provider must pronounce death; however, in some areas a coroner or a nurse may also perform this task.
- **The person who pronounces death must sign the death certificate.** In some agencies, the nurse is responsible for checking to see that it has been signed.
- **If the patient is donating organs,** review and make any necessary arrangements.
- **If an autopsy is to be performed,** as a rule, the provider (or other person designated by the institution) is responsible for obtaining signed permission from next of kin.

Care of the Body

- **Follow agency policies, and respect cultural and spiritual preferences.**
- **Wash the body if there has been any incontinence or drainage.** Place absorbent pads between the buttocks to absorb rectal drainage. Ask the family before washing the body. *In some cultures, the body is not washed, or family members arrange to have someone special do it.*
  - Special precautions must be observed in the handling of bodies of individuals who died from infectious disease (e.g., COVID-19). Nurses or other healthcare providers who handle the body should use standard precautions and wear appropriate personal protective equipment (PPE) (gloves, impermeable disposable gown, mask, eye protection) according to agency protocol. Educate the family to not touch the body without appropriate PPE; however, follow agency policy.
- **Dress the body in a clean gown, comb the hair, and straighten the bed linens.**
- **Place the body supine in a natural position.**
  - Place the dentures in the mouth before rigor mortis occurs.
- Close the eyes and mouth before rigor mortis occurs. Close the eyes by gently pressing on the lids with your fingertips. If they do not stay closed, place a moist compress on the eyelids for a few minutes and then try to close them again.
- Tie a strip of soft gauze (e.g., Kling) under the chin and around the head if your institution requires it (not all do). Alternatively, you can place a folded towel under the chin to keep the jaw closed. *This keeps the mouth set in a natural position in case there is a viewing later.*
- Place a pillow under the head and shoulders. *This prevents blood from settling there and causing discoloration.*
- **Be sure that dressings are clean, and unless an autopsy is to be done, remove all tubes and drains.** Be careful when removing tape or dressings. Apply small adhesive bandages to puncture sites. *After death, the skin loses its elasticity and can be torn easily.*
- **If the family asks about the coldness and color of the body, explain to them about algor mortis and livor mortis.**
- **After the family has spent time with the body, arrange to have it sent to the morgue,** where either an autopsy will be performed or, if not, the funeral home in charge of arrangements will arrive to transport the body.
  - Pad the wrists and ankles to prevent bruising; tie them together with gauze.
  - Wrap the body in a shroud or body wrap for transfer to the morgue.
  - If no relatives were present to receive patient belongings, bag them, label the bag, and send it with the patient to the morgue.
  - If possible, close doors to adjoining rooms before transport.
- **Make sure there are identification tags on the body, on the shroud or body bag, and on the patient's possessions, and, if necessary, hazard labels.** Follow agency policy for number and location of tags. They will usually include the patient's name, room and bed numbers, date and time of death, and the provider's name. Misidentification can create legal problems, for example, if the body is prepared incorrectly for a funeral.
- **Follow institutional policy if the patient has died of a communicable disease.** By law, there are special preparations to perform in such cases.
- **Handle the body with dignity.**

Documentation

Documentation varies among healthcare facilities. However, you will almost always document the time that you noted absence of heartbeat and respirations, any auxiliary equipment still present (e.g., mechanical ventilator), the disposition of the patient's possessions (especially money and jewelry), and the date and time the body is transported to the morgue or funeral home.

Practice Resources

de Swardt & Fouché (2017); Goncalves (2020); Williams (2016); World Health Organization (2020).

ASSESSMENT GUIDELINES AND TOOLS

You can use these guidelines for assessing dying patients as well as for other types of loss.

Focused Assessment

Assessing Grief and Loss

1. **Assess the patient and significant others for common grief reactions.**

Physical	Emotional	Behaviors	Cognition
Loss of appetite	Anger	Forgetfulness	Decreased concentration
Weight loss/gain	Sadness	Withdrawal	Forgetfulness
Fatigue	Guilt	Insomnia or too much sleep	Impaired judgment
Decreased libido	Relief	Dreaming of deceased	Obsessive thoughts of the deceased or lost object
Decrease in immune system	Shock	Verbalizing the loss	Preoccupation
Decreased energy	Numbness	Crying	Confusion
Possibly physical symptoms (e.g., headache, stomach pain)	Loneliness	Loss of productivity at work or school	Questioning spiritual beliefs
	Fear		Searching to understand
	Anxiety		Searching for purpose and meaning
	Powerlessness		
	Helplessness		
	Depression		

2. **Assess knowledge base of patient and significant others.**

   a. Can they make informed decisions about healthcare choices? You might ask the following questions:

   "Tell me what you understand about your illness."

   "Are there any questions about your illness that you would like me to answer?"

   "What are your options for treatment?"

   "Do you know how to reach your provider if you have questions about your care?"

   b. What and how much do the patient and family want to know? *Some people wish to have all the details of their condition and care. For others, the details cause anxiety.*

3. **Assess the history of loss.** Determine whether the patient or family has sustained recent losses or major changes (e.g., death, moving, divorce, retirement). Ask questions such as these:

   "Have you had any recent changes in your life?"

   "Tell me about your family."

   "Are your parents still living?" (as appropriate)

   "What experiences have you had with the loss of someone you loved (or with this or a similar condition)?"

4. **Assess coping abilities and support systems.**
   Questions to assess coping include the following:

   "What do you do to reduce stress?"

   "Which family/friends can you talk with?"

   "What or who would you say is your greatest support when going through difficult times?"

   "Tell me about a previous loss and what you did to cope with it."

   "What community resources can help you get through this? Have you contacted them?"

   The way individuals have coped in the past will affect how they cope with dying or with their current loss. It may also be therapeutic for them to identify their resources and support systems.

5. **Assess the meaning of the loss or illness.** Be alert for statements that may indicate the patient or family is struggling to find meaning, such as these:

   "I'm being punished."

   "They don't deserve this."

   "Why is this happening to me?"

   In trying to make sense of their loss or their dying, people try to attach a meaning to their suffering.

6. **Differentiate between grief and depressive disorder.**

   a. Symptoms common to both grief and depressive disorder are sadness, insomnia, poor appetite, and weight loss. Feelings of sadness and depression are a normal part of grief, provided the depression does not linger too long.

   b. Symptoms that indicate grief are not constant. For example, the person may feel relatively better in certain situations, such as when they are with friends and family. However, triggers, such as the deceased person's birthday, an anniversary, or holidays, cause the feelings to resurface more strongly.

   c. Symptoms that indicate depressive disorder are more intense. For example, the person is preoccupied with the loss and rarely gets any relief from the symptoms. Other symptoms include:

   Feelings of guilt not related to the loved one's death

Assessing Grief and Loss—cont'd

Thoughts about own death or of suicide (other than feelings the person would be better off dead now that the loved one is gone)

Preoccupation with own "worthlessness"

Sluggishness

Hesitant and confused speech

Prolonged and marked difficulty in carrying out activities of daily living

Hallucinations, other than thinking they hear the voice of or see the deceased person

7. **Perform a physical assessment.** Look for signs of increased stress, such as tension, forgetfulness, distraction, increased or decreased appetite and sleep, weight gain or loss, fatigue, and decreased self-care (e.g., deficient hygiene). *A thorough physical examination adds data to help you determine how well the patient is coping with the loss or illness.*

8. **Perform a cultural and spiritual assessment.**
   a. Assess the patient's and family's religious beliefs, any spiritual needs they may have (e.g., forgiveness, hope, meaning, love), and cultural influences that may affect the way they cope.

   Key Point: *Do not assume that a person adheres closely to the dominant values of their indicated religious or cultural group. Always assess. For example, ask, "To what religious and ethnic groups do you belong?" and "How closely do you identify with those groups?"*

   See Chapters 12 and 13 for details of cultural and spiritual assessment, if you need them.

9. **Perform these specific assessments for dying patients.** In addition to the other assessments in this guideline, you should assess the following:
   a. When the patient and family are ready, encourage them to talk about what the patient might want for burial or cremation or whether the person would like some tasks taken care of (e.g., giving away valuables, calling family members).
   b. Determine whether the dying person has a living will or advance directive.
   c. Discuss with the patient and family the possibility of organ donation if appropriate for the patient's circumstances.
   d. Observe for physical changes indicating the approach of death:

   1 to 3 months before death: Beginning withdrawal from others, increased sleep, decreased appetite, difficulty digesting food (especially meats), and preference for liquids. *Anorexia may be protective, as the resulting ketosis can diminish pain and increase the person's sense of well-being.*

   1 to 2 weeks before death: Cardiovascular deterioration brings decreased blood pressure, pulse and respiration changes (decreased or increased), a yellowish pallor to the skin, and extreme pallor of extremities. Observe for temperature fluctuations, increased perspiration, brief periods of apnea during sleep, rattling breathing sounds caused by congestion, and nonproductive cough.

   Days to hours before death: A brief surge of energy and mental clarity, with a desire to eat and talk with family members.
   - Dehydration, difficulty swallowing, decreasing blood pressure, weak pulse.
   - Mucous membranes dry and tacky; cracked lips. *Dehydration during the last hours of dying is thought to not cause distress and perhaps to stimulate endorphin release.*
   - Sagging of tongue and soft palate, diminished gag reflex, secretions accumulating in the oropharynx and/or bronchi.
   - Shallow, rapid, or irregular breathing; respiratory congestion; Cheyne-Stokes respirations; apnea of 10 to 30 seconds; "death rattle." *Cheyne-Stokes breathing is a cyclic pattern consisting of a 10- to 60-second period of apnea and then a gradual increase in depth and rate of respirations. Respirations gradually become slow and shallow, and then the cycle begins again with apnea.*
   - Decreased peripheral circulation, increased perspiration, clammy skin; extremities cool and mottled; dependent body parts darker than the rest of the body.
   - Decreased urinary output, concentrated and foul-smelling urine, secondary to decreased kidney function.
   - Slack facial muscles ("drooping").
   - Retained feces; bowel and bladder incontinence. *This condition is due to decreased peristalsis and relaxation of sphincters.*
   - Blurred vision; eyes open but unseeing.
   - Restlessness or agitation (check for impacted stool, distended bladder, pain, medications, cerebral hypoxia, unresolved emotional or spiritual issues).
   - Decreased communication, quiet, withdrawal. Some become more coherent and energized for a time.
   - Fatigue.

   Moments before death: Does not respond to touch or sound; cannot be awakened. There may be a short series of long-spaced breaths before breathing stops entirely and the heart stops beating. Auscultate to determine whether apical pulse and respirations are absent.

Sources: Burgess, L. (2020). What are the signs that someone is close to death? *Medical News Today.* https://www.medicalnewstoday.com/articles/320794

DerSarkissian, C. (2020). What to expect when your loved one is dying. WebMD. https://www.webmd.com/palliative-care/journeys-end-active-dying#2

Emanuel, L., et al. (2015). The last hours of living: Practical advice for clinicians. *Medscape.* http://www.medscape.com/viewarticle/716463

Galbadage, T., et al. (2020). Biopsychosocial and spiritual implications of patients with COVID-19 dying in isolation. *Frontiers in Psychology, 17.* https://doi.org/10.3389/fpsyg.2020.588623

Mayo Staff Clinic. (2020). End of life: Caring for someone who is dying. https://www.mayoclinic.org/healthy-lifestyle/end-of-life/in-depth/cancer/art-20047600

National Institute on Aging. (2017). Providing care and comfort at the end of life. *National Institute of Health.* https://www.nia.nih.gov/health/providing-comfort-end-life

CLINICAL REASONING
Applying the Full-Spectrum Nursing Model

PATIENT SITUATION

Marie is 84 years old and has had a right-side cerebrovascular accident (CVA, stroke, or brain attack). Doctors say she is unlikely to regain much physical function, even if she awakens from the coma. She was alert and active before her stroke and was able to maintain her independence with the help of a home health aide, who assisted her with ADLs and meal preparation three times a week. Kelly and Dan, her children, have met with the provider, who tells them that Marie's chance of survival is slim. He wants to put a feeding tube into Marie and has asked whether they want Marie to be resuscitated in case of cardiac or respiratory arrest. Kelly wants to do what is best for her mother, but she feels that Marie would not want to be kept alive in this condition. She is also concerned about putting her through uncomfortable procedures if there is no chance of recovery. Dan thinks Marie should have the feeding tube. Kelly asks to speak with you and wants to know the best thing to do for her mother.

THINKING

1. *Theoretical Knowledge (Recall of Facts and Principles):* If Marie and Dan agree that they do not want Marie to be resuscitated, the provider will complete a DNR prescription. What do the letters *DNR* represent?

2. *Critical Thinking (Problem-Solving):* At this stage of your education, you probably need more information about CVAs and tube feedings. Write a PICOT question you could use to search the literature for information about these two topics and how they are related. See Chapter 4 if you need to review PICOT questions.

DOING

3. *Practical Knowledge (Nursing Diagnosis):* Write a possible nursing diagnosis to describe Kelly's situation.

4. *Practical Knowledge (Basic Skills):* If Kelly and Dan agree to tube feedings for Marie, what basic nursing skills will you, as her nurse, need to perform? How will you learn to perform these skills, if you do not already know how to do them?

CARING

5. *Ethical Knowledge:* How do you think the situation came to this? What might Kelly, Dan, and Marie have done before the stroke to prevent this confusion and indecision?

6. *Self-Knowledge:* What are your responsibilities in this situation? What could you do to help Kelly and Dan?

Critical Thinking and Clinical Judgment

1. Jessie McCarthy is a 69-year-old woman who is terminally ill with multiple myeloma. She is currently hospitalized for a week of chemotherapy. Her husband of 49 years is recuperating from recent hip surgery and has difficulty getting around. Her daughter and son-in-law are very close to them, and her granddaughter, 14 years old, has a very special relationship with her "Gammie." The side effects of Mrs. McCarthy's chemotherapy include nausea and headaches. She does not like to have people around when she feels this way. Jessie's pastor comes to visit every other day and seems to bring her comfort. Her 50th wedding anniversary will occur when she is in the hospital. She verbalizes fear of "not making it home this time." You are her nurse in a hospital where palliative care is provided. Initiate a holistic plan of care for Mrs. McCarthy, addressing the main issues noted.

   a. What immediate physical problems does Mrs. McCarthy have? Do not use her medical diagnosis as an answer.

   b. What might you do to meet her physical needs?

   c. What psychological needs does Mrs. McCarthy have: (1) What are her fears? (2) What social and emotional issues is she facing? (3) How might you help meet her needs?

2. You are caring for Jack Wirtz, a 37-year-old man who was admitted to the hospital for a lumbar laminectomy (surgery of his lower spine). As you are doing Jack's preoperative assessment, he tells you that his 12-year-old son died 6 months ago in an automobile accident in which Jack was the driver. He is a builder and has been out of work since the accident. His wife now works to help support them. Jack's affect is flat, and he talks in a monotone.

   a. What losses has Jack experienced?

   b. What further assessments need to be made for Jack, and why?

3. A patient requests your participation in a plan for assisted suicide or passive euthanasia. What are your options as a nurse? Use the Internet to get information about this.

   a. List the URLs for the pages you found to be helpful in answering the question. Beside each URL, state the name of the organization, person, or agency to which the Web site belongs.

   b. For each URL, state what you believe to be the *purpose* of the Web site.

4. Find a partner. Take 5 minutes to describe to them a personal loss you have had (e.g., a person, a pet, an object, an aspect of health). The partner must listen silently and not speak at all during this time. When you have finished, answer the following questions:

   a. What did you feel when describing your loss?

   b. Did you feel that the listener was really listening to you?

   c. How did the listener respond to you?

5. Now reverse the process; you become the listener. When you have finished, answer the following questions:

   a. What did you feel while you were listening?

   b. Did the time go quickly or seem long?

   c. What did you learn from this listening experience?

6. John, 17 years old, is a volunteer at the hospital. He has just moved from another state because of his father's work, so he is a new senior at the local high school. As you chat with him, he reveals that his mother is getting radiation and chemotherapy treatments for breast cancer and has been very ill. What are some loss issues this young man is facing?

7. Sharon, 48 years old, is in the hospital for a hysterectomy (removal of her uterus) because of fibroids and heavy bleeding. With teary eyes, she shares with you that she is feeling "down" and doesn't want any visitors this evening. She says, "I really thought I would feel better after having this surgery done."

   a. Why do you think Sharon is teary and feeling down?

   b. What should you do to begin helping Sharon cope with her loss?

8. You are having lunch with a nursing colleague, who reveals to you that her mother has Alzheimer disease. Her mother has been placed in a nursing home because she is losing her memory and is not safe at home. Your friend describes feeling distracted, angry for no reason, and unable to shake her feelings of sadness.

   a. What might be causing your colleague to feel distracted and angry?

   b. How would you respond to her?

9. You are caring for Mr. Bishop, a 57-year-old man who is terminally ill with metastatic bone cancer. He wants to donate his organs for research after his death, but his wife is totally against this.

   a. What could you do or say to him to help resolve this issue? Go to the URL http://organdonor.gov and download information on organ donation and transplantation to use in this situation.

   b. Now go to the top of the Web page and look at the logo and other information. Who do you think provides and maintains the content for this Web site? What else would give you a clue about the source of the site?

   c. Look at the bottom of the Web page. What department of the U.S. government "owns" this page?

10. For each of the following concepts, use critical thinking to describe how or why it is important to nursing, patient care, or loss, grief, and dying. Note that these are *not* to be merely definitions.

   Physical loss

   Actual loss

   Dysfunctional or complicated grief

   Disenfranchised grief

   Significance of the loss

   Stages of grief

   Advance directives

   Assisted suicide

   Palliative care

What Are the Main Points in This Chapter?

- How people cope with loss directly affects their healing and well-being.
- Loss may be actual or perceived, physical or psychological, external or internal.
- Grief is the physical, psychological, and spiritual response to loss.
- People do not move neatly from one stage of grief or dying to the next; there is constant movement and overlap between and among them.
- Factors that affect the grieving process include the significance and circumstance of the loss, the timeliness of the death, the bereaved support system, spiritual beliefs, cultural values, the person's developmental stage, and conflicts existing at the time of death.
- Patients experience loss of independence, body image, self-esteem, and so on when they are ill and/or hospitalized. Recognizing these as losses, you can assist the patient with the grieving process, thus promoting physical, emotional, and spiritual healing.
- The Uniform Determination of Death Act states that death has occurred when "an individual . . . has sustained either (1) irreversible cessation of circulatory and respiratory functions, or (2) irreversible cessation of all functions of the entire brain, including the brainstem. . . ."

- Palliative care focuses on providing comfort care and symptom relief without further efforts to stop the disease process or prevent death.
- Hospice care is a movement and an approach to allow terminally ill persons to face death with dignity while surrounded by family in the comfort of their home.
- Healthcare providers are responsible for educating staff and patients about advance directives.
- A do-not-resuscitate (DNR) prescription is a specific prescription to *not* perform cardiopulmonary resuscitation.
- Nurses should be aware of what is involved with assisted suicide and euthanasia. You should think ahead about what your response might be if a patient wants to discuss these topics. You may find helpful the American Nurses Association (ANA) position statement on the nurses' roles and responsibilities in end-of-life care.
- An autopsy is a medical examination of the body to determine the cause of death.
- When a patient is dying or has experienced a loss, you should perform a thorough holistic assessment.
- Most grief is normal, not dysfunctional; you should not diagnose dysfunctional/complicated grieving for every person who is grieving a loss.

- You can facilitate grief work by validating feelings ("It's normal to feel that way") and providing an opportunity and encouragement to talk about the lost person for whom the person is grieving.
- Active dying usually occurs over a 10- to 14-day period, although it can take as little as 24 hours. During the final 4 to 48 hours, failure of body systems results in death.
- When the patient is very near death, focus on relieving physical symptoms and emotional distress. If the patient can communicate, ask about immediate concerns, such as whom the patient wants in the room.
- At the moment of death, do not interrupt or intrude on the family; give them as much time as they need to say good-bye to their loved one. Express your sympathy.
- Care of the body includes making it presentable for the family, carefully placing identification tags, and arranging to have the body sent to the morgue.
- The death certificate must be signed by the person who legally pronounced the death (usually a provider).

Knowledge Map

TYPES OF LOSS
- Actual
- External
- Physical
- Perceived
- Internal
- Psychological

TYPES OF GRIEF
- Complicated
- Uncomplicated
- Disenfranchised
- Anticipatory

- Chronic
- Masked
- Delayed

FACTORS AFFECTING LOSS
- Aspects of self
- Significant relationships
- Environment

LOSS

GRIEF

FACTORS AFFECTING GRIEF
- Significance of loss
- Support systems
- Existing conflicts
- Circumstances
- Prior losses
- Developmental stage
- Spirituality
- Culture
- Timeliness

THEORISTS
- Engel
- Worden
- Rando
- Bowlby

LEGALITIES
- Organ donation
- Autopsy
- Advanced directives
- Assisted suicide
- Euthanasia

DYING

SELF-CARE FOR NURSES
- Self-knowledge (fears, beliefs)
- Look for support
- Allow own grief

PHYSIOLOGICAL STAGES
- Withdrawal
- Systems deterioration
- Cheyne-Stokes breathing
- Mottling
- Organ failure
- Death

PSYCHOLOGICAL STAGES (Kübler-Ross)
- Denial
- Anger
- Bargaining
- Depression
- Acceptance

CARE
- Mobility
- Oxygenation
- Safety
- Nutrition
- Fluids
- Pain

PALLIATIVE CARE
- Holistic
- Comfort

HOSPICE CARE
- "Way" of care
- Dignity
- Quality of life
- Spiritual

CARE
- Honesty
- Therapeutic communication
- Spiritual and cultural support

UNIT 2 Factors Affecting Health

UNIT 3

Essential Nursing Interventions

15 **Communication & Therapeutic Relationships**
16 **Patient Education**
17 **Interprofessional Partnerships: Documenting & Reporting**
18 **Measuring Vital Signs**
19 **Health Assessment**
20 **Promoting Asepsis & Preventing Infection**
21 **Promoting Safety**
22 **Facilitating Hygiene**
23 **Administering Medications**

CHAPTER 15

Communication & Therapeutic Relationships

STUDENT RESOURCES

The questions and exercises in this book allow you to practice the kind of thinking you will use as a full-spectrum nurse. Critical-thinking questions usually have more than one right answer, so we do not provide "correct" answers for these features. Try to answer these questions yourself. It is more important to develop your nursing judgment than to just cover content. You will learn more by discussing the questions with your peers. If you are still unsure, see the Davis Advantage chapter resources for suggested responses.

To explore learning resources for this chapter,

Go to www.DavisAdvantage.com and find:

Answers and Suggested Responses for all questions in this chapter
Concept Map
Knowledge Map
References and Bibliography

Key Concepts

Communication
Communication techniques
Therapeutic relationships

Related Concepts

See the Concept Map on Davis Advantage.

Caring for the Williams Family

Following is a transcript of an interaction that occurred during Stanley Williams' first visit to the family healthcare clinic. As you may recall, Assad Johnson is a family nurse practitioner who is examining Mr. Williams. Analyze the interaction. Identify open-ended and closed questions and therapeutic communication techniques. Comment on responses that Assad might have improved on.

Assad: Are your parents still living?

Stanley: Yes, they're both alive. My father is 80 years old, and my mother is 76.

Assad: I'd like to hear a little more about your family history. Tell me about your father's cancer. How old was he when he was first diagnosed? Has he had treatment?

Stanley: He was probably about 60 when he first found out about it. I know he had some kind of surgery and takes medications, but I don't know the details. He seems all right, though.

Assad: Your father also has high blood pressure and heart disease. Please tell me a little more about that.

(Continued)

141

Caring for the Williams Family (continued)

Stanley: My father and mother both have high blood pressure and heart disease. They both take medication for their blood pressure. My father had a small heart attack about 10 years ago. My mother has never had a heart attack that I know of, but she sometimes has chest pain.

Assad: Your mother also has diabetes?

Stanley: She's had that for a long time. A lot of people in my family, especially on my father's side, have diabetes but nobody in my mother's family. Yet my mother is the one with diabetes!

Nadine: A lot of people in my family have diabetes, too. But so far, I'm okay, I think.

Assad: Have you had a health examination lately, Mrs. Williams?

Nadine: Not in about a year, but I'm going to schedule an appointment here.

Practical Knowledge clinical application

This section provides clinical insights and focused assessments for communication.

CLINICAL INSIGHTS

Clinical Insight 15-1 ▶ Collaborative Professional Communication

American Nurses Association (ANA) (2021)

Standards of professional performance stress the importance of communication to collegiality, leadership, and collaboration. The following are some of the competencies for these standards.

Standard 9. Communication

The registered nurse communicates effectively in all areas of practice.
- Assesses one's own communication skills and effectiveness
- Demonstrates cultural empathy when communicating
- Assesses communication ability, health literacy, resources, and preferences of healthcare consumers to inform the interprofessional team and others
- Uses language translation resources to ensure effective communication
- Incorporates appropriate alternative strategies to communicate effectively with healthcare consumers who have visual, speech, language, or communication difficulties
- Uses communication styles and methods that demonstrate caring, respect, deep listening, authenticity, and trust
- Conveys accurate information
- Maintains communication with interprofessional team and others to facilitate safe transitions and continuity in care delivery
- Contributes the nursing perspective in interactions with others and discussions with the interprofessional team
- Exposes care processes and decisions when they do not appear to be in the best interest of the healthcare consumer
- Discloses concerns related to potential or actual hazards and errors in care or the practice environment to the appropriate level
- Demonstrates continuous improvement of communication skills

Standard 10. Collaboration
- Communicates effectively with the healthcare consumer, the family, and healthcare providers regarding healthcare consumer care and the nurse's role in the provision of care

Standard 11. Leadership
- Communicates to manage change and address conflict
- Collaborates with the interprofessional team to implement quality improvement plans and interventions

Standard 15. Professional Practice Evaluation
- Provides peers with formal or informal constructive feedback regarding their practice or role performance

Source: American Nurses Association (2021). *Nursing: Scope and standards of practice* (4th ed.). Silver Spring, MD: Nursebooks.org; 71, 73, 79, 81.

Clinical Insight 15-1 ➤ Collaborative Professional Communication—cont'd

American Association of Critical-Care Nurses (AACN) (2016)

Standard 4: Communication

The following are competencies for skilled communication for nurses caring for acutely and critically ill patients:

- Assessing the preferred and most effective style for communicating with acutely and critically ill patients, families, and interprofessional team
- Seeking to protect and advance collaborative relationships among colleagues while exhibiting respect for the perspectives of others
- Contributing professional perspective and seeking the rationale and relevant perspectives supporting patient care decisions
- Continually improving professional communication and conflict resolution skills
- Reporting observations or expressing concerns related to the safety of patients, hazards in the healthcare environment, or possible errors in care
- Communicating clearly with other providers to minimize risks associated with patient handoffs, transfers, and transitions in care

The Joint Commission 2022 National Patient Safety Goals

Goal 2: Improve the effectiveness of communication among caregivers.

The 2022 National Patient Safety Goal 2 is to improve the effectiveness of communication among caregivers. More specifically, Goal 2.03.01 is to report critical results of laboratory and diagnostic procedures to the right person in a timely manner.

Source: American Association of Critical-Care Nurses (AACN). (2016). *AACN standards for establishing and sustaining healthy work environment: A journey to excellence.* American Association of Critical-Care Nurses.

Clinical Insight 15-2 ➤ Communicating With SBARQ*

Situation	Identify yourself and the patient and describe the present situation that prompted you to call. State the following: 　Your name 　Your unit 　The patient's name and room number 　Brief overview of the problem
Background	Give other information pertinent to the situation—not the patient's entire history since admission, but circumstances leading up to the situation.
Assessment	State the problem and what you think is causing it.
Recommendation	State what you think will correct the problem, or what you need from the provider.
Question	Allow an opportunity to ask or answer any questions. Review specific concerns.

Practice Resource

Leonard, M., Bornacum, D., Graham, S. (2017). SBAR tool: situation-background-assessment-recommendation. Institute for Healthcare Improvement. https://f.hubspotusercontent30.net/hubfs/241684/2020%20LPs%20-%20downloads/SBARTechniqueforCommunication-IHI%20v2.pdf; Eberhardt, S. (2014, November). Improve handoff communication with SBAR. *Nursing, 44*(11), 17–20. doi:10.1097/01.NURSE.0000454965.49138.79.

Clinical Insight 15-3 ▶ Communicating With Clients From Another Culture

General Guidelines

- Be aware of your own cultural beliefs and attitudes.
- Learn about other cultures, especially those in your area.
- Convey empathy and show respect.
- Be certain the communication strategies you usually use are culturally appropriate for the individual.
  - Is direct eye contact viewed as aggressive or impolite? Or is it perceived as engaged and caring?
  - How much space should you keep between yourself and the patient?
- Use touch cautiously.
- Proceed slowly. Rushing may cause the patient to be more anxious and is offensive to some.
- Smile and be polite, but not overfriendly or casual. Use the patient's title and last name when introducing yourself.
- Use short words and sentences. Do not give too much information in one sentence.
- Present one idea at a time.
- Provide written teaching materials.

If There Is a Language Barrier

- Written information provided must be appropriate to the population served and the language of the patient (The Joint Commission, 2010).
- Use a trained medical interpreter, if possible.
- To review guidelines for communicating with clients who speak a different language, refer to How Do I Communicate With Clients Who Speak a Different Language? in Chapter 12 of this book.

Some medical dictionaries or Web-based resources have a comprehensive list of English–Spanish phrases, such as these:

English	Spanish
How do you feel?	¿Como se siente?
Good	Bien
Bad	Mal
Have you any difficulty breathing?	¿Tiene dificultad al respirar?
Are you thirsty?	¿Tiene sed?
Have you any pain?	¿Tiene dolor?
Show me where	Enséñeme dónde
Is it worse now?	¿Está peor ahora?
Cough	Tosa
Open your mouth	Abra la boca
Take a deep breath	Respire profundamente
You may eat	Puede comer
Tea	Té
Coffee	Café
I will give you something for	Le dare algo para eso
A pill	Una píldora

Source: The Joint Commission. (2010). *Advancing patient-centered communication, cultural competence, and family-centered care: A roadmap for hospitals.* Joint Commission. https://www.jointcommission.org/assets/1/6/ARoadmapforHospitalsfinalversion727.pdf

ASSESSMENT GUIDELINES AND TOOLS

Focused Assessment

Communication

A focused assessment should identify factors that alter a patient's ability to receive, understand, and convey verbal and nonverbal messages.

Medications

- Is the patient taking medications that might interfere with speech, cognition, or level of consciousness?
- Does the patient use alcohol or other substances? Are they intoxicated?

Language, Vocabulary, Literacy

- What is the patient's primary language?
- Is the patient proficient with the English language?
- Is an interpreter (foreign language or sign language) required?
- Can the patient read and write? At what level and in what (preferred) language?

Cognitive Function

Communication difficulties may signal cognitive impairment. Look for history of developmental delays and pathology or injury of the central nervous system.

- What is the patient's level of consciousness?
- Is there short-term or long-term memory loss, or both?
- Is intellectual function at, below, or above expectations for age?
- Can the patient read simple instructions?
- Can the patient follow simple spoken instructions?
- Can the patient understand a yes-or-no choice?
- Are there symptoms or a diagnosis of mental illness or dementia?
- If the patient is unconscious, are there nonverbal responses that indicate that they can hear you (e.g., blinking, moving the head, squeezing your hand)?

Focused Assessment

Communication—cont'd

Hearing
- Ask the patient and observe whether there are hearing problems.
- Is the patient wearing a hearing aid? If so, is it working properly? Does the patient appear to be reading your lips?
- Does the patient use sign language to communicate?
- Refer to Chapter 19 for tests of hearing (e.g., ticking watch).

Vision
- Is the patient wearing glasses or contact lenses?
- Is the patient able to see adequately?
- Refer to Chapter 19 for vision tests.

Also see the Davis's Nursing Skills Video **Brief Bedside Assessment.**

Aphasia
- Is there a history of stroke or a diagnosis of aphasia?
- Is there receptive aphasia (inability to receive or interpret verbal or nonverbal messages)?
- Is there expressive aphasia (inability to express verbal or nonverbal messages)?

Physiological Barriers
Does the patient have conditions that cause difficulty speaking, such as the following?
- Dyspnea
- Artificial airway
- Oral problems, such as poorly fitted dentures
- Cleft palate or other structural problems

Communication Style
- Is it difficult to understand what the patient says (e.g., slurring words, stuttering, inability to pronounce certain sounds)?
- Does the patient speak readily or are they quiet?
- Does the patient speak slowly or rapidly, spontaneously, or hesitantly?
- Is the vocabulary adequate for the purpose needed?
- Has the person's normal vocabulary changed?

Other
- Are verbal and nonverbal communication congruent?

CLINICAL REASONING
Applying the Full-Spectrum Nursing Model

Choose two of the following communication techniques and plan to consciously use them with your next patient. Use the following thinking, doing, and caring questions to reflect on your interaction.

- Active listening
- Communicating assertively using "I" statements
- Restating a message
- Clarifying messages
- Validating messages
- Sharing observations about body language
- Asking open-ended questions
- Using silence
- Summarizing the conversation

THINKING

1. *Critical Thinking (Contextual Awareness):* Before you have the conversation, make a note of what is going on in the situation (e.g., values, environment, culture) that might influence the effectiveness of the two techniques you will be using.

DOING

2. *Nursing Process (Assessment/Recognizing Cues):* Before using the two techniques, assess for factors that might affect the patient's ability to communicate. Make a note of them.

3. *Nursing Process (Implementation/Taking Action):* As soon as possible after using the techniques, record the conversations. Try to remember the exact words.

4. *Nursing Process (Evaluation):* Evaluate your ability to use the two techniques you chose.

   a. Did you use them at an appropriate time in the conversation, for example, as an appropriate response to something the patient said?

   b. What effect did your communication have on the interaction? How did the patient respond to what you said?

   c. Do you think your communication was therapeutic for the patient?

CARING

5. *Self-Knowledge:*

   a. What were your thoughts and feelings before, during, and after the interaction?

   b. In what way has your comfort level with these two techniques changed?

   c. Describe the type of patient or situation in which you would be the least confident in your ability to communicate therapeutically.

Critical Thinking and Clinical Judgment

1. Mrs. Washington arrives at the clinic complaining of a painful lump in her left breast. She is 40 years old and appears very nervous. She tells you, "I was afraid to come in, but I guess I have to find out what this is."

   a. How might you acknowledge Mrs. Washington's feelings? Give examples.

   b. What might you say to clarify and validate her messages?

   c. Write a hypothetical conversation with Mrs. Washington that:

   - Acknowledges her feelings
   - Establishes trust
   - Explores the issue
   - Clarifies and validates her messages
   - Uses silence
   - Summarizes the conversation

2. Paramedics bring a 35-year-old man and his 14-year-old son to the ED. Both have been involved in a recreational vehicle gas explosion and have suffered burns. The son is placed in one of the trauma rooms adjacent to his father. He has partial- and full-thickness burns over his face, neck, chest, arms, and hands, and he is unresponsive. The father has partial-thickness burns on his right hand and forearm. He appears to be in a lot of pain and is yelling out for his son in Spanish. His wife soon arrives at the ED, crying and asking whether her husband and son will be okay. Her English is fluent.

   a. Identify at least two interventions to help you communicate with the father.

   b. What kind of body language would you expect from the father?

   c. How could you show acceptance and establish trust with the father?

   d. Identify at least two factors that will influence communication with the son.

   e. Identify at least two communication strategies to use with the son.

f. Explain or give an example of how to use the following techniques as you communicate with the anxious wife and mother:

Establishing trust

Using silence

Offering nonverbal support

3. For each of the following concepts, use critical thinking to describe how or why it is important to nursing, patient care, or communication. Note that these are not to be merely definitions.

Verbal communication	Therapeutic communication
Nonverbal communication	Therapeutic relationship
Intrapersonal communication	Barriers to therapeutic communication
Interpersonal communication	Distance between sender and receiver
Group communication	Communication strategies

What Are the Main Points in This Chapter?

- Communication is a dynamic, reciprocal process of sending and receiving messages.
- Communication occurs on three levels: intrapersonal, or self-talk; interpersonal (between two or more people); and group communication.
- The sender delivers a message to the receiver via verbal and/or nonverbal communication. The receiver provides feedback to the sender.
- Verbal communication is the use of spoken and written words.
- Nonverbal communication, sometimes called *body language,* communicates how someone is feeling and gives a more accurate account of an individual's true sentiment.
- Physical development, maturity, language skills, intellectual abilities, culture, gender, roles, and relationships influence the communication process.
- Collaborative professional communication is assertive without being aggressive.
- Communication is most successful in a comfortable environment. A favorable environment is quiet, private, free of unpleasant smells, and at a comfortable temperature.
- The distance between individuals engaged in communication is affected by the relationship of the individuals, the nature of the conversation, the setting, and cultural influences.
- Relationships affect the choice of vocabulary, tone of voice, use of gestures, and distance associated with the communication.

- Therapeutic communication is the use of communication skills that result in a positive effect on client care; it is the foundation of professional nursing practice.
- Therapeutic communication occurs in the context of a helping relationship. The helping relationship has four phases: preinteraction, orientation, working phase, and termination.
- Group communication occurs when you are interacting with a family, a community, or a committee. Groups may be focused on a task, self-improvement, coping skills, or work-related issues.
- To enhance communication, listen actively, establish trust, be assertive, restate messages, clarify and validate messages, interpret body language, share observations, explore issues, use silence, summarize the conversation, and make use of process recordings while you are learning.
- Barriers to communication include asking too many questions, asking why, firehosing information, changing the subject inappropriately, failing to listen, failing to probe, expressing approval or disapproval, offering advice, providing false reassurance, stereotyping, and using patronizing language.
- Language barriers, sensory perceptual alterations, impaired cognitive skills, and physiological barriers make therapeutic communication challenging, but nursing activities can enhance communication with these clients.

UNIT 3 Essential Nursing Interventions

Knowledge Map

PROCESS
- Sender
- Message
- Channel
- Receiver
- Feedback

factors affecting
- Environment
- Developmental level
- Gender
- Personal space
- Sociocultural facts
- Roles/relationships

CONTENT

SENDER → **COMMUNICATION** ← *RECEIVER*

Verbal communication

Nonverbal communication
- Gait
- Posture
- Facial expression
- Appearance
- Space
- Touch

nurses use → **THERAPEUTIC COMMUNICATION**

KEY CHARACTERISTICS
- Empathy
- Respect
- Genuineness
- Concreteness
- Confrontation

are phases of
- Pre-interaction
- Orientation
- Working
- Termination

enhance
- Active listening
- Mutual trust
- Assertive style
- Nothing body language

deter
- Asking questions: Too many; closed ended; "why"
- Failing to listen/explore
- Approving/disapproving
- Giving advice
- False reassurance
- Stereotyping

CHAPTER 16

Patient Education

STUDENT RESOURCES

The questions and exercises in this book allow you to practice the kind of thinking you will use as a full-spectrum nurse. Critical-thinking questions usually have more than one right answer, so we do not provide "correct" answers for these features. Try to answer these questions yourself. It is more important to develop your nursing judgment than to just cover content. You will learn more by discussing the questions with your peers. If you are still unsure, see the Davis Advantage chapter resources for suggested responses.

To explore learning resources for this chapter,

Go to www.DavisAdvantage.com and find:

Answers and Suggested Responses for all questions in this chapter
Concept Map
Knowledge Map
References and Bibliography

Key Concepts

Health literacy
Learning
Learning environment
Teaching

Related Concepts

See the Concept Map on Davis Advantage.

Caring for the Williams Family

Stanley Williams has medical diagnoses including hypertension, type 2 diabetes mellitus, obesity, and osteoarthritis. There is a positive history of tobacco abuse. Based on the information you know about Stanley and his family, consider the following questions:

A. What kinds of information does Stanley probably need?

B. What would be the best approach to teach Stanley about his healthcare conditions?

C. You have been asked to teach Stanley about weight loss. What theoretical knowledge must you have, and where can you obtain it?

(Continued)

Caring for the Williams Family (continued)

D. What patient information do you need to know before planning your teaching?

E. Stanley tells you that he feels overwhelmed with his recent diagnoses. He does not believe he can begin a weight-loss program or attend any teaching sessions. How might you handle this concern?

F. Stanley has been prescribed the following medications. Devise one or more teaching sessions focused on these drugs. You will need to use your pharmacology reference books to devise this plan. As you plan your teaching, recall that Stanley is overwhelmed by his recent diagnoses.

Lisinopril 20 mg PO daily
Hydrochlorothiazide 25 mg PO daily
Metformin 500 mg PO bid

Practical Knowledge clinical application

ASSESSMENT GUIDELINES AND TOOLS

Learning Assessment

Preassessment

Before assessing the client, think about the following:

- **Time constraints.** How much information do you need to present? How much time do you have to do it?
- **Available resources.** What equipment and supplies do you have to work with? Do you have audiovisual equipment? Internet access? A copier? Books?

Assessing the Client

A teaching/learning assessment should include the following:

- **Intended audience**
  Whom are you teaching?
  What is the person's age, occupation, developmental level, and cultural affiliation?
  Will you be teaching a person or a group?
- **Learning needs**
  What is the client's medical (or other) problem?
  What behavioral changes are needed?
  What self-care knowledge and skills do the client need?
- **Knowledge level.** Determine what the client already knows so that you can reinforce knowledge or adapt the teaching plan to the client's learning needs. Ask questions such as the following:
  What do you think caused your health problem?
  What are your concerns about it?
  How has the problem affected your usual activities?
  What are your concerns about treatment (e.g., tests, surgery)?

- **Health beliefs and practices**
  Ask the client to give a general description of her health:
  What do you usually do to stay healthy?
  What problems do you think you are at risk for?
  What lifestyle changes would you be willing to make to improve your health?
- **Physical readiness.** Check ability to concentrate, manual dexterity skills, and pain level.
- **Emotional readiness**
  Find out whether the client has anxiety or emotional distress that will interfere with the learning process.
  Ask the client whether they would like a family member or friend to be present during the learning.
- **Ability to learn**
  What are the client's cognitive and psychomotor developmental abilities?
  How does the client learn best (e.g., by memorization or recall, or by problem-solving or applying information)?
  How well does the client recall previously presented material?
- **Health literacy level**
  Can the patient understand basic health information and services needed to make appropriate healthcare decisions?
  Can the person read and write?
  Do the patient and healthcare provider speak the same language?

Focused Assessment

Learning Assessment—cont'd

- **Neurosensory factors**

  What is the client's ability to feel, see, hear, and grasp?

  Does the client have a medical condition that causes neurosensory compromise?

- **Learning styles.** Ask the person the following:

  How do you prefer to learn new things? For example, do you prefer to read about them, talk about them, watch a streaming video, be shown how to do it, listen to the nurse, or use a computer?

  Do you like to read?

  Where do you get information about your health—from the Internet, books, magazines, your family, your healthcare provider?

  Do you learn best alone or with other people?

CLINICAL REASONING
Applying the Full-Spectrum Nursing Model

PATIENT SITUATION

Katrina Peplowski, a 22-year-old college student from Poland, is transported to the ED after passing out in her dorm room. Before this episode, Katrina had a viral illness for 5 days, with fever, nausea, vomiting, and diarrhea. She had been drinking large amounts of an electrolyte replacement drink because of her insatiable thirst, thought to be related to the fever and vomiting. Even before the illness, Katrina's friends and family had commented about her remarkable weight loss since she started school 2 months earlier, especially despite her increased appetite. On arrival to the ED, Katrina's blood sugar is 585 mg/dL. She is diagnosed with type 1 diabetes mellitus (DM). After her blood sugar is stabilized with fluid therapy and insulin infusion, Katrina regains consciousness. Although Katrina speaks some English, her proficiency is limited.

THINKING

1. *Theoretical Knowledge (Recall of Facts and Principles):* Because Katrina is newly diagnosed with type 1 DM, there are many areas in which your patient will need healthcare education. List at least six important topics that are relevant to her care.

2. *Critical Thinking (Application of Knowledge):* What will you consider as you are devising a teaching plan for Katrina?

3. *Critical Thinking (Synthesis of Knowledge):* What factors are important for customizing her teaching plan, considering the communication limitations?

DOING

4. *Nursing Process (Assessment/Recognizing Cues):* What are some pertinent personal factors that you should assess for Katrina when adapting a teaching plan to suit her learning needs?

5. *Nursing Process (Planning/Prioritizing Hypotheses and Generating Solutions):* As you think about involving other members of the healthcare team in her care, how would you plan to optimize Katrina's motivation to learn about managing her diabetes after discharge?

CARING

6. *Self-Knowledge:* What areas of commonality do you have with Katrina around which you might form a caring relationship?

7. *Ethical Knowledge:* Suppose Katrina refuses to receive information from you about DM. She states she is not interested in knowing how to give herself insulin because she does not want to give herself injections at home or have to deal with an insulin pump. How should you respond to Katrina's requests?

Critical Thinking and Clinical Judgment

1. Recall that Heather (Meet Your Patient, in Volume 1) is a 20-year-old mother of a 4-year-old preschooler. They have come to a family practice clinic for a well-child checkup. You notice that the child speaks only in one- or two-word phrases. Heather is impatient with her and repeatedly tells her to "stop using that baby talk." Your nursing instructor tells you that you need to assess for teaching needs and provide anticipatory guidance to the mother regarding safety, nutrition, and normal preschool child growth and development.

   a. Heather says, "I don't know what I'm doing wrong. All her little friends are taller and talking more. She was small when she was born, so I suppose it's my fault." How do you assess Heather's learning needs without reinforcing her feelings of self-blame?

   b. Your assessment shows that although the child is below the 5th percentile for height and weight, she has grown appropriately since her last clinic visit. What teaching could you provide that might help address her mother's learning needs related to childhood growth and development?

   c. In addition to information on growth and development, your anticipatory guidance should include safety measures and nutrition for a 4-year-old. How can you evaluate whether your teaching has been effective and further promote Heather's retention of this new information?

2. Your instructor tells you that you need to begin teaching for discharge as soon as the client is admitted. You hear the nurses complaining that they just do not have time for any teaching. So where do you begin? You will need to use the teaching process for your assigned client.

   Your client is a 9-year-old girl who is being admitted to the outpatient procedures unit for testing because of chronic recurrent urinary tract infections. She receives on a daily basis an antibiotic, lisdexamfetamine dimesylate (Vyvanse) for attention-deficit hyperactivity disorder (ADHD), and an asthma inhaler to help her participate in sports activities. She is accompanied by her mother and father; a younger sister; and her big, pink teddy bear. She is scheduled for x-ray studies and blood work. Depending on the results of her tests, she may require surgery or dilation of her ureters. The parents appear very anxious and tell you that their daughter "has a hard time understanding things and needs a lot of repetition." You have an hour to prepare her for the procedures and testing.

   a. Assessment/Recognizing Cues

      (1) What information do you already have that will be significant for your teaching plan?

      (2) What other information will you need to gather?

   b. Nursing Diagnosis/Analyzing Cues

      (1) What possible nursing diagnoses are involved in this situation? Consider a diagnosis for your client and another one for at least one of her family members.

   c. Planning/Prioritizing Hypotheses and Generating Solutions

      (1) What information will you present first?

      (2) What teaching techniques would you use for this situation?

      (3) Who would you include in the teaching?

      (4) Where would you complete the teaching?

d. Implementation/Taking Action

   (1) Write an appropriate goal for your client (the child). Remember to make the goal client centered, timed, and realistic. You have only an hour to complete this teaching.

   (2) What content and methods would you include in your teaching plan?

   (3) How can you incorporate the client's teddy bear in your teaching?

e. Evaluation

   (1) How would you determine whether your teaching was effective?

   (2) What further teaching do you need to continue to prepare your client for discharge?

3. For each of the following situations, determine which teaching techniques would be most effective.

   a. A group of adolescents with diabetes are preparing for their prom. The after-prom party lasts until 6:00 a.m. and will interfere with their usual schedule for insulin administration. You need to help them decide how to manage this problem. They are all busy with after-school activities and attend three different schools.

   b. An 80-year-old man has had a cerebrovascular accident (CVA, also called stroke) with right-side weakness. He will need mobility training and assessment of his home situation for safety hazards. Currently he lives alone.

   c. A new mother must learn how to feed her infant, who has a cleft palate. She is in considerable pain after an emergency Caesarean section and unexpected blood loss.

4. You are assigned to a client with a diagnosis that you are unfamiliar with. You are expected to prepare a teaching session for this client and family and for your classmates. How should you prepare for this assignment?

5. Give an example of teaching content you might need to present to a 58-year-old patient who has been diagnosed with hypertension. What chapters in this text (Volume 1) might be useful if you need theoretical knowledge about hypertension to answer this question? Where would you look to find out where this information is located?

6. Do you think it is appropriate for a nurse to offer personal experiences in the teaching process? Explain your thinking.

7. A client refuses to make eye contact during a teaching session. This makes it difficult for you to determine whether they are paying attention to what you are saying. How can you assess whether they are focused on the teaching session?

8. For each of the following concepts, use critical thinking to describe how or why it is important to nursing, patient care, or teaching clients. Note that these are *not* to be merely definitions.

Role of teaching in nursing practice	Choice of techniques
Principles of teaching and learning	Relevance
Factors that affect the learning process	Learning styles
Factors that affect the teaching process	Amount of information to be presented
Timing	

What Are the Main Points in This Chapter?

- Teaching is an essential component of professional nursing.
- Nurses do formal and informal teaching for individuals and groups.
- To be effective, teaching requires cooperation between the learner and the teacher.
- Learning is a change in behavior, knowledge, skills, or attitudes that occurs because of exposure to environmental stimuli.
- Bloom and Krathwohl (1956) identified three domains of learning: cognitive, psychomotor, and affective.
- Krathwohl (2002) adapted Bloom's model describing learning using a more outcomes-based approach: remember, understand, apply, analyze, evaluate, and create.
- Teaching includes motivating the learner.
- Teaching is interactive and requires communication.
- Readiness means that the learner is both motivated and able to learn at a specific time.
- Other factors that affect learning include emotions, timing, active involvement, feedback, repetition, environment, amount and complexity of the content, communication, developmental stage, culture, and literacy.
- Common barriers to teaching in the hospital setting include failure to see teaching as a priority and lack of time, preparation, space, privacy, poor coordination, and third-party reimbursement for teaching.
- Barriers to learning include illness, physical discomfort and fatigue, anxiety, low health literacy, environmental distraction, overwhelming amount of behavioral change needed, lack of time, lack of positive reinforcement, and feelings of discouragement.
- The teaching process is similar to the nursing process.
- The NANDA-I nursing diagnosis of deficient knowledge may be the primary problem or the etiology of other problems; this diagnosis is often overused or used incorrectly.
- A teaching plan is similar to a nursing care plan, except that (1) interventions are actually teaching strategies and (2) the plan includes the content of the teaching, the sequencing of the content, and the materials to be used.
- Demonstration and return demonstration are the most effective strategies for teaching psychomotor skills.
- A certain amount of forgetting is normal. You can aid learner retention by using strategies that require learner participation and by providing printed materials to use at a later time.
- It is important to document specifically what teaching you did as well as your evaluation of the learning that occurred.

CHAPTER 16 Patient Education   155

Knowledge Map

STANDARDS
- ANA
- The Joint Commission
- Patient Care Partnership
- Pew Commission

INFORMAL — independent nursing action

FORMAL

TEACHING
Interactive process/activity intended to meet outcomes

using

TEACHING STRATEGIES
- Lecture
- Group/individual discussion
- Demo/return demo
- Multimedia
- Pamphlets, instruction sheets
- Simulation
- Role-playing
- Independent instruction
- Use of Internet
- Gaming

Use a combination of strategies to affect all three domains

COGNITIVE DOMAIN
Storage and recall

PSYCHOMOTOR DOMAIN
Physical skill

AFFECTIVE DOMAIN
Change in attitude, feeling, or belief

LEARNING
Change in behavior, knowledge, skill, or attitude

FACTORS AFFECTING LEARNING
- Motivation
- Readiness
- Environment
- Timing/scheduling
- Use of feedback, repetition
- Content and how it is communicated
- Developmental stage
- Culture
- Literacy

Is learning successful?

EVALUATE USING
- Written tests
- Oral interview/questionnaires
- Return demonstration
- Analysis of client report

CHAPTER 17

Interprofessional Partnerships: Documenting & Reporting

STUDENT RESOURCES

The questions and exercises in Volume 2 allow you to practice the kind of thinking you will use as a full-spectrum nurse. Critical-thinking questions usually have more than one right answer, so we do not provide "correct" answers for these features. Try to answer these questions yourself. It is more important to develop your nursing judgment than to just cover content. You will learn by discussing the questions with your peers. If you are still unsure, see the Davis Advantage chapter resources for suggested responses.

To explore learning resources for this chapter,

Go to www.DavisAdvantage.com and find:

Answers and Suggested Responses for all questions in this chapter
Concept Map
Knowledge Map
References and Bibliography

Key Concepts

Documentation
Oral reporting

Related Concepts

See the Concept Map on Davis Advantage.

Caring for the Williams Family

Nadine Williams arrives at the Family Medicine Clinic complaining of pain and drainage from her right eye. She requests an appointment. As part of your clinical experience working as a triage nurse at the clinic, you must evaluate the client's status and determine whether she needs to be seen today. What follows is your conversation with Mrs. Williams:

Mrs. Williams: I don't have an appointment, but I need to see someone today. My husband is a client here. I have an appointment in 2 weeks for a physical, but I've never been here before. I just can't wait 2 weeks.

You: What seems to be the problem?

Mrs. Williams: My eye is killing me. My right one. It burns and stings, and there's all this nasty gunk coming out. I think I need some medicine for it.

You: Tell me a little more about this problem. When did this start?

Mrs. Williams: I woke up yesterday with a painful, itchy eye. I used some saline drops, but

156

Caring for the Williams Family (continued)

the eye seems to be worse. I work at a preschool, and they won't let me work unless I take care of this. I also think I need to be checked for other things. I haven't had an appointment in a long time. I suppose I just need some tests. My husband just found out he has high blood pressure, but I don't think I do. I guess I'm not old enough. I'm 55, but my mother got high blood pressure when she was 70.

As she is talking, you notice a large amount of thick, yellow-green drainage in the corner of her right eye and the eye is reddened. She is rubbing this eye vigorously and dabbing at it with a tissue. The skin is puffy around the eye as well. Her left eye is slightly red, but there is no drainage.

Her vital signs are as follows: blood pressure, 132/76 mm Hg; heart rate, 88 beats/min; respirations, 18 breaths/min; and temperature, 37.2°C (98.9°F). Based on your brief assessment, you ask the receptionist to give Mrs. Williams an urgent appointment.

A. Document two entries to describe the events. First, make a brief narrative note.

B. Next, construct a SOAP(IER) note. Be sure to follow documentation guidelines when you prepare your note.

PracticalKnowledge clinical application

Material in this section will help you to assess and plan care for families.

CLINICAL INSIGHTS

Clinical Insight 17-1 ▶ Giving Oral Reports

For All Types of Report Formats

Remember the acronym CUBAN (Currie, 2002):
- **C**onfidential
- **U**ninterrupted
- **B**rief
- **A**ccurate
- **N**amed nurse

Use a Standardized Format Such as the Following

PACE

Client/Problem—Include client's name, room number, diagnosis, reason for admission, and recent procedures. State the present problem. Summarize medical history relevant to the current problem.

Assessment/Actions—Nursing assessments and interventions directed to the problem

Continuing/Changes—Continuing needs and potential changes include:
- Client care and treatments that must be monitored on other shifts (e.g., dressing changes)
- Changes in the client's condition or the care plan, recent or anticipated (e.g., new prescriptions, changes in discharge date)

Evaluation—Evaluation of responses to nursing and medical interventions, progress toward goals, and effectiveness of the plan

SBAR/SBAR-RQ

Identify yourself, the client, and the agency.
Situation—"Here's the situation..."
Background—"The supporting background information is..."
Assessment—"My assessment of the situation is that..."
Recommendation—"I recommend that you..."
[**R**ead back—"To repeat the information and..."]
[**Q**uestions—Questions asked and answered]

(Continued)

Clinical Insight 17-1 ▶ Giving Oral Reports—cont'd

IPASS

Illness severity—Describes the client's illness acuity level
Patient summary—A comprehensive overview of the client (e.g., history, diagnostic test results)
Action list—correlates with interventions (e.g., consultations, prescriptions, medications)
Situation awareness and contingency plans—Overall plan based on client's response (condition deteriorates or improves)
Synthesis by receiver—Confirmation of understanding; message sent is the message received (Clements, 2017; Coolen et al., 2020; The Joint Commission, 2017; Lo et al., 2021)

Include the Following Content

In a handoff report:
- Client's name, age, and room number
- Client's admitting diagnosis—One or several may exist. Status of identified outcomes
- Client's relevant medical history
- Treatments the client has received during this admission, such as surgery, line placements, breathing treatments. Include consultations completed with other disciplines.
- Upcoming consultations, diagnostic tests, surgeries, or treatments
- Client restrictions, such as diet, bedrest, isolation, activity limits
- Plan of care, such as IV therapy, pain management, current medications, wound care, client or family concerns, discharge planning
- Significant assessment findings from the previous shifts
- Teaching conducted

In a transfer report:
- Your name, facility, and phone number
- Client's name, age, sex, gender, and admitting and current diagnoses
- Client's providers(s), if still following client
- Procedures or surgeries performed
- Current medications and last date/time each was taken/time next dose is due
- Client status at present as well as progression since admission
- Last set of vital signs, plus any pertinent trends since admission
- Tubes in place, such as IVs, catheters, drainage tubes, along with the intake and output of each tube or drain
- Presence of wounds or open areas of the skin plus current interventions for each
- Names and contact numbers for family and significant others
- Special directives, such as code status, presence of advance directives, preferred intensity of care, or isolation required
- Reason the client is being transferred
- Location of the aforementioned information (on transfer form, in medical records, etc.)

When your report is finished
- Ask the receiving nurse whether they have any questions.
- Get the nurse's full name and then record it plus the transfer date and time in your transfer documentation.

Practice Resources
Ernst et al. (2018); Gore et al. (2015); The Joint Commission (2017); Coolen et al. (2020); Lo et al. (2021); Podder et al. (2020); Schroeder (2006); Shahid & Thomas (2018); Streeter & Harrington (2017).

Clinical Insight 17-2 ➤ Receiving Telephone and Verbal Prescriptions

✚ You should accept verbal and telephone prescriptions only in specific situations when the primary care provider is not able to electronically submit, write, or enter them personally.

- **Have a second nurse listen to the prescription,** if possible, to verify its accuracy.
- **Write or enter the prescription electronically only if you heard it yourself;** no third-party involvement is acceptable.
- **Repeat the written prescription** even if you believe you have clearly understood it.
- **Spell unfamiliar names** when repeating to be sure the spelling is correct.
- **Pronounce digits of numbers separately.** For example, instead of "seventeen," say "one, seven." Mishearing a number can lead to a serious error in medication dosage.
- **Make sure the prescription makes sense** given the client's current status.
- **Transcribe the prescription directly into the medical record as quickly as possible.** Writing it on a piece of paper and then copying it again onto a paper prescription form or into an EHR introduces an additional chance of error. If entering the prescription into an EHR, it's best to have the EHR's prescription entry area open and begin entering the prescription as the prescriber dictates it to you.
- **Write the prescription while the prescriber remains on the telephone or in the building** so that you can ask any necessary questions immediately without the need for a return call.
- **When writing on a paper prescription form, first document the date and time.** Next write the text of the prescription. Following the text of the prescription, depending on how you received the prescription, write "TO" (telephone order) or "VO" (verbal order) followed by the prescribing provider's name and then your name. The following is an example of a telephone prescription:

  00/00/0000   0815   Morphine 2 mg IV push x1 for pain now. TO Dr. Clayton Kent/Sarah Hogan, RN; prescription read back for verification and validated.

- **Sign electronically to activate the prescription.** If entering the prescription electronically, indicate during entry that it was given verbally or over the telephone, the date and time the prescription was given, and then search for and select the prescribing provider's name. Click "sign" or whatever option in your EHR indicates the prescription is signed and is now active.
- **Be sure you have the provider's phone number** so that you can reach them if future questions arise.
- **All verbal and telephone prescriptions must be countersigned** by the provider within 24 hours or according to agency policy.

Practice Resources

Clinical System Transformation (2022); National Coordinating Council on Medication Error Reporting and Prevention (2015); Institute for Safe Medication (2017); Kelly (2017); Gadre et al. (2022).

Clinical Insight 17-3 ➤ Guidelines for Documentation

GUIDELINE	HOW TO APPLY	RATIONALE OR EXAMPLE
\multicolumn{3}{c}{**When to Document**}
Documentation begins at the start of your shift.	■ *Hospital or long-term care facility*—Start of shift ■ *Home visit or outpatient facility*—When you first encounter the client ■ *On first observation*—Document the condition of your client when you first observed them. Were they awake? Were they in bed? Did they have any complaints? What did you do?	
Document immediately.	Discipline yourself to document as soon as possible after making an observation or providing care.	The longer you wait, the more likely you will forget important details.
Never document ahead.	Never document before performing an intervention.	It is impossible to see into the future and be sure that what you expect to happen will actually happen. Doing this threatens the credibility of the medical records.

(Continued)

Clinical Insight 17-3 ▶ Guidelines for Documentation—cont'd

GUIDELINE	HOW TO APPLY	RATIONALE OR EXAMPLE
Avoid "block" documentation.	Each entry needs to be made individually; record the time each was done.	Do not document an entry time as "From 1300 to 1500."
Document chronologically.	■ *On paper*—Document times in chronological order. ■ *EHRs*—Most automatically insert the current date and time when forms are opened. Follow the documentation system's guidelines for changing those dates and times before signing.	Chronological documentation communicates the changing status of the client.
Designate late entries (paper).	■ If you forget to make an important entry while documenting, you will later need to add "late entry" to the first available line. ■ Record the time and date you are making the addition; clearly designate it is a late entry.	■ Late entry example: 00/00/0000, 1400; late entry for 00/00/0000, 1200
	■ If you know legal action is pending, do not place a late note in the health record without notifying the nurse manager or risk management officer first.	■ It is a criminal offense to alter a client record after the organization's approved time limit for doing so has passed.
Designate late entries (EHR).	■ Open the appropriate form and change the automatically generated current date/time to the date/time your care was actually done; then sign. ■ Follow the agency policy regarding the time period for making a late entry.	

What to Document

Questions to aid your recall.	As your shift or visit progresses, you will perform assessments and nursing interventions. To remind yourself what to record, ask yourself these examples of questions.	■ What were your assessment findings? ■ Did any abnormalities exist? ■ What was the client's response to your intervention? Did any changes occur from the initial assessment?
Interventions, client responses, and evaluation of progress toward goals.	■ These are often recorded on an IPOC. ■ Clearly describe what your client is experiencing. ■ **Key Point:** *Do not document a symptom without also documenting what you did about it and how the client responded.*	(Symptom) Pt complained of pain, rated 6 on a 0–10 scale. (Intervention) Administered Tylenol 1000 mg, by mouth, at 0900. At 1030, client rated pain as 3.
Significant events or changes in condition.	When possible, quote the client's interpretation of the event or change.	Quoting the client directly gives all healthcare providers consistent data.
Informed consent.	■ If you are asked to obtain informed consent for a procedure, document your actions. ■ In most states, your signature (paper or electronic) confirms only that the client signed the consent. ■ For further discussion of informed consent, see Chapters 40 and 41.	The primary provider conducting the procedure is legally responsible for discussing the procedure and its risks and benefits.
Client teaching.	■ Include instruction about medications and client diagnoses. ■ Include discharge teaching. ■ If the client's physical or cognitive condition prevents teaching, explain that in your documentation.	Documenting client teaching can positively affect insurance and other payments to the institution.
Spiritual or other concerns expressed by the client and/or family.	Document your interventions.	Addressing spiritual concerns ensures that the client receives holistic healthcare.

Clinical Insight 17-3 ▸ Guidelines for Documentation—cont'd

GUIDELINE	HOW TO APPLY	RATIONALE OR EXAMPLE
Attempts made to contact the primary care provider.	■ Contacts may, for example, be to notify the provider of the client's condition or to clarify prescriptions. ■ If you are unable to contact the primary provider, document your contacts with your charge nurse, nurse manager, supervisor, medical director, and hospital administrator.	You must indicate that you made every effort to communicate your concerns.
Client leaving the facility against medical advice (AMA).	■ Document the client's condition, any explanations of risks and consequences given to the client, the client's destination (if known), and your notification of the client's care providers. ■ If your facility has specific forms for AMA departures, use the designated form. ■ If the form is hard-copy paper, have the client sign the form before leaving. ■ If the client refuses to sign, note this in your chart.	Your actions and responsibilities in the situation must be clear in the record.
Client's refusal of treatment.	■ Try to determine the reason for refusal. ■ Quote the exact language the client used in this situation whenever possible.	This helps to ensure documentation of facts instead of inferences.
Use of restraints.	■ Most facilities have a separate form that allows you to document the reason for restraint use, the type of restraint, and frequent checks of the client. ■ You must have contacted the primary care provider.	■ The primary care provider must place a signed prescription for restraints in the medical records. ■ Prescription for restraint must be reordered inside a specific timeframe set by the organization or the restraints are discontinued (see Chapter 21).
"Occurrences."	■ Document your findings accurately and objectively. ■ Fill out a separate occurrence form and send to the risk manager (paper forms). ■ Do not refer to the occurrence form anywhere in your documentation.	■ Examples of occurrences: falls and medication errors. ■ Occurrence forms are not part of the client's health record. ▸ Go to **Occurrence Reports,** in Volume 1.
Complete data about medications.	■ *Paper MAR*—Include the date, time, and medication given, and your initials. ■ *Electronic MAR*—Ensure your entry is accurate, then sign electronically the successful administration of the medication.	Accurate documentation is an essential component of the nurse's role.
prn, unscheduled, IV infusions, and STAT medications.	■ Document on the MAR. ■ Include comments regarding the medication in your narrative documentation or insert a comment in your electronic file. ■ Document a timely evaluation of client's response to the medication.	Certain prn medications require a follow-up response be documented within a specific time period set by the organization, usually 15 to 30 minutes after the medication is given.
Medications not administered.	■ Document omission on the MAR. ■ If the client states a reason for refusing the medication: *Paper notes*—Quote the client in your narrative notes. *Electronic MAR*—Use pull-down or other menu.	■ *Examples:* Client refuses medication; dose accidentally omitted. ■ Most electronic MARs include an explanation with a selection from a drop-down list such as "Client refused" or "Client not available." ■ Some MARs also contain a narrative section to type a comment regarding nonadministration of a medication.

(Continued)

Clinical Insight 17-3 ▸ Guidelines for Documentation—cont'd

GUIDELINE	HOW TO APPLY	RATIONALE OR EXAMPLE
\multicolumn{3}{c}{**How to Document**}

GUIDELINE	HOW TO APPLY	RATIONALE OR EXAMPLE
Know your organization's requirements for reimbursement.	■ Requirements typically specify frequency of documentation and the type of data to record. ■ Fulfilling documentation requirements helps to ensure appropriate reimbursement. ■ Home care, hospitals, clinics, office settings, and long-term care facilities have specific guidelines for documentation necessary for payment.	
Date and time all your documentation.	■ Most organizations use a 24-hour clock (military time) to avoid confusion between a.m. and p.m. ■ The day begins at 0001 (1 minute past midnight) and ends at 2400 (12 midnight). ■ *Morning hours*—Most people have little difficulty with early morning hours. Example: 9:00 a.m. is 0900. ■ *Hours after 12 noon*—To convert to military time after 12 noon, simply add 12 to the clock time. Example: 7:30 p.m. + 12 = 1930 in military time.	Many healthcare facilities use the 24-hour clock.
Document accurately and objectively, using nonjudgmental language.	■ Avoid labeling clients or team members. ■ Do not document judgments about decisions made by members of the care team. ■ Document objective facts so the reader can draw an informed conclusion. ■ Quote the client in their own words, when possible.	■ *Document:* "I'm not taking that medicine. Take it away." ■ *Do not document:* "Client obnoxious and refuses prescribed medication."
Avoid vague, subjective words.	■ When possible, give specific examples.	■ Terms such as *good, average,* or *normal* do not clearly define the status of the client. ■ Descriptive details allow caregivers to understand your client's individual needs.
Use only the abbreviations authorized by your organization.	See Tables, Abbreviations Commonly Used in Health Care, following Clinical Insight 17-4.	
Use correct spelling and grammar.	Incorrect spelling may raise questions about what you are attempting to communicate. Incorrect grammar implies carelessness on your part and creates a question of your competence if your documentation is reviewed.	
Document your own nursing actions.	■ Do not allow anyone to document for you. ■ Do not document the actions of others as though you had performed them.	Each nurse is responsible for documenting their own assessments, interventions, and evaluations. A deviation from this principle can imply cover-up, carelessness, or a blatant disregard of policy and standards of practice.
You may need to document the actions of someone else.	■ Try to avoid this, but if you must do it, be sure to clearly designate whose actions they are. ■ EHRs—You can indicate another person performed the action in an added comment or by searching for and selecting the other care provider in the appropriate field, then signing.	For example, if the UAP (unlicensed assistive personnel) helps the client ambulate: *Do not document:* "Client assisted to bathroom." *Do document:* "J. Scott, UAP, assisted client to bathroom."
Avoid documenting what someone else said, heard, felt, or smelled.	■ If the information is critical and you *must* document it, use quotations and attribute the remarks to the person who made them.	*Example:* "Wife stated, 'My husband told me that he is in a lot of pain but does not want to bother the nurses.'"

Clinical Insight 17-4 ▶ Guidelines for Paper Health Records

To comply with HIPAA requirements, paper health records need to be stored in designated areas accessible only to healthcare providers. To ensure your written paper documentation is effective, the forms used must be efficient, comprehensive, and relevant to the client's healthcare needs. The forms should guide you to document appropriately according to your organization's policies and procedures. Use the following guidelines to document appropriately.

- **Maintain confidentiality.** Do not provide written or verbal information to anyone not involved in the direct care of the client without the patient's consent.
- **Ensure you have the correct form** (e.g., I&O sheet, graphic record) before you begin writing.
- **Check that the medical record and documentation forms are clearly marked with the client's name and identification number.**
- **Write legibly, neatly, and in an organized manner.** This enables others to read your entries and use them to make clinical decisions. Sloppy or illegible handwriting creates errors or, at least, leads to poor communication.
- **Always use black ink for handwritten notes (some agencies do permit blue ink).** Inks other than black or blue are not legible when a patient record is photocopied. Do NOT use green or red pen. Remember that the patient record is a legal document.
- **Do not leave blank lines in the narrative notes.** If you need to leave space for clarity, draw a straight line through the area and begin on the next line. Open areas leave an opportunity for later tampering.
- **Draw a line through the incorrect documentation and initial it.** Never use a correction fluid, "ink over," or otherwise cover up written notes.
- **Sign all your paper documentation entries with your first name, last name, and professional credentials,** such as Judy Long, RN.
- **Don't write in "shorthand" or use your own abbreviated symbols.**
- **Use only abbreviations that are approved by your organization.**

TABLES

Abbreviations Commonly Used in Healthcare

ABBREVIATION	MEANING	ABBREVIATION	MEANING
ADL	Activities of daily living	CO_2	Carbon dioxide
ad lib	As desired, if the patient desires	CPR	Cardiopulmonary resuscitation
AKA	Above-knee amputation	CVA	Cerebrovascular accident (stroke)
Amb	Ambulation, ambulatory	D&C	Dilation and curettage
Amt	Amount	DM	Diabetes mellitus
ASAP	As soon as possible	dsg or drsg	Dressing
Bid	Twice a day	DX or Dx	Diagnosis
BM	Bowel movement	EBL	Estimated blood loss
BR	Bedrest	ECG/ECG	Electrocardiogram
BRP	Bathroom privileges	ED/ER	Emergency department, emergency room
BSC	Bedside commode	EEG	Electroencephalogram
c̄	With	EENT	Eyes, ears, nose, throat
Cal	Calories	ETOH	Alcohol
Cath	Catheter	F	Female
CBC	Complete blood count	FBS	Fasting blood sugar
CCU	Critical care unit or coronary care unit	Ft	Foot
c/o	Complaint of		

(Continued)

Abbreviations Commonly Used in Healthcare—cont'd

ABBREVIATION	MEANING	ABBREVIATION	MEANING
Fx	Fracture	NGT	Nasogastric tube
GI	Gastrointestinal	Noc	At night
gtt(s)	Drop(s)	NPO	Nothing by mouth
GU	Genitourinary	O_2	Oxygen
GYN	Gynecology	OB	Obstetrics
HA	Headache	OOB	Out of bed
HMO	Health maintenance organization	OPD	Outpatient department
h/o	History of	Ortho	Orthopedics
hob or HOB	Head of bed	OR	Operating room
HOH	Hard of hearing	Os	Mouth, opening
H&P	History and physical	OT	Occupational therapy
Hr	Hour	Oz	Ounce
Ht	Height	Pc	After meals
HTN	Hypertension	PCA	Patient-controlled analgesia
Hyper	Above or high	PO	By mouth
Hypo	Below or low	P, p̄	After
ICU	Intensive care unit	PPBS	Postprandial blood sugar
I&O	Intake and output	Prn	As needed
Isol	Isolation	Pt	Patient
IV	Intravenous	PT	Physical therapy
IVP	Intravenous push (caution: do not use to mean "IV piggyback")	Q	Every
		Qam	Every morning
L	Liter	Qh	Every hour
lb	Pound	Qid	Four times a day
LPN	Licensed practical nurse	RN	Registered nurse
LMP	Last menstrual period	R/O	Rule out
LVN	Licensed vocational nurse	RX or Rx	Treatment or prescription
Mcg	Microgram	s̄	Without
MD	Medical doctor	SCD	Sequential compression device
Med	Medication	SOB	Short of breath
Mg	Milligram	s̄s̄	One-half
mL	Milliliter	SSE	Soapsuds enema
MN	Midnight	Stat	Immediately
NAS	No added salt	STI or STD	Sexually transmitted infection or sexually transmitted disease
N/V/D	Nausea, vomiting, diarrhea		
NKA or NKDA	No known allergies or no known drug allergies	TB	Tuberculosis
		TO	Telephone order
NG	Nasogastric	TPR	Temperature, pulse, respirations

Abbreviations Commonly Used in Healthcare—cont'd

ABBREVIATION	MEANING	ABBREVIATION	MEANING
Tid	Three times a day	w/c	Wheelchair
VO	Verbal order	WNL	Within normal limits
VS	Vital signs	Wt	Weight
WBC	White blood count		

Key Point: *Abbreviations vary among healthcare agencies. Furthermore, they change rather often because of regulating agency guidelines (e.g., The Joint Commission). Therefore, you will need to be familiar with the abbreviations in the agency in which you work.*

DOCUMENTATION FORMS

Adult admission history electronic screen

CHAPTER 17 Interprofessional Partnerships: Documenting & Reporting

Nursing assessment flowsheets are comprehensive charting documents.

PATIENT CARE FLOW SHEET

Left side (Assessments/Interventions/Lab/Intake/Output/Respiratory columns by DATE/TIME):

- **VS**: TIME, BP, P R, TEMPERATURE
- **ASSESSMENTS / INTERVENTIONS**: ACTIVITY, PAIN LEVEL, INTERVENTION, RESPONSE, DR. VISIT
- **LAB**
- **INTAKE**: DIET / APPETITE, PO, IV, IV TUBE / SITE CONDITION
- **OUTPUT**: URINE, BM
- SAFETY, PERSONAL CARES
- **RESPIRATORY**: ☐ HEATED, ☐ COOL MIST, ☐ CROUP TENT, F1O2, LIST, O2, LPM, ADJ, O2 SAT, RA, O2, INC SPIRO
- INITIAL

Breath sound assessments (3 sets):
TIME ___ BREATH / PULSE Before / After / LU LL SOUNDS RU RL / ☐ ☐ CLEAR ☐ ☐ / ☐ ☐ CRACKLES ☐ ☐ / ☐ ☐ RHONCHI ☐ ☐ / ☐ ☐ WHEEZING ☐ ☐ / ☐ ☐ DIMINISHED ☐ ☐ / ☐ ☐ ABSENT ☐ ☐
After Treatment Eval: ☐ NO CHANGE ☐ IMPROVED ☐ ADVERSE
DRUG ___ ☐ P&PD ___ INITIAL

PUPIL SIZE
1 mm 2 mm 3 mm 4 mm 5 mm 6 mm 7 mm 8 mm

GLASGOW COMA SCALE

Child		Adult	
Eye Opening		**Eye Opening**	
Spontaneous	4	Spontaneous	4
To sounds	3	To speech	3
To painful stimulation	2	To pain	2
None	1	Nil	1
Motor Responses		**Motor Responses**	
Spontaneous Movement	6	Obeys commands	6
Localizes to pain	5	Localizes pain	5
Withdraws	4	Withdrawal	4
Reflex flexion	3	Abnormal flexion	3
Reflex extension (decerebrate)	2	Extensor rigidity	2
None (flaccid)	1	Nil	1
Verbal Responses		**Verbal Responses**	
Appropriate words or social smile; fixes and follows	5	Oriented	5
Cries, but consolable	4	Confused	4
Persistently irritable	3	Inappropriate	3
Restless, agitated	2	Incomprehensible	2
None	1	Nil	1

NEUROVASCULAR RATING SCALE
EXTREMITY: RA, LA, RL, LL CAP REFILL: NOR = <3 SEC * = >3 SEC
COLOR: NOR = NORMAL DU = DUSTY RED = RED PALE = PALE
SENSATION: NOR = INTACT NUMB = NUMBNESS TIN = TINGLING Ø = ABSENT
MOTION: FULL = FULL LTD = LIMITED Ø = NONE PAIN: RATE (0-10)
PULSES: NOR = NORMAL - = DIMINISHED Ø = NOT PALPABLE DOP = DOPPLER

STRENGTH (DESIGNATE EXTREMITY)
5 = NORMAL STRENGTH   2 = LIFTS, FALLS BACK
4 = LIFTS AGAINST RESISTANCE   1 = MUSCLE CONTRACTION, NO MOVEMENT
3 = LIFTS AGAINST GRAVITY   0 = NO MUSCLE CONTRACTION, NO MOVEMENT

ADJUCANTS FOR O2 ADMINISTRATION
NC Nasal Cannula M Mask NRB Non Rebreather
TT Trans Trach ET Endotracheal Tube

Activity	Personal Cares/Safety	Diet
AMB - Ambulating	AM - AM Care	R - Regular
ARMS - Being held	PA - PM/HS Care	S - Soft
BR - Bed rest	CLWR - Call Light Within Reach	NA - Low Sodium
CH - Chair		LF - Low Fat
L - Lavatory	OR - Oral Care	MS - Mechanical Soft
ROM - Range of motion	SH - Shower	ADA - Diabetic Diet
SLP - Sleeping	SP - Sponge	CL - Clear Liquids
T/P - Turned/Positioned	SK - Skin Care	FL - Full Liquids
↑c̄ - Up with assist	SR↑ - Side rails up	ICE - Ice Chips
↑s̄ - Up without assist	SR↓ - Side rails down	ø - Refused
DA - Dangle	L△ - Linen changed	
CO - Commode	PE - Peri care	
IV Site/Condition	FO - Foley care	**Wound Interventions**
✓ - No redness, swelling, leakage	SN - Snack	DDI - Dressing dry, intact
DC - Discontinued	BA - Backrub	DRNG - Drainage
INF - Infiltrated	**Lab Values**	D△ - Dressing change
SWL - Swelling	✓ - Physician notified	SSG - Serosanguinous
D△ - Dressing change		SWL - Swelling
T△ - Tubing change		O - Odor

PAIN ASSESSMENT IN ADULTS
0 (NO PAIN) 1 2 3 4 5 6 7 8 9 10 (WORST PAIN)

INIT.	SIGNATURE / TITLE	INIT.	SIGNATURE / TITLE

PATIENT NAME

CLINICAL REASONING
Applying the Full-Spectrum Nursing Model

PATIENT SITUATION

Ellen Smith is 85 years old and has sustained a right-sided cerebrovascular accident (CVA, stroke, or brain attack). Doctors say she is unlikely to regain much physical function, even if she awakens from the coma. Her children, Mary and Dale, have met with the provider, who tells them that Ellen is not likely to survive. The provider wants to insert a feeding tube and has asked whether Mary and Dale want Ellen to be resuscitated in case of cardiac or respiratory arrest. Mary tells you she wants to do what is best for her mother, but she feels that Ellen would not want to be kept alive in this condition. She is also concerned about putting her through uncomfortable procedures if there is no chance of recovery. Her brother, Dale, says, "Mom needs the feeding tube. I can't sit and watch her starve to death. As long as she's alive, there's hope."

THINKING

1. *Theoretical Knowledge (Recall of Facts and Principles):* You plan to use the Focus Charting format to document this interaction.

    a. Write the focus for this note.

    b. What does the acronym DAR stand for?

2. *Critical Thinking (Contextual Awareness):*

    a. What aspects of this situation have you experienced or observed before in your role as a caregiver?

    b. How might those past experiences affect your perception in this situation?

DOING

3. *Practical Knowledge (Handoff Report):* Ellen's last name is Smith; assume her children are also named Smith. Ellen is in room 820. Using the PACE format, what would you say to the oncoming nurse during handoff report? You will be able to address only a small amount of physiological information because the scenario does not provide it.

CARING

4. *Self-Knowledge:* In what way(s) can you identify with any of the people involved in this scenario?

Critical Thinking and Clinical Judgment

1. You are caring for a 96-year-old patient, James Wilson. Mr. Wilson has been admitted to the hospital for pneumonia. He is normally alert and oriented to place, time, and person. However, during this admission he has become confused and agitated. He frequently yells at staff and resists care by kicking and hitting. While you are providing morning care, Mr. Wilson becomes very agitated and yells and curses at you. When you attempt to provide oral hygiene, he throws his dentures at you. The dentures break when they hit the floor.

    a. Construct a nurse's note that documents this situation using the paper format you prefer.

    b. You will need to complete an occurrence report regarding the broken dentures. The report asks you to identify actions that you might have taken to prevent this incident. Brainstorm this question with your peers. Identify one or two actions that might have prevented this incident.

2. The primary care provider has written a prescription on your client's paper medical record that you find illegible. A veteran nurse states that they can read it, and they translate it for you. What factors should you consider before determining how to proceed?

3. For each of the following concepts, use critical thinking to describe how or why it is important to nursing, client care, or documenting and reporting. Consider both paper and electronic documentation in each. Note that these are *not* to be merely definitions.

Narrative documentation	Flowsheets
SOAP(IER) documentation	Charting by exception
Nursing admission database	Signing documentation forms
Medication administration record	Handoff report
Occurrence report	Late entry

What Are the Main Points in This Chapter?

- The client record is a collection of documents that form a legal record of the client's healthcare experience.
- The client record is used by health professionals to communicate about the client's care, to legally document the care delivered to the client and the client's responses to that delivered care, to document care for reimbursement, to educate students, to determine whether care is adequate, as a data source for health research, and as the basis for determining the cost of care.
- In source-oriented records, members of each discipline record findings in a separately labeled section.
- In problem-oriented records, members of each discipline document on shared notes, and the record is organized around a problem list.
- In electronic health records (EHRs), members of each discipline all document inside the same EHR. The EHR can be organized as source-oriented, problem-oriented, or a combination of the two.
- The EHR can be accessed by many members of the healthcare team at the same time.
- The narrative format tells the story of what has occurred in a chronological format.
- SOAP(IER) is an acronym for subjective data, objective data, assessment, plan (and intervention, evaluation, and revision). This format may be used to address a single problem or to document summative notes on a client.
- In Focus Charting, data are entered in a data–action–response (DAR) format.
- Charting by exception (CBE) uses preprinted or electronic flowsheets to document most aspects of care. CBE assumes that unless a separate entry is made—an exception—all standards have been met and the client has responded as expected.

- Paper and electronic flowsheets and graphic records are used to record recurring assessments, such as vital signs, intake and output, weight, hygiene, and ADLs.
- Paper progress notes, although not common due to the move to electronic records, may be used to document the client's responses to care. They may be in the form of narrative, SOAP(IER), PIE, or Focus-style notes.
- A discharge summary should be completed when the client is discharged from the organization. A transfer form should be completed when the client is transferred within the organization.
- An occurrence report, or incident report, is a formal record of an unusual occurrence or accident that is not part of the client's medical record.
- The most commonly used home health documentation form is OASIS, a federally required form that includes history, assessment, demographics, and information about the client's and caregiver's abilities.
- Federal law requires that a resident in long-term care be evaluated using the Minimum Data Set for Resident Assessment and Care Screening (MDS) within 14 days of admission. The MDS must be updated within the specified time frame and with any significant change in client condition.
- The handoff report is designed to alert the next nurse about the client's status, changes in the client condition, planned activities, tests or procedures, or concerns that require follow-up.
- A consistent, structured (standardized) format should be used in handoff reports that contain critical key items to minimize miscommunication and other errors.

- Nurses should not take verbal and telephone prescriptions unless the prescribing provider is in a situation in which the prescription cannot be entered electronically or the client is in a life-threatening situation.
- Telephone prescriptions offer more room for error because of unfamiliar terminology and differences in background noise.
- Documentation should be accurate and nonjudgmental.
- You should document as soon as possible after you make an observation or provide care.
- You should never share your electronic username or password with someone else.
- Document any significant events or changes in condition, teaching performed, use of restraints, and client refusal of treatment or medications.
- You are responsible for documenting the care you provided. Never document the actions of others as though you had performed them.
- You are legally and ethically required to question a provider's prescription that you believe is inappropriate or unsafe.

CHAPTER 17 Interprofessional Partnerships: Documenting & Reporting 171

Knowledge Map

DOCUMENTATION

Systems:
- **ELECTRONIC HEALTH RECORD** — All disciplines document in one record
- **PROBLEM-ORIENTED** — All disciplines chart to problems
- **SOURCE-ORIENTED** — Separate sections for each discipline

TYPES:
- Narrative
- SOAP(IER)
- PIE
- Focus
- CBE
- FACT

USE OF NURSING PROCESS

NURSES CHART ON:
- Admission data forms
- Flowsheets
- MAR
- Progress notes
- Kardex
- IPOC
- Discharge summary
- Occurrence report
- Graphic records
- Checklists
- I&O

PURPOSES:
- Communication
- Legal documentation
- Quality improvement
- Legislative requirements
- Professional standards of care
- Reimbursement
- Education
- Research

UNIQUE SETTINGS:
- Long-term care: MDS
- Home care: OASIS

Recording → PATIENT CARE

- Verbal orders
- Telephone orders

Communicating ← REPORTING

Handoff:
- SBAR
- PACE
  - Patient's name, diagnosis
  - PMH, treatments, tests
  - Significant assessments
  - Plan of care

Transfer:
- Unit-to-unit
- Facility-to-facility

CHAPTER 18

Measuring Vital Signs

STUDENT RESOURCES

The questions and exercises in this book allow you to practice the kind of thinking you will use as a full-spectrum nurse. Critical-thinking questions usually have more than one right answer, so we do not provide "correct" answers for these features. Try to answer these questions yourself. It is more important to develop your nursing judgment than to just cover content. You will learn more by discussing the questions with your peers. If you are still unsure, see the Davis Advantage chapter resources for suggested responses.

To explore learning resources for this chapter,

Go to www.DavisAdvantage.com and find:

Answers and Suggested Responses for all questions in this chapter
Concept Map
Knowledge Map
References and Bibliography

Key Concepts

Oxygenation
Perfusion (pulse, blood pressure)
Thermoregulation
Vital signs

Related Concepts

See the Concept Map on Davis Advantage.

Caring for the Williams Family

Recall that on Stanley Williams' preliminary visit to the Family Medicine Center, his blood pressure (BP) was 162/94 mm Hg. On subsequent visits, his BP was 168/100 mm Hg and 174/96 mm Hg, and he was continuing to gain weight. Mr. Williams was diagnosed with hypertension and prescribed an antihypertension medication to be taken each morning. This morning Mr. Williams has come to the clinic for follow-up. The following information is gathered as he checks in for his visit.

VS: BP, 168/92 mm Hg; pulse, 80 beats/min; respirations, 20 breaths/min; temperature, 98.4°F (36.9°C)
Weight: 210 lb (95 kg)

Caring for the Williams Family (continued)

Review the preliminary data and the preceding information to answer the following questions:

A. What patterns do you see in the data?

B. Do you have enough information to draw any conclusions? If not, what other information should you gather?

C. Identify three alternatives that may explain what is happening with Mr. Williams' vital signs.

D. How could you determine which of these alternatives provides the best explanation of what is happening?

E. Why is it important to intervene in this situation?

PracticalKnowledge clinical application

Use the Procedures, Clinical Insights, and tables in this section when assessing your clients' vital signs.

PROCEDURES

Procedure 18-1 ■ Assessing Body Temperature

▶ For steps to follow in *all* procedures, refer to the Universal Steps for All Procedures on the inside back cover.

Equipment
- Thermometer (an oral thermometer generally has a blue tip; a rectal thermometer generally has a red tip)
- Thermometer cover, if needed
- Procedure gloves, if taking a rectal temperature or if there is risk of contact with body fluids (e.g., saliva)
- Water-soluble lubricant, if taking a rectal temperature
- Towel, if needed, for taking an axillary temperature *(to dry the axillae)*
- Tissues

Delegation
You can delegate temperature measurement to unlicensed assistive personnel (UAP) if you conclude that the patient's condition and the UAP's skills allow. Perform the preprocedure assessments and inform the UAP of the route and type of thermometer used. Explain to the UAP any special considerations (e.g., patient's oral intake in the last 20 to 30 minutes; patient is confused). Ask the UAP to document and immediately report a temperature greater than 37.8°C (100°F) or lower than 36.6°C (97.9).

Preprocedure Assessments
- Determine the most appropriate site for the patient. Consider patient comfort, safety, and accuracy of measurements. For example, do not use the oral route for a patient who is unable to hold the thermometer properly, for children or others who cannot follow instructions (e.g., unconscious patients), or for patients who use mouth breathing.
- For an oral temperature: Determine how long it has been since the patient smoked, had anything to eat or drink, or chewed gum. If so, wait 20 to 30 minutes before taking the temperature.

Smoking, eating, drinking, and chewing gum can all affect an oral reading.

(continued on next page)

Procedure 18-1 ■ Assessing Body Temperature (continued)

- Assess for any contraindications to using the site you have chosen. For example:

  Tympanic: Assess for impacted earwax or hearing aid.

  Rectal: Check the patient record for diarrhea or impacted stool.

  Axillary: Check the patient record for presence of fever or hypothermia.

Skin: Assess for the presence of conditions that require a very precise, reliable reading (e.g., fever, hypothermia).
Some conditions increase the risk for patient injury; others contribute to inaccurate, unreliable temperature measurement.

- What were the previous recordings, if any?
Noting changes over time is important in all patient assessments.

- Assess for clinical signs and symptoms of temperature alterations.

Procedure 18-1A ■ Taking an Axillary Temperature

> When performing the procedure, always identify your patient according to agency policy, using two identifiers, and be attentive to standard precautions, hand hygiene, patient safety and privacy, body mechanics, and documentation.

Procedure Steps

1. **Position the client supine or sitting.**

2. **Dry the patient's axilla,** as needed.
Moisture from perspiration alters the temperature reading.

3. **Slide the thermometer into a protective sheath** (depending on type of thermometer).
A protective sheath provides a barrier to prevent transmission of organisms.

4. **Place the thermometer tip** in the middle of the axilla.

5. **Position the patient's upper arm down,** with the lower arm across the chest.
Puts the thermometer close to the axillary blood vessels, allowing it to better reflect the core temperature. >

6. **Hold the thermometer in place** for the recommended time.
   a. Leave an electronic probe in place until it beeps.
   b. Leave a nonelectronic thermometer in place for 8 minutes, or according to agency policy (usually 5 minutes for children).
   Study findings differ for accuracy of temperature measurements at the axillary site. Follow agency policy.

7. **Read the temperature.**
   a. **Electronic thermometer:** Read the digital display; remove the thermometer.
   b. **Glass thermometer:** Remove the thermometer, hold it at eye level, and rotate it until the markings are clear. Avoid using glass, if possible.

8. **After removing the thermometer,** discard the cover. If there is no cover, wipe the thermometer with a tissue.
Removes any moisture that may have accumulated.

9. **Clean and replace the thermometer** in the storage base, following agency policy.
Prevents microbial growth on thermometers and recharges the battery.

CHAPTER 18 Measuring Vital Signs   175

Procedure 18-1B ■ Taking an Oral Temperature

➤ When performing the procedure, always identify your patient according to agency policy, using two identifiers, and be attentive to standard precautions, hand hygiene, patient safety and privacy, body mechanics, and documentation.

Procedure Steps

1. **If you must use a glass or plastic thermometer,** shake down the liquid if necessary.
   a. Stand in an open area away from tables and other objects.
      Prevents thermometer breakage.
   b. Hold the end opposite the bulb between your thumb and forefinger, and snap your wrist downward.
   c. Shake the thermometer until the reading is less than 36°C (96°F).
      The reading must be lower than the anticipated temperature measurement.

2. **Slide the thermometer into** a protective sheath.
   Provides a barrier to prevent transmission of microorganisms.

3. **Place the thermometer tip** under the tongue in the posterior sublingual pocket (right or left of frenulum).
   Puts the tip close to the major blood vessels under the tongue, allowing the thermometer to reflect the core temperature. ➤

4. **Have the patient close their lips** around the thermometer, cautioning them not to bite down on it.
   Protects the thermometer from exposure to the air, which could alter the reading. Biting may break a glass thermometer, injuring the mouth.

5. **Leave the thermometer in place** for the recommended time.
   a. Glass or plastic thermometer: 5 to 8 minutes, according to agency policy.
   b. Electronic (digital) thermometer: Until it beeps.
      Research findings differ on the optimal time for measuring an oral temperature, so follow agency policy.

6. **Read the temperature.**
   a. **Glass thermometer:** Position the thermometer at eye level and rotate it until the markings are clear. ▼
   b. **Electronic thermometer:** Read the digital display.

7. **After removing the thermometer,** discard the cover. If there is no cover, wipe the thermometer with an antimicrobial or alcohol-based wipe.
   Wiping removes mucus that can make the markings on a glass thermometer difficult to read.

8. **Clean and replace the thermometer.** Follow agency policy.
   Prevents microbial growth on thermometers and recharges battery of electronic thermometers.

Procedure 18-1C ■ Taking a Rectal Temperature

➤ When performing the procedure, always identify your patient according to agency policy, using two identifiers, and be attentive to standard precautions, hand hygiene, patient safety and privacy, body mechanics, and documentation.

➤ *Note:* This procedure primarily describes use of an electronic (digital) thermometer.

Procedure Steps

1. **Slide the thermometer into a protective sheath.**
   A protective sheath provides a barrier to prevent transmission of microorganisms.

2. **Position an adult patient** in Sims position (on the side with the knees flexed); drape the patient so that only the anal area is exposed. ➤

Step Variation Taking a Rectal Temperature for a Small Child
Place the child in the prone position. You can lay the child face down across your lap or a parent's lap.
Flexing the knees helps relax the muscles to ease insertion and aid in visualization. Draping provides privacy and decreases embarrassment.

(continued on next page)

Procedure 18-1 ■ Assessing Body Temperature (continued)

3. **Lubricate the tip** of the thermometer by squeezing water-soluble lubricant onto a tissue and then applying it to the thermometer.
   Prevents injury to the rectal mucosa and eases insertion. Inserting the thermometer into the lubricant container would contaminate contents of the container.

4. **Don a procedure glove** on your dominant hand, or on both hands if necessary.

5. **With your nondominant hand,** separate the patient's buttocks to visualize the anus.

6. **Gently insert the thermometer** approximately:
   Adult: 1 to 1.5 in. (2.5 to 3.7 cm)
   Child: 0.9 in. (2.5 cm)
   Infant: 0.5 in. (1.5 cm)

The thermometer must be placed past the rectal sphincter.

a. Have the patient take a deep breath. Insert the thermometer as they exhale.
   Taking a deep breath helps relax the anal sphincter.

b. If you feel resistance, do not use force.
   Inserting the thermometer too far or forcing against resistance may injure the rectal mucosa. ▼

7. **Hold the thermometer in place** until it beeps. (For a plastic, or glass if you must use it, thermometer, hold the thermometer 3 to 5 minutes.)
   The thermometer must be held in place to prevent inadvertent injury to the patient. An electronic thermometer will beep when a constant temperature is reached. Research differs on the optimal time for measuring a rectal temperature, so follow agency policy.

8. **Remove the thermometer,** discard the cover, and read the digital display.

9. **Remove the procedure glove(s)** and discard in a biohazards container.

10. **Follow agency policy** for cleaning and storing thermometers.
    Prevents microbial growth on thermometers and recharges electronic thermometer battery.

Procedure 18-1D ■ Taking a Temporal Artery Temperature

➤ When performing the procedure, always identify your patient according to agency policy, using two identifiers, and be attentive to standard precautions, hand hygiene, patient safety and privacy, body mechanics, and documentation.

➤ *Note:* If the patient has been lying down, do not measure the temperature on the side that was lying on the pillow. Do not measure if a cap or hair has been covering the area over the temporal artery, as these can prevent heat dissipation and produce a falsely high reading.

Procedure Steps

1. **Remove the protective cap** from the instrument; clean the lens/probe according to the manufacturer's instructions.

2. **Place the probe flat** on the center of the forehead, midway between the eyebrow and the hairline. ▼

3. **Press and hold the button** while you stroke the thermometer medially to laterally across the forehead; keep the lens/probe flat and in contact with the skin and slide in a reasonably straight line until you reach the hairline. ▼

4. **Still holding the button,** touch the thermometer lens/probe behind the earlobe in the soft depression below the mastoid.
   This step is necessary for an accurate reading if there is any moisture at all on the patient's forehead. ▼

5. **Release the button for** the temperature reading. ▸

Procedure 18-1E ■ Taking a Tympanic Membrane Temperature

▸ When performing the procedure, always identify your patient according to agency policy, using two identifiers, and be attentive to standard precautions, hand hygiene, patient safety and privacy, body mechanics, and documentation.

Procedure Steps

1. **Make sure the thermometer** lens is intact and clean.
   Ensures an accurate reading.

2. **Place a disposable cover tightly** over the lens, making sure the clear film is smooth across the lens.
   Ensures an accurate reading and prevents cross-contamination.

3. **Position the patient's head** to one side. If you are right-handed, try to use the right ear; if you are left-handed, use the left ear.
   This allows you to better visualize the ear canal.

4. **Straighten the ear canal** or follow the manufacturer's instructions. As a rule: ▾

   a. **For an adult,** pull the pinna up and back. ▾

   b. **For a child,** pull the pinna down and back. ▾

   Some tympanic thermometers require you to straighten the ear canal; others do not. Some instruct, for adults, to pull the ear up, backward, and slightly away from the head. Some models instruct, for a child, to pull the pinna *straight back instead of down and back. The external auditory canal is curved upward in children younger than 3 years of age. In an adult, it is a slightly S-shaped structure.*

5. **Insert the probe into the ear** canal gently and firmly, directing it toward the tympanic membrane and inserting far enough to seal the opening.
   Creates a seal to obtain an accurate reading without causing trauma to the ear canal.

6. **Rotate the probe handle** toward the jaw (for some thermometer models). Follow the manufacturer's instructions; not all models require this.
   Aims the lens toward the tympanic membrane.

7. **Take the measurement.**
   a. Press and release the button to obtain the reading.
   b. Follow the instructions for the specific tympanic thermometer being used.
   Some tympanic thermometers record the reading immediately; for some you must wait for about 3 seconds.

(continued on next page)

Procedure 18-1 ■ Assessing Body Temperature (continued)

8. **Remove the thermometer** when you hear a beep and the display flashes. Note the reading in the display window.

9. **Repeat the measurement** in the other ear or, in the alternative, use the same ear for each measurement.

Research shows a significant difference in temperature in the left compared with the right ear due to individual variations, presence of dirt or earwax, or other factors (Levander & Grodzinsky, 2017; Microlife, 2022).

10. **Discard the probe cover** (usually you will press an "eject" button to do this) and replace the thermometer in its charging base.

Recharges the battery to ensure its usability during the shift and protects the instrument.

Procedure 18-1F ■ Taking a Skin Temperature Using a Chemical Strip Thermometer

▶ When performing the procedure, always identify your patient according to agency policy, using two identifiers, and be attentive to standard precautions, hand hygiene, patient safety and privacy, body mechanics, and documentation.

Procedure Steps

1. **Place the thermometer strip** (paper or tape) on the patient's skin, generally on the forehead or abdomen. *The thermometer strip must be in contact with the skin to work properly.* ▼

2. **Leave the thermometer strip** in place 15 to 60 seconds (or as the manufacturer directs).

3. **Observe for color changes.**
Chemical strips have indicators that change colors to indicate temperature changes.

4. **Read the temperature before** removing the strip from the patient's skin.
Ensures the most accurate reading.

5. **Remove and discard** the thermometer strip.

? What if . . .

- **The patient's temperature is not within normal range?**

  Identify whether the temperature reading indicates hypothermia, fever, or hyperthermia (e.g., heatstroke).

  Perform other assessments to determine the cause or severity of the findings.

  Assess for clinical signs to confirm an abnormal temperature reading.

  Institute interventions to raise or lower temperature, as appropriate.

  Provide comfort measures (e.g., change linens if they are wet from diaphoresis).

- **I must use a glass thermometer?**

  ✚ Be sure the thermometer does not contain mercury.

  Before and after using, shake down the thermometer as needed.

  Clean the thermometer with soap and water or approved solution before and after using; rinse.

  Use disposable covers, if available.

  When reading the thermometer, hold it at eye level and rotate it until the markings are clear and easy to read.

  Handle carefully and store in an appropriate container to avoid breakage.

Evaluation

- Compare to normal range for developmental stage, site used, and client's baseline data.
- Look for trends to identify potential concerns.
- Notify the appropriate healthcare provider of abnormal findings.

Patient Teaching

- Inform the patient of the temperature reading.
- Explain the significance of the temperature reading and any interventions that may be needed.

Home Care

- Patients commonly use chemical strip (disposable), glass, or tympanic membrane thermometers at home. Teach the following points:

  - ✚ Do not use an oral thermometer to take a rectal temperature. Use a specially shaped, more rounded, rectal thermometer to avoid injury to the rectum.
  - ✚ Do not use glass-and-mercury thermometers. If you discover a glass-and-mercury thermometer, or any kind of glass thermometer, urge the client to replace it with a safer instrument (e.g., a plastic thermometer). Arrange for an exchange if there is a procedure for this in your agency or community.

  Glass-and-mercury thermometers carry the risk of breakage, cuts, and exposure to toxic mercury.

- If you obtain a high or low reading using a chemical strip or a tympanic thermometer, retake the temperature using a plastic or digital thermometer.
- Teach the same procedures you have learned for measuring temperature. Observe as the patient takes a temperature to ensure correct technique.
- Patients often use the oral site. Remind them not to drink, eat, or smoke for 30 minutes before taking the temperature.
- Reinforce the following points about care of reusable thermometers:
  - If you use the same thermometer for more than one person, use disposable covers, if possible. Clean the thermometer well between uses.
  - If the person has an infection or communicable illness, soak the thermometer in 70% isopropyl alcohol between uses.
  - Clean the thermometer after each use, even if it is used for only one person. Wash with soap and water; rinse with cold water; dry well; and store in a clean, dry container.
  - If you store a thermometer in alcohol, rinse it with cold water before taking the temperature.
  - ✚ Do not use the same thermometer for both oral and rectal temperatures.

Documentation

You will usually document temperatures in the electronic medical record. In some situations (e.g., a fever), you may need to write a nurse's note. If so, follow these suggestions:
- Document the temperature, indicating the route of measurement, according to agency policy.
- Notify the appropriate provider of abnormal findings.
- Document supporting findings, such as "Skin is hot and dry," and state whether the temperature reading is consistent with the client's condition.

Sample documentation

00/00/0000   1230   Oral temperature 105°F: has risen steadily since the first elevation at 0630, when it was 100°F. Skin hot and dry. Patient is voiding only small amounts of dark, clear urine. Denies burning sensation on urination. No chills. I&O monitoring initiated. Administered Tylenol 650 mg by mouth and notified Dr. Anderson of patient's condition and medication. Will continue to monitor temperature.   ———Jill Reardone, RN———

Practice Resources

Amoore (2010); Levander & Grodzinsky (2017); Myatt (2021); Robertson & Hill (2019); Sapra et al. (2022).

Thinking About the Procedure

The video **Assessing Body Temperature,** along with questions and suggested responses, is available on the **Davis's** *Nursing Skills Videos* Web site at www.fadavis.com.

Procedure 18-2 ■ Assessing Peripheral Pulses

➤ For steps to follow in *all* procedures, refer to the Universal Steps for All Procedures on the inside back cover.

Equipment
- Watch with a second hand or digital readout
- Pen, pencil, and flowsheet or agency-approved smart device

Delegation

You can delegate measurement of pulses to the UAP if you conclude that the patient's condition and the UAP's skills allow. For example, if pedal circulation is critical and you suspect it may be difficult to palpate, you should not delegate assessment of the pedal pulse.
- If you do delegate, perform the preprocedure assessments and tell the UAP which site (e.g., radial, brachial) to use. Inform the UAP of any special considerations (e.g., to note what the patient's activity has been just before taking the pulse).
- Ask the UAP to document and report the pulse to you and to report immediately if it is outside normal limits (you must specify what is "normal" for each patient).

Preprocedure Assessments
- Determine why assessment of pulses is indicated.
  Conditions requiring an assessment of pulses include blood loss, cardiac or respiratory disease, diabetes mellitus, and other conditions that affect oxygenation.
- Assess factors that may alter the pulse, such as activity and medications. If the patient has been active recently, wait 5 to 10 minutes before measuring.
  Activity increases the pulse rate; increased intracranial pressure decreases the rate; medications such as digoxin decrease the rate; other medications, such as albuterol, increase the pulse rate.

(continued on next page)

Procedure 18-2 ■ Assessing Peripheral Pulses (continued)

Procedure 18-2A ■ Assessing the Radial Pulse

➤ When performing the procedure, always identify your patient according to agency policy, using two identifiers, and be attentive to standard precautions, hand hygiene, patient safety and privacy, body mechanics, and documentation.

Procedure Steps

1. **With the patient sitting or supine,** flex their arm, and place the forearm across their chest.

2. **Palpate the radial artery.**
   The radial site is the most frequently used to calculate the patient's heart rate because it is generally the easiest site to use.
   a. Place the pads of your index or middle fingers (or both) in the groove on the thumb side of the patient's wrist, over the radial artery.
   b. Press lightly but firmly until you are able to feel the radial pulse. Start with light pressure to prevent occluding the pulse, and gradually increase the pressure until you feel the pulse.
   The fingertips are the most sensitive parts of the hand to palpate arterial pulsations. Avoid using the thumb, because it has its own pulsation and may interfere with the accuracy of your count. ➤

3. **Note the rhythm and quality** of the pulse. Note whether the thrust of the pulse against your fingertips is bounding, strong, weak, or thready.
   The rhythm and quality of the pulse are a reflection of the patient's cardiac output. The strength of the pulse reflects the volume of the blood that is ejected against the arterial wall with each contraction of the heart. An irregular or weak pulse indicates decreased cardiac output. A bounding pulse indicates increased cardiac output.

4. **Count the pulse:**
   a. Count for 60 seconds the first time you take a patient's pulse. After that, you can count a pulse with a regular rhythm for 15 seconds and multiply by 4, or count for 30 seconds and multiply by 2 to get the beats per minute. If you do not know the patient well, count for a full minute to be certain to detect irregularities. See Step 4c rationale.
   b. Begin timing with the count of 0 (CDC, 2022), starting with the first beat that you feel.
   c. Count an irregular pulse for 1 full minute (60 seconds).
   You must count an irregular pulse for 1 full minute to be accurate.

5. **For an admission assessment** or peripheral vascular check, palpate the radial pulses on both wrists simultaneously. Note any difference in the quality of the pulse between arms. Is the pulse on one side weaker than on the other?
   Palpating simultaneously enables the recognition of small differences in the peripheral circulation.

Procedure 18-2B ■ Assessing the Brachial Pulse

➤ When performing the procedure, always identify your patient according to agency policy, using two identifiers, and be attentive to standard precautions, hand hygiene, patient safety and privacy, body mechanics, and documentation.

Procedure Steps

1. **Palpate the brachial artery.**
   a. Using firm pressure, press in the inner aspect of the antecubital fossa until you palpate the brachial artery.
   b. If you have difficulty palpating the pulse, ask the patient to pronate the forearm (i.e., turn the palm of the hand downward).
   This brings the brachial artery over a bony prominence and makes the pulse easier to feel. ▼

2. **Assess pulse rate, rhythm, and quality, and assess bilaterally** (see Procedure 18-2A).
   The brachial pulse is used most frequently to assess blood pressure and to identify the presence of a pulse during cardiopulmonary resuscitation (CPR) in an infant.

Procedure 18-2C ■ Assessing the Carotid Pulse

▶ When performing the procedure, always identify your patient according to agency policy, using two identifiers, and be attentive to standard precautions, hand hygiene, patient safety and privacy, body mechanics, and documentation.

✚ **Caution!** Do not palpate the carotid pulse except during CPR in an adult, or in certain situations to assess for circulation to the head. Persons not trained in CPR should not assess the carotid pulse.

Pressure on the carotid (especially in older adults) can stimulate the vagus nerve, causing the pulse and blood pressure to drop suddenly and potentially lead to fainting or circulatory arrest. It can also decrease circulation to the brain.

Procedure Steps

1. **Palpate the carotid artery lightly.** Place your fingers on the patient's trachea and slide them to the side into the groove between the trachea and the sternocleidomastoid muscle. *Compressing or massaging the carotid arteries can stimulate the carotid bodies and significantly decrease the patient's heart rate and blood pressure.* ▼

✚ NEVER compress the carotid artery on both sides of the neck at the same time.

2. **Assess the rate, rhythm, and quality,** and compare bilaterally.

Procedure 18-2D ■ Assessing the Dorsalis Pedis Pulse

▶ When performing the procedure, always identify your patient according to agency policy, using two identifiers, and be attentive to standard precautions, hand hygiene, patient safety and privacy, body mechanics, and documentation.

Procedure Steps

1. **Palpate the dorsalis pedis pulse.**
   a. Run your fingers up the groove between the great and first toes to the top of the foot.
   b. Palpate very lightly.
   The dorsalis pedis pulse is easily obliterated, so use very light pressure. The dorsalis pedis pulse is used to assess circulation of the foot.

   🍁 Because of atherosclerosis (hardening of the arteries), the dorsalis pedis may be difficult to palpate in older adults.

2. **Assess pulse rate, rhythm, and quality,** and assess bilaterally. ▼

3. **If you are unable to palpate the dorsalis pedis pulse,** use a Doppler ultrasound device to assess the pulse and circulation to the lower extremity.

(continued on next page)

Procedure 18-2 ■ Assessing Peripheral Pulses (continued)

Procedure 18-2E ■ Assessing the Femoral Pulse

➤ When performing the procedure, always identify your patient according to agency policy, using two identifiers, and be attentive to standard precautions, hand hygiene, patient safety and privacy, body mechanics, and documentation.

Procedure Steps

1. **Palpate the femoral pulse** by pressing deeply in the groin midway between the anterosuperior iliac spine and the symphysis pubis.
   The femoral artery lies very deep and requires significant pressure to palpate. You may need to use both hands to feel the pulse on an adult. ➤

2. **Assess pulse rate, rhythm, and quality,** and assess bilaterally.
   The femoral pulse is used to determine the presence of a pulse during CPR and to assess circulation to the leg.

Procedure 18-2F ■ Assessing the Posterior Tibial Pulse

➤ When performing the procedure, always identify your patient according to agency policy, using two identifiers, and be attentive to standard precautions, hand hygiene, patient safety and privacy, body mechanics, and documentation.

Procedure Steps

1. **Palpate the posterior tibial pulse** by pressing on the inner (medial) side of the ankle below the medial malleolus.
   The posterior tibial pulse is usually palpated easily, but it may be deeper in some people. So, press down moderately and then increase pressure until you feel the pulse. It is relatively easy to obliterate. ➤

2. **Assess pulse rate, rhythm, and quality,** and assess bilaterally.
   The posterior tibial pulse is used to assess circulation to the lower extremity; it is assessed along with the dorsalis pedis pulse.

Procedure 18-2G ■ Assessing the Popliteal Pulse

➤ When performing the procedure, always identify your patient according to agency policy, using two identifiers, and be attentive to standard precautions, hand hygiene, patient safety and privacy, body mechanics, and documentation.

Procedure Steps

1. **Palpate the popliteal pulse** by pressing behind the knee in the middle of the popliteal fossa.
   The popliteal pulse can be difficult to feel. It is used only when specifically indicated because of absence of pedal pulses or for taking a thigh blood pressure. ➤

2. **Assess pulse rate, rhythm, and quality,** and assess bilaterally.
   The popliteal pulse is used to assess circulation of the lower leg and auscultate a thigh blood pressure.

Procedure 18-2H ■ Assessing the Temporal Pulse

➤ When performing the procedure, always identify your patient according to agency policy, using two identifiers, and be attentive to standard precautions, hand hygiene, patient safety and privacy, body mechanics, and documentation.

Procedure Steps

1. **Palpate the temporal pulse** by pressing lightly lateral (outside area) and superior to (above) the eye. ▼

2. **Assess pulse rate, rhythm, and quality,** and assess bilaterally as for the radial pulse (see Procedure 18-2A). *The temporal pulse is easily accessible and is used frequently in infants.*

? What if . . .

- **The patient is an infant or a child younger than 3 years of age?**

  Auscultate an apical pulse rate. Rates are faster and small arteries are more difficult to feel in a child or infant. If a parent is present, encourage the parent to hold the child to reduce anxiety.
  Fear increases the pulse rate.

- **The patient is an older adult?**

  Have the patient rest for 15 to 20 minutes after activity and before assessing the pulse.
  The pulse tends to return to baseline more slowly in older adults.

  If the pulse is fast, take repeated measures; if a pattern of fast rate emerges, note this for the primary care provider for further evaluation.
  An elevated heart rate is related to increased mortality in older female adults, so it is a simple index of general health status.

- **The pulse is faint or weak?**

  Use a Doppler ultrasound device to detect blood flow.
  Lack of pulses indicates inadequate circulation to the lower extremities. If you cannot feel the pulse, you must determine whether the pulse is absent or whether you are having difficulty feeling. To draw the conclusion that the pulse is "absent," you must use a Doppler.

  Apply transmission gel to the end of the probe. Do not use water-soluble lubricant as a substitute for transmission gel.
  Place the probe lightly on the skin over the artery you are using.
  Turn on the instrument and set the volume control to the lowest setting. Tilting the probe to a 45° angle to the artery, move the probe slowly in a circular motion to locate the signal (a rhythmic hissing noise). Count for 60 seconds.
  Move the probe slowly to avoid distorting the signal.

  When you are finished, wipe the gel off the patient's skin. Clean the probe with soapy water or an antiseptic solution. Do not immerse the probe or bump it against anything hard.
  Clean the probe to prevent cross-contamination to other patients. Probes are fragile and may malfunction if bumped against a hard surface.

Evaluation

Especially if pedal pulses are decreased, observe for other indications of inadequate circulation, such as cool skin, decreased capillary refill, and bluish or ashen skin tone. You must provide supporting evidence if you document that pedal pulses are decreased or absent. The complete absence of a pulse requires immediate intervention.

Patient Teaching

- Teach the patient about the significance of any abnormalities in pulse rate or rhythm.
- Explain any interventions that may be needed.

Home Care

Assess the skill level of the person who will be assessing the client's peripheral pulses in the home and provide instruction if necessary.

Documentation

Usually you will document routine vital signs, including pulse, in the EHR. Documentation in the nurse's note must include the pulse rate, rhythm, quality, and site (e.g., "radial pulse 64 beats/min, regular, and strong bilaterally").

Practice Resources

Centers for Disease Control and Prevention (CDC) (2022); Lowry & Ashelford (2015); Pickering (2013); Sapra et al. (2022); Zimmerman & Williams (2021).

Thinking About the Procedures

The video **Assessing Peripheral Pulses,** along with questions and suggested responses, is available on the **Davis's *Nursing Skills Videos*** Web site at www.fadavis.com.

Procedure 18-3 ■ Assessing the Apical Pulse

▶ For steps to follow in *all* procedures, refer to the Universal Steps for All Procedures on the inside back cover.

Equipment
- Watch with a second hand or second readout
- Stethoscope
- Alcohol wipes (to clean stethoscope)

Delegation
You can delegate measurement of the apical pulse to the UAP if you conclude that the patient's condition and the UAP's skills allow.
- First perform the preprocedure assessments.
- Then inform the UAP of any special considerations (e.g., to note what the patient's activity was just before taking the pulse, or to mark the time exactly so you can compare it to the patient's ECG).
- Ask the UAP to document and report the pulse to you and to report immediately if it is outside normal limits (you must specify what is "normal" for each patient).

Preprocedure Assessments
- Determine why assessment of the apical pulse is indicated.
  Conditions that require assessment of the apical pulse include digitalis therapy, blood loss, cardiac or respiratory disease, or other conditions that affect oxygenation status.
- Assess factors that may alter the pulse, such as activity and medications. If the client has been recently active, wait 10 to 15 minutes before obtaining a measurement.
  Activity can increase the pulse rate. Relate the aforementioned factors to baseline pulse rate to determine their effect.

▶ When performing the procedure, always identify your patient according to agency policy, using two identifiers, and be attentive to standard precautions, hand hygiene, patient safety and privacy, body mechanics, and documentation.

Procedure Steps

1. **With the client supine or sitting,** expose the left side of the chest, but only as much as necessary.
   Prevents distortion of sound from the patient's gown rubbing on the stethoscope, while also protecting the patient's privacy. ▼

   Apex, PMI

2. ✚ **Clean the stethoscope with** a 70% alcohol or benzalkonium chloride wipe before and after examining the patient.
   Cleaning can reduce the bacterial count by up to 100%.

3. **Palpate the fifth intercostal space** at the midclavicular line for the apical pulse.
   The left ventricle of the heart and the point of maximum impulse lie in this area. The apical pulse is generally best heard at the PMI, over the apex of the heart.

   a. To locate the fifth intercostal space, slide your finger down from the sternal notch to the angle of Louis (the bump where the manubrium and sternum meet).
   b. Slide your finger over to the left sternal border to the second intercostal space.
   c. Now place your index or ring finger (depending on which hand you use) in the second intercostal space and count down to the fifth intercostal space by placing a finger in each of the spaces.
   d. Slide over to the midclavicular line, keeping your finger in the fifth intercostal space.
   The apical pulse is generally best heard at the PMI in the fifth intercostal space at the midclavicular line. The PMI is located over the apex of the heart.

   For an adult, this site is on the anterior chest at 3 inches (8 cm) or less to the left of the sternum, at the fourth, fifth, or sixth intercostal space at the midclavicular line.

4. **Palpate the apical pulse.**
   a. The palpated apical pulse (also called the PMI).
   b. The pulse area should be about the size of a quarter, without lifts or heaves.
   A larger-than-normal pulsation may indicate ventricular hypertrophy.

5. **Warm the stethoscope** in your hand for 10 seconds. Then place the diaphragm over the PMI and listen to the normal S_1 and S_2 heart sounds ("lub-dub"). Count each pair of sounds ("lub-dub") as one heartbeat.
   A cold stethoscope placed on the skin may startle the patient and increase the heart rate. Heart sounds result when blood moves through the valves of the heart. The first heart sound is louder at the apical area and should be audible when the pulse is auscultated.

6. **Count the apical heart rate** for 1 full minute.
   Ensures accuracy. Because the apical heart rate is needed as an assessment measure for the administration of some medications (e.g., digoxin), accuracy is essential. Some cardiac conditions cause either slow or irregular rates, both of which must be counted for a full minute to ensure accuracy.

7. **Clean the stethoscope** again with 70% alcohol or benzalkonium chloride wipe.

? What if...

- **The apical rate is less than 60 beats/min?**

   (**Note:** You may also see "bpm" as an abbreviation for "beats per minute" or for "beats/min.")
   If the patient is taking cardiac medications, withhold them and consult with a provider about whether to adjust dosage.
   Certain cardiac medications (e.g., digoxin) are given to slow the heart rate; bradycardia may indicate that blood levels are too high.
   Assess for chest pain, dizziness, and dyspnea.
   May indicate decreased cardiac output.

- **The apical rate is greater than 100 beats/min?**

   Obtain a complete set of vital signs. Assess for possible causes (e.g., pain, anxiety, fever, dehydration, decreased oxygenation, hypotension, decreased exercise).
   Addressing the cause of factors that increase pulse rate may help return it to a normal rate.

Evaluation

- Are the findings within normal limits?
- Are there other factors supporting the findings?
- What are the trends over time?
- Is the skin pink, warm, and dry?
- Is there any cyanosis?

Patient Teaching

- Teach the patient about the significance of any abnormalities in the pulse rate or rhythm.
- Explain any interventions that may be necessary.

Home Care

- Assess the skill level of the person who will be assessing the client's apical pulse in the home and provide instruction if necessary.
- Teach the home caregiver when to hold medications and/or to call the primary care provider (e.g., to hold the digitalis if the rate is <60).
- Before leaving the home, clean the stethoscope with detergent or disinfectant, when possible; or place it in a plastic bag for transporting to the reprocessing location.
- If the patient has a multidrug-resistant organism infection, reusable equipment such as stethoscopes should remain in the home. If the stethoscope cannot remain in the home, clean and disinfect it before leaving the home, using a low- to intermediate-level disinfectant. If this is not practical, place the stethoscope in a plastic bag and transport it to another site for cleaning and disinfection.

Documentation

Document the pulse rate, rhythm, and site.

Sample documentation

   mm/dd/yyyy   0800——Apical pulse regular rhythm, and strong, rate of 64 bpm———Jay Jones, RN

Practice Resources
Cleveland Clinic (2022); Lowry & Ashelford (2015).

Thinking About the Procedure

The video **Assessing Apical Pulse,** along with questions and suggested responses, is available on the **Davis's Nursing Skills Videos** Web site at www.fadavis.com.

Procedure 18-4 ■ Assessing for an Apical-Radial Pulse Deficit

➤ For steps to follow in *all* procedures, refer to the Universal Steps for All Procedures on the inside back cover.

Equipment
- Watch or clock with a second hand or second readout
- Procedure gloves, if indicated
- Stethoscope
- Alcohol wipes to clean the stethoscope

Delegation
Instead of delegating measurement of an apical-radial pulse to a UAP, you would most likely ask the UAP to assist you in this procedure because it is best performed by two persons working together.

Preprocedure Assessments
- Determine why assessment of pulse deficit is indicated.
  Conditions that require assessment of pulse deficit include digitalis therapy, blood loss, cardiac or respiratory disease, and other conditions that affect oxygenation status.
- Assess factors that may alter the pulse, such as activity and medications.
- Obtain another nurse to assist with the procedure.

➤ When performing the procedure, always identify your patient according to agency policy, using two identifiers, and be attentive to standard precautions, hand hygiene, patient safety and privacy, body mechanics, and documentation.

Procedure Steps

1. ✚ **Clean the stethoscope with a 70% alcohol or benzalkonium chloride wipe** before and after examining the patient.
   Cleaning can reduce the bacterial count by up to 100% and prevent the transmission of microbes.

2. **Expose the left side** of the patient's chest, minimizing patient exposure.
   Prevents distortion of sound from the patient's gown rubbing on the stethoscope and protects privacy.

3. **Place the watch so that the** second hand is visible to both nurses (if two nurses are performing the procedure).
   Using one watch increases accuracy of counts.

4. **Nurse 1 prepares to auscultate the apical pulse.** They palpate the fifth intercostal space at the midclavicular line, then hold the diaphragm of the stethoscope in place, using firm pressure until Nurse 2 says "Start."
   Aids in hearing high-pitched sounds and ensures good contact between the diaphragm of the stethoscope and the skin. ➤

5. **Nurse 2 palpates to locate the radial pulse,** preparing to assess rate, rhythm, and quality.

6. **Nurse 2 says "Start" when ready to begin** and "Stop" when finished. Both nurses count the pulse simultaneously for 1 full minute.
   Count simultaneously to ensure accuracy. Counting for 1 full minute is necessary for an accurate assessment of any discrepancies that may exist between the two sites.

7. **To obtain pulse deficit, subtract** the radial rate from the apical rate.

   Apical Rate – Radial Rate = Pulse Deficit

   Atrial and ventricular dysrhythmias may cause beats that do not perfuse, so although you hear an apical heartbeat, you do not feel a peripheral pulse. The pulse deficit is the number of heartbeats that do not perfuse.

? What if...

- **Another nurse is not available to assist?**
  Hold the stethoscope in place with the one hand while palpating the radial pulse with the hand wearing the watch. Even if you cannot manage to count both rates, you should be able to feel any differences between the apical and radial pulses.

- **There has been an increase in pulse deficit since the last measurement?**
  An increase in pulse deficit means that the patient's cardiac output has decreased. You should notify the provider of your findings.

Evaluation
- Identify the presence of an apical-pulse deficit, and compare to previous findings.
- Assess other measures of cardiopulmonary status to identify a decline in the patient's condition.
- Look for trends.

The presence of any apical-radial pulse deficit is abnormal.

Patient Teaching
- Teach the patient about the significance of an apical-radial pulse deficit.
- Explain any necessary interventions.

Home Care
- Assess the skill level of the person(s) who will be measuring the client's apical-radial pulse deficit in the home and provide instruction if necessary.
- Before leaving the home, clean the stethoscope as described in the Home Care section of Procedure 18-3.

Documentation
Document the apical-radial pulse deficit.

Sample documentation

mm/dd/yyyy ——— 0900——————Apical-radial pulse deficit is 4 beats/min.—————Jon Albertson, RN

Practice Resources
Cleveland Clinic (2022); Opio & Kellett (2017).

Thinking About the Procedures.

> The video **Assessing for an Apical Radial Pulse Deficit,** along with questions and suggested responses, is available on the **Davis's Nursing Skills Videos** Web site at www.fadavis.com.

Procedure 18-5 ■ Assessing Respirations

> For steps to follow in *all* procedures, refer to the Universal Steps for All Procedures on the inside back cover.

Equipment
- A watch with a second hand (or a wall clock)

Delegation
You can delegate the counting of respirations to the UAP if you conclude that the patient's condition and the UAP's skills allow.
- Perform the preprocedure assessments, and inform the UAP of any special considerations (e.g., the need to keep the patient in a certain position).
- Ask the UAP to document and report the respirations to you and to report immediately if they are not within the normal range for this patient (specify the range).

Preprocedure Assessments
- Observe for signs of respiratory distress—breathing faster or slower than normal, gasping breaths, confusion, circumoral (around the month) cyanosis.
  Signs of hypoxemia may indicate that the patient is not adequately oxygenated.
- Determine the baseline respiratory rate and character of respirations.
- Assess for factors that may affect the respiratory rate (e.g., pain, activity, fever, respiratory disorders).

> When performing the procedure, always identify your patient according to agency policy, using two identifiers, and be attentive to standard precautions, hand hygiene, patient safety and privacy, body mechanics, and documentation.

(continued on next page)

Procedure 18-5 ■ Assessing Respirations (continued)

Procedure Steps

1. **Position the patient.** With the patient in a sitting position (preferably), flex the patient's arm, and place their forearm across their chest.
   Aids in counting the patient's pulse rate by making the rise and fall of the chest more discernible and by making the patient less aware that you are measuring the respiratory rate. The patient's awareness might alter the respiratory rate and/or pattern because respirations are partially under voluntary control. ▼

2. **Palpate and count the radial pulse;** remember that number.

3. **Then, keeping your hand** on the patient's wrist, count the respirations.
   Allows you to count the respirations unobtrusively.

4. **Observe the respiratory rate, rhythm, and depth.**
   - *Rate:* Normal for patient's age, fast (tachypnea), or slow (bradypnea)
   - *Rhythm:* Regular or irregular
   - *Depth:* Normal, shallow, or deep (e.g., Kussmaul's)

   All of these characteristics are necessary to evaluate respiratory status. Different pathologies affect each of these characteristics differently. Changes in respiratory rate and characteristics can be an indicator of clinical deterioration.

5. **Count the number of breaths** per minute. Begin timing the respirations with a count of 1.
   a. If the respiratory rhythm is regular, count the rate (one inhalation and one exhalation is one respiration) for 30 seconds, and multiply by 2.
   b. If the rhythm is irregular, count the rate for 1 full minute (60 seconds).

6. Variations in rhythm may cause an inaccurate rate when counted for less than 1 minute.

? What if...

- **The patient is an infant?**
  Place your hand on the abdomen to assess the respiratory rate. Auscultate breath sounds with a stethoscope.
  Infants and young children breathe rapidly and are abdominal breathers, so it is difficult to see every rise and fall of the abdomen. Using a stethoscope increases the accuracy of the count and provides information about the breath sounds.

  For infants and very young children, count for 1 full minute.
  Infants and young children have irregular respirations. Counting for a full minute provides a more accurate rate for irregular respirations.

- **The patient is receiving oxygen therapy, or requires careful assessment of respiratory status?**
  Apply a pulse oximeter (see Procedure 33-2, Monitoring Pulse Oximetry [Arterial Oxygen Saturation]).
  Evidence suggests that pulse oximetry is useful for detecting deterioration of physiological function that might otherwise be missed (e.g., during the perioperative period or in seriously ill patients).

Evaluation

- Compare the respiratory rate and rhythm with previous readings.
- Note other vital signs, especially temperature.
- Look for trends, and note whether the respiratory rate and rhythm are changing in conjunction with changes in the other vital signs.

  If the patient has an elevated temperature, the respiratory rate will increase. Corresponding elevation in pulse with respiratory rate may indicate hypoxemia. If respirations are not within normal parameters, assess oxygenation with a pulse oximeter.

Patient Teaching

Teach the patient about factors that affect respiratory status, such as smoking and activity.

Home Care

Assess the skill level of the person(s) who will be measuring the patient's respiratory rate in the home, and provide instruction as needed.

Documentation

You will document routine vital signs (including respirations) in the EHR. When a nurse's note is needed, follow these guidelines:
- Document the respiratory rate, depth, and rhythm.
- Document that respirations are either labored or unlabored. If labored, describe in what way (e.g., intercostal retractions, use of accessory muscles, nasal flaring).

Example of electronic health record

Practice Resources
Hill & Annesley (2020); Rolfe (2019); Sapra et al. (2022); Wheatley (2018a).

The video **Assessing Respirations,** along with questions and suggested responses, is available on the **Davis's Nursing Skills Videos** Web site at www.fadavis.com.

Procedure 18-6 ■ Measuring Blood Pressure

➤ For steps to follow in *all* procedures, refer to the Universal Steps for All Procedures on the inside back cover.

Equipment
- Stethoscope

  ✚ **Do not wear a stethoscope around your neck.** *There is a slight risk that you can entangle it in an IV and other lines. There is also a risk that a psychotic or delirious patient could use it to harm you. Also, wearing a stethoscope can be a source of cross-contamination.*

- 70% alcohol or benzalkonium chloride wipes
  For cleaning stethoscope before and after use. Clean all parts.

- Sphygmomanometer with a cuff of the appropriate size (refer to Clinical Insight 18-1)
  A cuff that is too small will result in a false high reading; using a cuff that is too large will result in a false low reading.

- *Note:* This procedure describes the use of an aneroid manometer or an electronic measuring device.

Delegation
You can delegate measurement of BP to the UAP if you conclude that the patient's condition and the UAP's skills allow.
- Perform the preprocedure assessments.
- Inform the UAP of the site (e.g., radial, brachial) to use.
- Inform the UAP of any special considerations (e.g., not to place a BP cuff on the same side as the site of a mastectomy).
- Ask the UAP to document and report the BP to you, and to report immediately if it is outside normal limits (you must specify what is "normal" for each patient).
- Tell the UAP that if BP is elevated, to note which arm, the patient's position during measurement, and activity immediately preceding the measurement.

(continued on next page)

Procedure 18-6 ■ Measuring Blood Pressure (continued)

Preprocedure Assessments
- Check for factors or activities that may alter the readings.
  Caffeine, smoking, exercise, and stress can all elevate the BP. Be certain the patient has been lying or sitting for at least 5 minutes (30 minutes after strenuous exercise) and is relaxed.
- Check the previous recording, if any.
  Noting changes over time is important with all patient assessments. Because BP changes constantly and because so many factors affect it, you cannot draw conclusions from a single measurement.

▶ When performing the procedure, always identify your patient according to agency policy, using two identifiers, and be attentive to standard precautions, hand hygiene, patient safety and privacy, body mechanics, and documentation.

▶ *Note:* To improve the accuracy of your readings, also refer to Clinical Insights 18-1 and 18-2.

Procedure Steps

1. **Clean the stethoscope** before and after the procedure.
   Although only a small percentage of microorganisms are pathogenic, cleaning can reduce the bacterial count by 94% to 100%.

2. **Position the patient** comfortably, ensuring that:
   a. The legs are uncrossed, the back is supported, and the feet are resting on the floor (if the patient is sitting in a chair) or the patient is supine.
      This position allows for the most accurate reading. Crossing the legs may elevate the BP reading.
   b. The measurement arm is supported at heart level, slightly flexed, with the palm facing upward.
      The blood pressure will decrease if the arm is above the heart and increase if the arm is below the heart or not supported.

3. **Fully expose the arm,** being careful that clothing is not tight. Remove clothing rather than rolling up a sleeve.
   Clothing that is tight enough to restrict blood flow will alter the reading.

4. **Place the cuff** on the upper arm. ▼

   a. Wrap the cuff snugly.
   b. Ensure that the cuff is totally deflated and palpate the brachial artery.
   c. Place the bottom edge of the cuff approximately 1 in. (2.5 cm) above the antecubital space.
   d. Place the center of the cuff bladder directly over the brachial artery (the center is often indicated with an arrow on the BP cuff). The cuff has the appropriate tightness if one finger easily fits at the top and bottom of the cuff and two fingers are very snug (Muntner et al., 2019).
      The center of the cuff bladder needs to be directly over the brachial artery to obtain an accurate reading. Loose application of the cuff results in overestimation of the pressure.

5. **Place the stethoscope ear pieces** in your ears, pointing slightly forward.
   When the earpieces point slightly forward, they direct sound into the ear canal, making the sounds more audible.

6. **Palpate the brachial artery** on the arm with the cuff. (Use the radial artery for this step if you prefer.)
   For correct stethoscope placement.

7. **Inflate the cuff as follows:**
   a. Close the sphygmomanometer valve and inflate the cuff rapidly to about 80 mm Hg.
   b. Then palpate the pulse while you continue inflating in 10 mm Hg increments until you no longer feel the pulse.
   c. As you *inflate* the cuff, the artery is occluded as the pressure of the cuff exceeds the pressure in the artery. At that point, blood flow through the artery is halted, and no sound can be heard. Note the pressure at which the pulse disappears.
   d. Go to step 8 or the variation, as you prefer.
      Palpating the artery while inflating the cuff ensures that the cuff is inflated higher than the systolic BP. If the patient has an auscultatory gap, the systolic pressure can be mistakenly identified as lower than it actually is. Palpation is particularly important if the baseline systolic BP is unknown or if the patient is hypertensive.

8. **Continue inflating the cuff** to a pressure that is 20 to 30 mm Hg above the level at which the pulse disappeared. Move to Step 9.
   Helps ensure you will not miss an auscultatory gap or a faint first sound.

Variation: Cuff Inflation Technique
- Do not continue palpating after the pulse disappears; instead, deflate the cuff rapidly.
- Wait 2 minutes, then place the stethoscope over the brachial artery and inflate the cuff to a pressure that is 30 mm Hg above the palpated level.
- Continue with Steps 9 and 10.

9. **Place the stethoscope over** the brachial artery as follows: ▼

   a. Be certain that the stethoscope tubing is not touching anything and that the diaphragm is not tucked under the edge of the cuff.
   When the tubing rubs against clothing, for example, it produces artifact sounds that make it difficult to hear the BP sounds. Placing the bell or diaphragm under the cuff can partially occlude the brachial artery, delaying the appearance of the Korotkoff sounds.

   b. Using the bell will enable you to hear BP sounds more accurately, especially at diastolic pressures. However, most people use the diaphragm because it is easily placed and because some stethoscopes do not have a bell.

10. **Deflate the cuff slowly** (2 to 3 mm Hg per second or per beat), listening for the Korotkoff sounds as you deflate.
    Deflating the cuff slowly increases patient discomfort and may alter the reading. Deflating the cuff faster may cause errors in hearing the Korotkoff sounds.

    a. As you deflate the cuff, blood begins to flow rapidly through the partially open artery, producing turbulence that you will hear through the stethoscope as a tapping sound. Note the point on the manometer at which you hear the first sound. This is the *systolic BP*. (If you are using an electronic BP device, read the digital screen when the numbers appear. Follow the manufacturer's instructions.)
    The first Korotkoff sound is the systolic pressure.

    b. Continue deflating the cuff and note the level at which the sounds become muffled and disappear. The artery is no longer compressed and sound will disappear. Document the point at which the sound disappears as the diastolic pressure.
    The fifth Korotkoff sound (the disappearance of sound) is the diastolic BP. The American Heart Association recommends that the BP in children be taken in the right arm.

11. **If you need to repeat** the measurement, deflate the cuff completely, and wait 2 minutes before reinflating it.
    Prevents venous congestion and false high readings.

❓ What if . . .

- **I cannot feel the brachial pulse?**

  While supporting the arm at the elbow, have the patient pronate the forearm.
  This moves the brachial artery more over a bony prominence, making the pulsation easier to feel.

- **I have difficulty hearing BP sounds for many patients?**

  You may need a stethoscope with a built-in amplifier.

- **I am not certain of the systolic reading when beginning to deflate the cuff?**

  Do not stop cuff deflation to recheck the systolic reading. Deflate the cuff completely and wait 1 to 3 minutes before taking another measurement.
  Stopping deflation and retaking the BP too soon can lead to a muffling of the Korotkoff sounds and inaccurate results.

- **I am using an automatic blood pressure device?**

  Follow the same guidelines as for a manual BP (e.g., cuff size and placement, patient position).

  Turn on the machine; be sure the cuff is deflated.

  Apply the cuff.

  Press the button to start the measurement.

  At the tone, read the digital measurement.

- **I do not have a cuff size to fit the upper arm?**

  Use the forearm, thigh, or calf. See Procedure Variations A, B, and C, respectively.

- **The patient requires contact or isolation precautions?**

  Follow agency guidelines for equipment (e.g., stethoscope, BP cuff). Generally, the equipment remains in the room with the patient; otherwise, it must be disinfected before leaving the room. For information about contact precautions and protective isolation, see Chapter 20, Clinical Insights 20-2, 20-3, and 20-4.

Procedure Variation A: Measuring Blood Pressure in the Forearm

- Place a properly sized cuff on the forearm, midway between the elbow and the wrist. Auscultate over the radial artery.
- Note that a forearm reading is not interchangeable with an upper arm reading.

Procedure Variation B: Measuring Blood Pressure in the Thigh

- Use the thigh or the calf if the cuff will not fit either the upper or lower arm.
  Note: The thigh systolic measure may be 20 to 30 mm Hg higher than an arm BP reading. The diastolic reading is generally comparable.
- Place the patient in a prone position. If patient cannot be prone, place supine with knee slightly bent.

(continued on next page)

Procedure 18-6 ■ Measuring Blood Pressure (continued)

- Choose the correct cuff size. Wrap the cuff snugly around the thigh so that the lower edge of the cuff is approximately 1 in. (2.5 cm) above the popliteal fossa and the center of the cuff bladder is positioned directly over the popliteal artery (often indicated with an arrow on the blood pressure cuff).
- Palpate and auscultate over the popliteal artery. ▼

Procedure Variation C: Measuring Blood Pressure in the Calf
- Use the thigh or the calf if the cuff will not fit either the upper or the lower arm.
- Place the patient supine.
- Choose the correct size of cuff. Wrap the cuff snugly around the calf so that the lower edge of the cuff is approximately 2.5 cm above the malleoli or ankle.
- Place the stethoscope over either the dorsalis pedis or the posterior tibial artery.
  Note: Calf BP measurements are not equivalent to upper arm measurements in adults; they tend to produce a higher systolic BP.

Procedure Variation D: Palpating the Blood Pressure
- Apply the cuff and palpate for the radial or brachial pulse.
- Begin to inflate the cuff. When you can no longer feel the pulse, inflate the cuff about 30 mm Hg more.
- As you release the valve and slowly deflate the cuff, note the reading on the manometer at which you once again feel the pulse.
- Document the palpated blood pressure according to the way it was assessed (e.g., "Palpated, low Fowler's, left arm 86/——" [or "86 systolic"]).

Evaluation
- Compare the BP reading with previous readings.
- Look for trends. Is the BP slowly decreasing (e.g., impending shock) or slowly increasing (e.g., hypervolemia)?
- Look for a corresponding change in pulse rate, indicating potential hypoxemia.
- If this is the first BP measurement for the client, check readings in both arms.
  A difference of 10 mm Hg or less is normal. Document the higher of the readings.
- Report any significant changes in the BP reading.

Patient Teaching
- Teach the patient about:
  - Normal BP values (keep in mind that prehypertension is diagnosed at a lower level when using self-monitored readings).
  - Significance of the BP reading.
  - Further follow-up that may be necessary.

Home Care
- The American Heart Association (AHA) and other guidelines recommend self-monitoring of BP at home. Self-measurement of BP is thought to (1) provide more reliable data than office BP because of the availability of multiple readings, and (2) improve adherence to treatment regimens.
- If possible, use the same equipment each time to prevent false changes in measurement.
- Explain the need for frequent recalibration of the home-monitoring device.
- Assess the skill level of the person(s) who will be measuring the patient's BP in the home and provide instruction if necessary.
- Assess whether self-monitoring is causing the client to be anxious.
  Some clients do become overly anxious when they know they must monitor their BP, or when they obtain a high reading. Self-monitoring should not be used if it produces too much anxiety; this raises the BP even more.
- Teach clients not to change their medication dosage without consulting their primary provider when their BP goes up or down.
- ✚ Before leaving the home, clean the stethoscope and sphygmomanometer with detergent or disinfectant, when possible; or place them in a plastic bag for transporting to the reprocessing location.
- ✚ If the client has an infection with a multidrug-resistant organism, reusable equipment such as stethoscopes should remain in the home. If the stethoscope and sphygmomanometer cannot remain in the home, clean and disinfect them before leaving the home, using a low- to intermediate-level disinfectant. If this is not practical, place them in a plastic bag and transport them to another site for cleaning and disinfection.

Documentation
- You will usually document BP on a flowsheet in the EHR (such as in Procedure 18-5, Documentation).
- Document the blood pressure systolic/diastolic readings (e.g., 130/80).
- If you hear the fourth Korotkoff sound or muffling, document systolic/muffling/diastolic (e.g., 130/80/70). If you hear an auscultatory gap, document "systolic/diastolic with an auscultatory gap from…" For example, "170/90 with an auscultatory gap from 170 to 140."

- Follow agency policy regarding the recording of muffled sounds.
- If you chose an alternative site, document the site used and the reason for not using the upper arm.

Practice Resources
Alvarez et al. (2016); American Heart Association (2021); McEvoy (2019); Muntner (2019); Sapra et al. (2022); Weinfield et al. (2021).

Thinking About the Procedure

The video **Measuring Blood Pressure,** along with questions and suggested responses, is available on the Davis's *Nursing Skills Videos* Web site at www.fadavis.com.

CLINICAL INSIGHTS

Clinical Insight 18-1 ➤ Choosing a Blood Pressure Cuff Size

- The *width* of the bladder should cover approximately two-thirds of the *length* of the upper arm (or other extremity) for an adult, and the entire upper arm for a child.
- Another method for sizing:
  1. The cuff width should be 40% of the arm circumference.
  2. The *length* of the bladder should encircle 80% of the arm.
- Perhaps the easiest sizing method is to measure *arm circumference* and follow these guidelines:

For arm circumference	Cuff should be
22–26 cm (8½ × 10¼ in.)	small adult size: 12 × 22 cm (4¾ × 8¾ in.)
27–34 cm (10½ × 13½ in.)	adult size: 16 × 30 cm (6¼ × 11¾ in.)
35–44 cm (13¾ × 17¼ in.)	large adult size: 16 × 36 cm (6¼ × 14¼ in.)
45–52 cm (17¾ × 10½ in.)	adult thigh size: 16 × 42 cm (6¼ × 16⅝ in.)

Practice Resources:
Pickering et al. (2005); Mishra et al. (2017); Muntner et al. (2019); Sapra et al. (2022); Whelton et al. (2018).

Clinical Insight 18-2 ➤ Taking an Accurate Blood Pressure

To improve your technique and accuracy of measurement, use the following tips in addition to Procedure 18-6.
- Explain the procedure, particularly on admission or when changing the routine.
  Reduces patient anxiety
- Wait 30 minutes before assessing BP after patient has ingested caffeine, smoked, or exercised.
- Have the patient empty their bladder.
- Have the patient relax and sit in a chair, with feet on the floor, back supported for at least 5 minutes.
- Do not assess BP while the patient is in pain.
- Apply the cuff over bare skin. Advise patients who are home monitoring to remove all clothing covering the location of cuff placement and to apply the cuff over bare skin.
- Ensure the patient's arm is supported and that the middle of the cuff on the upper right arm is at the level of the right atrium.
- Instruct the patient not to talk during BP measurement. You should not talk, either.
- Keep environmental noise and patient movement to a minimum.
- Hold the stethoscope lightly but completely against the skin; do not put your thumb on top of the bell or diaphragm. Try not to allow the tubing to brush against your clothing or the bed.
- Do not be influenced by the patient's previous BP measurements.
- Use the same limb for each measurement, unless you are comparing arms or averaging readings from both arms.
- For the initial reading, measure the BP in both arms and use the arm with the higher reading for subsequent measurements.
- If you obtain an elevated reading, confirm in the other arm.
- Do not draw conclusions based on one reading. Take two or more readings, 1 to 2 minutes apart and average them. If the readings differ by more than 5 mm Hg, obtain an average of the additional readings.
- Provide the patient with their BP readings orally and in writing.

Practice Resources
Muntner (2019); Park et al. (2022); Sapra et al. (2022); Whelton (2018).

Clinical Insight 18-3 ➤ Teaching Your Patient About Hypertension

Teach the patient and family about lifestyle changes for preventing and managing hypertension.

- Limit salt intake to 1 teaspoon per day (2,400 mg of sodium).
- Consume a diet high in potassium (e.g., fresh fruits and vegetables such as bananas, potatoes, and acorn squash).
- Consume a diet high in calcium (e.g., milk and milk products [yogurt], sardines, molasses, tofu).
- Limit alcohol intake to 1 or 2 drinks per day for men, 1 for women. (One drink is 12 ounces of beer, 1.5 ounces of 80-proof spirits, or 6 ounces of wine.)
- Maintain ideal body weight; lose weight if overweight.
- For overall cardiovascular health, reduce saturated fat and cholesterol intake.
- Eliminate smoking.
- Engage in aerobic exercise (30 to 45 minutes several days a week, or a total of 150 minutes per week).
- Try to reduce stress and stressful situations.
- Teach the patient that even one lifestyle change has effects similar to treatment with a single antihypertensive drug. More than one change has an even more positive effect on BP.

Teach the patient about monitoring blood pressure at home.

- Monitor blood pressure at home to determine whether lifestyle modifications and/or medications are effective.
- Keep a record of your BP readings that contain the date, time, systolic and diastolic numbers, and any information that you want your provider to know.
- Take your BP whenever you have symptoms such as headaches or dizziness.
- Use an upper arm or wrist BP monitor that has been validated.
- When using a wrist BP monitor, place the sensor directly over the radial artery and ensure the wrist is at heart level.
- Take your BP equipment when you visit your healthcare provider to check your monitor for accuracy.
- Follow the researchers' and manufacturer's guidelines for arm position and recalibration. This is especially true for wrist monitors and aneroid sphygmomanometers (Muntner et al., 2019).
- Teach the importance of follow-up assessments.

➤ Refer to **Table 18-6: Classification of Adult Blood Pressure.**

Sources: Whelton, P., et al. (2018). 2017 ACC/AHA/AAPA/ABC/ACPM/AGS/APhA/ASH/ASPC/NMA/PCNA guideline for the prevention, detection, evaluation, and management of high blood pressure in adults. *Journal of the American College of Cardiology, 71*(19), e127-e248. DOI:10.1016/j.jacc.2017.11.006
Muntner, P., et al. (2019). Measure of blood pressure in humans: A scientific statement from the American Heart Association. *Hypertension, 73,* e35-e66. https://www.ahajournals.org/doi/pdf/10.1161/HYP.0000000000000087

CLINICAL REASONING
Applying the Full-Spectrum Nursing Model

PATIENT SITUATION

A patient in the critical care unit had a stable pulse and BP for the first few days. He has become more ill and now his pulse and BP are weak and difficult to palpate. His last BP reading was abnormally low, so it must be monitored frequently. He is receiving IV fluids in both arms.

THINKING

1. *Critical Thinking (Reflecting and Deciding What to Do):* Which of the patient's vital signs (temperature, pulse, respirations, and blood pressure) might you delegate to a UAP?

DOING

2. *Practical Knowledge:* How would you take the patient's BP? Be specific:
   a. What site would you use?
   b. What equipment would you use?

3. *Nursing Process (Assessment):*
   a. Will you need to validate any of the vital signs you obtain? If so, why?
   b. How could you validate those vital signs?

CARING

4. Assume that you are very busy. How would you demonstrate caring to this patient while you are assessing his vital signs (the ones you did not delegate to a UAP)?

Critical Thinking and Clinical Judgment

1. Recall the clients in the Meet Your Patients scenario (in your textbook, Volume 1). Two-year-old Jason's oral temperature was 38.8°C (101.8°F) and his skin was warm, dry, and flushed. His mother told you that he had been eating poorly and was very irritable. What cues alert you that something is wrong?

2. You have already established (in Think Like a Nurse 18-3, in your textbook, Volume 1) what, if any, additional information you need to determine the meaning of Jason's temperature elevation.

    a. What theoretical knowledge may account for Jason's temperature?

    b. Are there any actions you should take while meeting with Jason and his mother? If so, what?

    c. What biases do you have that affect your thinking about this situation? (This requires self-knowledge.)

3. Suppose you have the following data: In a long-term care center, where most patients are older, the average normal oral temperature of the patients is 36.2°C (97.1°F). In a local well-baby nursery, the average skin temperature of the newborns ranges from 36.5°C to 37.0°C (97.7°F to 98.6°F), but it fluctuates during the first 24 hours after birth. At a walk-in surgery center, the average oral temperature of the healthy clients is 36.7°C (98°F).

    a. What conclusion might you draw about what is causing the differences in average body temperature among these three groups? (*Clue:* First list the average temperatures in order, from highest to lowest.)

    b. What theoretical knowledge did you use to answer that question?

4. Suppose you have the following data about patients' temperatures:

    Patient A, 58 years old: 0600, 36.5°C (97.7°F); 1200, 37.1°C (98.8°F); 2100, 37.2°C (99°F)

    Patient B, 14 years old: 0600, 36.4°C (97.5°F); 1200, 36°C (97.9°F); 2100, 36.9°C (98.4°F)

    Patient C, 80 years old: 0600, 35.8°C (96.4°F); 1200, 37.1°C (96.8°F); 2100, 36.2°C (97.2°F)

    What conclusion can you draw about what is probably affecting the patients' temperatures? (*Clue:* Look at the pattern for each patient. How are the patterns similar?)

5. Organize a small group of classmates. Obtain several sizes of blood pressure cuffs for each member of the group. Practice checking blood pressures on each other. Vary the size of the cuffs used, and note the variation generated by the change in cuff size. List your findings here (for at least three different people and at least two cuff sizes).

BP READING	LARGE	MEDIUM	SMALL
Person A			
Person B			
Person C			

Cuff size

6. Analyze the following scenario. A 46-year-old man is hospitalized with multiple trauma injuries after a mountain bike accident.

    Vital signs on admission: BP, 138/90; pulse, 108 beats/min; respirations, 24 breaths/min; temperature, 37.2°C (98.9°F)

    8 hours later: BP, 162/100; pulse, 122 beats/min; respirations, 26 breaths/min; temperature, 100.2°F (37.9°C)

    He is restless, agitated, and in pain.

    a. What is going on in this situation that may be influencing the vital signs?

    b. Do you have enough patient information to determine what is happening?

c. What nursing actions should you consider?

d. Should you involve others in your discussion of possible actions? If so, who?

e. What can you delegate in this situation?

f. Should you report this change in vital signs to the primary care provider? Why or why not?

7. Ms. Alvin is an 80-year-old patient in a long-term care facility. Her BP readings have been in the range of 120/70 to 130/80 mm Hg for the past month. When she is newly assigned to your care, you see that according to her medical records, she has a history of hypertension. She is taking an antihypertensive medication. You observe that she is very thin, especially in her extremities. She weighs only 90 lb (40.8 kg), although she is of average height.

   a. Do you think the recorded BPs are probably accurate? Why or why not?

   b. How could you make sure that the recorded BP readings are accurate?

   c. After looking for a small BP cuff, you discover that there is only one size available in the agency: a standard adult size. What should you do?

8. For each of the following concepts, use critical thinking to describe how or why it is important to nursing, patient care, and measuring vital signs. Note that these are not to be merely definitions.

Vital signs	Radial artery
Circadian rhythm	Brachial artery
Metabolism	Apical pulse
Shivering	Diaphragm
Fever	Oxygen saturation and pulse oximetry
Pulse	Blood pressure
Stethoscope	Peripheral resistance

What Are the Main Points in This Chapter?

- Vital signs (temperature, pulse, respirations, and blood pressure) are indicators of a person's state of health and functioning of the body systems.
- Many factors, such as age, activity, smoking, and sex, cause normal variations in vital signs.
- Body temperature is the balance between heat production and heat loss.
- Fever is a symptom, but it is also beneficial to the immune response.
- A normal pulse rate varies widely according to age, from an average of 120 beats/min for newborns to 80 beats/min for adults.
- Assess the pulse for quality, bilateral equality, volume, and rate.
- Respiration is the process of supplying the body with oxygen and disposing of carbon dioxide.
- Assess respirations for rate, depth, rhythm, and associated clinical signs (e.g., breath sounds, chest movement, cough, pallor, and cyanosis).
- Blood pressure is the pressure of the blood as it is forced against arterial walls during cardiac contraction.
- Normal blood pressure in an adult is a systolic reading of less than 120 mm Hg and a diastolic reading of less than 80 mm Hg based on an average of two or more readings taken on two or more occasions.
- The "elevated" classification for blood pressure is a systolic reading of 120 to 129 mm Hg systolic and diastolic reading more than 80 mm Hg based on an average of two or more readings taken on two or more occasions.
- Hypertension stage 1 is a systolic reading of 130 to 139 mm Hg or a diastolic reading of 80 to 89 mm Hg based on an average of two or more readings taken on two or more occasions.
- Hypertension stage 2 is a systolic reading of equal to or greater than 140 mm Hg or a diastolic reading of 90 mm Hg or greater based on an average of two or more readings taken on two or more occasions.
- Patients can prevent or modify hypertension through certain lifestyle changes (e.g., exercise, weight control, diet, and stress management).
- Nurses can delegate the activity of taking vital signs, but the nurse is responsible for evaluating the meaning of the data.

Knowledge Map

CHAPTER 18 Measuring Vital Signs

VITAL SIGNS

Factors affecting (Temperature):
- Developmental level
- Environmental temperature
- Hormones
- Exercise
- Emotions/stress
- Circadian rhythm

Heat production — In adults: metabolism and skeletal muscle movement

TEMPERATURE:
- Degree of heat maintained by the body
- Difference between heat produced and heat lost

When?
- On admission
- Before/after surgery
- To monitor effect of med/s
- Change in patient condition
- Time frame depends on:
  - HC setting
  - Nursing judgment

What?
- Part of the data used to detect physiological changes
- Indicators of a person's state of health/function of body systems

In some facilities:
- Pain assessment
- Pulse oximetry

Factors affecting (Blood Pressure):
- Family history
- Lifestyle/exercise
- Pain/stress
- Race/sex
- Obesity
- Diurnal variations
- Disease/medications

SYSTOLIC: peak pressure, ventricular contraction/ejection

DIASTOLIC: minimum pressure, between contractions

BLOOD PRESSURE:
- Pressure of blood as it's forced against arterial wall: during cardiac contraction

PULSE:
- Rhythmic expansion of artery
- Produces when heart contracts/moves a bolus of blood

Assess rate, rhythm, quality
Compare bilaterally

Sites: Apical (apex of the heart)
Peripheral: radial, brachial, carotid, femoral, popliteal, dorsalis pedis, posterior tibial

Factors influencing (Pulse):
- Age/sex
- Exercise/position changes
- Food
- Stress
- Fever/disease
- Blood loss
- Medications

RESPIRATIONS: (mechanical)
- Pulmonary ventilation/breathing
- Active movement of air in and out
- Involves contraction/relaxation of thoracic muscles and diaphragm, changes in air pressure

Involves: Contraction/relaxation of thoracic muscles and diaphragm; changes in air pressure

Assess rate, rhythm, depth, effort
Abnormal sounds: rhonchi; crackles; stridor; stertor

Factors influencing (Respirations):
- Exercise
- Pain/stress
- Smoking
- Fever/pulse rate
- Hemoglobin
- Disease
- Medications

Can influence (between Temperature, Pulse, Respirations, Blood Pressure)

CHAPTER 19

Health Assessment

STUDENT RESOURCES

The questions and exercises in this book allow you to practice the kind of thinking you will use as a full-spectrum nurse. Critical-thinking questions usually have more than one right answer, so we do not provide "correct" answers for these features. Try to answer these questions yourself. It is more important to develop your nursing judgment than to just cover content. You will learn more by discussing the questions with your peers. If you are still unsure, see the Davis Advantage chapter resources for suggested responses.

To explore learning resources for this chapter,

Go to www.DavisAdvantage.com and find:

Answers and Suggested Responses for all questions in this chapter
Concept Map
Knowledge Map
References and Bibliography

Key Concepts

Health assessment
Nursing assessment
Physical examination

Related Concepts

See the Concept Map on Davis Advantage.

Caring for the Williams Family

Stanley Williams has had a comprehensive physical examination with Assad Johnson, the nurse practitioner. To review the note written by Assad,

Go to **Chapter 19, Documenting Physical Examination Findings,** in Volume 1.

Also, for laboratory data for Stanley Williams,

Go to **Chapter 19, Caring for the Williams Family, including Laboratory Data for Stanley Williams,** in Volume 1.

Caring for the Williams Family (continued)

A. Discuss how each of the following would differ from the examination Assad Johnson conducted and what would be expected if:
   - A registered nurse conducted the examination.
   - A nursing student performed the examination.

B. Review Assad's documentation of the examination. Identify the abnormal findings.

C. Review the laboratory work. Identify the abnormal findings.

D. What conclusions, if any, can you draw from these findings? What actions should you consider based on these conclusions?

E. Identify at least two nursing diagnoses based on these findings.

F. Assad Johnson has identified that Mr. Williams is overweight.
   - What information do you need to determine the etiology of this problem?
   - Because you do not have that information, write a two-part diagnostic statement describing Mr. Williams' nutrition status.

G. Now rewrite the nutrition statement as a three-part statement, using "as evidenced by."

H. Assad Johnson has identified the diagnosis pain (in knees) for Mr. Williams. If the pain is caused by the medical condition osteoarthritis, how would you write a two-part diagnostic statement to describe this health status?

I. How would the examination of Nadine Williams differ from the examination Stanley had?

J. How would the examination of Kayla Robinson, Stanley's 3-year-old granddaughter, differ?

K. If you were responsible for examining Stanley Williams, what aspects of the examination would you find most challenging? Explain why.

PracticalKnowledge clinical application

PROCEDURES

Key Point: *As the RN, you are responsible for (1) performing the initial assessment to establish a baseline and (2) performing follow-up assessments for any changes.* You can instruct unlicensed assistive personnel (UAPs) to report any changes to you. You can delegate measurement of height, weight, and vital signs to the UAP. However, you may want to obtain the first set of vital signs yourself, because they will serve as a baseline.

Together, the procedures in this section represent a comprehensive physical examination you can use for initial and ongoing physical assessments. Procedure 19-20 provides a brief bedside assessment. The following procedures are described mainly for adult patients. It is essential that you identify the *individual and special* needs of each patient. This is particularly important for patients with physical, intellectual, or developmental disabilities. Patients with disabilities have health conditions and factors affecting their health that can vary in kind, manifestation, severity, or complexity from those of others in the community. You should approach their care and interventions in a manner that is adapted to their individual needs. To review ways in which to modify your examination for people of different ages and abilities,

> Go to **Chapter 19, Modifications for Different Age Groups,** in Volume 1.

Also note the following:

- *Developmental modifications* for various age groups are given just before the procedure steps. Use these to help you adapt your examination techniques to the specific patient.
- *Developmental variations* are provided in the procedure in column 2, under Expected and Abnormal findings. Use these when you are analyzing assessment findings.

Key Point: *Compare side to side throughout the examination.*

UNIT 3   Essential Nursing Interventions

Procedure 19-1 ■ Performing the General Survey

▶ For steps to follow in *all* procedures, refer to the Universal Steps for All Procedures on the inside back cover.

Equipment
See Equipment Needed for Physical Examination, later in this chapter.

Equipment Needed for Physical Examination

Usual Equipment for Ongoing Assessment

Thermometer (for measuring temperature)

Stethoscope (for measuring blood pressure and listening to heart, lung, and bowel sounds)

Sphygmomanometer (for measuring blood pressure)

Tape measure (to measure circumference and length)

Pocket ruler (to measure size or distance)

Scale (to measure weight and height)

Gloves (to wear if there is any possible exposure to blood or body fluids)

CHAPTER 19 Health Assessment

Equipment Needed for Physical Examination—cont'd

Additional Equipment for a Comprehensive Assessment

Snellen acuity chart (for screening vision)

Ophthalmoscope (for inspection of the internal structures of the eye)

Otoscope (for examining the external auditory canal and tympanic membrane)

Nasal speculum (for examining the nasal turbinates)

Tuning fork (for auditory screening and assessment of vibratory sensation during the neurological examination)

Percussion hammer (for eliciting deep tendon reflexes)

Penlight (for visualizing the eyes and inside of mouth, or highlighting a skin lesion)

Vaginal speculum and lubricant (for examining the female pelvis; lubricant is also used for rectal examinations)

Cotton-tipped applicators (for obtaining specimens)

Cotton balls, tongue depressor, strong-smelling substance, a glass of water (for testing various cranial nerves)

(continued on next page)

Procedure 19-1 ■ Performing the General Survey (continued)

Positioning

- Have the client seated as you begin the examination (on an examination table or on the side of the bed). Face the client and make eye contact.
  Builds rapport and puts the client at ease. **Key Point:** *Keep in mind, though, that culture can influence whether it is considered polite or rude to make eye contact when addressing someone, and whether eye contact is necessary to indicate that one is listening. Understanding your patient's cultural preferences is key.*
- If the client is unable to sit, use Fowler's or semi-Fowler's position.
  An upright position allows the client to expand their lungs fully and is useful for assessing vital signs, head and neck, heart and lungs, back, and upper extremities.

Focused History Questions

- How are you feeling today?
- (If the client is an outpatient) What brings you to the clinic today?
- Are you in any discomfort or pain?
- Have you had any hospitalizations or surgeries?
- What medicines do you take? Name both prescribed and over-the-counter drugs.
- How much alcohol do you drink per day? Do you smoke cigarettes or use tobacco products (e-cigarettes, chew)? If so, how many per day? Do you use drugs for nonmedical purposes?
- Do you use any herbal products or natural remedies? If so, which ones and how often?
- Do you have any difficulty falling asleep or staying asleep?

Developmental Modifications for Infants and Children

- Encourage the parents to be present for the examination.
  Infants and toddlers usually feel most secure if a parent is present.
- Adolescents should be examined without parents or siblings present unless they request otherwise. Provide privacy.

Developmental Modifications for Older Adults

- *Older adults*—Assess the older adult's functional status. You can use the Lawton Instrumental Activities of Daily Living (IADL) found in the Assessment Guidelines and Tools in Chapter 3.
- *Older adults*—Work the SPICES assessment into the examination of various body systems: **s**leep disorders, **p**roblems eating or feeding, **i**ncontinence, **c**onfusion, **e**vidence of falls, **s**kin breakdown.

> When performing the procedure, always identify your patient according to agency policy, using two identifiers, and be attentive to standard precautions, hand hygiene, patient safety and privacy, body mechanics, and documentation.

Procedure Steps	Findings
Observe the client's general characteristics.	
1. **Identify cues of physical or emotional distress** (e.g., pain, fear, or anxiety). If cues of distress are present, perform a focused assessment, and address the immediate problem.	**Expected findings:** The client is in no apparent distress. The client appears relaxed, with no evidence of pain, fear, or anxiety. **Abnormal findings:** Pain, grimacing, breathing problems, skin color changes
2. **Observe apparent age, sex, gender, and race.** Ask the patient these questions: What racial or ethnic group do you identify with? What is your sex? What sex were you assigned at birth? ■ What is your gender? ■ Do you consider yourself transgender? Have you had any gender-confirming surgeries or treatments? Ask yourself these questions: ■ Is apparent age consistent with biological age? ■ Are there cultural or gender-related factors that influence the examination or findings?	**Expected findings:** Client appears stated age. Makes eye contact consistent with cultural norms. Is reasonably comfortable with being examined.

3. **Note facial characteristics**, including facial expression, symmetry of facial features, and the condition and color of the skin. Ask yourself these questions:
   - What is the client's face telling me?
   - Is the facial expression appropriate to the situation?
   - Are facial features symmetrical (palpebral fissure and nasolabial folds)?
   - Are there any changes in condition or color of skin?
   - Does the client maintain eye contact appropriate to their developmental and cultural preferences?
   - Does the client appear older than stated age?

   Expected findings: Face is symmetrical; visible skin is intact without excessive wrinkling, discoloration, or deformity.

   Abnormal findings: Excessive wrinkling may be from sun exposure, tobacco use, or illness.

4. **Note body type and posture.**

   Ask yourself these questions:
   - Is the body build stocky, slender, as expected, obese, or **cachectic** (very thin, wasted appearance)?
   - Are the body parts proportional to the client's overall size?
   - Is body fat distributed proportionally?
   - Does the client assume a specific position for comfort (e.g., sitting versus supine)?

   Expected findings: Posture is upright, and body appears proportionate.

5. **Observe gait**, and note any abnormal movements. If the client has altered mobility, determine ability to move and amount of assistance needed. Ask yourself these questions:
   - Does the client move in a coordinated manner?
   - Are there any obvious gait problems?
   - Does the client walk with a wide base of support or short stride length?
   - Does the client use assistive devices, such as a cane?
   - Are there any abnormal or spastic movements?

   Expected findings: Movements are coordinated; gait is steady; does not use assistive devices.
   For clients with a physical disability: safe and efficient use of assistive devices or wheelchair.

   Abnormal findings: Unstable or shuffling gait; spastic and stiff movements may be associated with joint, muscle, or neurological disorders. A slumped position may indicate fatigue, depression, osteoporosis, or pain.

6. **Listen to your client's speech pattern,** pace, quality, tone, vocabulary, and sentence structure while you are examining the body systems. Ask yourself these questions:
   - Are the responses appropriate (a) to the situation, and (b) for developmental stage?
   - Is there any difficulty with speech?
   - Does the client's tone of voice match their statements?
   - Is the voice hoarse?
   - Does the client have a language barrier from physical language disabilities (stuttering, articulation disorder, and hearing loss) or related to not sharing a common language with the provider?

   Expected findings: Client responds appropriately to questions either by voice or by use of assistive device. If using voice, tone matches responses; speech is clear and evenly paced and rises and falls based on content.

   Abnormal findings: Rapid speech, slow speech, slurred speech, illogical responses, language barrier.

(continued on next page)

Procedure 19-1 ■ Performing the General Survey (continued)

7. **Assess mental state and affect.**
   a. Determine level of consciousness.
   b. Determine orientation to time, place, and person.

   Ask yourself these questions:
   - If the client is disoriented, do they reorient easily?
   - What is the client's mood? Is it appropriate for the situation?

   NOTE: *If you note any abnormal findings, be sure to focus on them when you assess mental status during the sensory neurological examination.*

   Expected findings: Awake, alert, and oriented to time, place, person, and self. Mood is appropriate for the situation.

   Abnormal findings:
   - Confusion and irritability may indicate hypoxia or medication side effects.
   - Inability to recall information or provide history may indicate a neurological disorder.
   - Lethargy and somnolence may be due to medications; depression; or a neurological, thyroid, liver, kidney, or cardiovascular disorder.
   - Bizarre responses may signal a psychiatric problem.

8. **Observe dress and hygiene.**
   - Describe the client's attire (clothing).
   - Describe the client's hygiene.
   - Describe any unusual odors.

   Expected findings: Client is dressed appropriately for the climate. Skin is clean. No noticeable odor.

   Abnormal findings: Poor hygiene, dirty skin or nails, uncombed hair, visible soiling of clothing, mismatched or wrinkled clothing, objectionable odor. May indicate an impaired ability to care for oneself, chronic pain, fatigue, depression, or low self-esteem.

9. **Measure vital signs:** blood pressure, temperature, radial pulse, respiratory rate. If your initial observations and interview indicate that the client is in pain, perform a pain assessment, as well. (See Chapter 28.)

   Expected findings:
   BP: <120/80 mm Hg
   Temperature: 97.3°F–98.6°F (36.3°C–37°C) oral
   Pulse: 60–100 beats/min, regular, and easily palpated
   Respiratory rate: 12–20, regular and even

   Abnormal findings: See Chapter 18.

10. **Measure height and weight.**
    a. For adults: Calculate BMI, or use the accompanying table.

    $$\frac{Wt\ (lb) \times 703}{Ht\ (in.)^2} = BMI$$

    b. For children: Plot height and weight on growth chart.

    Expected findings: For adults: BMI is 18.5–24.9.
    For children: Height and weight are consistent with previous trend on growth chart.

    Abnormal findings: BMI <18.5 = underweight
    BMI 25–29.9 = overweight
    BMI >30 = obese
    BMI 30–34.9 = level I moderate obesity
    BMI 35–39.9 = level II severe obesity
    BMI >40 = level III morbid obesity

    NOTE: *For growth charts for males and females from birth to 20 years of age,*

    ▶ Go to the CDC National Center for Health Statistics Web site at http://www.cdc.gov/growthcharts/clinical_charts.htm

Developmental Modifications

Adults
- Use a platform scale with a sliding ruler, or a bed scale if the client cannot stand safely.

Infants and children
- Weigh infants without clothing; weigh older children in their underwear.
- For infants and children younger than 2 years, use a stationary measure (e.g., infant scale) if available. Position supine to measure height; be sure knees are extended.
- For infants and children younger than age 2 years, also measure head circumference.

❓ What if...

- **There is an apparent language barrier?**
  Obtain an interpreter; and refer to Clinical Insight 15-4 in Chapter 15 of this volume.

Use this table to find body mass index, based on height and weight, or use a BMI calculator such as the ones at http://www.nhlbi.nih.gov/health/educational/lose_wt/BMI/bmicalc.htm ▼

Weight (lb)

Height (ft/in)	120	130	140	150	160	170	180	190	200	210	220	230	240	250	260	270	280	290	300	310	320	330
4'5"	30	33	35	38	40	43	45	48	50	53	55	58	60	63	65	68	70	73	75	78	80	83
4'6"	29	31	34	36	39	41	43	46	48	51	53	56	58	60	63	65	68	70	72	75	77	80
4'7"	28	30	33	35	37	40	42	44	47	49	51	54	56	58	61	63	65	68	70	72	75	77
4'8"	27	29	31	34	36	38	40	43	45	47	49	52	54	56	58	61	63	65	67	70	72	74
4'9"	26	28	30	33	35	37	39	41	43	46	48	50	52	54	56	59	61	63	65	67	69	72
4'10"	25	27	29	31	34	36	38	40	42	44	46	48	50	52	54	57	59	61	63	65	67	69
4'11"	24	26	28	30	32	34	36	38	40	43	45	47	49	51	53	55	57	59	61	63	65	67
5'0"	23	25	27	29	31	33	35	37	39	41	43	45	47	49	51	53	55	57	59	61	63	65
5'1"	23	25	27	28	30	32	34	36	38	40	42	44	45	47	49	51	53	55	57	59	61	62
5'2"	22	24	26	27	29	31	33	35	37	38	40	42	44	46	48	49	51	53	55	57	59	60
5'3"	21	23	25	27	28	30	32	34	36	37	39	41	43	44	46	48	50	51	53	55	57	59
5'4"	21	22	24	26	28	29	31	33	34	36	38	40	41	43	45	46	48	50	52	53	55	57
5'5"	20	22	23	25	27	28	30	32	33	35	38	38	40	42	43	45	47	48	50	52	53	55
5'6"	19	21	23	24	26	27	29	31	32	34	36	37	39	40	42	44	45	47	49	50	52	53
5'7"	19	20	22	24	25	27	28	30	31	33	35	36	38	39	41	42	44	46	47	49	50	52
5'8"	18	20	21	23	24	26	27	29	30	32	34	35	37	38	40	41	43	44	46	47	49	50
5'9"	18	19	21	22	24	25	27	28	30	31	33	34	36	37	38	40	41	43	44	46	47	49
5'10"	17	19	20	22	23	24	26	27	29	30	32	33	35	36	37	39	40	42	43	45	46	47
5'11"	17	18	20	21	22	24	25	27	28	29	31	32	34	35	36	38	39	41	42	43	45	46
6'	16	18	19	20	22	23	24	26	27	29	30	31	33	34	35	37	38	39	41	42	43	45
6'1"	16	17	19	20	21	22	24	25	26	28	29	30	32	33	34	36	37	38	40	41	42	44
6'2"	15	17	18	19	21	22	23	24	26	27	28	30	31	32	33	35	36	37	39	40	41	42
6'3"	15	16	18	19	20	21	23	24	25	26	28	29	30	31	33	34	35	36	38	39	40	41
6'4"	15	16	17	18	20	21	22	23	24	26	27	28	29	30	32	33	34	35	37	38	39	40
6'5"	14	15	17	18	19	20	21	23	24	25	26	27	29	30	31	32	33	34	36	37	38	39
6'6"	14	15	16	17	19	20	21	22	23	24	25	27	28	29	30	31	32	34	35	36	37	38
6'7"	14	15	16	17	18	19	20	21	23	24	25	26	27	28	29	30	32	33	34	35	36	37
6'8"	13	14	15	17	18	19	20	21	22	23	24	25	26	28	29	30	31	32	33	34	35	36
6'9"	13	14	15	16	17	18	19	20	21	23	24	25	26	27	28	29	30	31	32	33	34	35
6'10"	13	14	15	16	17	18	19	20	21	22	23	24	25	26	27	28	29	30	31	32	34	35

Less risk ─────────────────────── More risk

Documentation

- Document BP as right or left arm, and note the patient's position: sitting, standing, or lying.
- Document temperature measurement route: oral, rectal, or tympanic membrane.
- If you need more information about documenting your findings,

▶ Go to **Chapter 19, Caring for the Williams Family**, including **Documenting Physical Examination Findings (Stanley Williams),** in Volume 1.

Practice Resources

Centers for Disease Control and Prevention (CDC) (last updated 2021); CDC (last updated 2022); National Guideline Clearinghouse (NGC) (2017, June 3); National Heart, Lung, and Blood Institute (n.d.).

Procedure 19-2 ■ Assessing the Skin

➤ For steps to follow in *all* procedures, refer to the Universal Steps for All Procedures on the inside back cover.

Equipment
- Nonlatex gloves (if exposure to body fluids is a possibility)
- Flexible transparent ruler
- Penlight
- Magnifier
- Pen and record form

✚ Clean stethoscope and rulers before and after use unless they are used for only one patient.

Focused History Questions
Ask the patient about the history or presence of any of the following:
- Rashes
- Allergies
- Areas of skin that have changed color
- Skin lesions
- Skin with rough or unusual texture
- Skin that is always warm or cool, regardless of room temperature

Developmental Modifications for Older Adults
- Assess the level of risk for pressure injury. For assessment tools (Braden scale, Norton scale), go to Chapter 32 in this volume.

  As adults age, the subcutaneous tissue layer thins. The dermal layer loses elasticity as a result of changes in collagen fibers, and the strong bond between the epidermal and dermal layers decreases. These changes make the skin prone to breakdown.

➤ When performing the procedure, always identify your patient according to agency policy, using two identifiers, and be attentive to standard precautions, hand hygiene, patient safety and privacy, body mechanics, and documentation.

Procedure Steps

1. **Inspect skin color, including mucous membranes, tongue, and conjunctiva.**
   To assess color changes of exposed and unexposed areas. Color changes and odors may indicate underlying disease and should be fully investigated.
   a. Provide good lighting.
   b. For clients with dark skin, look for color changes in the conjunctiva or oral mucosa, tongue, lips, nailbeds, palms of the hands, and soles of the feet.
   Skin color varies widely among individuals by age and ethnicity, but in each individual skin color is fairly uniform over the entire body. ▼

   c. Note any unusual odors.
   d. To assess for cyanosis, be sure to examine the tongue.
   Exposure to cold causes the lips to turn blue, but not the tongue. Cyanosis affects the color of the skin, mucous membranes, and tongue.

Findings

Expected findings: Skin color is uniform, with darker exposed areas. Mucous membranes and conjunctiva are pink and moist. No unusual odors.

Developmental Variations

Newborns—May be jaundiced for a few weeks. Blue-black dermal melanocytosis and pink-red capillary hemangiomas are common and fade with time. ✚ Differentiate congenital dermal melanocytosis with marking resulting from cupping, coining, or abuse, especially due to the location (lumbosacral region) and color (bluish).

Older adults—May have thin, translucent skin and wrinkles due to loss of elasticity. Fragile skin is not uncommon among lighter-skinned, older adults.

Abnormal findings: Pallor, jaundice (may require further investigation), cyanosis, erythema, hyperpigmentation, hypopigmentation.
- Café-au-lait spots, although usually normal, may sometimes signal a genetic disorder.
- If there are abnormal findings, ask the patient (or someone who knows the client well) about the baseline skin color.

For more information about skin color changes, see Table 19-2 in Volume 1.
Also see the following illustrations: Skin Color Changes.

Skin Color Changes

Jaundice

Cyanosis

Vitiligo

Port-wine stain (nevus flammeus)

2. **Palpate skin for temperature.**
   a. Wear procedure gloves and discard after examining any open areas of the skin.
   b. Use dorsal aspect of hand or fingers.
   c. Compare bilaterally.
   The dorsa of the hands and the fingers are most sensitive to temperature variations.
   d. Check the skin temperature over any area of erythema.
   e. If skin feels excessively warm, validate your data and assess for fever.

Expected findings: Skin is warm; temperature is the same bilaterally.

Abnormal findings: Local area(s) that are warmer or cooler than the rest of the skin; generalized temperature increase or decrease.
- Localized warmth with erythema can indicate an infection.
- Cool skin might be a sign of compromised circulation, shock, exposure to cold, hypothyroidism, or dehydration, particularly in older adults.

(continued on next page)

Procedure 19-2 ■ Assessing the Skin (continued)

3. **Palpate skin for turgor.** Test an unexposed area, such as the area below the clavicle, inner thigh, sternum, or forehead, by gently pinching up the skin, noting its return when you release it.

   Developmental Modifications

   Infants—Check skin turgor on the abdomen.

   Older adults—Check skin turgor over the sternum or clavicle. ▼

   Expected findings: Skin returns immediately to its original position.

   Developmental Variations

   🍁 *Older adults* have decreased skin turgor due to decreased elasticity.

   Abnormal findings: Decreased or increased turgor.
   - *Tenting (decreased turgor):* Skin takes several seconds to return to original position.
   - *Tenting* is seen with dehydration or normal aging. It predisposes the patient to skin breakdown.
   - *Increased turgor:* Skin tension does not allow the skin to be pinched up; may be due to edema or scleroderma.

4. **Palpate the skin for texture.**
   Texture varies, depending on the area being assessed and the age of the client.

   Expected findings: Skin is smooth and soft. Exposed areas and extensor surfaces (e.g., elbows and knees) are drier and coarser than other areas.

   Developmental Variations

   Infants and young children—Have smooth skin.

   Abnormal findings: Coarse, thick, rough, or dry skin; very smooth, thin, fine-textured, shiny skin

5. **Palpate skin for moisture/hydration.** Use the dorsum of your hand.

   Expected findings: Skin is warm and dry.

   Developmental Variations

   🍁 *Older adults*—Skin may be dry and flaky because of decreased activity of sebaceous and sweat glands.
   Adolescents—May have skin that is oilier than normal.

   Abnormal findings: Increased moisture (skin feels damp, visible diaphoresis); decreased moisture (skin feels dry)

6. **Inspect for edema.**
   a. Press firmly with your fingertip for 5 seconds over a bony area, such as the tibia.
   b. Release your finger and observe the skin for the reaction.
   c. If edema is present, note the location, degree, and type of swelling. For example, if you observe edema in the lower leg, how far up the leg does it extend?

   Expected findings: No edema. Normally there will be no evidence of the pressure once you release your finger. If pitting edema is present, you will see a depression in the skin.

   Grading System

   Trace: Minimal depression with pressure

   + 1:   2 mm depression; rapid return of skin to position

   + 2:   4 mm depression that disappears in 10–15 seconds

CHAPTER 19 Health Assessment   209

+ 3: 6 mm depression that lasts 1–2 minutes. Area appears swollen.

+ 4: 8 mm depression that persists for 2–3 minutes. Area is grossly edematous.

Abnormal findings: Edema is an abnormal finding.

7. **Identify any skin lesions.**
   a. Inspect and palpate lesions.
   b. When you notice bruises, be alert for signs of abuse (see Chapter 5).
   c. Ask the client, "Do you have any new moles or other lesions? Has there been any change in existing moles/lesions?"
   d. Assess for malignant lesions using ABCDE:
      A (asymmetry)
      B (irregular borders)
      C (color variations)
      D (diameter: 0.5 cm)
      E (elevation) ▼

Malignant melanoma

Expected finding: No lesions are present.

Normal variations include moles, freckles, birthmarks, striae (in pregnant women or clients who have lost much weight), and wrinkles.

Developmental Variations

Newborns—**Milia** (tiny collections of sebum, usually on the face) are common.

Adolescents—Acne is a common abnormal finding among adolescents.

Adults—**Acrochordon**s (skin tags) may be seen around the neck, axillae, skinfolds, or areas where clothing rubs.

Older adults—Flat beige or brown macules are common on exposed skin areas.

Abnormal findings: See the illustrations in the following Abnormal Skin Lesions section and the table Describing Skin Lesions at the end of this procedure.

Abnormal Skin Lesions

Herpes

Capillary hemangioma

Vesicles (blisters)

Venous star

Petechiae

Ringworm

(continued on next page)

Procedure 19-2 ■ Assessing the Skin (continued)

Describing Skin Lesions

When you observe a lesion, evaluate and describe the following:
- **Size.** Measure the length, width, and depth of the lesion.
- **Shape and pattern.** Describe the *shape* of individual lesions. If there are clusters or groups, describe the *pattern*. Is it linear or circular? Are the *borders* distinct, or do they run together? Is the border smooth or irregular?
- **Color.** Describe the color of the lesion, and determine whether there is any variation of color within the lesion.
- **Distribution.** Are the lesions distributed over the entire body? Are they confined to a specific region? What parts of the body are affected?
- **Texture.** The texture (e.g., smooth, rough, scaly) of a lesion helps with classification.
- **Surface relationship.** To assess surface relationship, you will need to palpate the lesion. Is it flat, raised, or depressed? Is it firmly attached to the surrounding skin or mobile?
- **Exudate.** Examine the lesion(s) for signs of drainage. Describe the color, appearance, amount, and odor of drainage, if present.
- **Tenderness, pain, or itching.** Press on the lesion, and determine the patient's reaction. Does touching the lesion cause pain or discomfort?

Patient Teaching

Teach the patient the signs and symptoms of skin cancer, the importance of the skin examination, and preventive measures.

Home Care

- Assess the skill level of the caregiver. Instruct the caregiver on the importance of skin assessment and measures to prevent skin breakdown.
- ✚ Be alert for lesions (e.g., burns, bruises) that may signal physical abuse. For more signs of abuse, refer to Procedure 6-1.

Documentation

- If lesions are present, describe the history: onset, duration, associated or aggravating factors (e.g., itching), factors that relieve symptoms, treatments that have been used, and responses to treatment.
- Sketch the location of skin lesions on body diagrams, if available (see example); or sketch a body if necessary. ▼

If you need more information about documenting your findings,

▶ Go to **Chapter 19, Caring for the Williams Family,** including **Documenting Physical Examination Findings (Stanley Williams),** in Volume 1.

Describing Skin Lesions

PRIMARY LESIONS

Types		Description
Macule (nonpalpable, <1 cm)	Macule (nonpalpable, <1 cm)	Flat and colored. Examples: freckle, petechiae, birthmark, Mongolian spot
Papule (palpable) <1 cm; plaque >1 cm	Papules (seborrheic keratosis)	Elevated and raised but superficial. Examples: mole, psoriasis
Vesicle (palpable), <1 cm; bulla, >1 cm	Vesicles (blisters)	Elevated and filled with serous fluid. Examples: blister, herpes simplex

(continued on next page)

CHAPTER 19 Health Assessment 211

Procedure 19-2 ■ Assessing the Skin (continued)

Describing Skin Lesions—cont'd
PRIMARY LESIONS

Types		Description
Cyst (palpable), <2 cm	Keratogenous cyst	Palpable, fluid-filled, and encapsulated. If not fluid-filled, called a nodule.
Pustule (palpable)	Pustules (acne)	Elevated and filled with pus. Examples: acne, folliculitis, impetigo
	Nodule (palpable)	Elevated, solid, and firm, with depth into dermis. Examples: wart, lipoma (fatty cyst)
Wheal	Hive	Elevated, superficial, with localized edema. Examples: insect bites, hives

CHAPTER 19 Health Assessment   213

Describing Skin Lesions—cont'd

SECONDARY LESIONS

Types		Description
Excoriation	Excoriation from pruritus	Abrasion or loss of skin that does not extend beyond the superficial epidermis. Examples: scratches, stasis dermatitis, atopic dermatitis
Erosion	Erosions	Loss of superficial epidermis, usually secondary to rupture of a blister. Examples: abrasions and impetigo
Fissure	Cheilitis	Linear break in the skin ("crack"); may extend to the dermis. Examples: athlete's foot, cheilitis
Ulcer	Stasis ulcer	Irregularly shaped with loss of tissue. Graded based on depth and tissue involvement. Examples: pressure injury, stasis ulcers

(continued on next page)

Procedure 19-2 ■ Assessing the Skin (continued)

Describing Skin Lesions—cont'd

SECONDARY LESIONS

Types		Description
Crust	Crust	Elevated, rough texture with dried exudate. Examples: impetigo, herpes simplex
Scales	Psoriasis	White to tan flaking, dead skin cells; may be adherent or loose. Examples: psoriasis and dandruff
Scar		Fibrous tissue at site of injury, trauma, or surgery. Examples: surgical site, trauma site
Keloid	Keloids	Raised and irregular scar due to excess collagen formation. Examples: surgical scars, ear piercing

Sources: Linton, C. P. (2011). Describing the configuration of skin lesions. *Journal of the Dermatology Nurses' Association, 3*(6), 379.
Reddy, M. (2008). Skin and wound care: Important considerations in the older adult. *Advances in Skin & Wound Care, 21*(9), 424–436.

Practice Resources
Linton (2011); Reddy (2008).

Procedure 19-3 ■ Assessing the Hair

▶ For steps to follow in *all* procedures, refer to the Universal Steps for All Procedures on the inside back cover.

Equipment
- Nonlatex procedure gloves (if exposure to body fluids is a possibility)
- Pen and record form

Focused History Questions
- Have you had any changes in hair texture?
- Have you had any hair loss?
- Do you use dyes or chemical treatments for curling or straightening?

▶ When performing the procedure, always identify your patient according to agency policy, using two identifiers, and be attentive to standard precautions, hand hygiene, patient safety and privacy, body mechanics, and documentation.

Procedure Steps

1. **Inspect the hair and scalp.** Check the color, quantity, and distribution of the hair and the condition of the scalp. Note the presence of lesions or pediculosis.
   Sex, genetics, and age affect hair distribution on the head, extremities, pubis, and axillae. With aging, melanocyte function declines and sebaceous gland function decreases. ▼

   Alopecia areata

   Pediculosis (lice)

Findings

Expected findings: The hair is evenly distributed on the scalp, and fine body hair is present over the body (male individuals often have more hair on face, chest, and back; alopecia is considered normal in males). The hair is clean and free of debris or pediculosis.

Developmental Variations

Infants—May have very little scalp hair.

Adolescents—May have oily hair. Puberty marks the onset of pubic hair growth and increased hair growth.

🍁 *Older adults*—Scalp, axillary, leg, and pubic hair may be dry and thin; hair of the ears, nostrils, and eyebrows may become coarse.

Abnormal findings:
- Generalized hair loss not attributed to genetics or aging; patchy hair loss
- **Hirsutism** (excess facial or trunk hair)
- White hair accompanied by very pale skin is seen in a condition known as albinism (lack of pigment).
- Alterations in hair distribution may be signs of disease.

2. **Palpate the texture of the hair.**

Expected findings: Hair texture varies (fine, medium, coarse) depending on genetics and treatments.

Abnormal findings: Very dry, coarse hair may indicate hypothyroidism; thinning and very fine hair may indicate hyperthyroidism.

(continued on next page)

Procedure 19-3 ■ Assessing the Hair (continued)

3. **Palpate the scalp for mobility and tenderness.**

Expected findings: Scalp is smooth, firm, symmetrical, nontender, and without lesions.

Abnormal findings: Common deviations include an asymmetrical or bumpy scalp due to trauma or lesions and scaly flakes or patches due to fungal infection (e.g., dandruff), dermatitis, or psoriasis. Tenderness, lesions

Developmental Variations

Infants: In newborns **cradle cap**—scaly white patches over the scalp due to secretion of sebum—is common. It can be removed with washing and gentle scrubbing.

Patient Teaching
If indicated, teach the patient to check for head lice, and provide preventive measures.

Documentation
If you need more information about documenting your findings,

▶ Go to **Chapter 19, Caring for the Williams Family,** including **Documenting Physical Examination Findings (Stanley Williams),** in Volume 1.

Procedure 19-4 ■ Assessing the Nails

▶ For steps to follow in *all* procedures, refer to the Universal Steps for All Procedures on the inside back cover.

Equipment
- Nonlatex gloves (if exposure to body fluids is a possibility)
- Pen and record form

Focused History Questions
- Have you had any recent changes in the way your nails grow or look?
- Have you had any recent trauma to your nails?
- Do you use acrylic nails?
- Do you have any medical problems, such as peripheral vascular disease or diabetes?

▶ When performing the procedure, always identify your patient according to agency policy, using two identifiers, and be attentive to standard precautions, hand hygiene, patient safety and privacy, body mechanics, and documentation.

Procedure Steps

1. **Inspect nails.**
   - Check nails for color, condition, texture, and shape.
   - Examine nails on both hands and feet. However, for efficiency you may defer examination of the toenails until the assessment of peripheral circulation. ▼

   Nail root
   Nail body
   Nailbed

   About 160°   Flattened angle (180°)   Angle > 180°

Findings
Expected findings: Healthy nailbeds are level, firm, and similar to the color of the skin. The shape is convex, with a nail plate angle of about 160°.

Developmental Variations

Newborns—Have very thin nails

Children—May bite their nails. Most children outgrow this habit.

🍁 *Older adults*—Nails grow more slowly, become thicker, and tend to split.

Abnormal findings:
- Black discoloration resulting from blood under the nail is seen after local trauma.
- Pale or cyanotic nailbeds are seen in circulatory or respiratory disorders that result in anemia or hypoxia.
- White spots may indicate zinc deficiency.
- Spoon-shaped (concave) nails are associated with iron deficiency.
- Crescent moon–shaped nails may indicate an endocrine disorder.

CHAPTER 19 Health Assessment   217

2. **Inspect and palpate for texture.**
Grooves or lines in the nails provide information about nutrition and health problems.

Expected findings: Nails are smooth and uniform in texture; surrounding tissue is smooth.

Abnormal findings: Thickened nails with yellowing may indicate fungal infection, known as *onychomycosis*.
- Brittle nails are seen with hyperthyroidism, malnutrition, calcium and iron deficiencies, and repeated use of harsh nail products.
- Soft, boggy nails are seen with poor oxygenation.
- Paronychia

3. **Assess capillary refill.** Briefly press the tip of the nail with firm, steady pressure; then release and observe for changes in color.
This test assesses circulatory adequacy rather than the nails themselves. However, circulatory insufficiency affects the nails and nailbeds. It is convenient to perform the assessment at this point in the examination. ▼

Expected findings: Normal capillary refill is <2 to 3 seconds.

Developmental Variations

Older adults—Capillary refill time (CRT) is slower.
Males—CRT is faster than in women.
Environment—CRT is slower in a cool environment.

Abnormal findings: Delayed capillary refill ▼

Fungal infection

Paronychia

Half-and-half nails

(continued on next page)

Procedure 19-4 ■ Assessing the Nails (continued)

Documentation
If you need more information about documenting your findings,

➤ Go to **Chapter 19, Caring for the Williams Family,** including **Documenting Physical Examination Findings (Stanley Williams),** in Volume 1.

Practice Resources
Lima & Bakker (2015); Linton (2012).

Procedure 19-5 ■ Assessing the Head and Face

➤ For steps to follow in *all* procedures, refer to the Universal Steps for All Procedures on the inside back cover.

Equipment
- Nonlatex gloves (if exposure to body fluids is a possibility)
- Penlight (to transilluminate the sinuses)
- Pen and record form

✚ Clean equipment before and after use unless used for only one patient.

Focused History Questions
- Have you had any recent headaches?
- Have you ever had a head injury or loss of consciousness?
- Have you ever had a seizure?
- Do you have jaw or facial pain?

Positioning
The client should be sitting, if possible.

➤ When performing the procedure, always identify your patient according to agency policy, using two identifiers, and be attentive to standard precautions, hand hygiene, patient safety and privacy, body mechanics, and documentation.

Procedure Steps

1. **Inspect the head. Check for size, shape, symmetry, and position.**
   If size seems unusual, measure it.

   Developmental Modifications
   Newborns and infants—Assess and transilluminate fontanels, and measure head circumference.

Findings

Expected findings: There is wide variation in head size and shape, although the shape should be symmetrical and rounded. The head should be erect, midline, and proportional to the body size based on age.

Developmental Variations
Newborns and infants—Cranial bones are not fused at birth, and head shape may reflect normal pressure or trauma during vaginal birth for several weeks. The anterior fontanel ("soft spot") fuses at about 18 months; the posterior, at about 8 weeks. Infants normally cannot hold their head up until about 2 months of age.

Abnormal findings: Larger or smaller than expected size for age, asymmetry of skull

2. **Inspect the face.** Note the client's facial expression. Ask yourself these questions:
   - Are the facial features symmetrical?
   - Are there any abnormal facial movements?
   - Are there any visible lesions or abnormal hair distribution?

Expected findings: Facial expression is appropriate for the situation. No visible lesions. Facial features and movement are symmetrical.

CHAPTER 19   Health Assessment   219

Helpful hint: Look for symmetry in the palpebral fissures and the nasolabial folds. ▼

Nasolabial fold
Palpebral fissure

Abnormal findings: Facial appearance inconsistent with sex, age, or racial/ethnic group; asymmetry of facial features or facial movement ▼

Bell's palsy

Cushing syndrome

3. **Palpate the head. Check for masses, tenderness, and scalp mobility.**

Developmental Modifications

Newborns and infants—Palpate anterior and posterior fontanels.

Expected findings: The head should be nontender, relatively smooth and symmetrical, and without unusual contours, bulges, or lesions.

Abnormal findings: Contour abnormalities (e.g., indentations, "bumps") or tenderness can result from trauma, congenital anomalies, or surgery.

4. **Palpate the face for symmetry, tenderness, muscle tone, and temporomandibular joint (TMJ) function.** ▼

Palpating the TMJ

Expected findings: Smooth, symmetrical movement with no pain, crepitus, or clicking of the jaw

Abnormal findings: Irregular or uneven movement of the jaw; pain or popping/cracking with movement may indicate TMJ syndrome.

Documentation

- If you need more information about documenting your findings,

▶ Go to **Chapter 19, Caring for the Williams Family,** including **Documenting Physical Examination Findings (Stanley Williams),** in Volume 1.

Procedure 19-6 ■ Assessing the Eyes

> For steps to follow in *all* procedures, refer to the Universal Steps for All Procedures on the inside back cover.

Equipment
- Nonlatex gloves—if exposure to body fluids is a possibility
- Visual acuity chart with color bars (Snellen)
- A card—to cover one eye during the acuity examination
- Penlight
- Cotton ball and cotton-tipped applicator
- Ophthalmoscope
- Pen and record form

✚ Clean equipment before and after use unless used for only one patient.

Positioning
The client should be sitting, if possible.

Focused History Questions
- Have you noticed any changes in your vision?
- Do you wear glasses or contact lenses?
- Have you ever had an eye injury?
- Have you ever had an eye infection or stye?
- Do you have problems with excessive tearing or dry eyes?
- Have you ever had eye surgery?
- Have you ever had blurred vision?
- Do you have difficulty with nighttime vision?
- Do you ever see halos of light, spots or floaters, or flashes of light?
- Do you have a history of eye problems, such as glaucoma, or medical problems, such as diabetes or hypertension?
- When was your last eye examination?
- Do you use any prescription or over-the-counter eye medications?

> When performing the procedure, always identify your patient according to agency policy, using two identifiers, and be attentive to standard precautions, hand hygiene, patient safety and privacy, body mechanics, and documentation.

Procedure Steps

1. **Test distance vision.**
   - Depending on client's age and literacy level, use the Snellen standard eye chart or Snellen E chart (for those who cannot read). Picture charts are available for preschoolers.
   - If the client wears corrective lenses, they should be worn during a test.
      a. Have the client sit or stand 6 m (20 ft.) from the chart. With a card, cover the eye not being tested; ask the client to read the smallest line of print that they can distinguish. Consider a line to be read correctly if the client makes no more than two mistakes in that line. If the client hesitates when reporting the letters or symbols, document "with hesitation."
      b. Test the opposite eye.
      c. Test both eyes together.

Findings

Expected findings: 20/20 vision in the right eye, left eye, and both eyes. The top number of the fraction indicates the distance the person was standing from the chart; the bottom number is the distance from which a person with normal vision would be able to read the chart.

Developmental Variations

Children—Distance vision does not reach 20/20 until around 6 or 7 years of age.

Middle adults—At about middle age, the lens of the eye begins to lose some ability to accommodate to near objects.

Abnormal findings: A smaller fraction (e.g., 20/100) indicates diminished distant vision (myopia). A larger fraction (e.g., 20/15) indicates diminished near vision, called hyperopia.

CHAPTER 19 Health Assessment 221

d. At the end of each line of the Snellen chart is a fraction—the top line is 20/200. After each test, record the resulting fraction: the number at the end of the smallest line the patient could read with no more than two errors. If there were more than two errors in a line, record the number of items missed. ▼

Preliterate chart Snellen standard chart Snellen E chart

2. **Test near vision.** Test the client's ability to read newsprint at a distance of 35.5 cm (14 in.) from the eyes. Use print-sized pictures if the patient is unable to read.

   Expected findings: The client reads newsprint at a distance of 35.5 cm (14 in.).

   Developmental Variations

   Adults: The lens of the eye naturally loses some ability to accommodate to near objects. In clients older than 45 years of age, diminished near vision is known as presbyopia.

3. **Test color vision.**
   a. Have the patient differentiate patterns of colors on color cards or identify the color bars on the Snellen eye chart.
   b. Inability to distinguish colors requires a thorough evaluation using the Ishihara cards to determine the scope of the color deficit. ▼

   Expected findings: Color vision is intact.

   Developmental Variations

   Older adults—Experience some decline in color vision, especially in the ability to see purples and pastels.

   Abnormal findings: Inability to distinguish colors

Ishihara card

(continued on next page)

Procedure 19-6 ■ Assessing the Eyes (continued)

4. **Test peripheral vision.**
   a. Seat the client 60–90 cm (2–3 ft) from you.
   b. Have client cover one eye and fix the gaze straight ahead while you bring an object in from the periphery to the center of the visual fields. Be sure to begin by holding the object well outside the range of normal peripheral vision. Instruct the client to identify when the object becomes visible.
   c. Repeat this in each of the four visual fields, moving clockwise. ▼

Expected findings: Expect no deficits in the visual fields.

Abnormal findings:
- **Strabismus** (crossed eye) is a condition in which one or both eyes deviate from the object they are looking at. Constant strabismus of one eye may result in **amblyopia** ("lazy eye"), in which the brain does not fully acknowledge the images seen by the amblyopic eye. This creates reduced vision in that eye, not correctable by glasses or contact lenses.
- **Loss of peripheral vision.** Report gross deficits to an ophthalmologist for further assessment.

Developmental Variations

Infants: Strabismus is normal during the first 1 or 2 months of life. After that, it may be caused by weak intraocular muscles or a lesion on the oculomotor nerve.

Positions for peripheral vision testing
Superior field 50°
Inferior field 70°
Nasal field 60°
Temporal field 90°-110°

5. **Assess extraocular movements (EOMs).**
   a. **Inspect the eyes for parallel alignment.**
   b. **Test the corneal light reflex** by shining a penlight at the bridge of the nose. Note where the light reflects on the cornea of each eye.

   a. **Expected findings:** The eyes should be in parallel alignment.
   b. **Expected findings:** Corneal light reflex appears at the same position in each eye.

   Abnormal findings: An asymmetrical corneal light reflex may indicate weak extraocular muscles or strabismus.

c. **Test the six cardinal fields of gaze.** Stand in front of the client, and have the client follow an object through the six cardinal fields without moving their head. ▼

Up left

Side left

Down left

Down right

Side right

Up right

d. **Perform the cover/uncover test.** Cover one eye and have the client gaze at a distant object. Uncover the eye. Repeat on the opposite side.

6. **Inspect the external structures.**
   a. **General appearance.** Check the color and alignment of the eyes.

   b. **Inspect the eyelids.** Note the presence of any lesions, edema, or lid lag. ▼

   Hordoleum (stye)

c. **Expected findings:** The eyes move through all six gaze positions.

   Abnormal findings: Inability to move through all gaze positions

d. **Expected findings:** The gaze should be steady when the eye is covered and uncovered.

   Abnormal findings: A shift in gaze indicates weak eye muscles.

a. **Expected findings:** Eyes clear, bright, and in parallel alignment

   Developmental Variations
   Older adults—A decrease in periorbital fat may give the eyeballs a sunken appearance.

   Abnormal findings: Glazed eyes may indicate a febrile state.

b. **Expected findings:** Eyelid margins moist and pink. No crusting, scales, or lesions present; lids move freely. Upper eyelid covers half of the upper iris; lower eyelid appears at bottom edge of iris.

   Developmental Variations
   Older adults—The lower lids may sag; skinfolds are prominent in the upper lids.

   Abnormal findings: Asymmetry of lids may result from CN III damage or from a stroke. Lesions may be benign (e.g., a stye) or pathological (e.g., basal cell carcinoma).

(continued on next page)

Procedure 19-6 ■ Assessing the Eyes (continued)

c. **Inspect the eyelashes.** Note symmetry and distribution.

d. **Inspect the lacrimal ducts and glands.** Note any edema, excessive tearing, or drainage.

e. **Inspect the conjunctivae.** Note the color, moisture, and contour of the conjunctivae.
   (1) The palpebral conjunctivae cover the lids. To assess, have the patient look up as you place a cotton-tipped applicator on the upper lid, gently grasp the upper lid and lashes, and evert the lid over the cotton-tipped applicator.
   (2) The bulbar conjunctiva covers the eyeball. To assess, pull the lower lid down. ▼

Examining the palpebral conjunctiva

Examining the bulbar conjunctiva

f. **Inspect the sclera.** Note the color of the sclera and whether lesions are present.

c. **Expected findings:** Eyelashes are evenly distributed and curve outward. No crustations or infestations are present.

   Abnormal findings: Inflammation of the eyelids, which may be caused by infection; inverted eyelashes (entropion); everted eyelashes (ectropion); visible sclera between the iris and upper lid

d. **Expected findings:** No periorbital edema or lesions are present. No drainage

   Abnormal findings: Swelling, redness, drainage, or tenderness

e. **Expected findings:** The palpebral conjunctivae are smooth, glistening, and peach in color. Minimal blood vessels are present. The bulbar conjunctivae are clear with few underlying blood vessels and white sclera visible.

   Developmental Variations
   Older adults—The conjunctivae may be pale or have a slightly yellow tint due to fat deposits.

   Abnormal findings: Pallor, dryness, edema; pterygium; subconjunctival hemorrhage ▼

Pterygium

Subconjunctival hemorrhage

f. **Expected findings:** The sclera should be smooth, white, and glistening. Patients with dark skin may have a yellowish cast to the peripheral sclera or small brown spots more centrally.

   Abnormal findings: Yellow (icteric) scler

g. **Inspect the cornea and lens.** As the client looks straight ahead, shine a penlight at an angle to the eye, and move it across the corneal surface. Note the color and whether any lesions are present.

h. **Test the corneal reflex.** Touch the cornea with a wisp of sterile cotton, or use a needleless syringe to shoot a small amount of air over the cornea.

   Note: This is not routinely performed on conscious patients. A conscious person can blink intentionally, so there is no need. In addition, there is a slight risk of corneal abrasion from cotton.

i. **Inspect the iris and pupils.** Note the color, size, shape, and symmetry.

j. **Test pupillary reaction.** In a dimly lighted room, have the client look straight ahead. Bring a penlight in from the side, and shine the light onto one eye. Note the reaction, equality, and speed of response of both eyes. (For example, when you shine a light onto the right eye, the right pupil reaction is direct; the left eye is consensual.) Repeat the test on the opposite eye. ▼

Testing pupillary reaction to light

g. **Expected findings:** The cornea and lens are clear, smooth, and glistening.

   Developmental Variations

   Older adults—Arcus senilis (white, gray, or blue opaque ring in the corneal margin) is a normal variant.

   Abnormal findings: Lens opacities (cataracts); roughness or irregularity of the cornea

h. **Expected findings:** Blink reflex is prompt.

   Abnormal findings: Failure to blink may result from neurosensory deficits.

i. **Expected findings:**
   - The iris is blue, green, brown, or a combination of these colors; its shape is circular.
   - The pupils are round and of equal size. Unequal pupils (anisocoria) can be a normal variation if the difference is less than 0.5 mm.

   Developmental Variations

   Older adults—Pigment degeneration may cause the iris to be pale with brownish discolorations.

   Abnormal findings:
   - Damage to one eye may cause the iris to be a different color.
   - Absence of part or all of the iris is a congenital problem.
   - Unequal pupils may result from CN III damage, stroke, brain herniation, or increased intracranial pressure (ICP).
   - Enlarged pupils (mydriasis); constricted pupils (myosis)
   - Cloudy pupils

j. **Expected findings:** Normal direct and consensual response to light is brisk, with equal constriction of both pupils.

   Developmental Variations

   Older adults—Pupil reaction may be slower but should be symmetrical.

   Abnormal findings: Sluggish or fixed pupils may result from CN II damage or brain injury. Absence of consensual response may result from nerve compression or anoxia.

(continued on next page)

Procedure 19-6 ■ Assessing the Eyes (continued)

k. **Test pupil accommodation.** Have the client look straight ahead and focus on an object about 30 cm (12 in.) from their face. Slowly bring the object in toward the client's eyes. Note pupil size and location.

k. **Expected findings:** The pupils constrict and the eyes cross as a person attempts to focus on a near object.

> **Developmental Variations**
> *Older adults*—Accommodation may be slow.

Abnormal findings: One or both pupils fail to accommodate, or they accommodate slowly.

l. **Inspect the anterior chamber.** Shine a penlight across the eye from the side as the patient looks straight ahead. Observe color, size, shape, and symmetry.

l. **Expected findings:** The chamber should be clear and symmetrically curved.

Abnormal findings: Blood or pus in the chamber

7. **Palpate the external structures.**
   a. Gently palpate the globe (eyeball) with your fingertips on the upper lids over the sclera. Note the consistency and any tenderness. ▼

Expected findings: The globe is firm and nontender. Lacrimal glands are nonpalpable; no tenderness is present.

Abnormal findings: Firm or tender globe; swelling and tenderness over the lacrimal glands

   b. Palpate the lacrimal glands and ducts by palpating below the eyebrow and below the inner canthus of the eye. Note tenderness and excessive tearing or discharge.

8. **Assess the internal structures via ophthalmoscopy.** This is an advanced physical assessment technique.
   a. Darken the room.
   b. Stand about 1 foot from the client at a 15° lateral angle.
   c. Dial the lens wheel to zero with your index finger. Hold the ophthalmoscope to your brow.
   d. Have the client look straight ahead while you shine the light on one pupil and identify the red light reflex. ▼

Expected findings: A positive red light reflex. On internal examination, the optic disk is round with sharp margins. There are no opacities and the cup-to-disk ratio is 1:2. The disk is yellow with a white cup.

Abnormal findings: Any findings not consistent with the aforementioned should be reported promptly. ▼

Red reflex over pupil area

Checking red reflex

e. Once you identify the red light reflex, move in closer to within a few inches of the eye and observe the internal structures of the eye. Adjust the lens wheel to focus as needed. Use your right eye to examine the patient's right eye, and use your left eye to examine the patient's left eye. ▼

Examining internal structures of the eye

Normal fundus

f. Repeat for the opposite eye.

Patient Teaching
Teach the importance of routine eye examinations.

Documentation
If you need more information about documenting your findings,

➤ Go to **Chapter 19, Caring for the Williams Family,** including **Documenting Physical Examination Findings (Stanley Williams),** in Volume 1.

Procedure 19-7 ■ Assessing the Ears and Hearing

➤ For steps to follow in *all* procedures, refer to the Universal Steps for All Procedures on the inside back cover.

Equipment
- Nonlatex gloves (if exposure to body fluids is a possibility)
- Tuning fork
- Watch that ticks (or a similar device)
- Otoscope with pneumatic tube
- Pen and record form

Positioning
Have the patient seated, if possible.

Focused History Questions
- Do you have any hearing problems?
- Have you ever had ringing in your ears?
- Have you had any changes in your hearing?
- Do you have any ear drainage? If yes, how much and what color?
- Do you have any ear pain?
- Do you have any balance problems, dizziness, or vertigo?
- Do you have a history of head trauma?
- Are you exposed to noise pollution at work or in your home environment?

(continued on next page)

Procedure 19-7 ■ Assessing the Ears and Hearing (continued)

▶ When performing the procedure, always identify your patient according to agency policy, using two identifiers, and be attentive to standard precautions, hand hygiene, patient safety and privacy, body mechanics, and documentation.

Procedure Steps

1. **Inspect the external ear.**
   a. Check the placement and angle of attachment of the ear. ▼

   Normal ear attachment | Deviated alignment | Low-set ear attachment

   b. Note the shape, size, and symmetry of the ears. ▼

   Helix, Antihelix, External auditory canal, Tragus, Antitragus, Lobule

   c. Observe the color of the ear.

   d. Observe the condition of the skin; observe for drainage and visible lesions.

2. **Palpate the external structures of the ear.** Note the consistency of the skin, the presence of lesions, and any signs of tenderness.

Findings

a. **Expected findings:** The normal angle of attachment is 10°.

   Abnormal findings: High or low placement of the ear may be a sign of hearing deficit or genetic problems (for example, Down syndrome).

b. **Expected findings:** The helix, antihelix, antitragus, tragus, and lobule are present. The ears are 4–10 cm in length and symmetrical in size and shape.

   🍁 *Developmental Variations*
   Older adults—The ear changes shape as the lobe elongates.

   Abnormal findings: Absence of any of the landmarks may indicate a hearing deficit. Ears that are <4 cm long or >10 cm long may indicate a genetic disorder.

c. **Expected findings:** Color is consistent with skin color.

   Abnormal findings: Redness may indicate inflammation or infection.

d. **Expected findings:** Skin is intact with no drainage or lesions. Piercings may be present.

   🍁 *Developmental Variations*
   Older adults—May have coarse hair on the helix, antihelix, and tragus; skin may be dry.

   Abnormal findings: Bloody drainage may result from trauma. Purulent drainage may be seen with infection. The ears are a common location for skin cancer.

Expected findings: Skin is soft, pliable, and nontender. No nodules or lesions are present.

Abnormal findings: Tenderness is often associated with infection (e.g., otitis externa, otitis media).

3. **Perform an otoscopic examination.**
   This is an advanced physical assessment technique.
   a. Use a speculum with the largest diameter and shortest length that the ear canal can accommodate; 4 mm is a common size for adults.
   b. Have the patient tilt the head to the side not being examined.
   c. For adults, grasp the pinna and gently pull upward and back. For a child, position the pinna down and back.
   Positions the ear canal with more direct alignment, allowing for improved visualization.
   d. Insert the speculum no farther than halfway into the ear canal. As you advance the speculum, examine the canal for redness, open areas, drainage, or foreign objects. ▼

Otoscope insertion with handle up

Otoscope insertion with handle down

   e. Look through the magnifying lens.
      (1) Observe the ear canal.
      (2) Observe the tympanic membrane.
   f. Test the mobility of the tympanic membrane by using the otoscope's pneumatic tube to gently "puff" air into the external ear canal while observing movement of the cone of light.

   NOTE: The ears are mirror images, with the cone of light at 7 o'clock in the left ear and 5 o'clock in the right ear.

Developmental Modifications

Children—Many young children fear the otoscopic examination. Demonstrating the procedure on a parent or a doll may relieve their anxiety.
   g. Carefully remove the otoscope from the ear canal, being careful not to traumatize the delicate tissue.

Expected findings: The ear canal is light in color and patent, with a small amount of cerumen (color may vary). Tympanic membrane (TM) is shiny and pearly gray with a cone of reflective light on the nasal aspect (this would be 7 o'clock in the left ear and 5 o'clock in the right ear). Bony landmarks are visible. The TM is mobile. No bulging or retraction of the TM. ▼

Normal TM left ear

Developmental Variations

Older adults—May have dry ear cerumen. The TM is translucent, and the light reflex may be diminished.

Abnormal findings: Excessive cerumen may occlude the canal. TM that is red, with a distorted light reflex, suggests otitis media. A change in the position or shape of the cone of light reflex indicates an imbalance in middle ear pressure. ▼

Otitis media   Perforated TM

(continued on next page)

Procedure 19-7 ■ Assessing the Ears and Hearing (continued)

4. **Test gross hearing.**
   a. Stand 1–2 ft behind the client. Have the client cover one ear as you whisper some numbers or letters. Repeat on the other side. Have the client repeat the words they heard.
   A test of hearing also indicates cranial nerve XIII is intact.

Developmental Modifications
Infants—For infants younger than 3 months of age, loudly clap your hands behind the infant and observe whether the infant startles. After 3 months of age, the infant should turn the head or eyes toward a sound, for example, when the parent stands behind the infant and calls their name.

Expected findings: The client is able to hear you whisper on both sides and repeat at least three out of six numbers or letters correctly.

Developmental Variations
Older adults—Often have a generalized loss of hearing. It first occurs in the high-frequency sounds (*f, s, sh,* and *ph*) and then progresses to include all frequencies.

Abnormal findings: Problems with the whisper test indicate low-tone hearing loss.

5. **Perform the Weber test.** Place a vibrating tuning fork on top of the client's head. Ask the client whether the sound is the same in both ears or louder in one ear. ▼

Weber test

Expected findings: The client hears the sound equally in both ears.

Abnormal findings: Sound is louder in one ear.
- If there is a *conductive hearing loss,* the vibration will be louder in the impaired ear. Conductive hearing loss may be caused by external or middle ear problems, such as infection, blockage of the canal by cerumen, or trauma to the TM.
- If there is a *sensorineural hearing loss,* the sound will be louder in the unaffected ear. Sensorineural loss may result from inner ear problems or from some medications.

6. **If the Weber test is positive: Perform the Rinne test.**
   a. Strike a tuning fork on the table. While it is still vibrating, place it on the client's mastoid process.
   Tests bone conduction of sound
   b. Measure the elapsed time in seconds that the client hears the vibration.
   c. Move the tuning fork to 2.5 cm (1 in.) in front of the ear, and measure the elapsed time until the client can no longer hear the vibration.
   Tests air conduction of sound

Expected findings: Normally, sound transmission through air (step 6c) is twice as long as transmission through bone (step 6b); that is,

$$AC = 2 \times BC$$

The ratio of AC to BC is similar in both ears.

d. Repeat for the opposite ear. ▼

Rinne test

Step 6c

Abnormal findings:
- *Conductive loss:* AC is less than 2 × BC.
- *Sensorineural loss:* AC is greater than BC but not 2× longer; or the client is unable to hear the tuning fork through BC.
- A difference between ears indicates unilateral hearing loss.
- Inability to hear the tuning fork through BC indicates sensorineural hearing loss.

7. **Perform the Romberg test.** Have the patient stand with feet together, hands at side, with eyes opened and then with eyes closed. Note the patient's ability to maintain balance.

   ✚ Stand nearby in case the client loses balance.

   Tests for balance. Strictly speaking, it does not assess the ears, but the vestibular nerve and other parts of the central nervous system. Therefore, you may prefer to perform the test during the neurological examination.

Expected findings: The patient maintains balance with minimal sway.

Abnormal findings: Positive Romberg (swaying) is seen with vestibular and cerebellar disorders.

Patient Teaching

Teach the client the importance of routine hearing examinations.

Documentation

If you need more information about documenting your findings,

➤ Go to **Chapter 19, Caring for the Williams Family,** including **Documenting Physical Examination Findings (Stanley Williams),** in Volume 1.

Procedure 19-8 ■ Assessing the Nose and Sinuses

> For steps to follow in *all* procedures, refer to the Universal Steps for All Procedures on the inside back cover.

Equipment
- Nonlatex procedure gloves (if exposure to body fluids is a possibility)
- Penlight
- Nasal speculum or otoscope with a wide-tipped speculum
- Pen and record form

Positioning
Have the client seated, if possible.

Focused History Questions
- Do you have any nasal congestion?
- Do you have a history of nose or sinus problems?
- Do you have problems with seasonal or environmental allergies?
- Do you have a history of sinus headaches?
- Do you have nosebleeds (epistaxis)?
- Have you ever broken your nose?
- Have you had any changes in your sense of smell or taste?
- Do you use any nasal sprays or allergy medications?

> When performing the procedure, always identify your patient according to agency policy, using two identifiers, and be attentive to standard precautions, hand hygiene, patient safety and privacy, body mechanics, and documentation.

Procedure Steps

1. **Position the client for the examination.** Sitting is the preferred position.

2. **Inspect the external nose.** Note the position, shape, and size. Observe for discharge and flaring.

   Expected findings: The nose is midline and symmetrical. No discharge or flaring

   Abnormal findings:
   - Asymmetry suggests congenital deformity or trauma.
   - Flaring suggests respiratory distress (especially in infants, who cannot breathe through the mouth).
   - Clear drainage suggests allergy; yellow or green drainage suggests upper respiratory infection; bloody drainage may result from trauma, hypertension, or a bleeding disorder.

3. **Check for patency of the nasal passages.** Ask the client to close their mouth, hold one naris closed, and breathe through the other naris. Repeat with the opposite naris.

   Expected findings: The client breathes freely through both nares.

4. **Inspect the internal structures.**
   a. Use a nasal speculum or an otoscope with a large speculum (or a penlight with a speculum) to assess the internal structures.
   b. Tilt the client's head back to facilitate speculum insertion and visualization.
   c. Brace your index finger against the client's nose as you insert the speculum.

   Expected findings: Nasal mucosa is pink and moist. Septum is intact and midline. No lesions

   > **Developmental Variations**
   >
   > *Older adults*—The sense of smell diminishes in older adults because of a gradual decrease in and atrophy of the olfactory nerve fibers.

d. Insert the speculum about 1 cm into the nares. Use the other hand to position the client's head and to hold the penlight if you do not have a lighted scope. ▼

Step 4d

e. Observe the nasal mucosa for color, edema, lesions, erosion or ulceration, blood, and discharge. Inspect the septum for position and intactness.
f. Check for sense of smell using commonly recognized objects, such as a lemon or vanilla. Do not use a noxious odor. You can defer this test until the sensorineurological part of the examination if you choose, but keep the same order for every examination.
Cranial nerve I is intact when the patient shows an ability to detect odor.

Developmental Modifications

Infants and children—You will not need a speculum to examine internal structures. Push the tip of the nose upward with your thumb, and direct a penlight into the nares.

5. **Transilluminate the frontal and maxillary sinuses.**
   First, darken the room.
   a. Frontal sinuses: Shine a penlight or the otoscope with speculum below the eyebrow on each side. ▼

   Step 5a

   b. Maxillary sinuses: Place the light source below the eyes and above the cheeks. Look for a glow of red light at the roof of the mouth through the client's open mouth. ▼

   Step 5b

Abnormal findings: Deviated septum; polyps
- Pale boggy mucosa is seen with allergies; bright red mucosa is associated with rhinitis, sinusitis, and cocaine use.
- Clustered vesicles suggest herpes infection. ▼

Frontal
Ethmoid
Sphenoid
Maxillary

Paranasal sinuses frontal, ethmoid, sphenoid, and maxillary

- Erosion of nasal mucosa should signal you to investigate further for other signs or history of crack/cocaine use.
- Blood in the nasal passage indicates trauma, nosebleeds, or polyps.

a. **Expected findings:** A red glow is seen above the eyebrow, indicating that the frontal sinus is patent.

b. **Expected findings:** A red glow may be (but is not always) seen in the roof of the mouth, indicating that the maxillary sinus is patent.

Abnormal findings: Absence of transillumination may result from mucosal thickening or sinusitis.

(continued on next page)

Procedure 19-8 ■ Assessing the Nose and Sinuses (continued)

6. **Palpate the external structures.**

   Expected findings: No tenderness, lesions, or deformity

7. **Palpate the frontal and maxillary sinuses.**

   Expected findings: No tenderness

   Abnormal findings: Tenderness may indicate infectious or allergic sinusitis.

Documentation

If you need more information about documenting your findings,

Go to **Chapter 19, Caring for the Williams Family,** including **Documenting Physical Examination Findings (Stanley Williams),** in Volume 1.

Procedure 19-9 ■ Assessing the Mouth and Oropharynx

➤ For steps to follow in *all* procedures, refer to the Universal Steps for All Procedures on the inside back cover.

Equipment
- Nonlatex procedure gloves
- Penlight
- Tongue blade
- Small gauze pad
- Pen and record form

Positioning
Have the client seated, if possible.

Focused History Questions
- Do you have any problems with your mouth or teeth?
- When was your last dental examination?
- Do you have any discomfort in your mouth or throat?
- Have you had any recent changes in your mouth or teeth?
- How often do you brush your teeth? Floss?
- Do you smoke or chew tobacco?
- Do you have any sores or irritation in your mouth? If so, when did you first notice this?

➤ When performing the procedure, always identify your patient according to agency policy, using two identifiers, and be attentive to standard precautions, hand hygiene, patient safety and privacy, body mechanics, and documentation.

Procedure Steps

1. **Inspect the mouth externally.** Locate the placement of the lips and their color and condition. Ask the client to purse the lips.

Findings

Expected findings: The lips are midline, symmetrical, moist, and intact with no lesions. Coloring is consistent with ethnic group/race. The client can purse lips.

Abnormal findings:
- Asymmetry may be due to congenital deformity, trauma, paralysis, or surgical alteration.
- Pallor; cyanosis; redness
- Inability to purse lips may indicate facial nerve damage.
- Lesions may be caused by bacteria, viruses, or trauma.

2. **Note the color and condition of the oral mucosa and gums.**
   a. **Don procedure gloves.**
   b. **Inspect and palpate the lower lip.** Pull the lower lip away from the teeth, and inspect the inner side of the lip. Palpate any lesions for size, mobility, and tenderness. ▼

   Step 2b

   Step 2b

   c. **Inspect the buccal mucosa,** top to bottom and back to front.
   - Ask the client to open mouth. Use a tongue depressor to retract the cheek, then shine a penlight onto the mucosa.
   - Using a tongue blade and penlight, inspect the Stensen's duct openings to the parotid glands.
   - Finally, **palpate inside each cheek** by placing a finger inside and thumb outside. Grasping the cheek between them, move the finger about. Repeat on both sides.

Expected findings: *Oral mucosa* is pink, moist, and intact; no lesions. *Gingiva* is consistent in color with the other mucosae and is intact, with no bleeding. *Buccal mucosa* is pink and moist, with no lesions. Mucosa is darker in clients with dark skin.

> *Developmental Variations*
>
> *Older adults*—Mucosa is drier than in young adults because of decreased salivary gland activity; brownish pigmentation of gums may be seen, especially in people with dark skin.

Abnormal findings: Pallor may indicate anemia or inadequate oxygenation. The following are types of abnormal lesions.
- **Gingivitis** is a sign of periodontal disease. You will see red, swollen, or spongy, bleeding gingiva and receding gumlines. The gums may be tender.
- **Parotitis** is an inflammation of the parotid salivary gland.
- **Stomatitis** is inflammation of the oral mucosa.
- **Leukoplakia** (thick, elevated white patches) that do not scrape off may be precancerous lesions; white, curdy patches that scrape off and bleed indicate **thrush** (a fungal infection).
- **Redness or abrasions** of the gingiva may be caused by poorly fitted dentures.
- **Aphthous ulcers** are small, painful vesicles with a reddened periphery and a white or pale-yellow base.
- **Canker sores** are a benign type of aphthous ulcer believed to be caused by viral infection, allergies, stress, or trauma. So-called *major* aphthous ulcers may be caused by herpes simplex virus, HIV, and bacterial infections.

(continued on next page)

Procedure 19-9 ■ Assessing the Mouth and Oropharynx (continued)

d. Also **examine the gums** as you are inspecting the buccal mucosa. Check for color, bleeding, edema, retraction, and lesions. Press gum tissue gently with gloved finger or tongue blade to assess firmness. ▼

Structures of the mouth and oropharynx

3. **Inspect the teeth.** You can do this while you are inspecting the oral mucosa and gums, in step 2.
   a. Observe the number, color, and condition of the teeth. Note the occlusion ("bite") and any loose teeth.
   b. If the client wears dentures, ask the client to remove them. Inspect for cracked or worn areas; assess the fit. ▼

Gingival recession

Expected findings: Most adults have 28 teeth, or 32 if the wisdom teeth have erupted. Children have 20 teeth. The teeth should be white, in good repair, with no caries and good occlusion. The top front teeth should slightly override the lower ones.

Developmental Variations

Older adults—May have receding gums, so teeth appear longer. Teeth may be chipped, eroded, or stained.

Abnormal findings: Missing or poorly anchored teeth, misalignment, and brown or black enamel (indicative of dental caries or staining, such as from taking tetracycline). White spots may indicate excessive fluoride intake.

4. **Inspect the tongue and the floor of the mouth.**
   a. Ask the client to stick out their tongue. Examine the upper surface for its color, texture, position, and mobility.
   b. Ask the client to roll their tongue upward and move it side to side.
   c. Have the client place the tip of their tongue on the roof of their mouth, as far back as possible. Using the penlight, inspect the underside of the tongue, the frenulum (which fastens the tongue to the floor of the mouth, in the center), and the floor of the mouth.
   d. Inspect the two Wharton's duct openings to the submaxillary glands, on either side of the frenulum.

Expected findings: Tongue is moist, with rough surface; coloring is consistent with the client's race. Mucosa has no lesions or discoloration. Papillae are intact. Tongue is midline with full mobility. The base of the tongue is smooth with prominent veins. No tenderness; no palpable nodules. A geographic tongue is a common normal variant.

Developmental Variations

Older adults—May have varicosities under the tongue

e. Use a tongue blade or gloved finger to move the tongue aside and examine the lateral aspects of the tongue and the floor of the mouth bilaterally. Use caution when placing your finger into the mouth of a noncompliant client. ▼

Abnormal findings:
- Limited mobility
- Deviation from midline—may be caused by damage to the hypoglossal nerve (CN XII)
- **Glossitis** (inflammation of the tongue)
- A dry, furry tongue—associated with dehydration
- A black, "hairy" tongue—associated with fungal infections
- Reddened mucosa, ulcerations, and absence of papillae—may indicate allergy, inflammation, or infection
- Swelling, nodules, or ulcers
- A smooth, red tongue—may occur in clients who have a deficiency of iron, vitamin B_{12}, or vitamin B_3

Geographic tongue

Red, beefy tongue

Black, hairy tongue

Leukoplakia

Cancer of the tongue

5. **Palpate the tongue and floor of the mouth.** Stabilize the tongue by grasping it with a gauze pad. Palpate top, bottom, and sides with your other index finger.

6. **Inspect the oropharynx (hard/soft palate, tonsils, and uvula).** Note the color, shape, texture, and condition.
   a. **Have the client tilt the head back** and open the mouth as widely as possible. Depress the tongue with a tongue blade, and shine a penlight on the areas to be inspected.
   b. **To inspect the uvula,** ask the client to say "ah," and watch the uvula as the soft palate rises.
   c. **Inspect the oropharynx** by depressing one side of the tongue at a time, about halfway back on the tongue.
   d. **Note the size and color of the tonsils;** note any discharge, redness, swelling, or lesions.
   e. **Look and palpate for cleft palate,** especially in infants.

Expected findings: Hard and soft palates are pink and smooth. Uvula is midline and rises symmetrically. Tonsils are pink, symmetrical, and without lesions or exudate.

Developmental Variations

Children—Until about age 12, the tonsils may extend beyond the palatine arch.

Abnormal findings:
- Redness, edema, lesions, plaques, drainage; yellow or greenish streaks on the posterior wall of pharynx (indicate postnasal drainage)
- Tonsils that are red, edematous, or enlarged or have white or pale patches of exudates
- Asymmetrical rise of the uvula may indicate a problem with CN IX or X.

(continued on next page)

Procedure 19-9 ■ Assessing the Mouth and Oropharynx (continued)

7. **Test the gag reflex** by touching the back of the soft palate with a tongue blade.

Expected findings: Positive gag reflex is present.

Developmental Variations
Older adults—May have a slightly slower gag response.

Abnormal findings:
- Absence of a gag reflex is seen with extreme sedation, head injury, or damage to CN IX and X.

8. **Ask the client to repeat the following words:** *Light, tight, dynamite*. Again, you may defer this test to the sensorineurological portion of the examination if you choose.

Expected findings: Ability to articulate words as requested

Abnormal findings: Inability to articulate the specified words indicates CN XII is not intact.

Patient Teaching
Incorporate SDOH screening when assessing the mouth and oropharynx, and discuss community resource or social service options for free or low-cost dental care. Instruct the client on the importance of dental care and the need for regular checkups.

Documentation
If you need more information about documenting your findings,

Go to **Chapter 19, Caring for the Williams Family,** including **Documenting Physical Examination Findings (Stanley Williams),** in Volume 1.

Procedure 19-10 ■ Assessing the Neck

▶ For steps to follow in *all* procedures, refer to the Universal Steps for All Procedures on the inside back cover.

Equipment
- Stethoscope and antiseptic wipe
- Pen and record form

Positioning
- Have the client seated, if possible.
- For infants and children, position supine.

Focused History Questions
- Do you have any difficulty swallowing?
- Do you have any neck pain or stiffness?
- Do you have any neck masses or lumps?
- Do you have any history of thyroid disease?

▶ When performing the procedure, always identify your patient according to agency policy, using two identifiers, and be attentive to standard precautions, hand hygiene, patient safety and privacy, body mechanics, and documentation.

Procedure Steps
1. **Inspect the neck.** Note symmetry, range of motion (ROM), and the condition of the skin.
   a. Inspect the neck in a neutral position.
   b. Inspect the neck when it is hyperextended.
   c. Inspect the neck when the client swallows water.

Findings
Expected findings: Neck is erect, midline, and symmetrical with full ROM. No masses are present; skin is intact. Larynx and trachea rise with swallowing. Thyroid is not visible.

Abnormal findings:
- Asymmetrical head position may result from damage to the muscles, swelling, or masses.
- Painful or erratic movement may be due to a benign condition, such as muscle spasm, or to significant problems, including meningitis, neurological injuries, or chronic arthritis.
- Swollen lymph nodes may be visible.
- An enlarged thyroid may be visible in the lower half of the neck.

2. **Palpate the cervical lymph nodes.** Note the size, shape, symmetry, consistency, mobility, tenderness, and temperature of any palpable nodes.
    a. Use light palpation with one or two fingerpads in a circular movement.
    b. Palpate the cervical nodes in the following order:
        (1) *Preauricular*—in front of the ear
        (2) *Posterior auricular*—behind the ear
        (3) *Tonsillar*—at the angle of the jaw
        (4) *Submandibular*—halfway up the lower jaw
        (5) *Submental*—under the tip of the chin
        (6) *Occipital*—at the base of the skull in the occipital area
        (7) *Superficial cervical*—below the tonsillar node over the sternocleidomastoid muscle
        (8) *Deep cervical*—under the sternocleidomastoid muscle
        (9) *Posterior cervical*—in posterior triangle along trapezius muscle
        (10) *Supraclavicular*—above the clavicle

    Note: Use the same sequence every time so that the steps will become automatic and you will not omit any area.

Expected findings: Lymph nodes are supple and nontender; no masses are palpable. ▼

Abnormal findings: Lymphadenopathy (palpable nodes 1 cm or greater). Immobile nodes may indicate malignancy, inflammation, or infection in the area they drain.

3. **Palpate the thyroid.**

To use the posterior approach:
   a. Stand behind the client, and ask the client to flex the neck slightly forward and to the left.
   b. Position your thumbs on the nape of the client's neck.
   c. Using the fingers of your left hand, locate the cricoid cartilage, which is located below the thyroid cartilage. Push the trachea slightly to the left with your right hand as you palpate just below the cricoid cartilage and between the trachea and sternocleidomastoid muscle.
   d. Ask your client to swallow (give small sips of water if necessary), and feel for the thyroid gland as it rises up.
   e. Reverse and repeat the same steps to palpate the right thyroid lobe by using the fingers of your left hand to displace the trachea to the right, while using the fingers of your right hand to palpate the thyroid to the right of the trachea.

To use the anterior approach:
   f. Stand in front of the client, and ask them to flex the neck slightly forward and in the direction you intend to palpate.
   g. Place your hands on the neck, and apply gentle pressure to one side of the trachea while palpating the opposite side of the neck for the thyroid as the client swallows.
   h. Reverse and repeat the same steps on the opposite side.

Expected findings: The thyroid is generally nonpalpable. If some tissue is palpable, the consistency is firm and smooth. There is no nodularity, enlargement, or tenderness.

Abnormal findings: An enlarged thyroid may signify a tumor or goiter (hypo- or hyperthyroidism). A tender thyroid is associated with inflammation. ▼

Steps 3a–d

(continued on next page)

Procedure 19-10 ■ Assessing the Neck (continued)

? What if...

- **The thyroid gland is enlarged or there is a mass?**

  Auscultate the thyroid for bruits using the bell portion of the stethoscope. Ask the client to hold their breath as you auscultate. There should be no bruits.

Patient Teaching

Teach the client how to perform a "neck check"—self-check the thyroid with a glass of water and a handheld mirror. Tell the patient: "Hold the mirror in your hand and focus on your neck just below the Adam's apple and above your collarbone. Tip your head back, take a drink of water, and swallow. As you swallow, look at your neck. Check for any bulges in this area as you swallow." To download Neck Check instructions, and for more information about thyroid health,

➡ Go to https://www.aace.com/disease-and-conditions/thyroid/how-check-your-thyroid

Documentation

- Describe enlarged nodes (greater than 1 cm in diameter) according to their location, size, shape, consistency, mobility, and tenderness.
- If you need more information about documenting your findings,

  ➡ Go to **Chapter 19, Caring for the Williams Family,** including **Documenting Physical Examination Findings (Stanley Williams),** in Volume 1.

Procedure 19-11 ■ Assessing the Breasts and Axillae

▶ For steps to follow in *all* procedures, refer to the Universal Steps for All Procedures on the inside back cover.

Equipment

- Nonlatex procedure gloves, if exposure to body fluids is possible
- Glass slide
- Culturette
- Pen and record form

Positioning

The patient must assume several positions during breast examination (see step 1).

Focused History Questions

- Do you have a lump or thickening in your underarm or breasts? For cisgender females: Do the lumps or thickening persist throughout your menstrual cycle?
- Do you have any breast pain or discharge?
- Have you noticed any changes in the skin on your breasts, nipples, or underarms?
- Have you had any changes in your nipples?
- Have your breasts changed in size, shape, or contour?
- Do you perform breast self-examination (BSE)?
- Are you taking any medications or hormones?
- If you are premenopausal, when was your last period?

▶ When performing the procedure, always identify your patient according to agency policy, using two identifiers, and be attentive to standard precautions, hand hygiene, patient safety and privacy, body mechanics, and documentation.

Procedure Steps

1. **Inspect the breasts.** Note size, shape, symmetry, and color. Inspect with the client in each of the following positions:
   a. Sitting or standing with arms at side
   b. Sitting or standing with arms raised slightly but not overhead
      Aids in detecting dimpling or retraction of breast tissue
   c. Seated or standing with hands pressed on hips
      Aids in detecting dimpling or retraction of breast tissue
   d. With the client leaning forward
      Helpful when examining large, pendulous breasts

Findings

Expected findings: The breasts are symmetrical; however, the dominant side may be more developed, resulting in a slightly asymmetrical appearance. Skin color is lighter than exposed areas, and there are no lesions, redness, or edema. Texture is smooth, with no dimpling or retraction. Striae are a normal variation.

Developmental Variations

Newborns—You may see breast enlargement and watery, white discharge from the nipples during the first 2 weeks of life.

Children—Breasts typically begin to develop between 8 and 13 years of age; the breasts may not develop at equal rates.

e. With the client supine with a pillow under the shoulder of the breast being examined
Helps spread the breast tissue over the chest wall

Pregnancy—Breast size increases; areolae and nipples darken; superficial veins become prominent; stretch marks may be present; colostrum (a thick, yellow precursor to breast milk) can sometimes be expressed as early as the second trimester.

Older adults—Breasts lose firmness and become flaccid and pendulous.

Abnormal findings:
- Asymmetry warrants further investigation.
- Swelling or erythema may be seen in infection (mastitis).
- **Peau d'orange** (dimpled skin texture): skin changes may be seen with lymphatic obstruction that is present in some forms of breast cancer.
- Puckering, lesions, and retraction may also be seen with breast cancer.
- **Gynecomastia** (enlargement of breasts in male individuals) may indicate hormone imbalance or for transmale patients may be a result of hormone therapy.

2. **Inspect the nipples and areolae.** Note color, shape, and symmetry. Observe for any discharge.

Expected findings: The areolae and nipples are darker in color than breast tissue. Nipples are everted and point in the same direction. No discharge is present, except in newborns and during pregnancy and lactation. No lesions or erosion is present.

Abnormal findings:
- Nipple discoloration that is not associated with pregnancy
- Nipples point in different directions. Such findings warrant follow-up as a potential sign of an underlying mass.
- Flat or inverted nipples, which are caused by shortening of the mammary ducts. May make breastfeeding difficult.
- Any nipple discharge not associated with newborns, pregnancy, or breastfeeding requires a thorough evaluation.
- Cracks and nipple redness may occur with breastfeeding.

3. **Inspect the axillae.** Note the color, condition of the skin, and hair distribution.

Expected findings: Skin is intact with no lesions or rashes. Presence of hair depends on the age of the client and personal preference. Axillary hair develops with puberty. Some clients may choose to shave the hair, whereas others will allow it to grow.

Abnormal findings:
- Rashes, redness, or unusual pigmentation may indicate infection or allergy to deodorants.
- Dark-pigmented, velvety skin may be seen with **acanthosis nigricans,** a condition associated with obesity and type 2 diabetes mellitus.

4. **Palpate the breasts, wearing procedure gloves if necessary.** Using the fingerpads of your three middle fingers, make small circles with light, medium, and deep pressure.
   Begin at an imaginary line drawn straight down the side from the underarm; move across the breast to the middle of the sternum. Check the entire breast area, moving down until you feel only ribs and up to the clavicle.

Expected findings: Breasts are soft and nontender with no lesions or masses.

Developmental Variations

Consistency depends on age; premenopausal clients have firm and elastic tissue, whereas postmenopausal clients have softer tissue that may be stringy or cordlike.

(continued on next page)

242 UNIT 3 Essential Nursing Interventions

Procedure 19-11 ■ Assessing the Breasts and Axillae (continued)

Use one of the following three patterns (evidence suggests the vertical strip method is best).

a. **Vertical strip method:** Start at the sternal edge, and palpate the breast in parallel lines until you reach the midaxillary line. Go up one area and down the adjacent strip (like "mowing the grass"). ▼

Vertical strip method

b. **Pie wedge method:** This method examines the breast in wedges. Move from one wedge to the next. ▼

Pie wedge method

c. **Concentric circles method:** Start at the outermost area of the breast at the 12 o'clock position. Move clockwise in concentric, ever smaller, circles. ▼

Concentric circle method

Abnormal findings: Breast lumps or masses may be benign or malignant and require follow-up.

Technique Hints
- Do not remove your fingers from the skin surface once you have begun palpating. Move from area to area by sliding the fingers along the skin.
- Most breast lesions in female individuals are found in the upper-outer quadrant.
- Most breast cancer in male individuals occurs in the areola.

5. **Palpate the nipples and areolae, wearing gloves if necessary.**
   a. If the client is supine, place a small pillow or folded towel under the shoulder of the breast you are examining.
   b. Squeeze the nipple gently between your thumb and finger to check for discharge.
   c. Note tissue elasticity and tenderness.

Expected findings: Nipples are elastic and nontender. No discharge is present.

Developmental Variations

Nipple tenderness is normal when establishing breastfeeding.

Abnormal findings: Loss of elasticity may indicate underlying malignancy. Bloody, purulent discharge may indicate infection. Other forms of drainage may indicate malignancy.

6. **Palpate the axillae and clavicular lymph nodes.**
   a. Have the client sitting with the arms at sides or supine.
   b. Using your fingerpads, move your fingers in a circular fashion.
      - *Central nodes:* located high in the midaxillary region
      - *Anterior pectoral nodes:* located on the lower border of the pectoralis major in the anterior axillary fold
      - *Lateral brachial nodes:* located high in the axilla on the inner aspect of the humerus
      - *Posterior subscapular nodes:* located high in the axilla on the lateral scapular border
      - *Epitrochlear nodes:* located above the elbow
      - *Infraclavicular nodes:* located below the clavicle
      - *Supraclavicular nodes:* located above the clavicle

Expected findings: Nodes are nonpalpable.

Abnormal findings: Palpable nodes may be seen with infection or malignancy. Enlarged lymph nodes caused by infection are tender. ▼

Location of normal lymph nodes

? What if...

- **There is a nipple discharge?**

If there is nipple discharge in a client who is not pregnant or breastfeeding, obtain a specimen by placing a glass slide up to the breast to capture a drop of discharge, following agency policy. Transport the slide to the laboratory as soon as possible. If there is ample discharge, obtain a swab of the discharge with a culturette.

Patient Teaching

You should demonstrate BSE procedure as part of client teaching for self-care, if the client chooses to perform BSE. Instruct clients that clinical breast examinations should be done annually for individuals aged 40 and older and every 1 to 3 years for female individuals aged 20 to 39 (American Congress of Obstetricians and Gynecologists [ACOG] [2017, reaffirmed 2021]). Guidelines vary regarding the best age to start clinical breast examinations (CBE) and mammograms to screen for breast cancer. Annual or biennial mammograms or breast thermography most commonly begin after age 45, or at a younger age and more often for those at high risk (American Cancer Society, n.d.b, revised 2018; 2022). Evidence at present does not support the need for a CBE if a mammogram is done (Monticciolo et al., 2021).

Documentation

- If you palpate a mass or lump, document its size, shape, symmetry, mobility, tenderness, and skin color changes. To document the location, divide the breast into four quadrants by intersecting vertical and horizontal lines. With the nipple as the center, locate the mass or lump as though the breast were a clock; state the distance in cm from the nipple (e.g., 4 o'clock, 2.5 cm from nipple).
- If you need more information about documenting your findings,

▶ Go to **Chapter 19, Caring for the Williams Family,** including **Documenting Physical Examination Findings (Stanley Williams),** in Volume 1.

Practice Resources

American Congress of Obstetricians and Gynecologists (ACOG) (2017, reaffirmed 2021);
American Cancer Society (n.d.b, revised 2018, 2022); Monticciolo et al. (2021).

Procedure 19-12 ■ Assessing the Chest and Lungs

> For steps to follow in *all* procedures, refer to the Universal Steps for All Procedures on the inside back cover.

Equipment
- Stethoscope and antiseptic wipe
- Felt-tipped marker and ruler
- Pen and record form

✚ Clean stethoscope and rulers before and after use unless they are used for only one patient.

Positioning
- Have the client sitting, if possible, and leaning forward for the posterior approach.
  If the client is unable to sit up, findings will be distorted.
- If the client is lying down, findings are more evident on the dependent side; help the client change positions so that you can assess with each side dependent.

Focused History Questions
- Do you have fatigue or activity intolerance?
- Do you have any current respiratory problems?
- Have you had any recent respiratory problems?
- Do you have a cough?
- Do you have any difficulty breathing?
- What, if anything, causes you to be short of breath?
- Have you had any chest pain?
- Do you have a history of allergies or asthma?
- Do you smoke (cigarettes, e-cigarettes, cigars)? If so, how much and for how long?
- If you smoke, have you tried to quit? Would you like to quit?
- Are you exposed to air pollutants at home or at work?

> When performing the procedure, always identify your patient according to agency policy, using two identifiers, and be attentive to standard precautions, hand hygiene, patient safety and privacy, body mechanics, and documentation.

Procedure Steps

1. **Count the respiratory rate and observe the rhythm and depth; observe the symmetry of chest and respiratory movements.**
   (See Chapter 18 if you need more information about counting respirations.)

Findings

Expected findings:
- Respirations are quiet with a regular rhythm and depth; rate 12–20 breaths/min for adults.
- Chest movement is symmetrical, rising and falling with each respiration.

Developmental Variations

Infants and children—The normal respiratory rate varies by age. A newborn may have a respiratory rate of 40–90. The rate gradually declines as the child matures. Newborns breathe abdominally, so you will see little chest movement. The chest in a young child is apple shaped.

🍁 *Older adults*—Rate changes very little; however, respirations decrease in depth as muscles become weakened.

Abnormal findings:
- Chest asymmetry may be seen with musculoskeletal disorders of the spine, such as kyphosis or scoliosis.
- Asymmetrical movement during breathing is seen in rib fractures, pneumothorax, and atelectasis; affected chest area may not move at all with respiration.
- Sternal and intercostal retractions are seen with hypoxia, respiratory distress, and airway obstruction.
- Respiratory rate may be increased with activity, smoking, fever, pain, or anemia.

CHAPTER 19   Health Assessment   245

2. **Inspect the chest.**
   a. Inspect the anteroposterior (AP)-to-lateral ratio.

a. **Expected findings:** Normal adult AP-to-lateral ratio is 1:2.

Developmental Variations

Infants—AP is equal to the lateral diameter.

Older adults—Kyphosis (excessive curvature of the thoracic spine), scoliosis (lateral curvature of the spine), and osteoporosis change the size and shape of the chest; weakening thoracic and diaphragm muscles allow the chest to widen and become more barrel-shaped, as does COPD.

Abnormal findings: AP-to-lateral ratio is increased in COPD (barrel chest).

   b. Inspect the costal angle. ▼

b. **Expected findings:** The costal angle is <90°.

Abnormal findings: Costal angle is >90° in COPD.

Clavicle
Manubrium of sternum
Body of sternum
Costal cartilage
Diaphragm
Xiphoid process
Costal angle

   c. Identify any spinal deformities. ▼

c. **Expected findings:** The spine is straight without lateral curvatures or deformity.

Abnormal findings: Scoliosis is a lateral curvature of the spine. Kyphosis is excessive thoracic curvature.

Scoliosis   Kyphosis

   d. Observe the effort required to breathe.

d. **Expected findings:** Respirations appear effortless. No retraction or use of accessory muscles.

Abnormal findings: Sternal and intercostal retractions are seen in severe hypoxia or respiratory distress.

(continued on next page)

Procedure 19-12 ■ Assessing the Chest and Lungs (continued)

e. Note the color and condition of skin.

e. **Expected findings:** Skin color and hair distribution are consistent with the client's sex, ethnicity, and exposure to the sun. The skin is intact with no scars.

Abnormal findings: Cyanosis of the chest wall (due to extreme hypoxia or cold temperature)

3. **Palpate the trachea.** Place your fingers and thumb on either side of the trachea and note its position. (In a comprehensive examination, you may have already done this with the neck examination.)

Expected findings: Trachea is in the midline.

Abnormal findings: Tracheal deviation may occur from a mass in the neck (e.g., thyroid enlargement) or from excess pressure in the lungs (e.g., **tension pneumothorax**).

Developmental Modifications
*Infants—*Neck is short, so it may not be possible to palpate the trachea.

4. **Palpate the chest.**
   - Observe for tenderness, masses, or **crepitus** (crackling skin due to air in the subcutaneous tissue).
   - Palpate the anterior, posterior, and lateral chest by placing your hands on the chest wall.

Expected findings: The chest is nontender. No masses or crepitus present.

Abnormal findings:
- Pain in the chest wall may be due to fracture, inflammation, or trauma.
- Crepitus results from air leaking into the subcutaneous tissue. It is most likely to occur around wounds, central IV line sites, chest tubes, or a tracheostomy.

5. **Palpate chest excursion** (expandability).
   a. Place your hands at the base of the client's chest with fingers spread and thumbs about 5 cm (2 in.) apart (at the costal margin anteriorly and at the 8th to 10th ribs posteriorly).
   b. Press your thumbs toward the client's spine to create a small skinfold between them.
   c. Have the client take a deep breath, and feel for chest expansion. This may be performed on the anterior or posterior portion of the chest, or both. ▼

Expected findings: Chest excursion is symmetrical on the anterior and posterior aspects of the chest (you should feel equal pressure on your hands; thumbs should move apart equal distances).

Abnormal findings:
- Limited chest excursion may occur with shallow breathing, restrictive clothing, or restrictive airway disease.
- Asymmetrical excursion may result from airway obstruction, pleural effusion, or pneumothorax.

6. **Follow the same pattern and sequence** for palpating fremitus, percussing, and auscultating the chest. See the accompanying diagram. ▼

7. **Palpate the chest for tactile fremitus.**
   a. Use the palmar surface of your hands, but raise the fingers off the client's chest so that you palpate with the bony metacarpophalangeal joints of your hands.
      Bony prominences are best for detecting vibrations.
   b. Palpate for vibrations as the client says "99." ▼

Expected findings: Tactile fremitus is equal bilaterally on the anterior and posterior chest; it is diminished at midthorax. Fremitus is normally diminished if the chest wall is very thick or the voice is very soft.

Developmental Variations

Children and thin adults—May have increased fremitus.

Abnormal findings:
- Increased fremitus occurs with conditions that cause fluid in the lungs (e.g., pulmonary edema).
- Decreased or absent fremitus occurs when there is decreased air movement or tissue consolidation (e.g., emphysema, asthma).

Developmental Modifications

Infants—Place your hand over the chest while the infant is crying.

8. **Percuss the chest.** Compare the right side to the left side.
   - Percuss over the intercostal spaces rather than over the ribs.
     Percussion over bone produces less resonance.
   - Use the indirect percussion method on the anterior, posterior, and lateral chest, following the diagram in step 6.

Expected findings:
- The anterior chest is resonant to the 2nd ICS on the left and to the 4th ICS on the right.
- The lateral chest is resonant to the 8th ICS.
- The posterior chest is resonant to T12.

Abnormal findings: Dullness is heard with fluid or masses in the lungs. Hyperresonance is heard with air trapping that occurs with emphysema.

(continued on next page)

Procedure 19-12 ■ Assessing the Chest and Lungs (continued)

9. **Percuss the posterior chest for diaphragmatic excursion.**
   a. Percuss the level of the diaphragm on full expiration. Have the client exhale completely and hold their breath while you percuss (beginning just below the scapula) from resonance over the lung downward toward the diaphragm. The sound will become dull at the diaphragm. Mark the area with a pen.
   b. Percuss the diaphragm level on full inspiration. Have the client take a deep breath and hold it as you percuss again. Mark the location.
   c. Measure the distance between the two marks. ▶

Expected findings: Diaphragmatic excursion (the distance between the two marks) is normally 3–6 cm.

Abnormal findings: Decreased excursion may indicate paralysis, atelectasis, or COPD with overinflated lungs.

10. **Auscultate the chest.**
    a. *Routine daily assessment:* Follow the pattern in Step 6, using fewer locations.
    b. *For a focused assessment,* auscultate more areas while still following the pattern in step 6.
    Following a pattern allows you to compare findings side to side.
    c. Use the diaphragm of the stethoscope.
    d. Have the client take slow, deep breaths through the mouth as you listen at each site through one full respiratory cycle.

    To review lung sounds, refer to the tables at the end of this procedure.

Expected findings: No abnormal or adventitious sounds are heard. Lung fields are clear to auscultation.
- *Bronchial* breath sounds are heard over the trachea.
- *Bronchovesicular* breath sounds are heard over the sternum anteriorly and between the scapulae posteriorly.
- *Vesicular* breath sounds are heard over most of the lung fields.

Developmental Variations

Infants—Breath sounds are louder than in adults.

Abnormal findings: Crackles or rales, rhonchi, wheezing, stridor, friction rub, grunting
- **Diminished breath sounds** are heard with poor inspiratory effort, in the very muscular or obese, or with restricted airflow.
- **Misplaced breath sounds** (e.g., bronchial breath sounds heard over the lung fields) indicate constriction of flow.
- **Adventitious breath sounds,** such as wheezes, rhonchi, and rales, are sounds heard over normal breath sounds.
  Key Point: *If an abnormal sound is heard, have the client cough, and listen again.*

11. **Auscultate for abnormal voice sounds if there is evidence of lung congestion.** Follow the pattern in Step 6.
    a. Assess for *bronchophony* by having the client say "one, two, three" as you listen over the lung fields.
    b. Assess for *egophony* by having your client say "eee" as you listen over the lung fields.
    c. Assess for *whispered pectoriloquy* by having your client whisper "one, two, three" as you listen over the lung fields.

Expected findings: No abnormal voice sounds are heard.

Abnormal findings:
a. **Bronchophony** is present if the words are clearly heard over the lungs.
b. **Egophony** is present if the sound you hear is "ay."
c. **Whispered pectoriloquy** is present if you hear "one, two, three" clearly.

Patient Teaching

Instruct the client about the dangers of tobacco use, especially smoking; exposure to air pollutants and environmental pollutants, such as radon or asbestos; and the signs and symptoms of lung cancer.

Home Care

- Instruct clients or caregivers to identify any pollutant within the home that may cause respiratory problems, such as radon, dirty heating/air-conditioning systems, or mold.
- Instruct caregivers or patients with allergies and/or asthma to eliminate potential allergens, such as cigarette smoke, dust, feathers, and pet dander.

Documentation

If you need information about documenting your findings,

> Go to **Chapter 19, Caring for the Williams Family,** including **Documenting Physical Examination Findings (Stanley Williams),** in Volume 1.

Normal Lung Sounds

NORMAL LUNG SOUNDS	LOCATION	DESCRIPTION	ILLUSTRATION
Bronchial or tubular	Heard over the trachea	Blowing, hollow sounds; inspiration is shorter than expiration and lower-pitched	Inspiration / Expiration
Bronchovesicular	Heard over the 1st and 2nd ICS anteriorly and over the scapula posteriorly	Medium-pitched, medium intensity, blowing sounds; inspiration and expiration are equal length and similar pitch	Inspiration / Expiration
Vesicular	Heard over the lung periphery	Soft, low-pitched sounds; inspiration is longer, louder, and higher-pitched than expiration	Inspiration / Expiration

Abnormal Lung Sounds

ABNORMAL LUNG SOUNDS	CAUSE	CHARACTERISTICS	EXAMPLES
Crackles (sometimes called rales)	Air bubbling through moisture in the alveoli	Bubbling, crackling, popping; soft, high-pitched, and very brief sounds, usually heard during inspiration	Pneumonia Congestive heart failure (CHF) Bronchitis Emphysema
Rhonchi	Mucous secretions in the large airways	Coarse, snoring, continuous low-pitched sounds heard during inspiration and expiration; may clear with coughing	Bronchitis Emphysema Narrowed airways Fibrotic lungs
Wheezes	Narrowing of small airways by spasm, inflammation, mucus, or tumor	High-pitched musical or squeaking sounds heard during inspiration or expiration	Acute asthma Emphysema

(continued on next page)

Procedure 19-12 ■ Assessing the Chest and Lungs (continued)

Abnormal Lung Sounds—cont'd

ABNORMAL LUNG SOUNDS	CAUSE	CHARACTERISTICS	EXAMPLES
Stridor*	Partial upper airway obstruction or tracheal or laryngeal spasm	High-pitched, continuous honking sounds heard throughout the respiratory cycle but most prominent on inspiration	Acute respiratory distress Foreign body in airway Epiglottitis
Friction rub	Rubbing together of inflamed pleural layers	A high-pitched grating or rubbing sound that may be heard throughout the respiratory cycle; loudest over lower lateral anterior surface	Pleuritis
Grunting	Retention of air in the lungs	A high-pitched tubular sound heard on expiration	Emphysema

*Patients with stridor need immediate medical evaluation.

Procedure 19-13 ■ Assessing the Heart and Vascular System

➤ For steps to follow in *all* procedures, refer to the Universal Steps for All Procedures on the inside back cover.

Equipment
- Combination stethoscope with bell and diaphragm
- Alcohol or other antiseptic wipes
- Two rulers
- Pen and record form

✚ Clean stethoscope and rulers before and after use unless they are used for only one patient.

Positioning
Place the client in three positions: sitting, supine, and left lateral (to facilitate hearing specific sounds).

Focused History Questions
- Have you had any fatigue or activity intolerance?
- Do you have a history of high blood pressure or stroke?
- Have you ever passed out or felt light-headed?
- Do you have any problems with your heart or circulation?
- Do you ever have chest pain? If so, describe the circumstances that triggered the pain.
- What was the pain like? What did you do to relieve it?
- Do you ever have palpitations or a rapid heartbeat?
- Do you ever feel short of breath?
- Do you ever wake up and can't catch your breath?
- Do you ever get swelling in your feet?
- What medications are you taking?

➤ When performing the procedure, always identify your patient according to agency policy, using two identifiers, and be attentive to standard precautions, hand hygiene, patient safety and privacy, body mechanics, and documentation.

Procedure Steps
1. **Inspect the neck.**
   a. With the patient *supine, inspect the carotid and jugular venous system* in the neck for pulsations.

Findings
Expected findings: Carotid pulsation is easily visible. A slight pulsation in the supraclavicular area or suprasternal notch indicates jugular venous pressure. The pulsation should be easily obliterated when you apply pressure to the area.

b. *Assess jugular flow:* Compress the jugular vein below the jaw. The vein collapses, and the jugular wave is more prominent at the supraclavicular area. ▼

Assessing jugular flow

The jugular venous pulse is easily obliterated with gentle pressure.

c. *Assess jugular filling:* Compress the jugular above the clavicle. The vein distends and the jugular wave disappears. ▼

Assessing jugular filling

Abnormal findings: Significant jugular vein distention suggests right-sided heart failure.

2. **Measure jugular venous pressure (JVP).**
   a. Elevate the head of the bed to a 45° angle.
   b. Identify the highest point of visible internal jugular filling.
   c. Place a ruler vertically at the sternal angle (where the clavicles meet).
   d. Place another ruler horizontally at the highest point of the venous wave.

Expected findings: Normal jugular venous pressure is <3 cm.

Abnormal findings: Elevated JVP (in chronic HF or constricted flow into the right side of the heart); low JVP (in hypovolemia)

(continued on next page)

Procedure 19-13 ■ Assessing the Heart and Vascular System (continued)

e. Measure the distance in centimeters vertically from the chest wall. ▼

Measuring jugular venous pressure

3. **Inspect the precordium for pulsations.** (Have the patient supine with tangential lighting.) You may have to lift breast tissue away from chest wall to visualize pulsations.

   Developmental Modifications
   Children—Look for the PMI more medially and at about the 4th ICS in children younger than age 8.

   Expected findings: Visible pulsation at the point of maximal impulse (PMI, the 5th ICS in the midclavicular line).

   Developmental Variations
   In thin adults and children, a pulsation may also be visible over the base of the heart.

   Abnormal findings:
   - A pulsation (a heave or lift) displaced toward the axillary line indicates left ventricular hypertrophy.
   - Pulsations to the right of the sternum may indicate an aortic aneurysm.

4. **Very gently palpate the carotid arteries.**

   ✚ **NOTE:** This step is not done for all patients. It is a part of a thorough cardiovascular assessment and is done only when indicated.
   a. ✚ Palpate each side separately, never at the same time.
      Bilateral pressure may impair cerebral blood flow.
   b. ✚ Avoid massaging the carotid artery as you palpate.
      Increased pressure on the carotid will lead to a drop in the heart rate and blood pressure.
   c. Note the rate, rhythm, amplitude, and symmetry of the pulse.
   d. Note the contour, symmetry, and elasticity of the arteries.
   e. Note any thrills.

   Expected findings:
   - *Rhythm* is regular with + 2 amplitude.
   - *Contour:* There should be a smooth upstroke with less acute descent.
   - *Symmetry:* Pulses are equal bilaterally.
   - *Elasticity:* Carotids are soft and pliable.

   Developmental Variations
   Pulse rate is age dependent.
   🍁 *Older adults*—The carotids may be stiff and cordlike.

   Abnormal findings: A thrill indicates turbulent flow.

5. **Palpate the precordium.**
   a. For this part of the examination, have the patient sit up and lean forward. If lying down, have the patient turn to the left side.
      Brings the apex of the heart closer to the chest wall
   b. Palpate in all five areas: apex, left lateral sternal border, epigastric area, base left, and base right.
   c. Feel for pulsations, lifts, heaves, and thrills.

   Helpful Hint: *Perform cardiac palpation and auscultation from the patient's right side, whenever possible.*
   This allows you to stretch the stethoscope during auscultation so that you minimize interference and static.

   Expected findings: PMI is palpable at the apex over a 1-cm to 2-cm area. Slight pulsation from the abdominal aorta may be felt at the epigastric area. No pulsations, lifts, heaves, or thrills are palpable.

   Abnormal findings: A pulsation, lift, or heave may be seen with left ventricular hypertrophy.
   - A **lift** is a pulsation that is forceful enough to seem to lift the examiner's fingers with palpation.
   - A **heave** is a pulsation that feels rolling under your fingers.
   - A **thrill** indicates turbulent flow and feels like a vibration over the PMI.

6. **Auscultate the carotids.**
   a. Place the bell portion of the stethoscope over the carotid artery to listen for bruits.
      Bruits are low-pitched sounds, best heard by the bell portion.
   b. Have the patient hold their breath as you listen.
      Breath sounds over the trachea are loud and could interfere with the ability to hear a bruit.

   NOTE: *If you hear a bruit, lightly palpate the neck for thrills (pulsations or vibrations), which further confirm turbulent flow.*

   Expected findings: No audible bruit is present.

   Developmental Variations

   Children—Bruit may be heard because of a high-output state.

   Abnormal findings: In adults, a bruit suggests carotid stenosis, increased cardiac output secondary to fluid overload, use of stimulants, or hyperthyroidism.

7. **Auscultate the jugular veins.**
   a. Place the bell portion of the stethoscope lightly over the jugular veins to listen for a low-pitched venous hum.
   b. Have the patient hold their breath as you listen.

   Expected findings: No venous hum is audible.

   Developmental Variations

   Children—A venous hum may be heard. This is a benign condition whereby blood travels to the brain and back down again to the heart, causing the vein walls to vibrate.

8. **Auscultate the precordium.** To review heart sounds, **Key Point:** *Be systematic. To keep from missing important parts of the examination, always auscultate in the same order to all the areas.*
   - Ask the patient to sit upright and lean forward a bit.
     This will position the heart closer to the chest wall for clearer auscultation.
   - Listen for the S_1, S_2, S_3, and S_4 sounds.
   - Listen for murmurs.
   - Listen with both the bell and the diaphragm at the sites in the following figure:
     These sites are located along the pathway the blood takes as it flows through the atria, ventricles, and valves of the heart.

   Expected findings: No extra sounds are heard. No murmurs, clicks, or rubs are present.

   An S_4 sound is normal in athletes.

   Developmental Variations

   Infants—You may hear a split S_2 when the child takes a deep breath.

   Children—The chest wall is thinner, so heart sounds are louder than in adults. An S_3 is normal in young children and adolescents when they are sitting or lying, but it disappears when they stand or sit up.

   Pregnancy—An S_3 is a normal variant in the third trimester of pregnancy.

   (continued on next page)

Procedure 19-13 ■ Assessing the Heart and Vascular System (continued)

Older adults—An S_4 sound is considered normal; extra systoles per minute are considered normal. ▼

Cardiac auscultation sites

Abnormal findings:
- A split sound at either S_1 or S_2 may occur if there is a delay in closure of one of the valves.
- An S_3 that does not disappear with position change is abnormal and represents heart failure or volume overload.
- An S_4 may be heard in adults with coronary artery disease, hypertension, and pulmonic stenosis.

---

a. *Base right (aortic valve).* Locate the angle of Louis (the prominence on the sternum, two to three fingerbreadths below the suprasternal notch). Slide your fingers laterally until you feel the 2nd ICS.
The right 2nd ICS is the best place to auscultate the aortic valve.

a. **Expected findings:** $S_1 < S_2$

---

b. *Base left (pulmonic valve).* Locate the angle of Louis (the prominence on the sternum, two to three fingerbreadths below the clavicular notch). Slide your fingers laterally until you feel the 2nd ICS.
The left 2nd ICS is the best place to auscultate the pulmonic valve. ▼

b. **Expected findings:** $S_1 < S_2$

c. *Apex (mitral valve).* You may be able to locate the apex by observing the pulsation at the PMI. It is at the 5th ICS in the midclavicular line.

c. **Expected findings:** $S_1 > S_2$

Developmental Variations

Children—You will hear S_3 at the apex in about 30% of children.

d. *Left lateral sternal border (LLSB) (tricuspid valve).* From the apex, *slide* your finger up to the 4th ICS, then move close to the sternum.

d. **Expected findings:** $S_1 \geq S_2$. You may hear a split S_1.

Abnormal findings: Extra sounds (S_3 or S_4), murmurs, clicks, or rubs

NOTE: *A diastolic murmur or a murmur greater than grade ³⁄₆ is never innocent.*

Developmental Variations

In infants, a split S_2 sound during normal respirations may indicate an atrial-septal defect.

Assessing Murmurs

Auscultating murmurs is an advanced technique that requires practice and experience. However, if you hear a murmur, assess its:
- Location
- Quality
- Frequency (high, medium, or low pitch)
- Intensity (loudness)
- Timing (in relation to S_1 and S_2)
- Duration
- Configuration (constant or crescendo/decrescendo)
- Radiation (can you hear this in other locations?)
- Respiratory variation (does it change with breathing?)

Classifying Murmurs

Grade

¹⁄₆ Very faint, comes and goes

²⁄₆ Quiet, but heard immediately

³⁄₆ Moderately loud

⁴⁄₆ Loud, associated with a thrill

⁵⁄₆ Heard with stethoscope half off the chest wall; thrill present

⁶⁄₆ Heard with stethoscope entirely off the chest wall; thrill present

9. **Inspect the periphery for color, temperature, and edema.** (You will probably already have done this when examining the integumentary system.)

Expected findings: Skin is warm. No edema is present. Color is appropriate for race.

Abnormal findings: Pallor, cyanosis, coolness, shininess, sparse hair growth, and clubbing of the nails (may indicate pulmonary oxygenation problems or impaired central or peripheral circulation).

10. **Palpate the peripheral pulses:** Radial, brachial, femoral, popliteal, dorsalis pedis, and posterior tibial.
    - Using the distal pads of your second and third fingers, firmly palpate pulses.
    - Palpate firmly but not so hard that you occlude the artery.
    - If you have trouble finding a pulse, vary your pressure, feeling carefully at the correct anatomical location.
    - Assess pulses for rate, rhythm, equality, amplitude, and elasticity.
    - Describe pulse amplitude on a scale of 0 to 4:
        0 = Absent, pulse cannot be felt.
        1 = Weak (thready): Pulse is barely palpable and can be easily obliterated by finger pressure.
        2 = Normal quality: Pulse is easily palpated, not weak or bounding, obliterated by finger pressure.
        3 = Full: Pulse is easily felt with little pressure, not easily obliterated.
        4 = Bounding, forceful, obliterated only by strong finger pressure.

Expected findings: All pulses are regular, strong, and equal bilaterally. Pulse amplitude is +2.

Developmental Variations

Older adults—Arterial pulses may be difficult to palpate because of decreased arterial perfusion.

Abnormal findings: Weak, absent, or asymmetrical pulses may indicate partial or complete occlusion of the artery. Other signs of arterial occlusion include pain, pallor, cool temperature, paresthesia, or paralysis.

(continued on next page)

Procedure 19-13 ■ Assessing the Heart and Vascular System (continued)

11. **Inspect the venous system.** If a client has varicosities, assess for valve competence with the manual compression test, following:
    a. With the client standing, compress the distal portion of the vein.
    b. Still holding the distal portion, compress the proximal portion.
    c. Feel for a pulsation with your lower (distal) hand.
       - **If the valves are competent,** you will not feel backflow when you compress the vein.
       - **If the valves are incompetent,** you will feel a wave pulsation with your lower hand as a result of backflow when you press on the proximal segment.

Expected findings: Veins are not distended. Superficial spiderlike veins, especially on the lower extremities, may occur with normal aging.

Developmental Variations
Older adults—Often have peripheral edema as a result of chronic venous insufficiency.

Abnormal findings: Ropelike, distended, tortuous, or painful veins **(varicosities)**.

? What if...

■ **The patient is obese and heart sounds are difficult to hear?**

The larger the body mass over the heart, the more difficult it is to hear heart sounds clearly. However, it may help to have the patient sit upright and lean forward as you auscultate.

■ **Findings from inspecting and palpating peripheral pulses are abnormal?**

If inspection or palpation findings are abnormal, perform the tests in the table More Extensive Tests for Abnormal Findings at the end of this procedure.

Patient Teaching
Instruct the patient in the risk factors of heart disease and stroke and in the signs and symptoms of heart disease.

Documentation
If you need information about documenting your findings,

▶ Go to **Chapter 19, Caring for the Williams Family,** including **Documenting Physical Examination Findings (Stanley Williams),** in Volume 1.

If you need more information about assessing apical and peripheral pulses and measuring blood pressure, go to

▶ The video **Vital Signs,** along with questions and suggested responses, on the **Davis's *Nursing Skills Videos*** Web site at www.fadavis.com.

More Extensive Tests for Abnormal Findings

TESTS	EXPECTED FINDINGS

1. **Perform the capillary refill test** anywhere you note signs of diminished blood flow.
  a. Press the skin with sufficient pressure to produce blanching.
  b. Release the pressure and observe the return of color.
	1. Color returns in less than 3 seconds.

2. **Perform Allen's test** to assess abnormal pulse findings and arterial flow in the hands.
  a. Have the client form a tight fist with one hand.
  b. With fist still clenched, compress radial and ulnar arteries.
  c. Ask the client to open hand; observe for pallor.
  d. Release the ulnar artery and watch for natural color to return.
  e. Then repeat the process, but release the radial artery.
	2. In a healthy individual, skin color returns rapidly with each maneuver. Failure to return to normal color indicates impaired flow through the open artery. Normally pallor resolves in 3–5 sec.

More Extensive Tests for Abnormal Findings—cont'd

TESTS	EXPECTED FINDINGS
3. **Check the ankle–brachial index (ABI)** to assess circulatory impairment of the feet. a. Use a Doppler (handheld ultrasonic device) to measure blood pressure at the posterior tibialis or dorsalis pedis pulse sites. b. Compare that pressure with blood pressure obtained over the brachial artery. c. To calculate the ABI, divide the systolic pressure at the ankle by the systolic pressure at the brachial site.	3. Normally ankle pressure is higher than brachial pressure. The following is a summary of ABI findings. Normal: 1 or greater Minimal disease: 0.8–0.95 Moderate disease: 0.79–0.4 Severe disease: 0.39–0 *Example:* If the systolic pressure at the ankle is 75 and at the brachial artery is 100, the ABI is 75/100, or 0.75. This indicates moderate peripheral vascular disease.
4. **Perform the color change test** to assess arterial circulation in the legs. a. While the client is lying supine, elevate the legs to increase venous return. b. Have the client quickly move to a sitting position with the feet dangling.	4. Normal color should return to the feet in less than 10 seconds. Pallor with the legs elevated and dependent **rubor** (reddish-purple color) are signs of arterial insufficiency.

Procedure 19-14 ■ Assessing the Abdomen

▶ For steps to follow in *all* procedures, refer to the Universal Steps for All Procedures on the inside back cover.

Equipment
- Stethoscope and antiseptic wipe
- Felt-tipped marker
- Tape measure and ruler
- Penlight or examination light
- Pen and record form

✚ Clean stethoscope and other equipment before and after using unless they are used for only one patient.

Positioning
Begin with the client supine, arms at sides, with small pillows under the head and knees.
Relaxes the abdominal muscles, allowing for more effective palpation.

Focused History Questions
- What types of foods do you typically eat?
- Are there any foods that you cannot eat? If so, why?
- How many cups of coffee, tea, cola, or caffeinated beverages do you drink per day?
- Do you smoke or use tobacco products (e-cigarettes, cigars, water pipes)? If so, how much and at what age did you start?
- Do you drink alcohol? If so, how many drinks per day? Per week?
- Do you use any drug for nonmedical purposes? If so, which ones and how often?
- Do you have any abdominal pain?
- How often do you have a bowel movement (BM)?
- Have you noticed any changes in your BMs?
- Are you having any problems with constipation, diarrhea, or getting to the bathroom in time to use the toilet?
- Have you ever seen blood in your stool or noticed blood when you wipe after a BM?
- Have you ever had black, tarry stools?
- How often do you use antacids, laxatives, enemas, aspirin, or anti-inflammatory medicines such as Anaprox or Motrin?
- What home remedy, herbal, or over-the-counter medicines do you use?
- What prescription medicines do you use?
- Have you ever been immunized for hepatitis?
- Have you ever had a blood transfusion?
- What is your occupation?
- Have you ever been diagnosed with an ulcer, hemorrhoids, hernia, bowel problem, cancer, hepatitis, liver problems, cirrhosis, or appendicitis?
- Have you ever had abdominal surgery? If so, when, what type, and what if any follow-up was done for the problem?
- Do you have any family history of abdominal problems, such as ulcers, gallbladder disease, bowel disease, or cancer?
- Do you ever have trouble with swallowing, heartburn, nausea, vomiting, diarrhea, bloating, excess gas, yellowing of the skin?

> **Developmental Modifications**
>
> *For older adults*, recall that problems with eating is a part of the SPICES assessment. Ask clients, for example:
> - Do you have difficulty chewing or swallowing your food?
> - How is your appetite?
> - Are you able to shop for and prepare your food?

(continued on next page)

Procedure 19-14 ■ Assessing the Abdomen (continued)

▶ When performing the procedure, always identify your patient according to agency policy, using two identifiers, and be attentive to standard precautions, hand hygiene, patient safety and privacy, body mechanics, and documentation.

Procedure Steps

1. **Have the client void before the examination.**
   Empties the bladder so that you do not mistake a full bladder for a mass

2. **Position the client supine with the knees slightly flexed.**
   Relaxes the abdominal muscles for more effective palpation

3. **Inspect the abdomen.**
   a. Observe the size, symmetry, and contour of the abdomen.
      (1) Stand at the client's side and view across the abdomen.
      (2) If distention is present, use a tape measure to measure girth at the level of the umbilicus.
      (3) Have the client raise their head and check for bulges.
         Accentuates hernia, if present.

   b. Observe the condition of skin and skin color. Look for lesions, scars, striae, superficial veins, and hair distribution (if you have not already done this in your examination of the integumentary system).

   c. Note abdominal movements.

Findings

a. **Expected findings:** Abdomen is flat, slightly rounded, scaphoid (concave), or slightly protuberant; sides are symmetrical. No visible masses or distention are present.

Developmental Variations

Infants and toddlers—Protuberant abdomen is normal.

Abnormal findings:
- Asymmetry may be caused by tumors, cysts, or scoliosis.
- Distention may be due to gas, fluid retention, or bowel obstruction.

b. **Expected findings:** Skin color is consistent with ethnicity but is usually lighter in color than exposed areas. No lesions are present. Hair distribution is appropriate for age and sex. Striae, superficial veins, and scars are common variations.

Abnormal findings:
- Skin color changes may be associated with bruising, internal bleeding, or jaundice.
- Striae occur after periods of rapid growth or weight gain. Pink striae are new. Older striae are silver-white in color.
- Dilated veins are associated with liver disease and obstruction of the vena cava.

c. **Expected findings:** On a thin client, peristalsis and aortic pulsations may be visible. Men tend to use their abdominal muscles for breathing.

Developmental Variations

Infants and children—Peristaltic waves are often visible. Abdominal breathing is common in infants and young children.

🍁 *Older adults*—Abdomen may be more rounded because of decreased muscle tone.

Abnormal findings:
- Peristaltic waves may be seen if there is intestinal obstruction.
- Abnormal respiratory movements may be seen with respiratory distress.
- Pulsations (in other than a thin client) may indicate an aortic aneurysm.

d. Note the position, contour, and color of the umbilicus. ▼

Umbilical hernia

d. **Expected findings:** Umbilicus is inverted and in the midline. No discoloration or discharge is present. ▼

Omentum, Fat, Bowel, Body wall

Abnormal findings: Protrusion of the umbilicus may result from a hernia or underlying mass.

4. **Auscultate the abdomen.**
   a. Ask the client when they last ate.
      Bowel sounds are loudest 5 or 6 hours after the person eats, when the small intestine contents empty through the ileocecal valve into the large intestine. They also increase immediately after eating.
   b. Listen for bowel sounds.
      (1) Using the stethoscope diaphragm, listen in several areas in all four quadrants (see the figure).
         The diaphragm of the stethoscope is used because bowel sounds are high-pitched.
      (2) If bowel sounds are infrequent or difficult to hear, listen to the right of the umbilicus over the ileocecal valve.
      (3) Listen for up to 5 minutes before concluding that bowel sounds are absent. ▼

   b. **Expected findings:** Audible bowel sounds, occurring every 5–15 sec or 5–30 times per min

      Abnormal findings:
      - **Hyperperistalsis** (hyperactive): >2 or 3 sounds per sec or >30 sounds per min
      - **Hypoperistalsis** (hypoactive): <5 sounds per min
      - **Absent** bowel sounds: none after listening for 5 min

The four abdominal quadrants (RUQ, LUQ, RLQ, LLQ) — Xiphoid process, Liver, Stomach, Transverse colon, Descending colon, Umbilicus, Small intestine, Ascending colon, Sigmoid colon, Bladder, Pubic symphysis

(continued on next page)

Procedure 19-14 ■ Assessing the Abdomen (continued)

c. Use the stethoscope bell to listen for bruits over the aorta and the renal, femoral, and iliac arteries.

c. **Expected findings:** No audible bruits are present.

Abnormal findings: A bruit is abnormal and may indicate an aneurysm or altered blood flow. ▼

Locating abdominal arteries

5. **Percuss the abdomen.** (See Clinical Insight 19-1.)
   a. Use indirect percussion to assess at multiple sites in all four quadrants.
   b. Estimate organ size by noting the change in sounds as you percuss over the liver, spleen, and bladder. ▼

Expected findings: Tympany, with dullness over organs or fluid, is present. No tenderness

Abnormal findings: Extremely high-pitched tympanic sounds are heard with distention. Extensive dullness indicates organ enlargement or underlying mass.

6. **Using fist or blunt percussion, percuss the costovertebral angle** (where the end of the rib cage meets the spine) bilaterally to assess for kidney tenderness. ▼

Expected findings: No costovertebral angle tenderness is present.

Abnormal findings: Pain or tenderness is associated with kidney infection or musculoskeletal problems.

7. **Palpate the abdomen.**
   a. **Begin with light palpation** throughout the abdomen. Identify surface characteristics, tenderness, muscular resistance, and turgor.
      (1) If the client is having pain in one area of the abdomen, palpate that area last.
      A guarding response to pain from palpation can interfere with your assessment of the other areas.
      (2) Using your fingertips, press down 1–2 cm in a rotating motion.
      (3) Lift your fingers and move to the next site.
      (4) Palpate the entire abdomen if possible.
      (5) Proceed in an organized fashion through all quadrants, using the same sequence in every examination.
      (6) Observe for grimacing, guarding, or verbal statements of tenderness or pain.

   Developmental Modifications

   Encourage a child to place their hand lightly over yours as you palpate.

   ⊕ Caution: Do not palpate the abdomen if the client has a Wilms' tumor, a large diffuse pulsation, or a history of organ transplant.

   b. **Use deep palpation** to palpate organs and masses. See the table Deep Palpation Techniques at the end of this procedure.

   c. **Palpate the liver.**
      (1) Stand at the client's right side.
      (2) Place your right hand at the client's right midclavicular line under the costal margin, parallel to the right costal.
      (3) Place your left hand under the client's back at the lower (11th to 12th) ribs, and press upward. This elevates the liver toward the abdominal wall.
      (4) Ask the client to inhale and deeply exhale while you press in and up, gently but deeply, with your right fingers.

   Alternative approach: Hooking technique. Place your hands over the right costal margin, and hook your fingers over the edge. Have the client take a deep breath, and feel for the liver's edge as the liver drops down on inspiration and then rises up over your fingers during expiration. ▶

   a. **Expected findings:** The abdomen is soft and nontender, with no masses. Muscles are easily palpated; no guarding is present.

   Abnormal findings: Guarding and rigidity may indicate peritonitis. Tenderness on light palpation indicates the need for further evaluation.

   b. **Expected findings:** Tenderness may be noted in a normal adult near the xiphoid process and over the cecum and sigmoid colon.

   Developmental Variations

   Older adults—May have a higher pain threshold, so they may not react to palpation even if there is an abnormality in the abdomen.

   Abnormal findings: A mass indicates the need for further evaluation.

   c. **Expected findings:** The liver is not normally palpable unless the client is very thin. If it is palpable, the edge should be smooth and nontender.

   Developmental Variations

   Children—Liver is relatively large and can be palpated 1–2 cm (0.5–1 in.) below the right costal margin.

   Abnormal findings: Palpation below the costal margin indicates enlargement.

(continued on next page)

Procedure 19-14 ■ Assessing the Abdomen (continued)

d. **Palpate the spleen.**
   (1) Stand at the client's right side.
   (2) Reach across the client to place your left hand under the costovertebral angle, and pull upward to move the spleen anteriorly.
   (3) Place your right hand under the left anterior costal margin, and have the client take a deep breath.
   (4) During exhalation, press your hands together (inward) to try to palpate the spleen. ▶

d. **Expected findings:** The spleen is not normally palpable.

Abnormal findings: Splenic enlargement or tenderness may result from infection, trauma, or cancer.

? What if...

- **The patient has a nasogastric (NG) tube attached to suction?**

Discontinue suction or clamp the tube while auscultating so that you will not mistake the sound of suction for bowel sounds.

- **The patient is ticklish or guarding when I palpate the abdomen?**

Distract the person by giving a task, such as "Count aloud to 10" or "Count backward from 100." Alternatively, have the client place their hand on their abdomen; place your hand on theirs and begin light palpation. When they begin to feel more relaxed, slip your hand underneath theirs and continue.

- **The patient complains of abdominal pain?**

Check for rebound tenderness: Place your hand perpendicular to the abdomen. Press firmly and slowly, then release quickly.

If pain increases when you remove your hand, this indicates peritoneal irritation. Rebound tenderness in the right lower quadrant may be a sign of appendicitis.

Patient Teaching

Instruct the patient on the importance of proper diet, the signs and symptoms of colorectal cancer, and the importance of colonoscopy screening.

Documentation

If you need more information about documenting your findings,

➡ Go to **Chapter 19, Caring for the Williams Family,** including **Documenting Physical Examination Findings (Stanley Williams),** in Volume 1.

Deep Palpation Techniques

DEEP PALPATION: ONE-HANDED TECHNIQUE

- Using your fingertips, press down 4–6 cm in a dipping motion.
- Proceed in an organized fashion through all four quadrants. ▼

DEEP PALPATION: BIMANUAL TECHNIQUE

- This technique is useful when palpating a large abdomen.
- Place your nondominant hand on your dominant hand.
- Depress your hands 4–6 cm (1.5–2 in.) in a dipping motion.
- Proceed in an organized fashion through all four quadrants. ▼

? What if...

- **I palpate a mass?**

Have the client tighten abdominal muscles.
If the mass is in the abdominal wall, it will become easier to palpate. If it is deep in the abdomen, it will be difficult to palpate.

Procedure 19-15 ■ Assessing the Musculoskeletal System

➤ For steps to follow in *all* procedures, refer to the Universal Steps for All Procedures on the inside back cover.

Equipment
- Tape measure
- Goniometer
- Pen and record form

Developmental Modifications

For older adults, recall that "problems with falls" is a part of the SPICES assessment. If your facility has a falls assessment tool, perform that focused assessment.

Focused History Questions
- Do you have any difficulty with coordination (e.g., folding clothes, brushing your teeth)?
- Do you now have, or have you ever had, musculoskeletal problems, pain, or disease? If so, what medications or treatments are you using?
- Have you ever injured your bones or joints?
- Do your joints, muscles, or bones limit your activities?
- Do you lose your balance or fall?
- Do you have any occupational hazards that could affect your muscles and joints?

➤ When performing the procedure, always identify your patient according to agency policy, using two identifiers, and be attentive to standard precautions, hand hygiene, patient safety and privacy, body mechanics, and documentation.

Procedure Steps

1. **Assess posture.**
   a. Note the body and head positions.

   b. Check the alignment and symmetry of the shoulders, scapulae, and iliac crests. Inspect from the front, back, and side.

Findings

a. **Expected findings:** Posture is erect, with the head in the midline.

b. **Expected findings:** The shoulders, scapulae, and iliac crests are symmetrical.

(continued on next page)

Procedure 19-15 ■ Assessing the Musculoskeletal System (continued)

Developmental Modifications

Newborns—Palpate clavicles for fractures that may have occurred at birth. Check for congenital hip dysplasia (dislocation) by examining for asymmetry of the gluteal folds or shortening of the femur.

   c. Assess the spinal curvature by:
      (1) Observing the client's profile while client is standing erect
      (2) Having the client bend forward at the waist with arms hanging free at the sides ▼

c. **Expected findings:** Cervical and lumbar curves are concave; thoracic and sacral curves are convex.

Developmental Variations

Children—**Lordosis** (exaggerated lumbar curve) is normal before age 5.

   Abnormal findings: Kyphosis, scoliosis, lordosis ▼

Cervical (concave)
Thoracic (convex)
Lumbar (concave)
Sacral (convex)

Assessing for normal curves

Assessing for kyphosis and scoliosis

Lordosis

Kyphosis

Scoliosis

d. Have the client stand upright with the feet together. Note the position of the knees. ▼

d. **Expected findings:** Patella is in the midline on an imaginary line drawn from the anterior superior iliac crest to the feet.

Developmental Variations

Children—**Genu varum** (bowlegs) is normal for 1 year after a child begins to walk.

---

2. **Assess gait by observing the client walking.**

Developmental Modifications

Children—Observe them at play.

Physical disability—Allow client to use assistive device (walker, cane) and proceed only if the gait is steady; stand nearby in case the client loses their balance.

   a. Pay attention to the base of support (distance between the feet) and stride length (distance between each step).

   a. **Expected findings:**
   Average base of support for an adult is 5–10 cm (2–4 in.).
   Average stride length is 30–35 cm (12–14 in.).
   The longer the legs, the longer the stride length.

   Abnormal findings:
   - *Abnormal gait* can be caused by muscle weakness, joint stiffness, pain, deformities, lumbar disc problems, central nervous system dysfunction, muscle atrophy or hypertonicity (e.g., from stroke or brain tumor), Parkinson's disease, cerebral palsy, multiple sclerosis, and spinal tumors.
   - A *wide base of support and shortened stride length* reflect a balance problem, placing the client at risk for falls.

   b. Observe the phases of the gait. ▼

   b. **Expected findings:** Movements are smooth and coordinated, weight is evenly distributed, arms swing in opposition, and toes point forward.

   Abnormal findings: Toeing in or out, jerky or shuffling movements, touching the floor first with the toe rather than the heel, arms held out to the side or front.

(continued on next page)

266　UNIT 3　Essential Nursing Interventions

Procedure 19-15 ■ Assessing the Musculoskeletal System (continued)

Stance Phase ▼

| Heel strike | Foot flat | Midstance | Push-off |

Swing Phase ▼

| Accelerate | Swing-through | Decelerate |

Abnormal Gaits

| Propulsive gait | Scissors gait | Spastic gait | Steppage gait | Waddling gait |

3. **Assess balance.**
   Key Point: *If the client was unsteady when walking, do not complete this portion of the examination. Proceed only if the gait is steady; stand nearby in case the client loses their balance.*
   a. Have the client tandem walk heel to toe.
   b. Have the client walk alternately on heels and toes.
   c. Ask the client to do a deep knee bend.
   d. Ask the client to hop in place on each foot several times.
   e. Perform the Romberg test (if you did not already do so when examining the ears): Have the client stand with feet together and eyes open. Then have the client close eyes and stand still. ▼

   Expected findings:
   - The client is able to perform each of these maneuvers smoothly.
   - The Romberg test (see Procedure 19-7) is negative—the client is able to maintain balance with minimal sway with eyes open and closed.

   Developmental Variations
   Infants—Should be able to sit alone by age 8 months.

   Abnormal findings: Balance problems may indicate a cerebellar disorder, an inner ear problem, or muscle weakness.

   Step 3a. Walking heel to toe

   Step 3b. Walking on heels

   Step 3b. Walking on toes

Developmental Modifications
Infants—Observe sucking, swallowing, and kicking movements.
Children—To assess a child's movement, coordination, ROM, and so on, watch the child at normal play. Cerebellar function cannot be tested on infants and toddlers because of their immature neuromuscular system.

4. **Assess coordination while the client is seated.**
   a. Test upper extremity coordination by having the client perform finger–thumb opposition. Test one side and then the other. ▼

   Expected findings: The client is able to perform these movements smoothly and in a coordinated fashion. The dominant side (usually the right) may be slightly more coordinated.

   Developmental Variations
   Older adults—Decreased coordination and reaction time may result from slower nerve conduction and loss of muscle tone.

   Abnormal findings: Slowness or awkwardness with movement may indicate a cerebellar disorder or muscle weakness.

   b. Test rapid alternating movements by having the client alternate between supinating and pronating hands.
   c. Assess lower extremity coordination by having the client perform rhythmic toe tapping, one side at a time.
   d. Have the client run the heel of one foot down the shin of the other leg. Repeat on the opposite side.

(continued on next page)

268　UNIT 3　Essential Nursing Interventions

Procedure 19-15 ■ Assessing the Musculoskeletal System (continued)

5. **Test accuracy of movements.** Have the client touch finger to nose with eyes open. Repeat with eyes closed.

   Expected findings: The movement is accurate with eyes open and closed.

   Abnormal findings: Inaccurate movements indicate cerebellar dysfunction.

6. **Measure the limbs.**
   a. Measure arm length from the acromion process to the tip of the middle finger.
   b. *Apparent leg length*—Measure from the umbilicus (a nonfixed point) to the medial malleolus.
   c. *True leg length*—Measure from the anterior superior iliac crest, crossing over the knee to the medial malleolus. ▼

   Expected findings: The differences in length between the right and left arm and leg are 1 cm or less.

   Abnormal findings: Leg length discrepancies may cause back and hip pain and gait problems. An *apparent leg length* discrepancy may result from a pelvic tilt or flexion deformity of the hip; a *true leg length* discrepancy results from unequal bone length.

   Apparent leg length　　　True leg length

   d. Measure the circumference of the forearms, upper arms, thighs, and calves.

   d. **Expected findings:** The differences in circumference between the right and left arm and leg are 1 cm or less.

   Abnormal findings: Circumference differences >1 cm may reflect atrophy or hypertrophy.

7. **Inspect muscles and joints bilaterally for symmetry and shape.**

   Developmental Modifications

   Older adults—Observe for surgical scars indicating joint replacement or joint surgeries. ▼

   Degenerative joint disease (Heberden's nodes)

   Expected findings: Size and shape are symmetrical. Muscles and joints are smooth, nontender, and similar in color and temperature to surrounding tissue.

   Developmental Variations

   Older adults—Muscle mass and tone decrease.

   Abnormal findings:
   - Hot, red, swollen, stiff, or painful joints may indicate injuries, arthritis, gout, bursitis, or other inflammatory diseases.
   - **Heberden's nodes** are hard, painless nodules over the distal interphalangeal joints—usually seen with degenerative joint disease (DJD), but they may be seen with rheumatoid arthritis (RA).
   - DJD most commonly affects weight-bearing joints (lower back, hips, knees, feet), causing deformity, pain, and stiffness. Crepitus may be heard in DJD.

Rheumatoid arthritis

- RA most often involves the small joints of the hands and feet but can involve other joints, including the jaw, causing misalignment and deformity. The joint involvement is usually *symmetrical*.

8. **Test active ROM by asking the client to move the following joints through ROM:**
   a. TMJ
   b. Neck
   c. Thoracic and lumbar spine
   d. Shoulder
   e. Upper arm and elbow
   f. Wrist
   g. Hands and fingers
   h. Hip
   i. Knee
   j. Ankles and feet

Expected findings:

TMJ—Able to flex, extend, move side to side, protrude, and retract the jaw

Neck—Flexes, extends, hyperextends, bends laterally, and rotates side to side

Spine—Able to bend at the waist, stand upright, hyperextend (bend backward), bend laterally, and rotate side to side

Shoulder—Able to move the arm forward and backward, abduct, adduct, and rotate internally and externally

Upper arm and elbow—Able to bend, extend, supinate, and pronate the elbow

Wrist—Flexes, extends, hyperextends, and moves side to side

Hands and fingers—Able to:
  Spread the fingers (abduct)
  Bring them together (adduct)
  Make a fist (flex)
  Extend the hand (extend)
  Bend fingers back (hyperextend)
  Bring thumb to index finger (palmar adduction)

Hip—Able to:
  Extend the leg straight
  Flex the knee to the chest
  Abduct and adduct the leg
  Rotate the hip internally and externally
  Hyperextend the leg

Knee—Able to flex and extend the knee

Ankles and feet—Able to dorsiflex, plantar flex, evert, invert, abduct, and adduct the feet and ankles

Key Point: *If a patient cannot move the limb, put the joint through passive ROM. Never force a joint against resistance or if it causes discomfort.*

(continued on next page)

Procedure 19-15 ■ Assessing the Musculoskeletal System (continued)

Joint Movements

Depression: lowering a body part
Elevation: raising a body part

Retraction: moving backward
Protraction: moving forward

Abduction: moving away from midline
Adduction: moving toward midline

Flexion: bending, decreasing joint angle

Extension: straightening, increasing joint angle

Circumduction: moving in a circular fashion

Opposition

Supination: turning upward

Pronation: turning downward

External rotation: turning away from midline

Internal rotation: turning toward midline

Inversion: turning inward

Eversion: turning outward

9. **Test muscle strength by repeating ROM against resistance.** Use the rating scale at the end of this step.
   a. **Test hand grip** by crossing your middle and index fingers and asking the patient to squeeze. *(Tip: If you are wearing rings, a strong hand grip on those fingers can be painful.)*
   b. **Test biceps strength.** Place one hand on the client's biceps and have the patient raise the forearm (flex the elbow) as you apply resistance at the wrist.
   c. **Test triceps strength** by having the client straighten the arm at the elbow (extend the elbow) as you apply resistance at the wrist.
   d. **Test leg strength** by having the patient raise a leg (straighten the knee) against your hand as you apply resistance.
   e. **Test ankle strength** by asking the patient to point the toes downward (plantar flexion) at the ankle while you apply resistance to the plantar surface of the foot.
   f. **Test ankle strength** by having the client point the toes toward the knee (dorsiflexion) as you apply resistance to the top of the foot.

Expected findings: Expect active motion against full resistance. There should be no crepitus (clicking) or pain with joint movement. ▼

Muscle Strength Rating Scale		
RATING	**CRITERIA**	**CLASSIFICATION**
5	Active motion against full resistance	Normal
4	Active motion against some resistance	Slight weakness
3	Active motion against gravity	Weakness
2	Passive range of motion	Poor range of motion
1	Slight flicker of contraction	Severe weakness
0	No muscular contraction	Paralysis

(continued on next page)

Procedure 19-15 ■ Assessing the Musculoskeletal System (continued)

? What if...

■ **There is limited range of motion in a joint?**

Use a goniometer to measure the limited motion in degrees. Place the goniometer over the joint, matching the angle of the joint. ➤

Using a goniometer

Documentation

If you need information about documenting your findings, ➤ Go to **Chapter 19, Caring for the Williams Family,** including **Documenting Physical Examination Findings (Stanley Williams),** in Volume 1.

Procedure 19-16 ■ Assessing the Sensory-Neurological System

➤ For steps to follow in *all* procedures, refer to the Universal Steps for All Procedures on the inside back cover.

➤ *Note:* This procedure provides guidelines for performing a comprehensive neurological examination. Steps 1–10 assess cognitive status, and the box at the end of the procedure contains questions that are useful for screening cognitive status.

Equipment

- Pen and record form
- Wisp of cotton
- Sharp object, such as a toothpick or sterile needle
- Objects to touch, such as a coin, button, or key
- Something fragrant, such as coffee or rubbing alcohol
- Something to taste, such as sugar, salt, or lemon
- Tongue blade
- Two test tubes
- Reflex hammer
- Ophthalmoscope

Developmental Modifications for Children

- For children younger than age 5 years, use the Denver Developmental Screening Test II to assess neurological and motor function.
- Check the child's ability to understand and follow instructions.

Developmental Modifications for Older Adults

You may need to perform the sensory-neurological examination over several sessions. The full examination is lengthy, and older adults fatigue easily. If the client seems to be getting tired, stop the test and finish at a later time.

Focused History Questions

- Do you have any neurological ("nerve") concerns?
- Have you ever had head trauma, loss of consciousness, dizziness, headaches, or seizures?
- Do you have memory problems, forgetfulness, or inability to concentrate?
- Have you noticed any changes in your ability to see, smell, taste, hear, feel, or maintain balance?
- Do you have any weakness, numbness, or paralysis?
- Do you have a history of Bell's palsy?
- Do you have any problems performing activities of daily living (ADLs)?
- Do you have any problems walking?
- Do you have mood problems or depression?
- Do you use alcohol or drugs for nonmedical purposes? If so, how much and how often?
- Have you ever been treated for neurological or psychiatric issues?
- Do you have a history of hypertension, diabetes, stroke, or circulation problems?

➤ When performing the procedure, always identify your patient according to agency policy, using two identifiers, and be attentive to standard precautions, hand hygiene, patient safety and privacy, body mechanics, and documentation.

Procedure Steps

1. **Assess behavior.** Note the client's facial expression, posture, affect, and grooming.

2. **Determine level of arousal (LOA):**
   a. Note the client's response to **verbal stimuli**.
   b. If the client does not respond to verbal stimuli, try **tactile stimulation:** Gently shake the client's shoulder. **Key Point:** *Clients who have hearing deficits lip-read to compensate. Catch the client's attention by combined auditory and visual stimuli (e.g., touch their hand).*
   c. If the client does not respond to tactile stimuli, try **painful stimuli:** Squeeze the trapezius muscle, rub the sternum, apply pressure on the mandible at the angle of the jaw, or apply pressure over the "moon" of the nail.

   NOTE: Clients who respond to painful stimuli withdraw when pressure is applied.

   The Glasgow Coma Scale and the FOUR Scale at the end of this procedure provide standard references for assessing LOA for a patient with head injury.

3. **Determine the level of orientation.**

   a. *Orientation to time:* Ask the client to state the year, date, and time of day.

   b. *Orientation to place:* Ask the client to state where they are (i.e., city, state, where they live).

   c. *Orientation to person:* Ask the names of family members. Ask, "Do you know who I am?" If the client cannot answer these questions, ask them to state their name. *Self-identity remains intact the longest.*

Findings

Expected findings: The client is dressed appropriately for the climate, with an erect posture, pleasant facial expression, and appropriate affect.

Abnormal findings: Inappropriate behavior may result from neurological or psychological problems as well as from a variety of medications, alcohol, and substance use.

Expected findings: The patient is awake and alert and readily responds to verbal stimuli.

Abnormal findings: Lethargy, stupor, or coma may result from trauma, neurological disorder, hypoxia, or chemical substances.

✚ A changing level of arousal (along with forgetfulness, restlessness, or sudden quietness) is one of the earliest indicators of increased intracranial pressure, which can be life threatening.

Expected findings: The client is awake, alert (see Step 2), and oriented to time, place, and person (AAO × 3).

a. **Expected findings:** Hospitalized patients commonly lose track of date and time of day, but they easily reorient. As a rule, they should at least know the year.

Abnormal findings: Older adults who become disoriented to time usually think it is an earlier date. If a client offers an extremely incorrect time or futuristic date, consider psychiatric concerns as the cause of disorientation.

b. **Expected findings:** Interpret data carefully. In some situations (e.g., after an automobile accident away from home), the patient may know they are in the hospital but not know which hospital or which city.

c. **Expected findings:** Patient should know you are a healthcare worker, but not necessarily your name.

🍁 *Developmental Variations*

Older adults—The stress of an unfamiliar situation can create confusion in an older adult.

Abnormal findings: Disorientation may result from physical or psychological disorders. Bizarre responses are usually associated with psychiatric disorders.

(continued on next page)

Procedure 19-16 ■ Assessing the Sensory-Neurological System (continued)

4. **Assess memory.**
   a. *Assess immediate memory* by asking the client to repeat a series of three numbers that you speak slowly (e.g., 1, 5, 8). Gradually increase the length of the series until the client cannot repeat the series correctly. Record the length of the last correct series (e.g., "Successfully repeats a series of 7 numbers correctly").
   b. *Repeat the test,* beginning with a series of three numbers, but ask the client to repeat them back to you in reverse order.
   c. *Assess recent memory* by naming three items (e.g., "mirror, truck, and the letter X") and asking the client to recall them later during the examination. Alternatively, you can ask questions such as these: "How did you get to the hospital? What did you have for breakfast?" However, you will need to verify the patient's answers.
   d. *Assess remote memory* by asking the client their birth date or the date of a major historical event.

   Developmental Modifications
   Children—Assess memory by using names of toys (e.g., truck, ball, puzzle), names of family members, or names of familiar cartoon characters.

   Expected findings: Immediate, recent, and remote memory are intact. Average series recall is 5–8 numbers in sequence and 4–6 numbers in reverse order.

   Developmental Variations
   Children—Number of objects recalled is usually fewer than the child's age in years.

   Older adults—Loss of immediate and recent memory is common; long-term memory is usually not impaired.

   Abnormal findings: Memory problems may be benign or may signal underlying neurological problems. Temporary memory loss may occur after trauma.

5. **Assess mathematical and calculation skills.**
   a. Have the client solve a simple mathematical problem, such as 3 + 3.
   b. If the client is able to solve that problem, present a more complex example, yet simple enough that regardless of math skills the client could still determine the appropriate response, such as "If you have $3 and you buy an item for $2, how much money will you have left?"
   c. To assess both calculation skills and attention span, ask the client to count backward from 100.
   d. A more difficult test is to have the client perform serial 3s or serial 7s. Ask them to begin at 100 and keep subtracting 3 (or 7).
   Consider the person's language, education, and culture in deciding whether this test is appropriate.

   Expected findings: Mathematical and calculation ability is appropriate for the patient's age, education level, and language ability. The average adult can solve simple mathematical problems and can complete serial 7s in about 90 seconds with 3 or fewer errors.

   Abnormal findings: Inability to calculate at a level appropriate for age and educational level may indicate neurological impairment or developmental delay.

6. **Assess general knowledge.**
   You can ask questions directly or work this into the overall interaction with the client.

   NOTE: Ask the client how many days in the week or months in the year.

   Expected findings: Vocabulary and general knowledge are intact.

7. **Evaluate thought processes.** Assess throughout the examination. Notice attention span, logic of speech, ability to stay focused, and appropriateness of responses.

   Expected findings: Thought processes are clear, client responds appropriately, and speech is coherent and logical.

   Abnormal findings: Alteration in thought processes may be due to physical disorders, such as dementia; psychiatric disorders, such as psychosis; or alcohol and drugs.

8. **Assess abstract thinking.** Ask the client to interpret a maxim (or saying), such as "A penny saved is a penny earned" or "A rolling stone gathers no moss."

Developmental Modifications

Children—The ability to think abstractly does not develop until the late school-age years or adolescence. To assess a child under the age of 12, ask the child to describe things that are like and unlike a named object (e.g., "Tell me something that is like a cup").

Expected findings: Abstract thinking is intact.

Abnormal findings: Inability to think abstractly is associated with dementia, delirium, intellectual disability, and psychoses.

9. **Assess judgment.**
   Ask the client to respond to a hypothetical situation, such as "If you were walking down the street and saw smoke and flames coming from a house, what would you do?"

Expected findings: Judgment is intact.

Abnormal findings: Impaired judgment may be associated with dementia, psychosis, or substance abuse.

10. **Assess communication ability.**
    a. **Listen to the client's speech.** Note the rate, flow, choice of vocabulary, and enunciation.

    a. **Expected findings:** Speech flows easily, and patient enunciates clearly. Vocabulary is consistent with the client's age, education, and language fluency.

    Abnormal findings: Problems with flow (e.g., halting speech, stuttering, very rapid speech, slurred words) may be due to language problems, nervousness, anxiety, or neurological problems.

    b. **Test spontaneous speech:** Show the client a picture, and have the client describe it.

    b. **Expected findings:** Spontaneous speech is intact.

    Abnormal findings: Impaired spontaneous speech is associated with cognitive impairment.

    c. **Test motor speech** by having the client say "Do, re, mi, fa, so, la, ti, do." Assess ability to swallow. Observe for clarity of speech, facial mobility, drooling, and oral hypotonia. Ask the client to repeat a short phrase 2 or 3 times and observe for lack of coordination.

    c. **Expected findings:** Motor speech is intact.

    Abnormal findings: Impaired motor speech is associated with problems with CN XII or with coordination of speech muscles.

    d. **Test automatic speech** by having the client recite the days of the week.

    d. **Expected findings:** Automatic speech is intact.

    Abnormal findings: Cognitive impairment or memory problems cause difficulty with automatic speech.

    e. **Test sound recognition** by having the client identify a familiar sound, such as clapping hands.

    e. **Expected findings:** Sound recognition is intact.

    Abnormal findings: Temporal lobe problems may be the cause of impaired sound recognition.

    f. **Test auditory–verbal comprehension** by asking the client to follow simple directions (e.g., "Point to your nose; rub your left elbow").

    f. **Expected findings:** Auditory–verbal comprehension is intact.

    Abnormal findings: Temporal lobe problems affect reception. Frontal lobe problems affect expression.

    g. **Test visual recognition** by pointing to objects and asking the client to identify them.

    g. **Expected findings:** Visual recognition is intact.

    Abnormal findings: Impaired visual recognition indicates parieto–occipital lobe problems.

    h. **Test visual–verbal comprehension** by having the client read a sentence and explain its meaning.

    h. **Expected findings:** Visual–verbal comprehension is intact.

    Abnormal findings: Impaired visual–verbal comprehension indicates cognitive impairment.

(continued on next page)

Procedure 19-16 ■ Assessing the Sensory-Neurological System (continued)

    i. **Test writing** by having the client write their name and address.

    j. **Test ability to copy figures** by having the client copy a circle, the letter X, a square, a triangle, and a star.

    i. **Expected findings:** Writing ability is intact.

    j. **Expected findings:** The client is able to copy figures.

11. **Test cranial nerve I—olfactory nerve.**

    NOTE: You can assess CN I with your examination of the nose and sinuses (see Procedure 19-8).
    a. Before testing, check the patency of the nostrils by gently occluding each nostril and having the client sniff.
    b. Have the client occlude one nostril and hold an aromatic substance (e.g., lemon, coffee, vanilla, alcohol) under the nostril.
    c. Repeat with a different substance under the other nostril. ▼

    Expected findings: The client can identify the substances.

    Developmental Variations
    Older adults—May have a decreased sense of smell.

    Abnormal findings: Anosmia is the loss of the sense of smell. It may be genetic, related to chronic nose or sinus problems, a virus (e.g., COVID), heavy tobacco use, snorting cocaine, or zinc deficiency.

Developmental Modifications
Children—Select a substance that you are certain the child is familiar with (e.g., bananas or apples).

12. **Test cranial nerve II—optic nerve.**

    NOTE: You can assess CN II with your examination of the eyes (see Procedure 19-6).
    a. Test visual acuity by asking the client to identify the smallest print readable on the Snellen chart.

    Developmental Modifications
    Use picture chart for small children, Snellen E for school-age children.

    b. Identify visual field by having the client describe the boundaries of the visual field while their eye is in a fixed position.
    c. Perform a fundoscopic examination. (See Procedure 19-6.)

    a. **Expected findings:** Visual acuity is 20/20 in the right eye, left eye, and both eyes.

    Abnormal findings: Many visual deficits are correctable with eyeglasses or contact lenses. They are not necessarily caused by optic nerve damage.

    b. **Expected findings:** Peripheral vision range is approximately 50° in the superior field, 70° in the inferior field, 60° in the nasal field, and 90°–110° in the temporal field.

    c. **Expected findings:** Disc margins are sharply demarcated. The cup is half the size of the disc or smaller.

    Abnormal findings: CN II deficits may be due to tumor or CVA.

CHAPTER 19 Health Assessment 277

13. **Test cranial nerves III, IV, and VI—oculomotor, trochlear, and abducens nerves.**
    a. Test EOMs by having the client move the eyes through the six cardinal fields of gaze while holding the head steady. ▼

    b. Test pupillary reaction to light and accommodation.

    NOTE: See Procedure 19-6 for further details on each of these tests.

Expected findings: Client can move their eyes through the six cardinal fields of gaze. Pupils are equal in size and react to light and accommodation.

Abnormal findings: Changes in intracranial pressure (ICP) may affect EOMs and pupillary reaction.

14. **Test cranial nerve V—trigeminal nerve.**
    a. **Test motor function** by having the client move their jaw from side to side, clenching the jaw, and biting down on a tongue blade.

    NOTE: You can assess this function in your examination of the mouth and oropharynx (see Procedure 19-9).

    b. **Test sensory function** by having the client close their eyes and identify when you are touching their face at the forehead, cheeks, and chin bilaterally—first with your finger and then repeat with a toothpick.
    c. **Test the corneal reflex** by touching the cornea with a wisp of cotton or puffing air from a syringe over the cornea.

    ✚ The corneal reflex is not usually tested on a conscious person because the procedure is unpleasant and a corneal abrasion can occur. A conscious person can blink intentionally, so there is no need to stimulate the blink.

    NOTE: You can assess the corneal reflex in your examination of the eyes (see Procedure 19-6).

Expected findings: The client is able to perform all motor functions and can perceive light touch and superficial pain bilaterally; corneal reflex is intact.

Abnormal findings: Inability to perceive light touch and superficial pain may indicate peripheral nerve damage. An absent corneal reflex is an ominous neurological sign.

15. **Test cranial nerve VII—facial nerve.**
    a. Test motor function by having the client make faces, such as smile, frown, or whistle.

    Note: You can assess this function in your examination of the head and face (see Procedure 19-5).

    b. Test taste on the anterior portion of the tongue by placing sweet (sugar), salty (salt), or sour (lemon) substance on the tip of the tongue. Do not test taste by using pungent, bitter, or markedly unpleasant flavors.

    Note: You can assess this function in your examination of the mouth and oropharynx (see Procedure 19-9).

Expected findings: The client is able to perform all movements and can distinguish sweet, salty, and sour tastes.

🍁 *Developmental Variations*
Older adults—Have decreased taste sensation, especially sweet and salty, due to taste bud atrophy and diminished sense of smell.

Abnormal findings: Asymmetrical movement may be seen with nerve damage from a CVA or Bell's palsy. Impaired taste may be associated with a virus (e.g., COVID), nerve damage, chemotherapy, or radiation to the face or neck.

(continued on next page)

Procedure 19-16 ■ Assessing the Sensory-Neurological System (continued)

16. Test cranial nerve VIII—acoustic nerve.

NOTE: You can assess this function in your examination of the ears (see Procedure 19-7).

a. Perform watch-tick test for hearing by holding a watch close to the client's ear.
b. Perform Weber and Rinne tests to assess air and bone conduction.
c. Test balance with the Romberg test, if it has not already been performed.

See Procedures 19-7 and 19-15 for further details on these tests.

Expected findings: Hearing is intact. Romberg test is negative.

Abnormal findings: Hearing loss, loss of balance, or vertigo may result from acoustic nerve damage.

Developmental Modifications

Children—Romberg test is appropriate only after age 3.

17. Test cranial nerves IX and X—glossopharyngeal and vagus nerves.

a. Observe ability to talk, swallow, and cough.
b. Test motor function by asking the client to say "ah" while you depress a tongue blade and observe the soft palate and uvula.
c. Test sensory function by taking a tongue blade and gently touching the back of the pharynx to induce a gag reflex.
d. Test taste (sweet, salty, and sour) on the posterior portion of the tongue. Avoid bitter or repulsive-tasting substances.

Expected findings: Swallow and cough reflex are intact. Speech is clear. The uvula and soft palate rise symmetrically, and the gag reflex is intact. Taste on the posterior tongue is intact.

Developmental Variations

Older adults—Have decreased taste sensation, especially sweet and salty, due to atrophy of the taste buds and a diminished sense of smell.

Abnormal findings: Damage to CN IX and X impairs swallowing. Damage to CN X changes voice quality.

Loss of taste may be caused by current or previous COVID infection.

18. Test cranial nerve XI—accessory nerve.

NOTE: You can assess this motor nerve function with your examination of the musculoskeletal system (see Procedure 19-15).

a. Place your hands on the client's shoulder, and have the client shrug shoulders against resistance.
b. Have the client turn head from side to side against resistance. ▼

Expected findings: Movement is symmetrical and pain-free. Full ROM of the neck with +5 strength.

Abnormal findings: Asymmetrical movement, pain, or absent movement indicates CN XI disorders.

19. Test cranial nerve XII—hypoglossal nerve.

a. Ask the client to say "d, l, n, t."
b. Have the client protrude the tongue and move it from side to side.

Expected findings: The client can articulate the sounds and move the tongue easily.

Abnormal findings: Tongue paralysis

20. **Test superficial sensations.**
    - Begin with the most peripheral part when testing the limbs (e.g., test the foot before the leg). ▶
      If the client can feel sensation in the most peripheral part, you can assume the sensory nerve is intact to that point.
    - If the client does not perceive the touch in an area, determine the boundaries of the dysfunction by testing at about every inch (2.5 cm). Sketch the area of sensory loss.
    - Wait about 2 seconds before moving to each site.
      Wait so that you can be sure that the patient is perceiving each stimulus separately.

    a. *Light touch:* With the patient's eyes closed, brush a cotton wisp on various areas of the body, comparing sides. Ask the client to say "Now" when they feel your touch and to point to the spot you are touching.

    b. *Pain:* With the patient's eyes closed, use a toothpick (or sterile needle) with dull and sharp ends. Touch various areas of the body (except the face), and have the patient identify whether the sensation is dull or sharp. Alternate the dull and sharp ends as you move from spot to spot. Compare sides of the body.

    c. *Temperature sensation:* Test only if the patient's perception of pain is abnormal. Use test tubes filled with hot and cold water. Touch the tube to various areas of the body, comparing sides; have the client say "Hot," "Cold," or "Don't know."
      If pain sensation is intact, temperature will be, too, because sensations for pain and temperature are transmitted along the same tracts.

Testing light touch

a. **Expected findings:** Able to identify areas of light touch.
   Abnormal findings: Diminished sensation or areas of absent perception

b. **Expected findings:** The client is able to identify the areas stimulated and the type of sensation.
   Abnormal findings:
   - **Hyperalgia:** increased pain sensation
   - **Analgesia:** no pain sensation
   - **Paresthesia:** numbness and tingling

   Developmental Variations
   Older adults—May have a decreased perception of temperature and deep pain.

21. **Test deep sensations.**
    Assess vibratory sensation by placing a vibrating tuning fork on a metatarsal joint and distal interphalangeal joint. Have the patient identify when the vibration is felt and when it stops. ▼

Expected findings: Vibratory sense is intact bilaterally in the upper and lower extremities.

Abnormal findings: Diminished or absent vibration sense is seen with peripheral nerve damage from vascular disease, diabetes, alcoholism, or damage to the posterior column of the spinal cord.

(continued on next page)

Procedure 19-16 ■ Assessing the Sensory-Neurological System (continued)

22. **Test kinesthetic sensation (position sense).**
    Hold the client's finger or toe on the sides and move it up or down. With the client's eyes closed, have them identify the direction of the movement. ▼

    Expected findings: Position sense is intact bilaterally in the upper and lower extremities.

    🍁 *Developmental Variations*
    Older adults—May lose position sense in the great toes.

    Abnormal findings: Diminished or absent position sense indicates nerve or spinal cord damage.

23. **Test discriminatory sensations.**
    a. *Assess stereognosis* by placing a familiar object (e.g., a coin or a button) in the palm of the client's hand and having them identify it.

    b. *Assess graphesthesia* by drawing a number or letter in the palm of your patient's hand and having the patient identify what was drawn.

    c. *Test two-point discrimination* with toothpicks. Have the patient close their eyes. Touch the client on the finger with two toothpicks simultaneously. Gradually move the points together, and have the client say "One" or "Two" each time you move the toothpicks. Document distance and location at which the client can no longer feel two separate points. ▶

    a. **Expected findings: Stereognosis** (the ability to recognize the form of solid objects by touch) is intact bilaterally.

    b. **Expected findings: Graphesthesia** (the ability to recognize outlines, numbers, or symbols written on the skin) is intact bilaterally.

    c. **Expected findings: Point discrimination** (recognizing whether 1 or 2 areas of the skin are being touched). Discriminates between two points on fingertips no more than 0.5 cm apart.

    d. *Test point localization* by having the client close their eyes while you touch them. Have the client point to the area you touched. Repeat on both sides and the upper and lower extremities.

    e. *Test sensory extinction* by simultaneously touching the client on both sides (e.g., on both hands, both knees, both arms). Have the client identify where they were touched. ▼

    d. **Expected findings: Point localization** (the ability to identify where one is being touched) is intact bilaterally in the upper and lower extremities.

    e. **Expected findings:** Extinction is intact: Client should feel the sensation on both sides of the body.

    Abnormal findings: Abnormalities in any of the discriminatory sensation tests may indicate a lesion or disorder of the sensory cortex or disorder of the posterior column of the spinal cord.

🍁 *Developmental Modifications*
Older adults—May need more time to respond to a stimulus, as reaction time may be slower.

CHAPTER 19 Health Assessment 281

24. **Test deep tendon reflexes.**
    Use the accompanying scale to grade responses.

Deep Tendon Reflex Grading Scale

0   No response detected
+1 Diminished response
+2 Response normal
+3 Response somewhat stronger than normal
+4 Response hyperactive with **clonus** (involuntary contractions that continue after the first contraction is elicited by the hammer)

Developmental Variations
Older adults—Reflex responses may not be as strong as in young adults. Reaction time is slower as well.

a. **Biceps reflex** (spinal cord level C5 and C6). Rest the patient's elbow in your nondominant hand, with your thumb over the biceps tendon. Strike the percussion hammer to your thumb. ▼

a. **Expected findings:** +2 response: You can feel the biceps contract with your thumb; slight flexion of the elbow.

b. **Triceps reflex** (spinal cord levels C7 and C8). Abduct the patient's arm at the shoulder, and flex it at the elbow. Support the upper arm with your nondominant hand, letting the forearm hang loosely. Strike the triceps tendon about 2.5–5 cm (1–2 in.) above the olecranon process. ▼

b. **Expected findings:** +2 response: Contraction of triceps with slight extension at elbow

(continued on next page)

Procedure 19-16 ■ Assessing the Sensory-Neurological System (continued)

c. *Brachioradialis reflex* (spinal cord levels C3 and C6). Rest the client's arm on her leg. Strike with the percussion hammer 2.5–5 cm (1–2 in.) above the bony prominence of the wrist on the thumb side. ▼

c. **Expected findings:** +2 response: Flexion at elbow and supination of forearm

d. *Patellar reflex* (spinal cord levels L2, L3, and L4). Have the client sit with legs dangling. Strike the tendon directly below the patella. ▼

d. **Expected findings:** +2 response: Contraction of quadriceps with extension of leg

e. *Achilles reflex* (spinal cord level S1, S2). Have the patient lie supine or sit with legs dangling. Hold the patient's foot slightly dorsiflexed, and strike the Achilles tendon about 5 cm (2 in.) above the heel with the percussion hammer. ▼

e. **Expected findings:** +2 response: Plantar flexion of foot

🍁 *Developmental Variations*
Older adults—May lose this reflex.

Abnormal findings:
- Absent or diminished responses are seen with degenerative disease, nerve damage, or lower motor neuron disease.
- Hyperactive reflexes are seen with spinal cord injuries and upper motor neuron disease.
- Rooting, palmar grasp, and tonic neck reflexes present after 6 months of age.

Developmental Modifications

Newborns—test the following reflexes:
- **Rooting reflex**—Stroke the cheek; the head should turn to the side you touched.
- **Palmar grasp**—Place one finger in the baby's hand; baby's fingers should curl around your finger.
- **Tonic neck reflex**—Position the baby supine; turn baby's head to one side. The arm and leg on that side should extend, and those on the other side will flex.

25. **Test superficial reflexes.**
    Plantar reflex (Babinski response): With your thumbnail or pointed object, stroke the sole of the client's foot in an arc from the lateral heel to medially across the ball of the foot. Record response as negative (normal) or positive (abnormal). ▼

    Expected findings: Babinski response is negative. All the toes curl downward or there is no response.

    Developmental Variations

    Infants and children—Positive Babinski is normal until age 2 or until the child begins walking.

    Abnormal findings: A positive Babinski response: dorsiflexion of the great toe and fanning of the other toes. Seen with drug or alcohol intoxication or upper motor neuron disease.

    Developmental Modifications
    Older adults—This reflex may be difficult to elicit.

26. **Mental status screening**
    The following questions may be used for a rapid evaluation of cognitive status. You may have already assessed for some aspects of mental status (e.g., orientation to time).

Questions for Evaluating Cognitive Status

This complete set of questions is included so you can use them for a mental status examination that is not part of a comprehensive assessment. In a comprehensive assessment, do not repeat questions you have already covered in other portions of the assessment.

QUESTION	FUNCTION ASSESSED
What is today's date?	Orientation to time
What time is it?	Orientation to time
Where are you?	Orientation to place
What is the reason for your visit? (If the patient is hospitalized, modify the question as Why are you in the hospital?)	Communication, vocabulary, thought processes, recent memory
Ask the patient to count backward from 100.	Word comprehension, abstract reasoning
Ask the patient to name several objects that you point to. Be sure to use common objects such as a pen, shoe, or window.	Vocabulary, general knowledge, and word comprehension
Write a brief command, such as "Clap your hands," on a slip of paper. Hand the paper to the patient and ask them to follow the instructions.	Reading comprehension
Ask the patient to write the names of family members, along with their relationship.	Writing, thought processes, memory, sound recognition
Ask the patient to name three things that begin with the letter D.	Auditory comprehension, thought processes
Ask the patient to draw a circle, square, and triangle next to each other on a sheet of paper.	Word comprehension, mathematical and calculation skills, communication (naming)
Difficulty with any of these questions requires further evaluation.	

(continued on next page)

Procedure 19-16 ■ Assessing the Sensory-Neurological System (continued)

? What if...

■ The patient is an older adult?

For a mental status examination for older adults, you may wish to use the following sites:

The Mini-Cog (mental status assessment of older adults)

https://mini-cog.com

Mini-Mental State Examination

https://www.ihpa.gov.au/what-we-do/standardised-mini-mental-state-examination-smmse

You should also assess older adults for dementia, which is characterized by these four features:
- Mental status change of sudden onset or fluctuating course
- Difficulty focusing attention, distractible
- Disorganized, illogical thinking
- Increased or decreased level of consciousness (e.g., hyper-alert, lethargic)

Delirium occurs in 15% to 60% of older hospitalized patients. You should assess them frequently to facilitate prompt identification and management of delirium.

For a reliable tool for assessing confusion and dementia in older adults, go to the following Web site or search in your browser for the Confusion Assessment Method Instrument:

https://www.va.gov/covidtraining/docs/The_Confusion_Assessment_Method.pdf

Home Care

Instruct caregivers on home safety if the client has cerebral function deficits or sensory or motor deficits.

Documentation

If you need more information about documenting your findings,

> Go to **Chapter 19, Caring for the Williams Family,** including **Documenting Physical Examination Findings (Stanley Williams),** in Volume 1.

Glasgow Coma Scale

EYE RESPONSE	SCORE	MOTOR RESPONSE	SCORE	VERBAL RESPONSE	SCORE
Opens spontaneously	4	Obeys verbal commands for movement	6	Oriented and converses	5
Opens to verbal commands	3	Reacts purposefully to localized pain	5	Disoriented but converses	4
Opens to pain	2	Withdraws in response to pain (generalized body response)	4	Uses inappropriate words	3
No response	1	Assumes flexor posture (decorticate posturing—arms flexed to chest, hands clenched and internally rotated) in response to pain. Indicates problem is at or above the brainstem	3	Makes incomprehensible sounds	2
		Assumes extensor posture (decerebrate posturing—arms extended, hands clenched and hyperpronated); indicates problem at the brainstem level	2	No response	1
		No response	1		
Totals					

Full Outline of UnResponsiveness (FOUR)

Eye Response
4—Eyelids open, tracing, or blinking on command
3—Eyelids open but not tracking
2—Eyelids closed but open to loud voice
1—Eyelids closed but open to pain
0—Eyelids remain closed with pain

Motor Response
4—Thumbs-up, fist, or peace sign
3—Localizing to pain
2—Flexion response to pain
1—Extension response to pain
0—No response to pain or generalized myoclonus status

Brainstem Reflexes
4—Pupil and corneal reflexes present
3—One pupil wide and fixed
2—Pupil or corneal reflexes absent
1—Pupil and corneal reflexes absent
0—Absent pupil, corneal, and cough reflexes

Respirations
4—Not intubated, regular breathing pattern
3—Not intubated, Cheyne-Stokes breathing pattern
2—Not intubated, irregular breathing
1—Respirations greater than ventilator rate
0—Respirations at ventilator rate or apnea

Note: **Education is necessary to use this scale properly.**
To see how to use it,

Go to https://www.myamericannurse.com/using-the-four-score-scale-to-assess-comatose-patients/. Further validation of the FOUR Score Coma Scale is found at https://www.ncbi.nlm.nih.gov/pmc/articles/PMC2719522/

Sources

Hanrahan, K., et al. (2015). Sacred cow gone to pasture: A systematic evaluation and integration of evidence-based practice. *Worldviews on Evidence-Based Nursing, 12*(1), 3–11.

Okasha, A.S. et al. (2014). The FOUR Score predicts mortality, endotracheal intubation and ICU length of stay after traumatic brain injury. *Neurocritical Care, 21*(3), 496–504.

Wijdicks, E.J.S. et al. (2015). Comparison of the Full Outline of UnResponsiveness score and the Glasgow Coma Scale in predicting mortality in critically ill patients. *Critical Care Medicine, 43*(2), 439–444.

Procedure 19-17 ■ Assessing the Male Genitourinary System

▶ For steps to follow in *all* procedures, refer to the Universal Steps for All Procedures on the inside back cover.

Equipment
- Nonlatex procedure gloves
- Penlight
- Pen and record form

Developmental Modifications for Children
- Obtain the parental permission to perform this assessment.
- Explain to the child what you are going to do, and expect some resistance or embarrassment.

Children are taught to not let strangers touch their genitals, and many children are modest.

Developmental Modifications for Older Adults
- Assess for incontinence.

Incontinence is one of the elements of the SPICES assessment model for older adults.

Focused History Questions
- What is your sex?
- What sex were you assigned at birth?
- What is your gender?
- Do you consider yourself transgender?
- Have you had any gender-confirming surgeries or treatments?
- Have you noticed any redness, swelling, discharge, or odor in your genital area?
- Have you noticed asymmetry, lumps, or masses in your genitals? If so, describe them, and show me where they are.
- Have you ever been told you have a hernia?
- Have you ever had trauma to your genitals?
- Are you having any problems urinating?
- Are you sexually active? If not, have you ever been?
- Do you have sex with men, women, or both?
- What types of sexual activity do you engage in? Oral, anal, genital?
- Do you have more than one partner? How many partners have you had in the past 6 months?

(continued on next page)

Procedure 19-17 ■ Assessing the Male Genitourinary System (continued)

- Do you use birth control? If so, what type and how often?
- Have you ever been treated for a sexually transmitted infection (STI)? If so, what type?
- Are you concerned about STIs or HIV?
- Do you take any precautions to avoid infections?
- Do you have any concerns about your sexual function?
- Do you have any difficulty achieving or maintaining an erection?
- Have you been taught to examine your testicles?
  In spite of the low prevalence of testicular cancer, clients should be aware that a lump in the testicle and/or a feeling of heaviness or swelling in the scrotum could be a sign of testicular cancer and should report these findings to their healthcare provider immediately (American Cancer Society, n.d.).
- How often do you do testicular self-examination?
- Have you had any surgery of your reproductive tract?

> When performing the procedure, always identify your patient according to agency policy, using two identifiers, and be attentive to standard precautions, hand hygiene, patient safety and privacy, body mechanics, and documentation.

Procedure Steps

1. **Instruct the client to empty the bladder and undress** to expose the groin area.

2. **Have the patient stand while you sit at eye level to the genitalia;** alternatively, the patient can lie supine on the examination table with legs slightly apart.

3. **Inspect the external genitalia.**

   a. *Hair.* Note the hair distribution pattern and condition of pubic hair. See the table discussing Tanner staging, at the end of this procedure.
   The appearance of the external genitalia depends on the client's developmental stage.

   b. *Skin:* Inspect the condition of the skin of the penis. Observe for the presence or absence of the foreskin. Note the position of the urethral meatus and any lesions or discharge.

   c. *Scrotum:* Observe the condition, size, position, and symmetry of the scrotal sacs.

Findings

Expected findings: Hair distribution is triangular and appropriate for age. No pediculosis is present.

Abnormal findings: Sparse or absent hair may result from genetic factors, aging, or local or systemic disease.

Expected findings: Skin is intact with no lesions or discharge. Color is consistent with ethnicity. The urethral meatus is midline. The foreskin may be absent (circumcised); if present, it covers the glans and easily retracts.

Developmental Variations

Infants—Foreskin is difficult to retract in the uncircumcised male until about age 3 months.

Older adults—Penis and testes decrease in size.

Abnormal findings: Ulcerations or lesions (may be seen with STIs, such as genital warts and genital herpes); **phimosis** (foreskin cannot be retracted and becomes swollen).

Expected findings: The skin should be free of lesions, nodules, swelling, rash, and erythema. The skin is rugated and deeper in color than the rest of the body. Size and shape vary greatly. The left scrotal sac is usually lower than the right.

Abnormal findings:
- A rash may be caused by **tinea cruris,** a fungal infection often called "jock itch."
- Swelling may indicate hernia, tumor, or infection.

d. **Inguinal area:** Note the condition of the inguinal areas. Look for swelling or bulges. The best way to do this is to have the client bear down while you palpate the inguinal canal.

Expected findings: The inguinal area should be free of swelling or bulges.

Abnormal findings: A bulge may indicate a hernia or enlarged lymph node.

Abnormalities: Male Genitourinary System

Syphilitic chancre

Genital warts

4. **Palpate the penis.**
   a. With a gloved hand, use your thumb and fingers to palpate the shaft of the penis. Note consistency, tenderness, masses, or nodules.
   b. Retract the foreskin if present.

Expected findings: The penis is nontender with no masses or nodules. Pulsations are present on the dorsal side. The foreskin, if present, easily retracts.

Abnormal findings:
- Inability to palpate a pulse may indicate vascular insufficiency.
- Difficulty retracting the foreskin or problems with its return to position need further evaluation.

5. **Palpate the scrotum, testes, and epididymis.**
   a. Don a procedure glove and use your thumb and fingers to palpate. ▼

   b. Note size, shape, consistency, mobility, masses, nodules, or tenderness.
   c. Transilluminate any lumps, nodules, or edematous areas by shining a penlight over the area in a darkened room. ▼

Expected findings:
- The scrotal skin is rough but without lesions.
- Each testicular sac contains a testicle and epididymis.
- The testes are rubbery, round, movable, and smooth. They are sensitive to pressure but nontender.
- The epididymis is comma shaped.
- The spermatic cord is smooth and round.
- There is no swelling or nodules.
- The left scrotal sac is usually lower than the right.

Abnormal findings:
- A unilateral mass.
- Painless intratesticular masses may indicate testicular cancer.
- A testicle that is swollen or tender may indicate infection or torsion.

(continued on next page)

Procedure 19-17 ■ Assessing the Male Genitourinary System (continued)

6. **Palpate the inguinal and femoral area for hernias.** ▼

   a. Assess for inguinal hernias with a gloved hand. Have the patient hold penis to one side. Place your index finger in the client's scrotal sac above the testicle, and invaginate the skin. Follow the spermatic cord until you reach a slitlike opening (Hesselbach triangle). Ask the client to cough or bear down as you feel for bulges.
   b. Palpate for femoral hernias by palpating below the femoral artery while having the client cough or bear down.

   Expected findings: No bulges or palpable masses are present in the inguinal or femoral area.

   Abnormal findings: A bulge or mass often represents a hernia.

   Direct hernia: protrusion through the abdominal wall.

   Indirect hernia: protrusion into the inguinal canal or into the scrotum. ▼

   Inguinal ligament
   Indirect inguinal hernia
   Direct inguinal hernia
   Femoral hernia

   Locations of direct and indirect hernias

7. **Palpate the lymph nodes** in the groin area and the vertical chain over the inner aspect of the thigh. ▼

   Expected findings: Nodes should be <1 cm in size and freely mobile.

   Abnormal findings: Enlarged or tender lymph nodes may indicate local or systemic disease.

Documentation

If you need more information about documenting your findings,

➤ Go to **Chapter 19, Caring for the Williams Family,** including **Documenting Physical Examination Findings (Stanley Williams),** in Volume 1.

Tanner Staging

STAGE	PUBIC HAIR	PENIS	TESTES AND SCROTUM
Stage 1: Preadolescent	No pubic hair except for fine body hair similar to that on abdomen	Same size and proportions as in childhood	Same size and proportions as in childhood
Stage 2	Sparse growth of long, slightly pigmented, downy hair, straight or only slightly curled, chiefly at base of penis	Slight or no enlargement	Testes larger, scrotum larger, somewhat reddened and altered in texture
Stage 3	Darker, coarser, curlier hair spreading sparsely over pubic symphysis	Larger, especially in length	Further enlarged
Stage 4	Coarse and curly hair, as in adult; area covered greater than in stage 3 but not as great as in adult	Further enlarged in length and breadth, with development of glans	Further enlarged; scrotal skin darkened
Stage 5 Adult	Hair same as adult in quantity and quality, spreading to medial surfaces of thighs but not up over abdomen	Adult in size and shape	Adult in size and shape

Adapted from Tanner, J. (1962). *Growth at adolescence* (2nd ed.). Oxford: Blackwell Scientific.

Procedure 19-18 ■ Assessing the Female Genitourinary System

> For steps to follow in *all* procedures, refer to the Universal Steps for All Procedures on the inside back cover.

Equipment
- Patient drape
- Additional light source
- Nonlatex procedure gloves (if exposure to body fluids is a possibility)
- Pen and record form

Positioning
Lithotomy position, if possible.

Developmental Modifications for Older Adults
- Assess for incontinence.
  Incontinence is one of the elements of the SPICES assessment model for older adults.
- Older clients may have arthritis, which, along with muscle weakness, may make it difficult for them to assume the lithotomy position. You may need to use Sims' position and/or provide support for them to maintain a position.

Developmental Modifications for Children
- Obtain parental permission for this examination.
- Explain to the child what you are going to do, and expect some resistance or embarrassment.
  Children are taught to not let strangers touch their genitals, and many children are modest.

Key Point: *Do not perform internal assessment of an adolescent unless the client is sexually active.*

Focused History Questions
- What is your sex?
- What sex were you assigned at birth?
- What is your gender?
- Do you consider yourself transgender?
- Have you had any gender-confirming surgeries or treatments?
- Are you having any problems urinating?
- Have you noticed any redness, swelling, discharge, or odor in your genital area?
- Have you ever been told you have a hernia?
- Have you ever had trauma to your genitals?
- Are you sexually active? If not, have you ever been?
- Do you have sex with men, women, or both?
- What types of sexual activity do you engage in? Oral, anal, or genital?
- How many partners do you currently have?
- How many partners have you had in the past 6 months?
- Do you use birth control? If so, what kind and how often?
- Have you ever been treated for a sexually transmitted infection (STI)? If so, what type?
- Are you concerned about STIs or HIV?
- Do you take any precautions to avoid infection?
- Do you have any concerns about your sexual function?
- Have you had any surgery of your reproductive tract?
- When was your last menstrual period?
- How often are your periods?
- Do you have any concerns with your periods, such as cramping, breast pain, or heavy flow?
- How often do you have a gynecological health examination?
- When was your last Pap smear?
- Have you ever had an abnormal Pap smear? If so, how was it treated?
- How many times have you been pregnant?
- How many children do you have?
- Have you ever had a miscarriage? An abortion?

> When performing the procedure, always identify your patient according to agency policy, using two identifiers, and be attentive to standard precautions, hand hygiene, patient safety and privacy, body mechanics, and documentation.

Procedure Steps

1. **Instruct the client to undress as needed to expose the pelvic area; position** in lithotomy or Sims' position, providing support as needed.

2. **Inspect the external genitalia.**
   a. Note the hair distribution pattern and the condition of pubic hair. See the table Maturation Status in Females at the end of this procedure.
   The appearance of the external genitalia depends on the developmental stage of the client.

Findings

a. **Expected findings:** Hair distribution in the pubic region is inverse triangular. Some hair may extend onto the abdomen and upper thighs. Hair distribution is appropriate for age.

   Abnormal findings: Sparse or absent hair (may result from genetic factors, aging, or local or systemic disease)
   Pediculosis pubis (lice), **nits** (white lice eggs), or flecks of dried blood on the skin

b. Inspect the condition of the skin of the mons pubis and labia. Observe for color, condition, lesions, and discharge.

b. **Expected findings:** Skin is intact with no lesions or discharge. Labia majora and minora are symmetrical, with smooth to moderate wrinkling. Skin color is consistent with ethnicity. No ecchymosis, excoriation, nodules, edema, rash, or lesions are present.

> *Developmental Variations*
> Older adults—Labia and vulva are atrophied.

Abnormal findings: Ulcerations or lesions may occur with STIs.

3. **Inspect the clitoris, urethral meatus, and vaginal introitus.**
   a. Wearing gloves, use your thumb and index finger to separate the labia and expose the clitoris. Observe the clitoris for size and position. ▼

a. **Expected findings:** The clitoris is about 2 cm long and 0.5 cm in diameter. No redness or lesions are present.

Abnormal findings: Enlargement of the clitoris may result from androgen excess or swelling related to trauma. Absence of the clitoris, along with parts of the labia, is seen with female circumcision.

   b. With the labia separated, observe the urethral meatus and vaginal introitus. Observe for color, size, and presence of discharge or lesions.

   c. Have the client bear down while you observe the introitus.

b. **Expected findings:** The urethral meatus is slitlike, midline, and free of discharge, lesions, swelling, or erythema. The mucosa of the introitus is pink and moist. Some clear to white discharge may be present and is odor-free.

c. **Expected findings:** The introitus is patent, and there is no bulging or discomfort with bearing down.

Abnormal findings:
- Discharge, redness, or swelling may result from infection.
- Pale and dry mucosa may result from aging or use of topical steroids.
- Bulging may indicate prolapse of the uterus, bladder, or rectum.

4. **Palpate Bartholin's glands, the urethral glands, and Skene's ducts.**
   a. Lubricate the index and middle fingers of your dominant hand with water-soluble lubricant.
   b. To palpate Bartholin's glands, insert your lubricated fingers into the vaginal introitus, and palpate the lower portion of the labia bilaterally between your thumb and fingers. ▼

Expected findings:
- No swelling, masses, or tenderness of the glands is present.
- No urethral discharge.
- Labia are uniform in texture, no discharge or pain with palpation.
- Perineum is smooth and firm in **nulliparous** clients (clients who have had no children), thinner in **parous** clients (clients who have had children).

Abnormal findings:
- Pain or discharge from the glands may indicate infection.
- Fissures or tears in the perineum are painful and require treatment.

(continued on next page)

Procedure 19-18 ■ Assessing the Female Genitourinary System (continued)

c. To palpate Skene's ducts, rotate your internal fingers upward, and palpate the labium bilaterally.
d. To milk the urethra, apply pressure with your index finger on the anterior vaginal wall, and observe for urethral discharge. Culture any discharge you see. ▶

5. **Assess vaginal muscle tone and pelvic musculature.**
   a. Insert two gloved fingers into the vagina.
   b. Ask the client to constrict the vaginal muscles and then to bear down as though having a bowel movement.

   Expected findings: Muscle tone should be strong in clients who have never given birth. With increasing **parity** (number of births), pelvic muscle tone diminishes. Diminished tone may also result from injury, age, or medication. No bulges should be noted.

6. **Palpate the inguinal and femoral area for hernias.**

   Expected findings: No bulges or palpable masses are present in the inguinal or femoral area.

7. **Palpate the lymph nodes** in the groin area and the vertical chain over the inner aspect of the thigh.

   Expected findings: Nodes should be <1 cm in size and freely mobile.

   Abnormal findings: Enlarged or tender lymph nodes may indicate local or systemic disease.

Documentation

If you need more information about documenting your findings,

▶ Go to **Chapter 19, Caring for the Williams Family,** including **Documenting Physical Examination Findings (Stanley Williams),** in Volume 1.

Maturation Status in Females		
STAGE OF DEVELOPMENT	BREASTS	PUBIC HAIR
Stage 1. Prepuberty	Elevation of papilla	No pubic hair except for fine body hair similar to hair on abdomen

CHAPTER 19 Health Assessment 293

Maturation Status in Females—cont'd		
STAGE OF DEVELOPMENT	**BREASTS**	**PUBIC HAIR**
Stage 2	Breast bud. Elevation of breast and nipple and increased diameter of areola	Sparse growth of long, slightly pigmented, downy hair, straight or only slightly curled, mostly along labia
Stage 3	Areola deepens in color and enlarges further; glandular tissue begins to develop beneath areola	Hair becomes darker, coarser, and curlier and spreads sparsely over pubic symphysis
Stage 4	Areola appears as a mound; breast appears as a mound; papilla and areola form a secondary mound.	Pubic hair is coarse and curly as in adults; it covers more area than in stage 3 but does not extend to the medial thighs.
Stage 5. Adult	Mature breast; areola recesses to general contour of breast; nipple projects forward	Quality and quantity are consistent with adult pubic hair distribution and spread over medial surfaces of thighs but not over abdomen.

Adapted from Tanner, J. (1962). *Growth at adolescence* (2nd ed.). Oxford: Blackwell Scientific.

Procedure 19-19 ■ Assessing the Anus and Rectum

▸ For steps to follow in *all* procedures, refer to the Universal Steps for All Procedures on the inside back cover.

Equipment
- Water-soluble lubricant
- Hemoccult test
- Nonlatex procedure gloves
- Pen and record form

Developmental Modification for Infants and Children
You will not usually perform a rectal examination on infants and children.

Focused History Questions
- Do you have any pain or discomfort around your anus?
- Do you ever have difficulty passing stool?
- Have you ever noticed blood in your stool or when you wipe?
- Do you have or have you ever been told you have hemorrhoids?
- Do you have receptive anal sex?
- For male patients, have you ever had a prostate examination or a prostate-specific antigen (PSA) blood test? If so, what were the results?

▸ When performing the procedure, always identify your patient according to agency policy, using two identifiers, and be attentive to standard precautions, hand hygiene, patient safety and privacy, and body mechanics.

Procedure Steps

1. **Inspect the anus.** Note the condition of the skin and the presence of any lesions.

Findings

Expected findings: Anal area is intact, with no inflammation or lesions. Anus is a darker color than surrounding tissue.

Abnormal findings:
- A fissure or tear may be due to trauma, severe constipation, or an abscess.
- External hemorrhoids or skin tags may be visible.

2. **Palpate the anus and rectum.**
   a. *For female clients,* change gloves to prevent cross-contamination. Insert a lubricated index finger gently into the rectum. Palpate the rectal wall, noting masses or tenderness.
   b. *For male clients,* have the client bend over the examination table or turn on the left side to recumbent. Insert a lubricated index finger gently into the rectum. Palpate the rectal wall, noting masses or evidence of tenderness. ▼

Expected findings: Good sphincter tone. Rectum is nontender. No palpable masses or hard stool. The stool is brown and negative for occult blood.

Abnormal findings:
- Hard stool in the rectum indicates impaction.
- Positive occult blood indicates bleeding in the GI tract.
- A palpable mass or enlarged prostate gland requires further evaluation.
- Internal hemorrhoids may be present.

Prostate gland

   c. Test any stool on the gloved finger for occult blood. See Procedure 26-1.

Patient Teaching
Instruct the client on the importance of colonoscopy and prostate examination.

Documentation
If you need more information about documenting your findings,

> Go to **Chapter 19, Caring for the Williams Family,** including **Documenting Physical Examination Findings (Stanley Williams),** in Volume 1.

Procedure 19-20 ■ Brief Bedside Assessment

Note: This assessment is not as detailed as in Procedures 19-1 through 19-19. You might perform such an assessment when admitting a patient to a hospital unit. You can also use it for ongoing assessments. For daily patient assessments, you will modify the procedure to fit the patient's health status. You may be able to omit some portions, and you may need to add in-depth, focused assessments of some body systems. The entire assessment should take no more than 15 minutes after you become skilled.

➤ For steps to follow in *all* procedures, refer to the Universal Steps for All Procedures on the inside back cover.

Equipment
- Thermometer, stethoscope, sphygmomanometer
- Procedure gloves

Focused History Questions
- Ask about cultural norms that may require a modification in standard care.
- Ask about sexual identity and gender.
  - What was your sex assigned at birth?
  - What is your gender identity?
  - What pronouns do you prefer?
- Ask about any health problems, allergies, or medications.
- Ask your patient how they feel currently and during the previous month and year.
- Ask other questions as you assess each body system.

➤ When performing the procedure, always identify your patient according to agency policy, using two identifiers, and be attentive to standard precautions, hand hygiene, patient safety and privacy, body mechanics, and documentation.

Procedure Steps
1. **Greet the patient and explain what you need to do.** Ask the patient their name and confirm by checking the identity band.
   Ensures that you have the correct patient and also allows you to assess mental status and communication

2. **Observe the environment** (e.g., IV lines, oxygen, urinary catheter) and patient's general appearance (including signs of distress).
   This allows you to identify any immediate actions you may need to take before performing the assessment.

3. **Begin by measuring the vital signs (patient supine or sitting):**
   a. Temperature, pulse, respirations, blood pressure
   b. Pain status
   c. Pulse oximetry

4. **Now assess each body system.**
   a. Use a systematic approach such as head to toe.
   b. As you assess each system, observe for mobility, range of motion (ROM), balance, and coordination.
   c. As you talk with the patient, observe thought processes and level of consciousness.

5. **Assess the integument.**
   a. Ask about any hair, nail, or skin changes, including rashes.
   b. With each body system, inspect skin color, rashes, and lesions; palpate for temperature, turgor, and texture. Also inspect the hair and nails in that area (e.g., when assessing the legs and feet).
   c. Assess wounds: appearance, size, drainage, dressings, drains.
   d. Inspect and palpate the hair and scalp.

6. **Assess the head and neck.**
   a. Ask the patient about any problems with the head and neck.
   b. **Key Point:** Remember to continue assessing mental status and orientation to time, place, and person.
   c. Inspect the external ears; observe for apparent hearing deficit.
   d. Check the eyes for pupil reaction and cardinal fields of gaze. Ask about and observe for any problems with vision.
   e. Inspect the color of the lips, mucous membranes, and conjunctiva.
   f. Inspect the tongue and oropharynx.
   g. Inspect for hydration, color, and lesions of the mucous membranes.
   h. Lightly palpate the carotid pulse (only if indicated by patient's condition) and listen for carotid bruits.

   ✚ Do not palpate both carotid arteries at the same time. See Procedure 19-13.

7. **Assess the heart.**
   a. Have the patient sit up and lean forward a bit.
   b. Ask about any cardiovascular problems.
   c. Auscultate heart sounds. Note rate, rhythm, S_1, S_2, and extra sounds.

(continued on next page)

Procedure 19-20 ■ Brief Bedside Assessment (continued)

8. **Assess the back while patient is in the sitting position.**
   a. Inspect skin.
   b. Auscultate breath sounds; compare side to side and apex to base.
   c. Assess respiratory rate, rhythm, and effort.
   d. Note cough, secretions, how many pillows used to sleep on, and whether head of bed is elevated for breathing.
   e. Check oxygen order, SaO_2, ability to use incentive spirometer.

9. **Assess the anterior chest.**
   a. Ask about any respiratory problems.
   b. Palpate skin turgor, temperature, and PMI.
   c. Auscultate breath sounds.

10. **Assess the abdomen with the patient supine.**
    a. Inspect the size, shape, symmetry, and condition of the abdominal skin.
    b. Observe abdominal movements including respirations, pulsations, and peristalsis.
    c. Auscultate bowel sounds in all four quadrants and the aorta for bruits.
    d. Palpate all four quadrants for tenderness, guarding, and masses; inspect for rebound tenderness.
    e. Ask the patient about any weight changes, GI complaints, and change in appetite or diet.
    f. Review the pattern for bowel movements; when examining a female client, ask the last menstrual period.

11. **Assess urinary status.**
    a. Review voiding pattern with the patient (including frequency and dysuria).
    b. If there is an indwelling catheter, observe for patency, kinks in the tubing, and color of urine; monitor intake and output.
    c. Palpate for bladder distention.

12. **Assess the upper extremities.**
    a. Ask about any problems with the hands and arms, such as weakness, arthritis, change in sensation, temperature, or color.
    b. Inspect the condition of the skin and nails.
    c. Palpate skin temperature and bilateral brachial and radial pulses.
    d. Check capillary refill.
    e. Note any stiffness or limited ROM of the hands and arms.
    f. Test muscle strength by having the patient grip your hands or two fingers.
    g. Note whether the patient has any casts, traction, splints, or slings.
    h. Observe for edema.

13. **Assess the lower extremities.**
    a. Ask about any problems with the legs, such as weakness, numbness, tingling, arthritis, edema, change in sensation, and temperature or color.
    b. Observe ROM and ability to ambulate or move about in bed.
    c. Inspect the condition of the skin and nails.
    d. Palpate skin temperature and pedal pulses; check capillary refill.
    e. Test for leg strength by asking the patient to raise the leg against your counterpressure. (This is more easily done with the patient sitting.)
    f. Check sensation through light touch, proceeding to pain as needed.
    g. Observe for problems such as paralysis.
    h. Observe for edema.

14. **Ask the patient to stand, and inspect for:**
    a. Gross spinal deformities
    b. Balance and coordination of movements
    c. ROM and gait

15. **With the patient seated in bed, legs extended, check for:**
    a. Babinski reflex
    b. Homans' sign

Documentation

■ Document your findings and report any significant changes or findings to the primary care provider. As a student, report your findings to the instructor and the patient's assigned RN for validation and action.

   ■ If you need more information about documenting your findings,

   ➤ Go to **Chapter 19, Caring for the Williams Family,** including **Documenting Physical Examination Findings (Stanley Williams),** in Volume 1.

Thinking About the Procedure

To practice applying clinical reasoning to this procedure,

➤ The video **Brief Bedside Assessment** along with questions and suggested responses is available on the **Davis's Nursing Skills Video** Web site at www.fadavis.com.

CLINICAL INSIGHTS

Clinical Insight 19-1 ► Performing Percussion

Direct Percussion
Tap lightly with the pads of the fingers directly on the skin.

Direct percussion over the sinuses

Indirect Percussion
- Keep your fingernails short.
- Strive for a quiet environment: Turn off all entertainment media and music, shut the door, and so on.
  This allows you to better perceive the subtle differences in percussion notes.
- One hand is considered the stationary hand; the other is the striking hand.
- Hyperextend the middle finger of your stationary hand, and place its distal portion firmly against the client's skin over the area you wish to percuss.
- Lift the rest of your fingers off the patient's skin.
  Prevents dampening the sounds produced
- Be sure both of your hands are relaxed to best perform the technique.
  Stiff hands will not effectively produce the percussion sounds for assessment.
- Use the middle finger of your dominant hand as the striking finger **(plexor)**, and tap the distal portion of the middle finger of the stationary hand using a quick motion from your wrist.

Indirect percussion

- Use enough force to elicit a clear sound.
- Percuss two times over each location, then move to a new body location and repeat.

Describing Sounds
Use the terms in the following list to describe the sounds you hear. The terms are based on the components of the sounds produced by percussion:
- **Amplitude**—The loudness or softness of a sound
- **Pitch**—The number of vibrations per second, either high or low in nature
- **Quality**—A distinctiveness about the sound produced
- **Duration**—How long the sound lingers

Percussion Notes

SOUND	AMPLITUDE	PITCH	QUALITY	DURATION	EXAMPLE
Resonant	Medium-loud	Low	Hollow	Medium	Normal lung
Hyperresonant	Louder	Lower	Booming	Longer	Hyperinflated lung (as in emphysema)
Dull	Soft	High	Muffled thud	Short	Liver/spleen
Flat	Very soft	High	Absolute dullness	Very short	Thigh or tumor
Tympany	Loud	High	Musical	Longest	Gastric air bubble, intestinal air

Clinical Insight 19-2 ▶ Performing Auscultation

- Provide a quiet environment to facilitate auscultation.
- ✚ Clean your stethoscope with a 70% alcohol or benzalkonium chloride wipe before and after using it to examine a patient. Most stethoscopes are colonized by bacteria, although only a small percentage are pathogenic. Cleaning can reduce the bacterial count by 94% to 100%.
- Use the diaphragm to listen to high-pitched sounds that normally occur in the heart, lungs, and abdomen. Press the diaphragm hard enough to produce an obvious ring on the patient's skin.
- Use the bell to hear low-pitched sounds, such as extra heart sounds (murmurs) or turbulent blood flow (bruits). Apply the bell lightly with just enough pressure to produce an air seal with its full rim.
- Place the earpieces facing forward. *Seals the ear canal and improves detection of sounds.*
- Warm the stethoscope before you place it on the client's skin.
- Place the stethoscope directly on the client's skin. Do not listen through clothing. *Clothing can create artifact or reduce the quality of auscultation.*
- If body hair prevents good contact with the skin, dampen the hair before you listen.
- Close your eyes as you listen through the stethoscope. This helps improve your focus.
- Concentrate on one sound at a time. Do not try to evaluate breath and heart sounds at the same time. This improves the quality of the data.

Practice Resources
Centers for Disease Control and Prevention (2009, updated 2019); Holleck et al. (2017); Messina et al. (2017).

Clinical Insight 19-3 ▶ Assisting With a Speculum Examination

Equipment
- Patient drape
- Nonsterile gloves
  Vaginal speculum (see accompanying figure)
  The speculum may be plastic or metal.
  The size of the speculum depends on the patient's history and is not tied to patient weight or body size.
  If a culture or a Pap smear is to be obtained, lubricate the speculum with warm water. Otherwise, use a water-soluble lubricant.
- Lubricant
- Pap smear slide, spatula, brush, or specimen broom and container with solution
- Fixative, if the smear technique is used
- Genital culture supplies
- Additional light source

Preparing the Patient
- Explain to the patient that an internal examination of the vagina and pelvic organs will be performed. The examination usually takes only a few minutes, and although it might not be comfortable it should not be painful.
- Have the patient urinate before the examination if needed. *Emptying the bladder helps the patient to feel more comfortable during the examination.*
- Provide privacy and keep the patient warm during the procedure.
- Assist the patient to the lithotomy position, and cover exposed area with a drape.

Inserting the Speculum
The speculum is inserted into the vagina to visualize the cervix (see accompanying figure). Once the speculum is inserted, you may need to adjust the light source for the examiner.

Clinical Insight 19-3 ▶ Assisting With a Speculum Examination—cont'd

A. A vaginal speculum examination: placement of the speculum in the vagina

B. View through the speculum

Collecting Specimens
If a routine screening for cervical and uterine cancer is being done, a specimen will be collected. Additional cultures or screenings may be required if there is unusual discharge or risk of sexually transmitted infection (STI). Genital cultures are endocervical smears.

Pap Smear Procedure
Most commonly, the examiner inserts a small brush through the cervical os and rotates it to obtain cells from within the cervical canal (endocervical smear). The brush is then rolled onto the slide.

Using a specimen broom to obtain endocervical cells

A second specimen may be obtained by lightly scraping the cervix with a wooden spatula to obtain cells from the ectocervix (the lowest portion of the cervix that protrudes into the vagina).

Using a spatula to obtain ectocervical cells

The spatula is then smeared on the slide. Some examiners use both specimen sources and then apply a fixative, usually a spray or liquid, on top of the specimen to preserve it for examination. After the samples are obtained, the speculum is removed.

Pap Smear, Alternative Method
The examiner inserts a specimen broom into the cervical os and rotates it. The broom is then inserted into a fixative solution and rotated to disperse cells into the solution. This technique is gaining popularity because it is considered more sensitive for detection of cervical changes. After the samples are obtained, the speculum is removed.

Bimanual Examination
After removing the speculum, the examiner inserts lubricated gloved fingers into the vagina while pressing down on the lower abdomen and suprapubic area. This is known as a **bimanual examination.** It is used to assess the consistency of the cervix and the size of the uterus, and to detect tenderness over the ovaries and fallopian tubes or with movement of the cervix.

Postprocedure
- Assist the patient to a sitting position at the end of the examination.
- You may need to assist the patient with perineal care.
- If there is any bleeding or discharge, provide a perineal pad.
- Document the date and time of the procedure, the name of the examiner, the patient's tolerance of the procedure, and any nursing assessments or interventions performed.

Practice Resources
American Congress of Obstetricians and Gynecologists (2017, reaffirmed 2021); Bibbins-Domingo et al. (2017).

What Are the Main Points in This Chapter?

- A physical examination may be conducted to obtain data about the patient, to further investigate an identified health problem, to monitor a client's health status, or to screen for health problems.
- A comprehensive physical assessment includes a complete head-to-toe examination of every body system. Data from a comprehensive physical assessment provide guidance for care and determine the need for further assessment.
- A focused physical assessment is performed to obtain data about an actual, potential, or possible problem that has been identified. A focused examination adds to the database created from the comprehensive assessment.
- An ongoing assessment is appropriate for periodic reassessment of the client and reflects the dynamic state of the client. This is a less detailed examination than a comprehensive assessment.
- Before a physical assessment, you will need to gather equipment, prepare the environment, review the skills you will use, familiarize yourself with the patient situation, review the nursing plan of care, and assist the patient to relax by taking the time to learn more about the individual patient (culture, race, gender, sex).
- *Inspection* is the use of sight to gather data. Inspection begins the moment you meet the client.
- *Palpation* is the use of touch to gather data. Use palpation to assess temperature, skin texture, moisture, anatomical landmarks, and abnormalities such as edema, masses, or areas of tenderness.
- *Percussion*, tapping on the skin with short strokes from your fingers, produces vibrations that allow you to determine the location, size, and density of underlying structures.
- *Auscultation* is the use of hearing to gather data. Direct auscultation is unassisted listening. Indirect auscultation is listening to the sounds produced by the body with the help of a stethoscope.

Knowledge Map

PHYSICAL EXAMINATION

Health Assessment → Physical Assessment

PURPOSE:
- Obtain baseline data
- Identify nursing diagnoses, PCs, Wellness dx
- Monitor status of identified problems
- Screening

TYPES:
- Comprehensive:
  - interview
  - head-to-toe
- Focused:
  - data gathered on particular topic, body part/functional ability
- Ongoing:
  - prn with every pt. contact

APPROACHES:
Ways to gather data
- head to toe
- body systems

PREPARATION

SELF
- Know A&P
- Know purpose of exam
- Know pt. situation & plan of care
- Be familiar with equipment
- Exam technique
- Therapeutic communication
- How to document

ENVIRONMENT
- Provide privacy
- Decrease extraneous noise
- Adequate lighting
- Comfortable temperature

PATIENT
- Promote relaxation
- Develop a rapport
- Position patient properly
- Have patient void prior
- Alert patient to touch
- Attend to cultural preferences

AGE MODIFICATIONS:
Infant: have parent hold
Toddler:
- allow to sit on parent lap
- allow choices; use praise
- invasive assessments last

Preschooler:
- demo assessment on doll
- let child help
- give reassurance

School-age Child:
- develop rapport
- allow independence
- demo equipment

Adolescent:
- no parent/sibling present
- respect privacy during exam
- emphasize healthy lifestyle habits
- assess for suicide potential

Young/Middle-Aged Adult:
- no specific modifications unless acute/chronic disease

Older Adult:
- tailor exam to energy and mobility levels
- adapt techniques for vision & hearing changes

ASSESSMENT SKILLS:
Inspection:
- use of sight/observation

Palpation:
- use of touch: fingertips, dorsum/palm of hand, finger/thumb grasp

Percussion:
- vibrations elicited through tapping
- sound indicates location, size, density of underlying structure

Auscultation:
- use of hearing
- direct via stethoscope

Olfaction: not a formal skill
- use of sense of smell

GENERAL SURVEY:
- Appearance/behavior
- Body type; posture
- Dress; grooming; hygiene
- Mental status
- Vital signs/height/weight assessment

Proceeding to: **Assessment of all body systems**

CHAPTER 20

Promoting Asepsis & Preventing Infection

STUDENT RESOURCES

The questions and exercises in this book allow you to practice the kind of thinking you will use as a full-spectrum nurse. Critical-thinking questions usually have more than one right answer, so we do not provide "correct" answers for these features. Try to answer these questions yourself. It is more important to develop your nursing judgment than to just cover content. You will learn more by discussing the questions with your peers. If you are still unsure, see the Davis Advantage chapter resources for suggested responses.

To explore learning resources for this chapter,

Go to www.DavisAdvantage.com and find:

Answers and Suggested Responses for all questions in this chapter
Concept Map
Knowledge Map
References and Bibliography

Key Concepts

Body defenses
Infection
Infection prevention and control
Medical asepsis
Surgical asepsis

Related Concepts

See the Concept Map on Davis Advantage.
Sample Problems
Multidrug-resistant organism (MDRO) infections

Caring for the Williams Family

Nadine Williams works as a preschool teacher in her community. Kayla, her grandchild, has been attending the preschool since she came to live with her grandparents. Mrs. Williams tells you at a recent visit to the clinic that Kayla has had "a lot of problems with colds and a runny nose since she started preschool."

A. Based on your theoretical knowledge of asepsis and immunity, what is the most likely explanation for Kayla's symptoms?

B. Do you have enough patient data to make any conclusions? If not, what other information should you gather?

C. Identify three alternatives that may explain what is happening.

D. What strategies could you recommend that Mrs. Williams implement at the preschool to help limit the number of infections? Identify at least two strategies.

Practical Knowledge clinical application

As a nurse, you play a vital role in preventing the transmission of infection. Most infection control measures are independent nursing activities that do not require a medical prescription. You do need theoretical knowledge and scrupulous medical and surgical asepsis technique. The Procedures and Clinical Insights in this volume provide the guidance you will need to implement your infection-control concepts in providing safe, effective nursing care.

PROCEDURES

Procedure 20-1 ■ Hand Hygiene

▶ For steps to follow in *all* procedures, refer to the Universal Steps for All Procedures on the inside back cover. For this procedure, also refer to Clinical Insight 20-1.

Equipment
- Liquid soap
- Paper towels
- Warm, running water
- Hand moisturizer (recommended)

Preprocedure Assessments
- Check your hands for breaks in the skin.
  Breaks in the skin provide a route for microbial entry.
- Inspect the condition of your nails.
  - Nails should be no longer than ¼ inch from the fingertips.
  - Do not wear artificial nails or extensions.
  - Nail polish should not be chipped.
  - Preferably, do not use nail polish.

  The area under the nails, artificial nails/extensions, and chipped polish act as reservoirs for microorganism for the transmission of infection. If your glove were to tear or perforate, microorganisms could enter the surgical wound.

Procedure 20-1A ■ Using Soap and Water

▶ When performing the procedure, always identify your patient according to agency policy, using two identifiers, and be attentive to standard precautions, hand hygiene, patient safety and privacy, body mechanics, and documentation.

Procedure Steps

1. **Bare your hands and forearms.** Push your sleeves above your wrists; remove your wristwatch and rings.
   Moist clothing facilitates transfer of microorganisms; jewelry harbors bacteria and creates a moist area on the skin, which facilitates bacterial growth.

2. **Turn on the water. Use electronic faucet when possible.** Adjust water to warm, not hot.
   Hands-free electronic faucets lessen risk of recontamination of hands after washing as there is no need to manually turn off the water. Warm water opens pores and helps remove microorganisms without removing skin oils. Hot water irritates the stratum corneum (outer layer of the skin) and can lead to chapping and subsequent skin infections.

3. **Wet your hands and wrists with clean, running (warm or cold) water.** Keep your hands below your wrists and forearms.
   Prevents water from running from hands to the wrists and forearms. Hands are considered more contaminated than the wrists and arms.

   a. Avoid splashing water onto clothing.
   b. Avoid touching the inside of the sink.
      Microorganisms travel in moisture. The inside of the sink is considered contaminated. ▼

4. **Apply enough liquid soap to cover all hand surfaces** (typically three or four pumps from a dispenser).
   3 to 5 mL of liquid soap provides adequate amounts to completely cover the hands for maximum effectiveness to remove transient microorganisms. Harsh soaps will clear microbes from the skin but can irritate the skin and disrupt the acid balance in the skin, leading to drying and chapping, which can harbor microbes.

5. **Vigorously rub your hands together** for at least 20 seconds (CDC, 2020, January 30). Lather all surfaces, interlacing fingers, rubbing around each finger and thumb into the web spaces, rubbing the backs and palms of the hands in a circular motion with knuckles against palms of the hands.
   It takes at least 20 seconds for mechanical removal of microorganisms and for

(continued on next page)

Procedure 20-1 ■ Hand Hygiene (continued)

antimicrobial products to be effective. The areas of the hands most often missed are the thumb, the wrist, and areas between the fingers. ▼

6. **Clean under your fingernails,** using a disposable nail cleaner.
   Areas under the nails harbor high concentrations of microorganisms.

7. **Rinse your hands thoroughly.** Keep your hands below your wrists and forearms.

8. **Dry your hands thoroughly,** moving from your fingers up to your forearms and blotting with a clean paper towel or air dry.
   Move from the area you wish to keep cleanest (hands). Blotting decreases skin irritation.

9. **Turn off the faucet.** If faucet is not motion-operated, hold a dry paper towel in your hand to turn it off. Do not handle the paper towel with the opposite hand.
   A paper towel acts as a barrier to prevent contamination of hands from the faucet. After the towel has contacted the contaminated faucet, it can transfer microorganisms to your clean hand. Many pathogens can live on faucets and countertops.

10. **Apply a hand moisturizer** at least twice daily; use hand care products recommended by infection preventionists. (Many agencies use soaps that contain moisturizers.)
    Hand moisturizer helps prevent skin from drying and chafing, which may lead to transmission of infection. Petroleum-based products compromise latex gloves, resulting in permeability.

Procedure 20-1B ■ Using Alcohol-Based Handrubs

➤ When performing the procedure, always identify your patient according to agency policy, using two identifiers, and be attentive to standard precautions, hand hygiene, patient safety and privacy, body mechanics, and documentation.

Procedure Steps

1. **Use 60% to 95% alcohol-based handrubs** when hands are not visibly soiled and when certain pathogens are suspected.
   Antiseptic solutions are not effective when organic material or dirt from hands is present. Alcohol-based handrubs cannot remove spores and therefore should not be used for hand hygiene when Clostridium difficile or Bacillus anthracis is suspected of being present.

2. **Bare your hands and forearms.** Push your sleeves above your wrists. Remove your jewelry and wristwatch.

3. **Apply antiseptic solution** in a quantity sufficient (at least 3 mL) to cover the hands and wrists.
   All surfaces must be covered with sufficient product to effectively remove microorganisms. ▼

4. **Vigorously rub antiseptic solution** into your hands for 20 to 30 seconds (or as long as it takes to sing "Happy Birthday" if no clock is available). Cover all surfaces of the hands: interlacing fingers, rubbing around each finger and thumb, and rubbing the backs and palms of the hands in a circular motion including under the nails until the solution is completely dry.
   A period of 20 to 30 seconds is required for effective disinfection by alcohol handrubs (World Health Organization, 2009). All surfaces must be thoroughly covered with product to effectively remove microorganisms.

Evaluation
Hands are free of handrub and dry.

Documentation
Hand hygiene is a responsibility of all healthcare providers. It usually does not require documentation.

Thinking About the Procedure
To practice applying clinical reasoning to this procedure,

The video **Hand Hygiene: Using Soap and Water** and **Using Alcohol-Based Handrubs,** along with questions and suggested responses, is available on the **Davis's Nursing Skills Videos** Web site at www.fadavis.com.

Practice Resources
Association of periOperative Registered Nurses (AORN) (2022); Association of Surgical Technologists (AST) (2008); Boyce & Pittet (2002); CDC (2020, January 30, reviewed); CDC (2021, December 13, reviewed); CDC (2019, April 29, updated); Pittet et al. (2017); Siegel, Rhinehart, Jackson, et al. (2022, May, updated); Wood et al. (2016, September); World Health Organization (WHO) (2009).

Procedure 20-2 ■ Donning Personal Protective Equipment (PPE)

➤ For steps to follow in *all* procedures, refer to the Universal Steps for All Procedures on the inside back cover.

Equipment

Following CDC recommendations, you will usually use some combination of gloves, gown, mask, and eye protection, depending on the organism and level of precaution. In certain situations, you may need hair covers and shoe covers (e.g., when full barrier precautions are needed). Determine the availability of appropriate PPE.

- Disposable gloves of the proper size
- Disposable isolation gown
- Face mask (or N-95 respirator mask, as indicated)
- Face shield or goggles
- Hair cover (if needed)
- Shoe covers (if needed)

➤ When performing the procedure, always identify your patient according to agency policy, using two identifiers, and be attentive to standard precautions, hand hygiene, patient safety and privacy, body mechanics, and documentation.

Procedure Steps

1. **Assess the need for PPE.**
   a. **Gloves:** When you may be exposed to body secretions directly or indirectly
   Gloves provide a barrier against body fluids. All patients are considered potentially infected per Standard Precautions (see Clinical Insight 20-3).
   b. **Gowns:** When your uniform (e.g., scrubs) may become exposed to potentially infective secretions
   Key Point: *Do not substitute a patient gown for a disposable isolation or protective gown. Isolation gowns must be made of moisture-repelling materials to prevent contamination of underlying clothing and skin.*
   Examples of such situations include excessive wound drainage, fecal incontinence, or other discharges from the body, or when fluids may be splashed (as in eye irrigation).
   c. **Face mask:** When splashing may occur during close contact (3 ft or less) and potentially contaminate your mouth or nose
   Surgical masks provide a barrier to large-particle droplets (>5 microns in diameter), helping prevent transmission of pathogens to the nurse's mucous membranes.
   d. **Face shield or eye goggles:** When splashing might occur and fluids enter your eyes (e.g., blood splashes, respiratory droplets, or wound dbridement). To protect the entire facial area, wear a face shield (for maximum protection, it should protect the crown and chin and wrap around the face to the ear).
   Helps prevent pathogens from entering the conjunctiva directly or indirectly
   e. **N-95 respirator:** When caring for clients infected with airborne organisms (<5 microns) such as tuberculosis bacillus or COVID-19
   This device prevents the airborne transmission of the tuberculosis bacterium. The respirator mask shown is disposable; some are reusable. ▼
   f. **Hair covers:** When there is a potential for spraying or splashing of body fluids
   Although this is not in the CDC report (Siegel, Rhinehart, Jackson, et al., 2022, updated), agency policy may advise hair covers in certain situations.
   g. **Shoe covers:** When there is a potential for contamination of shoes with body fluids
   The floor (and anything in contact with it) is considered contaminated. However, certain categories of pathogens require full protective gear, and in those circumstances shoe covers are necessary.

2. **Don the isolation gown.**
   a. Pick up the gown by the shoulders, allowing the gown to fall open without touching the floor or other surfaces.
   Touching the floor or other surfaces will contaminate the gown with environmental pathogens. ▼

(continued on next page)

Procedure 20-2 ■ Donning Personal Protective Equipment (PPE) (continued)

b. Slip your arms into the sleeves. ▼

c. Fasten ties at the neck.
d. Position the gown so that it covers the back and fasten the ties at the waist. Do not bring ties around to the front of the gown.
   The front of the gown is considered contaminated after you enter the patient's room. If the ties are at the front of the gown, they will be contaminated, making it difficult to remove the gown safely.
e. If the gown does not completely cover your clothing in the back, wear two gowns.
   - Don the first gown so that the opening is in the front.
   - Then place the second gown over the first so that the opening is in the back.

3. **Don the N-95 respirator.**
   a. Determine how the mask is secured. Identify the top edge of the mask by locating the thin metal strip (nosepiece) that goes over the bridge of the nose.
      Surgical masks may be secured by ties at the back of the head and neck, loops around the ears, or elastic bands.
   b. Pick up the mask with the top ties or ear loops. Place the mask over your nose, mouth, and chin. Press the flexible metal strip so that it conforms to the bridge of your nose.
      The mask must fit snugly to the face for maximum barrier protection. Correct positioning will also keep your glasses or goggles from fogging. ▼

   c. Tie the upper ties to the back of your head and the lower ties to the back of your neck, or slip the loops around your ears or place the elastic bands as with the ties.

   d. Place the lower edge of the mask below your chin and tie the lower ties.
      Covering the nose and mouth creates a barrier to prevent droplet pathogens from entering through the nasal and oral mucous membranes or the respiratory system.

4. **Don the face shield or goggles.**
   a. *Face shield:* Place the shield over your eyes, adjust the metal strip over the bridge of your nose, and tuck the lower edge below your chin. Secure the straps behind your head.
   b. *Safety glasses or goggles:* Set them over the top edge of the mask. See Step 1c, d, e for rationale.

5. **Don hair cover, if indicated.**
   Hair covers can be worn to protect from contamination when you anticipate sprays or airborne exposure.

6. **Don shoe covers, if indicated.**

7. **Don gloves.**
   a. Select nonsterile disposable gloves of the appropriate size. See Clinical Insight 20-3.
      The correct size will prevent gloves from falling off or ripping while you are working with the client.
   b. If you are wearing a gown, make sure that the glove cuff extends over the cuff of the gown. If skin is visible between the gown and the glove, tape the glove cuff to the gown cuff, covering all visible skin.
      To provide complete protection of hands and wrists, no skin should be visible between the glove and gown.

Patient Teaching
Answer questions the patient may have and educate about the need for PPE, their disease process, and the purpose of isolation.

Home Care
- Identify the type of PPE needed and ensure that the necessary supplies are available.
- Develop a plan with the client and family for using and disposing of personal protective equipment and contaminated items.
- Teach family members to don PPE as needed.
- Obtain referral for a home health agency to provide support.

Documentation
The use of personal protective equipment is generally assumed and does not require documentation.

Practice Resources

AORN (2022); CDC (n. d. b.; 2016, January 26; 2019; 2022); Cowperthwaite & Holm (2015, February); Ortega, Bhadelia, Obanor, et al. (2015, March 19); Siegel, Rhinehart, Jackson, et al. (2022, May, updated); World Health Organization (WHO) (2015, January 28).

Thinking About the Procedure
To practice applying clinical reasoning to this procedure,

The video **Donning Personal Protective Equipment (PPE),** along with questions and suggested responses, is available on the **Davis's** *Nursing Skills Videos* Web site at www.fadavis.com.

Procedure 20-3 ■ Removing Personal Protective Equipment (PPE)

➤ For steps to follow in *all* procedures, refer to the Universal Steps for All Procedures on the inside back cover. For this procedure, also refer to Clinical Insights 20-2 and 20-3 if you need more information.

Key Point: *Considered contaminated: front areas, sleeves, mask, and gloves of the PPE, and head and shoe covers, if you are wearing them*

Key Point: *Considered clean: inside of the gown, gloves, ties on the mask and at the back of the gown, and the inside of the head and shoe covers, if you are wearing them*

➤ When performing the procedure, always identify your patient according to agency policy, using two identifiers, and be attentive to standard precautions, hand hygiene, patient safety and privacy, body mechanics, and documentation.

Procedure Steps

1. **Remove gloves first** (unless the gown ties in front; in that case, see "What If...").
   Gloves are the most contaminated PPE and must be removed first to avoid contamination of clean areas of the PPE during their removal.

   a. **Remove the first glove:**
      - Grasp the outside cuff of the glove with the opposite gloved hand.
      - Pull downward so that the glove turns inside out.
      - Do not touch the skin of your wrist or hand with your gloved hand.
      The outside of both gloves is contaminated. To prevent contamination, touch only the outside (contaminated) surface of first glove to outside (contaminated) surface of second glove. "Dirty touches dirty" and "clean touches clean." ▼

   b. **Remove the second glove:**
      - Hold the removed glove in the palm of your gloved hand.
      - Slip two ungloved fingers inside the cuff of the remaining glove.
      - Pull the glove off, inside out, over the glove that hand is holding. Do not touch the outside of the soiled glove with your bare fingers.
      The insides of gloves are considered "clean" because they have not been in contact with client or contaminated surfaces. Therefore, you can touch the insides with your bare hands. ▼

(continued on next page)

Procedure 20-3 ■ Removing Personal Protective Equipment (PPE) (continued)

   c. **Dispose of gloves** in a designated waste container, keeping them away from your body.
2. **Remove the gown:**
   a. **Release the waist ties** and the neck ties of the gown, bending slightly forward to allow the gown to fall forward.
      Allowing the gown to fall forward exposes the clean area for the hands to grasp more readily.
   b. **Slip your hands inside the neck** and peel the gown away from the shoulders.
      - Reach inside to pull off the cuff and remove your arm from the sleeve.
      - Repeat the maneuver to remove the second sleeve.
      - Do not touch the front of the gown, even if it is not visibly soiled.
      The inside of the gown is clean and will not contaminate your hands. The front of the gown and the sleeves are considered contaminated. ▼

3. **Fold the gown so the inside of the gown is to the outside.** Holding the gown away from your uniform, roll it up with the contaminated front and sleeves in the center, and place in the designated waste container.
   Folding the gown prevents contamination of your hands, the clothing, and the environment. ▼

4. **Remove goggles.**
   a. Grasp only the earpieces (or headband) of the goggles and pull off the face.
   b. If the goggles are not disposable, place in the container provided for disinfection.
      Earpieces are considered clean. Some goggles are cleaned and reused.

5. **Remove your mask or face shield,** unless the mask is a respirator. In that case, remove it after leaving the patient room and closing the door.
   a. Untie the lower ties first.
   b. Untie the upper ties next, being careful not to let go of the ties.
   c. Touch only the ties; do not touch the front of the mask.
   d. Dispose of the mask by holding on to the ties and placing it in a designated waste container.
      Ties are considered clean. Touching the outside of the mask would contaminate your hands.

6. **Remove your hair covering.**
   a. Slip your bare fingers under the edge of the hair cover, being careful not to touch the outside of it.
   b. Lift it up and away from your hair.
   c. Touching only the inside of it, place it in a designated waste container.
      The inside of the hair covering is considered clean, so you may touch it with your bare hands.

7. **Remove shoe covers.** Be careful to touch only the insides of the covers.

8. **Perform hand hygiene** immediately after removing PPE.
   Even if wearing gloves, hands may become contaminated.

9. ✚ **Close the door.**
   Keeping the door closed contains contaminants and makes signage more visible.

? What if...

■ **The gown is tied in front?**

Untie the front gown ties before removing your gloves; then remove the gloves and untie any back ties (e.g., at the neck). (This would be an unusual circumstance.)
Because the front of the gown (including a front tie) is considered contaminated, once you remove your gloves, you could not use your bare hands to untie a front tie.

■ **I am wearing two gowns (top one tied in back, inner one tied in front)?**

Remove gloves; untie waist ties of outer gown, remove the gown, and fold it inside out. Remove the inner gown by untying it in front. Fold inner gown inside out. Take off goggles and face mask or shield.

Patient Teaching
See Procedure 20-2.

Home Care
See Procedure 20-2.

Documentation
The removal of personal protective equipment is generally assumed and does not require documentation.

Practice Resources
AORN (2022); CDC (n.d.); Cowperthwaite & Holm (2015); Ortega, Bhadelia, Obanor, et al. (2015); Siegel, Rhinehart, Jackson, et al. (2022, updated); World Health Organization (2015, January 28).

Thinking About the Procedure
To practice applying clinical reasoning to this procedure,

The video **Removing Personal Protective Equipment (PPE),** along with questions and suggested responses, is available on the **Davis's** *Nursing Skills Videos* Web site at www.fadavis.com.

Procedure 20-4 ■ Surgical Hand Washing: Traditional Method

➤ For steps to follow in *all* procedures, refer to the Universal Steps for All Procedures on the inside back cover. For this procedure, also refer to Clinical Insights 20-2, 20-3, and 20-4 if you need more information.

Equipment
- Antimicrobial soap (FDA-approved for surgical hand asepsis)
- Soft, nonabrasive scrub sponge
- Disposable single-use nail cleaner
- Deep sink with foot or knee controls or motion-operated faucet
- Surgical shoe covers, cap, and face mask
- Sterile gloves of the correct size
- Surgical pack containing a sterile towel

➤ When performing the procedure, always identify your patient according to agency policy, using two identifiers, and be attentive to standard precautions, hand hygiene, patient safety and privacy, body mechanics, and documentation.

Procedure Steps

1. **Determine that sterile gloves,** gown, and towel are set up for use after the scrub.
   To maintain sterility, the sterile towel, gown, and gloves must be ready for use immediately after you scrub. If you need to gather supplies after the scrub, you must start the scrub procedure over again.

2. **Determine the agency policy for** the duration of the surgical scrub and the type of cleansing agent used.
   The type of cleansing agent determines how long to scrub. Typically, an alcohol-based antimicrobial soap requires 2 to 6 minutes.

3. **Avoid nail polish and artificial nails.** Trim so nails do not extend beyond fingertips. Remove rings, watches, and bracelets.
   Rings are a substantial risk factor for harboring moisture and gram-negative bacilli and *Staphylococcus aureus; artificial nails and chipped polish are more likely to carry gram-negative pathogens, including Pseudomonas, because water collects between the artificial and natural nails.*

4. **Don surgical shoe covers, cap,** and face mask before the surgical scrub.

5. **Perform a prewash** before the surgical scrub (see Procedure 20-1).
   The prewash removes any visible soil, reduces the number of microorganisms on your skin, and allows you to begin the surgical scrub with clean hands (Boyce & Pittet, 2002; Ellingson et al., 2014; Wood et al., 2018; World Health Organization [WHO], n.d.).

6. **Remove debris from under your nails** using a single-use nail file under running water.
   Decreases the number of microorganisms. ▼

7. **To begin the surgical scrub,** turn on the water, using the knee or foot controls or motion sensors. Adjust the temperature so that the water is warm.

(continued on next page)

Procedure 20-4 ■ Surgical Hand Washing: Traditional Method (continued)

Hot water removes the skin's protective oils. Knee and foot controls or motion-operated faucet help to prevent contamination of the hands. Do not touch any unsterile surface once you begin the surgical hand wash. ▼

8. **Wet your hands and forearms** from elbows to fingertips, keeping hands above elbows and away from your body. If using a scrub sponge, wet the sponge.
   Prevents water running down from your "dirty" elbows and forearm over "clean" rinsed hands.

9. **Apply a liberal amount of antimicrobial soap** to your hands and the sponge.
   - Lather well to 2 inches above the elbow.
   - Do not touch the inside of the sink with your fingers, hands, or elbows.
   - Avoid splashing your surgical attire.
   Scrub brushes are harsh on the skin. Soft, nonabrasive sponges are recommended instead. Antimicrobial soap reduces the number of microorganisms.

10. **Scrub one hand and arm,** all surfaces, using a circular motion.
    - Start at the fingers. Scrub at least 10 strokes each on nail, all four sides of each finger, hands, and arms.
    - When scrubbing the arm, use 10 strokes each for the lower, middle, and upper areas of the forearm.
    - Keep hands higher than elbows.
    Cover all surfaces to remove maximum number of microorganisms from the skin. Keep hands higher than elbows so that water from the area nearest the unscrubbed skin does not run downward and contaminate the hands. ▼

    10 circular motions over each area

11. **Rinse the brush and reapply** antimicrobial soap. Repeat the scrub on the second hand and arm. Normally the scrub takes 2 to 6 minutes.
    The length of the scrub depends on the time needed for the scrub agent to be effective in removing microorganisms on the hands.

12. **Rinse your hands and arms,** keeping your fingertips higher than your elbows.
    Prevents contamination of hands from water running from the upper arm down onto hands. ▼

13. **Repeat Steps 8 through 12** if directed to do so by the soap manufacturer or agency policy.

14. **With arms flexed and your hands** held higher than your elbows, move to the area with the sterile towel and gown.
    Avoids contamination of hands from water runoff.

15. **Grasp the sterile towel** and step back while not turning your back or your eyes from sterile field.
    Backing away keeps the sterile field dry and prevents you from inadvertently brushing against the table, which would contaminate the field. ▼

16. **Lean forward slightly,** and allow the towel to fall open, being careful not to let it touch your clothing.
    The towel would be contaminated if it brushed against your clothing.

17. **Use one end of the towel** to dry one hand and arm. Use the opposite end to dry the other hand and arm. Be certain your skin is thoroughly dry before donning sterile gloves.

Drying skin prevents maceration and allows gloves to go on much more easily. Use a separate section of the towel to prevent rewetting the skin or contaminating an already clean area.

? What if . . .

- **The agency uses an alcohol-based surgical hand antiseptic product?**
  a. Perform Steps 1 through 6. Omit Steps 7 through 17.
  b. Using the indicated amount of hand antiseptic, rub all surfaces of the hands, including the nails, and up the arm to 2 inches above the elbow, according to the manufacturer's recommendations and agency policy.
  Many different products are available. Be careful to follow the manufacturer's guidelines for use for maximum effectiveness.
  c. Allow the hand scrub to dry completely before you don sterile gloves.

Patient Teaching

If the patient is able to observe the procedure, explain the purpose of the surgical scrub and sterility.

Practice Resources
AORN (2022); AST (2008); Boyce & Pittet (2002); Gaspar et al. (2018); Pittet et al. (2017); Siegel, Rhinehart, Jackson, et al. (2022, updated).

Documentation

A surgical hand scrub does not require documentation. Instead, chart the procedure (or surgery) and how the patient tolerated it.

Procedure 20-5 ■ Surgical Hand Washing: Brushless System

➤ For steps to follow in *all* procedures, refer to the Universal Steps for All Procedures on the inside back cover. For this procedure, also refer to Clinical Insights 20-2 and 20-3 if you need more information.

Equipment

- Antimicrobial soap (60% to 95% alcohol, or other FDA-approved product for surgical hand asepsis)
- Disposable single-use nail cleaner
- Deep sink with foot or knee controls or motion-operated faucet
- Surgical shoe covers, cap, and face mask
- Sterile gloves of the correct size
- Surgical pack containing a sterile towel

➤ When performing the procedure, always identify your patient according to agency policy, using two identifiers, and be attentive to standard precautions, hand hygiene, patient safety and privacy, body mechanics, and documentation.

Procedure Steps

1. **Determine agency policy** for the type of cleansing product to be used and for duration of the surgical scrub (typically 2 to 6 minutes).
   Policies vary from institution to institution, although all should be based on sound principles for infection control designed in accordance with CDC and the Association of periOperative Registered Nurses (AORN) guidelines and follow manufacturer's directions for product use. The type of cleansing agent determines how long to scrub. Typically, alcohol-based handrub is rubbed onto hands and arms until dry.

2. **Before starting the scrub,** gather supplies and set up sterile gloves, gown, and towel for use after the scrub.
   To maintain sterility of the hands after the scrub, the sterile gloves, gown, and towel must be ready before washing.

3. **Observe recommended hygiene.**
   a. Do not wear artificial nails. Nails should be free of polish and not extend beyond the ends of the fingers.
   Especially important when in direct contact with patients or in high-risk situations, such as the perioperative setting or among those receiving immunosuppressant therapy. Artificial nails have been shown to harbor more pathogenic organisms in the subungual area than natural nails, particularly gram-negative bacilli (especially Pseudomonas) and various strains of yeast. Long nails can tear gloves.
   b. Remove rings, watches, and bracelets before starting the scrub.
   Hand jewelry can prevent the hand scrub from reaching all skin areas and increase the spread of potential pathogens. Risk of infection from microorganisms increases exponentially in relation to the number of rings worn.

(continued on next page)

Procedure 20-5 ■ Surgical Hand Washing: Brushless System (continued)

4. **Don shoe covers, a cap, and a mask.** Tuck hair completely under the cap.
   Masks filter out possible airborne pathogens carried in the nose or mouth, preventing contamination of sterile areas. Covering the hair reduces the transmission of pathogenic organisms that adhere to the hair shaft or scalp.

5. **Perform a prewash** before the surgical scrub. Use a pick to remove dirt and debris from under the nails; discard.
   Prewash removes any visible soil, reduces the number of microorganisms on your skin, and allows you to begin the surgical scrub with clean hands. The area under the nails harbors dirt, debris, and microorganisms.

6. **Turn on the water,** using the knee or foot controls or motion controls or motion-sensitive faucet. The temperature usually adjusts automatically in a surgical scrub sink. If it does not, adjust to warm.
   Water that is too hot can cause injury to the skin, making it prone to disruption in the skin integrity. It can also remove the skin's normal flora and natural oil, which has a protective effect.

7. **Wet hands and forearms** from the fingertips to elbows, always keeping hands above the elbows and away from the body.
   Prevents water running down from your elbows and forearm over washed and rinsed hands.

8. **Dispense a palm full of** antibacterial cleansing solution into your dominant hand.
   a. Insert the fingertips of your nondominant hand into the cleansing solution using a twisting motion to apply the product to the fingertips and nails.
   b. Then rub the hands together to distribute the soap over the hands. ▼

9. **Vigorously rub all surfaces** of your nondominant hand and fingers, adding water as needed.
   - Do not touch the inside of the sink during the cleansing procedure.
     Complete contact and friction are necessary for removal of microorganisms adherent to the skin's surface. The inside of the sink is considered contaminated with microbes. Incidental contact necessitates repeating the cleansing procedure.
   a. Rub the hands together palm to palm.
   b. Using your dominant palm, clean the back of your nondominant hand.
   c. Then rub your nondominant palm over your dominant hand.
   d. Then rub your palms together with your fingers interlaced, cleansing the web of skin between each finger.
   e. Rub the back of your fingers on your closed right hand back and forth across your nondominant palm, with your curved fingers interlaced. Do the same with your other hand. ▼
   f. With your nondominant hand, clasp your dominant thumb and make rotational movements to cleanse the thumb. Repeat on the other hand.
   g. Hold your fingers together on the dominant hand and move them back and forth and in a circular pattern against your other palm.
      Although the palmar surface carries more organisms than the back side of the hands and arms, this area nonetheless should be cleansed thoroughly to reduce microbial count.

10. **Rinse using deep basin sink** with knee-, foot-, or motion-operated controls. Dispense soap into the hands each time when cleansing a new area.
    Improved adherence to sterile technique commonly results from use of motion-, foot-, or knee-operated controls for faucets.

11. **Next cleanse the remaining** ⅔ of the arms, beginning at the wrist, to 2 inches above the elbow. Cover every aspect of the middle and upper third of the forearm.

12. **Dispense cleansing solution** into the hands each time you cleanse a new area.

13. **First, scrub the nondominant arm** wrist to elbow. Then repeat the wrist-to-elbow scrub on the dominant arm. Rinse each arm thoroughly and independently.

14. **This completes one washing cycle.**
    a. Using the same motions, beginning with Step 8, perform a second cycle.

b. Then finish with a third cycle in which you scrub only the hands. The scrub is complete after cleansing every aspect of the hands and forearms for 3 full minutes.
The AORN promotes a 2- to 3-minute scrub time using an antiseptic detergent to achieve maximal microbicidal activity while avoiding irritant-contact dermatitis associated with use of an abrasive sponge. Reduced time required to perform the surgical scrub often results in increased compliance with the prescribed technique.

15. **With arms flexed and hands** held higher than the elbows away from the body, move to the area with the sterile towel and gown.
This position prevents water running down from your elbows and forearm over rinsed hands.

16. **Grasp the sterile towel,** and back away from the sterile field. Lean forward slightly, and allow the towel to fall open, being careful not to let it touch clothing or gown.
This motion is performed to maintain a dry sterile field and prevent inadvertent brushing against the table and contaminating the field.

17. **Use one end of the towel** to dry one hand and arm using a dabbing motion. Dry the other hand and arm with the opposite end of the towel.
Use of a separate section of the towel guards against inadvertently rewetting the skin or contaminating an already clean area.

18. **Allow time for the skin to dry** thoroughly before donning sterile gloves.
Dry skin prevents maceration and allows the gloves to go on more easily. Moisture left on the skin can be a source of further microbial contamination.

19. **Once the brushless scrub is complete,** keep your hands in front of your body and above the waist. It may be necessary to enter backward through the door of the surgical suite.
These actions help prevent contamination of the hands and forearms when moving from the scrub sink.

Documentation

A brushless surgical hand scrub does not require documentation in the patient's medical record, although there may be a checklist. However, you must adhere to the institution's policy for performing the technique.

Patient Teaching

If the patient is able to observe the procedure, explain the purpose of a diligent approach to surgical scrub for promoting a low-risk environment for infection.

Home Care Adaptations

Sinks in the home environment typically do not have knee- or foot-operated controls or motion-sensor on/off devices. Therefore, when scrubbing for a sterile procedure in the home, contact with the faucet handles is performed with barrier objects (e.g., a paper towel or a sterile towel for a sterile scrub) between the clean hands and the environmental surface.

Practice Resources
AORN (2022); AST (2017, revised); AST (2008); Boyce & Pittet D. (2002); Cowperthwaite & Holm (2015).

Thinking About the Procedure

To practice applying clinical reasoning to this procedure,

The video **Surgical Hand Washing: Brushless System,** along with questions and suggested responses, is available on the **Davis's** *Nursing Skills Videos* Web site at www.fadavis.com.

Procedure 20-6 ■ Sterile Gown and Gloves (Closed Method)

➤ For steps to follow in *all* procedures, refer to the Universal Steps for All Procedures on the inside back cover. For this procedure, also refer to Clinical Insights 20-2 and 20-3 if you need more information.

Equipment
- Sterile gloves of the right size
- Sterile gown

You should find these items lying on a sterile field. If they are not, you will need to create a sterile field to place them on.

➤ When performing the procedure, always identify your patient according to agency policy, using two identifiers, and be attentive to standard precautions, hand hygiene, patient safety and privacy, body mechanics, and documentation.

Procedure Steps

1. **Grasp the gown at the neckline.**
   a. Hold the gown up and allow it to fall open as you step back from the table.
   b. Do not allow the gown to contact nonsterile areas while you are lifting it off the table and opening it.
   The gown will be contaminated if it touches unsterile objects. ▼

2. **Slide both arms into the sleeves,** but do not extend your hands through the cuffs.
   Sleeve cuffs are considered unsterile when your hands pass beyond the cuff (they are sterile if you don gloves using the closed method).

3. **Keep the sleeves of the gown** above waist level.
   Hands will contaminate the sleeve edge if allowed to pass through the cuff. ▼

4. **Ask a coworker** (or the circulating nurse if you are in the surgical suite) to stand behind you and pull the shoulders of the gown up and tie the ties at the neck. The coworker touches only the inside of the gown while pulling it up.
   Touching only the inside prevents contamination of the gown with the nurse's hands.

5. **Don sterile gloves** using the closed method. Open the sterile glove wrapper, keeping your fingers inside the sleeve of the gown. The outer wrapper has already been discarded.

   Glove the dominant hand first.
   a. With your nondominant hand, keeping your hands inside the gown sleeves, grasp the cuff of the glove for your dominant hand. Turn your dominant hand palm up.
   Keeping the hand inside the cuff ensures that you are contacting the sterile gown; sterile is touching sterile.
   b. Lay the glove on the dominant gown cuff, thumb side down, with the glove opening pointed toward the fingers and thumb of glove positioned over the thumb side of the dominant hand. ▼

   c. Keeping your dominant hand inside the sleeve, grasp the inside of the glove cuff. ▼

CHAPTER 20 Promoting Asepsis & Preventing Infection

d. With your other hand (inside its sleeve), grasp the upper side of the glove cuff and stretch it over the gown cuff.
e. Pull the sleeve of your gown up to pull the glove cuff over your wrist as you move your fingers into the glove fingers.

Glove the nondominant hand.

f. Place the fingers of your gloved hand under the cuff of the second glove.
   - Lay the glove on the forearm of your nondominant hand, thumb side down, with glove opening pointing toward the fingers.
   - Grasp and anchor the inside glove cuff with your nondominant (ungloved) hand through the gown, being careful to keep fingers inside the gown.
g. With your dominant (gloved) hand, pull the glove cuff over the cuff of the gown as you move your fingers into the glove. ▼

h. **Adjust the fingers in both** gloves for a snug fit over the fingers. *Maintains sterility of the gown and gloves by maintaining a closed system. The final adjustment of the gloves is done when both gloves are in place to prevent contaminating the gloves. Taut gloves, especially over the fingertips, allow better feel and dexterity.*

6. **Grasp the waist tie on the gown;** then hand the tie to the circulating nurse or a coworker who is wearing a hair cover and mask. Your coworker will grab the tie with sterile forceps. *The tie is considered sterile. You will need help pulling it around you. A coworker can help you. Using sterile forceps keeps the tie sterile.* ▼

7. **Make a three-quarter turn,** then receive the tie from your coworker. *Because only areas within your field of vision are considered sterile, a coworker must pull the waist tie around you.*

8. **Secure the waist tie.** *Ensures that the gown is secured and will not expose clothing to a sterile field.*

Patient Teaching

If the patient is alert during the procedure, explain:

- The need for the sterile procedure
- Why they must not touch the drapes
- Why they must not move or talk once the drapes are in place
- Any special precautions during the procedure

Documentation

- Donning sterile gown and gloves does not require documentation.
- You will need to chart the procedure performed and how the patient tolerated it.
- In the surgical suite, the circulating nurse charts about the surgery and the patient's response.

? What if . . .

- **My hand inadvertently comes through the cuff opening when putting on the gown?**

  Change gowns. The cuff would have been contaminated and would then contaminate your glove.

Practice Resources
AORN (2022); Boyce & Pittet (2002); Cowperthwaite & Holm (2015).

Thinking About the Procedure

To practice applying clinical reasoning to this procedure,

➤ The video **Sterile Gown and Gloves (Closed Method),** along with questions and suggested responses, is available on the **Davis's *Nursing Skills Videos*** Web site at www.fadavis.com.

Procedure 20-7 ■ Sterile Gloves (Open Method)

▶ For steps to follow in *all* procedures, refer to the Universal Steps for All Procedures on the inside back cover. For this procedure, also refer to Clinical Insights 20-2, 20-3, and 20-4 if you need more information.

Equipment
- Sterile gloves of the correct size

▶ When performing the procedure, always identify your patient according to agency policy, using two identifiers, and be attentive to standard precautions, hand hygiene, patient safety and privacy, body mechanics, and documentation.

Procedure Steps

1. **Determine the correct size** of sterile glove. The gloves should be snug but not tight.
   Gloves that are too loose are more easily contaminated and make handling equipment or supplies difficult. Gloves that are too tight are uncomfortable and may tear during use.

2. ✚ **Assess the glove package** for intactness and expiration date. Do not use the gloves if the package is torn, has become moist, or is past the expiration date.
   Torn packaging may allow the gloves to become contaminated. Moisture allows wicking and may cause contamination. Expired gloves are not considered sterile. ▼

3. **Assess the patient's environment** for a clean, flat space with enough room to allow you to open the glove package. Don the gloves without touching a nonsterile item.
   Inadvertently touching a nonsterile item will contaminate the gloves.

4. **Open the outer wrapper** and place the inner glove package on a clean, dry surface.

5. **Open the inner glove package** so that the glove cuffs are closest to you. Be careful to fully open the flaps of the package so that they do not fold back over and contaminate the gloves.
   The outer 1-inch border of the glove package is considered contaminated. ▼

6. **With your nondominant hand,** grasp the inner surface of the glove for the dominant hand.
   - Lift the glove up and away from the table, keeping it away from your body.
   - Do not touch anything else on the sterile field.
   The inside of the glove is not considered sterile because it is in contact with your skin. Lifting the glove up and away from the table prevents you from accidentally touching the table or clothing while donning it.

7. **Slide your dominant hand** into the glove, keeping your hand and fingers above your waist and away from your body.
   The area below the waistline is considered contaminated. Keeping gloves away from your body prevents accidental contamination. ▼

8. **Slide your gloved fingers under** the cuff of the glove for the nondominant hand, keeping your gloved thumb well away from your ungloved hand. Lift the glove up and away from the table and away from your body.
   The outside of the glove is sterile and may be touched with your sterile gloved hand. ▼

9. **With gloved fingers still under the cuff,** slide your nondominant hand into the glove and pull it on, being careful to avoid contact with your gloved hand, especially the thumb.

   A general rule when applying the second glove is to touch glove to glove and skin to skin. The already gloved hand may touch any of the sterile surfaces of the second glove. The second hand may touch only the inside of the glove (the portion that will have contact with the skin). ➤

10. **Adjust both gloves to fit your fingers.** If necessary, pull the fingers of the gloves down so that no excess is at the fingertips.

    Adjusting your gloves after both have been donned decreases the risk of contamination and allows for greater dexterity during the procedure.

11. **Keep your hands between shoulder** and waist level in front of you.

    Keeps the gloves within your field of vision to avoid contamination.

    NOTE: *To remove soiled gloves after the procedure, refer to Procedure 20-3.*

Patient Teaching
Explain the reason sterile gloves are needed for the procedure.

Home Care
- Many home care procedures are clean rather than sterile. The client is in his own environment and not surrounded by other patients, who may serve as hosts for infection.
- You may need to teach caregivers how to apply sterile gloves for some procedures. No modifications are required. Demonstrate the procedure, and have the caregiver do a return demonstration.

Documentation
- No special documentation is needed for sterile gloving.
- Chart the procedure you performed and the patient's response to the procedure.

Practice Resources
AORN (2022); CDC (n.d.); Cowperthwaite & Holm (2015).

Thinking About the Procedure
To practice applying clinical reasoning to this procedure,

➤ The video **Sterile Gloves (Open Method),** along with questions and suggested responses, is available on the **Davis's** *Nursing Skills Videos* Web site at www.fadavis.com.

Procedure 20-8 ■ Sterile Fields

➤ For steps to follow in *all* procedures, refer to the Universal Steps for All Procedures on the inside back cover. For this procedure, also refer to Clinical Insights 20-2 and 20-3 if you need more information.

Equipment
- Package of sterile supplies required for the procedure
- Sterile gloves of the correct size

Procedure 20-8A ■ Setting Up a Sterile Field

➤ When performing the procedure, always identify your patient according to agency policy, using two identifiers, and be attentive to standard precautions, hand hygiene, patient safety and privacy, body mechanics, and documentation.

Procedure Steps

- Close doors and limit the number of people in the area.
  Air currents can carry dust and microorganisms.
- Prepare a sterile field as close as possible to the time of use.
  To minimize the opportunity for contamination via air currents.

1. **Check all packaging of supplies and equipment** to be sure all are intact and expiration dates are current.
   Only sterile items should enter a sterile field. Any compromise in packaging means that the item is assumed not to be sterile.

2. **Arrange the environment** for performing the sterile procedure.
   a. Remove all items from the surface you will use to set up the sterile field.
      Inadequate space causes inadvertent contamination during sterile procedures.
   b. Position the patient as needed for the procedure before setting up the sterile field.
      Allows you to efficiently proceed with the procedure. Once the sterile field is established, air movement can create contamination of the sterile items.

Procedure Variation: Using Sterile Packaged Equipment

3. **Place the sterile package** on a clean, dry surface.
   Prevents contamination of the sterile item. If a surface is damp, strike-through may occur, making the item unsterile. ▼

4. **Open the flap away from you first** to prevent passing an unsterile arm over the sterile items.
   If you move an unsterile item over a sterile field, the field is no longer considered to be sterile. ▼

5. **Open the side flaps.** ▼

6. **Pull the final flap toward you.** The wrapper is now the sterile field. Touch the inside of the wrapper only after you don sterile gloves.
   - The area 1 inch from the edge of the wrapper and 1 inch from the table edge is considered unsterile.
   - Do not readjust the sterile area after the package has been opened. Only the horizontal surface of the draped area is considered sterile. Any part of the sterile wrapper that falls below the level of the sterile area (e.g., top of the table) is considered unsterile. If you move the field after opening, the field shifts and places unsterile areas of the wrapper on the surface. ▼

Procedure Variation: Opening a Fabric- or Paper-Wrapped Sterile Package

7. **Check and remove** the chemical indicator strip.
   Confirms that the package was sterilized. The pack usually is also dated.

8. **Remove the outer wrapper** and place the inner wrapped package on a clean, dry surface.
   The outer wrapper is not considered sterile and is discarded.

9. **Open the inner wrapper** following the same technique described in Steps 3 through 6.

Procedure Variation: Using a Sterile Drape
Omit Steps 3 through 6.

10. **Place the package on a clean, dry surface.**
    a. With the outer wrapper still on the package, hold the edge of the package flap down toward the table.
    b. Grasp the top edge of the package and peel back.
    The sterile drape is inside the outer wrapper. This maneuver opens the package without contaminating the sterile drape. ▼

11. **Pick up the sterile drape by the corner.**
    - Allow the drape to fall open away from your body and away from unsterile surfaces.
    - Place it on a clean, dry surface by touching only the edge of the drape.

    - Do not fan the drape.
      A 1-inch border around the sterile drape is considered unsterile.

12. In some situations, when placing a sterile drape (e.g., under a patient) you may need to protect your gloved hands by cuffing the drape over your hands. ▼

Procedure 20-8B ■ Adding Supplies to a Sterile Field

➤ When performing the procedure, always identify your patient according to agency policy, using two identifiers, and be attentive to standard precautions, hand hygiene, patient safety and privacy, body mechanics, and documentation.

Procedure Steps

1. ✚ Before adding items to a sterile field, inspect them for proper packaging, integrity, and inclusion of a sterilization indicator. Never assume an item is sterile. If there is any doubt about its sterility, consider it contaminated.

2. **Hold the sterile package in your** dominant hand. Grasping the corner of the wrapper, peel each corner back with your nondominant hand.
   The inside of the wrapper is sterile and will be used as a barrier when placing the sterile item onto a sterile field.

3. **Holding the contents several** inches above the field, allow the supplies to drop onto the field inside the 1-inch border of the sterile field. Do not let your arms pass over the sterile field.
   By holding the package upside down, you ensure that the sterile part of the package is facing the sterile field and that you deposit the item onto the sterile field. ▼

4. **Dispose of the wrapper,** then continue opening any needed supplies for the procedure.

   Key Point: *Once sterile gloves are on, you will not be able to add items without contaminating the gloves.*

(continued on next page)

UNIT 3 Essential Nursing Interventions

Procedure 20-8 ■ Sterile Fields (continued)

Procedure 20-8C ■ Adding Sterile Solutions to a Sterile Field

➤ When performing the procedure, always identify your patient according to agency policy, using two identifiers, and be attentive to standard precautions, hand hygiene, patient safety and privacy, body mechanics, and documentation.

Procedure Steps

1. **Use a sterile bowl or container.** Place it on the side of the sterile field closest to you.
   Prevents you from reaching over and thereby contaminating the field.

2. **Check that the sterile solution** is correct, then confirm that the solution concentration is correct and that the expiration date has not passed. ▼

3. **Remove the cap from the solution** bottle by lifting it directly up. Throw it away.
   The edge of the container is considered contaminated after the contents have been poured and the sterility of the contents cannot be ensured if the cap is replaced.

4. **Hold the bottle 4 to 6 inches** above the bowl and pour the needed amount of the solution into the bowl.
   Prevents you from inadvertently touching the sterile bowl with the bottle and thereby contaminating the bowl. Limited height reduces the risk of splashing, which strikes through and contaminates a cloth or permeable sterile field. A disposable sterile drape generally has a plastic membrane in the middle to prevent strike-through. ▼

5. **Discard the remaining solution.**
   Reusing open containers may cause contamination due to drops contacting the unsterile areas and running back over the container opening.

6. **Before donning sterile gloves** to perform the procedure, double-check that all supplies have been added to the field using sterile technique.
   - Do not leave the sterile field unattended.
   - Do not turn your back to the sterile field.
   If a sterile item is out of your field of vision, it is no longer considered sterile because airborne particles, insects, or liquids could contaminate the field.

Home Care

- Most sterile procedures in the home are done by visiting nurses.
- Procedures performed by clients or family members are usually clean rather than sterile.

Documentation

- You will not document the actual setup of the sterile field.
- Document the procedure, your assessment of the patient's tolerance for the procedure, and your assessment of the area being treated by the procedure.

? What if . . .

- **I observe a breach in sterility by the surgeon?**
  As a nurse, it is your duty to protect the patient above all else, even when the situation is uncomfortable for the healthcare provider. The nurse is obligated to follow the institution's policy and advocate for patient safety.

Practice Resources
AORN (2022); Simko (2012).

Thinking About the Procedure
To practice applying clinical reasoning to this procedure,

> The videos **Setting up a Sterile Field—Sterile Packaged Equipment; Setting up a Sterile Field—Fabric- or Paper-Wrapped Sterile Package; Setting up a Sterile Field—Sterile Drape; Adding Supplies to a Sterile Field—Sterile Packaged Equipment; Adding Supplies to a Sterile Field—Fabric- or Paper-Wrapped Sterile Package; Adding Supplies to a Sterile Field—Sterile Drape; Adding Sterile Solutions to a Sterile Field—Sterile Packaged Equipment; Adding Sterile Solutions to a Sterile Field—Fabric- or Paper-Wrapped Sterile Package;** and **Adding Sterile Solutions to a Sterile Field—Sterile Drape,** along with questions and suggested responses, are available on the **Davis's Nursing Skills Videos** Web site at www.fadavis.com.

CLINICAL INSIGHTS

Clinical Insight 20-1 ➤ Guidelines for Hand Hygiene

Hand Washing

When to Wash
- When hands are visibly dirty or soiled with blood or body fluids
- When arriving on and leaving the patient care unit
- Before direct contact with a patient, even if you intend to wear procedure gloves
- Before donning gloves (either procedure or sterile)
- When gloves are changed during a procedure
- After removing gloves
- After contact with a patient's intact skin (e.g., when lifting a patient or taking blood pressure)
- After contact with body fluids, mucous membranes, nonintact skin, and wound dressings even if hands are not visibly soiled
- When moving from a contaminated body site to a clean body site during patient care
- Before and after contact with objects and equipment in the patient's immediate vicinity
- Before eating and after using a restroom (use soap and water)
- Before and after touching any area on your face and hair

What to Use
- Use alcohol-based handrub (at least 60% alcohol) for routine hand hygiene and if hands are not visibly soiled.
- Use soap and water:
  When hands are dirty or visibly soiled
  After using a restroom

  ✚ If there is potential for exposure to *Bacillus anthracis* (or other spore-producing bacteria such as *C. difficile*). *Alcohol-based solutions are not effective against spores.*

- Use warm, not hot, water.
- Use disposable paper towels.

How to Wash
Refer to Procedure 20-1: Hand Hygiene.

Fingernails
- Keep natural fingernails short (¼ inch or less) and avoid wearing fingernail polish or artificial nails in the perioperative setting (AORN, 2022; AST, 2008; CDC, 2022, June 15, reviewed). Chipped nail polish can contaminate a sterile environment when gloves are not worn or are punctured or torn. Artificial nails, including gels, acrylics, and resins, harbor microorganisms and impede proper hand hygiene. Nail polish can contaminate a sterile environment when gloves are not worn or are punctured or torn. Most bacterial growth occurs along the proximal 1 mm of the nail, adjacent to subungal skin (WHO, n.d.).
- Scrub the undersides of fingernails with soap and water and nail brush every time you wash your hands.
- Clean nail grooming tools before use.
- Avoid biting or chewing nails or cuticles. Trim hangnails with a sanitized nail trimmer (CDC, 2016, July 26, reviewed).

Jewelry
- Remove all jewelry before beginning hand hygiene or surgical hand scrub (AORN, 2022; AST, 2008; CDC, 2022, June 15, reviewed). Hand jewelry may make donning gloves more difficult and cause gloves to tear more readily.
- The WHO (n.d.) prohibits any jewelry or watches on the hands of the surgical team. Skin underneath rings is more heavily colonized than comparable areas of skin on bare fingers.
- It is recommended that you not wear a watch or rings in the clinical setting, especially rings with stones. If your agency permits you to wear jewelry, clean it thoroughly and often.

Practice Resources
AORN (2022, 2018); AST (2008); Boyce & Pittet (2002); CDC (2002; 2019, April 29, updated; 2022, January 30, reviewed; 2022, June 15, reviewed); Pittet, Boyce, & Allegranzi (eds.) (2017); Rupp, Fitzgerald, Puumala, et al. (2008); Siegel, Rhinehart, Jackson, et al. (2007; 2023, May); WHO (2009).

Clinical Insight 20-2 ▸ Providing a Clean Patient Environment

Use the following guidelines along with standard precautions for all patients.

Supplies and Equipment

- Do not stock rooms with unnecessary supplies.
- Consider supplies that are brought into a patient's room contaminated. Do not return them to the linen or supply cart; instead, handle them according to agency policy.
- Items brought from the patient's home and gifts from visitors are considered unclean.
- Mobile devices should be cleaned (e.g., pagers, smartphones, point-of-care keyboards, and medication administration devices). Be sure to perform hand hygiene after using such a device.
- Wipe stethoscopes with alcohol before using on a patient. Do not wear stethoscope around your neck.
- Disinfect reusable equipment that is soiled with blood or body fluids according to agency policy—typically, autoclaving, ethylene oxide gas, or dry heat.
- Do not reuse equipment for the care of another patient until it has been cleaned and reprocessed appropriately.
- Dispose of single-use equipment that is soiled with blood or body fluids in appropriate biohazard containers.
- Wear gloves when handling equipment that is visibly contaminated. Perform hand hygiene.

Linens

- While wearing gloves, carefully handle contaminated linens. *To prevent skin and mucous membrane exposure, contamination of clothing, and transfer of microorganisms to other patients or the environment.*
- Bag and remove soiled linens from the room immediately. *Linens may harbor microorganisms that may transfer to your clothing, open skin, or mucous membranes, which could then be carried to other clients or environment.*

Uniforms and Laboratory Coats

- Do not wear a uniform (e.g., scrubs) or a laboratory coat for more than 1 day without laundering. *Care provider clothing is often contaminated when moving from patient to patient. The traditional laboratory coats are typically laundered less often than scrubs (Goyal, Khot, Ramachandran, et al., 2019, August) and considered vehicles for the transfer of pathogens (AST, 2008, 2017, April 14, revised).*
- Visibly soiled, wet, and/or contaminated scrub attire must be changed as soon as possible.
- (Scott, Goodyear, Nicoloro, et al., 2015).
- If you wash your scrubs at home, use warm or hot water and detergent. However, if exposure to multidrug-resistant organisms is possible, then add bleach.
    - Home laundering of surgical attire is not recommended. *Significantly higher bacteria counts were isolated from home-laundered scrubs than from hospital-laundered scrubs (Nordstrom et al., 2011).*

Spills and Waste

- Empty and clean bedpans, urinals, and emesis basins immediately after use.
- Place soiled dressings, drains, and so forth in appropriate waterproof bags for disposal, never in an open trash can.
- Wipe up small spills from tabletops and floors. Notify the housekeeping or environmental services department for large spills.

Needles and Sharps

✚ Do not recap, bend, break, or hand-manipulate used needles. If recapping is necessary, use a one-handed "scoop" technique. Place used sharps in puncture-resistant containers.

Practice Resources
AORN (2022); AST (2008, 2015, 2017, revised); CDC (2002); Nordstrom, et al. 2011; Siegel, Rhinehart, Jackson, et al. (2022, updated).

Clinical Insight 20-3 ➤ Following CDC Standard Precautions

Key Point: Standard precautions (Tier 1) apply to all clients and should be used whenever there is a possibility of coming in contact with blood, body fluids (except sweat), excretions and secretions, mucous membranes, and breaks in the skin.

These precautions protect you from exposure to potential pathogens, decrease the likelihood that you will transmit pathogens among patients, and protect the patient from microorganisms that you may carry.

✚ Assume that every person may be infected or colonized with an organism that could be transmitted to others.

STANDARD PRECAUTIONS	RECOMMENDATIONS
Hand Hygiene	▪ Perform hand hygiene after touching blood, body fluids, secretions, excretions, or contaminated items; immediately after removing gloves; and between patient contacts. Refer to Clinical Insight 20-1 for details.
Respiratory Hygiene/Cough Etiquette for Patients	▪ Instruct symptomatic persons to cover mouth/nose when sneezing/coughing.
	▪ Provide and use tissues and dispose in a no-touch container.
	▪ Perform hand hygiene after soiling hands with respiratory secretions or after using a tissue or covering the mouth/nose.
	▪ Wear a surgical mask if tolerated or do not come within 3 feet of another person if possible. Some patients may not be able to tolerate the decreased oxygen that is available when breathing room air through a mask.
Masks and Eye Protection (for the Nurse)	▪ Wear a mask and eye protection or a face shield to protect mucous membranes of the eyes, nose, and mouth during patient care activities that are likely to generate splashes or sprays of blood, body fluids, secretions, and excretions.
Patient Placement	Pace in a single-patient room if:
	▪ The patient is at increased risk of transmitting or acquiring infection.
	▪ Does not maintain appropriate hygiene
	▪ Is likely to contaminate the environment
	▪ Is at increased risk of developing an adverse outcome after infection
Gowns	▪ Wear a clean, nonsterile, nonpermeable gown during procedures and activities when you anticipate contact of clothing or exposed skin with blood or body fluids, secretions, and excretions (e.g., when there is a risk of spray or splash onto clothing).
	▪ Promptly remove the gown once it is soiled. Avoid contaminating clothing when removing the gown.
	▪ Perform hand hygiene after removing the gown.
	▪ See Procedures 20-2 and 20-3, Donning PPE and Removing PPE.
Needles and Sharps	▪ ✚ Never recap, bend, or break used needles; or otherwise manipulate them using both hands; or use any other technique that involves directing the point of a needle toward any part of the body. Instead, use either a one-handed "scoop" technique or a mechanical device designed for holding the needle sheath (see Procedure 26-10, Recapping needles).
	▪ Use safety features when available.
	▪ Place sharps in puncture-resistant containers for disposal.

(Continued)

Clinical Insight 20-3 ▶ Following CDC Standard Precautions—cont'd

STANDARD PRECAUTIONS	RECOMMENDATIONS
Patient Resuscitation	▪ Use one-way valve mouthpieces, resuscitation bags, or other ventilation devices as an alternative to mouth-to-mouth resuscitation methods in situations when the need for resuscitation is predictable. *To prevent contact between rescuer's and client's mucous membranes and airflow, preventing transmission of microorganisms.*
Soiled Patient Care Equipment, Environment, Textiles, and Laundry	▪ Wear gloves if the equipment or laundry is visibly contaminated. ▪ Handle equipment, textiles, and laundry in a manner to prevent transfer of microorganisms to others and the environment. ▪ Perform hand hygiene. ▪ Develop procedures for routine care, cleaning, and disinfection of environmental surfaces, especially frequently touched surfaces in patient care areas.
Gloves	**When to Wear** ▪ If you have an area of irritation or a break in the skin, wear gloves or apply an occlusive dressing during patient contact. ▪ Wear gloves when contact with blood or other potentially infectious materials, mucous membranes, and nonintact skin could occur. **When to Remove or Change** ▪ Remove gloves immediately after caring for a patient. Avoid touching clean items, environmental surfaces, or another patient. ▪ Do not wear the same gloves for care of more than one patient; do not wash gloves and reuse gloves between patient contact. ▪ Change gloves during patient care if moving from a contaminated body site to a clean site. ▪ Change gloves between tasks or procedures on the same patient if you have made contact with material that may contain a high concentration of microorganisms. **Use and Storage** ▪ When preparing for a procedure, first collect equipment and place at the bedside ready for use; then perform hand hygiene and don gloves just before performing the procedure. Donning gloves ahead of time increases the risk for contamination before the procedure. ▪ Do not carry gloves in your pocket. Keep them in their original box and remove them when and where required. ▪ Do not store gloves on top of trash containers or on windowsills. ▪ ✚ Hand washing or disinfection is required regardless of whether gloves are used or changed. Gloves are not completely impermeable to microorganisms; furthermore, they may leak or tear. Hands can be easily contaminated when removing gloves as well.

Practice Resources

Boyce & Pittet (2002); CDC (n.d.b.; 2016, January 26; 2017, January 16); Pratt, Pellowe, Wilson, et al. (2007); Siegel, Rhinehart, Jackson, et al. (2022, updated).

Clinical Insight 20-4 ▶ Following Transmission-Based Precautions

When to Use: Use transmission-based (Tier 2) precautions when the routes of transmission are not completely interrupted using standard precautions alone. Refer to Clinical Insight 20-3 if you need to review standard precautions.

Pathogens may be transmitted by contact, droplet, or air. Each mode of transmission requires a unique approach to prevent infection and has a unique set of precautions.

Contact Precautions

When to Use: Use contact precautions when **direct contact** with the patient or the patient's environment (e.g., draining wounds, dressings, patient supplies, and secretions) can lead to spread of the pathogen. **Indirect contact,** or contact with fomites, can also transmit pathogens that spread by this method.

Patient Placement and Transport
- Consult with an infection preventionist for patient placement.
- Place in a private room when possible.
- If no private room is available, place patient in a room with a patient with an active infection caused by the same organism and no other infections.
- When transporting the patient, ensure that infected or colonized areas of the body are contained and covered.
- *Ambulatory care:* Place the patient in an examination room or cubicle as soon as possible.

Personal Protective Equipment
- Don clean, nonsterile gloves for any contact with the patient's intact skin. Put them on when entering the room.
- Wear a clean gown if you anticipate your clothing may contact the patient or any contaminated items in the room.
- Remove PPE and observe hand hygiene before leaving the room. Be careful that your skin and clothing do not contact environmental surfaces on the way out of the room.

Equipment, Supplies, and Environment
- Keep contact precaution supplies on a cart just outside the patient's room.
- Double bag all linen and trash (or use a single waterproof bag), and clearly mark as contaminated.
- Use disposable equipment (e.g., blood pressure cuffs) if possible; otherwise, clean and disinfect the equipment per institutional policy before removing them from the room and before using on another patient.
- Ensure that the patient room is cleaned and disinfected at least daily.
- *Home care:* Limit the amount of nondisposable equipment brought into the home. If possible, leave the equipment in the home until discharge from home care. If not, disinfect items or place them in a plastic bag for sanitation and transport to a reprocessing area.

Other
- Follow any additional precautions specific to the microorganism.
- Discontinue contact precautions according to pathogen-specific recommendations.

Droplet Precautions

When to Use: Droplets can spread infection by direct contact with mucous membranes or through indirect contact—for example, suctioning or touching a bedside table that was contaminated with droplets and then rubbing your eyes. Use droplet precautions when the pathogen can be spread via moist, large droplets (e.g., sneezing, coughing, talking).

Patient Placement and Transport
- If no private room, ensure that the patients are physically separated by more than 3 feet. Keep the privacy curtain closed. Consult with an infection preventionist for patient placement. *A private room provides the most effective protection.*
- Limit transport outside the room to medically necessary purposes; if transport is necessary, the patient should wear a mask.

Personal Protective Equipment
- Keep droplet precaution supplies on a cart just outside the patient's room.
- Wear a mask when working within 3 feet of the patient. Don the mask on entry into the room. Whether to wear goggles is an unresolved issue. Follow agency policy.
- Change PPE and perform hand hygiene between contact with patients in the same room, regardless of whether one or both patients are on droplet precautions.

Other
- Instruct patients to cough or sneeze in an elbow or cover nose and mouth with tissue.
- Discontinue droplet precautions according to pathogen-specific recommendations.

(Continued)

Clinical Insight 20-4 ▶ Following Transmission-Based Precautions—cont'd

Airborne Precautions

When to Use: Use airborne precautions to control the spread of infections that are transmitted person to person on air currents (e.g., ventilation system, fanning sheets, sweeping the floor).

Patient Placement and Transport
- Place the patient in an airborne infection isolation room (AIIR)—one with negative pressure that discharges and exchanges the air outside or through a high-efficiency particulate air (HEPA) filtration system. Monitor air pressure daily (usually this is via an electronic device with an alarm).
- If such a room is not available, transfer the patient to a facility where one is available.
- Keep the room door closed when not required for entry and exit (to maintain the negative pressure and contain the airborne organisms).
- In the event of an outbreak involving large numbers of patients who require airborne precautions, consult with infection preventionists for patient placement.
- Limit moving the patient outside the room to medically necessary purposes. If transport is necessary, cover any infectious skin lesions and have the patient wear a mask. Notify the receiving department to take airborne precautions.
- *Ambulatory or emergency care:* Triage and identify patients with suspected airborne precautions upon entry to the agency. Place the patient in an AIIR as soon as possible. If one is not available, place a mask on the patient and place them in an examination room. Do not reuse the room for at least an hour after the patient leaves it, or according to agency policy.

Personal Protective Equipment
- Keep airborne isolation supplies on a cart just outside the patient's room.
- Don a mask on entering the room. Wear a special, fit-tested, approved mask (e.g., N-95 respirator) if the patient is suspected of having pulmonary tuberculosis or smallpox.
- Remove your respirator/mask outside the room after closing the door. If the respirator is not disposable, clean and store according to the manufacturer's instructions.
- When using a respirator mask, check the seal. Hold your hands over the respirator and exhale. If you feel air around your nose, adjust the nosepiece; if you feel air at the edges, adjust the straps.
- When the patient has rubeola, chickenpox, or disseminated zoster, CDC makes no recommendation about use of PPE if, based on your history of vaccination or disease, you think you are presumed immune to the disease. If the hospitalized patient has or is suspected of having rubeola or varicella, only immunized caregivers should provide care.

Other
- Discontinue airborne precautions according to pathogen-specific recommendations of the CDC.
- Tape a waterproof bag to the bedside. *To facilitate proper disposal of tissues.*

Practice Resources
CDC (2017, March 15, updated); CDC (2017, March 15, updated); Pratt, Pellowe, Wilson, et al. (2007); Siegel, Rhinehart, Jackson, et al. (2022, May, updated).

DIAGNOSTIC TESTING

Common Tests for Evaluating the Presence of or Risk for Infection

TEST	DESCRIPTION
White blood cell (WBC) count with differential	A breakdown of the number and types of WBCs; normal WBC count is 5,000–10,000/mm^3.
Blood cultures	A sample of blood placed on culture media and evaluated for growth of pathogens. Normally should show no growth of infectious microorganisms.
Urine cultures	Urine is normally sterile with no microorganism growth.
Throat cultures, wound cultures	Presence of microorganisms is normal, but there should be no growth of infectious microorganisms. To yield the most reliable results, blood cultures should be obtained from peripheral sites, using venipuncture by trained phlebotomists, unless a culture is specifically ordered from a central catheter or peripherally inserted central catheter.
Disease titers	Blood tests for specific disease immunity (e.g., to rubella)
Panels to evaluate specific disease exposure	Blood tests to evaluate exposure to specific diseases (e.g., HIV, hepatitis)
Immunoglobulin (IgG, IgM) levels	Blood tests to evaluate humoral immunity status
C-reactive protein (CRP)	A blood test to measure inflammatory change or bacterial infection
Agglutinins, warm or cold	Used to diagnose atypical infections by detecting antigens in the blood
Erythrocyte (red blood cell) sedimentation rate (ESR or sed rate)	A measure of inflammatory changes. Sed rate increases with inflammation. Normally it is at 15 mm/hr for men and <20 mm/hr for women.
Iron level	Normally 60–90 grams/100 mg. Lower in chronic infection

CLINICAL REASONING
Applying the Full-Spectrum Nursing Model

PATIENT SITUATION

Mr. Long, a frail older man, is in the hospital because he has become dehydrated and needs intravenous fluids and other supportive care. The nurse administered intravenous fluids. Mr. Long also has a large pressure injury, which was cultured recently and found to be infected with **Staphylococcus aureus**. The nurse wore gloves to treat the injury. While doing so, she noticed that the IV was infusing too fast and, without thinking, regulated the IV without removing her soiled gloves. The next nurse to regulate the IV did so with her bare hands, and then, without realizing it, rubbed her neck. Later, the nurse developed a boil on her neck, which was infected with S. aureus.

THINKING

1. *Theoretical Knowledge:*

   a. What are the six links in the chain of infection?

   b. Why do you think the *S. aureus* was able to thrive in Mr. Long's pressure injury?

   c. What are the three modes of transmission of microorganisms? Which one is the most frequent mode of transmission?

2. *Critical Thinking (Reflecting):*

   a. What was the reservoir for the *S. aureus*?

   b. What was the exit from Mr. Long?

   c. What was (were) the fomite(s) for transmission to the nurse?

   d. What was the portal of entry into the nurse?

DOING

3. *Nursing Process (Implementation):* In addition to wearing gloves, what other PPE (if any) does the nurse need if she is performing decubitus care and changing Mr. Long's bed linens?

CARING

4. *Self-Knowledge and Ethical Knowledge:* Think of one instance in the clinical setting in which you did *not* follow standard precautions. Why do you think that happened?

Critical Thinking and Clinical Judgment

1. You notice that your clinical instructor is not washing their hands between patients. What should you do?

2. As you are gowning and gloving for your first experience in the operating room, you become nervous and forget the proper procedure for applying sterile surgical garb. How should you handle this situation?

3. What action should you take if you contaminate yourself while gowning and gloving?

4. Refer to Procedure 20-7, the open method for donning sterile gloves. In the photograph at Step 7, you can see that the nurse has a sterile glove on her right hand and is touching the glove with her bare left hand. Is the nurse breaking the "sterile-touches-sterile" principle? Explain your thinking.

5. Refer to Procedure 20-6, the closed method of donning a sterile gown and gloves. Examine the very last photograph, in which one nurse is preparing to turn and receive her gown tie from a coworker. The gowned nurse has already donned sterile gloves using the closed method. When the gowned nurse turns to receive the tie, what must she take care not to touch? What can she touch?

6. For each of the following concepts, use critical thinking to describe how or why it is important to nursing, patient care, or promoting asepsis and preventing infection. Note that these are *not* to be merely definitions.

Chain of infection	Standard precautions
Pathogens	Transmission-based precautions
Asepsis	Protective isolation
Healthcare-related infections	Sterile
Multidrug-resistant organisms (MDROs)	Medical asepsis
Contamination	Surgical asepsis

What Are the Main Points in This Chapter?

- The chain of infection consists of six links that must all be present for infection to be transmitted from one individual to another: infectious agent, reservoir, portal of exit, mode of transmission, portal of entry, and susceptible host.
- Pathogens are strains of bacteria, viruses, fungi, protozoa, helminths, and prions that cause disease.
- Drug-resistant and multidrug-resistant organisms (MDROs) have mutated to develop resistance to one or more classes of antimicrobial drugs. They are a serious problem because (1) options for treating MDRO infections are limited; (2) they are associated with serious illness, increased hospitalization, and higher death rates; and (3) they are associated with serious illness and increased mortality.
- Many emerging pathogens are airborne and widely spread before the carrier shows any symptoms. They have the potential for causing epidemics and pandemics.
- Infectious illnesses typically follow five predictable stages: incubation, prodromal stage, illness, decline, and convalescence.
- Primary body defenses, such as intact skin and mucous membranes, block entry of pathogens into the body.
- Invading microorganisms trigger the body's secondary defenses, which include phagocytosis, the complement cascade, the inflammatory response, and fever.
- The humoral immune response results in the production of antibodies that neutralize pathogens or trigger their destruction.
- The cell-mediated immune response results in the production of T cells that destroy infected body cells.
- Nutrition, hygiene, rest, exercise, stress reduction, and immunization protect the body against infection.
- Anything that weakens the body's defenses or increases the person's exposure to pathogens makes the person more susceptible to infection. Such factors include illness, injury, medical treatment and certain medications, infancy or advanced age, frequent public contact, and various lifestyle habits.
- Medical asepsis requires that objects and surfaces in the healthcare environment be disinfected.
- Thorough hand washing markedly decreases the transmission of infection and is the most important aspect of medical asepsis.
- Standard precautions are used with all clients whenever there is a possibility of contact with blood, body fluids (except sweat), excretions and secretions, mucous membranes, and break in the skin.
- Transmission-based precautions are added to standard precautions when there is concern about transmission of infection via contact, droplets, or air currents.
- Isolation precautions are designed to prevent the spread of disease, not to isolate the person who has the disease.
- Surgical asepsis reduces patient contact with *any* microorganisms.
- Sterile technique is required in many patient treatments, such as administering an injection, starting an intravenous line, or performing a sterile dressing change.
- Exposure to blood, body secretions, or body tissues containing blood or secretions requires immediate action. Minimize the exposure by washing hands or flushing the area thoroughly. Contact the infection preventionist or employee health nurse as soon after the exposure as possible, complete an incident report, and seek medical care.
- The task of the infection preventionist is to minimize the number of infections in the healthcare facility.
- A key factor in minimizing infectious outbreaks is recognizing unusual disease patterns.

Knowledge Map

RISK FACTORS
- Developmental stage
- Break in 1st line defense
- Illness/injury
- Chronic illness
- Lifestyle choices:
  - Smoking
  - Substance abuse
  - Sex practices
- Environment
- Medications
- Medical/nursing procedures

TYPES:
- Local
- Systemic
  - Bacteremia
  - Septicemia
- Primary
- Secondary
- Nosocomial
  - Endogenous
  - Exogenous
- Acute
- Chronic
- Latent

STAGES:
- Incubation
- Prodromal
- Illness
- Decline
- Convalescence

MULTIDRUG-RESISTANT ORGANISMS (MDROs)
- MRSA
- VRE
- Clostridium difficile

AGENT → RESERVOIR → PORTAL OF EXIT → TRANSMISSION → PORTAL OF ENTRY → SUSCEPTIBLE HOST → INFECTION

PROMOTING ASEPSIS

PREVENTING INFECTION

MEDICAL ASEPSIS:
- Clean environment
  - Disinfect
- Handwashing
  - Time
  - Water
  - Soap
  - Friction
  - Drying
- Protective environment
- Preventing MDROs

CDC TIERS:
Tier One:
- Standard precautions

Tier Two:
- Transmission-based precautions
  - Contact
  - Droplet
  - Airborne

SURGICAL ASEPSIS:
- Sterile environment
- Surgical scrub
- Surgical attire
- Sterile technique
- Sterile field

SUPPORTING HOST DEFENSES:
- Adequate nutrition
- Hygiene
- Rest and exercise
- Decrease stress
- Immunizations

HOST DEFENSES:
Primary: skin, respiratory tree, eyes, GI/GU tract
Secondary: phagocytosis, complement, inflammatory response, fever
Tertiary: humoral/cell-mediated immune responses

CHAPTER 21

Promoting Safety

STUDENT RESOURCES

The questions and exercises in this book allow you to practice the kind of thinking you will use as a full-spectrum nurse. Critical-thinking questions usually have more than one right answer, so we do not provide "correct" answers for these features. It is more important to develop your nursing judgment than to just cover content. You will learn more by discussing the questions with your peers. If you are still unsure, see the Davis Advantage chapter resources for suggested responses.

To explore learning resources for this chapter,

Go to www.DavisAdvantage.com and find:

Answers and Suggested Responses for all questions in this chapter
Concept Map
Knowledge Map
References and Bibliography

Key Concepts
Safety
Patient safety

Related Concepts
See the Concept Map on Davis Advantage.

Example Client Condition
Falls

Caring for the Williams Family

Refer to the assessment data for Stanley Williams in Volume 1 of this book. Use full-spectrum thinking to identify safety hazards for Mr. Williams; his 3-year-old grandchild Kayla Robinson, who lives with him; and his older sister, Naomi Jackson, who lives alone.

(Continued)

331

Caring for the Williams Family (continued)

A. Without even using any of Mr. Williams' patient assessment data (except ages), what theoretical knowledge do you have that will help you to identify risks that commonly occur in the developmental stages represented by these three clients?
Mr. Williams
Mr. Williams' 3-year-old grandchild, Kayla
Mr. Williams' older sister, Naomi

B. From Mr. Williams' assessment, what data can you put with your theoretical knowledge to identify the most likely safety risks for him? What are those risks?

C. From the risks and possible risks you have identified, for which one do you definitely need more data before deciding whether it increases his risk for accidents? That is, which piece of data is especially vague? What do you need to find out?

D. You know the theoretical (or possible) risks for Mr. Williams' sister, Naomi. What data do you need in order to determine her *actual* safety risks?

E. What, if any, data do you have that would help you to identify any *actual* safety risks for Mr. Williams' grandchild? What, if any, are those risks?

F. What would you want to assess at the child's preschool to be sure that safety measures exist for preventing falls?

Practical Knowledge clinical application

Nursing interventions to promote safety in the home focus mainly on patient teaching. In inpatient facilities, however, you will take a more proactive role in preventing injury to patients. You will need skills and techniques to prevent falls and to apply and manage restraints safely.

PROCEDURES

Procedure 21-1 ■ Using Bed and Chair Monitoring Devices

▶ For steps to follow in *all* procedures, refer to the Universal Steps for All Procedures on the inside back cover.

Equipment

Bed or chair exit monitoring device

At least four types of notification systems are used to warn caregivers that a patient is leaving a bed or chair: (1) pressure sensitive, (2) posture indicators, (3) motion sensors, and (4) pull-cord and combination alarms.

Delegation

As the nurse, you must determine whether a monitoring device is needed. You must also select the appropriate device and provide ongoing evaluation of its effectiveness. You may delegate to an unlicensed assistive personnel (UAP) the installation of the device after verifying the UAP has the necessary knowledge and skill.

Preprocedure Assessments

Assess for intrinsic factors that increase the risk for falls:
- Older than age 75
- History of falling
- Bowel and bladder incontinence (particularly urge bladder incontinence)
- Cognitive impairment
- Mood changes, lability
- Dizziness
- Functional impairment
- Medications (especially new medications or changes)
- Comorbidities (diseases such as dementia, hip fracture, type 2 diabetes, Parkinson disease, arthritis, and depression)
- Identify factors that increase risk for more severe injury in the case of a fall. These include use of anticoagulants (e.g., Coumadin, Plavix, or aspirin) and osteoporosis.

Assess for extrinsic (environmental) factors that increase the risk for falls:
- Use of an assistive device
- Equipment in the room
- Wet or uneven floors
- Use of physical restraints
- Poorly fitting footwear
- Poor lighting
- Lack of grab rails and bars in the bathroom
- Furniture and adaptive aids that are in disrepair or unstable (e.g., bed rails, IV poles)
- Clothing that may cause tripping
- Check the alarm on the monitoring device to ensure that it is working properly.

➤ When performing the procedure, always identify your patient according to agency policy, using two identifiers, and be attentive to standard precautions, hand hygiene, patient safety and privacy, body mechanics, and documentation.

Procedure Steps

1. **Apply the device.**

Variation: Bed or Chair Monitor
Place sensor pads under the patient's buttocks.
The sensor will alarm when the patient attempts to get out of the bed or chair; it alarms when there is no weight on it for more than a few seconds. For some devices, you may need to set the alarm sensitivity. For example, you may set the system to alarm when the patient exits the bed, when the patient attempts to exit the bed, or even when the patient moves in the bed. ▼

Variation: Leg Sensors
Place sensors on the patient's thigh.
The alarm will sound when the leg assumes a near-vertical position. ▼

Variation: Infrared Beam Detector
Attach next to the bed or on the wall. ▼

Variation: Cord-Activated Sensor
Attach one end of the cord (clip) to the patient's garment. Attach the other end to the control unit. The cord should be long enough to allow moderate movements but short enough to prevent false alarms. Be sure the cord is free to pull straight out from the monitor and is not blocked by pillows, bedding, or bed rails. *The alarm is activated when the patient's movement causes the cord to be detached from the control unit. Some patients will deactivate the alarms, including removing the alarms clipped to their garments.* ▼

2. **Connect the control unit to the sensor pad.**

Variation: Bed or Chair Monitor
Mount the control unit on the bed or chair.

(continued on next page)

Procedure 21-1 ■ Using Bed and Chair Monitoring Devices (continued)

Variation: Leg Sensor
Mount the control unit directly on the leg sensor.

Variation: Infrared System
Mount the control unit next to the bed or on the wall.

Variation: Cord-Activated System
Mount the control unit next to the bed or on the wall.

3. **Connect the control unit** to the nurse call system, if possible.
   Allows for a quicker response; however, not all call systems will accommodate this

4. **Before assisting the patient out of the bed** or chair, disconnect or turn off the alarm.
   Prevents false alarms. Some systems have a standby setting to allow the alarm to be temporarily suspended.

5. **Reactivate the alarm** after assisting the patient back to the bed or chair.
   Helps improve the timeliness of staff response, which may prevent patient falls

6. **Be sure the patient can access** the nurse call light easily.

Evaluation

- Assess the sensitivity of the monitoring device, and adjust as needed to ensure that the alarm is activated if the patient tries to get out of the bed or chair.
- Continue to assess fall risk per agency policy and as indicated by the patient's physical and/or mental status.
- In the event of a fall, perform a postfall assessment to identify possible causes. Monitor patients closely for 48 hours after a fall.

Patient Teaching

- Explain to the patient and family that a bed or chair exit monitoring device alerts the staff when the patient tries to get out of the chair or bed.
- To reassure the patient and family, explain that the purpose of the device is to help prevent falls using the least restrictive method possible.
- Explain to the patient that they will need to call for assistance when they want to get up.
  Calling for assistance will prevent the alarm from sounding. Summoning for help can prevent the patient from falling.

Documentation

- Document the initial sensor placement, including type of sensor used and the location of placement.
- After documenting initial placement, follow agency policy for documenting the use of bed exit monitor. Usually, the minimum documentation for exit monitors is every 8 hours.
- Place the patient on fall risk precautions according to agency policy.
- Document on the fall risk assessment sheet, restraint flowsheet, and nursing notes according to agency policy.

Sample Documentation

mm/dd/yy   1230.   Continues to be confused and to stand up without assistance. Wheelchair exit alarm placed on wheelchair and monitoring clip attached to back of client's gown. Notified client's daughter, June Kennedy, via telephone. Daughter agreed the exit alarm would help keep her mother from falling. ———— Mary Clinton, RN

Practice Resources
Agency for Healthcare Research and Quality (AHRQ). (2018); Gray-Micelli, D., & Quigley, P. (2016).

Thinking About the Procedure

The video **Using Bed and Chair Monitoring Devices**, along with questions and suggested responses, is available on the **Davis's Nursing Skills Videos** Web site at www.fadavis.com.

Procedure 21-2 ■ Using Restraints

▶ For steps to follow in *all* procedures, refer to the Universal Steps for All Procedures on the inside back cover.

▶ **Caution:** This procedure describes Medicare standards, but state and agency policies may be more restrictive.

Equipment

- Restraint of the appropriate size: belt, vest, wrist or ankle, or mitt
- Soft gauze or cotton padding for bony prominences

Delegation

As the nurse, you must determine whether restraints are needed in each specific situation. You must also select the least restrictive type of restraints, evaluate their effectiveness, and continue to assess for complications that may occur. You may delegate to UAPs the application and periodic removal of ordered restraints after verifying that the UAP has the knowledge and skill to do so.

Preprocedure Assessments

- Assess the patient's risk for falls, including mobility status and level of awareness.
- Assess for need for restraints: the immediate physical safety of the patient, a staff member, or others is threatened.
  If a patient must be temporarily restrained so that a procedure may be performed, this is not considered restraint.
- Determine that all less restrictive interventions have been tried unsuccessfully.
- Identify the appropriate restraint:
  - Is the least restrictive possible
  - Does not interfere with care or exacerbate patient's medical condition
  - Does not pose a safety risk to the patient
  - Can be changed easily to keep it clean

> When performing the procedure, always identify your patient according to agency policy, using two identifiers, and be attentive to standard precautions, hand hygiene, patient safety and privacy, body mechanics, and documentation.

Procedure Steps

1. **Determine whether dangerous** behaviors continue despite attempts to eliminate causal factors using less restrictive interventions.

2. **Obtain a physician's prescription** for restraint, including type of restraint, indications for use, site of restraint application, and duration. Determine whether the restraint is being used for medical-surgical or behavioral reasons.
   Federal and state regulations and laws permit healthcare facilities to use restraints only when they are medically needed. Restraints can be used only with a physician's or advanced practice nurse's order for a specified and limited time. When you apply restraint in an emergency, obtain the order as the restraint is being applied or as quickly as possible afterward. When the restraint prescription expires (maximum 24 hours), physician assessment and a new prescription are needed.

3. **Notify the family of the change** in patient status and the need for restraints. Obtain patient and family consent when clinically feasible.
   Patients have the right to refuse treatment. Consent may not be necessary if there is an immediate threat to patient safety; however, as a rule, the family must be notified of the use of restraints if the patient has cognitive impairment. Many times family members prefer to sit with the patient as an alternative to restraint.

4. ✚ **Pad bony prominences** and apply the appropriately sized restraint using appropriate knotting techniques.
   - Use a quick-release knot, such as the half-bow, when tying restraints to the bed frame or wheelchair.
   - Do not tie restraints to the side rails. ▼

A quick-release knot is used to prevent patient injury and for ease of caring for the patient. Tie the knot on an immovable part of the bed to prevent injuring the patient if the side rails or head of bed is lowered. A quick-release knot will not tighten or slip when the patient moves about, but it unties quickly when you pull on the loose end.

Variation: Belt Restraint

a. Place the belt restraint at the patient's waist, removing any wrinkles.
b. Make sure that the belt is snug but does not constrict the patient's waist.
c. Some belts have a key-locked buckle to prevent slipping.
   A belt restraint is used mainly to prevent a patient from falling when getting up from a chair or wheelchair and may be used to remind a patient not to get out of bed unassisted. ▼

(continued on next page)

Procedure 21-2 ■ Using Restraints (continued)

Variation: Vest or Jacket Restraint

d. Place the patient in the vest restraint. A zipper-style vest is preferred.
   A vest restraint with a rear zipper is less likely to accidentally strangle the patient.
e. Attach the vest straps to the bed or wheelchair.
   A vest restraint is used mainly to prevent a patient from falling out of a chair or wheelchair and sometimes to prevent a patient from getting out of bed unassisted. ▼

Variation: Wrist or Ankle Restraint

f. Apply the padded portion of the wrist or ankle restraint around the patient's wrist or ankle.
g. Make the restraint snug enough to prevent the patient from being able to slip it off but not tight enough to impair circulation.
h. Attach the restraint strap to the bed frame. Do not attach to bed rails.
   A wrist restraint is used mainly to prevent an agitated patient from pulling at tubes, such as IV sites and nasogastric tubes. ▼

Variation: Mitt Restraint

i. Place patient's hand in the mitt restraint, ensuring that fingers are slightly flexed in the mitt.
j. Attach restraint strap to the bed frame if necessary.
   A mitt restraint is used mainly to prevent a patient from pulling at tubes, such as IV sites and nasogastric tubes. Mitt restraints limit the use of the fingers, which may be enough to prevent the patient from grasping the tube. If this is the case, mitts that are not tied to the bed frame are the least restrictive restraint. ▼

Variation: Enclosed Bed

k. Place patient in the bed and zip all sides. Be sure zippers are completely closed and zipper tabs are positioned in the upper aspects of the net panels out of the patient's reach.
l. Adhere to the manufacturer's minimum height and weight recommendations.
m. Never leave the bed in the high position with the patient unattended.
   An enclosed bed is a canopy-like padded bed that is used mainly to keep a patient from wandering or from falling out of bed. The bed has nylon netting on all four sides, with zippered panels that can be opened to provide care. The patient has full freedom of movement and access to all parts of their body. Patients in enclosed beds have a higher risk of becoming entrapped between the bed rails and the mattress, risking suffocation. The dangers are greater for smaller patients and when the bed is left in a high position.

5. **Adjust the restraint** to maintain good body alignment, comfort, and safety. You should be able to slide two fingers under a wrist or ankle restraint.
   The restraint should be snug enough to prevent it from slipping off but not tight enough to impair circulation.

6. **Check restraint every 30 minutes, and release restraints at least** every 2 hours to provide skin care, passive and active range of motion (ROM), ambulation, toileting, hydration, and nutrition. Assess for the continued need for restraint.
   Prevents impaired circulation and injury. Medicare- and Medicaid-certified healthcare agencies must ensure that a patient's abilities do not decline unless the decline cannot be avoided because of the patient's medical condition. Patients often lose the ability to bathe, dress, walk, toilet, eat, and communicate when they are regularly restrained. If restraints are necessary, they must be used in a way that does not cause these losses.

7. **Place the patient on fall risk precautions according to agency policy.**
   Patients who are restrained have a higher incidence of falls.

? What if...
- I must apply a restraint in an emergency for the safety of the patient or others?

In such an emergency, an RN may initiate a restraint. When you apply restraint in an emergency, obtain the order as the restraint is being applied or as quickly as possible afterward.

Evaluation
- Assess the initial restraint placement, circulation, and skin integrity. Observe for pallor, cyanosis, and coolness of extremities when extremities are restrained.
- Check the restraint every 30 minutes (more often for a behavioral restraint).
- Reassess the restraint, circulation, the patient's response to the intervention, and the need for continuing the use of the restraint every 2 hours; remove it when it is no longer needed.
- **Key Point:** *Patients in behavioral restraints require more frequent monitoring and in some circumstances require continuous observation.*
  Ensures that the restraint is still functioning as intended. Monitoring and reassessment are critical components of caring for patients in physical restraints. Frequency of monitoring is determined by the type of restraint (behavioral vs. medical-surgical).
- Check every 24 hours to see that the restraint prescription has been renewed.
- Remove the restraint as soon as possible.
- Modify the plan of care to reflect the application of restraints and the plan for monitoring.

Patient Teaching
- Explain to the patient and family the need for the restraints.
- Explain that the restraints will be removed as soon as possible.

Home Care
- The same guidelines apply to clients in the home.
- Evaluate caregivers' knowledge and skill in using restraints, and provide teaching as needed (e.g., regarding padding bony prominences and the need to periodically release restraints).
- If an enclosed bed is used in the home, instruct the caregiver in safe use.

Documentation
Document the following:
- All nursing interventions that were done to eliminate the need for the restraint (e.g., moving patient closer to the nurses' station, asking a family member to remain with the patient, reorienting the patient)
- Reasons for placing the restraint (e.g., patient behaviors)
- The initial restraint placement, location, circulation, and skin integrity
- The teaching session with the patient and family members
- Circulation checks, ROM, and restraint removal per agency protocol
- Entries on fall risk assessment sheet, restraint flowsheet, and nursing notes according to agency policy

Sample Documentation
mm/dd/yyyy   1230.   Continues to be confused, pulling at IV lines. Physician notified and evaluated patient. Mitt restraints ordered and placed on bilateral hands. Fall risk precautions initiated. Mitt restraints explained to patient and wife. Wife agreed that mitt restraints would help keep her husband from removing IV line. ——— Mary Clinton, RN

Practice Resources
American Nurses Association (ANA). (2012); Centers for Medicare & Medicaid Services (2006, revised 2020).

Thinking About the Procedure

The video **Using Restraints: Belt Restraint, Mitt Restraint, Vest Restraint, and Wrist/Ankle Restraint**, along with questions and suggested responses, is available on the **Davis's *Nursing Skills Videos*** Web site at www.fadavis.com.

CLINICAL INSIGHTS

Clinical Insight 21-1 ▸ Choking Rescue Maneuver

For adults or children over age 12 months: If you suspect airway obstruction in an adult, do the following:
1. Determine whether the victim is able to speak or cough forcefully (other signs include noisy breathing; loss of consciousness; and dusky skin, lips, and nailbeds).
2. Ask, "Are you choking?"
3. If the person cannot speak or indicates they are choking, perform the Heimlich or choking rescue maneuver.

Infants under 1 year: Management of choking is for adults and children. Do not use the Heimlich maneuver for infants under 1 year of age.
1. Determine that the infant is choking. Before performing the choking maneuver, be certain that the airway is completely blocked: the infant cannot cough, breathe, or cry. The infant might also have high-pitched, noisy breathing; rib and sternal retractions; and bluish lips or skin.
2. Call 911. Send someone to do that for you, if possible.
3. Deliver back blows:
   - Sit and rest your forearm on your thigh.
   - Place the infant facedown along your forearm, head lower than the body. Support the chest and jaw in your hand. Don't cover the infant's mouth.
- With the heel of your other hand, deliver five rapid blows to the infant's back between the shoulder blades.
- For a summary and illustration of choking first aid for an infant under 1 year, go to MedlinePlus at this URL:

  ▸ https://medlineplus.gov/ency/presentations/100221_1.htm

- You can obtain a summary and illustration of the Heimlich maneuver at the U.S. National Library of Medicine, MedlinePlus, at this URL:

  ▸ https://medlineplus.gov/ency/imagepages/18152.htm

- There is also a YouTube video:

  ▸ https://youtu.be/XOTbjDGZ7wg

Clinical Insight 21-2 ▸ Preventing Needlestick Injury

Use needleless systems (e.g., retractable needles) when possible. More than 80% of needlestick injuries can be prevented with the use of safe needle devices (ANA, 2002).

For more discussion on handling needles safely,

▸ Go to Chapter 26, **Procedure 23-10B: Recapping Sterile Needles,** in Volume 2.

Before beginning a procedure:
- Provide adequate lighting and space to perform the procedure.
- Place the sharps container near the work area, if it is moveable.
- Obtain assistance if there is a risk the patient may be uncooperative, combative, or confused.
- Inform the patient about the procedure and explain the importance of avoiding any sudden movement.

During the procedure:
- Be sure you can see the sharps container at all times.
- When handling a sharp, be aware of other persons in the immediate area.
- Do not hand-pass exposed sharps from one person to another.
- When using a safety needle, observe for audio or visual cues that the feature has engaged.

Handling needles:
- Do not shear or break contaminated needles.
- Avoid recapping, bending, or removing contaminated needles and other sharps unless there is no feasible alternative.
- When you must recap a sterile needle, use a mechanical recapping device or a modified "scoop" technique (see Procedure 23-10).
- Never carry syringes in your uniform pocket.

Sharps containers:
- Keep puncture-proof needle disposal containers in every room.
- Place sharps containers at eye level; do not overfill the container.
- Make sure the container is large enough to hold the entire sharp device.

Clinical Insight 21-2 ➤ Preventing Needlestick Injury—cont'd

- Dispose of sharps immediately. Do not wait until you have finished the procedure.
- Inspect sharps and waste containers for protruding sharps. If found, notify safety personnel for removal of the hazard.

If your agency does not use needleless systems or protective devices, you should do the following:

- Explain the OSHA Bloodborne Pathogens Standard (BPS) to your employer, including the need to provide needleless systems or protective devices for blood products and parenteral medication administration.

   ➤ Refer your employer to the OSHA Web site at https://www.osha.gov/bloodborne-pathogens/quick-reference.

- OSHA requires worker involvement in evaluating, selecting, and implementing the use of safer needle products; volunteer to serve on that committee.
- Ask your agency for a copy of their exposure control plan, which is required by the BPS for monitoring compliance with the new law.
- Keep a record of needlestick injuries on your unit and of "near-misses" (e.g., overfilled sharps containers, sharps left on bed or overbed table).
- Submit written concerns to your employer.
- If your employer refuses to purchase safety devices, you may want to file an OSHA complaint. If you do so, refer to whistleblowing in Chapter 41. Complaints can be filed anonymously.
- For complaint filing,

   ➤ Go to http://www.osha.gov/as/opa/worker/complain.html.

Practice Resources
Adapted from ANA (2002); Centers for Disease Control and Prevention (n.d..); National Institute for Occupational Safety and Health (NIOSH) (n.d., updated 2012.); U.S. Department of Labor, Occupational Safety and Health Administration (OSHA) (n.d.c.).

Clinical Insight 21-3 ➤ What You Should Know About Using Restraints

- **Agency policy,** professional guidelines, and state laws should guide use of restraints.
- **Use restraints only for safety** to ensure the immediate physical safety of the patient or others.
- **You must obtain a medical prescription** from a physician or other licensed care provider.
- **No standing orders** or "as needed" orders for physical restraint are allowed.
- **You must renew restraint prescriptions every 24 hours** (more often for behavioral restraints).
- **You must modify the plan of care** to reflect the application of restraints and the plan for monitoring.
- **Explain the need for the restraints** if you must use them.
- **Obtain consent** from the patient and family when feasible.
- **Medications are considered a restraint** when they are used to restrict the patient's freedom of movement or to manage behavior.
- **Physical holding of a patient is not always considered restraint.** Sometimes it is necessary to use devices or methods that involve the physical holding of a patient for routine physical examinations or tests.
- **Monitor and reassess.** These are critical components of caring for patients in physical restraints. Assess restraints every 30 minutes (more frequently for patients with behavioral restraints, who may need continuous monitoring).
- **Remove restraints for assessment, feeding, toileting, and skin care every 2 hours.** Patients in medical-surgical restraints should be evaluated by an RN at least every 2 hours. Those in behavioral restraints require more frequent monitoring.
- **Always use the least restrictive restraint that ensures safety.**
- **Remove the restraint as soon as possible.**

ASSESSMENT GUIDELINES AND TOOLS

Focused Assessment

SAS Safety Assessment Scale

CLSC CÔTE-DES-NEIGES

Name _____

S.A.S.   SAFETY ASSESSMENT SCALE

CAREGIVER AND LIVING ENVIRONMENT (1)

a) This person lives on her own.   Yes [1]   No [0] _____

b) This person is alone at home.
Always [4]   Most of the time [3]   Occasionally [2]   Never [1] _____

SMOKING (2)
This person leaves cigarette burn marks on the floor, furniture, or clothing.
Yes [1]   No [0] _____

FIRE AND BURNS (3)
a) The stove on/off buttons are located...
on the front of the stove [1]   on the top of the stove [2]
behind the hotplates [3] _____

b) This person is capable of turning on the stove him/herself
Yes [1]   No [0]   Doesn't know [1] _____

c) This person cooks his/her own food.
Always [4]   Most of the time [3]   Occasionally [2]   Never [1] _____

d) This person forgets a pan on the stove.
Very often [4]   Often [3]   Sometimes [2]   Never [1] _____

e) The heating system uses...
electricity [1]   natural gas [2]   wood [3] _____

NUTRITION (4)
a) This person receives meals-on-wheels or other prepared meals.
More than once a day [1]   Once a day [2]
A few times a week (2 to 6 times a week) [3]   Once a week or less [4] _____

b) This person's meals contain foods from different food groups
(dairy products, meat or fish, cereals, fruit and vegetables).
Always [1]   Most of the time [2]   Occasionally [3]   Never [4] _____

FOOD POISONING AND TOXIC SUBSTANCES (5)
This person can tell the difference between food that is fresh and food
that is spoiled.   Yes [0]   No [1] _____

MEDICATION AND HEALTH PROBLEMS (6)
a) This person takes, on a regular basis...*
1 to 3 medications [2]   4 to 6 medications [3]
7 medications or more [4]   Does not take any medication [1]
*prescribed medications only _____

b) This person takes medication to help him/her sleep or relax.
Yes [1]   No [0] _____

c) Does this person suffer from any physical health problem?
None [1]   Minor [2]   Moderate [3]   Severe [4] _____

d) This person accepts treatment for his/her physical health problems.
Yes [0]   No [1]   Does not apply [0] _____

WANDERING AND ADAPTATION TO CHANGING TEMPERATURE (7)
a) This person gets lost in familiar surroundings.
Very often [4]   Often [3]   Sometimes [2]   Never [1] _____

b) Has this person ever gotten lost?   Yes [1]   No [0] _____

c) Can this person find his/her way home?   Yes [0]   No [1] _____

d) Does this person dress appropriately according
to the changing temperature, both indoors and outdoors?
Yes [0]   No [1] _____

An Affiliated University Centre
Affiliated with McGill University

Assessed by _____

SCORE   47

Source: Dr. Louise Poulin de Courval © CLSC Côte-des-Neiges. Used with permission.

Focused Assessment

SAS Safety Assessment Scale—cont'd

Get Up and Go Test

As a nurse, you can perform this test. If the patient has difficulty or unsteadiness, you will need to assess further, so

▸ Go to **Example Client Condition: Falls,** in Volume 1.

Timed Up and Go

For more information about the Timed Up and Go Test,

▸ Go to **Example Client Condition: Falls,** in Volume 1.

You can also see this tool if you

▸ Go to the CDC Web site at https://www.cdc.gov/steadi/pdf/TUG_Test-print.pdf.

CLINICAL REASONING
Applying the Full-Spectrum Nursing Model

PATIENT SITUATION

Recall your patient Alvin Lin from Meet Your Patients scenario in Volume 1. Mr. Lin is a 79-year-old man who was just transferred from a long-term care facility to your medical unit. His admitting diagnoses are dehydration and pneumonia. In the handoff report you were told he had rested well during the night and was alert and oriented. When you enter his room, he is confused and does not know where he is. He is becoming combative and is trying to get out of bed.

THINKING

1. *Theoretical Knowledge:*

    a. What is the pathophysiology of pneumonia?

    b. When the oxygen level of the blood falls, what is the effect on the central nervous system? If you don't know the answer to this question, consult a reliable reference.

    c. What are the major characteristics for the diagnosis fluid volume deficit?

2. *Critical Thinking (Considering Alternatives):*

    a. Which of the three major characteristics (in 1c) may increase Mr. Lin's risk for falls? Why?

    b. What else may be increasing his confusion and his risk for falls?

DOING

3. *Practical Knowledge:* Suppose you have tried all the less restrictive restraints, but Mr. Lin still attempts to get out of bed. He has even pulled out his intravenous line. You decide you must apply restraints to keep him safely in bed. You have called the physician, but he has not returned your call. You cannot wait any longer because you have other patients who need you, yet you must stay with Mr. Lin to keep him from falling. What should you do right now?

4. *Nursing Process (Diagnosis/Analyzing Cues):* Which nursing diagnosis seems more useful to you in planning care for Mr. Lin?

    a. Confusion related to disease process

    b. Risk for falls related to confusion and possibly r/t weakness

CARING

5. *Self-Knowledge:*

    a. Do you think having a restraint-free facility is a valuable goal or not? Explain your thinking.

    b. How did you come to believe that?

6. *Ethical Knowledge:* Suppose Mr. Lin is too confused to give consent for restraints, and you cannot reach his family by telephone. How can you justify applying restraints, and what must you do later to follow up?

Critical Thinking and Clinical Judgment

1. Recall from Meet Your Patients, in Volume 1, the clients you encountered in the community setting. Teresa was caring for her 2-year-old daughter and her elderly grandmother. The grandmother has a fear of falling. In Volume 1, we addressed some of the issues related to childproofing the home. You would like to suggest ways for Teresa to safeproof the home for her frail grandmother.

    a. Refer to the critical-thinking model and questions on the inside back cover of Volume 1 of your textbook. What questions in the Inquiry section should you ask before making suggestions to Teresa?

    b. What specific information do you need about the grandmother? About the home?

    c. Once you have the necessary information, what suggestions could you make about home safety measures?

    d. Consider alternatives. What types of assistive devices might be helpful in preventing falls?

    e. Explore the alternatives. For example, are they practical? What do you need to know about this family to determine whether it is practical for them to obtain such devices?

    f. Think now about Teresa. Given the situation, what might create a safety risk for her?

2. Recall Alvin Lin (Meet Your Patients, in Volume 1), the 79-year-old man you were assigned to care for on your first day on the medical unit. The initial report you received was that he was alert and oriented, but you find that he is now confused and is becoming combative.

    a. What should be your first two priorities in this situation?

    b. What specific patient data do you need to determine what might have caused this change in behavior? How could you get those data?

    c. What alternatives to restraints might you consider?

3. A friend calls to tell you she thinks her 18-month-old daughter swallowed some of your friend's sleeping pills. The child is very sleepy, and your friend is having difficulty rousing her. Your friend has ipecac in her medicine cabinet and wonders whether she should try to get her awake enough to take it.

    a. What is the first thing you would recommend that the mother do?

    b. What is a major concern with inducing vomiting, given that you must assume from the mother that the child is very drowsy? What could go wrong if the child vomits?

    c. If the mother decides to take the daughter to the hospital instead of taking time to call the poison control center (PCC), what should you remind her to take with her?

4. An older couple has health problems, and both are taking several medications. The husband has assumed care for himself and his wife, Ethyl, because Ethyl has been exhibiting confusion at times. He says he sometimes becomes overwhelmed with everything he has to do, and he is not sure that he always gives the medications at the right times.

    a. What information do you need to know to be able to help with this situation? About the medications? About resources? How would you obtain the information?

    b. What suggestions can you make to help the husband organize the medications?

5. You are caring for a patient 12 hours postsurgery after an abdominal hysterectomy for cancer. She asks you to help her to walk to a chair. You note that she has IV fluids infusing and is receiving narcotics via a patient-controlled analgesia (PCA) pump. She states that she has not been out of bed since surgery and that she has just administered some medication and would like to get up while she has pain relief. You also notice that there is a Foley (indwelling urinary) catheter connected to a bedside drainage.

   a. What environmental factors could be safety hazards when this patient gets out of bed?

   b. What assessments and other interventions would help to ensure safe ambulation despite those obstacles?

6. For each of the following concepts, use critical thinking to describe how or why it is important to nursing, patient care, or promoting safety. Note that these are *not* to be merely definitions.

   Environmental hazards
   Pathogens
   Poisoning
   Scald injuries
   Falls
   Teaching firearm safety to children
   Pollution
   Radiation
   Restraint
   Ambularm

   Choking rescue maneuver
   Refrigeration
   Mosquito control
   Rodent control
   Reduce, reuse, recycle, respond
   Back injuries
   Needlestick injuries
   Time, distance, and shielding
   Gang culture
   Morse Fall Scale

What Are the Main Points in This Chapter?

➤ Safety is a basic human need.
➤ Unintentional injuries are the third leading cause of death in the United States.
➤ Major causes of unintentional deaths in the United States are poisoning, motor vehicle accidents, and falls.
➤ The environment includes the physical and psychosocial factors that contribute to the life and well-being of each person. It may be identified as any setting where the nurse and client interact.
➤ A person's safety is influenced by developmental factors as well as individual factors, such as lifestyle, cognitive awareness, sensoriperceptual status, ability to communicate, mobility status, and sensory losses, particularly hearing and vision losses.
➤ The main safety hazards in the home are poisoning, carbon monoxide poisoning, scalds and burns, fires, falls, firearm injuries, suffocation and drowning, and take-home toxins.
➤ Most fatal home fires occur while people are asleep, and most deaths result from smoke inhalation.
➤ More than half of all falls occur in the home; about 80% involve people older than age 65.
➤ Community hazards include motor vehicle accidents, pathogens, improper sanitation, pollution (air, water, noise, and soil), and electrical storms.

➤ Safety hazards in the healthcare agency include falls, equipment-related accidents, fires and electrical hazards, restraints, mercury exposure, and biological hazards.
➤ When possible, nurses should use alternative interventions instead of restraints.
➤ Medical prescriptions for restraints must be renewed at least every 24 hours.
➤ Workplace hazards to nurses include back injuries, needlestick injuries, radiation injury, and violence.
➤ All inpatients should be assessed for their risk for falls.
➤ Identifying anxiety may allow the nurse to intervene before a patient becomes aggressive.
➤ The Heimlich maneuver differs from the American Red Cross choking rescue maneuver in that the Heimlich does not include back blows.
➤ Nursing interventions for promoting safety in the home focus on client teaching.
➤ Nursing interventions for promoting safety in the healthcare facility focus on assessing for risk and creating a safe environment.

Knowledge Map

- Developmental age/stage
- Lifestyle
- Cognitive awareness
- Sensory perceptual status
- Ability to communicate
- Mobility status
- Physical/emotional health
- Awareness of safety measures

Factors affecting ↓

SAFETY

HAZARD IN THE HOME
- Poisoning: household chemicals; medicines; lead
- Carbon monoxide poisoning
- Scalds/burns
- Fires
- Falls
- Firearm injuries
- Suffocation/asphyxiation
- Toxins from workplace

HAZARDS IN THE COMMUNITY
- Motor vehicle accidents
- Environmental pathogens
  - Foodborne
  - Vectorborne
  - Waterborne
- Pollution
- Electrical storms

HAZARDS IN THE HEALTHCARE FACILITY
- Never events
- Falls
- Equipment-related accidents
- Fire hazards
- Electrical hazards
- Restraints
- Mercury poisoning

HAZARDS TO HEALTHCARE WORKERS
- Back injury
- Needlestick injury
- Radiation injury
- Violence in the workplace

GLOBAL NURSING INTERVENTIONS
- Complete fall risk assessment on ALL patients
- Perform a home safety assessment
- Assess for potential violence
- Ongoing assessment for safety issues in the environment
- Modify the environment to minimize hazards
- Ongoing assessment of patient safety needs
- Teach clients about specific safety measures
- SPEAK UP

CHAPTER 22

Facilitating Hygiene

STUDENT RESOURCES

The questions and exercises in this book allow you to practice the kind of thinking you will use as a full-spectrum nurse. Critical-thinking questions usually have more than one right answer, so we do not provide "correct" answers for these features. Try to answer these questions yourself. It is more important to develop your nursing judgment than to just cover content. You will learn more by discussing the questions with your peers. If you are still unsure, see the Davis Advantage chapter resources for suggested responses.

To explore learning resources for this chapter,

Go to www.DavisAdvantage.com and find:

Answers and Suggested Responses for all questions in this chapter
Concept Map
Knowledge Map
References and Bibliography

Key Concepts
Activities of daily living
Hygiene
Self-care ability

Related Concepts
See the Concept Map on Davis Advantage.
Example Client Condition
Hygiene Self-Care Deficit

Caring for the Williams Family

Nadine Williams works as a preschool teacher. She schedules a clinic visit to discuss a variety of concerns. For each of the concerns she mentions, answer the following four questions:

1. What theoretical knowledge do you need?
2. Where could you find it?
3. What, if any, additional patient information do you need?
4. How would you respond to Mrs. Williams' concerns?

(Continued)

Caring for the Williams Family (continued)

A. Nadine tells you that her skin is very dry and irritated.

B. Nadine tells you that several of the children at the preschool have recently been diagnosed with head lice. She would like to know how to assess for pediculosis.

C. Nadine tells you that her 3-year-old granddaughter, Kayla, frequently refuses to bathe. She asks for advice on handling this.

Practical Knowledge
clinical application

The following procedures and clinical insights provide the practical knowledge you will need to assist patients with personal cleanliness and grooming. Patient Teaching and Home Care content in Procedures help you to promote increased activity and independence for patients.

PROCEDURES

Procedure 22-1 ■ Bathing: Providing a Complete Bed Bath Using a Prepackaged Bathing Product

▶ For steps to follow in *all* procedures, refer to the Universal Steps for All Procedures on the inside back cover.

Equipment
- Prepackaged bathing product with disposable wipes (e.g., Comfort Bath)
- Bath blanket
- Clean patient gown (with shoulder snaps or Velcro closures if the patient has an IV line)
- Clean bed linen
- Orangewood stick
- Deodorant, lotion, and/or powder as needed
- Emollient (if not included in prepackaged bathing product)
- Procedure gloves (for anal and perineal care)
- Bedpan or urinal
- Laundry bag
- Plastic trash bag for used wipes and other disposable soiled items ▶

Delegation
You can delegate this procedure to the UAP if you conclude that the patient's condition and the UAP's skills allow. Perform the preprocedure assessments and inform the UAP of the specific type of bath (e.g., packaged bath, basin and water bath); the amount of help the patient needs; and any special considerations, such as IV lines, drains, and so on. Ask the UAP to report the condition of the patient's skin, level of self-care, and ability to tolerate the procedure.

Preprocedure Assessments
- Assess mobility, activity tolerance, type of bath needed, and level of ability to perform bathing self-care.
  A patient who has decreased activity tolerance or mobility (e.g., chest pain or shortness of breath with exertion) may have limited ability to assist with the bath. Having the patient assist as much as possible increases mobility and sense of control and comfort.

- Check for positioning or activity restrictions (e.g., maintaining hip abduction after a total hip replacement).
  Prevents injuring the patient during the procedure.
- Determine the number of people you need to safely bathe and reposition the patient.
  Helps prevent injury to the patient or the nurse.
- Assess for personal and cultural issues that may be of concern to the patient regarding the bath.
  Bathing may conflict with the patient's sense of privacy or modesty. Cultural norms and individual preferences must be considered.
- Assess for specific patient needs and preferences during a bath, such as lotions and extra wipes or towels.
  Advanced age, certain skin conditions, or skin breakdown may require special soaps and/or lotions. Incontinence or drainage may require additional wipes, towels, and precautions. Meeting patient preferences helps prevent depersonalization and promotes patient cooperation with the procedure.

➤ When performing the procedure, always identify your patient according to agency policy, using two identifiers, and be attentive to standard precautions, hand hygiene, patient safety and privacy, body mechanics, and documentation.

➤ *Note:* You may find that you need to adapt the bathing order and other steps to meet individual needs.

Procedure Steps

1. **Provide for patient privacy** and comfort.
   a. Close the door or privacy curtains, adjust room temperature, and assist the patient with elimination as needed.
   b. Assist the patient with elimination before beginning the bath.
      Helps prevent interruptions during the procedure.
   c. Ask the patient and family if they wish family members to assist with the bath.
      Bathing practices differ among cultures and individuals but are often private. The patient or family may wish to have a family member assist with the bath, or the patient may prefer that they leave the room.

2. **Peel open the label on the commercial bath** without completely removing it.
   Allows for steam to escape as contents heat without spilling the contents.

3. **Heat the package** in the microwave for no longer than 1 minute. The temperature of the contents should be approximately 105°F (41°C). This is controversial. Some references suggest, for safety, using the commercial bag bath at room temperature.
   Heating to 105°F (41°C) brings contents to a safe and comfortable temperature. This must be done with caution to prevent burning, especially in patients who have fragile skin.

If Using a Warmer Unit
You do not need Step 3 because the bags are always warm.

4. **Adjust the bed** to working height, lower the side rail nearest you, and position the patient supine close to the side of bed you will be working on.

   ✚ Raise the side rail before you leave that side of the bed.
   Prevents patient falls and keeps you from having to lean over the patient or reach across the side rail, which can cause back strain or injury.

5. **Remove the bedspread** and spread the bath blanket over the top sheet; then ask the patient to hold the bath blanket in place while you remove the top sheet.
   Maintains modesty and prevents chilling. If no bath blanket is available, you can use the top sheet in its place. However, if the sheet becomes damp, it may chill the patient. ▼

Note: Before proceeding, assist the patient with oral hygiene as needed. See Procedures 22-6 and 22-7.

6. **Remove the patient's gown,** keeping the patient covered with the bath blanket. During the bath, expose just the part of the body you are bathing.
   Maintains the patient's modesty and prevents chilling.

Patient With an IV Line

If the patient has an IV and is wearing a gown that has snap-open sleeves:
Some systems include a needle-free 2-way connector that allows you to disconnect the tubing while still maintaining a closed line. In that case, you simply open the connection, remove the gown, and then reconnect the tubing. After the bath, follow the same procedure to place the clean gown on the patient.

If there is no 2-way, needle-free connector on the tubing,
   a. Remove the gown first from the arm without the IV.

(continued on next page)

Procedure 22-1 ■ Bathing: Providing a Complete Bed Bath Using a Prepackaged Bathing Product (continued)

b. Lower the IV container and pass the gown over the tubing and the container, taking care to keep the container above the level of the patient's arm. ▼

c. 🟢 Never disconnect this type of IV tubing connection; this breaks the sterile system and provides a portal of entry for pathogens.

d. Rehang the container; check the flow rate.
Manipulating the IV equipment may change the flow rate; flow rate must be maintained as prescribed.

e. After the bath, replace the gown by threading the IV equipment from inside the arm of the gown and onto the affected arm. Then place the unaffected arm through the other gown sleeve.

7. **Don clean procedure gloves** if exposure to body fluids is likely or if either you or the patient has any breaks in the skin.
Follows universal precautions; helps prevent transfer of microorganisms.

8. **Wash the patient's face, neck, and ears.**
 a. Fold the wipe around the hand to make a mitt, tucking in loose corners.
 Keeps loose ends from dragging across the skin. This is uncomfortable because loose ends cool quickly.
 b. Wash the face using one wipe.
 c. Use a different corner of the wipe to gently wipe each eyelid outward from the inner canthus.
 Some wipes contain chlorhexidine gluconate (CHG), an antimicrobial, which can be irritating to the eyes and mucous membranes. Use pH-balanced prepackaged wipes for the face, or use gauze squares moistened with agency-approved water or normal saline. **Key Point:** *A major principle is cleaning from "clean to dirty" to prevent contamination of a cleaner area. The inner canthus is considered the cleanest area. Prevents moving debris toward the nasolacrimal duct, which is located near the inner canthus.* ▼

 d. Wash the rest of the patient's face, neck, and ears.
 Move sequentially through the bath to make it less tiring for the patient and more efficient for the nurse.
 e. Allow areas to air dry. Do not rinse.
 Prevents the emollient and surfactant skin protectants from being removed.

9. **Discard each wipe after use.**
Ensures following the "clean to dirty" principle.

10. **Wash the patient's arms** using a new, clean wipe.
 a. Fold the bath blanket off one arm at a time and place a folded bath towel under the arm. Beginning with the patient's far arm, support the arm and wash the arm from the hands upward using long strokes.
 Long strokes increase circulation in the extremity. Washing from distal to proximal increases venous return from the periphery. Lifting the arm provides range of motion (ROM) to preserve joint mobility.
 b. Continue to support the arm while washing the axilla.
 Prevents potential injury to the joints. A sprain, subluxation, or dislocation of the joint can occur when an extremity is not properly supported, especially in older adults.
 c. Allow the areas to air dry; do not rinse.
 Prevents the emollient and surfactant skin protectants from being removed.
 d. Apply deodorant and/or powder if desired.
 Follow patient preferences whenever possible to increase comfort.
 e. Clean under the nails with an orangewood stick as needed.
 f. Repeat the preceding Steps 10a–d for the arm nearest you.

11. **Wash the patient's chest,** using a new, clean wipe.
 a. Cover the patient's chest with a bath towel, and lower the bath blanket to the patient's waist.
 Maintains patient comfort and modesty.
 b. For women, gently lift each breast to wash the skinfold. Keep the chest covered between the wash and rinse.
 Skinfolds are a source of odor and can become irritated because of skin-to-skin irritation and dampness from perspiration.
 c. Cover to maintain privacy and warmth.
 d. Allow the areas to air dry; do not rinse.
 Prevents the emollient and surfactant skin protectants from being removed.

12. **Wash the abdomen,** using a new, clean wipe.
 a. Fold the bath blanket down to the perineal area and cover the chest with a bath towel.

b. Wash the abdomen, including the umbilical area; allow to air dry. Pay special attention to skinfolds.
Perspiration and moisture do not evaporate well from skinfolds, predisposing them to maceration.

c. Cover the abdomen and chest with the bath blanket.
Prevents chilling; maintains privacy.

13. **Wash the legs and feet,** using a new, clean wipe for each leg.
 a. Uncover one leg at a time, beginning with the leg farthest from you. Place the bath towel under the leg.
 Keeps the sheet dry; prevents chilling.

 b. Wash the leg from distal to proximal with long, gentle strokes. Allow the leg to air dry.

 ✜ Do not massage the calves of the legs.
 Washing from distal to proximal may help to promote venous return. If a venous thrombus is present, massaging might dislodge the clot and cause an embolus. ▼

 c. Thoroughly wash the foot and toes. Allow the foot to air dry. Apply lotion if the prepackaged bath product does not include emollient and as needed, but not between the toes.
 Disease processes frequently decrease circulation to the feet and lower legs, increasing the likelihood that minor skin irritations may become more severe. Applying emollient between the toes can lead to skin breakdown.

 d. Repeat the procedure on the other leg and foot.

14. **Wash the back and buttocks,** using a new, clean wipe.
 a. Position the patient on their side with back facing you, or in the prone position. Make sure the side rail on the far side of the bed, facing the patient, is still up.
 Provides for clear visualization of back and access to the area.

 b. Exposing only the back and buttocks, place the bath towel under the back and buttocks. Wash the back first and then the buttocks. Observe for redness and skin breakdown in the sacral area.
 Maintains the principle of "clean to dirty." The sacral area is a common site of pressure injuries. ▼

 c. Unless contraindicated, give the patient a back rub, applying lotion to the back and buttocks (see Chapter 31, Procedure 31-1: Giving a Back Rub).
 Stimulates circulation and maintains the health of the skin. Because the patient is in bed, they are at risk for skin irritation and breakdown from immobility and friction. A back rub may be contraindicated for patients with musculoskeletal injuries or cardiovascular disease.

 d. Don procedure gloves if you have not already done so, and wash the rectal area, removing any fecal matter with tissues before washing with the wipe. Wash from front to back.
 Washing the rectal area at this time removes the need for the patient to turn to their side again and helps prevent soiling clean linen when changing the linen in an occupied bed. Fecal matter usually contains microorganisms. Washing from front to back helps prevent transferring bacteria from the rectum to the vagina and urethra. ▼

 e. Discard the soiled wipe. If linens are soiled, cover them with a clean sheet before repositioning the patient.

 f. Remove soiled gloves and perform hand hygiene. Don new procedure gloves before providing perineal care.
 Prevents transferring microorganisms from anal to genital area—cleansing the gluteal and anal areas contaminates the wipe. Maintains standard precautions during the bath and prevents soiling of clean linens during bed change and cross-contamination to other body sites.

15. **Cleanse the perineal area.** See Procedure 22-4: Providing Perineal Care.

16. **After providing perineal care, reposition and cover the patient with the bath blanket.** Remove soiled gloves and perform hand hygiene. Help the patient put on a clean gown, and attend to other hygiene needs (e.g., hair grooming).
Prevents contaminating clean linen with soiled gloves. Ensures proper body position and warmth.

17. **Change the bed linen** as needed, including soiled linen or linen that became damp during the bath. Properly dispose of soiled items by placing them in a linen bag. See Procedure 22-14: Making an Occupied Bed.
Ensures patient safety, comfort, and privacy.

(continued on next page)

Procedure 22-1 ■ Bathing: Providing a Complete Bed Bath Using a Prepackaged Bathing Product (continued)

? What if...

- **I am bathing the patient without assistance, or I am not tall enough to comfortably reach across the patient?**

These situations put you at risk for back strain. Thus, you may want to bathe one side of the body—that is, the right arm, trunk, right leg—and then move to the other side of the bed to bathe the opposite side of the body (instead of the order given in Steps 8 and 9). Move the patient close to you before beginning the bath.

- **I am bathing a patient in leg traction?**

You may decide to bathe the arms and trunk first. Then have the patient sit forward so that you can cleanse the back. Then have the patient lift up slightly so that you can wash the buttocks. Finally, wash the lower extremities.

- **I am bathing a patient with dementia?**

Use your knowledge of the person's bathing practices and preferences to determine a time of day and a routine the person will accept. Keep stimulation to a minimum. Turn on some calming music, speak softly and reassuringly, and don't rush. Keep the patient warm. If the patient becomes agitated and you cannot calm them, do not force the patient to bathe. Also,

▶ Go to **iCare Box 22-2, Caring Tips for Bathing a Patient With Dementia**, in Volume 1.

Many steps in the bathing process may be misinterpreted or stressful for the person, who may become disruptive or agitated. If forced to bathe, the patient may be upset for hours.

- **My patient becomes agitated and uncooperative during the bath?**

Speak calmly and softly. Give the patient a few minutes to calm down. Discontinue the bath if the patient remains upset.

- **My patient is an older adult?**
  a. Some clinicians recommend bathing older adults every other day instead of daily, and it is generally agreed that they should not bathe more than once a day unless soiling occurs.
  Helps prevent skin dryness.
  b. Ensure that the wipes are warm before use, but not hot.
  Prevents burns (older adults may have decreased sensation in their extremities).
  c. If you are not using a commercial packaged bath, use antibacterial soap or a mild soap substitute. If you must use soap, it should be nonperfumed and should be rich in moisture. If you use soap, rinse the skin well.
  To avoid skin irritation.
  d. Pat the skin dry or air dry; do not rub.
  e. Immediately after drying, wash your hands and apply moisturizer while there is still moisture in the skin.
  f. Cleanse the skin immediately after every incident of soiling (e.g., when the patient has a bowel movement).
  Prevents maceration and irritation from enzyme activity.

Evaluation

- Assess how well the patient tolerated the procedure. Was there any discomfort, shortness of breath, and so on?
- Observe the patient's mobility (both ROM and ease of movement).
- Note the condition of the patient's skin, including redness and other abnormal findings, especially in skinfolds.
- Ask the patient whether they are comfortable and satisfied.
- If someone other than the nurse performs the procedure, the nurse must still evaluate the care to be certain that it was done and performed satisfactorily.

Patient Teaching

- Discuss the need for activity (e.g., moving about in bed) and the hazards of immobility.
- Discuss usual skin care and how to increase the health of the skin.
- Demonstrate bathing procedure to family or other caregivers.

Home Care

NOTE: (1) Many of the following apply to older adults and others with self-care deficits. (2) The following refer to all types of home bathing, not just to Procedure 22-1:

- ✚ Evaluate the home for bathing safety considerations (not limited to bed bath), such as the following:
  Safety bars in the bathroom?
  To facilitate transfers and provide support while washing.
  A safe water supply for bathing?
  Bathing supplies that are available and accessible?
  Nonskid mat or abrasive strips for shower or tub?
  Stool for shower; transfer bench or stool for getting into the tub?
  Handheld shower spray?
  Long-handled brush or sponge?

- Assess the client's ability to help with the bath or to bathe independently.
- Ask how the client usually bathes (e.g., shower, at the sink). Follow the client's preference as much as possible.

- Ask what supplies the client usually uses for the bath, and ask where they are stored. You will need to adapt the procedure depending on the available equipment and supplies.
- Suggest the use of large plastic trash bags or a shower curtain to protect the mattress during a bed bath.
- Instruct caregivers to wear gloves when handling linens that are soiled with blood or other body fluids. Linens should be washed in cold water, separately from other household laundry, and then washed again, using hot water, detergent, and bleach.

Hot water coagulates proteins in the blood and makes it more difficult to remove. Detergent and bleach are used to destroy pathogens.

Documentation

Chart the type of bath given, how much patient was able to help with the bath, how well the patient tolerated the procedure, the patient's mobility, and any abnormal findings. Hygiene care is charted on checklists and flowsheets in most agencies.

Sample electronic documentation

0630   Complete bed bath given, pt. unable to assist in care. Patient tolerated procedure well, VSS, denied pain. Patient turned side to side with assist of one. Skin warm, dry, and intact. Emollient applied to dry areas. Encouraged patient to shift weight while in bed to prevent injury to skin. ——————————————— K. Barnett, RN

Practice Resources
Denny & Munro (2017); Fauth et al. (2016); Groven et al. (2017); Hørdam et al. (2018); Wolf (2022).

Thinking About the Procedure

The videos **Bathing: Providing a Complete Bed Bath Using a Prepackaged Bathing Product, Providing Perineal Care, Brushing and Flossing the Teeth,** and **Providing Foot Care,** along with questions and suggested responses, are available on the **Davis's** *Nursing Skills Videos* Web site at www.fadavis.com.

Procedure 22-2 ■ Bathing: Using a Basin and Water

Key Point: *Evidence indicates that (1) bath basins can become a reservoir for microorganisms and for cross-contamination of the immediate environment and healthcare personnel and (2) biofilm is commonly present in hospital water lines and faucets. Use this method only when a patient is grossly contaminated or a patient refuses other types of bath.*

➤ For steps to follow in *all* procedures, refer to the Universal Steps for All Procedures on the inside back cover.

Equipment
- Disposable water basin for single-patient use
- Tap, distilled, filtered, or sterile water (depending on facility policy)
- CHG and water solution (for bathing the patient and cleaning the basin)
- Lotion, deodorant, and/or powder as needed
- Bath blanket
- Clean patient gown (gown with shoulder snaps or Velcro closures if the patient has an IV line)
- Clean linen
- Procedure gloves

Delegation
You can delegate this procedure to the UAP if you conclude that the patient's condition and the UAP's skills allow. Perform the preprocedure assessments and inform the UAP of the amount of help the patient needs and of any special considerations, such as IV lines and drains. Ask the UAP to report the condition of the patient's skin, level of self-care, and ability to tolerate the procedure.

Preprocedure Assessments
Assessments are the same as in Procedure 22-1: Bathing: Providing a Complete Bed Bath Using a Prepackaged Bathing Product.

➤ When performing the procedure, always identify your patient according to agency policy, using two identifiers, and be attentive to standard precautions, hand hygiene, patient safety and privacy, body mechanics, and documentation.

Procedure Steps

1. ✚ **Fill the disposable basin** with warm water (approximately 41°C [105°F]). Check the temperature with a thermometer or your hand. If possible, ask the patient to test the water temperature.

Using tap water for bathing exposes patients to waterborne pathogens; use distilled, filtered, or sterile water if available. This differs among institutions, so follow agency requirements. Use water that is comfortable for the patient. Hot water removes protective skin oils and can injure the patient. If the water is too cool, the patient may become chilled.

(continued on next page)

Procedure 22-2 ■ Bathing: Using a Basin and Water (continued)

2. **Prepare a solution of 60 mL CHG** solution diluted in 3 qt (2.85 L) of water for bathing the patient (Petlin et al., 2014).
   Evidence indicates that use of CHG is effective in preventing the bath basin from becoming a reservoir for microorganisms and in helping to prevent HAIs.

3. **Prepare the patient for the bath** by doing the following (refer to Procedure 22-1 for rationales):
   a. Adjust the bed to working height.
   b. Remove the bedspread and spread bath blanket over top sheet.
   c. Remove the patient's gown, keeping the patient covered with the bath blanket.

   Patient With an IV Line
   - For a needle-free 2-way connector, open the connection, remove the gown, and reconnect the tubing.
   - If there is no 2-way needle-free connector, remove the gown first from the arm without the IV, lower the container, and pass gown over the container and tubing, taking care to keep the container above the level of the patient's arm. Rehang the container and check the flow rate.
   - After the bath, replace the gown by threading the container from inside the arm of the gown and onto the affected arm. Then place the unaffected arm through the other gown sleeve.
   d. Don clean procedure gloves if exposure to body fluids is likely or if either you or the patient has any breaks in the skin.

4. **Using a clean, rinsed washcloth, wash the patient in the following sequence:**
   Face, neck, ears
   Eyes
   Chest
   Abdomen
   Legs and feet
   Back and buttocks
   Rectal area
   Perineum
   Rinse and wring water from the washcloth as you move from each body area. Change water and use a clean washcloth to wash the perineal area.
   Rinsing keeps washcloth warm and clean. Changing water prevents cross-contamination and contamination of wounds with dirty bath water.

5. **Rinse body areas as needed** (i.e., if you use soap) and pat dry.
   Preserves skin integrity by preventing the drying effect of the soap on the skin.

6. **Apply deodorant, lotion, and/or powder as desired or as needed.**

7. **Put used washcloths in the laundry** for future use.

8. **Help patient don a clean gown.**

9. **Provide a back rub,** if not contraindicated.

10. **Reposition patient,** as needed.

11. **Change linens,** as needed, and bag soiled linen for laundering.

12. **Clean and dry the basin** according to agency policy.

    Evidence supports single-patient use of a disposable basin, cleaning it with chlorhexidine solution, drying the basin after each use, storing it upside down, not storing anything (e.g., bathing supplies) in it, and not reusing it (Powers, Peed, Burns, et al., 2012; Sturgeon et al., 2019).

> For Evaluation, Documentation, and Patient Teaching, see Procedure 22-1: Bathing: Providing a Complete Bed Bath Using a Prepackaged Bathing Product.

Practice Resources
Hørdam et al. (2018); Konno et al. (2021); Lewis et al. (2019); Powers, Peed, Burns, et al. (2012); Sturgeon et al. (2019); Wolf (2022).

Procedure 22-3 ■ Providing Perineal Care

➤ For steps to follow in all procedures, refer to the Universal Steps for All Procedures on the inside back cover.

Equipment
- Procedure gloves
- Prepackaged bathing product (i.e., Comfort Care)
- Bedpan or portable sitz tub (optional)
- Bath towel
- Toilet paper
- Plastic trash bag for used wipes and other disposable soiled items
- Perineal ointment or lotion if needed

If prepackaged bathing product is not available:
- Sterile, filtered, distilled, or tap water according to agency policy
- Disposable basin or perineal wash bottle, if needed
- Perineal cleansing solution or no-rinse soap
- Washcloths

Delegation

You can delegate perineal care to the UAP if the patient's condition and the UAP's skills allow. Perform the preprocedure assessments and inform the UAP of the amount of help the patient needs and any special considerations (e.g., presence of a urinary catheter, vaginal drainage). Ask the UAP to report the condition of the patient's perineum (skin, drainage), level of self-care, and ability to tolerate the procedure.

Preprocedure Assessments

- Assess the patient's mobility and activity tolerance.
  Determine whether the patient will be able to assist with the perineal care. Doing as much self-care as possible increases the patient's sense of independence and maintains modesty.
- Check for positioning or activity restrictions, such as maintaining hip abduction after a total hip replacement.
  Prevents injuring the patient during the procedure.
- Assess for psychosocial issues related to perineal care.
  Consider personal and cultural norms to ensure that the perineal care is appropriate for the patient. For example, in some cultures a woman would find it completely unacceptable for a male nurse to perform her perineal care (pericare).
- Assess for any specific patient needs, such as presence of a urinary catheter, perineal surgery, lesions, incontinence, or skin breakdown.
  You may need to adapt the procedure (e.g., clean around an indwelling urinary catheter or surgical incision, use special soaps). Incontinence requires assessment and follow-up to prevent impaired skin integrity.

➤ When performing the procedure, always identify your patient according to agency policy, using two identifiers, and be attentive to standard precautions, hand hygiene, patient safety and privacy, body mechanics, and documentation.

Procedure Steps

1. **Adjust the room temperature** and assist with elimination as needed.
   Assisting the patient with elimination before perineal care helps prevent interruptions during the procedure and allows for thorough cleansing. Adjusting room temperature prevents chilling.

2. **Warm the perineal bathing** product (disposable wipes).

   Variation: If Using a Microwave

   ✚ Heat the package in the microwave using manufacturer's recommendation. The temperature of the contents should be approximately 41°C (105°F). This step is controversial. Some references suggest, for safety, using the commercial bag bath at room temperature.

   Variation: If Using a Warmer Unit
   You do not need Step 2 because the bags are always warm.

3. **Prepare the patient.**
   a. Position the patient on their back (supine). Place waterproof pads under the patient if they are not already in place. You may wish to place the patient on a bedpan or portable sitz tub, especially if the perineum is excessively soiled. Place a waterproof bag within reach to discard wipes.
   Placing the patient on a bedpan raises the hips to increase visualization and allows for more thorough cleansing. A bedpan also allows for using water when needed.
   b. Wear procedure gloves (and other PPE as needed) when providing perineal care. If you are using a basin and water, you may wear a procedure gown and goggles if you are concerned about splashing (e.g., if the patient is confused and may be unable to follow instructions).
   When providing perineal care, there is a possibility of coming in contact with urine, vaginal secretions, or fecal material.
   c. Drape the patient to protect privacy.
      - Place the bath blanket over the patient's chest.
      - Fold the bed linens down to expose only the patient's perineum.
   d. Remove any fecal material with toilet paper.
   Prevents contamination of the perineum with feces, which can lead to bladder or incisional infections. If you are providing perineal care as part of giving a bed bath, you will have cleaned the anal area when the patient was in the lateral position.

4. **Wash the perineum** using a warm disposable wipe. In both males and females, cleanse the skinfolds of the groin area thoroughly. Examine the skin creases for redness or excoriation.

   Variation: For Female Patients
   Wash the perineum from front to back, using a clean portion of the wipe for each stroke. Cleanse the labial folds and around the urinary catheter, if one is in place.
   Prevents contaminating the urethra with fecal material. Any fecal particles that are left can cause skin breakdown due to enzyme activity and may increase the risk of a urinary tract infection because of the presence of Escherichia coli in the feces. ▼

(continued on next page)

Procedure 22-3 ■ Providing Perineal Care (continued)

Variation: For Male Patients

Retract the foreskin, if present, and gently cleanse the head of the penis using a circular motion. Replace the foreskin and finish washing the shaft of the penis, using firm strokes. Then wash the scrotum, using a clean portion of the wipe with each stroke. Handle the scrotum with care because the area is sensitive.

To adequately clean the head of the penis in an uncircumcised male, you must retract the foreskin. After cleaning, replace the foreskin to prevent constriction and edema of the penis. Firm strokes may help to prevent an erection. Using a clean portion of the wipe for each stroke prevents fecal contamination of the urethra and perineum. ▼

Detects and prevents excoriation in skinfold areas, where moisture accumulates.

5. **Allow body areas to air dry;** do not rinse.
   Prevents the emollient and surfactant skin protectants from being removed.

6. **Discard each wipe after use,** or place on the waterproof pad to discard when finished.
   Ensures following the "clean to dirty" principle.

7. **If perineal care is not being done** as part of the bath, clean the anal area. Ask the patient to turn to the side; wipe the buttocks and anal area as needed.
   Fecal contamination of the perineum can lead to urinary tract infections and skin irritation. Therefore, the anal area is cleansed last.

8. **Apply skin protectants** as needed. Powder only if the patient requests it.
   If urinary or fecal incontinence is present, skin barriers may be used to prevent urine, feces, or other drainage from contacting the skin. This helps prevent skin breakdown. For female patients, powder is a medium for bacterial growth. In the presence of moisture, it also creates a paste, which irritates the skin.

9. **If the patient has an indwelling** catheter and if agency policy requires special catheter care, you will usually provide the care at this point. Don clean gloves before providing catheter care and follow the agency's procedure. For more information about catheter care, see Clinical Insight 25-1: Caring for a Patient With an Indwelling Catheter.

10. **Reposition and cover the patient** with the bath blanket. Remove soiled gloves, discarding in a waterproof bag.
    Prevents contaminating clean linen with soiled gloves.

11. **Change linen as needed,** including soiled linen or linen that became damp during perineal care.
    Ensures patient safety, comfort, and privacy.

? What if...

- **The patient is unable to control bowel and/or bladder?**

  Gently cleanse the perineal/perigenital area after each incontinence/soiling and apply a moisture barrier according to agency protocols.
  Minimizing contact with irritants such as moisture, urine, and stool can decrease the development of incontinence-associated dermatitis.

  Use a spray no-rinse cleanser and soft wipes.
  These aid in preventing irritation from friction and reducing drying effects on the skin.

  Follow agency policy and use skin assessment tools (some geared particularly to perineal skin).

  Assess for signs of secondary infection in addition to irritation and report as needed.

  Consider bowel and bladder retraining and scheduling to reduce frequency of incontinence.

- **My patient is postpartum?**

  Educate the patient about perineal care. Include the importance of handwashing before and after cleansing the perineum, measures to keep the perineum clean, frequent changing of sanitary pads, and checking for signs and symptoms of abnormal lochia. If the patient had an episiotomy, laceration, or tear, teaching should also include management of discomfort and signs of wound infection.

Evaluation

- Assess the patient's responses to the procedure (e.g., any discomfort?).
- Observe for difficulty with movement or ROM during the procedure.
- Note the condition of the skin, including redness and other abnormal findings.
- Ask the patient if they feel more comfortable now.

Patient Teaching

- Discuss adaptations to perineal care. For example, if the area is tender, (1) instead of using toilet paper, wash the area with a warm moistened wipe after using the toilet, or (2) use a skin protectant on the area.
- Review the importance of handwashing after elimination.
- As needed, teach the caregiver how to provide perineal care, including the major concept of cleaning front to back ("clean to dirty"). Stress the importance of wearing gloves and washing hands.

- Advise female patients not to douche because it disturbs the balance of normal vaginal flora and can irritate or injure mucosal cells.
- Explain that scented and deodorant feminine hygiene products are not necessary for cleanliness and may even be harmful. Daily cleansing is the most effective means of odor control.

Home Care

- Evaluate the ability of the client or caregiver to provide perineal care.
- Determine the availability of supplies needed for perineal care.
- You will need to adapt the procedure depending on the available equipment and supplies. Major issues involved in perineal care in the home are the lack of clean water and/or linens. In some instances, you may need to use bottled water or boiled water for the procedure. One option is to use prepackaged moistened towelettes to provide the care (e.g., Comfort Bath towelettes).

Documentation

Usually perineal care is part of routine hygiene care and is charted on a flowsheet. If you need to write a narrative note, chart that perineal care was given, any patient responses to the procedure, and the condition of the perineal area.

Sample documentation

8/16/xx   1430   Perineal care given. Patient had no complaint of discomfort. No redness or discharge noted. ——————————————— Nora Noyes, RN

Practice Resources
Martin, Haider, Palleschi, et al. (2017); Pather & Hines, S. (2016).

Thinking About the Procedures

> The video **Providing Perineal Care,** along with questions and suggested responses, is available on the **Davis's Nursing Skills Videos** Web site at www.fadavis.com.

Procedure 22-4 ■ Providing Foot Care

➤ For steps to follow in *all* procedures, refer to the Universal Steps for All Procedures on the inside back cover.

➤ *Note:* This procedure describes foot care using a basin and water. It may also be done with prepackaged wipes, along with the bath.

Equipment

- Procedure gloves (if there are open lesions)
- Pillow (if procedure is done with the patient in bed)
- Disposable basin for water (distilled, sterile, or filtered tap water, per agency requirements)
- Liquid no-rinse soap
- Bath towel and washcloth
- Waterproof pad
- Orangewood stick
- Toenail clippers and nail file
- Lotion or prescribed ointment or cream

Delegation

You can delegate foot care to the UAP if the patient's condition and the UAP's skills allow. For example, as a rule you should not delegate care if the patient has impaired peripheral circulation or foot ulcers. Perform the following preprocedure assessments and inform the UAP of the amount of help the patient needs and any special considerations (e.g., ability to sit in a chair). Ask the UAP to report the condition of the patient's skin and nails, level of self-care, and ability to tolerate the procedure.

Preprocedure Assessments

- As you assess the feet and toenails, compare findings for both feet.
- Assess bilateral dorsalis pedis pulses, capillary refill, skin color, and warmth. Compare right and left feet. Palpate pulses at the same time bilaterally to determine whether one side is weaker than the other.

  Decreased circulation to the feet increases the risk for tissue injury and infection. A variety of diseases can cause poor circulation. For example, cardiac or renal disease may cause pedal edema, which impairs circulation to the skin, and diabetes causes vascular changes leading to poor circulation to the lower extremities.

- Assess for diseases (e.g., diabetes mellitus and peripheral vascular disease) that create risks for foot problems.
- Thoroughly assess all areas of the feet for skin integrity, edema, condition of toenails, and any abnormalities. Check carefully between the toes.

  Decreased circulation in the feet commonly causes such problems as thickened toenails, dry skin, and increased risk of infection. Changes in vision and mobility can increase the risk for injuries to the feet. Patients with diabetes also may have neuropathy, which

(continued on next page)

Procedure 22-4 ■ Providing Foot Care (continued)

prevents them from knowing when they have injured their feet. Identifying abnormalities enables you to provide interventions to help prevent potential problems. ▼

- Check institutional policy to verify whether a nurse is allowed to trim nails. Obtain a primary provider's prescription for trimming the patient's nails, if necessary.
  Patients who have diabetes or impaired circulation to the lower extremities require a prescription for trimming their nails. Refer the patient to a podiatrist if the circulation is severely compromised or if edema would make the procedure difficult.

- Assess the patient's usual footwear.
  Improperly fitting shoes, especially if they are too tight, are a common cause of foot problems (e.g., bunions, ingrown toenails).
- Assess the patient's ability to provide foot care. Evaluate the need for a referral. Determine whether the patient has the necessary vision and mobility for their own foot care.
- Assess the patient's knowledge about foot care, including usual foot care practices.
  ✚ Identify potential deficits in understanding that may require additional teaching or referral to a podiatrist, general practice physician, or advanced practice nurse.
  Many home remedies for foot problems can damage the tissue. For example, corn pads can increase pressure on the tissue, compromising circulation and causing local tissue ischemia. Cutting the sides of the toenails can lead to ingrown toenails.

➤ When performing the procedure, always identify your patient according to agency policy, using two identifiers, and be attentive to standard precautions, hand hygiene, patient safety and privacy, body mechanics, and documentation.

Procedure Steps

1. **Wear procedure gloves** and other PPE as needed when providing foot care.
   Follows standard precautions. The heel is a common place for skin breakdown, so use gloves if you are unable to see the area without lifting the foot. If the patient has significant drainage to the area, such as a draining wound, you may need to wear a protective gown.

2. **Ask the patient to sit in a chair** with a waterproof pad or bath towel under the feet, if possible. If the patient is unable to sit in a chair, place the patient in semi-Fowler's position in bed; place a pillow under the knees.
   It is easier to perform the procedure with the patient in a chair. The pillow supports the knee joints and prevents muscle fatigue.

3. ✚ **Fill the basin halfway** with warm water (approximately 105°F to 110°F [40°C to 43°C]).
   Recent research recommends the use of filtered, distilled, or sterile water. Using tap water for bathing exposes patients to waterborne pathogens that may be contained in biofilm in water lines and faucets. Hot water can injure the skin. Warm water promotes circulation. Filling the basin halfway prevents spilling when the patient places a foot in the water.

4. **Help the patient place one foot** in the water, first checking with the patient that the temperature is comfortable.
   a. If the patient is in a chair, place the basin on the floor (on the waterproof pad).
   b. If the patient is in bed, place the basin near the foot of the bed on the waterproof pad; pad the basin with a towel.
   The waterproof pad keeps the bed dry. Padding the basin prevents pressure on the back of the leg, which could cause discomfort and interfere with circulation.

5. **Allow the foot to soak** for 5 to 20 minutes, depending on the patient's tolerance and the condition of the feet.

   ✚ Soaking is not recommended for patients with diabetes or peripheral vascular disease (PVD).
   Soaking softens the skin and helps relax the patient. For patients who have diabetes or PVD, soaking is not recommended because it may remove natural oils, cause cracking of the skin, and cause burns even if the water is at the recommended temperature.

6. **Cleanse the foot** with mild or no-rinse soap.
   Removes loose debris. No-rinse soaps do not dry the skin. ▼

7. **Clean under the nails** with an orangewood stick while the foot is still in the water.
   Water softens the nails and makes cleaning easier.

8. **Remove the foot from** the water and dry it gently and thoroughly.
   Remaining moisture, especially between the toes, can cause maceration and promotes development of fungal infections.

9. **Change the water.**
   Ensures proper temperature and prevents cross-contamination.

10. **Soak the opposite foot** while performing Steps 11 through 14 for the first (clean) foot.
    Efficient use of time.

11. **Gently push the cuticles back** with the orangewood stick or towel.
    Increases cuticle health. Do not damage the cuticle; doing so can increase the risk of infection.

12. **Trim the nails straight across** with toenail clippers, if not contraindicated by the patient's condition and if permitted by agency policy. Note whether the nail has cut into the skin of the toe being trimmed or the adjacent toes. If the nails are brittle or thick, allow the foot to soak for 10 to 20 minutes before trimming.
    Trimming straight across prevents ingrown toenails. Early recognition and treatment of problems will prevent further complications, such as infection. ▼

Yes   No

13. **File the nails** with an emery board.
    Smooths the edges to prevent scratching the skin with the toenails.

14. **Apply cream, lotion,** or foot powder lightly to the feet and toes.
    Cream hydrates the skin; however, excess cream can cause maceration. Foot powder absorbs moisture and functions as a nonirritating deodorant for patients whose feet perspire heavily.

15. **Repeat Steps 11 through 14** with the second foot.

16. **Check the patient's footwear** for rough edges that may injure feet.

❓ What if ...

- **My patient has impaired bed mobility?**
  Apply protective devices (e.g., lamb's wool) as needed.

- **My patient has an injury, lesions, or pain?**
  You may need to use a bed cradle to keep the pressure of the bedding off the patient's feet. Refer to Chapter 32 for other measures to preserve skin integrity.

- **My patient has diabetes mellitus?**
  In addition to controlling blood glucose levels, adhering to a specific foot care plan is essential for people with diabetes. Include the following in your teaching:
  - The importance of inspecting the feet daily
  - Ways to protect the feet (e.g., by wearing shoes when out of bed)
  - Potential complications involving the feet
  - Management of symptoms
  - When to seek advice from a healthcare professional
  - What to include in the foot care regimen (apply moisturizing lotion on tops and soles of feet but not between toes)—and what not to do (cut corns and calluses, use topical corn removers, or soak the feet)
  - 🍁 Elderly patients with diabetes are especially at risk for development of foot-related complications. Visual changes and loss of flexibility could make it challenging to bend and visualize the feet. Plastic mirrors may be helpful in this regard.

  Early detection and treatment of problems can minimize foot-related complications.

Evaluation

- Observe that feet are clean, smooth, and intact; nails are trimmed and smooth; and normal pigmentation on the feet and soles (based on skin tone diversity).
- Be sure that foot problems are identified and interventions provided.
- Ask the patient to demonstrate or describe correct foot care.

Patient Teaching

For patient teaching,

▶ Go to the **Self-Care box, Teaching Your Client About Foot Care,** in Volume 1.

Home Care

The procedure does not vary in the home. The nurse must:
- Work with the client and care provider to determine the availability of supplies needed for foot care (e.g., clean water).
- Identify home care practices and teach the client and/or caregiver proper foot care techniques. Influencing older adults can be especially difficult if they have usual routines, such as walking barefoot, that put them at risk for injury. For clients with diabetes, the biggest risk to foot health is inadequate regulation of their blood glucose levels.

(continued on next page)

Procedure 22-4 ■ Providing Foot Care (continued)

Documentation

In most agencies you will not document routine foot care (except, perhaps, on a checklist) unless there are problems. If you do document, chart that foot care was given, and chart assessment findings.

Sample documentation

09/22/xx 0900. Foot care given. 2 cm circular reddened area on right heel. Skin abrasion outer lateral aspect of 5th toe, left foot —biooclusive dressing applied. ——————————————— Ann Hopkins, RN

Practice Resources

Bonner, Foster, & Spears-Lanoix (2016); CDC (2021); National Guideline Clearinghouse (n.d.); Powers et al. (2012); Siegel et al. (2007, updated 2018).

Thinking About the Procedure

The video **Providing Foot Care,** along with questions and suggested responses, is available on the **Davis's Nursing Skills Videos** Web site at www.fadavis.com.

Procedure 22-5 ■ Brushing and Flossing the Teeth

> For steps to follow in all procedures, refer to the Universal Steps for All Procedures on the inside back cover.

Equipment

- Toothbrush or sponge toothettes
- Toothpaste
- Dental floss (two pieces, each about 10 in. long) and floss holder (optional)
- Tonsil-tip suction connected to suction source (if aspiration is a concern)
- Emesis basin
- Towel
- Glass of water (distilled, sterile, or filtered water, according to agency requirements)
  Key Point: Recent studies recommend that hospitalized patients at high risk for infection avoid exposure to hospital water. Follow agency policy.
- Mouthwash and/or lip moisturizer, if desired
- Procedure gloves; mask and goggles if splashing may occur

Delegation

You can delegate oral hygiene to the UAP if the patient's condition and the UAP's skills allow. Perform the following assessments and inform the UAP of the specific type of oral care and the amount of help the patient needs. Ask the UAP to report the condition of the patient's mouth, level of self-care, and ability to tolerate the procedure.

Preprocedure Assessments

- Assess the patient's ability to assist with oral care.
  Having the patient assist whenever possible promotes independence and supports a positive self-image.
- Determine whether the patient has dentures, bridgework, or partial plates.
  Determines how you will provide oral care.
- Assess general oral health, including gag reflex and the condition of the teeth, gums, and mucous membranes. If a patient has dentures, examine the mouth with and without the dentures.
  (a) If the patient has a hypoactive or absent gag reflex, you will need a suction setup to prevent aspiration. (b) Inflammation or lesions in the mouth increase the patient's risk of infection and may make eating difficult or painful, leading to malnutrition. (c) Poorly fitting dentures can cause irritation of the gums.
- Assess the patient's usual oral care, including cultural practices.
  Helps determine the type of oral care you will provide and identifies areas of patient teaching needed.

> When performing the procedure, always identify your patient according to agency policy, using two identifiers, and be attentive to standard precautions, hand hygiene, patient safety and privacy, body mechanics, and documentation.

Procedure Steps

1. **Position the patient in a high Fowler's** position or in a chair, if possible. Position the patient on their side if the head of bed cannot be elevated.
   Prevents aspiration and makes the procedure easier.

2. **Set up suction, if needed.** Attach suction tubing and tonsil-tip suction; check suction.
   Suctioning equipment may be needed to prevent aspiration of secretions during the procedure, especially if the gag reflex is decreased.

3. **If the patient is able to perform self-care:**
   a. Arrange supplies within the patient's reach.
      Promotes the patient's ability to do self-care and therefore independence.

CHAPTER 22 Facilitating Hygiene   359

b. Assist the patient with brushing and flossing as needed.
Ensures that the teeth are thoroughly cleaned.

Procedure Variation: For Nurse-Administered Brushing and Flossing

Follow the remaining steps.

4. **Place the towel across the patient's chest.**
Prevents getting the patient's gown or linen wet during the procedure.

5. **Don procedure gloves as needed.** Wear gown and goggles if splashing might occur, such as with a confused patient.
Follows standard precautions.

6. **Adjust the bed to working height;** lower the side rail nearest you.
Prevents you from having to lean over the patient or reach across the siderail, possibly causing back strain or injury.

7. **Moisten a small, soft toothbrush** and apply a small amount of toothpaste. See Equipment for type of water to use.
A small toothbrush fits more easily into the mouth and reaches more areas. The soft bristles can be used to brush the tongue and also the gums if the patient is edentulous. Excessive toothpaste does not increase the cleaning, and toothpaste residue has a drying effect on the mucosa. Moistening the toothbrush increases patient comfort because patients frequently have dry mouths.

8. **Place, hold, or ask the patient** to hold the emesis basin under the chin.
Collects oral secretions and protects clothing and linens.

9. **Brush the teeth,** holding the bristles at a 45° angle to the gumline.
   a. Using short circular motions, gently brush the inner and outer surfaces of the teeth, from the gumline to the crown of each tooth.
   b. Brush the biting surface of the back teeth by holding the brush bristles straight up and down to the teeth and brushing back and forth.

This is the most effective technique for removing all food particles and plaque from the teeth and gums. Removing debris and subsequent plaque helps to decrease microbial colonization.

   c. If the patient is frail, perform oral suctioning when fluid accumulates in the mouth.
Prevents choking and aspiration. ▼

Brush teeth, holding bristles at a 45° angle to the gumline. Using short circular motions, gently brush the inner and outer surfaces of the teeth, including the gumline.

Clean front teeth.   Clean both inner and outer surfaces of the teeth.

Brush the biting surfaces of the back teeth with the brush bristles straight up and down.   Brush the surface of the tongue.

10. **Gently brush the patient's tongue.**
Removes coating and accumulated debris that can be a reservoir for bacteria. Brush gently to prevent gagging or vomiting.

11. **Floss the teeth.** Grasp dental floss in both hands or use a floss holder. ▼

Variation: If You Are Not Using a Floss Holder

   a. Wrap one end of the floss around the middle finger of each hand. ▼

   b. Stretch the floss between your thumbs and index fingers and move the floss up and down against each tooth. ▼

   c. Floss between and around all teeth.
Moving the floss up and down instead of back and forth prevents damaging the gums. ▼

12. **Assist the patient in rinsing** mouth, suctioning as needed. Or ask the patient to rinse vigorously and spit the water into the emesis basin.
Removes food particles from mouth. Suction if the patient has a decreased or absent gag reflex.

(continued on next page)

Procedure 22-5 ■ Brushing and Flossing the Teeth (continued)

13. **Offer a mild or dilute mouthwash** and apply lip moisturizer, if desired.
   Prevents irritation of the mucous membranes. Apply lip moisturizer for dry lips, for unconscious patients, or for those on a ventilator, or per patient preference.

14. **Reposition the patient** as needed and return the bed to the low position.
   Ensures patient comfort and safety.

? What if...

- **My patient has an excessively dry oral cavity?**

  You may need to use a saliva substitute. *Aging, adverse medication effects, and illness often lead to decreased salivary production.*

- **My patient has viscous (thick) mucus?**

  Use appropriately diluted sodium bicarbonate to dissolve viscous mucus.

- ✚ **My patient has a high risk of gum bleeding (e.g., such as associated with thrombocytopenia), my patient has painful mouth lesions, or teeth brushing is otherwise contraindicated?**

  You may use foam or cotton mouth swabs instead of a toothbrush. Do not use glycerin swabs, lemon glycerin swabs, or gauze squares. Use normal saline mouthwash.
  Foam swabs are less effective in removing debris and plaque and should be used only when brushing is contraindicated. Lemon glycerin swabs are drying to the mucosa and may cause decalcification of tooth enamel. Mouthwashes may be painful.

- **My patient has dementia or is uncooperative and agitated for other reasons?**

  Use dementia-focused behavior management strategies:
  - 🍁 Older adults with dementia frequently accumulate greater amounts of plaque and calculus, exhibit a higher incidence of periodontal gingival bleeding, and demonstrate a greater prevalence of denture-related oral mucosal lesions, yet they often resist oral care.
  - Provide oral hygiene at the same time every day, not necessarily at bathing time.
  - Use as many staff members as necessary.
  - Give care in a quiet, distraction-free environment. Keep stimulation to a minimum; turn on some calming music if desired.
  - Speak softly; give one-step directions in short, simple sentences.
  - Use a relaxed, slow approach; be sure your facial expression does not reflect tension.
  - Give reassuring body contact and use gentle touch.
    Promotes trust. Quick or forceful touch may frighten the patient.
  - Provide diversion.
    Occupies the patient's hands and prevents grabbing.

  ✚ *Never place your fingers between the teeth.*

  - Try placing a spare toothbrush or a rolled facecloth in the patient's hands while you provide oral care.
    Minimizes grabbing.
  - Use the "hand over hand" technique to gently guide the patient's own hand.
  - Try starting the task (e.g., brushing), then having the patient help finish it.
  - If the procedure is not going well, find another caregiver to come in and attempt the task.
  - Use modified equipment and aids, if available (e.g., mouth props, backward-bent and suction toothbrushes).

- **My patient is on a ventilator, is a frail older adult, or has undergone cardiac surgery?**

  Be certain the teeth are brushed twice a day.

  In addition to brushing, use moisturizer on lips and oral mucosa every 2 to 4 hours.

  Apply a 0.12% chlorhexidine gluconate solution twice daily to complement oral care.

- **My patient is receiving chemotherapy?**

  Stress the importance of good oral hygiene, including brushing the teeth after meals and before going to bed.
  Chemotherapy can cause neutropenia (reduced white blood cell count), predisposing the patient to infections. The oral cavity is a common site for infections in patients with neutropenia.

  Routine rinses of mouthwashes with chlorhexidine are not recommended. Instead, use a bland rinse of diluted salt and/or sodium bicarbonate. Patients should swish for a minimum of 30 seconds and then expectorate the residue.
  Chlorhexidine products have not proved superior to bland rinses in preventing or reducing either chemotherapy/radiation-induced mucositis or yeast colonization. In addition, chlorhexidine products may contain alcohol, cause discomfort, alter taste sensations, and stain teeth. Bland rinses containing 1 teaspoon of salt or sodium bicarbonate per pint of water reduce the acidity of oral secretions, lessen mucus accumulation, and discourage yeast colonization.

  An antifungal agent or a multiagent rinse (sometimes labeled "magic" or "miracle" rinse) may be used, followed by a short NPO period of 30 to 60 minutes. If other mouthwashes or rinses are also being used, allow 30 minutes to pass between their use and the use of an antifungal agent.

  ✚ *Multiagent rinses typically contain lidocaine. The resulting numbing effect may pose risks for a biting injury or aspiration. These rinses can neutralize antifungal agents.*

Evaluation

- Inspect the teeth, gums, and mucous membranes to verify that they are free of food particles.
- Inspect for abnormalities, such as bleeding, that may have been stimulated by the brushing or flossing.
- Observe for patient discomfort or gagging during the procedure.
- If the procedure was performed by the UAP, the nurse should still perform an evaluation of the care. This includes a physical assessment of the oral cavity as well as objective and subjective cues related to the patient's tolerance of and satisfaction with the care.

Patient Teaching

- Discuss the importance of daily oral care.
- Review any areas of brushing or flossing that the patient has not been performing adequately.
- Discuss any cues that need further follow-up, such as inflammation, bleeding, dryness, caries, missing teeth, or broken or missing dentures.

Home Care

The procedure does not vary in the home. The nurse must:
- Work with the client and care provider to determine supplies needed for the home.
- Determine whether suction is needed (e.g., if the client is unconscious or has a decreased gag reflex). Explain to the client and/or caregiver how to obtain a portable suction unit.
- Demonstrate how to position the client and perform the procedure if the height of the bed is not adjustable or if both sides of the bed are not accessible.

Documentation

Document that oral care was given, the patient's response, any abnormal findings, and nursing interventions. Oral care is usually charted on a flowsheet.

Sample documentation

12/16/xx   0815   Oral care given. Mucous membranes intact, pink, and dry. No choking or complaints of discomfort. Patient encouraged to increase fluid intake. ———————————— Nancy Botha, RN

Practice Resources

AACN (2017); Berry et al. (2011); Coker et al. (2017); Delwel et al. (2018); Hong et al. (2019).

Thinking About the Procedure

The video **Brushing and Flossing the Teeth,** along with questions and suggested responses, is available on the Davis's *Nursing Skills Videos* Web site at www.fadavis.com.

Procedure 22-6 ■ Providing Denture Care

▶ For steps to follow in *all* procedures, refer to the Universal Steps for All Procedures on the inside back cover.

Equipment

- See Procedure 22-5: Brushing and Flossing the Teeth.
- Denture cup

Delegation

You can delegate denture care to the UAP if the patient's condition and the UAP's skills allow. Perform the preprocedure assessments and inform the UAP of the specific care and the amount of help the patient needs. Ask the UAP to report the condition of the patient's mouth and dentures, level of self-care, and ability to tolerate the procedure.

Preprocedure Assessments

See Procedure 22-5: Brushing and Flossing the Teeth.

(continued on next page)

Procedure 22-6 ■ Providing Denture Care (continued)

> When performing the procedure, always identify your patient according to agency policy, using two identifiers, and be attentive to standard precautions, hand hygiene, patient safety and privacy, body mechanics, and documentation.

Procedure Steps

1. **Don gloves and remove dentures** (if the patient cannot do so).
   a. **Upper denture:** With a gauze pad, grasp the denture with your thumb and forefinger and move it gently up and down. Tilt the denture slightly to one side to remove it, without stretching the lips. Place the denture in the denture cup.
   The gauze gives you a better grip. Breaking the seal on the top dentures can be difficult; movement breaks the suction. Always place dentures in a denture cup as soon as you remove them to prevent accidental breakage.

   b. **Lower denture:** Use your thumbs to push up gently on the denture at the gumline to release from the lower jaw. Grasp the denture with your thumb and forefinger and tilt it to remove it from the patient's mouth. Place the denture in the denture cup.
   A gauze pad is not usually needed to grasp the lower dentures; however, you can use one if the dentures are difficult to grasp. Pushing up on the dentures breaks the seal. Rotating the dentures is necessary to remove the dentures from the patient's mouth. ▶

2. **Place the towel in the sink,** hold the dentures in your hand, and pour cool water (in accordance with agency policy) over the dentures to cleanse them.
   Heat can damage some dentures. It's best to cleanse in the sink under running water and over a plastic pan or towel. Running water facilitates cleansing; the towel/pan helps keep dentures from breaking. Dentures are expensive and usually not reimbursed by insurance. Institutions vary regarding the existence of biofilm in the water lines.

   a. Apply a small amount of special denture paste to a soft-bristled toothbrush.
   Denture paste assists in cleaning. Toothpaste and stiff-bristled brushes may be too abrasive for dentures. However, follow the patient's preference in use of denture cleaner. Some patients prefer to soak their dentures in a cleanser overnight. If dentures have been soaking, rinse them well before placing them in the patient's mouth.

   b. Brush all surfaces of each denture.
   Loosens all food particles and any old denture adhesive.

   c. Rinse thoroughly with cool water.
   Removes loosened particles and the cleaning agent. Do not use hot water with dentures, because hot water can react to make the denture material sticky. Hospitalized patients at high risk for infection should avoid exposure to hospital water and use distilled, sterile, or filtered water instead.

   Note: You can soak stained dentures in a commercial cleaner following the manufacturer's instructions. Do not soak the denture overnight if the appliance has metal parts.
   Soaking can cause corrosion of the metal parts.

3. **Inspect dentures** for rough, worn, or sharp edges.
   These can irritate the tongue, gums, or mucous membranes of the mouth.

4. **Inspect the mouth** under the dentures for redness, irritation, lesions, or infection.
   If these conditions are present, refer to a dentist to check the fit of the dentures or to make needed repairs.

5. **Apply denture adhesive** as needed (ask the patient whether they use denture adhesive).
   Adhesives are needed to "seal" some dentures and prevent slipping and irritation of the gums.

6. **Moisten the top denture** if it is dry. Then insert the top denture, at a slight tilt, and press it up against the roof of the mouth.
   Moistening the dentures eases insertion. You can tell when you have securely seated the dentures by checking to feel for any slippage or to confirm that the dentures stay in place. Because the top denture is larger, it is removed first and inserted first for ease of insertion.

7. **Moisten the bottom denture** if it is dry. Then insert bottom denture, rotating it as you put it in the patient's mouth.
Because it is smaller, the bottom denture is inserted after the top one. ▼

8. **Ask the patient whether** the dentures are comfortable.
Ensures that the dentures are properly placed.

9. **If the patient does not wish to wear the dentures,** cover them with water in a clean denture container with a lid. Label the container with the patient's name and the agency identifying number. Place denture container in bedside drawer rather than on top of bedside table for safekeeping.
Drying can cause dentures to warp. Hospitalized patients at high risk for infection avoid exposure to hospital water and use sterile water instead. Having the denture out of the mouth for several hours a day relieves pressure on the oral tissues, allows saliva to clean the tissues, and helps to minimize gingival irritation.

10. **Offer mouthwash.**

? What if...

- **My patient develops *Candida*-related denture stomatitis?**

Follow agency protocols. Microwave disinfection of complete dentures has been documented as an effective treatment of *Candida*-related denture stomatitis and can reduce the recurrence of infections.

Denture stomatitis ranges in severity. Treatment includes good oral and denture hygiene and administration of antifungal agents. Recurrence of infection after treatment can be due to colonization of Candida on the dentures.

Evaluation

- See Procedure 22-5: Brushing and Flossing the Teeth.
- Check to see that dentures are comfortable and fit properly.

Other

For Documentation, Patient Teaching, and Home Care, see Procedure 22-5: Brushing and Flossing the Teeth.

Practice Resources
Aslanimehr et al. (2018); Coker et al. (2017); Papadiochou et al. (2018); Siegel et al. (2007, updated 2018).

Thinking About the Procedure

The video **Providing Denture Care,** along with questions and suggested responses, is available on the **Davis's Nursing Skills Videos** Web site at www.fadavis.com.

Procedure 22-7 ■ Providing Oral Care for an Unconscious Patient

➤ For steps to follow in *all* procedures, refer to the Universal Steps for All Procedures on the inside back cover.

Equipment

- Toothbrush with soft bristles or sponge oral swabs
- Toothpaste
- Denture cup if the patient has dentures
- 4 in. × 4 in. gauze pad to remove dentures if present
- Tonsil-tip suction connected to suction source (you may use a product that combines the toothbrush or oral swab with the suction device)
- Tongue blade (padded) or bite block
- Towel

(continued on next page)

Procedure 22-7 ■ Providing Oral Care for an Unconscious Patient (continued)

- Waterproof linen protector
- Disposable emesis basin
- Water-soluble lip moisturizer
- Procedure gloves and goggles

Delegation

As a rule, you probably should not delegate oral hygiene for an unconscious patient to a UAP. However, in some situations it may be acceptable—for example, when agency policy permits, when the UAP has a great deal of experience caring for unconscious patients, and when the UAP's ability to perform oral hygiene safely for the agency is documented. Perform the preprocedure assessments and inform the UAP of any special considerations for care (e.g., if the patient must have the head of the bed elevated to facilitate breathing). Ask the UAP to report the condition of the patient's mouth and the patient's ability to tolerate the procedure (e.g., ask the UAP to take vital signs before and after the procedure or to note the oxygen saturation if it is being monitored).

Preprocedure Assessments

- Determine whether the patient has dentures or partial plates.
  The presence of these appliances determines how you will provide oral care.
  - *You may leave dentures out for an unconscious patient to decrease the risk that the dentures will be damaged or block the airway. However, when possible, keep the dentures in place to help ensure they will fit adequately later.*
  - *Remove partial plates in an unconscious patient to prevent the plate from causing aspiration or damage to the mouth if it becomes loosened.*
- Assess the patient's gag reflex.
  If the patient has an intact gag reflex, the risk of aspiration is lower.
- Assess the patient's general oral health, including the condition of the teeth and gums, and hydration of the mucous membranes. If the patient has dentures, examine the mouth with and without the dentures.
  Unconscious patients tend to breathe through the mouth, so oral mucosa are often dry. Because the oral mucosa acts as a barrier against microorganisms, inflammation or lesions in the mouth increase the risk for infection. The lips, gums, and mucous membranes should be pink, moist, and intact. The teeth should be intact and clean. Assess the fit of dentures and the condition of the skin under the dentures to determine whether the fit is proper and whether any irritation is present. The condition of the mouth determines what you will use to provide oral care.

➤ When performing the procedure, always identify your patient according to agency policy, using two identifiers, and be attentive to standard precautions, hand hygiene, patient safety and privacy, body mechanics, and documentation.

Procedure Steps

1. **Position the patient side-lying** with head turned to the side and, if possible, with the head of the bed down.
   Secretions will pool in the dependent side of the mouth. This position helps prevent aspiration and facilitates the removal of secretions by gravity.

2. **Don procedure gloves and eye goggles.**
   Follows standard precautions. Eye protection is needed when suctioning because of the risk of splashing.

3. **Place a waterproof pad** and then a towel under the patient's cheek and chin.
   The towel and pad will absorb water and keep the bed linens dry.

4. **Set up suction.** Attach suction tubing and tonsil-tip suction; check suction.
   Suctioning helps ensure that the patient does not aspirate oral secretions during mouth care.

5. **Place an emesis basin under the patient's cheek.**
   Catches the secretions draining from the patient's mouth.

6. **Brush the patient's teeth.**
   a. With one hand, hold the patient's mouth open. Use a padded tongue blade or bite block, as needed, to hold the patient's mouth open.
   The mouth is held open so you can visualize and reach all the areas of the mouth without injuring the oral mucosa. It also keeps the patient from biting your fingers. ▼

b. Moisten the toothbrush and apply a small amount of toothpaste. Use hospital-approved water (e.g., sterile, distilled, or filtered tap water).
   Excessive toothpaste does not enhance the cleaning. Brushing the teeth with a soft-bristled brush stimulates the mucosa, which improves the health of the gums.

c. Brush the teeth, holding the bristles at a 45° angle to the gumline.
   (1) Using short, circular motions, gently brush the inner and outer surfaces of the teeth, including the gumline.
   (2) Brush the biting surface of the back teeth by holding the brush bristles vertical to the teeth and brushing back and forth.
   (3) Brush the patient's tongue.
      This is the most effective technique for removing plaque and debris from the teeth and gums. The tongue can be a reservoir for bacteria.

d. ✚ Perform oral suctioning when fluid accumulates in the mouth.
   Removing fluid prevents choking and aspiration.

e. Draw about 10 mL of distilled, sterile, or filtered water or mouthwash (e.g., dilute hydrogen peroxide) into a syringe; eject it gently into the side of the mouth. Allow the fluid to drain out into the basin, or suction as needed.
   Removes any toothpaste residue, which may have a drying effect. Remove all fluid from the mouth to prevent aspiration into the lungs. Use a minimal amount of solution to prevent aspiration.

7. **Provide denture care,** if necessary. See Procedure 22-6: Providing Denture Care.

8. **Clean the tissues in the oral** cavity according to agency policy. Use foam swabs or a moistened gauze square wrapped around a tongue blade. Use a clean swab for each area of the mouth: cheeks, tongue, roof of the mouth, and so on.
   Oral tissues may be dry and sticky from mouth breathing. Using separate swabs prevents transfer of microorganisms from one area to another.

9. **Remove and dispose of the basin,** dry the patient's face and mouth, and apply water-soluble lip moisturizer.
   ✚ *Petroleum-based lip moisturizers (e.g., mineral oil, petroleum jelly) are not recommended because of the possibility of aspiration, which might cause pneumonia. Never use petroleum-based jelly for patients receiving oxygen therapy; it can cause burns.*

10. **Remove the waterproof pad** and towel; turn off suction equipment; discard gloves and used supplies.

11. **Reposition the patient** as needed.
    Maintains good body alignment.

12. **Cleanse and store reusable** oral hygiene tools in clean containers, separate from other articles of personal hygiene.
    Prevents possible contamination from the environment and other personal hygiene tools.

? What if...

- **I am providing oral care to a patient receiving mechanical ventilation?**

  Provide oral cleansing, including subglottic suctioning, at least every 2 hours and prn. Brush the teeth at least twice a day.
  Keeping the oral cavity clean and clear of secretions has proved to decrease the incidence of ventilator-associated pneumonia (VAP). Pooled oral secretions become rapidly colonized with pathogens that contribute to VAP.

  Avoid tap water. Use normal saline or a half-strength solution of saline for oral rinses.
  Studies show hospital plumbing and tap water are often colonized with microbial organisms.

  Apply a 0.12% chlorhexidine gluconate solution 2 to 4 times daily (check agency policy) to complement oral care.

- **It is difficult to floss the patient's teeth, or the patient doesn't tolerate flossing?**

  Handheld interdental tools may be used instead of floss. These devices are special small brushes, picks, or sticks.
  Toothbrush bristles can't reach between teeth to dislodge food particles and bacteria. Interdental cleaners can be as effective as floss in keeping these areas clean.

- **Oral tissues are dry and sticky?**

  Use appropriately diluted sodium bicarbonate to dissolve viscous mucus.

Evaluation

- Inspect the teeth, gums, and mucous membranes for cleanliness.
- Observe the oral mucosa and gums for hydration, inflammation, bleeding, or infection.
- Observe the patient's overall responses to the procedure (e.g., gagging, coughing, vital signs, skin color).

Patient Teaching

- Discuss with family members any problems that need further follow-up.
- Teach oral hygiene measures, as needed.

(continued on next page)

Procedure 22-7 ■ Providing Oral Care for an Unconscious Patient (continued)

Home Care
The procedure steps do not vary in the home.
- Work with the client and caregiver to determine supplies needed for the home.
- Determine whether suction is needed and explain to caregivers how to obtain a portable suction unit.
- Demonstrate how to position the client and perform the procedure if the height of the bed is not adjustable or if both sides of the bed are not accessible.

Documentation
Document that oral care was given, any abnormal findings, and nursing interventions. Typically, though, oral care is documented on a checklist or flowsheet.

Sample documentation
11/22/xx   0730   Oral care given. Mucous membranes pink and moist. White coating on tongue—physician notified. Patient had no coughing during procedure. Gag reflex intact. Respiratory rate 18. ————————— Pamela Giordano, RN

Thinking About the Procedure

The video **Providing Oral Care for an Unconscious Patient,** along with questions and suggested responses, is available on the **Davis's** *Nursing Skills Videos* Web site at www.fadavis.com.

Practice Resources
AACN (2017); American Dental Association (n.d.); Chipps et al. (2016); Khasanah et al. (2019).

Procedure 22-8 ■ Shampooing the Hair

➤ For steps to follow in *all* procedures, refer to the Universal Steps for All Procedures on the inside back cover.

Delegation
You can delegate this procedure to the UAP if the patient's condition and the UAP's skills allow. Perform the preprocedure assessments and inform the UAP of the specific type of procedure needed (e.g., in bed, at sink, disposable shampoo equipment) and the amount of help the patient needs. Inform the UAP of any special considerations, such as positions the patient cannot assume or presence of scalp lesions. Ask the UAP to report the condition of the patient's scalp and hair, level of self-care, and ability to tolerate the procedure.

Preprocedure Assessments
- Assess for contraindications to a shampoo (e.g., scalp sutures or limited head or neck movement). A rinse-free shampoo would be more appropriate in these cases.
- Determine the patient's ability to assist with the procedure.
  Promotes independence and provides active ROM.
- Assess the condition of the patient's hair and scalp. Note any dryness or irritation.
  Dry and brittle hair may indicate hypothyroidism or malnutrition and may require special shampoos or conditioners.
- Determine the need for special hair care products.
  Dandruff, lice, and dry hair are examples of conditions that require medicated shampoos or conditioners.
- Ask the patient how they normally care for their hair.

Procedure 22-8A ■ Shampooing the Hair for a Patient on Bedrest Using Rinse-Free Shampoo

➤ When performing the procedure, always identify your patient according to agency policy, using two identifiers, and be attentive to standard precautions, hand hygiene, patient safety and privacy, body mechanics, and documentation.

Equipment
- Rinse-free shampoo (no water is needed); conditioner is optional
- Bath towel
- Brush or hair pick and comb
- Procedure gloves (if scalp lesion or infestation present)

Procedure Steps
1. **Elevate the head** of the bed, if possible.
   Makes it easier to maintain good body mechanics during the procedure.

2. **Place a protective pad** or bath towel under the patient's shoulders.
   Prevents the linen from getting wet.

3. **Don procedure gloves** if lesions or infestations are present.
   Helps prevent transmission of disease.

4. **Work your fingers through the hair,** or comb the hair to remove tangles before washing. If the patient has their hair in small braids, do not take out the braids to wash the hair.

5. **Apply rinse-free shampoo.** Apply enough shampoo to thoroughly wet the hair. One application is usually sufficient to clean the hair.

6. **Work the shampoo through the hair** from scalp down to ends.
   Helps prevent pulling on and damaging the hair.

7. **Dry the hair** with a bath towel.
   Removes the shampoo. Leaves the hair feeling clean.

8. **Comb or brush hair** to remove tangles, starting at the ends and working toward the scalp.
   Prevents excessive pulling on the patient's hair, which may cause breakage.

9. **Dry the hair** with a hair dryer at a medium temperature, if desired.
   Use a medium temperature to prevent burning the patient.

10. **When you are finished,** be sure that the patient's clothing and bed linens are dry. Wash and store brushes and combs.

Procedure 22-8B ■ Shampooing the Hair Using Rinse-Free Shampoo Cap

▶ When performing the procedure, always identify your patient according to agency policy, using two identifiers, and be attentive to standard precautions, hand hygiene, patient safety and privacy, body mechanics, and documentation.

Procedure Steps

1. **Warm the shampoo cap** using a water bath or microwave according to package instructions. Be careful not to overheat. Check the temperature before placing on the patient's head to prevent burns.

   A commercial no-rinse shampoo cap is a microwavable cap that contains no-rinse shampoo and conditioner. Various products are available. Be sure to follow the directions on the package.

2. **Place the cap on the patient's hair** and gently massage.

3. **Remove the cap** and towel-dry the patient's hair.
   Removes the shampoo and excess water.

4. **Complete hair care** according to the patient's needs (see Procedure 22-8A, Steps 7–10, preceding).

Procedure 22-8C ■ Shampooing the Hair Using a Basin and Water

Key Point: *The use of prepackaged shampoo products is recommended. However, some patients prefer the traditional shampooing technique or may have excessive soiling of the hair and scalp requiring the use of water and basin. This traditional method of hair hygiene can result in significant variation from caregiver to caregiver and increase the risk of hospital-associated infection from contaminated basins and/or tap water. Such techniques also take longer so they require more nursing time and may be more tiring for the patient.*

Equipment

- Shampoo; conditioner is optional
- Disposable shampoo tray or commercial system, if available
- Disposable washbasin, plastic pail, small easy-to-handle plastic container
- Towels (2), washcloth, bath blanket
- Waterproof pads or plastic trash bag
- Brush and comb
- Procedure gloves, if indicated by the presence of lesions or infestation
- Hair dryer
- For inpatients, filtered tap, distilled, or sterile water is recommended (see Key Point before this section). Follow agency policy, as conditions vary among institutions.

▶ When performing the procedure, always identify your patient according to agency policy, using two identifiers, and be attentive to standard precautions, hand hygiene, patient safety and privacy, body mechanics, and documentation.

Procedure Steps

1. **If lesions or infestation is** present, don procedure gloves.
   Observes standard precautions.

2. **Unless contraindicated** (e.g., by a neck condition), lower the head of the bed, take the pillow from under the patient's neck, and place it under the shoulders.
   Hyperextends the neck and helps keep water from the eyes.

3. **Place the waterproof pad** or plastic trash bag under patient's shoulders and cover with towels. A commercial system will have a drain hose to use.
   Protects the bed from getting wet.

4. **Collect warm, not hot, water** (see Equipment) in a container and bring to the bedside.

5. **Place the shampoo tray** under the patient's shoulders (or head, depending on the type of tray). If you are using a hard plastic tray, pad the neck area with a towel. An inflatable shampoo tray needs minimal padding, but you will need to inflate it with an air pump before beginning the procedure.
   Protects the patient from lying on a hard surface and prevents water from leaking onto the bed.

6. **Ensure that the tray will drain** into the washbasin or plastic pail.
   Prevents water draining onto the bed or floor.

7. **Fold the top linens down** to the patient's waist and cover the upper body with a bath blanket.
   Keeps the linen dry; keeps the patient warm.

(continued on next page)

Procedure 22-8 ■ Shampooing the Hair (continued)

8. **Work your fingers through** the patient's hair, or comb the hair to remove tangles before washing.
   It is easier to remove tangles from dry hair. Note that very tangled or matted hair may sometimes indicate a lice infestation.

9. **Wash the hair.**
   a. Wet the hair, pouring warm water from the pitcher. Do not get water in the patient's eyes or ears.
   b. Next, apply shampoo and lather well, working from the scalp out and from the front to the back of the head.
   c. Gently lift the patient's head to rub the back of the head.

10. **Rinse thoroughly.**
    Shampoo is drying if left in the hair. ▼

11. **Apply conditioner to the hair,** if desired, especially for patients with hair that tangles easily, such as dry, long, curly, or kinky hair. Rinse if needed. Leave-in conditioner can be used and is recommended for curly hair.

12. **Remove the tray** and blot-dry the hair with the towel. Do not use circular motions to dry the hair.
    Circular motions will increase tangles.

13. **Comb or brush hair** to remove tangles, starting at the ends and working toward the scalp.
    Prevents excessive pulling on the patient's hair, which may cause breakage.

14. **Dry the hair** with a hair dryer at a medium temperature, if desired.
    Use a medium temperature to prevent burning the patient.

15. **When you are finished,** be sure that the patient's clothing and bed linens are dry. Wash the shampoo tray and the brushes and combs.

Procedure Variation: Shampooing the Hair of Black Patients

16. **If the hair is in cornrows or braids,** do not take out the braids to wash the hair. You may need to apply a cloth or net cap to the head before shampooing.

17. **Handle the patient's hair very gently,** being careful not to pull on the hair.
    Patients may have fragile hair that breaks easily. Because it is fragile, apply moisturizer, if needed, to untangle the hair.

18. **When shampooing,** thread your fingers through the hair from the scalp out to the ends. Do not massage the hair in circular motions.

19. **Rinse thoroughly,** then apply a conditioner to the hair if the hair is dry and fragile.
    A leave-in conditioner helps minimize tangles and breakage.

20. **Comb through the hair.**
    a. Use a wide-toothed comb or hair pick. Do not use a brush or fine-toothed comb.
    b. Part the hair into four sections and begin combing near the ends of the hair, working through each section.
    c. Use additional moisturizer to help soften and ease combing.
    Never pull on the hair because it will break easily.

21. **Apply a natural oil to the hair,** if desired. Examples of natural oils are coconut, sweet almond, shea butter, and avocado. Many commercial products use these oils.
    Mineral oil and Vaseline tend to clog pores and damage the hair, so use them only if the patient still prefers them after receiving this information.

22. **Let the hair air dry** if possible.
    A high temperature, such as from a hair dryer, may damage the hair.

❓ What if...

■ **I discover head lice or nits as I begin the shampoo?**

Stop the procedure. Discuss your findings with the patient and offer reassurance. Leave the patient in a position of comfort and safety. Perform hand hygiene. Report the findings and obtain an order for a prescription shampoo.

■ **I do not have a shampoo tray?**

Improvise by using a new, unused bedpan, and reserve it only for washing the hair. Pad it liberally with towels.

Evaluation

- Observe that the hair is clean, dry, and free of tangles.
- Observe for patient discomfort or fatigue during the procedure.
- Ask the patient how the hair and scalp feel.

Patient Teaching

- Educate patients and their families about how bathing technology has changed to improve patient care and reduce risk of infection. Products such as rinse-free shampoos or a shampoo cap can make shampooing easier to accomplish for a bedridden patient.
- Advise patients with coarse hair to wash it less frequently (every 3 to 7 days, depending on dryness). Leave-in conditioners are often recommended for dry, curly, or kinky hair.

Home Care

- In the home care setting, determine how the client usually washes their hair.
- If the client is confined to bed, work with the caregiver to develop an effective plan for washing the client's hair. For example, if a shampoo tray is not available, you can make one by using a plastic garbage bag and pillows or rolled towels.
- The newer rinse-free products or the inflatable shampoo tray may be good choices for the client.
- If the client cannot afford the adaptive equipment needed, refer the caregiver to local resources, such as senior services.
- If the client is ambulatory, recommend a shower stool. The stool needs to fit into the shower or bathtub securely, without wobbling, to prevent the client from falling.
- If the client has only a bathtub, an adaptor for the faucet can be used to attach a handheld showerhead. Using a shower stool will make the procedure easier.

Documentation

Chart that hair was shampooed, the condition of the hair and scalp, and the patient's responses to the procedure.

Sample documentation

mm/dd/yyyy   2045   Hair shampooed. Scalp without signs of irritation. Hair dry. Conditioner applied. No c/o discomfort. Pt states "My hair feels wonderful now, and my head doesn't itch anymore."   — Alicia Nelson, RN

Practice Resources

EZ-Shampoo Instructions for Use (2021); Thompson Healthcare, Inc. (2022). (Caveat: These are not research articles; they are manufacturers' recommendations.)

Procedure 22-9 ■ Providing Beard and Mustache Care

▶ For steps to follow in *all* procedures, refer to the Universal Steps for All Procedures on the inside back cover.

Equipment

- Scissors or beard trimmer
- Wide-toothed comb
- Mild shampoo; conditioner for coarse and/or dry hair
- Basin (single-patient use, disposable)
- Bath towel
- Procedure gloves (if skin nicks occur, contact with blood may occur)

Delegation

You can delegate beard and mustache care to the UAP if the patient's condition and the UAP's skills allow. Perform the preprocedure assessments and inform the UAP of the specific type of care needed (e.g., in bed, at sink, safety razor, electric razor). Inform the UAP of any special considerations, such as skin irritation or activity intolerance. Ask the UAP to report the condition of the patient's skin and beard, level of self-care, and ability to tolerate the procedure.

Preprocedure Assessments

- Ask the patient or family about preferences for beard and mustache care.
  Beards and mustaches may have personal and/or cultural meaning. In some cultures, beards are never cut or trimmed. Some patients use a comb and scissors to do a slight trim of their beard and/or mustache, whereas others use a beard trimmer for a closer trim.
- Assess the patient's skin and hair condition.
  Determine whether the skin has any reddened or dry areas and whether skin treatments are needed.

▶ When performing the procedure, always identify your patient according to agency policy, using two identifiers, and be attentive to standard precautions, hand hygiene, patient safety and privacy, body mechanics, and documentation.

Procedure Steps

1. **Drape the towel around** the patient's shoulders.
   Protects the patient's clothing from falling pieces of hair and water from shampooing the beard or mustache.

2. **Trim the beard and mustache** when they are dry.
   The beard and mustache are often shorter when dry. If they are cut when wet, they may be shorter than desired after they dry.

Variation: If Using a Comb and Scissors

a. Comb through the beard and cut the hair on the outside of the comb. Be conservative; cutting too little is better than cutting too much.
   Trimming too much off the beard can be upsetting for the patient, whereas if you cut too little, you can always trim off more.

b. Trim from the front of the ear to the chin on one side, and repeat on the other.
   Keeps the beard equal on both sides of the face.

Variation: If Using a Beard Trimmer

c. Select the trimming guide to the correct length. Adjust the guide to a longer length rather than a shorter length.
   Ensures that you do not cut the beard too short.

(continued on next page)

Procedure 22-9 ■ Providing Beard and Mustache Care (continued)

  d. Trim from the front of the ear to the chin on one side, and repeat on the other.

3. **Trim the mustache.**
   a. Comb the mustache straight down.
   Cuts the length equally so that the mustache is just above the upper lip. ▼

   b. Using either scissors or a beard trimmer, start in the middle and trim toward one side of the mouth and then toward the other. Do not trim the top of the mustache.
   Trimming from the center out toward each side helps you cut both sides equally.

4. **Define the beard line** by one of the following methods:
   a. Using either the scissors or a beard trimmer, trim the line of the beard so that it is well defined. Trim very little to ensure that you only define the beard and do not change the length. ▼

   b. Shave the neck to define the beard line, particularly for short beards.

5. **Apply procedure gloves,** if needed, and shampoo the beard and mustache using warm sterile, distilled, or tap water and a mild shampoo.
   The skin under a beard or mustache can be tender, so treat it gently with a mild shampoo. Follow standard precautions because it is possible to nick the skin and cause bleeding. Policies about use of tap water vary among institutions.

6. **Rinse well; pat and wipe** the beard and mustache dry with the towel.
   Any shampoo left can irritate the skin, as can rubbing motions with the towel.

7. **Apply conditioner,** if desired.

8. **Comb the beard and mustache** with a wide-toothed comb or a brush.
   Do not use a fine-toothed comb because it will pull the hair.

Evaluation
- Make sure that the beard and mustache are trimmed to the desired length and are clean.
- Verify that skin problems are identified and treatment initiated.

Home Care
No adaptations are required in the home. The patient's usual supplies are sufficient, as a rule.

Documentation
Chart that beard and mustache were trimmed and shampooed; chart the condition of the skin.

Practice Resources
Procter & Gamble (n.d.). (Caveat: This is not an evidence-based practice article. It is a manufacturer's recommendation.)

Procedure 22-10 ■ Shaving a Patient

▶ For steps to follow in *all* procedures, refer to the Universal Steps for All Procedures on the inside back cover.

Equipment
- Safety razor or electric razor
- Shaving cream or soap; after-shave lotion, if desired
- Shaving brush, if desired
- Warm water (sterile, distilled, or tap water per agency policy)
- Face towel and bath towel
- Procedure gloves

Delegation
You can delegate shaving to the UAP if the patient's condition and the UAP's skills allow. Perform the preprocedure assessments and inform the UAP of the amount of help and specific type of care (e.g., safety or electric razor, in bed, or at the sink) the patient needs. Inform the UAP of any special considerations, such as skin irritation or activity intolerance. Ask the UAP to report the condition of the patient's skin, level of self-care, and ability to tolerate the procedure.

Preprocedure Assessments
- Determine how much assistance the patient needs.
  Aids you in promoting as much independence as possible.
- ✚ Assess the patient's skin and hair condition for redness, skin lesions, or moles.

CHAPTER 22 Facilitating Hygiene 371

Identifies skin problems and determines whether skin treatments are needed or the procedure must be modified. To prevent abrading the skin, do not shave any areas that have skin lesions or moles.

- Assess the patient's usual shaving method, including use of electric razor or safety razor.
  When possible, follow the patient's routine. The patient may or may not use shaving cream or shaving soap, shaving brush, and after-shave lotion.

- ✚ Check for any contraindications to shaving, such as an increased risk of infection or bleeding (e.g., because of neutropenia, thrombocytopenia, or the administration of anticoagulants, such as warfarin or heparin).

➤ When performing the procedure, always identify your patient according to agency policy, using two identifiers, and be attentive to standard precautions, hand hygiene, patient safety and privacy, body mechanics, and documentation.

Procedure Steps

1. **Don procedure gloves.**
   To prevent exposure to blood if skin is nicked or scratched.

2. **Place a warm, damp face towel** on the patient's face for 1 to 3 minutes.
   Opens the pores and softens the beard to prevent pulling. Do not use hot water because it will dehydrate the skin and can burn sensitive skin.

3. **Apply shaving lotion** to the face with your fingers or a shaving brush. Lather well for 1 to 2 minutes.
   Lathering well further softens the beard. Do not use shaving creams that contain numbing agents because they close the pores and stiffen the beard.

4. **Shave the patient.**
   a. Pull skin taut with your nondominant hand, and gently pull the razor across the skin. If you are using a safety razor, hold the blade at a 45° angle to the skin.
   b. Shave the face and neck in the same direction of hair growth (the direction is not the same for all people). Using short strokes, start shaving at the sideburns and work down to the chin on each side and then the neck.
   c. Last, shave the chin and upper lip.
   Usually the hair on the face will grow down toward the chin and on the neck up toward the chin. The hair is generally thickest on the chin and upper lip, so shaving them last allows more time for the shaving cream to soften the hair. Shave in the same direction as the hair is growing to prevent skin irritation. ▼

5. **Rinse the razor** frequently while you are shaving.
   Avoids clogging the blade.

6. **When you are finished shaving,** rinse the patient's face with cool water (per agency policy), and gently pat it dry.
   Cool water helps close the pores. Pat dry, do not rub, to prevent irritating the skin.

7. **Apply after-shave lotion,** if desired.
   After-shave lotions that contain alcohol are not recommended because alcohol stings and dries out the skin. A moisturizer is recommended.

8. **Dispose of the single-use razor** in the sharps container.
   Prevents cutting injury to others.

Variation: If Using a Multiuse Razor
Shake the razor to remove excess moisture. Do not bang the razor against objects or dry with a towel. Store the razor in a covered container.
Banging or wiping the razor edge will dull the razor and may damage the holding mechanism. A covered container protects others from a cutting injury.

? What if . . .

- My patient has a condition that predisposes them to bleeding (e.g., thrombocytopenia) or infection (e.g., neutropenia)?

- ✚ Such patients must be shaved carefully using an electric razor, if at all.
   A razor scratch or cut causes a break in skin integrity, providing a portal of entry for pathogens. This could be especially serious for a patient whose defenses against infection are compromised. For a patient with a delayed clotting time, a cut could cause excessive blood loss.

(continued on next page)

Procedure 22-10 ■ Shaving a Patient (continued)

Evaluation
- Inspect the patient's face for closeness of the shave and for nicks or cuts.
- If the procedure was performed by the UAP, ask the patient about their satisfaction with and tolerance of the care.

Patient Teaching
Teach patients about changes that need to be made in their shaving technique as a result of changes in health status. For example, a patient who has begun taking anticoagulants may need to change from a blade to an electric razor because of an increased risk of bleeding.

Home Care
The procedure does not vary in the home. The nurse must:
- Determine the availability of supplies
- Assess the client's or caregiver's ability to perform the procedure.

Documentation
Chart that the patient was shaved and the condition of the skin. There will probably be a flowsheet or checklist for this information.

Practice Resources
Dunkley & McLeod (2015); Procter & Gamble (n.d.); *Men's Health* (2022). (Caveat: Not all of the preceding are not evidence-based resources. They are information from manufacturers.)

Procedure 22-11 ■ Removing and Caring for Contact Lenses

▶ For steps to follow in *all* procedures, refer to the Universal Steps for All Procedures on the inside back cover.

Equipment
- Contact lens wetting solution
- Contact lens soaking solution
- Sterile saline (optional)
- Contact lens case
- Contact lens remover (optional)
- Procedure gloves

Delegation
You can delegate this procedure if the patient's condition and the UAP's skills permit. For example, if the patient is unconscious, you must determine whether contact lenses are present, and you should not delegate their removal.

Preprocedure Assessments
- Determine whether the patient is wearing contact lenses. If the patient is unconscious, examine the eyes for the presence of contact lenses by shining a penlight across the eye. You should be able to see the edge of the lens.
- Determine the type of contact lenses in place.
  Each type of contact lens has unique care requirements. **Soft lenses** *are very thin and pliable and conform to the front surface of the eye.* **Silicone hydrogel lenses** *are an advanced type of soft contact lenses that are more porous than soft lenses and allow more oxygen to reach the cornea. Gas-permeable (GP or RGP) lenses are rigid contact lenses that are porous and allow oxygen to pass through them. Hard contact lenses have mostly been replaced by GP lenses and are rarely prescribed today.*

  Key Point: *Lenses are classified by wearing time: Daily wear must be removed nightly. Extended wear are worn overnight and up to 7 days consecutively without removal. Continuous wear are for 30 consecutive nights of wear (the maximum wearing time approved by the FDA for certain brands of extended-wear lenses).*
- Ask the patient whether they are able to remove their contact lenses.

▶ When performing the procedure, always identify your patient according to agency policy, using two identifiers, and be attentive to standard precautions, hand hygiene, patient safety and privacy, body mechanics, and documentation.

▶ *Note:* It is difficult to remove a contact lens when wearing procedure gloves. For hard lenses, you can use a suction cup device if one is available. ✚ If you must use ungloved hands (e.g., in an emergency situation), it is extremely important to perform hand hygiene before and after the procedure. *Do not* use your fingernails.

▶ *Note:* Lens cases are marked L and R to indicate left and right lenses. Clean, rinse, and place the lens you remove first into its designated cup before removing the second lens.

Procedure Steps

1. **Perform hand hygiene** and don gloves.
2. **Instill 1 or 2 drops** of contact lens multipurpose solution to moisten the lenses.
   Aids in lens removal.
3. **Remove the lenses.**

Variation: For Gas-Permeable Contact Lens (or Hard Lenses)

- *Alternative 1:* If the lens is not centered over the cornea, place your finger on the patient's lower eyelid and apply gentle pressure to move it into position. Place your index finger at the outer corner of the eye and gently pull sideways toward the ear; position your other hand below the eye to "catch" the lens. Ask the patient to blink. As the skin tightens, the palpebral fissure narrows and the lids catch on the edge of the lens to pop it out. ▼

- *Alternative 2:* Gently pull the top eyelid up and the lower lid down beyond the top and bottom edges of the lens. Then gently press the lower eyelid up against the bottom of the lens. When the lens is slightly tipped, move the eyelids together. This should cause the lens to slide out. ▼

Variation: For Soft Contact Lens

a. Hold the eye open with your nondominant hand.
   Allows you to visualize the contact lens.
b. Gently place the tip of your index finger on the contact lens and slide it down off the pupil to the white area of the eye.

To prevent potential damage to the eye, do not pinch a lens directly over the pupil. ▼

c. Using your thumb and index finger pads, gently pinch the lens and lift it straight up off the eye. If the edges stick together, moisten with a few drops of wetting solution. Rub gently until edges separate.
   A soft contact lens is very flexible and pinches easily. ▼

4. **Clean the lens** according to the instructions on the cleaning solution bottle. If there is no lens cleaner, use sterile saline. Be careful not to tear soft lenses.
5. **Rinse the lenses** with contact lens solution or sterile saline.
   Removes any particles from the lenses.
6. **Place the lenses in a contact** lens case containing soaking solution or sterile saline (see previous note regarding lens cases). ✚ Never use water.
   Prevents bacterial growth on the lenses and keeps them from drying out.

Evaluation

Examine the eyes for redness or irritation.

Patient Teaching

- Review with the patient and/or family the importance of keeping the contact lenses clean and moist.
- ✚ Teach the patient that contact lenses should not be worn or stored in water. If water touches the lens, remove and discard the lens.
- If hard contact lenses are used, they must be removed at bedtime to prevent hypoxia of the cornea.

Documentation

Chart that contacts were removed, what type of lenses they are, what solution they are stored in, and the condition of patient's eyes.

Practice Resources

All About Vision (n.d.); American Academy of Ophthalmology (2022); Bausch & Lomb (2022); Massachusetts Eye and Ear Infirmary (2022).

Procedure 22-12 ■ Caring for Artificial Eyes

> For steps to follow in *all* procedures, refer to the Universal Steps for All Procedures on the page facing the inside back cover.

Equipment
- Procedure gloves
- Normal saline solution
- Labeled container filled with saline or sterile, distilled, or filtered water
- Cotton balls

Delegation
You can delegate this procedure to the UAP if the patient's condition and the UAP's skills allow. Perform the preprocedure assessments and inform the UAP of any special considerations. Ask the UAP to report the patient's ability to tolerate the procedure.

Preprocedure Assessments
Assess the patient's activity tolerance and whether you will need another caregiver to assist.

> When performing the procedure, always identify your patient according to agency policy, using two identifiers, and be attentive to standard precautions, hand hygiene, patient safety and privacy, body mechanics, and documentation.

Procedure Steps

1. **Perform hand hygiene and don gloves.**

2. **Position the patient lying down.**
   If you drop the eye when removing it, it will fall onto the bed instead of the floor.

3. **To remove the artificial eye:**
   a. Raise the upper eyelid with your nondominant hand and depress the lower lid with your dominant hand.
   b. Apply slight pressure below the eye to release the suction holding it in place.
   c. Catch the eye in the palm of your dominant hand.
   d. Alternatively, you can use a small bulb syringe, place it directly on the eye, and squeeze to create suction and lift the eye straight up from the socket. ▼

4. **Clean the eye with saline** and store it in a labeled container filled with saline or sterile, distilled, or filtered water. ✚ Do not use solvents, disinfectants, or alcohol. These chemicals may irritate the socket or damage the artificial eye.

5. **Wipe the edge of the patient's** eye socket with a moistened cotton ball, wiping from outer canthus toward the nose.

6. **Inspect the socket** for redness, swelling, or drainage.
   Irritation or infection can occur if debris has entered the socket.

7. **To reinsert the eye:**
   a. Remove the prosthetic eye from the container, but do not dry it.
   b. Hold the eye between your thumb and the index finger of your dominant hand.
   c. With your nondominant hand, pull down on the lower lid while lifting the upper lid and guide the eye into the socket.
   The prosthesis will slide into place more easily when it is wet.

Evaluation
- Observe that the eye has been placed correctly in the socket.
- Ask the patient how the eye area feels.
- Observe the eye area for redness or irritation.

Patient Teaching
- Advise the patient to periodically inspect the eye area.
- Review the importance of hand hygiene and proper handling of the eye.
- If the eye wearer has dryness or irritation, a lubricant made for ocular prosthetics can be used.
- If the eye needs to be wiped but not removed, wipe from outer canthus toward the nose.
  Wiping outward may dislodge the prosthesis.
- Encourage the patient to sleep in the prosthesis at night and remove it every 1 to 3 weeks for cleaning (follow prosthesis specialist's advice). Some patients do find that it is necessary to remove and clean the prosthesis every day.
  Frequent removal irritates the lining of the socket and increases the amount of discharge produced by the eye socket.
- The eye should be professionally polished every 6 to 12 months. Symptoms that may indicate the need for a polish are irritated or itchy lids, increased drainage or discomfort, or changes in the appearance of the artificial eye.

Home Care
- In the home care setting, determine how the client usually performs eye care.
- Discuss ways to promote the safety of the artificial eye.
- Work with the client or caregiver to develop a plan of care for cleaning the eye and care of the area associated with the socket.

Documentation

Chart that the artificial eye was cleaned, the condition of the socket, care given to the area around the socket, and the patient's responses to the procedure.

Practice Resources

Artificial Eyes (2019); Erikson Labs Northwest (n.d.).

Procedure 22-13 ■ Caring for Hearing Aids

▶ For steps to follow in *all* procedures, refer to the Universal Steps for All Procedures on the page facing the inside back cover.

Equipment
- Face cloth, dry towel
- Damp cloth
- Cotton applicators
- Wax loop and wax brush, if available
- Pipe cleaner or toothpick, if wax loop and wax brush unavailable
- Procedure gloves (to prevent contact with earwax or ear drainage)

Delegation

You can delegate hearing aid care to the UAP if the patient's condition and the UAP's skills allow. Perform the preprocedure assessments and inform the UAP of the specific type of care needed (e.g., type of hearing aid) and the amount of help the patient needs. Inform the UAP of any special considerations, such as skin irritation or usual volume setting. Ask the UAP to report the condition of the patient's ears, level of self-care, ability to tolerate the procedure, and ability to hear in a normal conversation.

Preprocedure Assessments

- Determine how much assistance the patient needs.
  Aids you in promoting independence as much as possible.
- Determine the type of hearing aid in use. The three common types of hearing aids are (1) postaural hearing aid, (2) in-the-canal hearing aid, and (3) in-the-ear hearing aid.
  The cleaning procedure varies according to the type of hearing aid.
  To review the types of hearing aids,

  ▶ Go to Volume 1, Figure 22-7.

- Assess the patient's ear and outer canal for redness, skin lesions, earwax buildup, or drainage.
  Identify skin problems and determine whether any symptoms of infection exist. Earwax buildup increases with age and doesn't necessarily indicate a health problem.

▶ When performing the procedure, always identify your patient according to agency policy, using two identifiers, and be attentive to standard precautions, hand hygiene, patient safety and privacy, body mechanics, and documentation.

Procedure Steps

1. **Don procedure gloves.**
   The hearing aid may contain earwax buildup or drainage.

2. **Place a towel on a nearby table** or flat surface.
   The towel helps prevent the hearing aid from breaking if it is accidentally dropped.

3. **To remove the hearing aid:**
   a. Turn the hearing aid off by applying slight pressure against the volume control wheel and turning it backward (away from the nose).
      Stops the hearing aid from whistling.
   b. Rotate the earmold slightly forward (toward the nose) and gently pull it out. Do not pull on the battery door or the volume wheel.
      Pulling on the battery door or the volume wheel may damage the faceplate.
   c. Place the hearing aid on the towel.
      The towel will prevent the hearing aid from rolling off the table or banging against the table.

4. **Clean the hearing aid.**
   a. Wipe all external surfaces with a damp cloth.
   b. Clean the canal portion of the hearing aid using the wax loop and wax brush, cotton-tipped applicator, pipe cleaner, or toothpick. Clean the top portion only. Do not insert anything into the hearing aid itself.
      Poking utensils into any part of the hearing aid except for the canal portion may damage the hearing aid.

   Variation: Detachable Earmold
   c. Disconnect the earmold and soak it in soapy water. Rinse and dry well and then reattach it. Do not use alcohol. Never immerse a hearing aid in water, only the earmold.
      Detaching an earmold that is glued or fastened by a small metal ring will break the hearing aid. Alcohol will damage the earmold material.
   d. Check the hearing aid and any tubing for cracks and loose connections.
      A damaged hearing aid will be less effective and may cause injury to the ear. Early detection of hearing aid damage may allow for repair rather than replacement of the device.

5. **Cleanse the outer ear** using the corner of a washcloth or a cotton-tipped applicator. Inspect the outer ear for redness, abrasions, swelling, drainage, or other irregularities.
   Poorly fitting or improperly positioned hearing aids may cause trauma to the ear.

(continued on next page)

Procedure 22-13 ■ Caring for Hearing Aids (continued)

6. **Insert the hearing aid.**
   a. Check that the battery is functioning. Hold the hearing aid in your hand. Close the battery compartment door if open. Turn the power on, turn the volume high, and listen for a whistling sound.
   Whistling indicates proper power level and functioning of the battery.
   b. Set the volume control to "off."
   Prevents whistling during insertion and a sudden loud noise.
   c. Handle the hearing aid by the edges using your thumb and forefinger.
   Prevents whistling during insertion.
   d. Holding the hearing aid in your dominant hand, use your non-dominant hand to gently pull the ear up and back.
   Opens the ear canal slightly for an easier insertion and better fit.
   e. Insert the canal portion of the hearing aid into the ear. Apply slight pressure and gently rotate the hearing aid back and forth until the canal portion rests flat in the ear.
   Allows a better fit and prevents hearing aid from falling out.

Variation: When Inserting a Postaural Hearing Aid
Insert the earmold first and then place the earmold over the ear.

Variation: When Inserting an In-the-Canal Hearing Aid
Insert with the volume control at the top. The canal should be facing away from your hand.

Variation: When Inserting an In-the-Ear Hearing Aid
Insert with the volume control at the bottom.

7. **Turn the hearing aid on** and adjust the volume by turning the volume control wheel toward the nose. Set the volume control as low as possible.

   Normal setting requires a one-third to two-thirds turn of the volume control wheel. A noisier environment requires less volume, or one-fourth turn.

8. **Protect the hearing aid** from curling irons, hair dryers, and hair spray and other hair products.
   Heat and moist aerosols will damage the hearing aid.

Procedure Variation: Storing the Hearing Aid

9. **Open the battery compartment** and place the hearing aid in a closed container labeled with the patient's name.
   Saves battery power and allows any moisture to evaporate. Protects the hearing aid from accidental damage and loss.

10. **If the hearing aid is to be stored** and not worn for a week or more, remove the battery completely.
    Prevents battery acid from leaking and damaging the hearing aid.

11. **Store the hearing aid** in a cool, dry place, preferably in the bedside drawer. Keep the hearing aid away from children and pets.
    Moisture and heat will damage the hearing aid. Hearing aids and containers are easily lost. A child may choke on the hearing aid. Dogs and cats are attracted to the whistling noise and odor of the hearing aid and sometimes attempt to eat the device.

Procedure Variation: Replacing the Battery

12. **Use your finger** to swing the battery door open. Never force the door.

13. **Peel the tab off the new battery.**

14. **Hold the battery with the** positive (+) side up and slide it into the door, not into the hearing aid itself.

15. **Gently close the battery door.** Never force the door.

16. **Dispose of the old mercury-free battery** in the regular trash.
    NOTE: If the battery contains mercury, refer to the package for disposal instructions.

Guidelines for Care of the Batteries

- Always dispose of old batteries. Do not throw into a fire.
  Minimizes damage from leaking battery acid and prevents mistaking fresh battery from used battery. Heat and fire may cause the battery to explode.

- Store batteries in a cool, dry place. Do not place zinc-air batteries in the refrigerator.
  Heat shortens the life of the battery. Cold batteries warming to room temperature are exposed to condensation and subsequent corrosion.

- Do not store batteries near coins or other metals.
  Contact with other metals can short-circuit the batteries.

- Do not remove the tab from the battery until the battery is ready for use.
  The tab keeps air out of the battery. Once the tab is removed, the battery is activated. Early removal decreases the life of the battery.

- Keep batteries away from children, adults who are confused, and pets.
  Minimizes accidental swallowing.

? What if...

- **The hearing aid becomes wet?**
  If the hearing aid becomes exposed to moisture, dry it as thoroughly as possible. Remove the battery and throw it away. Keep the battery door open. Place the hearing aid in its container and allow it to dry overnight. Do not place a new battery in the hearing aid until the next morning.
  Moisture will cause the battery to corrode.

- **The patient wears bilateral hearing aids?**

Be sure to identify which hearing aid is for the left ear and which hearing aid is for the right ear. Most hearing aids have a color marking for easy identification (red is for right ear and blue is for left ear).

Attempting to force a hearing aid into the wrong ear may cause trauma to the ear.

- **The patient continues to have hearing difficulties despite hearing aids?**

Hearing aids will not restore full hearing. General tips when communicating with a person with a hearing deficit are listed in Clinical Insight 27-3: Communicating With Hearing-Impaired Clients.

Hearing aids will not block out background noise. A clear, distinct, low-pitched voice helps the client to understand what is being said.

Evaluation

- Assess how well the patient tolerated the procedure. Was there any discomfort, difficulty with insertion, and so on?
- Note the condition of the patient's skin, including pain, redness, and abnormal discharge.
- Note the condition of the hearing aid itself.
- Assess the patient's ability to hear normal speaking voices.
- Ask the patient whether they feel comfortable and hear satisfactorily.

Patient Teaching

- Discuss the importance of daily hearing aid care.
- Review any areas of care that the patient has not been performing adequately.
- Discuss any problems that need further follow-up, such as earwax buildup, faulty or broken hearing aid, or ill-fitting hearing aid.

Home Care

- The procedure does not vary in the home.
- Work with the patient and care provider to determine supplies needed for the home.

- Determine whether further knowledge is required (e.g., if the patient must expose hearing aids to prevailing weather conditions, uses a telephone extensively, must make several adaptations from quiet to noisy environments throughout the day).
- Provide a list of available resources (e.g., AARP, National Institutes of Health, Better Hearing Institute).

Documentation

Chart that the patient is wearing a hearing aid, the condition of the ear, and the ability to hear. There will probably be a flowsheet or checklist for this information.

Practice Resources

National Institute on Deafness and Other Communication Disorders (2015); Senior Living (2022); U.S. Food and Drug Administration (2021).

Procedure 22-14 ■ Making an Unoccupied Bed

▶ For steps to follow in *all* procedures, refer to the Universal Steps for All Procedures on the inside back cover.

Equipment

- Bottom and top sheets, possibly drawsheet
- Pillowcase for each of the pillows
- Linen bag or hamper
- Procedure gloves (if exposure to body fluids is possible)
- Moisture-proof gown (if heavy soiling of linens with body fluids is possible).

Delegation

You can delegate this procedure to the UAP. You are responsible for supervising to ensure that the procedure is performed correctly.

Preprocedure Assessments

- Check to see whether the linen (including the mattress pad, blanket, and bedspread) needs to be changed and what linens are needed.
- Assess whether the patient is able to be out of bed during the linen change.
- Assess for drainage or incontinence to determine whether personal protective equipment, such as procedure gloves and gown, is needed.

Note: This procedure describes bed making by one person. It is more efficient for two people to work together on opposite sides of the bed.

(continued on next page)

Procedure 22-14 ■ Making an Unoccupied Bed (continued)

➤ When performing the procedure, always identify your patient according to agency policy, using two identifiers, and be attentive to standard precautions, hand hygiene, patient safety and privacy, body mechanics, and documentation.

Procedure Steps

1. **Assist the patient to a chair.** Provide a robe and/or blanket if needed.
   Ensures that the patient is comfortable and will be warm enough during the bed change.

2. **Prepare the environment:**
   - Position the bed flat, raise to appropriate working height, engage the bed brakes, and lower the side rails.
   - Move the overbed table and other furniture as needed.
   - Place the linen bag or hamper conveniently near the bed.
     Maintains good body mechanics and prevents back strain during the procedure.
   - Remove obstacles to allow easy access to the bed. Place all items so you can work efficiently, saving time and energy.

3. **Don protective gloves** and other PPE as needed. Loosen all the bedding.
   This follows standard precautions and reduces the risk of contaminating your clothing.

4. **If the blanket or bedspread** is clean, fold it and place it on a clean area (e.g., on the back of a chair). Do not place on another patient's bed or furniture.
   Reuse the blanket and/or bedspread if it is not soiled. Placing the item on a clean area prevents cross-contamination.

5. **Remove the bottom and top sheet,** drawsheet, and pillowcases.
   a. Do not shake the linens.
      Minimizes dispersal of dust, skin cells, and microorganisms into the environment.
   b. ✥ Holding the items away from your body, place them in a laundry bag or hamper. Never place linen on the floor. Place the pillows on a clean area (e.g., on a chair).

   Hold dirty linen away from your uniform to prevent contamination. Cross-contamination can occur if you place linens on the floor. ▼

6. **Working from one side of bed,** to save steps:

   Variation: For a Contour-Bottom Sheet
   a. Fit the contour-bottom sheet on one side of the bed, and smooth it out over half the mattress.

   Variation: For a Flat-Bottom Sheet
   b. Fold the flat bottom lengthwise with the center crease in the middle of bed and unfold with the rough side facing down.
   c. Position the bottom sheet so that approximately 10 inches hang over at the top and sides. The hem of the bottom sheet should be just even with the bottom edge of the mattress.
   d. Tuck in the sheet, mitering the sheet at the top corner (see Step 11).
      When using a flat-bottom sheet, having extra sheet at the top helps keep it in place when the head of the bed is raised and lowered. Unfold the sheet rather than shake or fan to reduce dispersing microorganisms into the air. The sheet will not be long enough to tuck in at the bottom.

7. **Place the drawsheet with** the center fold in the middle of the mattress and unfold. Tuck the side in under the mattress and smooth out over half of the mattress.

   Ensures that all wrinkles are out of the bottom sheet and drawsheet. ▼

8. **Go to the other side of the bed,** straighten the linen, and finish tucking in the bottom sheet and drawsheet.
   a. Make the drawsheet tight and smooth any wrinkles in the bottom sheet and drawsheet.
      Pulling the drawsheet tight helps prevent wrinkles from developing under the patient when moving around in bed. ▼

   b. If desired, place a waterproof pad on or under the drawsheet.

9. **Place the top sheet and bedspread** along one side of the mattress. Center the top sheet and bedspread so that when you straighten them from the other side of the bed they fall equally over each side of the bed.
   Putting the linen on one side of the bed saves steps.

10. **At the foot of the bed,** make a small pleat in the top sheet and bedspread.
    Prevents the top covers from placing pressure on the patient's toes. ▼

11. **Tuck in the top sheet** and bedspread at the same time, mitering the corners.
    a. Tuck in the sheet and bedspread at the bottom of the mattress. ▼

    b. Bring the edge of sheet and the bedspread up to make a right angle. ▼

    c. Tuck the lower edge of sheet and bedspread under the mattress.
    Mitered corners help secure the linen at the foot of the bed. ▼

12. **Move to the other side of the bed,** smooth top linens, and repeat Step 11. At the head of the bed, fold the edge of sheet down over the bedspread.
    Prevents the bedspread from rubbing against the patient's skin. ▼

13. Fanfold the top sheet and bedspread back to the foot of the bed.
    Makes it easier for the patient to get into bed. ▼

14. **Change pillowcases.**
    a. Turn the pillowcase wrong-side out.
    b. Grasp the middle of the closed end of the pillowcase.
    c. Reaching through the pillowcase, grasp the end of the pillow. ▼

    d. Continuing to grasp the end of the pillow, pull the pillowcase down over the pillow.
    Do not hold the pillow under your arm or chin to put on pillowcase because contamination can occur. ▼

15. **Assist the patient back to bed,** return the bed to the low position, place the call signal within reach, and place the bedside table and overbed table so that they are accessible to the patient.
    Provides for patient comfort and safety.

(continued on next page)

Procedure 22-14 ■ Making an Unoccupied Bed (continued)

? What if...

- **The linens have been contaminated by body fluids?**
Follow recommended infection control procedures for laundering of linens (e.g., wear procedure gloves, place linen in moisture-proof bags, and so on).

- **The mattress has become contaminated by body fluids?**
Follow agency policies for cleaning the mattress before putting on clean linens. This often involves notifying another department, such as housekeeping or environmental services, whose members are trained in this procedure.

- **The mattress cover is damaged or worn?**
Regularly check each mattress cover for any visible signs of damage or wear such as cuts, tears, cracks, pinholes, snags, or stains. Routinely remove the mattress cover and check its inside surface for wet spots, staining, or signs of damage or wear. Check all sides and the bottom of the mattress. Remove any damaged, worn, or visibly stained medical bed mattress according to the healthcare facility's procedures and immediately replace any damaged mattress cover to reduce the risk of infection to patients.

- **The patient has a specialty bed or specialty mattress?**
Several products are available with specific criteria to match patients' needs regarding movement and comfort, prevention, or treatment of pressure ulcers (e.g., specialty beds designed for bariatric patients). Follow the manufacturer's directions (e.g., a recommendation for a specific mattress may be to use only one layer of sheet over the mattress for maximum benefit). If you find the sheets are not large enough to accommodate a specialized mattress, you may need to use two flat sheets to cover it.

Home Care

The only adaptations at home depend on the type of bed the patient has. If the height of the bed is not adjustable or the bed is not accessible from both sides, the procedure may be more difficult.

Documentation

Linen changes are generally recorded on a checklist, if at all. Additional charting would need to be done only if something abnormal occurred, for example, "The drawsheet had a 20-cm circular area of serosanguineous drainage."

Practice Resources

Doll et al. (2018); Mitchell et al. (2012); Siegel et al. (2007, updated 2017); U.S. Food and Drug Administration (2017).

Procedure 22-15 ■ Making an Occupied Bed

▶ For steps to follow in *all* procedures, refer to the Universal Steps for All Procedures on the inside back cover.

Equipment

- Bottom and top sheets; drawsheet
- Pillowcase for each of the pillows
- Bath blanket (as needed)
- Linen bag or hamper
- Procedure gloves (if exposure to body fluids is possible)
- Moisture-proof gown (if heavy soiling of linens with body fluids is possible).

Delegation

You can delegate this procedure if the patient's condition and the UAP's skills permit. For example, if the patient is very ill or in pain or requires two people for turning and repositioning, you should assist with or perform the linen change yourself.

Preprocedure Assessments

- Determine the patient's ability to assist with the procedure and whether additional help or assistive devices are needed.
- Make other assessments listed in Procedure 22-14.

▶ When performing the procedure, always identify your patient according to agency policy, using two identifiers, and be attentive to standard precautions, hand hygiene, patient safety and privacy, body mechanics, and documentation.

▶ *Note:* If linen change is done at the same time as the bed bath, some of these steps will vary.

Procedure Steps

1. **Prepare the environment:** Move the overbed table and other furniture, as needed, to allow access to the bed. Place the linen bag or hamper conveniently near the bed.
   To allow easy access to the bed and enable you to work efficiently, saving time and energy.

2. **Don protective gloves** and other gear if necessary.
   This follows standard precautions and reduces the risk of contaminating your clothing.

3. **Position the bed flat,** if possible, and raise it to working height. Lower the side rail nearest you.
   Maintains good body mechanics and prevents back strain during the procedure. Having the head of the bed flat makes it easier to smooth the bottom sheet. To prevent the patient from falling out of bed, lower the side rails only on the side where you are standing.

4. **Disconnect the call device** and remove the patient's personal items from the bed.
   Prevents items from getting lost.

5. **Check that no tubes** (e.g., IV, nasogastric) are entangled in the bed linens.
   Prevents dislodging tubes accidentally.

6. **If the blanket or bedspread** is clean, fold it and place it on a clean area (e.g., the back of a chair); do not place it on another patient's bed or furniture.
   Reusing the blanket and/or bedspread if it is not soiled conserves resources.

7. **Cover the patient** with a bath blanket, if available, or leave the top sheet over the patient.
   Covering the patient prevents chilling and preserves modesty.

8. **Slide the patient to the far side** of bed and place him in a side-lying position, facing the side rail. Place a pillow under his head. If needed for support, place a pillow between the patient and the side rail.
   Placing the patient close to the side rail will allow you to place the clean linen over a larger area, making it easier to roll the patient back onto the clean linen. Patients who cannot maintain the side-lying position should have a pillow placed between their chest and the side rail to prevent them from accidentally rolling into the side rail.

9. **Roll or tightly fanfold** the soiled linens toward the patient's back. Tuck the roll slightly under the patient. Cover any moist areas with a waterproof pad.
   Covering moist areas prevents contact with the clean linen or patient. ▼

10. **Remove soiled gloves,** perform hand hygiene, and don clean gloves.

11. **Place the clean bottom sheet** and drawsheet (or pad) on the near side of the mattress with the center vertical fold at the center of the bed. Fanfold the half of the clean linen that is to be used on the far side, folding it as close to the patient as possible and tucking it under the dirty linen. Tuck the lower edges of clean linen under the mattress. Smooth out all wrinkles.
    Wrinkles under the patient can cause skin irritation. ▼

12. **Roll the patient over the clean and dirty linen,** turning them toward you. Explain to the patient that they will be rolling over a "lump," and then gently pull the patient toward you so that the patient rolls onto the clean linen. ▼

13. **Raise the side rail** on the clean side of the bed.
    Prevents the patient from falling.

14. **Move the pillows** to the clean side. Position the patient comfortably on their side, near the side rail.
    Always ensure patient comfort and safety before going to the other side of the bed.

15. **Go to the opposite side of bed** and lower the rail. Pull the soiled linen away from under the patient and clean linen and place it in laundry bag or hamper. Never place linen on the floor.
    Prevents cross-contamination. ▼

(continued on next page)

Procedure 22-15 ■ Making an Occupied Bed (continued)

16. **Remove soiled gloves and** don clean gloves. Pull clean linens through and tuck them in. Pull taut, starting with the middle section.
Ensures that no wrinkles will be under the patient. ▼

17. **Assist the patient to a supine** position close to center of the mattress.

18. **Place the top sheet** and bedspread along one side of the mattress, and continue making the bed as in Procedure 22-14, Steps 9 through 14, *except* remove the bath blanket from under the top linens before tucking them in. ▼

19. ✚ **Return the bed to the low** position, raise the side rails, and attach the call light within patient's reach. Position the bedside table and overbed table within patient's reach.
Ensures patient safety and comfort.

? What if . . .

- **I am making the bed with a patient in leg traction?**

It may be easier to make the bed from top to bottom, as follows:
  - Loosen all bed linens and bring the dirty linens from the top of the bed to hip area. Put the clean bottom sheet on the top corners of the mattress, bring down to hip level, and tuck under the dirty linen. Cover any moist areas with a waterproof pad.
  - Ask the patient to grasp the trapeze and raise the buttocks. If the patient is unable to raise the buttocks, use an assistive device per agency policy.
  - Bring the dirty bottom sheet along with the clean bottom sheet toward the foot of the bed. Remove dirty linen and place in the laundry bag.
  - Tuck the clean sheet under the mattress. Cover with the top sheet. To accommodate traction equipment, do not tuck in the top sheet.

- **I need to move or reposition a patient in bed who is not able to assist or is obese?**

  ✚ Before making the occupied bed, assess the patient's ability to move. Use assistive equipment such as friction-reducing devices, mechanical lifts, air-powered mattresses, or lateral transfer devices.
  These are essential tools in preventing work-related injuries. Limit the need to use your own strength while lifting, turning, or repositioning the patient in bed because of the stress placed on the weaker muscles in the arms and shoulders.

  Follow agency policies and use of patient moving devices appropriately.
  Many healthcare facilities have adopted safe lifting and patient-handling policies to protect both the patient and the healthcare worker.

Evaluation
- Assess how well the patient tolerated the procedure. Was there any discomfort, shortness of breath, and so on?
- Ask the patient whether they feel comfortable.

Home Care
The only adaptations at home depend on the type of bed the patient has. If the height of the bed is not adjustable or the bed is not accessible from both sides, the procedure may be more difficult.

Documentation
Linen changes are usually recorded on a checklist. Additional charting needs to be done only if something abnormal occurred.

Practice Resources
Doll et al. (2018); Centers for Disease Control and Prevention (2009); Pegram & Bloomfield (2015); Siegel et al. (2007, updated 2017).

Thinking About the Procedure

➡ The video **Making an Occupied Bed,** along with questions and suggested responses, is available on the **Davis's Nursing Skills Videos** Web site at www.fadavis.com.

CLINICAL INSIGHT

Clinical Insight 22-1 ➤ Assisting With a Shower or Tub Bath

Inpatient Care

- Assess the patient's self-care abilities: sensorimotor, musculoskeletal, and cognitive function; activity tolerance; level of knowledge.
- Ensure that the patient has the necessary supplies (e.g., soap, washcloth, towel, clean gown).
- If using prepackaged bath product, be sure to warm bathing products before use.
- Hang a sign on the door to ensure privacy and place the call device within reach.
- Help wash and dry any areas that the patient cannot reach (e.g., feet, back).

Preventing Nosocomial Infections

- If using tap water for bath, check agency policy regarding the safety of the tap water for general use in bathing patients, including the following:
    - The hot water temperature is maintained above 55°C (131°F).
    - Routine sampling for bacteria is done.
- ✚ Avoid showers and exposure to faucet water for inpatients who are immunocompromised, the frail elderly, newborns, the critically ill, those having recent surgery or other loss of skin integrity, and patients requiring mechanical ventilation. Use prepackaged wipes instead.
- Verify water temperature for patients with impaired cognition or decreased sensory perception. Bath water should be 43°C to 46°C (110°F to 115°F) to avoid burns.
- Tubs should be stringently maintained and cleaned, preferably with a chlorhexidine gluconate (CHG)–based product, to prevent nosocomial infections related to the use of tubs (e.g., biofilm).

Preventing Falls

- ✚ Assist the patient to the shower or bathroom as needed.
- Ensure that there is a nonskid surface or mat in the shower or tub.
- Use a shower chair in the shower or tub for patients who have impaired mobility or activity intolerance.
- Be sure that the shower or tub is safe (e.g., with grab bars and handrails).
- Provide a call device for the patient to obtain help if needed; point out the emergency call device if there is one in the bathroom (usually it is a red button or cord on the wall).

Home Care

- ✚ Encourage patients and families to install grab bars on the sides of the bathtub and on the wall next to the tub.
- Advise parents never to leave a child alone in the tub or shower and to have a way to unlock the bathroom door from outside the room.
- Advise older adults or those who are ill not to lock the bathroom door while bathing so that help can be summoned if needed (e.g., if they fall).
- Help families to obtain benches for transferring into the bathtub, or use a plastic chair in the shower.
- Ensure that there is a nonskid surface or mat in the shower or tub.

Use a shower chair.

ASSESSMENT GUIDELINES AND TOOLS

Guidelines for Assessing Hygiene

Assess Functional Status

Assessment of Functional Abilities for ADL
The Katz Index of Independence in Activities of Daily Living (ADL) is used extensively to assess functional abilities in activities of daily living (bathing/hygiene, dressing/grooming, feeding, toileting). To use the Katz ADL Index,

➡ Go directly to https://consultgeri.org/try-this/general-assessment/issue-2.pdf

Observe Self-Care Abilities
When bathing, dressing, eating, and toileting, which of the following best describes the patient's ability?

- Is completely independent; requires no assistance.
- Requires a device or special equipment (e.g., a walker, a large-handle spoon).
- Requires help, supervision, or teaching from another person.
- Requires help from another person as well as from a device or special equipment.
- Is totally dependent; does not participate in the activity (e.g., total bed bath).

The Environment
- Is the room temperature comfortable?
- Are the side rails up, when indicated? Is the bed in low position?
- Are bed wheels locked?
- Are bed linens clean and wrinkle free?
- Is the patient's call device within reach?
- Is the overbed table clean and uncluttered?
- Is the walking space uncluttered?
- Are there unpleasant odors?

Skin

Subjective Data

♥ **iCare** Patients may be sensitive about skin problems or poor hygiene practices, so direct your questions to the patient in a nonjudgmental, respectful manner. General questions to ask include the following:

- How often do you prefer to bathe?
- How do you usually care for your skin?
- What soaps, lotions, or other skin care products do you use?
- Do you have difficulty controlling body odor?
- Have you ever had an allergic skin reaction to food, medications, plants, skin care products, or other materials?
- What problems have you had with your skin in the past?
- What problems are you having with your skin now?
- For each problem identified, ask the following:
    What symptoms are you having (e.g., any rash or itching)?
    Where is the problem located?
- How long have you had this problem?
- What have you done to provide relief from the symptoms?
- Do you use any prescription, over-the-counter (OTC), or herbal remedies to treat this problem?
- Have you seen a healthcare provider about this problem?
- Was a diagnosis made? If so, what was it?
- How has this problem affected your life?
- How can I best help you with your skin care?
- Also ask about the presence of diseases or other factors that are known to cause skin problems (e.g., decreased mobility, decreased circulation, incontinence, inadequate nutrition, or deficient knowledge).

Objective Data
- Note the skin's overall cleanliness, condition, color, texture, turgor, hydration, and temperature.
- Observe for rashes, lumps, lesions, and cracking.
- Look for drainage from wounds or around tubes.
- Observe for four significant color changes: pallor, erythema, jaundice, and cyanosis.

Feet

Subjective Data
Ask the patient the following questions or obtain the data from the records:

- What is your normal foot care routine?
- What type of footwear do you usually wear? Observe what the patient is wearing.
- Have you had any foot problems? If so, what treatments have you had for them?
- Do you examine your feet on a regular basis?
- Do you have diabetes mellitus or peripheral vascular disease?

Objective Data
Compare findings for both feet:

- Observe for cleanliness and skin integrity. Note open areas, drainage, or redness.
- Inspect for swelling, inflammation, or infection.
- Palpate for edema.
- Check the skin between the toes for cracks or signs of a fungal infection.

Focused Assessment

Guidelines for Assessing Hygiene—cont'd

- Notice the color and temperature of the feet; are they the same bilaterally? The color and temperature provide data about circulation and oxygenation. For example, cold, dusky feet may indicate impaired circulation or tissue perfusion secondary to a peripheral vascular disease.
- Check capillary refill. How many seconds does it take for the color to return after you apply pressure?
- Note the presence of foot odors, if any.

Nails

Subjective Data

Ask about the patient's usual nail care practices, history of nail problems, and their treatments.

Objective Data

Inspect the nails for the following:

- Shape, contour, and cleanliness
- Presence of broken nails, hangnails, or cracked cuticles
- Hands: Do the fingernails appear neatly manicured, or does the patient bite the nails?
- Feet: Are the toenails trimmed appropriately, straight across?
- Presence of redness or swelling at the nail base or sides

Oral Cavity

Subjective Data

- Usual hygiene practices
- History of periodontal disease or other oral problems
- Financial or insurance problems that limit access to dental care
- Nutrition status and dietary habits (e.g., intake of refined sugar)
- Medications, such as anticonvulsants or diuretics
- Medical treatments, such as radiation therapy, oxygen therapy, and nasogastric tubes
- Other factors known to cause oral problems (smoking, alcohol use, NPO status, dehydration, mouth breathing)
- Self-care deficits (e.g., cognitive impairment, activity intolerance, impaired mobility, depression, lack of knowledge, lack of motivation)

Objective Data

- Observe the lips, which should be pink and moist without lesions.
- Inspect the oral mucosa and gums, which should also be pink, moist, smooth, and free of lesions.
- Healthy gums should have a well-defined margin at each tooth. There should be no visible bleeding.
- Instruct the patient to stick out the tongue and to move it around. It should move freely. The tongue should be symmetrical and pink, with a slightly rough surface.
- Assess the teeth for the presence of any loose, missing, or decaying teeth.
- Examine the hard and soft palates for color, lesions, patches, or petechiae.
- Note any unusual mouth odors or halitosis.

Hair

Subjective Data

- Use of special products or medicated shampoos
- History of hair problems or current conditions needing treatment (e.g., pediculosis)
- History or presence of disease or therapy that affects the hair (e.g., chemotherapy)
- Factors influencing the patient's ability to manage hair and scalp care (e.g., impaired mobility)
- Personal or cultural preferences for styling of the hair

Objective Data

- Note the condition, cleanliness, texture, and oiliness of the hair.
- Inspect the scalp for dandruff, pediculosis (head lice), alopecia (hair loss), secretions, or lesions.

Eyes

Subjective Data

- If the patient wears glasses, ask when they use them (e.g., for reading, for driving) and ask how well they see without them.
- If the patient wears contact lenses, determine the following:
  - The type of lens (hard, soft, long-wearing, disposable).
  - How often they wear them (daily, occasionally) and for how long at a time (worn during sleep?)
  - History of or present problems with lens use (e.g., cleaning, removal)
  - Usual practices for cleaning and storage
- History of or current problems with the eyes (e.g., redness, tearing, irritation, dryness, or scratchy feeling)

Objective Data

- Inspect the eyes for redness, lesions, swelling, crusting, excessive tearing, or discharge.
- Check the color of the conjunctivae.

CLINICAL REASONING
Applying the Full-Spectrum Nursing Model

PATIENT SITUATION

Alice Baker is a frail woman, 93 years old, who lives in a nursing home. She has almost total self-care deficit related to her weakness, painful joints, and dementia. Her mental and physical conditions are not likely to improve. Imagine that your charge nurse has instructed you to provide a complete bed bath and other hygiene care for Ms. Baker. When you enter her room with bath supplies and say, "Good morning, Ms. Baker; it's time for your bath," she screams, "Go away from me. I just had a bath. I don't want a bath." You discuss this with the charge nurse, who says, "She has not had a bath, and she needs one today. You will need to do it whether she likes it or not." You tend to agree that Ms. Baker needs a bath because her clothing and linens have food stains, and she smells of urine and perspiration.

THINKING

1. *Theoretical Knowledge:*

   a. What benefits does a bath have for Ms. Baker?

   b. What are the disadvantages of bathing a patient with dementia who is resisting the bath?

2. *Critical Thinking (Considering Alternatives, Deciding What to Do):*

   a. What do you think Ms. Baker is feeling and experiencing, and how does that help you know what to do?

   b. What are some alternatives to a complete bed bath that would achieve the same purposes?

DOING

3. *Practical Knowledge:* Imagine that you have, indeed, decided that Ms. Baker needs a bath. Which type of bath will you give her? What supplies will you need, and where will you find them in the clinical agency you have attended most recently?

CARING

4. *Self-Knowledge:* What is your greatest concern about bathing Ms. Baker? What is the cause of your concern?

Critical Thinking and Clinical Judgment

1. You are caring for Mrs. Little, a 57-year-old woman who has had severe arthritic pain for the past 2 years. She rates her pain at an 8 or 9 on a 10-point pain-rating scale. During your assessment, you notice that Mrs. Little has a moderate body odor, long and untrimmed fingernails and toenails, oily hair, and unshaven legs and axillae. Mrs. Little readily admits that she has neglected her hygiene practices.

   a. What is the first hygiene-related nursing diagnosis (problem and etiology) that comes to your mind for Mrs. Little?

   b. What data do you have to support a diagnosis of self-care deficit: bathing? What data do you have to support an etiology of immobility secondary to pain?

   c. With the information in the scenario, how would you rate her self-care deficit: mild, moderate, severe, or total?

   d. Anything you could do to help relieve Mrs. Little's pain would facilitate her self-care abilities. However, to plan interventions in which you will assist with her hygiene care, what further patient data do you need?

   e. Suppose you assess Mrs. Little further and determine that she has arthritis in multiple joints, including her hands, shoulders, back, knees, and feet. You also determine that she will need a complete bath, either tub or shower, but that she can brush her own teeth if someone provides the necessary supplies. Could you delegate her hygiene care to an experienced UAP? If so, what instructions would you give the UAP?

2. Mr. Thomson is an 87-year-old Black man admitted 2 days ago after being found unconscious in his small apartment. Although Mr. Thomson denies having diabetes, his admission blood sugar was 653 mg/dL. His lower legs are swollen, red, and weeping a clear fluid. His toenails are long, thick, and yellow, and there is a small open sore on the great toe of his left foot. Mr. Thomson's skin is dry and scaly, and his hair is matted; he has a strong odor of perspiration and urine. He is uncircumcised. He refuses help with hygiene, saying, "I've taken care of myself for 87 years, and I'll keep doing it. I take my bath once a week on Saturday evening. Now go away!"

   a. What *theoretical* knowledge will you need in order to know what to assess and how to provide his hygiene care?

   b. Self-knowledge is important in this case as well. What things in this situation would make caring for Mr. Thomson especially difficult for you? What biases, values, or attitudes might interfere with your ability to give your best care?

3. Recall the Meet Your Patients scenario in Volume 1 of your textbook. The remaining critical-thinking questions refer to that scenario:

   Scenario: Your instructor has assigned you to assist the following patients with their hygiene. You must assess the needs of each person, gather information on their bathing habits and preferences, plan nursing measures necessary to meet individual needs, and (together with a UAP) provide care.

   The first person on your assignment is Mrs. Rosha, a 76-year-old woman of Indian heritage who was admitted yesterday after suffering a stroke that paralyzed her right side. Since the stroke, she has been unable to speak clearly and becomes frustrated as she attempts to communicate her needs. Her daughter says Mrs. Rosha is a proud and tidy woman who has been living alone and caring for herself independently since her husband's death last year, even maintaining the yard and garden. She wears eyeglasses for reading and driving and has a hearing aid.

   The second person on your assignment is Mr. Fuller, a 68-year-old Orthodox Jewish man, admitted last week after a massive heart attack. Although his eyes are open, he does not respond to external stimuli. Because of impaired swallowing, Mr. Fuller is unable to take food or fluid orally. A feeding tube was placed to ensure adequate nutrition and hydration. His oral mucous membranes and lips are dry and crusty. He is incontinent of urine and stool. Mr. Fuller's son, John, tells you that Mr. Fuller adheres to Orthodox Jewish law and requests that you respect this in his care.

   The following questions are about Mrs. Rosha:

   a. To assess Mrs. Rosha's self-care abilities, what important patient data do you still need?

   b. What problem has resulted from her stroke that will make it difficult for you to find out about Mrs. Rosha's hygiene preferences and practices?

   c. From what you know of the patient situation, why do you think Mrs. Rosha is becoming frustrated?

   d. How do you think you would react if this were to happen to you?

   e. How could you provide opportunities for Mrs. Rosha to maintain her independence?

4. **The following questions are about Mr. Fuller:**

   a. What additional theoretical knowledge do you need to meet Mr. Fuller's religious and cultural needs when providing hygiene care?

   b. Where could you obtain such information?

   c. If you decide to delegate Mr. Fuller's bed bath to a UAP, how could you incorporate his religious and cultural needs into your delegation decisions?

5. For each of the following concepts, use critical thinking to describe how or why it is important to nursing, patient care, or facilitating hygiene. Note that these are *not* to be merely definitions.

Personal hygiene
Delegation of tasks
Cultural differences
Skin integrity
Life span variables
Self-care deficits
The nursing process

Patient teaching
Bathing
Oral care
Environment and comfort
Hair care
Nail care

What Are the Main Points in This Chapter?

- Recent recommendations for hygiene care include (1) the use of disposable, single-patient-use basins to reduce risk of bacterial contamination and (2) avoiding the use of unfiltered tap water in hospitals, unless the water lines are known to not contain biofilm. Alternatives include prepackaged bathing products and the use of sterile or distilled water or filtered water from faucets.
- Personal hygiene contributes to physical and psychological well-being by promoting comfort, improving self-image, and decreasing infection and disease.
- Although a patient may need assistance with hygiene measures, the goal is to encourage as much independence with these tasks as possible.
- Numerous factors influence individual hygiene practices, including personal preferences, cultural/religious/spiritual values and beliefs, economic status, living environment, developmental or knowledge level, and physical and emotional health.
- Maintain a respectful, nonjudgmental attitude about cultural and spiritual differences. Avoid the temptation to impose personal values about hygiene practices onto patients.
- Consider patients' personal hygiene preferences and incorporate them into the care plan whenever possible. This reflects caring and promotes maximum participation and independence with ADLs.
- Although many hygiene measures can be delegated to the UAP, the nurse retains full responsibility for each patient and must instruct the UAP about the patient's limitations and restrictions, amount of assistance necessary, use of any assistive devices, any specific safety precautions to be undertaken, and any other factors influencing the patient's hygiene practices.
- The nurse should assess a patient's functional status regularly.
- Teaching patients about hygiene is a primary function of the professional nurse.
- Intact skin is the body's first line of defense to keep pathogenic microorganisms from entering the body and causing infection.

- Bathing removes perspiration and bacteria from the skin surface. It promotes relaxation and comfort, improves circulation, reduces odor, and enhances well-being by increasing self-image. However, it can be stressful for some patients.
- You should choose the type of bath to meet the patient's needs (e.g., assist bath, total bed bath, and so on).
- Bathing is stressful to some patients (e.g., the frail elderly, people with dementia, people with morbid obesity). You should focus on the patient's needs for warmth, safety, and comfort and adapt the bathing procedure to help reduce stress.
- Despite common myths, it does not take a lot of water to get a person clean, and not all patients need a complete bath every day.
- A complete bath includes perineal care.
- Careful assessment of the feet allows for early detection of common foot problems, such as calluses, corns, tinea pedis, ingrown toenail, or foot odor.
- Because dirt and debris can collect under the nails and be a source of infection, nail care is an important part of hygiene, especially in patients with diabetes mellitus or peripheral neuropathy.
- To maintain healthy mucous membranes, teeth, and gums, and to prevent tooth loss and gum disease, regular dental checkups and daily mouth care, including brushing and flossing the teeth, are necessary.
- For critically ill and frail elderly patients, as well as those using ventilators, special attention to oral hygiene helps to reduce the risk for pneumonia.
- Oral hygiene is challenging for patients with dementia, but it must not be neglected.
- The condition of the hair is a measure of an individual's overall health. Shampooing and daily brushing of the hair massage the scalp, stimulate the circulation, and distribute the natural oils.
- The eyes normally require very little care; however, when necessary, they may be gently cleansed from the inner to the outer canthus.

- Unconscious or critically ill patients who no longer have a blink reflex may need eye care every 2 to 4 hours. Keeping the eyes lubricated protects them from corneal abrasions and drying.
- Some contact lenses can be worn for only about 12 hours at a time; others may be worn for up to 30 days. Some are disposable; some are not. All types must be cleaned carefully and regularly.
- Hearing aids are expensive and should be properly handled and stored. They should not be immersed in water.
- When reinserting an artificial (prosthetic) eye, first be certain that it is wet.
- Usually no special care is required for the nose. Excess secretions can be removed by gentle blowing with both nostrils open.
- Clean, wrinkle-free bed linens help to promote comfort and a sense of well-being.
- Room temperature, adequate ventilation, low noise level, and neat and clean surroundings all contribute to a comfortable patient environment.

Knowledge Map

UNIT 3 Essential Nursing Interventions

HYGIENE

Affected by → FACTORS AFFECTING SELF-CARE
- Pain
- Limited mobility
- Sensory alteration
- Impaired cognition
- Emotional dysfunction

FACTORS AFFECTING HYGIENE
- Preference
- Culture
- Religion
- Economic status
- Developmental level
- Knowledge

SKIN PROBLEMS:
- Pruritus
- Dryness
- Maceration
- Excoriation
- Abrasions
- Pressure ulcers
- Acne

PERINEAL CARE

SKIN CARE: BATHING
- Removes bacteria
- Prevents odor
- Friction/warmth dilate surface vessels
- Promotes relaxation
- Enhances well-being
- Type of bath chosen based on nursing judgment

TYPES OF CARE
- Early AM
- AM-morning
- PM
- HS
- Bed; shower; tub
- Assist; partial, complete

HAIR CARE:
- Brushing
- Combing
- Shampoo
- Culturally specific
- Includes shaving

HAIR/SCALP PROBLEMS
- Dandruff
- Pediculosis
- Alopecia
- Infestation

FOOT CARE: FOCUS ON DIABETIC PATIENTS
- Prevent infection/odor
- Prevent trauma
- Daily inspection
- Wash, rinse, dry
- Water-soluble lotion

FOOT PROBLEMS:
- Corns/calluses
- Tinea pedis
- Ingrown toenail
- Plantar warts
- Odor
- Bunion

NAIL CARE:
- Daily inspection
- Trim or file
- Remove hangnails
- Clean under nails
- Moisturizing lotion

ORAL HYGIENE:
- Brushing
- Flossing
- Teaching self-care

SPECIAL CONSIDERATIONS:
- Denture care
- Oral care for the unconscious patient: preventing aspiration
- Oral care for the critically ill and frail elderly patient

ORAL PROBLEMS:
- Halitosis
- Caries/plaque
- Gingivitis
- Pyorrhea
- Stomatitis
- Glossitis
- Cheilosis
- Oral malignancy

NAIL PROBLEMS:
- Thickened
- Ridged
- Discolored
- Brittle
- Trauma

CHAPTER 23

Administering Medications

STUDENT RESOURCES

The questions and exercises in this book allow you to practice the kind of thinking you will use as a full-spectrum nurse. Critical-thinking questions usually have more than one right answer, so we do not provide "correct" answers for these features. Try to answer these questions yourself. It is more important to develop your nursing judgment than to just cover content. You will learn more by discussing the questions with your peers. If you are still unsure, see the Davis Advantage chapter resources for suggested responses.

To explore learning resources for this chapter,

Go to www.DavisAdvantage.com and find:

Answers and Suggested Responses for all questions in this chapter
Concept Map
Knowledge Map
References and Bibliography

Key Concepts

Medication administration
Medication safety
Pharmacology

Related Concepts

See the Concept Map on Davis Advantage.

Caring for the Williams Family

Because these are clinical judgment questions, they usually do not have a single answer. Discuss the questions with your peers—discussion can stimulate critical thinking.

Kayla Robinson, the 3-year-old granddaughter of Stanley and Nadine Williams, has been tired and observed to be sitting down a great deal at preschool. Last week, she developed coughing, wheezing, shortness of breath, nasal congestion, and extreme fatigue. The pediatrician at the Family Medicine Center diagnosed asthma. He prescribed a 5-day tapering course of prednisone, a leukotriene inhibitor (Singulair) 4 mg orally daily at bedtime, and periodic treatments with albuterol through a home nebulizer system.

Stanley's mother, Charlene Williams, became very upset when she saw the bottle of prednisone elixir. She was even more upset when she learned that Kayla received an injection of the medicine in the office. She advised Nadine not to give Kayla the medicine because, she said, it causes weak bones and stunts growth. Nadine has called the clinic asking for advice on how to handle this problem. (Look up the medications, and use your knowledge of different routes of administration.)

(Continued)

Caring for the Williams Family (continued)

A. What theoretical knowledge do you need to answer these concerns?

B. What are some reliable sources where you might find this information?

C. What rationale could you offer to Nadine to explain the safety of the prednisone prescription? You will need to use a variety of references to answer this question.

D. Nadine asks you to explain why Kayla received both a shot and pills. How would you respond?

E. Why is Kayla receiving a leukotriene inhibitor (Singulair) orally and albuterol by nebulizer?

Practical Knowledge clinical application

The practical knowledge you will need to administer medications safely and effectively includes procedures, clinical insights, and guidelines for calculating and measuring dosages and administering medications by a variety of routes.

PROCEDURES

Procedures in this section will assist you to prepare, measure, and administer various types of medications, locate injection sites, and handle needs safely.

Use the following Medication Guidelines for all types and routes.

Medication Guidelines: Steps to Follow for All Medications (Regardless of Type or Route)

➤ For steps to follow in *all* procedures, refer to the Universal Steps for All Procedures on the inside back cover.

Key Point: *Regardless of the type or route of the medication you are giving, you should always follow these steps.*

Equipment
- Medication administration record (MAR)
- Medication drawer or portable cart with, as needed, keys to the medication drawer
- Gloves for the procedure, as needed
- Other supplies and equipment needed for the specific procedure (e.g., water, antiseptic wipes)

Delegation
As a registered nurse (RN), you can usually delegate administration of medications (except for IV medications) to a licensed practical nurse/licensed vocational nurse (LPN/LVN). You cannot delegate this task to unlicensed assistive personnel (UAP). You can instruct a UAP in the therapeutic effects and side effects of medications and to report any effects observed.

Nurse practice acts (NPAs) governing medication administration vary from state to state, as do policies in healthcare agencies. In some states, with additional education and training, LPN/LVNs can administer IV medications and UAPs can administer some medications. You must know the scope of practice described in your state's NPA. **Key Point:** *The RN is always responsible for evaluating patient responses, which include both therapeutic effects and side effects.*

Preprocedure Assessments
- Assess your environment to ensure that it is conducive to the safe administration of medication.
 Environmental factors (e.g., noise, competing demands) can interfere with the astute focus and attention to detail required by the nurse in medication administration.

- Assess your knowledge of the medication (e.g., drug action, purpose, recommended dosage, time of onset and peak action, common side effects, contraindications, drug interactions, and nursing implications).
 Safe medication administration extends beyond the performance of the five rights of administration. You must have the pharmacological knowledge, clinical knowledge of your patient, and clinical reasoning to manage a situation as it emerges (Hanson & Haddad, 2021).

- Determine whether the prescribed dosage is appropriate for the patient's age and weight.
 Dosages are generally decreased for children because of both age and weight. Usually dosing for older patients is not based on weight

but on renal function. Both groups have less efficient liver and renal function compared with other age groups, increasing the length of time a drug stays in the body before being excreted.
- Check for any history of allergies to medications or food.
- At least the first time you administer medications to a patient, assess their knowledge of the medications being given.
 The patient will be more likely to take the medication correctly if they understand the reason for taking the medication.
- Assess for factors that could interfere with drug absorption (e.g., diarrhea, inadequate circulation, foods, impaired liver function, edema, inflammation, age-related changes, and other medication).
- Assess vital signs and check laboratory studies specific to the medication to determine whether the medication can be safely administered.
 Medications are metabolized more slowly in a person with decreased liver function.
- Assess for situations in which it would not be reasonable to administer the medication (e.g., oral medications prescribed for a patient who is NPO [nothing by mouth], vomiting, or sedated or has swallowing difficulties).
 If the medication does not seem reasonable, question the prescriber.

➤ When performing the procedure, always identify your patient according to agency policy, using two identifiers, and be attentive to standard precautions, hand hygiene, patient safety and privacy, body mechanics, and documentation.

Procedure Steps

1. **Check the MAR** for the patient's name and identification number, medication, dose, route, time, and drug allergies. The rights of medication administration are the right patient, right drug, right dose, right route, right time, and right documentation. At the beginning of your shift, check the MAR to determine when medications are due **(first check)**.
 Medication prescriptions may change even during your shift; checking the MAR helps ensure that you do not miss medication changes.

2. **Verify the prescription.** It should include the patient's name, patient identifier, medication name, dose, route, time, and patient allergies.
 You must note whether the prescription has changed (e.g., since the last time you gave the drug). Clarify any discrepancies before giving the medication.

3. **Follow agency policies** for medication administration, including the time frame. Most agencies allow medications to be given 30 minutes before or 30 minutes after the time indicated on the MAR. Do not pre-pour medications.
 The time of administration is important for some medications. For example, if an anti-infective agent is given early or late, a therapeutic blood level may not be maintained.

4. **Perform hand hygiene.**
 Hand hygiene minimizes transmission of microorganisms.

5. **Access the patient's medication** drawer, unlock the medication cart, or log onto the medication dispensing computer.

6. **Obtain the narcotic cabinet code (or input your ID number)** when administering a narcotic or barbiturate and sign out the medication, including the patient's name, drug, dose, and other pertinent information per agency policy. Note the drug count when removing a narcotic.
 Federal law governs administration of controlled substances. All narcotics and barbiturates are counted and signed for by an outgoing and oncoming nurse every shift.

7. **Select the prescribed medication.** Read the label and compare medication with the MAR for the first five rights (patient, drug, dose, route, time); check for drug allergies:
 - An inpatient should be wearing an identification band with the drug allergies identified.
 - Allergies should be clearly marked in the medical record and on the MAR or in the electronic health record (EHR).
 - Ask the patient about allergies the first time you administer a medication and before giving a newly prescribed medication.

 These actions ensure that the correct drug is being given to the correct patient at the correct time in the correct dose by the correct route and that any allergies are identified. Do not administer the medication if the patient states an allergy to it.

 Key Point: *Correct drug includes the correct form of the drug (e.g., oral, IV).*

8. **Calculate the medication dosage.** Double-check it. If you are unable to measure the dose exactly, contact the pharmacist.

9. **Check the expiration date** (on the label or on the box) of all medications.
 A medication that has expired is no longer guaranteed to be effective.

10. **Do a second check** after preparing the medications, to verify the correct patient medication, dose, route, and time **(second check)**.
 Verifies the first five rights of medication administration.

11. **Lock the medication cart.** Never leave an unlocked medication cart unattended.
 This guards against pilferage and protects children, older adults with dementia, or anyone wanting to open the cart.

(continued on next page)

Medication Guidelines: Steps to Follow for All Medications (Regardless of Type or Route) (continued)

12. **Administer the medications.**

   a. Take the medication and MAR or a handheld portable device with the EHR into the patient's room.
   You must be able to do the final check in the patient's room and verify that you are administering the correct medication to the correct patient.

   b. Identify the patient using two forms of identification, according to agency policy: Check the identification bracelet, have the patient state their name, compare the patient to their posted picture, and check the patient's date of birth against the MAR.
   Agencies have different means of identifying patients. The Joint Commission requires two forms of identification. ▼

   c. Do a check of the rights of medication: right patient, right medication, right dose, right route, and right time **(third check).**
   Checks for the rights of medication are always required to prevent medication errors. Although it is not actually an "error" until the patient has taken a medication, you may be required to file a report for a "near miss" that was detected during the preadministration checking process.

   d. Perform any necessary assessments, such as checking the pulse or blood pressure.
   Some medications can be given only if physical findings or vital signs are within certain parameters. For example, antihypertensive medications may need to be held if the blood pressure is lower than the patient's normal baseline.

   e. Explain to the patient that you are there to administer the medication; teach them about the medication.
   Patient teaching increases understanding of and compliance with treatment. The patient may then be able to identify potential errors in medication administration.

   ✚ *If the patient questions a medication, double-check the medication to be sure you are giving the correct drug and dosage.*

   f. Administer the medication using appropriate technique (see the procedures for administering medications by the specified route).

   g. Remain with the patient until you are sure that the patient has taken the medication.
   If you leave a medication at the bedside, someone else (e.g., another patient or a child) might take it, or the patient might discard it.

   h. Document the medication administered in the patient's medication record (date, dose, route, and your name).
   Your initials on the MAR mean that you administered the medication to the patient. If the documentation is not in the patient's record, there is a risk that another nurse will assume the medication was not given and administer it again.

? What if . . .

- **The patient tells me the tablet I am ready to give them is a different color from what they normally take of a certain prescribed medication?**

   Determine why the tablet is different from what the patient normally takes to be sure you are administering the correct drug and dose. Always verify the identity of the drug, especially when it is called into question by the patient who is familiar with their usual routine medications.
   Double-checking whenever you are uncertain about a medication you are about to administer or if the patient questions the drug helps prevent medication errors—it is possible you have the wrong drug or dosage.

- **The label on the medication shows an expiration date that has passed?**

   Do not give the medication. Send it back to the pharmacy for replacement.
   Expired medication can lose its potency.

- **The patient refuses to take the prescribed medication?**

   Discuss with the patient any concerns about the medication. Hold the dose and notify the prescriber of the patient's refusal and explain the patient's concerns.
   The patient has a right to refuse medication. You must document the patient's reason for refusal.

- **The patient's medication is not available from the pharmacy at the time the dose is due?**

   Do not borrow the medication from another patient's supply. Administer only medication prescribed for that particular patient. Notify the pharmacy of the need to immediately dispense the medication.
   Using another patient's medication increases the risk for error because drug dilution or dosage might vary among patients; or the drug names might sound similar, but they might be different medications. Also, the safety system for charges and refills is bypassed when doses are borrowed from other patients, resulting in missing doses or erroneous charges.

Evaluation

- Evaluate the therapeutic effects of the medication (e.g., check blood pressure after administering an antihypertensive medication, or check pain level after an analgesic).
- Be alert for any adverse reactions, side effects, or allergic reactions. If present, notify the appropriate care provider.

Patient Teaching

- Describe how the drug is prescribed and when the patient should take the medication.
- Discuss the importance of taking the medication as prescribed.
- Explain the need for any laboratory tests for monitoring the medication, such as tests to measure drug level in the blood, if appropriate.
- Explain the purpose, common side effects, and drug interactions of the medications the patient is taking.
- Teach the patient to observe for side effects that signal the need to contact the prescriber.
- Discuss ways to minimize the side effects of a medication, such as avoiding the sun when taking a medication that causes photosensitivity or rising slowly when taking a medication that causes orthostatic hypotension.
- Discuss potential cultural issues related to taking the medication (e.g., a patient may refuse a medication that is considered "hot" if they believe a "cold" treatment is needed).
- Teach the patient to self-administer medications (e.g., ear drops), as appropriate.

Home Care

- Assess the patient's ability to safely self-administer medications.
- Determine the patient's financial ability to obtain medications.
- Instruct the patient about safe storage of medications.
- Provide instructions for use of each medication.
- Determine whether the patient or caregiver has had past problems or present concerns about taking the medications as prescribed.
- If problems have occurred in the past or there are present concerns, discuss possible remedies. For example, you might teach the patient or caregiver to use a medication storage container with compartments for the times and days of the week.

Documentation

- Document the medication, time, dose, and route given, pre-administration assessments, and your signature.
- Do not document before giving the drug; do not document for anyone else; do not ask another nurse to document a drug you have given. Document only *after* administering the medication.
- Document all therapeutic and adverse effects of the medication. Also document your nursing interventions and teaching of potential adverse effects.
- Record the scheduled medications on the MAR. Record prn medications in the nursing notes and on the MAR, including the reason the medication was given and the patient's response to the medication.
- If the patient is unable or refuses to take the medication, document on the MAR that the medication was not administered and the reason and inform the provider.
- For parenteral medications, document the site of injection.

Sample EHR documentation

(continued on next page)

Medication Guidelines: ■ Steps to Follow for All Medications (Regardless of Type or Route) (continued)

Practice Resources
Hanson & Haddad (2021); Institute for Safe Medication Practices (2021); Agency for Healthcare Research and Quality (2019b); Tariq & Scherbak (2021).

Thinking About the Procedure

Go to the video **Medication Guidelines: Steps to Follow for All Medications (Regardless of Route)**, along with questions and suggested responses, available on the **Davis's** *Nursing Skills Videos* Web site at www.fadavis.com.

Procedure 23-1 ■ Administering Oral Medications

➤ For steps to follow in *all* procedures, refer to the Universal Steps for All Procedures on the inside back cover. Also refer to Medication Guidelines: Steps to Follow for All Medications (Regardless of Type or Route).

Equipment
- Desired liquid for swallowing medications
- Disposable medication cup
- Drinking straw, if needed
- Procedure gloves, if you will need to place a tablet in the patient's mouth
- For enteral medications:
  Water (for diluting and flushing the feeding tube)
  60-mL catheter-tip syringe
  Clean gloves
- Stethoscope
  Check the apical pulse before administering some cardiac medications.
- Blood pressure machine
  Check the blood pressure before administering antihypertensive medications.

Preprocedure Assessments
- Assess the patient's condition to determine whether there are contraindications to oral medications or to the specific medication (e.g., the ability to swallow).
  Impaired swallowing increases the risk for aspiration.
- Check fluid needs and restrictions. If the patient is NPO (nothing by mouth), check with the prescriber to determine whether the medication should be given by another route or can be given with small sips of water.
  A prescriber may decide it is medically necessary to administer oral medication to a patient who is NPO. If there is a fluid restriction, you need to consider how much fluid you can give with medication. Give additional fluid to a patient with dehydration; offer only sips for the patient with a fluid restriction.
- For enteral medications, check that the NG tube is in the stomach and is patent.

Delegation
- As a rule, you can delegate this skill to an LPN/LVN, depending on the medication, but not to a UAP, except under special policies and situations.

➤ When performing the procedure, always identify your patient according to agency policy, using two identifiers, and be attentive to standard precautions, hand hygiene, patient safety and privacy, body mechanics, and documentation.

Procedure Steps

1. **Prepare the medication** for administration.

For Tablet or Capsule
  a. If you are pouring from a multi-dose container, do not touch the medication. Pour the tablet into the cap of the container, then into the medication cup.
  b. If the medication is unit-dose, do not open the package. Place the entire unit-dose package into the cup.
  c. Many institutions allow combining all tablets or oral caplets scheduled for the same time for the same patient into the same cup. However, even if the agency protocol permits dispensing from a single container, you will need separate cups for medications that require preadministration assessment (e.g., checking the apical pulse rate before administering digoxin).
  If a medication is held because of a preadministration assessment finding, you can identify it more readily when it has been poured into a separate cup.
  d. You may break scored tablets with a knife or a tablet cutter if necessary.
  Only scored tablets may be broken. Breaking an unscored tablet would deliver an imprecise dose.
  e. If a patient has difficulty swallowing, check to see whether the medication can be crushed. If so, use a mortar and pestle to grind it. If the medication is in a unit-dose package, grind it while

it is still inside the package. Mix the ground medication with a small amount of soft food, such as applesauce or pudding.

Crushing some medications (e.g., capsules, enteric-coated tablets, and sustained-release formulas) may alter their effectiveness or result in an overdose due to rapid absorption.

For Liquid Medications

f. Check to see whether you must shake the liquid before opening the container.
Some liquids, such as suspensions, will precipitate and need to be shaken to mix the active ingredient with the suspension liquid.

g. Remove the bottle cap and place it flat side down on the cart or counter.

h. Hold the bottle with the label in the palm of your hand.
Keeping the label on the upward side of the bottle prevents the liquid from dripping down onto the label and obscuring it. ▼

i. Hold or place the plastic medication cup at eye level and pour the desired amount of medication. Read the dosage where the lowest part of the concave surface (meniscus) of the fluid is on the line. You can, instead, place the cup on a level surface, pour the medication, then hold the cup at eye level to read the amount.
Measuring liquids above or below eye level will cause you to read the dose incorrectly and pour too much or too little medication.

j. As you finish pouring medication, slightly twist the bottle to prevent the medication from dripping down the lip of the bottle. If medication does drip down over the lip, wipe the outside of the lip with a tissue or paper towel.
Wiping the outside of the bottle helps prevent contamination, particularly for thicker solutions, such as elixirs or syrups containing sugar.

2. **Administer the medication.**
   a. Assist the patient to a high-Fowler's position, if possible.
   An upright position facilitates swallowing and prevents choking.

   b. **Powder:** Mix with liquid at the bedside and give the mixture to the patient to drink.
   Some powders thicken very quickly and must be mixed immediately before administration.

   c. **Lozenge:** Instruct the patient not to chew or swallow it whole.
   Medication is absorbed through the oral mucosa and is generally inactivated by the acidity in the stomach.

   d. **Tablet or capsule:**
   1) If the patient is able to hold the medication in their hand, place the tablet or medication cup in their hand.
   Promotes independence and is easier for the patient.

   2) Give the patient water or other liquid.
   Giving the medication with liquid moistens the mouth and helps the patient swallow the tablet or capsule.

   3) If the patient is unable to hold the tablet, don procedure gloves and place the medication cup up to the lips, and tip the tablet or capsule into the mouth.
   Encourage the patient to do as much as possible. Getting the tablet or capsule to the back of the mouth will assist in swallowing.

   e. **Sublingual medications:** Have the patient place the tablet under the tongue and hold it there until it is completely dissolved.
   Sublingual medications are made to be rapidly absorbed through the oral mucosa. The area under the tongue is very vascular, so sublingual medications act very rapidly. Sublingual medications are inactivated by gastric acid if swallowed. ▼

   f. **Buccal medications:** Have the patient place the tablet between the cheek and gums.
   Buccal medications act by being absorbed through the oral mucosa or by being dissolved and swallowed in the saliva. ▼

3. **Stay with the patient until** all medications have been swallowed or dissolved.
   Some patients will "chipmunk" the medication in the side of the mouth without swallowing it, or spit it out. Staying at the bedside until the patient swallows oral medication ensures that the patient receives the dose.

(continued on next page)

Procedure 23-1 ■ Administering Oral Medications (continued)

Procedure 23-1A ■ Administering Medication Through an Enteral Tube

▶ For steps to follow in *all* procedures, refer to the Universal Steps for All Procedures on the inside back cover. Also refer to Medication Guidelines: Steps to Follow for All Medications (Regardless of Type or Route).

Preparation
- If the patient is receiving a continuous tube feeding, disconnect it before giving the medications. Leave the tube clamped for a few minutes after administering, according to agency protocol.
- If the enteral tube is connected to suction, you will usually discontinue the suction for 20 to 30 minutes after administration, and keep the tube clamped, to allow time for the drug to be absorbed.

▶ When performing the procedure, always identify your patient according to agency policy, using two identifiers, and be attentive to standard precautions, hand hygiene, patient safety and privacy, body mechanics, and documentation.

▶ *Note:* Follow Steps 1a through 1h of Procedure 23-1: Administering Oral Medication. Also, follow precautions for administering enteral medications.

Procedure Steps

1. **Prepare the medication.**
   a. Give the liquid form of medication, if possible. If the solution is hypertonic, be sure to dilute with 10 to 30 mL of sterile water before instilling through a feeding tube.
   Hyperosmolar substances administered too rapidly into the gut can cause bloating, nausea, and osmotic diarrhea.
   b. If tablets must be given, verify that the medication can be crushed and given through an enteral tube.
   Some tablets (e.g., sustained-release or enteric-coated tablets) should not be crushed or capsules opened because doing so changes their action.
   c. Crush the tablet and mix it with approximately 20 mL of water or obtain a liquid medication. If you are giving several medications, mix and administer each one separately.
   If you are using a small-bore tube, such as a percutaneous endoscopic gastrostomy (PEG) tube, Keofeed NG feeding tube, or jejunostomy tube, always obtain the liquid form of the medication, because small-bore tubes clog easily. Ensure that the medication is diluted enough to pass easily through the tube. Instilling drugs one at a time allows you to identify each medication.

2. **Don nonsterile procedure gloves.**
   Gloving maintains standard precautions.

3. **Place patient in a sitting (high-Fowler's) position,** if possible.
   An upright position reduces the risk for aspiration and choking.

4. **For NG tubes, check tube placement** (see Chapter 24, Clinical Insights 24-5 and 24-6) by x-ray, aspirating stomach contents or measuring the pH of the aspirate, if possible. Other, less accurate methods are injecting air into the feeding tube and auscultating, or asking the patient to speak; however, these are not confirmatory methods (Gardner & Wallace, 2021). **Key Point:** *Never rely on only one bedside method for checking tube placement; use a combination of methods.*
   NG tubes can become displaced or positioned in the lungs. If medications are given through a misplaced NG tube, the patient may develop aspiration pneumonia.

5. **Check for residual volume** (see Chapter 24, Procedure 24-3).

6. **Flush the tube.** Depending on the type of tube, use a piston tip or luer-lock syringe (usually a 30- to 60-mL syringe). Remove the bulb or plunger, attach the barrel to the tube, and pour in 20 to 30 mL of water.
   Flushing ensures patency of the tube and clears the tube of feeding solution that could clump with medication.

7. **Instill the medication by depressing** the syringe plunger or using the barrel of the syringe as a funnel and pouring in the medication. A smaller tube or thicker medication will require instilling the medication with a 30- to 60-mL syringe, but when larger tubes are used, the medication can be poured ▼

For Viscous Medication
Instill the medication by depressing the syringe plunger.

8. **Flush the medication through** the tube by instilling an additional 20 to 30 mL of water.
   Flushing ensures that all the medication has been administered and prevents the tube from clogging.

9. **If there is more than one medication,** give each separately, flushing after each.
   It is easier to validate the medication given if problems are encountered during the administration process.

10. **Have the patient maintain a sitting position** for at least 30 minutes after you administer the medication.
    An upright position minimizes the risk of aspiration. It takes at least 20 minutes for liquids to pass through the stomach.

? What if...

- **My patient vomits shortly after taking oral medication?**

  Notify the prescriber for instructions about whether to repeat the dose.

- **My patient is unable to sit upright to take oral medication?**

  Assist the patient into a side-lying position and offer a straw to take water with capsules or tablets.

- **My patient has difficulty drinking from a cup?**

  Use a syringe without a needle to place the medication in the patient's mouth. Place the patient in a side-lying or upright position. Place the syringe between the gum and cheek in the back corner of the mouth, and slowly push the plunger to administer the liquid.

- **My patient is NPO (nothing by mouth)?**

  Check with the prescriber to determine whether the medication should be given by another route or can be given with small sips of water.

- **My patient is on fluid restriction?**

  Use the smallest amount of water needed to swallow or dissolve tablets and to flush enteral tubes.

- **My patient is cognitively impaired?**

  Check level of consciousness, mentation, or alertness. Check for potential aspiration risk by checking the patient's swallow and gag reflexes. Request the patient open their mouth to see whether they have swallowed the medication; look under the tongue or side pocket near the inside of the cheek.

- **My patient is a child who is to receive medication through an enteral tube?**

  Use only medications that are prepared in liquid form.
  Helps prevent occlusion of the tube.
  Position an infant in a prone, side-lying, sitting, or reverse Trendelenburg position for 30 minutes to 1 hour after medication administration.
  These positions facilitate peristalsis and transport of medication through the intestine.

- **The prescribed medication should be given on an empty stomach?**

  Stop the feeding 30 minutes before giving the drug. Resume 30 minutes later.
  These times allow for the stomach to empty and for drug absorption to occur before the feedings resume.

Evaluation

For medications administered orally:
- Note whether the patient has difficulty swallowing, gags, or coughs while swallowing oral medication.
- Evaluate for gastric discomfort, nausea, vomiting, or diarrhea.
- Assess for signs of drug allergy or intolerance to the medication.

For medications administered through a feeding tube:
- In addition to the preceding assessments, assess that the NG tube is correctly placed and patent before and after administering the medication.

Patient Teaching

- Refer to **Medication Guidelines: Steps to Follow for All Medication (Regardless of Type or Route).**
- Discuss drug safety measures with the patient, including use of child-safety caps (or using an easy-open cap for older adults or with those likely to have difficulty opening containers of this type); keeping the medication in its original container; discarding expired medications; avoiding transferring medication to another container; and carefully reading the label and directions for each medication.
- Discuss the relationship between food and the medication, if needed. For example, is the medication to be taken with food or not? Does taking medication on an empty stomach contribute to nausea or gastric irritation? Does the medication interact with any foods?

For Enteral Medications

Cover the preceding topics for patient teaching about oral medications, plus the following:
- Discuss the importance of upright positioning for 20 to 30 minutes after taking medication through an enteral tube.
- Instruct the patient to immediately notify their healthcare provider if they choke or have difficulty breathing during or shortly after medication is given by enteral tube. The patient should stop the medication immediately, and emergency care might be necessary.

Home Care

Advise patients who are receiving enteral medication at home to do the following:
- Notify the healthcare provider (1) if any of the following lasts for more than a day: diarrhea, constipation, nausea, dark urine, bad-smelling urine, or dry mouth; (2) if the tube becomes clogged or seems to be moving farther out or in; or (3) if the feeding tube falls out or you cannot confirm that the end of the tube is in the stomach.
- To prevent a clogged feeding tube, flush the tube with water each time after giving a medication or a feeding.
- Brush your teeth at least twice daily if an NG tube remains in place continuously.

(continued on next page)

Procedure 23-1 ■ Administering Oral Medications (continued)

- Clean daily the area where the NG tube goes into the nostrils. Use a cotton-tipped applicator moistened with warm water. If your nose is sore, you might apply water-soluble lubricant.
- Change the nasal tape every other day or when it is loose or soiled.

Documentation

- Scheduled medications are often recorded only on the MAR.
- Document the drug, dosage, time, route, and your name as the healthcare provider administering the medication.
- Document any suspected drug reaction, intolerance, or patient response to the medication.
- For patients whose intake and output are being measured, document the amount of liquid medication and the water intake. Some patients may be on fluid restrictions, so record *all* intake. Follow your clinical facility protocol.

For Enteral Medications

Document the following:
- Patency, residual volume, and verification of placement.
- Any difficulty with administering the medications through the feeding tube.

- On the intake and output record, record the amount of liquid medication and the water used for flushing. Some providers prescribe a specific amount of water to flush with each medication administration or feeding. Some healthcare facilities use a protocol amount of water to flush gastrostomy tubes. Follow the protocol in your clinical facility.

Thinking About the Procedure

Go to the videos **Administering Oral Medications: Tablet or Capsule, Administering Oral Medications: Sublingual, Administering Oral Medications: Buccal,** and **Administering Oral Medications: Liquid Medications,** along with questions and suggested responses, available on the **Davis's Nursing Skills Videos** Web site at www.fadavis.com.

Practice Resources
Judd (2020); Kim & DeJesus (2022).

Procedure 23-2 ■ Administering Ophthalmic Medication

➤ For steps to follow in *all* procedures, refer to the Universal Steps for All Procedures on the inside back cover. Also refer to the Medication Guidelines: Steps to Follow for All Medications (Regardless of Type or Route).

Equipment

- Eye drops or ointment
- Tissue

For irrigation, add:

- Prescribed eye irrigation solution (e.g., 500 to 1,000 mL of normal saline or lactated Ringer's solution are commonly used)
- IV tubing or eye irrigation insert, such as the Morgan lens (follow manufacturer's directions for this specialized equipment)
- Ocular anesthetic, according to protocol or provider's prescriptions
- pH paper
- Basin and towel

Delegation

An RN can usually delegate eye instillations to an LPN/LVN. You usually cannot delegate this task to a UAP, unless the UAP has special training for a specific, defined situation (e.g., "medication aides" in some long-term care settings). See **Delegation in Medication Guidelines: Steps to Follow for All Medication (Regardless of Type or Route).**

Preprocedure Assessments

- Assess the patient's eyes for redness, discharge, or other signs of irritation.
- Determine whether the eyes need to be cleansed before administration of the medication.
  Excess tearing, debris, or excess mucus in the eye could interfere with the absorption, and thus effectiveness, of the medication.

✚ Check the prescription for where to instill medication

*(NOTE: **We do not advise using these abbreviations**—they have been disallowed by The Joint Commission—but you may still see them written in prescriptions.) Clarify with the provider the correct site.*

OD = right eye OS = left eye OU = both eyes

For irrigations also assess the following:

- Determine the cause of the eye problem—acid, alkaline, or other chemical burn or body fluid splash; or nonembedded foreign body.
  Irrigations are generally used to remove chemical or physical irritants, but they may be done after surgery or to treat a severe infection. Normal saline (NS) or lactated Ringer's is the solution generally

recommended for high-volume eye irrigations because the pH of 6 to 7.5 is closest to the normal tear pH of 7.1. Volumes of 500 to 1,000 mL are generally used.

- **Assess the patient's eyes for swelling, redness, drainage, or complaints of pain.**
  A baseline assessment is useful for determining the need for and effectiveness of irrigation. Sclera should be smooth, white, and glistening.

- **Determine the patient's ability to cooperate with the procedure.**
  Combative or otherwise uncooperative patients refusing instillation of medication can interfere with the efficiency of the procedure. If the patient cannot hold still for the procedure, the patient may need to be sedated.

- **Assess the pain level.**
  Debris, chemicals, and some liquids in the eye can be extremely painful. The eye may need to be anesthetized before irrigation or a general systemic pain medication is given.

▶ When performing the procedure, always identify your patient according to agency policy, using two identifiers, and be attentive to standard precautions, hand hygiene, patient safety and privacy, body mechanics, and documentation.

Procedure Steps

1. **Assist the patient to a** high-Fowler's position with head slightly tilted back, if possible.

   ✚ Do not tilt the head back if the patient has a neck injury or other contraindication. The medication can be given with the patient supine.

   An upright position keeps eye drops in the eye and helps prevent eye drops from draining into lacrimal duct.

2. **Don procedure gloves.**
   Gloving complies with standard precautions.

3. **Cleanse the edges of the eyelid** from the inner to outer canthus, if needed.
   By following the principle of "clean to dirty," you avoid transferring debris into the nasolacrimal duct.

Procedure Variation: Instilling Eye Drops
(Follow Steps 1–3. Note, however, that some sources recommend that the patient lie supine for eye drops.)

4. **Gently rest your dominant hand** (the one with the eyedropper) on the patient's forehead.
   Stabilizes the hand in the event the patient moves—prevents accidental injury to the eye.

5. **With your nondominant hand,** pull the lower lid down to expose the conjunctival sac.
   Allows visualization of the area where you will administer the medication.

6. **Position the eyedropper** about 1.5 to 2.0 cm (½ to ¾ in.) above the patient's eye. Ask the patient to look up, and drop the prescribed number of drops into the conjunctival sac. Do not let the dropper touch the eye.
   Keeping the dropper away from the globe of the eye reduces the risk of accidental injury to the eye and avoids contamination of the dropper. Having the patient look up helps to decrease the blink reflex. ▼

   Inner canthus — Outer canthus

7. **Ask the patient to gently close** their eyes.
   Closing the eyes helps to distribute the medication.

8. **If the medication has systemic** effects, press gently against the same side of the nose for 1 to 2 minutes to close the lacrimal ducts.
   Reduces systemic absorption through the lacrimal duct. ▼

Procedure Variation B: Administering Eye Ointment
(Follow Steps 1–3, then move to Step 9.)

9. **Gently rest your dominant** hand, the one with the eye ointment, on the patient's forehead.
   Stabilizing your hand helps to prevent accidental injury to the eye.

10. **With your nondominant hand,** pull the lower lid down to expose the conjunctival sac.
    Allows visualization of area where you will administer the medication.

(continued on next page)

Procedure 23-2 ■ Administering Ophthalmic Medication (continued)

11. **Ask the patient to look up** as you apply a thin strip of ointment—usually about 2 to 2.5 cm (1 in.)—in the conjunctival sac; twist your wrist to break off the strip of ointment. Do not let the tube touch the eye.
   If the medication ribbon is not broken off, lifting the tube will pull the medication out of the conjunctival sac. ▼

   a. Ask the patient to gently close their eyes for 2 to 3 minutes. Alternatively, release the eyelids and have the patient blink several times.
      Helps to distribute the medication.
   b. Explain to the patient that their vision will be blurred for a short time after administration of the ointment.
      The viscosity of the ointment can cause blurring.

? What if...

■ **My patient is a child who won't open their eye for the application?**
Try distracting the child by turning on the television or offering an age-appropriate toy in view.

Distraction and bribery are effective techniques for coaxing a child when cooperation is essential.

Ask a family member to help you gain cooperation of the child.
It might be fear or mistrust that is causing the patient to be unwilling to open their eyes.

■ **My patient wears soft contact lenses?**
Have the patient remove contact lenses before administering the medication and wait at least 15 minutes after instilling eye drops before reinserting the lenses.

Procedure 23-2A ■ Irrigating the Eyes

➤ When performing the procedure, always identify your patient according to agency policy, using two identifiers, and be attentive to standard precautions, hand hygiene, patient safety and privacy, body mechanics, and documentation.

Procedure Steps

1. **Assist the patient to a low-Fowler's position,** with the head tilted toward the affected eye, if possible.
   This position helps to drain the irrigating solution from the eye and prevents contamination of the unaffected eye.

2. **Place the towel and basin** under the patient's cheek to absorb the drainage.
   The patient will be more comfortable when clean and dry.

3. **Check the pH** by gently touching the pH paper to secretions in the conjunctival sac.
   A litmus test determines the correct irrigating solution and whether the irritant is alkaline or acidic. The normal pH of tears is approximately 7.1.

4. **Follow the agency protocol** or prescriber's prescription regarding use of ocular anesthetic drops.
   The ocular anesthetic will be washed out by the irrigation fluid, so it needs to be reinstilled every 2 to 3 minutes, or it can be added to the irrigation solution.

5. **Connect the solution and** tubing, and prime the tubing.
   Priming the tubing prevents blowing air across the cornea, which would be uncomfortable.

6. **Irrigate the eye.**
   a. Hold the tubing about 2.5 cm (1 in.) from eye.
      A safe distance helps prevent accidental trauma to the eye.
   b. Separate the eyelids with your thumb and index finger.
      It is easier to irrigate the cornea when the eyelids are separated.
   c. Direct the flow of solution over the eye from the inner canthus to the outer canthus.
      The inner canthus is considered clean primarily because of the open duct in this area. Flowing irrigation solution in this manner follows the principle of "clean to dirty." ▼

7. **Recheck pH, and continue** to irrigate the eye as needed.
   With alkaline or acidic chemical injuries, the pH of the eye needs to be returned to normal as soon as possible to prevent further eye injury.

Evaluation
- Examine the eyes for redness or drainage.
- Observe the patient's ability to follow instructions during the procedure.
- Observe the pain level during the procedure.
- After an irrigation, check for decrease in eye pain.

Patient Teaching
- Discuss how to prevent contaminating eye drops or ointment.
- Teach the best technique for instilling eye drops or ointment.
- Discuss the use of an eye drop guide if the patient needs assistance with instilling drops.
- Discuss the signs and symptoms to report to the provider, including eye pain, increased redness or drainage, and vision changes.

For irrigations:
- Discuss the cause and prevention of eye injuries, including use of protective goggles.
- Discuss the need for follow-up treatment. If the patient will be instilling eye medications or applying eye patches, ensure that he demonstrates the correct technique.

Home Care
If a splash occurs to the eyes in the home, teach the patient to immediately flood the eyes with cool water (as follows):
- Hold your eyelids open and put your head under a faucet or pour water from a clean container.
- Roll your eyes as much as possible while running water across your eyes.
- Flood your eyes for at least 20 minutes.
- Get medical help immediately after rinsing your eyes.

Documentation
- *For instillations:* Document assessment data before, during, and after instillation. Document the instillation on the MAR, as for all medications.
- *For irrigations:* Document the condition of the patient's eyes before the irrigation, including complaints of pain or burning. Document the eye pH, instillation of anesthetic drops, the type and amount of irrigation fluid used, the eye pH after irrigation, and the patient's response. Also document other treatment (e.g., instillation of lubricating and/or antibiotic ointment, application of eye patches).

Thinking About the Procedure

Go to the video **Administering Ophthalmic Medication,** along with questions and suggested responses, available on the **Davis's *Nursing Skills Videos*** Web site at www.fadavis.com.

Practice Resources
Bore (2018); Gao (2018), Gwenhure (2020); Lampert (2019); Stevens (2016).

Procedure 23-3 ■ Administering Otic Medication

➤ For steps to follow in *all* procedures, refer to the Universal Steps for All Procedures on the inside back cover. Also refer to the Medication Guidelines: Steps to Follow for All Medications (Regardless of Type or Route).

Equipment
- Ear drops
- Dropper with flexible rubber tip
- Cotton-tipped applicators
- Cotton ball

Delegation
The RN can usually delegate administration of otic medications to an LPN/LVN. You usually cannot delegate this task to a UAP unless allowed by the state's nurse practice act.

Preprocedure Assessments
- Assess the external ear and canal for erythema, drainage, and cerumen.
  You may need to clean the external ear to remove obstructions so that the medication can be distributed throughout the ear canal. Use the otoscope to evaluate the tympanic membrane if the drainage is bloody or the patient complains of pain or decreased hearing acuity. Use sterile technique if the tympanic membrane is ruptured.
- Assess for ear pain or hearing impairment.
  Establishes a baseline that can be used to evaluate the effects of treatment.

(continued on next page)

Procedure 23-3 ■ Administering Otic Medication (continued)

> When performing the procedure, always identify your patient according to agency policy, using two identifiers, and be attentive to standard precautions, hand hygiene, patient safety and privacy, body mechanics, and documentation.

Procedure Steps

1. **Hold the ear drop bottle** in your hand to warm it, or place it in warm water (not hot). Gently shake the bottle before using the drops.
   Warm solution is more comfortable than cool. Also, placing cool solutions in the ear can cause dizziness. Gently shaking the bottle disperses the medication throughout the solution.

2. **Assist patient to a side-lying** position (or turn the patient's head to the side if the patient cannot assume this position), with the appropriate ear facing up.
   Facilitates administering the drops and prevents drops from escaping from the ear.

3. **Clean the external ear** with a cotton-tipped applicator, if necessary.
   Cleaning the ear allows ear drops to reach all areas of the ear canal without trauma. Be careful not to push cerumen farther into the ear canal.

4. **Fill the dropper** with the correct amount of medication.

5. **For infants and young children,** ask a parent or another caregiver to immobilize the child while you administer the medication.
   Immobilization and restraint reduce the risk for injury for the child who struggles during the procedure.

6. **Straighten the ear canal.**
   a. For a child younger than 3 years old, pull the pinna down and back. ▼

   b. For children 3 years and older and adults, pull the pinna up and back. ▼
   These positions straighten the ear canal for proper channeling of the medication.

7. **Instill the prescribed number** of drops along the side of the ear canal, being careful not to touch the end of the dropper to any part of the ear.
   Avoiding contact between the dropper and the ear reduces the risk of contamination of the dropper.

8. **Gently tug on the external ear** after drops are instilled.
   Facilitates flow of medication into the auditory canal.

9. **Instruct the patient** to keep their head turned to the side for 5 to 10 minutes.
   Assists in distributing the medication and prevents drops from escaping the ear canal.

10. **Place a cotton ball,** or a piece of it, loosely at the opening of the auditory canal for 15 minutes.
    A cotton ball will absorb excess fluid and keep the medication from flowing out.

    ✚ *Keep in mind that cotton left near an infant can be a choking hazard and must be carefully supervised.*

? What if . . .

- **My patient is a child and rolls over so most of the otic medication flows back out of the ear?**
  Estimate the amount of the dosage that was lost. Replace it by repeating the procedure for instillation of the medication, except next time position the child securely until you are confident the medication has had time to penetrate the ear canal.

- **There is too much cerumen (earwax) in the canal to instill otic drops?**

  ✚ You can use special drops for softening the cerumen and allow for easier removal. Gentle irrigation with warm saline is effective unless the patient has perforation of the tympanic membrane or myringotomy tubes.
  - **You should not use a metal syringe** (Pomeroy syringe) for the removal of cerumen (1) because this type of syringe is heavy and difficult to control and (2) because of the pressure exerted, it may be associated with a higher risk of perforations of the tympanic membrane.
  - **Oral jet irrigators have been associated with some trauma,** including tympanic membrane perforation.
  - **You should not attempt to remove impaction by "ear candling,"** which is the application of hot candle wax.

Evaluation
- Assess for discomfort or pain during the procedure and for relief afterward.
- Evaluate for wax buildup, redness, swelling, or drainage.

Documentation
- Assess the amount, color, character, and odor of drainage, if present.
- Note any swelling or redness in the ear canal.
- Document pain or discomfort and hearing loss.

Thinking About the Procedure

Go to the video **Administering Otic Medication,** along with questions and suggested responses, available on the **Davis's *Nursing Skills Videos*** Web Site at www.fadavis.com.

Procedure 23-4 ■ Administering Nasal Medication

➤ For steps to follow in *all* procedures, refer to the Universal Steps for All Procedures on the inside back cover. Also refer to the Medication Guidelines: Steps to Follow for All Medications (Regardless of Type or Route).

Equipment
- Medication drops, spray, or aerosol
- Tissues

Delegation
As an RN, you can usually delegate administration of nasal instillations to an LPN/LVN. You usually cannot delegate this task to a UAP.

Preprocedure Assessments
- Check for nasal obstruction and congestion.
  Nasal obstruction or congestion can prevent the medication from reaching the nasal mucosa.
- Assess nasal discharge for color, consistency, and odor.
  The appearance of drainage is not always diagnostic of infection, especially for people with chronic sinus problems or polyps. Color can be indicative of the body's response to viral, bacterial, and allergic sources.
- Assess nasal mucous membranes for redness, color, moisture, excoriation, or trauma.
- ✚ Check the dropper tip to be sure it is not cracked or chipped.
  A cracked or chipped tip might interfere with drawing up the medication and scratch the nasal mucosa.

➤ When performing the procedure, always identify your patient according to agency policy, using two identifiers, and be attentive to standard precautions, hand hygiene, patient safety and privacy, body mechanics, and documentation.

Procedure Steps
1. **Explain to the patient** that the medication may cause some burning, tingling, or unusual taste.
   The taste of nasal medications can cause nausea or vomiting. The medication is more likely to cause burning or tingling if the nasal mucosa is inflamed.

2. **Ask the patient to gently blow** their nose and perform hand hygiene afterward.
   Removing nasal discharge allows the medication to come into contact with the mucous membranes without traumatizing already inflamed mucosa.

3. **Don procedure gloves.**
   Prevents transmission of microorganisms.

4. **Position the patient.**

   When Medicating the Frontal Sinuses With Spray
   "Head down and forward." Remember: "To spray your nose, look at your toes!" If the patient can comfortably assume this position, ask them to lean forward or kneel on the bed with their head down. Administer the medication, and then ask the patient to tilt their head back to medicate the nasal passages.
   Radionuclide studies have demonstrated that using nasal drops or sprays with the patient sitting and leaning the head back causes poor distribution of the medications into the nasal complex and sinuses. ▼

   Wrong position

   Correct positions
   (continued on next page)

Procedure 23-4 ■ Administering Nasal Medication (continued)

When Medicating the Ethmoid and Sphenoid Sinuses

Assist the patient into a supine position, tilted back with their head over the edge of the bed. Support the patient's head. Alternatively, place a towel roll behind the patient's shoulders, and allow the head to drop back.
These positions help to prevent straining of the neck muscles and facilitate distribution of the medication to the ethmoid and sphenoid sinuses. ▼

Ethmoid sinuses
Sphenoid sinus
Nasopharynx

When Medicating the Frontal and Maxillary Sinuses With Drops

With patient supine, tilt the head back over the edge of the bed or place a pillow under the head and turn toward the affected side.
Titling the head promotes gravity to distribute the medication to the frontal sinuses. ▼

Maxillary sinuses
Frontal sinuses

5. **Ask the patient to exhale** and then close one nostril. Place the tip of the sprayer into the nostril, pointing toward the outside of the nose.
   Blocking one nostril provides for deeper inhalation. Not pointing the tip toward the middle of the nose (septum) or straight up toward the sinus prevents accidental injury.

6. **Then ask the patient to breathe in** deeply through the nose and while they are breathing in, press down firmly and quickly once on the applicator. Ask patient to breathe out through the mouth. After spraying, lean head backward for a few seconds. If a dropper is used, do not touch the sides of the nostril.
   Inhaling through the mouth prevents aspiration of the drops into the trachea and bronchi. Touching the dropper to the nostril will contaminate the dropper.

7. **Repeat for the other nostril.**

8. **If nose drops are used,** ask the patient to stay in the same position for 1 to 5 minutes (depending on the manufacturer's guidelines).
   Maintaining this position promotes better absorption by using gravity to disperse the medication throughout the nasal passages and sinuses instead of draining out the nose.

9. **Instruct the patient not to blow** their nose for several minutes.
   To prevent expelling the medication.

? What if...

- **My patient cannot assume the "head down and forward" position?**

  Help them to hold their head upright to administer the drops or spray.

- **My patient can taste the medicine after it is administered?**

  That means their head was not down enough or they did not inhale long enough. Instruct them to put their head back down and sniff again without the medicine.

- **My patient has an excoriated area on the inside septum?**

  Assess further, examining other areas of the nasal mucosa. Determine whether the patient has a history of substance abuse or frequent nasal inhalations. Report the findings to the prescriber before administering nasal medication.

- **My patient begins to have nosebleeds after using nasal medication?**

  First, control the nosebleed. Then hold the medication and notify the prescriber. Assess for other signs of bleeding, bruising, or other petechiae.

Evaluation

Assess for a reduction of symptoms 15 to 20 minutes after administration.

Patient Teaching

- Teach the procedure for administering nasal drops or sprays, including proper positioning.
- Discuss the correct use of the medication and the adverse effects of overusing nasal decongestants.
- Explain the implications of the color of nasal secretions.

Documentation

Document according to Medication Guidelines: Steps to Follow for All Medication (Regardless of Type or Route). For example, document the administration of the medication on the MAR.

For nasal instillation, document:

- Premedication assessment
- Type and amount of solution administered
- Discomfort the patient experienced during the procedure
- Patient's report of response to nasal administrations, such as nasal discharge, obstruction of nasal passage, bleeding, or other complications after the procedure

Thinking About the Procedure

Go to the video **Administering Nasal Medication,** along with questions and suggested responses, available on the **Davis's** *Nursing Skills Videos* Web site at www.fadavis.com.

Practice Resources
Kim & DeJesus (2020); Mundlia et al. (2015).

Procedure 23-5 ■ Administering Vaginal Medication

➤ For steps to follow in *all* procedures, refer to the Universal Steps for All Procedures on the inside back cover. Also refer to the Medication Guidelines: Steps to Follow for All Medications (Regardless of Type or Route).

Equipment

- Medication: foam, jelly, cream, suppository, douche, or irrigating solution
- Applicator (if indicated)
- Perineal wash solution or wipes for perineal care as needed
- Water-soluble lubricant
- Toilet tissue
- Perineal pad
- Bath blanket
- **For irrigation:** you will also need a waterproof pad, bedpan, vaginal irrigation set (consists of a solution container, nozzle, tubing, and clamp; may be disposable), and IV pole.

Delegation

An RN can usually delegate the administration of vaginal medications to an LPN/LVN. Delegation of this task to a UAP will vary depending on the state's nurse practice acts and the healthcare facility policies. However, the RN is always responsible for evaluating patient responses, both therapeutic effects and side effects. You can instruct the UAP on the expected therapeutic effects and the side effects she should report.

Preprocedure Assessments

- Assess for vaginal burning, pruritus, and pain.
  A baseline assessment helps to determine the patient's level of comfort and later the effectiveness of treatment. Infections can cause vaginal burning, itching, and pain.
- Inspect the labia and vaginal orifice for redness and lesions.
  This is a good time to assess the perineal area for signs of sexually transmitted infection or other findings requiring healthcare.
- Check for vaginal discharge, including color, amount, consistency, and odor.

➤ When performing the procedure, always identify your patient according to agency policy, using two identifiers, and be attentive to standard precautions, hand hygiene, patient safety and privacy, body mechanics, and documentation.

Procedure Steps

1. **Ask the patient to void** before you insert the vaginal medication.
   A full bladder could cause discomfort during the instillation of vaginal medications.

2. **Position the patient** in a dorsal recumbent or Sims' position; drape the patient with a bath blanket so that only the perineum is exposed.

   a. **Dorsal recumbent position**—supine with knees flexed and legs rotated outward.
   b. **Sims' position**—semiprone on the left side with the right hip and knee flexed.
   These two positions allow for visualization during administration and promote retention of the medication after administration. Draping respects the patient's modesty.

3. **Prepare the medication.**
   - *Suppository:* Remove the wrapper and place the suppository on the wrapper or in a medication cup.
   - *Applicator:* Fill the applicator according to the manufacturer's instructions.

(continued on next page)

Procedure 23-5 ■ Administering Vaginal Medication (continued)

- **For irrigation:** Use a warm solution of approximately 105°F (40.5°C).
  Some suppositories come with applicators. Using a warm irrigation solution promotes patient comfort and prevents injury to the vaginal tissue. ▼

Invert cap and pierce end of medication tube

Attach applicator

Squeeze medication into applicator

4. **Don procedure gloves.**
   Prevents contaminating your hands and spreading microorganisms.

5. **Inspect and clean around vaginal orifice.**
   Prevents the introduction of microorganisms into the vagina during medication administration.

6. **Administer the medication.**

For a Suppository
   a. Apply water-soluble lubricant to the rounded end of the suppository and to your gloved index finger on your dominant hand.
      Eases insertion and prevents injury to the vaginal tissue.
   b. Separate the labia with your nondominant hand.
      Allows visualization of the vaginal orifice.
   c. Insert the suppository as far as possible along the posterior vaginal wall (about 8 cm, or 3 in.). If using an applicator, insert the applicator into the vagina and press the plunger.
      The posterior vaginal wall is about 2.5 cm (1 in.) longer than the anterior wall. ▼

   d. Ask the patient to remain in a supine position for 5 to 15 minutes. You may wish to elevate her hips on a pillow.
      Lifting the hips promotes retention and absorption of the medication.

For Applicator Insertion of Cream, Foam, or Jelly
   e. Separate the labia with your nondominant hand.
   f. Insert the applicator approximately 8 cm (3 in.) into the vagina along the posterior vaginal wall.
   g. Depress the plunger on the applicator, inserting the medication into the vagina.
   h. Dispose of the applicator, or place it on a paper towel if the applicator is reusable. You will later wash it in the appropriate solution.
   i. Instruct the patient to remain in a supine position for 5 to 15 minutes.
      A flat position promotes retention and absorption of the medication.

For Irrigations
   j. Hang the irrigation solution approximately 30 to 60 cm (1 to 2 ft) above the level of the patient's vagina.
      Uses gravity to create enough pressure for continuous irrigation without increasing the pressure so much that it causes the patient discomfort and possibly damages the vaginal tissue. ▼

   k. Assist the patient into a dorsal recumbent position, and position a waterproof pad and bedpan under the patient.
      Positioning the patient on the bedpan and using a waterproof pad protect the bedding.
   l. If using a vaginal irrigation set with tubing, open the clamp to allow the solution to completely fill the tubing.
      Flushing the tubing prevents introducing air into the vagina, which can cause discomfort.
   m. Lubricate the end of the irrigation nozzle.
      Lubrication reduces discomfort and irritation to the vaginal mucosa.
   n. Insert the nozzle approximately 8 cm (3 in.) into the vagina, directing it toward the sacrum.
   o. Start the flow of the irrigation solution, and rotate the nozzle intermittently as solution flows.
      The rotation ensures even distribution of the solution throughout the vagina.

CHAPTER 23 Administering Medications   409

p. After all irrigating solution has been used, remove the nozzle.
q. Assist the patient to a sitting position on the bedpan.
Promotes removal of all the irrigating solution by gravity.

solution and a washcloth or wipes. Dry the perineum.
Drainage could cause skin irritation.

8. **Apply a perineal pad** if necessary for excessive drainage.

? What if...

- **The labia are reddened?**
Pour warm water (bottled or specially filtered tap water) over the labia with an irrigation bottle to soothe irritation and cleanse the area.

7. **Remove the bedpan and clean** the perineum with perineal wash

Evaluation
- Assess for complaints of vaginal burning, pruritis, or pain.
- Assess for purulent vaginal discharge.

Patient Teaching
- Discuss with the patient personal hygiene and pericare.
- ✚ Teach women that douching may be harmful because it disturbs the normal pH and healthy balance of microorganisms in the vagina. Research has revealed a relationship between douching and ovarian cancer (Gonzalez, et al., 2016; Kim & DeJesus, 2020; Office on Women's Health, 2021).

Documentation
- **For vaginal medications,** document according to **Medication Guidelines: Steps to Follow for All Medication (Regardless of Type or Route).**
- **For vaginal irrigations,** document your assessment; the type and amount of solution administered; discomfort the patient experienced during the procedure; and the patient's report of decreased vaginal pain, itching, and/or burning after the procedure.

Practice Resources
Gonzalez et al. (2016); Kim & DeJesus (2022).

Procedure 23-6 ■ Inserting a Rectal Suppository

➤ For steps to follow in *all* procedures, refer to the Universal Steps for All Procedures on the inside back cover. Also refer to the Medication Guidelines: Steps to Follow for All Medications (Regardless of Type or Route).

Equipment
- Suppository Water-soluble lubricant
- Toilet tissue

Delegation
An RN can usually delegate administration of rectal medications to an LPN/LVN. Although in some institutions you can delegate the administration of a glycerin suppository (nonmedicated) to a UAP, you generally cannot delegate administration of rectal medications to a UAP. You cannot delegate the insertion of a Macy catheter to a UAP.

Preprocedure Assessments
- Determine the presence of contraindications for rectal administration, such as recent rectal surgery, rectal bleeding, or cardiac disease.
- Assess the rectal area for hemorrhoids or irritation.

➤ When performing the procedure, always identify your patient according to agency policy, using two identifiers, and be attentive to standard precautions, hand hygiene, patient safety and privacy, body mechanics, and documentation.

Procedure Steps

1. **Ask whether the patient needs** to defecate before the suppository insertion.
Stool in the rectum interferes with insertion of medication against the rectal wall and therefore with retention of the medication.

2. **Assist patient to Sims' position**—lying on the left side with the right hip and knee flexed. Drape the patient, keeping them covered as much as possible.

Sims' position allows visualization of the anus and promotes retention of the medication because the descending colon is on the left side. It also helps relax the external anal sphincter. Keeping the patient covered prevents chilling and maintains privacy.

3. **Don procedure gloves.**
Gloving prevents exposure to feces and spread of microorganisms; maintains standard precautions.

4. **For an uncooperative patient,** such as a confused patient or a young child, ask someone to help immobilize the patient while you insert the suppository.
Help with holding the patient allows proper instillation of medication and prevents injury to the rectal mucosa.

(continued on next page)

Procedure 23-6 ■ Inserting a Rectal Suppository (continued)

5. **Prepare the suppository:** Remove the wrapper. Using a water-soluble lubricant, lubricate the smooth end of the suppository and the tip of the glove on the index finger. If no lubricant is available, apply cool tap water to the rectal opening.
   Lubrication eases insertion and prevents friction damage to the rectal mucosa during insertion.

6. **Explain that there will be a cool feeling** from the lubricant and a feeling of pressure during insertion.
   The patient should not feel severe pain with the insertion of a suppository, but they will feel the coolness of the lubricant and pressure as the suppository is inserted past the rectal sphincter.

7. **Using your nondominant hand,** separate the buttocks.
   Separation of the buttocks allows you to visualize the anus.

8. **Ask the adult patient to take deep breaths** in and out through the mouth.
   Deep breathing helps relax the rectal sphincter. Pushing a suppository through a constricted sphincter produces discomfort.

9. **Insert the suppository:**
   a. Using the index finger of your dominant hand, gently insert the lubricated smooth end first, or follow the manufacturer's instructions.
      Lubrication eases insertion. ▼

   b. ✚ Never force the suppository during insertion.
      Forcing the insertion of the suppository into a fecal mass would affect absorption. Forcing anything into the rectum may cause rectal irritation.

   c. Push the suppository past the internal sphincter and along the rectal wall (½ to 1 in. in infants and 1 to 3 in. in adults).
      The suppository must be in contact with the rectal wall for the medication to be absorbed. Inserting the suppository past the internal sphincter promotes retention. For a child, inserting the suppository too far could damage the rectal mucosa. ▼

   Suppository — Rectum
   Anal-rectal ridge
   Anal sphincter

10. **Ask the patient to try to retain** the suppository if they are able. If they have difficulty retaining the suppository, hold the buttocks together for a short time.

11. **Wipe the patient's anus** with toilet tissue.
    Wiping maintains hygiene and comfort.

12. **Explain to the patient the need** to remain in the side-lying position for at least 10 minutes, if possible.
    Sims' position promotes retention and absorption of the medication. Explanation promotes compliance.

13. **Discard used materials** into a biohazard receptacle and wash hands thoroughly.

14. **Leave the call device within** reach and bedpan handy if the suppository was a laxative. Instruct the patient to call for assistance getting out of bed.
    In case the patient has a sudden urge to defecate or cannot retain the suppository for the recommended time, they can call for help. Providing assistance promotes safety.

Procedure 23-6A ■ Inserting a Macy Catheter

Equipment
- Macy catheter
- 20-mL syringe filled with tap water
- Water-soluble lubricant
- Toilet tissue

Macy catheter with callouts showing arrows, balloon port, balloon, medication port.

Delegation
An RN can usually delegate administration of rectal medications to an LPN/LVN. You cannot delegate the insertion of a Macy catheter to a UAP.

Preprocedure Assessments
- Determine the presence of contraindications for rectal administration, such as recent rectal surgery, rectal bleeding, or cardiac disease.
- Assess the rectal area for hemorrhoids or irritation.
- Check to ensure the catheter balloon is intact.

➤ For steps to follow in *all* procedures, refer to the Universal Steps for All Procedures on the inside back cover. Also refer to the Medication Guidelines: Steps to Follow for All Medications (Regardless of Type or Route).

Procedure Steps

1. **Ask whether the patient needs** to defecate before the catheter insertion.
   Stool in the rectum interferes with insertion of the catheter.

2. **Assist patient to supine with the knees bent or the Sims' position.** These positions provide easy visibility of the rectum. Drape the patient, keeping them covered as much as possible.
   Keeping the patient covered prevents chilling and maintains privacy.

3. **Don procedure gloves.**
   Gloving prevents exposure to feces and spread of microorganisms; maintains standard precautions. This is a nonsterile procedure.

4. **For an uncooperative patient,** such as a confused patient or a young child, ask someone to help immobilize the patient while you insert the catheter.
   Help with holding the patient allows proper insertion of the catheter and prevents injury to the rectal mucosa.

5. **Prepare the Macy catheter:** Remove the catheter tip. Using a water-soluble lubricant, lubricate the distal end of the catheter to the first arrow.
   Lubrication eases insertion and prevents friction damage to the rectal mucosa during insertion.

6. **Explain that there will be a cool feeling** from the lubricant and a feeling of pressure during insertion.
   The patient should not feel severe pain with the insertion of a catheter, but they will feel the coolness of the lubricant and pressure as the catheter is inserted past the rectal sphincter.

7. **Using your nondominant hand,** separate the buttocks.
   Separation of the buttocks allows you to visualize the anus.

8. **Ask the adult patient to take deep** breaths in and out through the mouth.
   Deep breathing helps relax the rectal sphincter.

9. **Insert the catheter to** between the first and second arrow.

10. **Remove the balloon cap and insert 15 mL of tap water.**
    Inflating the balloon secures the catheter in place.

11. **Gently pull back to ensure the catheter is secure against the rectal sphincter.**
    This validates that the catheter is secure against the inside portion of the rectal sphincter.

12. **Secure the tubing to the thigh or lower abdomen.**
    Prevents accidental dislodgment.

13. **Wipe the excess lubricant** from the patient's anus using the toilet tissue.

14. **Reinforce that the catheter will remain in place.**

15. **Discard used materials** into a biohazard receptacle and wash hands thoroughly.

16. **Position the patient for safety** and leave the call bell within reach.

(continued on next page)

Procedure 23-6 ■ Inserting a Rectal Suppository (continued)

? What if...

- **The prescribed dose is only half of the suppository?**
  Cut the suppository lengthwise with a clean cutting device, per agency policy, or a single-edge razor blade.

- **My patient is a child? What is the best way to give a rectal suppository so the child doesn't expel it?**
  For pediatric patients, it may be necessary to gently hold the buttocks together for 5 to 10 minutes.

- **My patient is an older adult? Is there anything special I should know?**
  Older adults may have difficulty retaining a suppository because of poor sphincter control. You may need to put the bedpan under the patient while you are inserting the suppository.

- **The Macy catheter becomes dislodged?**
  Assess the rectal area for injury, bleeding, or signs of irritation. Notify the provider. The catheter can be replaced unless contraindicated by irritation or injury to the rectal area.

Evaluation
- Assess for pain or burning during and after insertion of the medication.
- Determine that the patient retained the suppository for the desired time after insertion (reinsertion may be required).

Patient Teaching
Explain that suppositories may take up to 30 minutes to be absorbed, depending on the medication.

Documentation
- Refer to **Medication Guidelines: Steps to Follow for All Medication (Regardless of Type or Route).**
- Document the condition of anal tissue if abnormalities are present, any complaints of discomfort that are outside of the expected feelings and experience, and the length of time that the suppository was retained.
- Document responses to medication (e.g., symptom relief, side effects).

Practice Resources
Hua (2019); Kim & DeJesus (2022); Lowry (2016).

Thinking About the Procedure

Go to the video **Inserting a Rectal Suppository,** along with questions and suggested responses, available on the **Davis's** *Nursing Skills Videos* Web site at www.fadavis.com.

Procedure 23-7 ■ Applying Medication to Skin

▶ For steps to follow in *all* procedures, refer to the Universal Steps for All Procedures on the inside back cover. Also refer to the Medication Guidelines: Steps to Follow for All Medications (Regardless of Type or Route).

▶ Note: Follow agency policy or provider's prescription regarding whether to use prepackaged wipes or soap and water to cleanse the skin.

Delegation
An RN can usually delegate administration of most topical medications to an LPN/LVN. In some institutions, you can delegate the administration of an over-the-counter medication to a UAP. Refer to agency policy regarding administration of topical medication.

Preprocedure Assessments
- Assess for skin irritation, open lesions, area of hypersensitivity, or other skin abnormality.
- Determine the presence of contraindications for dermal application. Document and report these before administering medication.

Procedure 23-7A ■ Applying Topical Lotion, Cream, and Ointment

➤ When performing the procedure, always identify your patient according to agency policy, using two identifiers, and be attentive to standard precautions, hand hygiene, patient safety and privacy, body mechanics, and documentation.

Procedure Steps

1. **Don clean procedure gloves.**
   Complies with universal precautions and protects your skin from the topical medication.

2. **Cleanse the skin** with cleansing wipes or soap and water (according to agency policy) and pat dry before applying
   Clean skin enhances absorption. Moisture on the skin can interfere with adherence of topical ointment, depending on the product used to suspend the medication.

3. **Warm the medication** in your gloved hands.
   This will be more comfortable for the patient and make the preparation easier to apply.

4. **Use gloved hands or an** applicator to apply and spread the medication evenly, following the direction of hair growth when coating the area.
   Excessive application may irritate the skin. Gloves will protect you so that you will not absorb the medication through your own skin. ▼

Procedure 23-7B ■ Applying Topical Aerosol Spray

➤ When performing the procedure, always identify your patient according to agency policy, using two identifiers, and be attentive to standard precautions, hand hygiene, patient safety and privacy, body mechanics, and documentation.

Procedure Steps

1. **Don clean procedure gloves.**

2. **Cleanse the skin** with cleansing wipe or soap and water (according to agency policy) and pat dry before applying to enhance absorption.

3. **Shake the container to mix** the contents.
   To ensure that active ingredients are evenly distributed throughout the aerosolized suspension.

4. **Hold the container** at the distance specified on the label (usually 6 to 12 in.), and spray over the prescribed area.
   Prevents excess application to a local area.

5. **Hold most containers** upright when spraying. If you are spraying near the patient's head, cover their face with a towel.
   This will prevent the patient from inhaling the spray.

Procedure 23-7C ■ Applying Prescribed Powder

➤ When performing the procedure, always identify your patient according to agency policy, using two identifiers, and be attentive to standard precautions, hand hygiene, patient safety and privacy, body mechanics, and documentation.

Procedure Steps

1. **Don clean procedure gloves.**

2. **Cleanse the skin** with a cleansing wipe or soap and water and pat dry before applying to enhance absorption.
   Powder applied to a moist surface creates a pasty solution, which may irritate the skin.

3. **Spread apart skinfolds,** and apply a very thin layer.

4. **Be careful that the patient does** not inhale the powder.
   Particulate matter, such as powder, can irritate lung tissue and lead to pneumonitis or other inflammatory processes.

Procedure 23-7D ■ Applying Transdermal Medication

➤ When performing the procedure, always identify your patient according to agency policy, using two identifiers, and be attentive to standard precautions, hand hygiene, patient safety and privacy, body mechanics, and documentation.

Procedure Steps

1. **Don clean procedure gloves.**
   Complies with universal precautions and protects your skin from the topical medication.

2. **Remove the previous patch,** folding the medicated side to the inside.
   This helps to prevent unintentional contact of the medication on a different area of the patient's skin.

3. **Dispose of the old patch** carefully in an appropriate receptacle, keeping it away from children and pets.
   Even a used patch has some active medication on it. Proper disposal is important to prevent medication exposure to others.

(continued on next page)

Procedure 23-7 ■ Applying Medication to Skin (continued)

4. **Cleanse the skin of traces** of remaining medication. Allow the skin to dry.
   A clean, dry surface optimizes the effectiveness of adherence and absorption of the medication.

5. **Remove the new patch from** its protective covering, and then remove the clear, protective covering without touching the adhesive or the inside surface that contains the medication. ▼

6. **Apply the patch to** a clean, dry, hairless (or little hair), intact skin area, pressing it down for about 10 seconds with your palm. Be sure the area is free of scars, lesions, and irritation.
   A smooth surface maximizes the contact between medication and the skin. Skin that is disrupted can become irritated by topical medication. Lesions involving thickened layers of skin can compromise absorption.

7. **Rotate application sites** with each new application. Common sites are the trunk, lower abdomen, lower back, and buttocks.
   Rotating sites prevents irritation to local areas of the skin.

8. **Advise the patient** *not* to use a heating pad over the area.
   Heat can cause some ointments to irritate or even burn the skin.

9. **Write the date, the time,** and your initials on the new patch.
   Complete documentation helps to reduce medication errors.

10. **Remove your gloves and** perform hand hygiene.

11. **Observe for local side effects,** such as skin irritation, itching, and allergic contact dermatitis.
    If an adverse response occurs at the local site, remove the patch, wipe the skin clean, and notify the prescriber.

? What if . . .

- **The medication is packaged as an ointment form with calibrated paper?**

  Wear gloves; apply the ointment in a continuous motion along those marks to measure the required dose. Fold the paper in half to distribute the ointment evenly on the patch.

- **My patient is a child who does not want the medication to be applied?**

  Hold the child securely while medication is applied. Then cover the site with a dressing to keep the child from disrupting the application of medication.

- **My patient is an older adult and has fragile skin?**

  Avoid areas where penetration of the cream or ointment is likely to be reduced or cause irritation. Be gentle with application of anything to the skin and diligent with your assessment of the skin response to medication. Avoid using tape; use tape alternatives.

Evaluation

- Assess for rash, excoriation, hives, redness, swelling, or signs of allergy or skin sensitivity to topical medication.
- Ask the patient whether they feel burning, itching, pain, tenderness, or other sensation to skin where medication was applied.
- Assess for improvement in the patient's condition.

Patient Teaching

- Explain that topical medication may take up to 30 minutes to be absorbed, depending on the medication.
- Tell the patient to never ingest or inhale topical medication.
- Advise the patient to avoid touching their eyes after handling topical medication.
- Inform the patient not to use more medicine than prescribed or directed.

Documentation

- Refer to **Medication Guidelines: Steps to Follow for All Medication (Regardless of Type or Route).**
- Document the skin condition if abnormalities are present and complaints of discomfort during or after administration.
- Document responses to medication (e.g., symptom relief, side effects).

Sample Documentation

mm/dd/yyyy   0835   Transdermal nitroglycerin 74.6 mg patch applied to upper chest. Pt instructed to leave patch intact for 12 hours. Patient reported mild, transient headache approximately 45 minutes after application of patch. No evidence of flushing, faintness, or dizziness. Patient denies chest pain. ——M. Finegold, RN

mm/dd/yyyy   0830   Fentanyl patch dated 06/17/2021 removed from upper left arm. Skin intact, no irritation noted. Fentanyl patch applied to the left anterior chest wall below the clavicle. Patient stated, "This patch really helps my back feel better." ——M. Finegold, RN

Thinking About the Procedure

Go to the video **Applying Transdermal Medication**, along with questions and suggested responses, available on the **Davis's** *Nursing Skills Videos* Web site at www.fadavis.com.

Procedure 23-8 ■ Administering Metered-Dose Inhaler (MDI) Medication

➤ For steps to follow in *all* procedures, refer to the Universal Steps for All Procedures on the inside back cover. Also refer to the Medication Guidelines: Steps to Follow for All Medications (Regardless of Type or Route).

Equipment
- Metered-dose inhaler
- Spacer
- Tissues

Preprocedure Assessments
Assess the respiratory status before administration of medication to establish a baseline for evaluating the effects of treatment.

Delegation
An RN can usually delegate administration of MDI medications to an LPN/LVN. You usually cannot delegate this task to a UAP, unless the UAP has special training for a specific defined situation (e.g., "medication aides" in some long-term care settings in some states). If the patient is having respiratory distress, you should not delegate this task. Refer to **Medication Guidelines: Steps to Follow for All Medications (regardless of Type or Route).**

➤ When performing the procedure, always identify your patient according to agency policy, using two identifiers, and be attentive to standard precautions, hand hygiene, patient safety and privacy, body mechanics, and documentation.

Procedure Steps

1. **Determine the number of** remaining inhalations of medication in the canister based on the start date and instructions for use. **Key Point:** *Do not use the old method of floating the canister in water, because it is not an accurate estimate.* Replace the canister promptly when it is nearly empty.

   ✚ Do not float the canister in water as a method to determine how much medication remains. The effect of propellants on the weight of the canister may lead to false indication that there is medication in an empty container.

   ✚ Always have medication available for use, especially for MDI medications that are used as rescue agents during asthma attacks or periods of dyspnea.

2. **Assist the patient to a seated** or high-Fowler's position if in bed.
   Facilitates the ability to take a deep inhalation when medication is administered.

3. **Ask the patient to rinse** out their mouth and spit the fluid out (not to swallow it).
   Helps prevent transfer of bacteria from the mouth to the inhaler.

4. **Shake the inhaler.** Then remove the mouthpiece cap of the inhaler and insert the mouthpiece into the spacer while holding the canister upright.
   A spacer is the most efficient method to deliver inhaled medications. It should be used if the patient has difficulty coordinating the use of the inhaler, if the patient is using a corticosteroid, or if the spacer is prescribed.

5. **Remove the cap from the spacer.**

6. **Ask the patient to breathe out** slowly and completely. If a patient is unable to use the MDI independently, time the use of the device with the patient's own respirations.
   Deep breathing helps the patient to time the dose with their natural breathing.

7. **Place the spacer mouthpiece** into the patient's mouth and have them seal their lips around the mouthpiece. Sharply press down on the inhaler canister to discharge one puff of medication into the spacer. ▼

   If No Spacer Is Used
   If a spacer is not used, place the canister 1 to 2 inches (2.5 to 5.0 cm) from or directly into the mouth.
   A good seal allows proper delivery of medication.

8. **Ask the patient to slowly inhale** and then hold their breath for as long as possible. Encourage the patient to hold their breath for 10 seconds if possible.
   When the patient holds their breath, the medication can be delivered deep into the distal bronchioles of the lungs.

9. **If a second puff is needed,** wait at least 1 minute before repeating Steps 6 through 8.
   Allows the medication to be absorbed and the canister to recharge.

10. **If a corticosteroid inhaler** was used, assist the patient to rinse out their mouth with water and spit out the rinse.
    Prolonged exposure of this medication to the oral mucosa is irritating and can lead to thrush in some patients.

11. **Wipe the mouthpiece** with a tissue or moist cloth and replace the cap. Periodically rinse the spacer, mouthpiece, and cap with water.
    Proper cleaning of the MDI keeps the dispenser from clogging.

(continued on next page)

Procedure 23-8 ■ Administering Metered-Dose Inhaler (MDI) Medication (continued)

The following illustrations summarize the steps for using an MDI. ▼

A Shake canister.

B Remove cap. Discharge 2 puffs.

C Deep breath out.

D Press top. Inhale med slowly.

E Hold breath. Exhale slowly.

F Remove inhaler from mouth. Wait 1 minute before next puff.

? What if...

- **My patient is a small child or frail older adult who is unable to assist with taking medication from the inhaler?**

    You will need to time discharge of the medication with the patient's inspiration if the patient is unable to administer the medication with their own deep breaths.

- **My patient is using a dry-powder inhaler (DPI)?**

    Instruct the patient that the DPI is breath-activated, so they should breathe in very fast and deep to fill the lungs with medication (Stuart, 2021).

Evaluation

Assess for change in respiratory status after medication administration.

Patient Teaching

- Explain when to use the inhaler and what side effects to anticipate.
- Teach and demonstrate to patients how to correctly use a spacer and MDI.
- Explain how to determine whether the MDI canister is nearly empty.
- Explain that some inhalers are used in combination with others and must be used in correct order to receive the desired effect.

Home Care

General Information to Tell Patients

- Show your healthcare professional how you're using your MDI. If you're having trouble, ask for tips or to recommend another device.
- Never puncture or break the canister.
- Do not immerse the MDI in water.
- Keep the MDI where you can get it quickly when needed but out of children's reach.
- Store the MDI at room temperature. If it gets cold, warm it by rubbing the canister between your palms. Never use anything else to warm it.

Determining the Number of Remaining Doses

- When you begin using a new MDI, write the start date on the canister.
- The only reliable method for determining the number of doses remaining in a canister is to subtract the number of doses used from the number available. Some devices are equipped with counters. Floating MDIs in water is not accurate for assessing remaining doses and often will clog the valve.

Cleaning the MDI

- Clean your apparatus regularly to avoid drug buildup that might keep the medication from reaching the lungs. Specific maintenance procedures may vary with the manufacturer.
- Remove the metal canister that contains the medication by pulling it out.

Documentation

- Refer to **Medication Guidelines: Steps to Follow for All Medications (regardless of Type or Route).**
- Document the response to medications.

Sample documentation

09/25/2021   0800   Pt. c/o shortness of breath. RR 26 and labored. Combivent MDI 2 puffs administered with spacer. ———————————————— S. Smythe, RN

0815   RR 20,   regular, even, pt states he is comfortable. ———————————————— S. Smythe, RN

Thinking About the Procedure

> Go to the video **Administering Metered Dose Inhaler (MDI) Medication,** along with questions and suggested responses, available on the **Davis's** *Nursing Skills Videos* Web site at www.fadavis.com.

Practice Resources
Buddiga (2015); Glesson et al. (2020); Rodríguez-Martínez et al. (2017); Scullion (2018).

Procedure 23-9 ■ Preparing, Drawing Up, and Mixing Medication

> For steps to follow in *all* procedures, refer to the Universal Steps for All Procedures on the inside back cover. Also refer to the Medication Guidelines: Steps to Follow for All Medications (Regardless of Type or Route).

Equipment

- Medication vials, ampules, and/or prefilled syringe
- Alcohol prep pad (70% alcohol) or chlorhexidine gluconate (CHG)–alcohol product
- Syringe of the appropriate size for medication volume and viscosity
- Needle of the appropriate size for the site and viscosity to be aspirated through the vial access device (VAD)
- VAD, filter needle, or safety needle
- Gauze pad or ampule snapper, if you are using ampules ▼

Top: Syringe with a regular needle.
Bottom: Filter needle.

Vial access device.

Delegation

An RN can delegate administration of some parenteral medications to an LPN/LVN. You usually cannot delegate this task to a UAP. Nurse practice acts governing medication administration vary from state to state, and policies vary further among healthcare agencies. Nevertheless, the RN is always responsible for supervising and evaluating delegated care. You can instruct a UAP in the therapeutic effects expected from the medication.

(continued on next page)

Procedure 23-9 ■ Preparing, Drawing Up, and Mixing Medication (continued)

Preprocedure Assessments

- Check the ampule or vial for intactness, cloudiness, particles, and color.
  A change in color, cloudiness, particles, or cracks indicate the medication is altered or contaminated and should not be used.
- Check the compatibility of the medications to be mixed.
  Some medications are either chemically or physically incompatible and cannot be mixed. Medications are more likely to become incompatible the longer they are mixed together, so administer them promptly after they are mixed. Although physically incompatible medications can frequently be identified by a change in appearance, such as precipitation, no such indication exists for chemically incompatible medications.
- Determine the total volume of medications and whether the total volume is appropriate for the administration site.
  Although the reason for mixing medications is to limit the number of injections a patient receives, the total volume of the injections must not be greater than what is appropriate for the site.

Procedure 23-9A ■ Drawing Up Medication From Ampules

> When performing the procedure, always identify your patient according to agency policy, using two identifiers, and be attentive to standard precautions, hand hygiene, patient safety and privacy, body mechanics, and documentation.

Procedure Steps

1. **Gently flick or tap the top** of the ampule with your index finger to remove medication trapped in the top of the ampule. Alternative method: Shake the ampule by quickly turning and snapping your wrist, like shaking down a mercury thermometer.
   Medication left in the top of the ampule may lead to administering an inadequate dose. All the medication must be in the bottom of the ampule before you open it.

2. **Use an ampule snapper,** if available. Alternatively, wrap a 2 in. × 2 in. gauze pad (or an unopened alcohol wipe) around the neck of the ampule. Snap the top off, breaking it away from you.
   Prevents you from accidentally cutting your fingers or spraying glass fragments toward you. Do not use an opened alcohol wipe to break the ampule, because it is not thick enough to prevent injury. ▼

3. **Attach a filter needle** or filter straw to the syringe. If the syringe has a needle in place, remove both the needle and the cap, and place them on a sterile surface (e.g., a newly unwrapped alcohol pad still in the open wrapper), and attach the filter needle or straw.
   Opening a glass ampule produces a spray of tiny fractured glass particles, which can enter the ampule and contaminate the contents. The filter needle or straw filters the solution drawn up from glass ampules to remove glass particles.

4. **Withdraw the medication** from the ampule with a filter needle by using one of the following techniques. Be careful not to touch the neck of the ampule with the filter straw or needle while withdrawing medication.
   Touching the neck of the ampule with the needle or straw increases the risk of contamination.

   a. *Invert the ampule,* place the filter needle or straw tip in the liquid, and withdraw the prescribed amount of medication. Be careful not to insert the needle through the medication into the air at the top of the inverted ampule.
   This method is particularly useful with small ampules. The medication's surface tension prevents the liquid from leaking from the inverted ampule. However, if you insert the needle too far (into the air pocket above the medication), the medication will run out. ▼

b. *Alternatively, tip the ampule,* place a filter needle or straw in the liquid, and withdraw all medication. Reposition the ampule so that the needle or straw tip remains in the liquid.
This method allows for easier stabilization of the ampule while you withdraw the medication and may help keep you from contaminating the needle on the edge of the vial opening. ▼

5. **Hold the syringe vertically,** and draw 0.2 mL of air into the syringe (also see Clinical Insight 23-4). Draw up and measure the exact medication dose, plus 0.2 mL of air (the syringe plunger should be at 0.2 mL more than the prescribed dose).

6. **Remove the filter needle** or straw, and reattach the "saved" needle for administering the injection.

7. **Eject the 0.2 mL of air, and read** the dose. After all of the air is removed, if you need to eject some medication to make the dose correct, tip the syringe until it is horizontal to push out the medication.
   - Pulling air into the syringe allows for an exact dose when the medication is injected; the air will clear the needle (after the medication) so that the patient receives all the medication that is in the syringe.
   The syringe must be vertical to eject air. However, if you eject the medication while holding the syringe vertically, the drug will run down the needle and then track through the patient's tissue during the injection.

For a Filter Needle
Use a filter needle only to withdraw, not to measure, medication. Do not eject medication through it.
Pushing the medication out through the filter needle could cause the filter to break and release the glass fragments.

Key Point: *This is not the old "air lock" technique; you will eject the air before administering the medication to the patient.*

For Medications That Are Irritating to Tissues (e.g., parenteral iron)
You can leave the 0.2 mL of air in the syringe for injection. But be sure to account for the air when you read the dose markings on the syringe.

8. **Dispose of the top and bottom** of the ampule and the filter needle in a sharps container.
Disposal into a puncture-proof container prevents accidental needlestick injury.

Procedure 23-9B ■ Drawing Up Medication From Vials

➤ When performing the procedure, always identify your patient according to agency policy, using two identifiers, and be attentive to standard precautions, hand hygiene, patient safety and privacy, body mechanics, and documentation.

➤ This procedure assumes you are using a vial access device (VAD), since that is preferred. Use a needle only when a filter needle is required.

1. **Mix the solution in the vial,** if necessary, by gently rolling the vial between your hands.
Aqueous suspensions will settle to the bottom of the vial, so they need to be mixed. Rolling the vial between your hands will mix the medication without forming air bubbles. Shaking the vial traps air in the medication.

2. **Place the vial on a flat** work surface and thoroughly scrub the rubber top of the vial with an alcohol prep pad or CHG–alcohol product.
The alcohol prep pad removes dust, grease, and microorganisms.

3. **If a needle is attached** to the syringe, remove it and place it on a sterile surface (e.g., sterile, opened alcohol pad). Replace with a VAD.
   a. Uncap the VAD without touching the tip or shaft and attach the device to the syringe.
   VADs can be used only with single-use vials, unless the vial is designed for use with access pins, such as a Life-Shield vial.

4. **Place the VAD cap** on a clean surface, or hold the cap open-side out between two fingers of your nondominant hand.
This method prevents contamination of the cap and the needle during recapping.

5. **Draw air into the syringe** equal to the amount of medication to be withdrawn from the vial.
Injection of air into the vial makes withdrawing the medication easier. For small unit-dose vials, you may not have to instill air before withdrawing the medication, but you will need to maintain backward pressure on the plunger until the needle is completely withdrawn. If you release the plunger, the negative pressure in the vial will pull the medication back into the vial.

6. **Insert the VAD** into the vial without coring and while maintaining sterile technique. Use a filter needle *only* if it is required for the type of medication. If required, the filter needle becomes the VAD.
   a. Place the tip of the VAD in the middle of the rubber top of the

(continued on next page)

420   UNIT 3   Essential Nursing Interventions

Procedure 23-9 ■ Preparing, Drawing Up, and Mixing Medication (continued)

vial, with the bevel up at a 45° to 60° angle. ▼

b. While pushing the VAD into the rubber top, gradually bring the syringe (and VAD) upright to a 90° angle.
This method helps prevent coring, which occurs when a small piece of the rubber top is trapped inside the VAD during insertion. Coring is more likely to occur with large-gauge needles and VADs. ▼

7. With the tip of the VAD above the fluid line, inject the air in the syringe into the air in the vial.
The air creates positive pressure in the vial, making the medication easier to withdraw. Injecting the air into the medication will create air bubbles, which interfere with dosage measurement. ▼

"Air to air."

8. Invert the vial, keep the VAD vertical in the medication, and slowly withdraw the medication. Keep the tip of the VAD in the medication.
The vial needs to be inverted so that all the medication can be withdrawn. Keeping the VAD in the medication and slowly drawing the medication will help prevent you from drawing excess air into the syringe. ▼

9. Keeping the VAD in the vial, remove any air from the syringe by injecting it into the air in the vial:
When the VAD is connecting the vial and syringe, a sterile unit is formed. The volume of air in the hub of the syringe and inside the needle/VAD, dead space, will be drawn back into the syringe. Air bubbles alter the dose of medication being administered, so they must be expelled. You can use a pen to tap the syringe if extra force is needed. Injecting air to air prevents bubbles in the medication. ▼

A, **Incorrect**—If syringe is not vertical, air is trapped near the hub.

CHAPTER 23 Administering Medications 421

B, **Incorrect**—If tip is down, air is trapped at the plunger.

C, **Correct**—Syringe is vertical.

a. Carefully stabilize the vial and syringe, and firmly tap the syringe below the air bubbles. When air bubbles are at the hub of the syringe, make sure the syringe is vertical (straight up and down), and push the air back into the air in the vial.
Remember that air rises, so if the syringe is tilted, air will be trapped in it.

b. If additional medication is necessary to obtain the correct dose, withdraw it before removing the VAD from the inverted vial.
When working with only one vial, you can withdraw and eject medication into the vial as many times as needed to expel bubbles from the syringe and obtain the correct dose.

10. **When the dose is correct,** withdraw the VAD from the vial at a 90° angle.
A vertical angle prevents accidental contamination or bending of the needle.

11. **Hold the syringe upright** at eye level to recheck the medication dose.
Reading the syringe at an angle can result in inaccurate measurement.

12. **Recap the VAD** using a recapping device or the one-handed method. See Procedure 23-10.
Although recapping a sterile needle does not present a threat of bloodborne pathogen exposure, using a mechanical recapping device or the one-handed method helps develop safe habits.

13. **Change the VAD** before you inject the medication:
    a. Before changing the VAD or filter needle, draw back on the syringe plunger to remove all medication from dead space in the old needle (or VAD).
    b. Remove the old needle (or VAD) and reattach a sterile needle for injection (see Clinical Insight 23-4).
    You cannot eject medication through a filter needle or inject a patient with a VAD.
    c. Hold the syringe vertically and expel the air. If it is necessary to expel some medication, hold the syringe horizontally to do so.
    The difficulty with changing the needles is that you may slightly alter the dose. If you are planning to change the needles, draw slightly more than the prescribed dose unless you are combining in one syringe. After changing the needle, remeasure the dose. Holding the syringe horizontally prevents medication from running down the needle and tracking into the patient's skin.

14. **Dispose of the vial, VAD,** or any recapped needles in a sharps container.
This prevents sharps injury to healthcare workers or others in the vicinity. Proper disposal also reduces the risk of transmitting infectious organisms.

Procedure 23-9C ■ Mixing Medication From Two Vials

➤ First review the **Medication Guidelines: Steps to Follow for All Medications (Regardless of Type or Route),** Procedure 23-9B (Drawing Up Medication From Vials), and Procedure 23-10A (Recapping Contaminated Needles).

➤ Always use a VAD instead of a needle whenever possible. If you must use a needle, use a safety needle.

➤ When performing the procedure, always identify your patient according to agency policy, using two identifiers, and be attentive to standard precautions, hand hygiene, patient safety and privacy, body mechanics, and documentation.

(continued on next page)

UNIT 3 Essential Nursing Interventions

Procedure 23-9 ■ Preparing, Drawing Up, and Mixing Medication (continued)

Procedure Steps

1. **Scrub the tops of both vials** with an alcohol pad or CHG–alcohol product.

   NOTE: Some experts omit this step for single-dose vials.
   Not all pharmaceutical companies ensure the sterility of the rubber top on vials, even when they are first opened. However, be aware that once your fingers touch the alcohol pad, it is no longer sterile; therefore, you are not sterilizing, but rather are cleaning the vial top.

2. **Draw air into the syringe** in the same amount as the total medication doses for both vials (e.g., if the prescription is for 0.5 mL for vial A and 1 mL for vial B, then draw up 1.5 mL of air). ▼

3. **Inject air into the vials.**
   a. Maintaining sterility, insert the vial access device or safety needle into the vial in the middle of the rubber top of the vial with the bevel up at a 45° to 60° angle. While pushing the VAD (or needle) into the rubber top, gradually bring the needle upright to a 90° angle. ▼

   Vial A
   This method helps prevent coring of the rubber top.

   b. Keeping the tip of the VAD (or safety needle) above the medication, inject an amount of air equal to the volume of drug to be withdrawn from the first vial (e.g., 0.5 mL for vial A in Step 2); then inject the rest of the air into the second vial (1.0 mL for vial B). Take care to prevent coring. ▼

   Vial B
   Medication is easier to withdraw from a vial with positive pressure. For small unit-dose vials, it may be possible to withdraw the medication without instilling air, but you will need to maintain a slight backward pressure on the plunger until the needle is completely withdrawn. If you release the plunger, the negative pressure in the vial will pull the medication back in. Therefore, it is always safer to instill air.

Using One Multidose Vial and One Single-Dose Vial

You must withdraw medication from the multidose vial before withdrawing from the single-dose vial. However, the needle tip should stay above the medication at all times in Steps 2 and 3.
This is an extra precaution to prevent contamination of the multidose vial with medication from the single-dose vial.

When Mixing Two Types of Insulin

If you are mixing two types of insulin at Step 3, put air into the regular insulin last (see Clinical Insight 23-5 for mixing two types of insulin).

4. **Without removing the VAD** (or needle) from the second vial (B), invert it and withdraw the prescribed amount of medication. Expel any air bubbles and measure the dose. Remove the VAD from the vial, then pull back on the plunger enough to pull all medication out of the VAD into the syringe (see Clinical Insight 23-4). Read the dose at eye level. Tip the syringe horizontally if you need to eject any medication.
   Allows you to withdraw all the medication. Keeping the needle in the medication and withdrawing the medication slowly will help prevent drawing excess air into the syringe and prevent bubbles. ▼

   Vial B (Step 4)

5. **Insert the VAD (or needle)** into the first vial (A), invert, and withdraw the exact prescribed amount of medication, holding the syringe vertical.
   - When you are finished, the plunger should be at the line for the total/combined dose for vials A and B. (Using the example in Step 2, you would have 1.5 mL of the mixed medications in the syringe.)
   - Be very careful not to withdraw excess medication; keep your index finger or thumb on the flange of the syringe to prevent medication from being forced back by pressure. If this occurs, you must discard the medication in the syringe and start over.

   ✚ *Because the medications are mixed, withdrawing extra from the second vial makes the entire mixture incorrect. If you draw up too much of the second drug or if your final measurement of the total for both drugs is incorrect, you cannot eject medication, because you cannot know how much of that is medication A and how much of it is medication B you are ejecting. You must discard the syringe and medication and begin again.*

   You do not need to change the needle before Step 5 because even if one vial is a multidose vial, you would have withdrawn the medication from it first (in Step 4). It will not matter if you track medication into the single-dose vial. ▼

   Vial A (Step 5)

6. **Recap the VAD (or needle)** using a needle-capping device or the one-handed scoop method (see Procedure 23-10: Recapping Needles Using a One-Handed Technique).

   Although recapping a sterile needle does not present a threat of bloodborne pathogen exposure, using a mechanical recapping device or the one-handed method helps develop safe habits. As a rule, we do not recommend using the one-handed scoop for sterile needles; however, this needle will be discarded anyway, so if it is accidentally contaminated with a one-handed scoop, it will not be a major error.

7. **Remove the VAD** (or needle) and attach a new sterile needle on the syringe for the injection.

   Obviously, you must replace a VAD with a needle for injection. In addition, if you used a needle instead of a VAD, by the time you are finished withdrawing both medications you will have put it through a rubber vial top at least three times. This dulls the needle. A sharp needle causes less trauma to the patient on injection. A new needle also prevents tracking of the medication through the skin and subcutaneous tissues.

8. **Hold the needle vertically** to expel all air and recheck the dosage (the total for both medications).
   Allows for more accurate accounting of the dose.

9. **If you have used a VAD or filter** needle, refer to Clinical Insight 23-4.

Procedure 23-9D ■ Mixing Medications From One Ampule and One Vial

➤ First review the **Medication Guidelines: Steps to Follow for All Medications (Regardless of Type or Route),** Procedure 23-9A (Drawing up Medications from Ampules), Procedure 23-9B (Drawing Up Medication From Vials), and Procedure 23-10A (Recapping Contaminated Needles).

➤ When performing the procedure, always identify your patient according to agency policy, using two identifiers, and be attentive to standard precautions, hand hygiene, patient safety and privacy, body mechanics, and documentation.

Procedure Steps

1. **Begin with the vial.** Scrub the stopper of the vial using an alcohol wipe or CHG–alcohol combination product.
   Protects against microbial contamination.

2. **Attach a VAD** and draw **the same volume of air** into the syringe as the dose prescribed for the medication in the vial.

3. **Keeping the tip of the VAD** (or safety needle) above the medication, inject the amount of air equal to the volume of drug to be withdrawn from the vial. The needle should be injecting air to air within the vial.
   Draw from the vial first because you do not need to add air to ampules before drawing up the medication. In addition, if it is a multidose vial, you would contaminate it with the medicine if you withdrew from the ampule first.

   Injecting air into the vial creates a positive pressure that makes withdrawing the medication easier. For small unit-dose vials, it may be possible to withdraw the medication without instilling air, but you will need to maintain a slight backward pressure on the plunger until the needle is completely withdrawn. If you release the plunger, the negative pressure in the vial will pull the medication back into the vial. Therefore, it is always safer to instill air.

   (continued on next page)

Procedure 23-9 ■ Preparing, Drawing Up, and Mixing Medication (continued)

4. **Invert the vial.** Withdraw the prescribed volume (dosage) of medication, keeping the VAD tip in the fluid. See Procedure 23-9B.

5. **Expel any air bubbles** and measure the dose at eye level. Recheck the dosage, and withdraw more or eject the drug as needed.
   This prevents air from entering into the needle or VAD.

6. **After safely recapping** the VAD, remove it from the syringe. You may place it on an opened, sterile alcohol pad if you need your hands to open the filter needle packaging.
   Keeps the needle sterile, if you are using one; you will reuse it. **Key Point:** *You would not reuse a VAD from this step on.*

7. **Attach a filter needle** or filter straw to the syringe.
   The use of a 5-micrometer (μm) filter minimizes the possibility of withdrawing small glass fragments.

8. **Flick or tap the top** of the ampule (or snap your wrist) to remove medication from the neck of the ampule.
   Flicking the neck of the ampule will help the fluid to drain down into the main part of the ampule, thus reducing waste.

9. **Open the ampule** by wrapping the neck with a folded gauze pad or an unopened alcohol wipe or use an ampule snapper. Snap open away from you.
   Snapping outward prevents you from cutting your fingers or spraying glass fragments toward your face. Do not use an opened alcohol wipe to break the ampule, because it is not thick enough to prevent injury.

10. **Withdraw the exact prescribed** amount of medication from the ampule into the syringe (see Procedure 23-9A). **Key Point:** *Be very careful in drawing up the second medication; if the total amount of the two medications is incorrect, you must discard the syringe contents and start over.*

11. **Draw 0.2 mL of air into the syringe.**
    The extra bit of air clears the filter needle (see Clinical Insight 23-4).

12. **Confirm the dose is correct** by holding the syringe vertically and checking the dose at eye level.
    Ensures the total volume in the syringe equals the prescribed amount of both medications plus 0.2 mL of air from the needle.

13. **Recap the filter needle** using a needle capping device or the one-handed technique recommended in Procedure 23-10B.
    Although recapping a sterile needle does not present a threat of bloodborne pathogen exposure, using a mechanical recapping device or the one-handed method helps develop safe habits. Nevertheless, some scoop techniques pose a significant risk of contaminating the needle, so you must watch carefully that you maintain sterile technique.

14. **Remove the filter needle** or straw and discard it in a sharps container. Replace with a new sterile safety needle for administering the medication to the patient.
    This needle-recapping method prevents accidental needlestick injury. You cannot measure the dose accurately with a filter needle. You should not eject medication through the filter needle because of risk of breaking the filter. See Clinical Insight 23-4.

15. **After placing the administration** needle on the syringe, eject the 0.2 mL of air and check for the correct dose. If there is excess medication in the syringe, you must discard it and start over.

16. **Discard used needles and ampules** in a puncture-proof sharps container.

Procedure 23-9E ■ Using a Prefilled Cartridge and Single-Dose Vial—For Intravenous Administration

▶ Note: It is best not to use this technique with multidose vials because there is a risk of contaminating the multidose vial with the cartridge medication.

▶ First review the **Medication Guidelines: Steps to Follow for All Medications (Regardless of Type or Route).** Review Procedures 23-9 and 23-10, as needed.

▶ When performing the procedure, always identify your patient according to agency policy, using two identifiers, and be attentive to standard precautions, hand hygiene, patient safety and privacy, body mechanics, and documentation.

Procedure Steps

1. **Scrub the rubber stopper** of the vial thoroughly with an alcohol prep pad or CHG–alcohol product.

2. **Assemble the prefilled cartridge** and holder (see Clinical Insight 23-2).

3. **Remove the needle cap** from the prefilled cartridge, expel the air, and measure the correct dose of medication.
   You must confirm that the dose of the first medication is correct before you mix it with the second medication.

4. **Holding the cartridge with** the needle up, draw in an amount of air equal to the volume of medication you need from the vial.

5. **While continuing to hold** the syringe with needle straight up (vertically), invert the vial and insert the

needle into it until the tip of the needle shows in the air above the medication. Then inject the air into the vial. Maintain counterpressure on the plunger so that air and/or medication do not flow back into the syringe.

Injecting air into the vial makes the medication easier to withdraw. ▼

6. **While maintaining counterpressure** on the plunger, pull the needle down into the fluid and allow the pressure in the vial to push the medication into the syringe. Withdraw the prescribed amount of vial medication, being careful not to withdraw any excess.

7. **The pressure will generally push** a little less than you need, so carefully withdraw the amount you need for a correct dose—again, do not withdraw any excess.
Withdrawing excess medication will result in an altered mixed dose, so you would need to discard the syringe and start over.

8. **Recap the needle** (use a one-handed method) and if possible remove the needle from the prefilled syringe and replace it with a sterile injection cannula for IV administration.

For an intramuscular (IM) injection, if the prefilled cartridge does not have a safety needle, you would need to transfer the medication to a new syringe with a sterile safety needle for injection.

VADs and injection cannulas prevent needlestick injury. Unless there is a needle safety device for the prefilled syringe, it is not recommended for IM injections.

? What if...

- **I note particulate matter in the ampule or vial?**

  Discard the medication and obtain a new one.

Documentation
Document on the MAR.

Practice Resources
Bentley et al. (2015); CDC (2019).

Thinking About the Procedure

➤ Go to the videos **Drawing Up Medication From Ampules, Drawing Up Medication From Vials, Mixing Medication From Two Vials,** and **Mixing Medications From One Ampule and One Vial,** along with questions and suggested responses, available on the **Davis's *Nursing Skills Videos*** Web site at www.fadavis.com.

Procedure 23-10 ■ Recapping Needles Using a One-Handed Technique

➤ For steps to follow in *all* procedures, refer to the Universal Steps for All Procedures on the inside back cover. Also refer to **Medication Guidelines: Steps to Follow for All Medications (Regardless of Type or Route).**

Equipment
- Mechanical recapping device, if available
- Needle cover
- Safety syringe, if available
- Other supplies depending on the method used. ▼

Needle recapping device.

Safety syringe. A, Before injection. B, Cover slides up after injection.

Safety syringe. A, Before injection. B, Needle retracted after injection.

Delegation
Delegation is not usually an issue because recapping needles is done in conjunction with administering parenteral medications, which you will usually not delegate. If you do delegate administration of parenteral medications to an LPN/LVN, you must supervise and evaluate recapping to ensure that the nurse uses proper technique.

Preparation
- **Assess the need to recap the needle.**
  The Occupational Safety and Health Administration (OSHA) position is that recapping used/contaminated needles is inappropriate.
  ✚ *As a rule, place a contaminated syringe and needle directly into a puncture-proof sharps container, without capping, bending, or breaking the needle.*
- **Identify whether the needle is sterile or dirty.**
  Although a one-handed technique is used to recap both sterile and dirty needles, different considerations exist.

  Sterile needle—When you use the one-handed method for recapping a sterile needle, it is easy to contaminate the needle without realizing it. You should modify the technique to help prevent that—the main consideration is to "protect" the needle.

  Contaminated needle—The danger in recapping a dirty needle is that you will stick yourself with it, exposing yourself to pathogens. The main consideration is to protect yourself.

- **Determine the availability of mechanical recapping device or safety syringe.**
  Key Point: Always use a mechanical recapping device or safety syringe, if one is available.

Procedure 23-10A ■ Recapping Contaminated Needles

➤ When performing the procedure, always identify your patient according to agency policy, using two identifiers, and be attentive to standard precautions, hand hygiene, patient safety and privacy, body mechanics, and documentation.

➤ The following procedures should be used only in limited and specific situations (e.g., sharps or other appropriate container is not available).

Procedure Steps

1. **If you are using a safety needle,** engage the safety mechanism to cover the needle. (See Equipment.)
   OSHA regulations require the use of safety syringes to prevent needlestick injuries. You must engage the safety mechanism before placing the needle and syringe into the sharps container.

2. **Alternatively, place the needle** cap in mechanical recapping device, if one is available. (See Equipment.)

3. **If a mechanical recapping device** is not available, use the one-handed scoop method to recap the needle.
   a. Place the needle cover on a flat surface.
   Keeps the needle cover from rolling during the needle capping procedure. ▼

   b. Then, holding the syringe in your dominant hand, scoop the needle cap onto the needle. Tip the syringe vertically to slip the cover over the needle. Do not hold on to the needle cap with your non-dominant hand while scooping.
   A mechanical recapping device protects against accidental needlestick injury. If it is unavailable, the one-handed method of recapping will prevent accidental injuries when your own or the patient's safety is a concern. ▼

   c. Secure the needle cap by grasping it near the hub.
   Prevents an accidental stick if the needle goes through the needle cap. Needles are sharp enough to go through the needle cap if inserted at an angle. ▼

Procedure 23-10B ■ Recapping Sterile Needles

➤ When performing the procedure, always identify your patient according to agency policy, using two identifiers, and be attentive to standard precautions, hand hygiene, patient safety and privacy, body mechanics, and documentation.

Use one of the following techniques to ensure that you do not contaminate a sterile needle. If you contaminate the needle, microorganisms will be introduced with the injection.

Procedure Steps

1. **Place the needle cap** in a mechanical recapping device, if one is available.
   The device is specially developed to provide safe recapping.

2. **Alternative method: Medication cup.** Place the cap into a small liquid medication cup with the open end facing up. You can then insert the sterile needle into the cap, keeping your free hand well away from the cup.
   This step performs the same function as a mechanical recapping device. The needle and cover need to be taller than the cup you are using so that the open end of the cap protrudes above the cup. ➤

(continued on next page)

Procedure 23-10 ■ Recapping Needles Using a One-Handed Technique (continued)

3. **Alternative method: Scoop technique.** Place the cap on a clean surface so that the end of the needle cap protrudes over the edge of the counter or shelf, and scoop with the needle; keep your free hand well away from the needle and cap as you are recapping.

   This method prevents you from inadvertently hitting an unsterile surface with the needle. ▼

4. **Alternative method: Tubular container.** If the syringe is packaged in a hard plastic tubular container, stand the container on its large end; invert the needle cap; and place it in the top of the hard container. Insert the needle downward into the cap. ▼

5. **Alternative method: Alcohol wipe.** Place the needle cap on a sterile surface, such as on an open alcohol prep pad, and use the one-handed scoop technique. Be very careful not to touch anything with the needle other than the inside of the needle cap.

   The alcohol prep pad provides a sterile barrier. Because you must bring the needle parallel to the flat surface, and because the alcohol pad is so small, it is easy to contaminate the needle using this method. ▼

Documentation

No documentation needed for recapping needles.

Practice Resources

National Institute for Occupational Safety and Health (2018); U.S. Food and Drug Administration (2018).

Procedure 23-11 ■ Administering Intradermal Medication

▶ For steps to follow in *all* procedures, refer to the Universal Steps for All Procedures on the inside back cover. Also refer to Medication Guidelines: Steps to Follow for All Medications (Regardless of Type or Route).

Equipment
- Alcohol prep pad or CHG–alcohol product
- 2 in. × 2 in. gauze pad
- Pen (ink or felt)
- 1-mL syringe (tuberculin) with intradermal needle (25- to 28-gauge, ¼ to ⅝ inch with short bevel) ▼

Regular bevel | Intermediate bevel | Short bevel

Delegation

As an RN, you can usually delegate administration of parenteral medications to an LPN/LVN. You usually cannot delegate this task to a UAP.

Preprocedure Assessments

- Assess for allergies, previous reaction to skin testing, and the skin for signs of irritation (e.g., bruising, swelling, tenderness).

  Some skin tests, such as the tuberculin test, should not be repeated after positive test results. Do not give intradermal skin tests if skin abnormalities are present. Also avoid giving them in areas where reading the results may be difficult, such as areas of heavy hair growth.

Preparation

- Have appropriate antidotes (usually epinephrine hydrochloride, a bronchodilator, and an antihistamine) readily available before the start of the procedure.

  This is an important consideration because many intradermal injections are used for allergy testing.

- Know the location of resuscitation equipment (artificial airway, Ambu bag, and code cart).

  Allergic reactions can be fatal.

> When performing the procedure, always identify your patient according to agency policy, using two identifiers, and be attentive to standard precautions, hand hygiene, patient safety and privacy, body mechanics, and documentation.

Procedure Steps

1. **Draw up the medication** from the vial (see Procedure 26-9B). The usual dose is 0.01 to 0.1 mL.
   Intradermal sites can accommodate only small volumes of medication.

2. **Select the site for injection.** Usual sites are the ventral surface of the forearm and upper back. The upper chest may also be used. If you need to review site locations, see Figure 23-23.
   Use areas where subcutaneous fat is less likely to interfere with administration and absorption. The forearm is the standard initial starting point because it has the least amount of subcutaneous tissue. The forearm and upper back usually have little hair, permitting easier visualization to interpret results accurately.

3. **Assist the patient to a** comfortable position. If you are using the forearm, instruct the patient to extend and supinate their arm on a flat surface. If you are using the upper back, ask the patient to lie prone or lean forward over a table or the back of a chair.
   This method stabilizes the injection site. The procedure will be more comfortable if the patient is able to relax their muscles. Tension, in general, increases pain perception.

4. **Don procedure gloves.**
   Procedure gloves are recommended by the CDC to prevent accidental exposure to bloodborne pathogens.

   ✚ Remember, gloves cannot prevent needlestick injuries.

5. **Scrub the injection site** with an alcohol prep pad or CHG–alcohol product pad. For an alcohol product, circle from the center of the site outward. For CHG products, use a back-and-forth motion. Allow the site to dry before administering the injection.
   Cleansing to remove microorganisms follows the principle of "clean to dirty." Alcohol can interfere with the test results if a small amount is introduced during the injection. If the alcohol has not evaporated, it may cause the skin to sting during the injection.

6. **Grasp the syringe between** the thumb and index finger of your dominant hand, and uncap the needle.
   Enables you to administer the solution at the correct angle.

7. **Hold the patient's skin taut** with your nondominant hand by using one of the following methods:
   a. If using the forearm, you may be able to place your hand under the patient's arm and pull the skin taut with your thumb and fingers.
   b. Stretch the patient's skin between your thumb and index finger.
   c. Pull the patient's skin toward the wrist or down with one finger.
      A downward motion while stretching the skin eases needle insertion. Holding the skin taut can be difficult because of the low angle of administration.

8. **Continuing to hold the patient's skin** taut with your nondominant hand, hold the syringe in your dominant hand with the needle bevel up and parallel to the patient's skin at a 5° to 15° angle. Slowly insert the needle. The CDC recommends the needle bevel face upward.
   The low angle of insertion is necessary to place the needle tip in the intradermal layer instead of the subcutaneous tissue. Having the bevel up likely decreases the chance of injecting the medication deeper into the subcutaneous tissue. Patients receiving intradermal injections report bevel up more comfortable. ▼

   Epidermis
   Dermis
   Subcutaneous tissue

9. **Advance the needle** approximately 3 mm (⅛ in.) so that the entire bevel is covered. The bevel should be visible just under the skin.
   If the entire bevel is not inserted, the solution will leak out of the tissue. If you can see the bevel under the surface of the skin, you can be sure that the bevel is not in the subcutaneous tissue.

10. **Do not aspirate.** Hold the syringe stable with your nondominant hand and release the tightened skin.

11. **Slowly inject the solution.** You should feel firm resistance. A pale wheal, about 6 to 10 mm (¼ in.) in diameter, will appear over the needle bevel.
    The dermis does not have room to absorb the solution, so a wheal forms, stretching the skin. Slow administration gives you time to terminate the injection should a systemic reaction occur. If a bleb (wheal) forms, you have administered the drug properly. The size of the bleb depends on the amount of medication you injected. ▼

(continued on next page)

Procedure 23-11 ■ Administering Intradermal Medication (continued)

12. **Remove the needle** from the skin, engage the safety device, and dispose of the needle in a biohazard, puncture-proof container. If there is no safety device, place the uncapped syringe and needle directly in a biohazard, puncture-proof container.
   Prevents needlestick injuries.

13. **Gently blot any blood** with a dry gauze pad. Do not rub the skin or cover it with an adhesive bandage.
   Rubbing may cause the drug to leak out and alter absorption. An adhesive bandage can cause irritation and interfere with the skin test.

14. **With a pen, draw a 1-inch circle** around the bleb/wheal.
   Marking the site helps you to identify any change in the size of the wheal at a later time.

? What if . . .

- **My patient has a history of a skin reaction to PPD testing?**
  Obtain details about the type and severity of the reaction. If the previous reaction involved ulceration at the site, further Mantoux testing is contraindicated. Report this to the prescriber.

- **My patient is pregnant, is receiving chemotherapy, or has severe eczema?**
  Defer tuberculosis skin testing and inform the prescriber.

- **My patient received a live vaccine at the time of tuberculosis skin testing?**
  Tuberculosis skin testing should be deferred for 1 month after live viral vaccines or other major viral infection.

- **My patient has topical anesthetic cream on the skin?**
  Use a site where the topical anesthetic cream was not applied or reschedule tuberculosis skin testing for another date.

Evaluation

- Reassess the patient 5 and 15 minutes after administration for allergic reactions that may subsequently occur.
- Read the site within 48 to 72 hours of injection, depending on the test.
- Observe that a wheal (about 6 to 8 mm in diameter) forms at the site and that it gradually disappears.
- Observe for minimal bruising that may develop at the site of injection.

Patient Teaching

- Explain when the patient needs to have the intradermal injection read to determine whether the result is positive or negative.
- Explain that mild itching, swelling, or irritation may occur at the injection site and is normal.
  If the patient has antigens to the injected solution, a histamine response occurs, causing itching, swelling, or irritation. This response generally subsides within a week.
- Discuss the significance of a positive or negative skin test result. Explain that some signs of irritation may occur that do not mean a positive test result.
- Instruct the patient not to scratch, apply lotions or creams, cover the site with a bandage, or scrub the site.
  This might cause irritation and interfere with the test, which may produce false-positive results.

Documentation

- See the information in **Medication Guidelines: Steps to Follow for All Medication (Regardless of Type or Route).**
- Some medications require documentation of lot numbers (check agency policy).
- Document when the test is to be read.

Thinking About the Procedure

Go to the video **Administering Intradermal Medication,** along with questions and suggested responses, available on the **Davis's *Nursing Skills Videos*** Web site at www.fadavis.com.

Practice Resources

Becton Dickinson (2017); Centers for Disease Control and Prevention (2022); Shrestha (2018).

Procedure 23-12 ■ Administering Subcutaneous Medication

➤ For steps to follow in *all* procedures, refer to the Universal Steps for All Procedures on the inside back cover. Also refer to Medication Guidelines: Steps to Follow for All Medications (Regardless of Type or Route).

Equipment
- Syringe and needle appropriate for volume and site
- Alcohol prep pad or CHG–alcohol product
- Gauze pad (optional)

Delegation
As an RN, you can usually delegate administration of parenteral medications to an LPN/LVN. You usually cannot delegate this task to a UAP.

Preprocedure Assessments
- Check the selected site for inflammation, bruising, lumps, or other abnormalities that may contraindicate use of the site.
- Check the area for previous injection sites.
  Alternating among the arms, thighs, abdomen, and back changes the absorption rate of the medication. Absorption is fastest from the abdomen, then the arms, and then the thighs and back. Rotate sites within the same extremity or location, approximately 1 inch from the previous injection. Rotating the site helps prevent fat deposits and skin lumps.
- Do focused assessments for the specific medication being administered.

  Insulin—Check capillary blood sugar level, and determine when the patient will be having the next meal; check for signs of hypoglycemia or hyperglycemia.
  Insulin must be balanced with food intake to prevent the patient from developing hypoglycemia or hyperglycemia. Different insulins have specific rates of absorption, peak action, and duration. Some insulins, such as Humalog and regular insulin, are rapid acting. Before you administer rapid-acting insulin, the capillary blood sugar must be within the normal range or higher, and the patient must be ready to eat. With Humalog, the food tray should be in front of the patient before you administer the insulin.

  Heparin—Check activated partial thromboplastin time (aPTT) and for signs of overt bleeding (e.g., bleeding from gums, IV injection sites) and covert bleeding (e.g., blood in urine and stool).
  Heparin is an anticoagulant, so the major side effect is bleeding.

  NOTE: The aPTT will not be monitored as frequently with the low-molecular-weight heparins (LMWHs), because bleeding is less likely to occur.

➤ When performing the procedure, always identify your patient according to agency policy, using two identifiers, and be attentive to standard precautions, hand hygiene, patient safety and privacy, body mechanics, and documentation.

Procedure Steps

1. **Select an appropriate syringe** and needle.
   a. For insulin administration, you must use an insulin syringe—typically 0.3, 0.5, or 1.0 mL. Most insulin needles are 28 to 31 gauge. Needle length is often ³⁄₁₆ to 1 inch. For more information about giving insulin, see Clinical Insight 23-5.

      ✚ Although both insulin and tuberculin (TB) syringes come in a 1-mL size, they are not interchangeable. Insulin syringes are calibrated in units; they have a permanent (nonremovable) needle and a very small amount of dead space.

   b. For other medications, for volumes less than 1 mL, use a tuberculin (TB) syringe with a 25- to 27-gauge, ³⁄₈- to ⁵⁄₈-inch needle.
      Because of the small increments on the TB syringe, small doses can be measured more accurately. ➤

   Top: Insulin syringe. *Bottom:* TB syringe.

   c. For administering a volume of 1 mL, you may use a 3-mL syringe with a 25- to 27-gauge, ³⁄₈- to ⁵⁄₈-inch needle.

      ✚ Subcutaneous injections are typically 1 mL or less.

      Although you can measure 1 mL with a TB syringe, it will be difficult to handle the syringe because the plunger will be pulled back as far as it can go. It is easy to pull it inadvertently out of the end of the syringe. Some medications are supplied in prefilled syringes. Examples are enoxaparin sodium (Lovenox) and the other LMWHs.

2. **Draw up the medication.** See Procedure 23-9.

3. **Select an injection site** with adequate subcutaneous tissue. If you need to review site locations, see Figure 23-25.
   Helps you avoid accidentally injecting into the muscle.

   a. The usual sites are the outer aspect of the upper arms, abdomen (at least 2 inches away from the umbilicus), anterior aspects of the thighs, and high on the buttocks near waist level.
      These areas usually have good circulation and are easily accessible. The buttocks are a more convenient site if the injection is administered by someone else (i.e., when it is not self-administered).

   b. The anterolateral and posterolateral abdomen ("love handles") sites are the only subcutaneous site used for administering heparin or LMWHs. For more information

(continued on next page)

Procedure 23-12 ■ Administering Subcutaneous Medication (continued)

about giving heparin, see Clinical Insight 23-6.
The tissue 2 inches away from the umbilicus poses less risk of bleeding when an anticoagulant is administered.

4. **Position the patient** so that the injection site is accessible and the patient is able to relax the appropriate area. Check the site for inflammation, bruising, lumps, or other abnormalities.
Avoid areas with skin abnormalities, which may alter the absorption rates or increase patient discomfort during the injection.

5. **Don procedure gloves.**
To prevent exposure to bloodborne pathogens. You may prefer to don gloves before Step 4.

6. **Scrub the injection site** with an alcohol prep pad or CHG–alcohol product. Allow the site to dry before administering the injection. For alcohol, circle from the site outward; for CHG, use a back-and-forth motion. Do not go back over already-scrubbed areas.

7. **Remove the needle cap.**
The needle cap is more difficult to remove when using a one-handed technique.

8. **With your nondominant hand,** pinch the tissue at the injection site, and determine the angle at which to inject the needle. Insert the needle using a 45° to 90° angle, depending on the amount of adipose tissue (the less adipose tissue, the lower the angle). If the adipose tissue pinches 2 inches or more, use a longer needle and spread the skin taut instead of pinching.
Grasping and lifting the tissue prevent you from accidentally injecting into the muscle. The subcutaneous injection must be given in the fatty tissue and not into an intradermal layer. Traditionally, injections had been given using a 45° angle to ensure medication was deposited into the subcutaneous layer. ▼

9. **Holding the syringe between** the thumb and index finger of your dominant hand like a pencil or dart, insert the needle at the appropriate angle into the skinfold.
Quickly inserting the needle through the skin minimizes discomfort.

10. **Using the thumb or index finger** of your dominant hand, press the plunger slowly to inject the medication while stabilizing the syringe with your other hand. Alternatively, after inserting the needle, you can continue to hold the barrel with your dominant hand and use your nondominant hand to depress the plunger.
Slow administration allows the medication to disperse and decreases discomfort. Subcutaneous injections do not need to be aspirated beforehand because accidental entry into a blood vessel is rare. Stabilize the syringe to avoid discomfort and tissue damage from the needle.

11. **Remove the needle** smoothly along the line of insertion.
Prevents pulling against the skin and tissue and thus minimizes discomfort.

12. **Gently blot the site with gauze** if needed. Do not massage the site unless directed to do so by prescription or policy.
Occasionally there will be blood at the site after the needle is removed. You might have nicked a surface blood vessel when you injected, and blood is following the needle track out to the surface. Massaging or rubbing the site will alter the rate of absorption of the medication.

13. **Engage the needle safety device,** and dispose of the needle in a biohazard container. If there is no safety device, place the uncapped syringe and needle directly into a biohazard, puncture-proof container.
A sharps container prevents needlestick injuries.

Evaluation

- Observe for minimal bruising that may develop at the site of injection.
- Reassess the patient for anticipated response and adverse reaction to medication.

For insulin, observe for signs that patient's blood sugar level has returned to normal and for signs of hypoglycemia.

For heparin, observe that patient has no signs of bleeding.

For other medications, observe for side effects.

Patient Teaching

- Discuss possible lifestyle adaptations that the patient may need to undertake while receiving the medication (e.g., diet and exercise recommendations for managing diabetes mellitus).

Home Care

- Discuss with the patient or caregiver the options for insulin administration to determine the most appropriate choice for the person administering the injections.
Many options are available, including specially designed syringes that are easier to handle and read, pen injectors, and prefilled syringes.

- In the home environment, the patient might not routinely use an alcohol wipe to cleanse the site. This is acceptable as long as the skin is clean.
In the home environment there is less risk for superinfection with resistant strain organisms and other hospital-acquired infections.

- Do not encourage reusing needles and syringes.
- ✚ The very small insulin needles (30-gauge) bend very easily and are not recommended for reuse.

Determine whether reusing syringes is appropriate for the patient. Contraindications include inadequate hygiene, immunocompromised status, and difficulty handling equipment to prevent contamination of the needle.

- ✚ Discuss safety concerns regarding subcutaneous medication administration in the home, such as how to dispose of biohazardous wastes correctly and where to obtain a puncture-proof biohazard container.

The patient or caregiver may use a large plastic bottle or a coffee can. Local regulations regarding disposal must be followed.

- Discuss with the patient the need to rotate sites and reasons for doing so. Recommend that injections be given at the same time of the day, in the same body location, about 1 inch from the previous injection site.

Repeatedly giving the medication in the same site can cause abnormalities in the tissue and alter absorption rates.

- Remind the patient that when changing sites (thigh, arm, abdomen), the absorption rate may be altered.

- If the patient is receiving heparin or LMWHs, discuss the need to avoid nonsteroidal anti-inflammatory (NSAID) medications, such as acetylsalicylic acid (aspirin) and ibuprofen (Motrin, Advil).

These drugs increase the risk of bleeding.

- For patients receiving heparin or LMWHs, discuss home safety and the need to avoid falls.

The patient is at risk for bleeding and needs to follow safety guidelines to prevent injury. Older adults have an increased risk of developing bleeding problems with anticoagulant therapy. Nurses should carefully assess for abdominal bruising and complaints of abdominal pain.

Documentation

- Document according to **Medication Guidelines: Steps to Follow for All Medication (Regardless of Type or Route).**
- Some agencies have a specific code for documenting subcutaneous injections, which allows exact site documentation on an outline of the body.
- In the nursing notes, document any related patient assessment findings, such as capillary blood sugar, signs of hypoglycemia or hyperglycemia, bruising, and so on.
- Document in the nursing notes as well as MAR any medication that was given prn.

Sample EHR documentation

(continued on next page)

Procedure 23-12 ■ Administering Subcutaneous Medication (continued)

Thinking About the Procedure

➤ Go to the video **Administering Subcutaneous Medication,** along with questions and suggested responses, available on the **Davis's** *Nursing Skills Videos* Web site at www.fadavis.com.

Practice Resources
Centers for Disease Control and Prevention. (2019a); Kim et al. (2017); Kim & DeJesus (2022); Sexton et al. (2016); Shepherd (2018b).

Procedure 23-13 ■ Locating Intramuscular Injection Sites

➤ For steps to follow in *all* procedures, refer to the Universal Steps for All Procedures on the inside back cover. Also refer to **Medication Guidelines: Steps to Follow for All Medications (Regardless of Type or Route).**

Delegation
As an RN, you can usually delegate administration of parenteral medications (including locating injection sites) to an LPN/LVN. You usually cannot delegate this task to a UAP. If you delegate the skill, you are responsible for evaluating the LPN/LVN's ability to locate injection sites correctly.

Preprocedure Assessment
Always palpate the landmarks and the muscle mass to ensure correct placement of the needle. Because patients' body shapes vary, the site locations will differ slightly.

Procedure 23-13A ■ Locating the Ventrogluteal Site

➤ When performing the procedure, always identify your patient according to agency policy, using two identifiers, and be attentive to standard precautions, hand hygiene, patient safety and privacy, body mechanics, and documentation.

Procedure Steps

1. **Ask the patient to assume a side-lying** position with the legs straight, if possible.
   This position makes the site easier to locate.

2. **Locate the greater trochanter,** anterior superior iliac spine, and iliac crest.

3. **Place the palm of your hand** on the greater trochanter, your index finger on the anterior superior iliac spine, and your middle finger pointing toward the iliac crest. (Use your right hand on the patient's left hip; use your left hand on the patient's right hip.) Note that if your hands are very large or very small, the location of the "triangle" will be higher or lower on the hip. Be sure you locate it well in the muscle mass. ▼

4. **The middle of the triangle** between your middle and index fingers is the injection site.
   This is a safe site for IM administration because it is not close to any major blood vessels or nerves. The landmarks are easy to find. This large muscle can take volumes up to 5 mL in the average adult. It is safe for patients of all ages and the preferred site for adults and children older than 7 months; research supports this age and younger (Yapucu, 2016). Always palpate to assess adequacy of muscle mass, regardless of age. ▼

Procedure 23-13B ■ Locating the Deltoid Site

> When performing the procedure, always identify your patient according to agency policy, using two identifiers, and be attentive to standard precautions, hand hygiene, patient safety and privacy, body mechanics, and documentation.

Procedure Steps

1. **Completely expose the patient's** upper arm. Remove the garment; do not roll up the sleeve.
   Incomplete exposure of site and landmarks creates a risk of injecting into other than muscle tissue. This is a small site, and it is easy to make an error in location.

2. **Locate the lower edge** of the acromion process (which forms the base of a triangle), and go two to three fingerbreadths down. Your bottom finger will form the base of an upside-down triangle. ▼

3. **Next, draw an imaginary line** from each end of the triangle base downward 3 to 5 cm (1 to 2 in) to the midpoint of the lateral arm. The midpoint forms the apex of the triangle.

4. **The deltoid site is in the center** of the resulting inverted triangle.

5. **An alternative approach** is to place four fingerbreadths across the deltoid muscle, with your top finger on the acromion process. The injection goes three fingerbreadths below the process in the midline of the upper arm.
   Locates the appropriate site while avoiding the radial nerve and deep brachial artery. Because it is a fairly small muscle, only 0.5 to 1 mL of medication can be administered.

Procedure 23-13C ■ Locating the Vastus Lateralis Site

> When performing the procedure, always identify your patient according to agency policy, using two identifiers, and be attentive to standard precautions, hand hygiene, patient safety and privacy, body mechanics, and documentation.

Procedure Steps

1. **Position the patient** lying supine or sitting.
   The patient may perceive the injection as less painful if supine because they cannot see the needle enter the leg. For some people this provokes anxiety and intensifies pain.

2. **Locate the greater trochanter** and the lateral femoral condyle.

3. **Place your hands on the thigh,** with one hand against the greater trochanter and the other against the lateral femoral condyle.

4. **Visualize a rectangle** between your hands across the anterolateral thigh.
   - The index fingers of your hands form the smaller ends of the rectangle.
   - The long sides of the rectangle are formed by (a) drawing an imaginary line down the center of the anterior thigh and (b) drawing another line along the side of the leg, halfway between the bed and the front of the thigh.

(continued on next page)

Procedure 23-13 ■ Locating Intramuscular Injection Sites (continued)

- This box marks the middle third of the anterolateral thigh, which is the injection site.

The rectus femoris lies on the top (or anterior) portion of the thigh and partially covers the edge of the vastus lateralis. Therefore, do not inject too near the midline of the anterior thigh. Because it is not near any major blood vessels or nerves, the vastus lateralis site is safe for patients of all ages and is the recommended site for children younger than 7 months. ▼

Procedure 23-13D ■ Locating the Rectus Femoris Site

➤ When performing the procedure, always identify your patient according to agency policy, using two identifiers, and be attentive to standard precautions, hand hygiene, patient safety and privacy, body mechanics, and documentation.

Procedure Steps

✚ **Key Point:** *Use this site only if no other sites are accessible and no other medication routes are feasible.*

1. **Position the patient** in a supine or sitting position.
2. **Divide the top of the thigh into thirds** from the groin to the knee, and identify the middle third.
3. **Visualize a rectangle** in the middle of the anterior surface of the thigh. This is the location of the injection site. Also, refer to the drawing of the adult thigh in Procedure 23-13C. ▼

? What if...

- **My patient is a child? What is the best site to give an IM injection?**

    Because an infant's muscles are not fully developed, site selection is limited. Always access the adequacy of the muscle mass at the selected site. As a general rule:
    For children who are walking, use the ventrogluteal site.
    For children who are not yet walking, use the vastus lateralis. Once the gluteal muscles are developed further, which occurs with walking, the ventrogluteal site can be used.

Thinking About the Procedure

➤ The videos **Locating the Ventrogluteal Site, Locating the Deltoid Site,** and **Locating the Vastus Lateralis Site,** along with questions and suggested responses, are available on the **Davis's Nursing Skills Videos** Web site at www.fadavis.com.

Procedure 23-14 ■ Administering an Intramuscular Injection

➤ For steps to follow in *all* procedures, refer to the Universal Steps for All Procedures on the inside back cover. Also refer to Medication Guidelines: Steps to Follow for All Medications (Regardless of Type or Route).

➤ **Key Point:** *The Z-track method is preferred for all IM injections, except in a rare instance in which it is contraindicated.*

Equipment
- Syringe and needle appropriate for volume and site
- Alcohol prep pad or CHG–alcohol product
- Gauze pad or adhesive bandage
- Medication
- Procedure gloves
- Biohazard (sharps) container
- Small piece of gauze or cotton ball
- Small adhesive bandage

Delegation
As an RN, you can usually delegate administration of parenteral medications to an LPN/LVN. You cannot delegate this task to a UAP.

Preprocedure Assessments
- Identify the site of the previous injection.
- Assess the site for adequate muscle mass, bruises, edema, tenderness, redness, or other abnormalities.
  Muscle mass must be large enough to absorb the amount of medication prescribed. Abnormalities at the site increase patient discomfort and alter the absorption rate of the medication.
- Assess for factors that might affect absorption of the medication, such as decreased IM blood flow, as found in shock or muscle atrophy.
  Decreased peripheral circulation or muscle atrophy decreases the absorption of the medication.

Procedure 23-14A ■ Intramuscular Injection: Traditional Method

➤ When performing the procedure, always identify your patient according to agency policy, using two identifiers, and be attentive to standard precautions, hand hygiene, patient safety and privacy, body mechanics, and documentation.

Procedure Steps

1. **Select the appropriate syringe and needle.**
   a. The usual syringe size is 1 to 3 mL, depending on volume of medication to be given. For doses less than 1 mL, you can use a tuberculin syringe with an IM needle.
   b. The needle size is usually 21 to 25 gauge, 1½ inch in length for adults (or 1 in. for deltoid site). If there is excess adipose tissue, a longer needle (3 in.) might be necessary to penetrate the muscle.
      For IM administration, the needle gauge must be appropriate for the viscosity of the medication, and the needle must be long enough to deliver the medication into the muscle.
   c. Some medications are supplied in prefilled syringes, which are used for administration.

2. **Draw up the medication** (see Procedure 23-9A) or obtain prescribed unit dose, and verify medication. If the volume for injection is more than 3 to 5 mL, depending on the site, divide the dose for separate injections.

3. **Don procedure gloves.**
   Procedure gloves are required by OSHA to prevent exposure to bloodborne pathogens. You may prefer to don gloves at Step 6, while waiting for the antiseptic to dry.

4. **Position the patient** so that the injection site is well exposed and the patient is able to relax the appropriate muscles. Be sure the lighting is adequate.
   When the patient's muscles are relaxed (and not tense), it is easier to perform the injection, and patient discomfort during the injection is reduced. You must be able to fully visualize and safely access the site.
   a. **Deltoid site:** Position the patient with the arm relaxed at the side or resting on a firm surface, and completely expose the upper arm.
   NOTE: *This site is for small amounts of medication only (0.5 to 1 mL).*
   b. **Ventrogluteal site:** Position the patient on the opposite side, with the upper hip and knee slightly flexed.
   This position may cause the trochanter to become more prominent, making it easier to locate the site.
   c. **Vastus lateralis:** Position the patient supine or sitting, as the patient prefers.
   d. **Rectus femoris:** Position patient ♥ **iCare** supine. Because this site often causes more discomfort than others, use it only if all other sites are inaccessible and no other route is feasible.
   e. ✚ **Dorsogluteal:** Do not use this site because of the muscle's proximity to the sciatic nerve and major blood vessels.

5. **Using appropriate landmarks,** identify the injection site (see Procedure 23-13). If the patient is to receive more than one injection, rotate sites.
   Volumes of 1 to 5 mL may be given, depending on the muscle size (for adults, 0.5 to 1 mL in the deltoid, and typically 1 to 3 mL but up to 5 mL in the vastus lateralis site). If the volume for injection is more than 3 to 5 mL, depending on the site, then divide the dose for a separate injection. Rotating sites reduces discomfort and tissue trauma.

(continued on next page)

Procedure 23-14 ■ Administering an Intramuscular Injection (continued)

6. **Gently but thoroughly scrub the injection site.** Do not go back over already cleansed areas.
   a. If using an alcohol prep pad, thoroughly clean the site by circling from the center of the site outward.
   b. If using a CHG-based antiseptic, use a back-and-forth motion.
   Cleanse to remove microorganisms; follow the principle of "clean to dirty."

7. **Place the wipe on the patient's** skin outside the injection site, with a corner pointing to the site. Allow the site to dry before administering the injection. Do not fan the site.
   Leaving the antiseptic prep pad on the skin with a corner pointing to the injection site helps identify the location for the injection. If the antiseptic has not evaporated, it may cause the skin to sting during injection.

8. **Remove the needle cap.**

9. **With your nondominant hand,** spread the skin taut between your thumb and index finger.
   It is quicker, easier, and less painful to insert a needle through skin that is taut.

10. **Tell the patient what** you are going to do and that they will feel a prick as you insert the needle. Then hold the syringe between the thumb and fingers of your dominant hand like a pencil or dart and insert the needle at a 90° angle to the skin surface. Insert fully.
    Quickly inserting the needle through the skin minimizes discomfort. A 90° angle is needed for the needle to penetrate through the subcutaneous and adipose tissue to the muscle.

11. **Stabilize the syringe** with your nondominant hand.
    This prevents the needle from moving around in the tissue, thereby causing discomfort and possible tissue trauma.

12. **(If required by the agency policy) Aspirate by pulling back** on the plunger and waiting for 5 to 10 seconds. If you obtain a blood return, remove the needle, discard the syringe, and prepare the medication again. If there is no blood return, continue with Step 13.
    Aspirating blood indicates that the needle is in a blood vessel. Injecting would result in administering the medication intravenously instead of intramuscularly. If the needle is in a small vessel, it may take a few seconds for the blood to appear in the syringe. **Key Point:** *There are variations in practice regarding the requirement to aspirate for blood. Be sure to check with your instructor or the institution's protocol for the recommended method.*

13. **Using the thumb or index** finger of your dominant hand, press the plunger slowly to inject the medication (5 to 10 sec/mL).
    Slow administration allows the medication to disperse and decreases discomfort.

14. **Remove the needle** smoothly along the line of insertion.
    Removing the needle in this way prevents pulling against the skin and tissue and minimizes discomfort.

15. **Engage the safety needle device,** and dispose of the entire syringe in a biohazard container. If there is no safety device, place the uncapped syringe and needle directly into a biohazard, puncture-proof container.
    The biohazard sharps container prevents needlestick injuries.

16. **Gently blot the site** with a gauze pad, and apply an adhesive bandage as needed.
    Apply pressure to stop the bleeding but do not massage or rub the site after IM injection. This can cause medication to disperse into the subcutaneous tissue where the needle was injected, which might be irritating to the tissue.

Procedure 23-14B ■ Intramuscular Injection: Z-Track Method

➤ When performing the procedure, always identify your patient according to agency policy, using two identifiers, and be attentive to standard precautions, hand hygiene, patient safety and privacy, body mechanics, and documentation.

Procedure Steps

1–8. Follow Procedure 23-14A, traditional method, preceding.

Step 5 Variation. For Z-track method, use the larger muscles:
   a. *Ventrogluteal site:* Position patient on the side with upper hip and knee slightly flexed.
   b. *Vastus lateralis:* Position patient supine or sitting.

9. **With the side of your nondominant hand,** displace the skin away from the injection site, about 2.5 to 3.5 cm (1 to 1.5 in.).
   This displaces the skin and subcutaneous tissue over the muscle so that when it is released after the injection, the medication is sealed in the muscle. ▼

10. **Holding the syringe between** the thumb and fingers of your dominant hand like a pencil or dart, insert the needle at a 90° angle to the skin surface. Insert smoothly, quickly, and fully.
    Quickly inserting the needle through the skin minimizes discomfort. A 90° angle is needed for the needle to penetrate through the subcutaneous and adipose tissue to the muscle.

CHAPTER 23 Administering Medications   439

11. **Stabilize the syringe** with the thumb and forefinger of your non-dominant hand while continuing to displace the skin with your other three fingers. Do not release the skin to stabilize the syringe.
Stabilizing the needle reduces discomfort and possible tissue injury. You must keep the skin retracted to create a seal after the medication is injected and the skin released.

12. **(If required by the agency policy) Aspirate by pulling back slightly** on the plunger for 5 to 10 seconds. If you obtain a blood return, remove the needle, discard the syringe, and prepare the medication again. You should follow your institution's policy regarding aspiration with parenteral injections.
Aspirating blood indicates that the needle has penetrated a vein. Continuing could result in administering the medication intravenously instead of intramuscularly. ▼

13. **Using the thumb or index** finger of your dominant hand, press the plunger slowly to inject the medication (5 to 10 sec/mL).
Slow administration allows the medication to disperse and decreases discomfort.

14. **Wait for 10 seconds,** then withdraw the needle smoothly along the line of insertion, then immediately release the skin.
Waiting before withdrawing the needle leaves a zigzag needle track that traps the medication in the muscle, preventing it from leaking up into the subcutaneous tissue.

15. **Engage the safety needle device,** and dispose of it in a biohazard container. If there is no safety device, place the uncapped syringe and needle directly in a biohazard, puncture-proof container.

16. **Hold a cotton ball** or gauze pad with light pressure over the injection site. Do not massage the site. Apply an adhesive bandage if necessary.
Light pressure will stop superficial bleeding at the injection site. Massaging and rubbing can force medication into the subcutaneous tissues.

? What if...

- **My patient is unable to cooperate during the procedure?**
  Ask another healthcare provider or family member to help keep the patient from moving during the injection or to help position the patient.

- **My patient is a child; is there anything different about giving an IM injection?**
  Adapt the procedure to decrease pain: Apply topical anesthetic cream (e.g., EMLA [lidocaine-prilocaine]) or a topical cooling spray if time permits. If not, distract the child with conversation, or give them something to do, such as squeeze a hand, or apply a cold compress over the site.
  Adapt the way you spread the skin to inject: In infants and small children, grasp the muscle with your thumb and index finger; in children with excess adipose tissue, spread the skin and then grasp the muscle.
  Adapt the medication volume: Inject no more than 1 mL in a single injection, 0.5 mL in a small infant.
  The CDC recommends 1- and 1¼-inch needles for children 1 year old or younger. Follow agency procedures.

- **My patient is an older adult?**
  Many older adults have decreased muscle mass, so use a shorter needle; spread the skin and grasp the muscle to localize and stabilize the site for injection.
  Older adults tend to bleed from the site after injection because of reduced tissue elasticity. Apply a small pressure bandage if needed.

Evaluation

- Observe for minimal bruising or oozing that may occur at the site of injection.
- Observe for local reactions at site (e.g., pain, swelling, redness).

Home Care

- Discuss safety concerns with administering medication intramuscularly in the home, such as correct disposal of biohazardous wastes and where to obtain a puncture-proof biohazard container.
The caregiver or patient can use a large plastic bottle. The local regulations must be followed for disposal.

- Discuss with the patient the need to rotate sites.
Repeatedly giving the medication in the same site can cause abnormalities in the tissue and alter absorption rates.

Documentation

- Refer to Medication Guidelines: Steps to Follow for All Medications (Regardless of Type or Route).
- Document related assessment findings, such as pain level or presence of nausea.
- Unless the medication is prn, you will typically document it only on the MAR.

(continued on next page)

Procedure 23-14 ■ Administering an Intramuscular Injection (continued)

Practice Resources
Becton Dickinson (2017); Kim & DeJesus (2022); Ogston-Tuck (2014a); Sepah et al. (2017); Strohfus et al. (2018)

Thinking About the Procedure

Go to the videos **Intramuscular Injection: Traditional Method** and **Intramuscular Injection: Z-Track Method,** along with questions and suggested responses, available on the **Davis's *Nursing Skills Videos*** Web site at www.fadavis.com.

Procedure 23-15 ■ Adding Medications to Intravenous Fluids

▶ For steps to follow in *all* procedures, refer to the Universal Steps for All Procedures on the inside back cover. Also refer to Medication Guidelines: Steps to Follow for All Medications (Regardless of Type or Route).

Equipment
- Prescribed IV solution
- Syringe for measuring medication
- Needleless access device or safety needle (if a VAD is not available)
- Antimicrobial swab
- Label with medication, dose, date, time, and your initials

Delegation
As an RN, you would not usually delegate adding medications to IV fluids to LPN/LVNs. Nurse practice acts governing IV medication administration vary from state to state, and policies can further vary among healthcare agencies regarding which additives may be added by LPN/LVNs. Even if you delegate the skill, you are always responsible for evaluating the patient's responses, both therapeutic effects and adverse effects.

Preprocedure Assessments
- Assess the patency of the IV site.
- Assess the appearance of the IV site.
- Check the medication insert or *Physician's Desk Reference* (*PDR*) for appropriate time or rate for infusion and for compatibility.

▶ When performing the procedure, always identify your patient according to agency policy, using two identifiers, and be attentive to standard precautions, hand hygiene, patient safety and privacy, body mechanics, and documentation.

Procedure Steps

1. **Determine** whether the medication(s) are compatible with the IV solution and with each other.
   Not all medications or other additives can be mixed with the glucose or saline normally found in the primary IV bag. Multiple additives increase the possibility of incompatibility.

2. **Calculate or verify the amount of medication** to be instilled into the IV solution, and the rate of administration.
   Verifying the dose and the rate of infusion prevents medication errors.

3. **Remove any protective covers,** and inspect the bag or bottle for leaks, tears, or cracks. Inspect the fluid for clarity, color, and presence of any particulate matter. Check the expiration date.
   Double-checking the IV solution reduces the risk of infusing contaminated or expired solutions.

4. **Using the appropriate technique,** draw up the prescribed medication (see Procedure 23-9, as needed). Alternatively, insert a VAD transfer device into the medication vial.
   Medications can come in vials, ampules, or bags, with differences in administrations techniques.

5. **Gently and thoroughly clean all surfaces of the IV** additive port with an alcohol or CHG–alcohol combination product.
   Diligent cleaning with antimicrobial products reduces the transmission of microorganisms and helps maintain the sterility of the solution.

6. **Remove the cap from the syringe,** insert the needle or the needleless access device into the injection port, and inject the medication into the bag, maintaining aseptic technique. ▼

7. **Mix the IV solution and medication** by gently turning the bag from end to end.
   Ensures even distribution of the medication or additive into the solution.

8. **Place a label on the bag** so that it can be read when the bag is hung. Include the medication name, dose, route, and your name. Be sure the label does not cover the solution label or volume marks.
   A label informs you and others of additives to IV solutions. ➤

9. **Dispose of used equipment,** syringe, or the VAD appropriately.

Evaluation

- Check the IV line at least once every hour to ensure that the prescribed or calculated rate is maintained.
- Assess the patient for complaints of pain or signs of infiltration at the infusion site (e.g., redness, swelling).

Patient Teaching

- Discuss reasons the medication is being given intravenously.
- Explain whether it is a continuous or intermittent infusion.
- Explain the need to report immediately any reactions to the medication, such as breathing problems, rashes, or pain at the IV insertion site.

Documentation

- Document information according to Medication Guidelines: Steps to Follow for All Medications (Regardless of Type or Route).
- Document any findings on an IV flow record rather than in the nursing notes. Document only unexpected findings (e.g., if the IV has infiltrated) in the nurses' notes.

Practice Resources
Gorski L. et al. (2021)

Procedure 23-16 ■ Administering IV Push Medication

➤ For steps to follow in *all* procedures, refer to the Universal Steps for All Procedures on the inside back cover. Also refer to Medication Guidelines: Steps to Follow for All Medications (Regardless of Type or Route).

➤ The Institute for Safe Medication Practices identified several unsafe practices associated with IV push medications, including (1) using prefilled syringes or cartridges as vials, (2) unnecessary dilution of medications, and (3) failing to properly label medications not prepared at the patient's bedside (ISMP, 2018).

Equipment

- Syringe appropriate for medication volume and the type of line (e.g., peripheral IV, PICC)
- If you are administering through an intermittent device:
  - Two 5- to 10-mL syringes, or one 10-mL syringe with 2 to 10 mL of normal saline or heparin for flushing the line
    Although either is acceptable, separate syringes pose less risk of contamination.
  - Depending on site and facility policy, one 5- to 10-mL syringe containing 2 to 5 mL of heparin flush (or saline) solution
    Research found little evidence to conclude heparin was more effective than saline flush for CVC maintenance (Sharma et al., 2019;). The IHI (2020) recommends the elimination of heparin flush for peripheral IV lines. The INS society recommends preservative free normal saline for short and long peripheral IV catheters and for midline catheters (Gorski et al., 2021).
- Alcohol prep pad, or CHG–alcohol combination product and gauze pad
- Procedure gloves

Delegation

As an RN, you may, in some situations, be able to delegate administration of parenteral medications to an LPN/LVN. However, this is not a common practice.

Preprocedure Assessments

- Determine the type and amount of dilution needed for the medication.
- Check the compatibility of the medication with the existing IV solution if it is infusing.
  Medications can be physically or chemically incompatible with the IV solution. Physical incompatibility is often obvious because precipitation may occur. Chemical incompatibility is not obvious and may result in the medication's having a weaker or a stronger effect than anticipated.
- Assess the patency of the IV line.
  If the line is occluded, you will not be able to instill the medication.
- Check the site for redness, swelling, tenderness, and other signs of infiltration or phlebitis.
  Some medications are irritating and may be toxic to the tissue. If the IV line is infiltrated, the medication may leak into the tissue and cause injury. IV medications can also irritate the veins and cause phlebitis. Do not infuse a medication into a compromised site.

(continued on next page)

Procedure 23-16 ■ Administering IV Push Medication (continued)

Procedure 23-16A ■ Administering IV Push Medications Through a Primary IV Line

> When performing the procedure, always identify your patient according to agency policy, using two identifiers, and be attentive to standard precautions, hand hygiene, patient safety and privacy, body mechanics, and documentation.

Procedure Steps

1. **Determine how fast the medication** may be administered and whether the medication needs to be diluted for administration. Also, check to be sure the medication is compatible with the solution infusing. *IV push medications are frequently injected over 1 minute. Some must infuse over a longer period, and some require diluting before administration. Giving an IV push medication too fast and/or undiluted can result in local or systemic adverse reactions.*

2. **Prepare the medication** from a vial or ampule or obtain the prescribed unit dose and verify medication with the prescription (refer to Procedure 23-9). Dilute as needed. Temporarily pause the infusion pump to administer the medication. If the primary bag is infusing by gravity, simply clamp the tubing.

3. **Don procedure gloves** and vigorously scrub all surfaces of the injection port closest to the patient with an alcohol prep pad or CHG-alcohol combination product (Gorski et al., 2021).
   (a) Scrub time: *Follow agency policy. Some facilities require nurses to cleanse the port for 1 minute when accessing venous access devices.*
   (b) The port: *Using the port closest to the patient minimizes the distance the medication must travel and gets it into the patient's circulation faster. You must use an injection port, which is self-sealing because if you puncture the plastic IV tubing, it will leak.*
   (c) Scrub agent: *Use povidone–iodine solution (Betadine) only if the patient is sensitive to alcohol or CHG–alcohol combination.*

4. **Insert the medication syringe** into the injection port. If a needleless system is not available, use a syringe with a safety needle.
   Using a needleless system prevents needlestick injuries.

5. **Pinch or clamp the IV tubing** between the IV bag and the port.
   Occluding the tubing upline of the port prevents the medication from being injected back toward the IV bag. ▼

6. **Gently aspirate** by slowly pulling back on the plunger to check for a blood return.

   NOTE: *Some newer connectors do not require or allow for aspiration. Follow institutional policy.*
   (a) A blood return is one indication that the IV catheter is in the vein. An IV site may still be patent if no blood is returned, and an infiltrated IV line may have a blood return. Use the blood return as one indication of patency (Gorski, 2018).
   (b) Injecting an IV medication into an IV site that is not patent administers the medication into the local tissue at the IV site. Some medications will cause tissue irritation and even necrosis if infused into the subcutaneous tissue. In addition, the patient would not receive the immediate therapeutic benefit from the drug.

7. **If you have aspirated and obtained a blood return,** administer a small increment of the medication while observing for reactions to the medication.
   Slow injection allows you to observe adverse reactions to the medication before all the medication has been injected. Administering IV push medications carries the highest potential risk to the patient because immediate, life-threatening reactions can occur.

8. **Administer another increment** of the medication (you may pinch the tubing while injecting medication and release it when not injecting; this is optional).

9. **Repeat Steps 7 and 8 until** the full dose of medication has been administered over the prescribed time.
   Medications require different administration times. Follow agency guidelines, provider prescriptions, and pharmaceutical information regarding whether the medication needs to be diluted and the rate of administration.

10. **If you clamped the IV tubing** during the infusion, open it now and reset the pump at the correct infusion rate, if necessary.

11. **Dispose of used supplies safely** and according to agency procedures.

Procedure 23-16B ■ Administering IV Push Medications Through an Intermittent Device (IV Lock) When No Extension Tubing Is Attached to the Venous Access Device

> When performing the procedure, always identify your patient according to agency policy, using two identifiers, and be attentive to standard precautions, hand hygiene, patient safety and privacy, body mechanics, and documentation.

Procedure Steps

1. **Determine how fast the medication may be administered** and whether it needs to be diluted for administration.
   IV push medications are frequently injected over 1 minute. Some medications must be administered over a longer period, and some medications must be diluted before administration. Giving an IV push medication too fast and/or undiluted can result in an adverse local or systemic reaction.

2. **Prepare the medication** from a vial or ampule. Dilute as needed. Refer to Procedure 23-9.

3. **Select the appropriate size of syringe** for flush solution.
   Smaller syringes exert more pressure against the wall of the IV catheter than do larger syringes. Check with the IV catheter manufacturer for specific recommendations, and follow agency policy.

4. **Don procedure gloves.**

5. **Thoroughly scrub all surfaces** of the injection port closest to the patient with an alcohol prep pad or CHG–alcohol combination product (Gorski et al., 2021).
   Follow agency policy. Some facilities require nurses to scrub all surfaces of the port with an alcohol-based antimicrobial product for 1 minute when accessing venous access devices. (a) Port: Using the port closest to the patient minimizes the amount of medication in the IV line. (b) Scrub: Use povidone-iodine solution (Betadine) only when the patient cannot tolerate an alcohol-based disinfectant.

6. **Insert the flush syringe** into the injection port and gently aspirate by pulling back on the plunger to check for a blood return.

   NOTE: Some newer connectors do not require or allow for aspiration. Follow institutional policy.

   A blood return is an indication that the IV catheter is in the vein. An IV site may still be patent if no blood is returned; conversely, an infiltrated IV may have a blood return. Use the blood return as only one indication of patency.

7. **Administer a flush solution** (usually 1 to 3 mL) to clear the line if you aspirated and blood was returned. Use a forward pushing motion on the syringe, with a slow, steady injection technique. If blood is not returned, see the What if...? section at the end of this procedure.
   (a) Flush syringes may be prefilled, and in some cases the amount to inject may be a part of agency policy. (b) Avoid rapid flushing that creates a jet effect that can cause the catheter tip to migrate to other venous locations. (c) Injecting an IV medication into an IV site that is not patent administers the medication into the local tissue at the IV site. Some medications will cause tissue irritation and even necrosis if infused into the subcutaneous tissue.

8. **Continue to hold the injection port,** remove the flush syringe, and again scrub the port with the alcohol prep pad or CHG–alcohol combination product.
   Cleansing the port reduces the risk of introducing microorganisms into the bloodstream. Scrub: Use povidone-iodine only when the patient is sensitive to alcohol-based disinfectants.

9. **Attach the medication** syringe and inject the medication in small increments over the correct time interval. Use a slow, steady injection technique until the correct dose is instilled over the prescribed time.
   For example, if 1 mL of the medication is to be given over 1 minute, inject approximately 0.25 mL every 15 seconds. ▼

10. **Continuing to hold the injection port,** remove the medication syringe and gently but thoroughly scrub all surfaces of the port with alcohol prep pad or CHG–alcohol product for at least 15 seconds. Attach the flush syringe.
    Gently but thoroughly cleaning/scrubbing reduces the chance of contamination of the port.

(continued on next page)

Procedure 23-16 ■ Administering IV Push Medication (continued)

11. **Administer the flush solution** usually 1 to 3 mL, or according to prescription or agency policy.
   Use the amount of flush solution that will clear the medication from the administration set and catheter. Flushing ensures that all the medication has been administered and prevents occlusion of the IV catheter.

12. **Use a slow, steady injection pressure technique** when removing the syringe by placing your thumb or index finger to avoid movement of the plunger. (Follow equipment guidelines; you may not always need to do this.) Continue to administer the flush solution while withdrawing the syringe cannula from the injection port.

   This positive-pressure technique prevents blood backflow into the IV catheter, which might cause an occlusion. Follow equipment guidelines because some injection ports maintain positive pressure by removing the syringe and then closing the clamp. ▼

   1. Give flush solution
   2. Give medication
   3. Give flush solution

13. **Discard the flushing syringe** from the needleless connector into a safety disposal container.

Procedure 23-16C ■ Administering IV Push Medications Through an Intermittent Device With IV Extension Tubing

➤ When performing the procedure, always identify your patient according to agency policy, using two identifiers, and be attentive to standard precautions, hand hygiene, patient safety and privacy, body mechanics, and documentation.

Procedure Steps

1. **Determine how fast the medication** may be administered and whether the medication needs to be diluted for administration.
   IV push medications are frequently injected over 1 minute. Some must be administered over a longer period, and some require diluting before administration. Giving an IV push medication too fast and/or undiluted can result in a local or systemic adverse reaction.

2. **Prepare the medication** from a vial or ampule. Dilute as needed. Refer to Procedure 23-9.

3. **Determine the volume of any extension tubing** attached to the access port.
   The volume of extension sets can be greater than the IV push medication being given. If not accounted for, all the medication may be injected into the patient's bloodstream at once when the second flush solution is given.

4. **Don procedure gloves.**

5. **Clean/scrub all surfaces of the injection** port with an antiseptic wipe.

6. **Insert the flush syringe** into the injection port. If a needleless system is not available, use a syringe with a safety needle. Depending on the equipment, you may then need to aspirate for a blood return as one sign of vein patency. Some equipment does not require or allow aspiration. (a) In tubing that allows for or requires aspiration, a blood return is a sign that the IV catheter is in the vein. However, an IV site may still be patent if no blood is returned. (b) Using a needleless system prevents needlestick injuries.

7. **Administer the flush** (commonly 1 to 3 mL) after establishing patency of the IV line. If blood appears in the tubing during aspiration, administer the rest of the flush. If blood is not returned, assess patency by administering a small amount of the flush solution and monitoring for ease of administration, swelling at the IV site, or patient complaint of discomfort at the site.

8. **Again clean/scrub the port.** Attach the medication syringe and inject a volume of medication equal to the volume of the extension set at the same rate as the flush solution.
   - When using a 5-mL syringe for peripheral lines and a 10-mL syringe for central lines, administer the flush solution briskly.
   - When you use a smaller syringe, use a slower rate to prevent excess pressure damaging the vein or shearing of the IV cannula.
   The medication clears the line of saline solution and fills it with medication; it also flushes the IV catheter with saline as the medication pushes the saline through the catheter. ▼

   Baxter Extension Set: Volume = 1.3 mL (1.3 mL before medication gets to the patient)

9. **Using a slow, steady injection** technique, administer the remainder of the medication over the prescribed time interval for the specific medication.

    Rapid flushing can create a jet effect that can cause the catheter tip to migrate to an unintended venous location.

10. **Continuing to hold the injection port connector,** remove the medication syringe, gently, but thoroughly scrub all surfaces of the connector for at least 15 seconds, then attach the flush syringe. **Key Point:** *The only time you should open the catheter hub is when the needleless connector or primary continuous IV set must be changed, usually at 96-hour intervals or as otherwise prescribed.*

11. **Administer the same amount** of flush solution at the same rate as the medication, using a slow, steady injection technique. For example, if the extension tubing has a volume of 1.3 mL, give the first 1.3 mL of the flush solution at the same rate as the medication. Then administer the remainder of the flush solution.

    (a) At this step, the extension tubing contains all the medication. Administering the flush solution all at once pushes the medication too fast (it will enter the vein all at once). (b) Once you have incrementally cleared the medication from the extension tubing and all the medication is already in the vein, then the rate no longer matters as far as the medication is concerned.

12. **Use a slow, steady injection pressure technique** when removing the syringe. Continue to administer the flush solution while withdrawing the syringe cannula from the injection port. Follow equipment instructions regarding the method and order of removing the syringe, closing the clamp, and maintaining positive pressure.

13. **Discard the flushing syringe** from the needleless connector into a safety disposal container.

? What if . . .

- **When using equipment requiring aspiration, no blood is returned?**

    Do not give IV push medication until you can verify the patency of the IV site.

    If the patency of the IV site is questionable, restart the IV at another site.

    Further assess the patency of the IV line by administering a small amount of the saline flush and monitoring for ease of administration, swelling at the IV site, or patient complaint of discomfort at the site.

    Another technique to determine patency is to lower the IV bag below the level of the IV site—a blood return should occur.

    If the IV catheter is a small gauge, a blood return may not always be aspirated.

- **There is resistance when flushing the line?**

    Never force the flush solution into the VAD; look for a closed clamp on the catheter or tubing. Or you may check to see if an inline filter is clogged. Do not proceed with the medication infusion until you are sure the catheter is still positioned correctly and that the fluid pathway is unobstructed.

- **The IV infusing a dextrose solution infiltrates into the surrounding tissue of a peripheral catheter?**

    Immediately stop the intravenous infusion, remove the catheter, and elevate the site. Initially apply a cool, moist compress to the site for vasoconstriction to limit dispersion. Later, alternate cool and warm compresses for 15 to 20 minutes every 4 hours (Kim et al., 2020) to promote comfort.

    Infiltration can cause tissue injury, inflammation, and edema and may even lead to tissue necrosis and sloughing.

    Some medications, such as vasopressors (e.g., dopamine), might need intradermal injection of an antidote, such as phentolamine (Regitine), to reverse the effects of extravasation.

    If the IV fluid contains dextrose at greater than 10% concentration, calcium salts, potassium salts, sodium bicarbonate, blood, and parenteral nutrition, contact the primary care provider, who will likely prescribe injection of hyaluronidase (Amphadase) into the surrounding tissue.

Evaluation

- Assess the patient for complaints of pain or discomfort at the site.

Patient Teaching

- Discuss why the medication is being administered intravenously.
- Explain the need to immediately report any reaction to the medication.

Home Care

- Discuss with the patient and/or caregiver how to care for the IV site, including flushing. Many IV push medications need to be administered by a nurse. However, cost-cutting efforts have led to short hospital stays, and some patients are now being taught to administer their own IV antibiotics at home.
- Explain how to identify problems with the IV site, such as infiltration and phlebitis.
- Determine whether the patient has adequate facilities for storing the medication, such as refrigeration, if needed.
- Discuss safety issues, such as keeping medications and needles and syringes secure and away from children and pets.

Documentation

In addition to documenting according to Medication Guidelines: Steps to Follow for All Medications (Regardless of Type

(continued on next page)

Procedure 23-16 ■ Administering IV Push Medication (continued)

or Route), document related patient assessment findings, such as the appearance of the IV site and patient complaints of pain or discomfort during IV administration. You will usually document on an IV flow record and/or the MAR rather than in the nursing notes. Document a nursing note only if there is a problem (e.g., IV infiltration, patient experiences during medication administration).

Practice Resources
Gorski (2018); Gorski et al. (2021).

Thinking About the Procedure

Go to the videos **Administering IV Push Medications Through a Primary IV Line, Administering IV Push Medications Through an Intermittent Device (IV Lock) When No Extension Tubing Is Attached to the Venous Access Device,** and **Administering IV Push Medications Through an Intermittent Device With IV Extension Tubing,** along with questions and suggested responses, available on the **Davis's** *Nursing Skills Videos* Web site at www.fadavis.com.

Procedure 23-17 ■ Administering Medication by Intermittent Infusion

➤ For steps to follow in *all* procedures, refer to the Universal Steps for All Procedures on the inside back cover. Also refer to Medication Guidelines: Steps to Follow for All Medications (Regardless of Type or Route). For step-by-step instructions in using volume-control devices (pumps), see Procedure 35-3.

Equipment
- Correct size syringe for measuring medication
- Needleless access cannula or safety needle
- Volume-control IV set (e.g., Buretrol, Volutrol, Soluset) or small bag of diluted medication with piggyback tubing
- Primary IV solution and tubing (unless one is already infusing)
- Antimicrobial swabs
- Labels for the IV tubing and medication administration system

Delegation
Nurse practice acts governing IV medication administration vary from state to state, and policies can further vary among healthcare agencies regarding which medications or methods of administration the LPN/LVN may perform. You cannot delegate this procedure to a UAP.

Preprocedure Assessments
- Check the compatibility of the medication with the IV solution.
  Medications can be physically or chemically incompatible with the IV solution. Physical incompatibility will be obvious if precipitation occurs. Chemical incompatibility is not obvious and may result in the medication having a weaker or stronger effect than anticipated.

- Assess the patency of the IV line.
  If the line is occluded or if the fluid has infiltrated, the medication will not infuse.

- Check the site for redness, swelling, tenderness, and other signs of infiltration or phlebitis.
  Some medications are irritating to the tissue. If the IV fluid has infiltrated, medication would leak into the tissue and cause injury. IV medications can also irritate the veins and cause phlebitis. Do not infuse a medication into a compromised site.

- Determine the amount of IV solution needed to administer the specific medication.
  Most medications state (on the prescription or on the label) specific dilution to prevent potential harm to the patient.

- Determine the period over which the solution needs to be infused.
  Infusing a medication too slowly may result in an inadequate blood level to achieve therapeutic levels, and infusing a medication too rapidly can cause harm.

- Perform assessments that will provide a basis for evaluating the drug's effectiveness, such as checking blood pressure after administering an antihypertensive agent.

Procedure 23-17A ■ Using a Piggyback Administration Set With a Gravity Infusion

➤ When performing the procedure, always identify your patient according to agency policy, using two identifiers, and be attentive to standard precautions, hand hygiene, patient safety and privacy, body mechanics, and documentation.

Procedure Steps

1. **Obtain the medication.** IV medications usually are premixed and labeled in small bags by the pharmacy. You will rarely need to draw up the medication and inject it into the piggyback solution (see Procedure 23-15). Date and initial the medication bag label. Verify that it has the patient's name, amount of medication, date, and time given.

2. **Obtain and attach** the piggyback tubing to the medication bag. Do not touch the spike.
   Tubing connects the piggyback to the primary line. The piggyback tubing is short. Prevents contamination of tubing and solution.

3. **Be sure the slide clamp is closed.** Squeeze the drip chamber, filling it one-third to one-half full.
   Clamping prevents excess air coming into the line when you are priming the tubing.

4. **Open the clamp and prime** the tubing, holding the end of the tubing lower than the bag of fluid. Do not let more than one drop of fluid escape from the end of the tubing. Close the clamp.

Alternative: Backflushing the Piggyback Line
   a. Clamp the piggyback tubing.
   b. Scrub all surfaces of the primary Y port, and attach the piggyback setup with the needleless connector.
   c. Open the clamp on the piggyback tubing, and lower the bag below the primary bag to prime the piggyback line.
   d. Once all the air is expelled from the piggyback tubing, clamp the tubing and finish the procedure.
   Priming removes air from the tubing and maintains sterility of the system. Medications are diluted in small amounts of fluid (usually 50 to 100 mL), so you cannot waste any medication. The backflush method ensures you will not do so.

Note: The INS recommends pack priming the secondary administration set from the primary infusion container for secondary intermittent infusions with compatible medications (Gorski et al., 2021).

5. **Label the piggyback tubing** with the time, the date, and your initials.
   Tubing used for intermittent infusions can be used for 48 to 72 hours, depending on facility policy; labeling allows the nurse to know when it must be changed.

6. **Hang the piggyback container** on the IV pole. Lower the primary IV container to hang below the level of the medication bag.
   Gravity causes the higher bag (the piggyback IV setup) to flow instead of the primary IV setup. When the piggyback IV solution has infused, the primary IV line will resume infusing.

7. **Open the clamp** of the piggyback line, and regulate the drip rate with the roller clamp on the primary line. Regulate to the prescribed infusion rate for the medication. ▼

Because the piggyback is the only bag running, the primary roller clamp regulates the speed of the piggyback bag.

8. **When the medication is all infused,** clamp the piggyback tubing, and move the primary bag back to its original height. Use the roller clamp to reset the primary bag to its correct infusion rate.
   This ensures that the primary fluids infuse at their prescribed rate rather than flowing at the rate the piggyback medication was flowing—which would probably be either faster or slower than the prescribed primary fluid rate.

Procedure 23-17B ■ Using a Piggyback Administration Set With an Infusion Pump

➤ For step-by-step instructions in using intermittent infusion devices (pumps), also see Procedure 35-3.
➤ *Note:* This procedure describes the use of a one-piston infusion pump. The steps for using a two-piston pump vary slightly.
➤ When performing the procedure, always identify your patient according to agency policy, using two identifiers, and be attentive to standard precautions, hand hygiene, patient safety and privacy, body mechanics, and documentation.

Procedure Steps

1. **Obtain the medication.** IV medications usually are premixed in small bags and labeled by the pharmacy. If this is not the case, inject the medication into the prescribed piggyback solution (see Procedure 23-15). Date and initial the medication bag label. Verify that it has the patient's name, amount of medication, date, and time given.

2. **Be sure you have the correct secondary infusion tubing.** Hang the piggyback container on the IV pole. Attach the piggyback tubing to the medication bag. Do not touch the spike.

(continued on next page)

Procedure 23-17 ■ Administering Medication by Intermittent Infusion (continued)

Piggyback tubing is short. Secondary tubing connects the piggyback to the primary line. Touching the spike would contaminate the tubing and solution.

3. **Be sure the slide clamp** is closed. Squeeze the drip chamber, filling it one-third to one-half full.
   Clamping prevents excess air coming into the line when you are priming the tubing.

4. **Open the clamp and prime** the tubing, holding the end of the tubing lower than the bag of fluid. Do not let more than one drop of fluid escape from the end of the tubing. Close the clamp.

Alternative: Backflushing the Piggyback Line
   a. With the drip chamber one-third filled, air will be in the secondary tubing.
   b. Pause the infusion pump.
   c. Scrub all surfaces of the Y port on the primary line and attach the piggyback setup with a needleless connector.
   d. Open the clamp on the piggyback tubing, and lower the bag below the primary bag to prime the piggyback line. The fluid from the primary line will flow up through the secondary tubing until all air is removed from the tubing. Restart the pump.
   e. Once the line is primed, clamp the tubing and finish the procedure.

Priming removes air from the tubing and maintains sterility of the system. Medications are diluted in small amounts of fluid (usually 50 to 100 mL), so you cannot waste any medication. The backflush method ensures you will not do so.

Note: The INS recommends pack priming the secondary administration set from the primary infusion container for secondary intermittent infusions with compatible medications (Gorski et al., 2021).

5. **Label the piggyback tubing** with the time, the date, and your initials.
   Tubing used for intermittent infusions can be used for 48 to 72 hours, depending on facility policy. Labeling allows the nurse to know when it must be changed.

6. **Hang the piggyback container** on the IV pole. Lower the primary IV container to hang below the level of the piggyback medication bag.
   The tubing system works such that the higher bag (the piggyback IV setup) flows instead of the primary IV setup.

7. **Program the pump** by selecting the secondary infusion button.
   This converts the fluid infusing from the primary line to the secondary line.

8. **Program the rate and total volume** to be infused. (Some pumps allow you to select the medication and dose.)
   Ensures accurate infusion amount and restart of primary fluids.

9. **Vigorously scrub the port** of the primary line.
   Minimizes the introduction of microorganisms.

10. **Remove the cover from** the secondary tubing and connect it to the connection port of the primary line. (This was done at Step 4 if the blackflush priming method was used.)

11. **Open the clamp** on the secondary tubing.

12. **Press "start"** on infusion pump.

13. **Check drip chambers** to ensure that the secondary solution is infusing and the primary solution is not.
    This ensures that medication is infusing and patient does not receive an overload of fluids.

14. **Check the pump information** again to ensure the correct rate and volume.

15. **At the end of the infusion,** the primary IV line will resume infusing. Once the secondary infusion is complete, the pump programming will reset to the previously programmed primary rate.
    This ensures that the primary fluids infuse at their prescribed rate rather than flowing at the rate the piggyback medication was flowing—which would probably be either faster or slower than the prescribed primary fluid rate.

Procedure 23-17C ■ Using a Volume-Control Administration Set

▶ For step-by-step instructions in using volume-control devices (pumps), see Procedure 35-3. If you have not already done so, affix a label to the secondary bag indicating the name and amount of medication, date and time given, and your name or initials.

▶ When performing the procedure, always identify your patient according to agency policy, using two identifiers, and be attentive to standard precautions, hand hygiene, patient safety and privacy, body mechanics, and documentation.

Procedure Steps

1. **Prepare the volume-control set.**
   a. Close both the upper and lower clamps on the tubing, if they are not already closed.
      Clamping prevents air bubbles from forming in the tubing.
   b. Open the clamp of the air vent on the volume-control chamber.
      Venting allows air to escape, which lets the IV solution enter the chamber.
   c. Maintaining sterile procedure, attach administration spike of the volume-control set to the primary IV bag.
   d. Fill the volume-control chamber with the desired amount of IV solution by opening the clamp between the bag and the volume-control chamber. When the correct amount of solution is in the chamber, close the clamp.
      The drip chamber provides solution for priming the tubing and diluting the IV medication.
   e. Prime the rest of the tubing by opening the clamp below the chamber and running the IV fluid until all the air has been expelled.
      Priming clears the IV tubing of air.

f. Recheck the amount of fluid in the volume control chamber and add more fluid to the desired amount, if needed.
Priming the tubing alters the volume in the chamber. You must fill to the desired amount.

2. **With an alcohol or CHG–alcohol swab,** gently but thoroughly scrub all surfaces of the injection port closest to the patient.
Thorough cleansing is necessary to remove microorganisms and particles from the IV port, which could potentially enter the patient's bloodstream.

3. **Connect the end of the volume-control IV line** to the patient's IV site (e.g., directly to the IV catheter, to the extension tubing, or to the injection port closest to patient).

4. **Thoroughly scrub the injection port** on the volume-control chamber, attach the medication syringe (preferably with a blunt, needleless device), and inject the medication into the solution in the chamber.

5. **Gently rotate the chamber** to mix the medication in the IV solution.
Distributes the medication within the IV solution.

6. **Open the lower clamp,** and start the infusion at the correct flow rate.
Unclamping allows the infusion of the medication. A correct flow rate infuses the medication over the correct length of time and prevents a toxic reaction to it.

7. **Label the volume-control chamber** with the date, time, medication and doses added, and your initials, according to agency policy.

8. **When the medication has finished infusing,** add a small amount of the primary IV fluid to the chamber, and flush the tubing. For the flush volume, use twice the volume in the dead space of the tubing; check the tubing package for the amount.
Flushing the line ensures all the medication is given to the patient and does not adhere to the tubing. ▶

Evaluation
- Assess for pain or discomfort at the site.
- Intermittent infusions via a pump are generally infused over 30 to 60 minutes; therefore, you need to assess the patient as soon as the medication begins infusing and every 15 to 20 minutes until it is absorbed.

Patient Teaching
- Discuss why the medication is being administered intravenously.
- Explain the need to report immediately any reaction to the medication.
- Ask the patient to activate the call device if the infusion pump starts to alarm. Explain common reasons for the alarm to minimize anxiety.

Home Care
- Discuss with the patient and/or caregiver how to care for the IV site. Only a nurse should add medications to the IV.
- Explain how to identify problems with the IV site, such as infiltration and phlebitis.
- Assess whether the patient has adequate facilities for storing the medication, such as refrigeration if needed.
- Discuss safety issues, such as keeping medications, needles, and syringes secure and away from children and pets.

Documentation
- Document information according to Medication Guidelines: Steps to Follow for All Medications (Regardless of Type or Route).
- Document related patient assessment findings, such as the appearance of the IV site and patient complaints of pain or discomfort during the administration.

Thinking About the Procedure

▶ Go to the videos **Using a Piggyback Administration Set With a Gravity Infusion, Using a Piggyback Administration Set With an Infusion Pump,** and **Using a Volume-Control Administration Set,** along with questions and suggested responses, available on the Davis's *Nursing Skills Videos* Web site at www.fadavis.com.

Practice Resources
Gorski et al. (2021); Hamilton (2019).

PROCEDURE 23-18 ■ Administering Medication Through a Central Venous Access Device (CVAD)

▶ For steps to follow in *all* procedures, refer to the Universal Steps for All Procedures on the inside back cover. Also refer to Medication Guidelines: Steps to Follow for All Medications (Regardless of Type or Route).

Equipment

See Figures 23-36A (Implantable device) and 23-36B (Multilumen catheter with blunt cannula, split septum, needleless access device).

- Syringe appropriate for medication volume (10 mL or larger)

  ✚ *Use of syringes smaller than 10 mL when flushing a CVAD can cause increase pressure and may rupture the CVAD.*

- Needleless device or safety syringe with a filter needle for drawing up the medication (you would also need a sterile needle for injection)
- Two syringes for the flush solution
  - Saline or heparin flush solution, as prescribed; research found little evidence to conclude heparin was more effective than saline flush for CVC maintenance (IHI, 2020; López-Briz et al., 2018; Sharma et al., 2019; Zhong et al., 2017)
- Prep pad: CHG–alcohol combination product or appropriate antiseptic solution and gauze pad
- One pair nonsterile procedure gloves

Preprocedure Assessment

- Carefully palpate the area around the insertion site through the dressing. If the patient has tenderness, assess further for other signs of infection. Check the surrounding catheter insertion site for intact sutures, redness, swelling, warmth, or drainage.
  This can indicate catheter-related infection.
- Assess the patient's external chest wall for engorged veins at the surface of the skin. If the jugular's site is used, also assess for difficulty moving the neck or jaw, headache, or ear pain.
  This can indicate vein thrombosis.
- PICC line sites should be observed daily for swelling, tenderness, drainage, or streaking. Take site measurements at regular intervals during dressing changes and compare to preinsertion arm circumference.
  May indicate problems with phlebitis and/or catheter sepsis.
- Conduct a comprehensive pain assessment, looking for unusual pain or discomfort.
  Pain can be associated with the catheter's position in the vein, especially if the line is not in an optimal position.

▶ When performing the procedure, always identify your patient according to agency policy, using two identifiers, and be attentive to standard precautions, hand hygiene, patient safety and privacy, body mechanics, and documentation.

Procedure Steps

1. **Prepare the medication.**
   a. Check compatibility of the medication with the existing IV infusion.
   b. ✚ Verify the medication that can safely be administered through a central site. Double-check the infusion rate as well.
      Some medication might be incompatible with infusion solution or additives. Because dosage may be different for medications given centrally versus peripherally, and because the medication enters the heart almost instantly, any error is potentially life threatening.
   c. Draw up the medication using a needleless device or needle with a filter. Then change to a sterile safety needle or needleless device for administering the medication.
      Filter needles prevent small particles from entering into the line.
   d. Recap any needles throughout, using a needle-capping device or approved one-handed technique that has a low risk of contaminating the sterile needle (see Procedure 23-10B).
      Recapping prevents needlestick injury and, performed correctly, maintains the sterility of the needle.
   e. Dilute the medication, if needed. Fill the medication syringe to the exact volume to be infused; expel excess volume.
   f. Label the syringe with the contents, including medication name, dilution, time to be administered, route, and name of person constituting the medication.
      Excess volume of medication in the syringe is a risk for inadvertent overdosing.

2. **Flush the line.**
   a. Obtain heparinized or saline solution for flushing the CVAD, following the institution's protocol or the prescription.
      The usual concentration for heparin is 10 to 100 units/mL of solution for adults. The recommended volume of flush varies by institution. Most facilities recommend 3 to 5 mL of solution to flush the catheter, although some are flushed with 10 mL. Some medication might be incompatible with infusion solution or additives.

      ✚ *Dosage for centrally administered drugs is critical because the medication enters the heart almost instantly, so any error is potentially life threatening.*

Using heparin flush in venous access devices is becoming more controversial because of the potential for heparin-induced thrombocytopenia. Be sure to follow the manufacturer's guidelines, prescriber's prescription, and the policy of your institution.

b. Before flushing the CVAD, examine the syringe for bubbles. Remove them by flicking the syringe. Eject the air and bubbles, but be sure you have enough flush solution remaining in the syringe.
Flicking causes the bubbles to rise to the top. Remove bubbles from the syringe before giving medication through the CVAD port to avoid injecting air into the patient's vein and causing an embolus.

c. With clean procedure gloves, using pressure and friction, vigorously scrub all surfaces of the CVAD connectors as well as the luer-locking threads, and the luer-lock, including the extension "tail," with an alcohol wipe, CHG–alcohol combination product, or other antimicrobial product for at least 15 seconds. Then let it dry for 15 seconds. Do not touch this connector after cleansing.
Antimicrobial swabs reduce the risk of line-related infection by decreasing colonization of the port and tubing.

d. Insert the flush syringe at a vertical (90°) angle into the port using a needleless system or safety syringe.
A 90° angle reduces stress on the access port, which may cause shearing or mechanical trauma to the material.

e. Open the clamp between the syringe and the patient.
The clamp between the access port and the tubing that goes to the patient must be patent for medication to be injected through the CVAD.

f. Check for blood return, if necessary. Equipment differs regarding the need to aspirate, so follow agency protocols.
In some administration systems, aspiration is one indication that catheter placement is in the vein.

g. Inject saline or heparinized flush solution into the line, per agency protocol or provider's orders and type of catheter. Some catheter types (e.g., Groshong) do not require heparin in the flush solution. *Flush slowly when using a pre-filled flush syringe.* Close the clamp.
Saline or heparin flush is used, depending on the type of CVAD, institutional protocol, and manufacturer recommendations.

- Saline is generally indicated when simple clearing of the line is needed.
- If blood is likely to backflow into the line, then heparin might be used in the flush solution to reduce the risk of clot formation.
- Most often heparin is used for implanted CVADs to reduce the risk of occlusion from a clot forming on the device.
- Different catheters require different volumes of flush solutions. Some are more prone to clot formation, depending on whether they are open- or closed-system devices. The initial flush maintains patency of the line and removes any heparin that was left if the catheter was used previously.

h. Never force the flush solution into the venous access device if you feel resistance. Look for a closed clamp on the catheter or tubing. Check to see if an inline filter is clogged.
Forcing fluid creates a risk of rupturing the catheter.

i. Disconnect the flush syringe.

CAUTION: Techniques of flushing and clamping may vary depending on the type of connector you are using. Consult agency protocols and manufacturer's instructions.

If using a needleless connector, in general, do the following:

If Using Negative Fluid Displacement Device
Use a positive-pressure technique:
- For a blunt cannula with split septum, or mechanical valve, withdraw the cannula before the syringe is completely empty, keeping your thumb on the syringe plunger.
- For a mechanical valve device with negative displacement, maintain pressure on the syringe plunger, close the clamp on the IV line between the needleless connector and the patient, and then disconnect the syringe.

If Using a Positive Fluid Displacement Device
Do not use a positive-pressure technique. Flush using a push-pause technique. Wait 10 seconds (or per manufacture guidelines) to allow fluid displacement to occur. Remove syringe, and only then may you clamp the catheter.
The positive-pressure technique would keep the internal mechanism from functioning properly.

For Neutral Fluid Displacement Devices
Any flushing technique can be used. The clamping and disconnecting sequence does not matter.
The clamping sequence is directly dependent on the needleless connector being used and is critical for the final locking solution.

j. After removing the flush syringe from the port, discard it into a safety disposal container.

3. **Administer medication** through the CVAD.
   a. Scrub all surfaces of the external ports, tubing, and connectors with a CHG–alcohol combination product for at least 15 seconds. Allow the port to dry for 15 more seconds or follow manufacturer's guidelines.
   Antimicrobial swabs reduce the risk of line-related infection by decreasing colonization of the port and tubing.
   b. Close the clamp to the infusion if a primary IV is running.
   The medication could travel back up the line rather than infuse into the patient if the clamp is open.
   c. Inject medication into the port, according to the medication prescription (infusion time).
   Some medication is infused as a bolus; other medication is given over time.

(continued on next page)

Procedure 23-18 ■ Administering Medication Through a Central Venous Access Device (CVAD) (continued)

4. **After scrubbing all surfaces** of the port again with a CHG–alcohol product or other approved antiseptic, administer the second syringe of flush solution.
   The flush prevents incompatible medication or fluid from mixing at later administrations and ensures that all of the medication clears the catheter and enters the bloodstream. Flush slowly when using a prefilled flush syringe.

5. **Clamp the tubing** between the syringe and the CVAD port. If there is an infusing primary IV, make sure the tubing is open between the IV fluid and the patient.

? What if...

- **My patient is a child; how should I secure the line?**

  Dress infants and younger children in a one-piece undershirt that fastens between the legs and tape the line to the shirt, leaving a little bit of slack to allow for movement.

- **The line does not flush easily?**
  - Make sure all clamps are unclamped.
  - Check to see if the central line is kinked or twisted.
  - After straightening lines, attempt to flush the central line again. If the flush solution cannot be injected easily from the syringe into the CVAD, do not force the flush. *Too much flush pressure may dislodge a clot that has formed in the central line.*
  - Check to see if an inline filter is clogged.
  - Assess the insertion site to see if the stabilization device or dressing may be causing the occlusion.
  - Try to reposition the patient to lying down and turned to one side.
  - You might also have the patient lift their arms above their head and then attempt to flush the central line.
  - If it is still difficult to flush after repositioning, notify the provider.

- **The central line inadvertently comes out?**

  Hold firm, constant pressure on the site to control bleeding. Have a colleague notify the provider immediately.

- **The central line is cracked or leaking?**

  Close the clamp between the break or leakage in the line and the patient's line insertion site. Wrap an alcohol wipe and gauze around the broken part of the line. Immediately change the tubing.

- **The clamp on the line is broken?**

  Change the tubing. Ensure the clamp works properly on the new tubing. This is essential for patient safety.

- **The central line gets caught on or pulled by the patient's clothing?**

  Loop the tubing over the dressing and secure with tape.

- **My patient is short of breath or complains of chest pain?**

  Notify the provider immediately. *These symptoms could be a sign of fluid overload or other complications, such as a dislodged clot or embolism.*

- **My patient feels pain in the neck or ear on the side where an implantable CVAD is located? Or the patient hears swishing noises or has palpitations?**

  Notify the provider immediately. *In this case, the implanted device might be dislodged. Placement must be confirmed by x-ray.*

- **My patient complains of nausea, changes in appetite, or other disturbances in odor and taste after the CVAD is flushed?**

  Educate the patient that this may be due to the use of a prefilled syringe used for flushing and that these are not permanent sensations/changes. *Substances from the plastic syringe due to the sterilization methods may be the causative factor (Gorski et al., 2021).*

Patient Evaluation

- Monitor for signs of catheter complications (e.g., shortness of breath, chest pain, and palpitations).
- Monitor for signs of catheter dislodgement (e.g., neck swelling or pain, bleeding at the site or within the line, palpitations, or gurgling noise).
- Assess for signs of catheter-related infection (e.g., fever, increased WBC count, redness, warmth at the site).
- Observe for leaking or blood backup at the injection ports, tubing connections, and the site.
- Observe for bleeding at the CVAD site.
- Assess for signs of allergic response or adverse effects to medication.

Patient Teaching

- Teach patients, families, and caregivers that the overall goal is to maintain a patent CVAD or PICC line that is free of infection, occlusion, or dislodgement.
- Avoid obtaining blood pressure readings in the arm where a PICC line is inserted.
- If a PICC line is in place, do not immerse the arm in water. The patient may shower if the site is covered by an occlusive dressing.
- Follow prescribed activity restrictions.
- Teach signs of catheter complications including line-related infection, thrombosis, and accidental dislodgement.
- Teach signs of catheter dislodgement to include pain or swelling in the neck or area near the ear of the affected side of the CVAD. Gurgling sounds might also indicate a problem with the placement of the CVAD.

Home Care

- The goals of home care for a patient receiving medication through a CVAD or PICC line are medication safety and maintaining an infection-free line.
- Candidates for home IV therapy through a CVAD or PICC line are those who:
  - Have a family member or other caregiver who can competently provide or assist with care of the line.
  - Have telephone access—either via landline or via cell phone.
  - Have access to reliable transportation in case of a line-related emergency.
  - Have caregivers who are able to read instructions for home care.
- Procedures in the home environment are similar to those for the hospital setting, except clean technique is used instead of sterile.
- Home health supplies may be different than the ones used in the hospital.
- After discharge, follow-up care in the home environment is important to ensure safety.

Documentation

- Document any signs of allergic response to or adverse effects of medication.
- Note any signs of catheter complications or dislodgement.
- Document signs of catheter-related infection.
- Document the date and time tubing and port cap are changed.
- Document all medications infused through the CVAD.

Thinking About the Procedure

Go to the videos **Administering Medication Through a Central Venous Access Device,** along with questions and suggested responses, available on the **Davis's *Nursing Skills Videos*** Web Site at www.fadavis.com.

Practice Resources
Gorski (2018); Gorski et al. (2021).

PracticalKnowledge
clinical application

CLINICAL INSIGHTS

Clinical Insight 23-1 ▸ Taking Action After a Medication Error

✚ First, check the patient. Take their vital signs and perform assessments related to the medication that was given. Note any changes from previous assessments

- If you are unfamiliar with the side effects of the medication, consult a drug reference source.
- Verify that you have made a medication error, and identify the type of error.
- Notify the charge nurse of the error. Request guidance if this is your first error.
- Notify the prescriber and follow the prescriptions for intervention.
- Document in the medical record that the medication was given, but do not indicate that it was given in error. This alerts anyone reviewing the records that an error was made.

- Complete an incident report according to the facility's policies. Ask for assistance if you are unfamiliar with the format or requirement of this form. It is important that the information you provide be factual and accurate.
- **Key Point:** *Do not document in the patient's medical record that an incident report was filed. This alerts anyone reviewing the record that an error was made and makes the incident report available for legal review in the event of a lawsuit.*

♥ **iCare** ▪ When you are calmer and can think clearly, critically reflect on the error. Identify the influences that led to the error. Were you rushed? Did you check the prescription? Did you follow the rights of medication? Whatever the reason, use this situation as a learning experience to improve your practice.

Clinical Insight 23-2 ➤ Using Prefilled Unit-Dose Systems

Prefilled systems are commonly used in a variety of healthcare settings and in self-administration.

Technique

1. Check each medication cartridge and dose carefully, because all of the cartridges look alike.
2. No medication preparation is necessary.
3. Insert the cartridge into the holder.
4. Swing or twist the plunger into place, depending on the type of syringe you use. Lock it securely at the needle end.
5. Attach the plunger, if necessary. (The system may come with plunger attached.) ▼

6. Expel air and excess medication.
7. Don gloves.
8. Administer the medication.
9. Dispose of the empty cartridge. Some types are available for reuse.

Technique Variations

The needle gauge or length is not correct for the patient. You can transfer the medication into a regular disposable syringe, maintaining sterile technique. There are two ways you can do it.

Cartridge without removable needle:
1. Pull back on the plunger of the regular disposable syringe and keep a capped, sterile needle ready.
2. Insert the cartridge needle through the open tip of the disposable syringe.
3. Eject the medication into the regular syringe.
4. Replace the capped needle onto the regular syringe.
5. Eject the air and check for the correct dosage.

Cartridge with removable needle:
The capped needle can be removed from some prefilled cartridges, allowing the cartridge to be used as a vial. This allows you to safely draw the medications into a different (disposable) syringe, using a vial access device or safety needle. Do not inject air into a cartridge, because the excess pressure may eject the movable bottom. ▼

Clinical Insight 23-3 ➤ Reconstituting Medication

1. **Remove the caps of both the medication and diluent vials.**
2. **If a multidose vial is used, scrub the tops of both vials** with alcohol or other antiseptic wipe.
   To clean the cap of dust and reduce the number of microorganisms.
3. **Attach a VAD to the syringe.**
4. **Draw up the diluent into the syringe.**
   a. Draw air into the syringe in a volume equal to the amount of diluent you will be withdrawing.
   b. Insert the VAD needle carefully through the center of the rubber cap and, keeping the bevel of the needle (or cannula) above the diluent, inject the air.
   The air prevents negative pressure inside the vial when you withdraw the diluent, allowing you to withdraw the diluent easily. Keeping bevel above diluent helps prevent bubbles.
   c. Withdraw the diluent in the specified amount, holding the syringe at eye level.
   d. Pull a little more air out of the vial and withdraw the needle from the vial. Remove the extra air from the diluent.
   This depressurization technique prevents the diluent from squirting out when the needle is removed from the vial.
5. **Inject diluent into the medication vial** by inserting the VAD carefully through the center of the rubber cap and then injecting the diluent. ▼

6. Remove and recap the VAD (see Procedure 23-10A). Alternatively, you can place the syringe and VAD on a sterile field (e.g., the wrapper the syringe came in).

7. **Mix the medication, taking care not to create bubbles** (e.g., roll, do not shake, the vial). ▼

8. **Reinsert the VAD.** Add air equal to the amount of medication to be withdrawn, inject the air into the vial, and withdraw the reconstituted medication into the syringe. Use the depressurization technique.
9. **Replace the VAD** with a sterile needle of the appropriate size before measuring the medication.
   This ensures that the dose is correct and minimizes discomfort. It also prevents tracking of medication through the tissues. You should not eject fluid through a filter needle since it is used to filter out particulates.
10. **Hold the syringe vertically, and carefully eject all air** from the syringe, but do not eject the medication. Read the dosage.
11. **If necessary, hold the syringe horizontally to eject unneeded medication** from the syringe to reach the prescribed dose.

Clinical Insight 23-4 ▶ Measuring Dosage When Changing Needles

Using a Nonfilter Needle
When drawing medication from a multidose vial, you may sometimes need to use two regular needles. Alternatively, you may use a needleless reconstitution device that is designed with a dispensing spike instead of a needle on one end and a luer-lock port on the other end that attaches to the syringe.

Equipment
One needle (or needless reconstitution device) for drawing up the medication, and one needle for injecting the medication into the patient.

1. **Using needle 1, draw up the prescribed amount of medication.** When using a vial, inject air into the air pocket within the vial. Then withdraw the correct amount of medication from the vial. Be sure to keep the tip of the needle in the fluid to avoid aspirating air bubbles into the syringe.
2. **Remove bubbles; eject the air.** After drawing up the medication, tap on the barrel of the syringe to remove air bubbles, if necessary. Then eject the air from the syringe (keeping the syringe vertical) while retaining the correct amount of medication in the syringe. Check the volume closely at eye level.
3. **Remove needle 1 and discard it** into a needle-safe container. Put on a fresh needle (needle 2) for injection.
4. **Using needle 2,** pull back on the plunger and draw an extra 0.2 mL of air to account for the air within the needle.
5. **Check the medication dosage.** Your plunger should be 0.2 mL more than the prescribed dose.
6. **Still using needle 2, when you inject the patient,** they will receive the correct dose. The air will drive the medication from the needle into the patient's tissues. This is important when giving irritating medications, such as iron. (This is called an air lock.) ▼

Steps 1 and 2 Withdraw medication. Eject air.
Step 3 Change needle.
Step 4 Pull back medication to clear needle of medication.
Step 5 Give injection.

Nonfilter needles

Using a Filter Needle
Always use a filter needle to withdraw medications, if one is available. You must change needles to give the injection because:
- Filter needles are large. To give the injection, you must use a needle of the correct gauge and length.
- You should not push medication out of the syringe through the filter needle because it can break the filter and release glass and other fragments. However, you cannot measure dosage accurately with air in the syringe.

In the following method, pulling air into the syringe allows for exact dosage when the medication is injected. When ejected, the air will clear the needle so that the patient receives all the medication that is in the syringe.

Equipment
One filter needle (or filter cannula) and one regular needle.
1. **With the filter needle (or cannula), withdraw** the exact amount of medication, keeping the syringe vertical as needed to obtain the correct dose. Remember, you must not eject fluid through the filter needle.
2. **Pull back on the plunger to withdraw all the medication from the filter needle (or filter cannula) into the syringe.** Depending on the size of the access cannula, this may be as much as 0.2 mL. It will now appear that you have more than the prescribed dose in the syringe (but you do not; the air is taking up some of the space).

Clinical Insight 23-4 ▶ Measuring Dosage When Changing Needles—cont'd

3. **Change to the needle you will use for injection.** Needle 2 has air in it instead of medication.
4. **Hold the syringe vertically, and eject air** until you see a drop of medication at the tip of the needle ("drop to the top").
5. **Measure the medication.** It should be at the correct syringe marking. If it is not, then tip the syringe horizontally, and eject the medication until the dose is correct.
6. **When you inject the patient, they will receive the correct dose** even though some medication will remain in the needle.
7. **If you are giving an irritating medication** (e.g., iron), draw 0.2 mL of air into the syringe before giving the injection. (This is called an air lock.) ▼

Step 1 Withdraw medication. Eject air.
≈ 0.2 mL medication
1.0 mL medication

Step 2 Pull back plunger to clear needle of medication.
≈ 0.2 mL air
0.2 mL medication from needle
1.0 mL medication

Step 4 Eject air.
≈ 0.2 mL medication
1.0 mL medication

Step 6 Give injection.
1.0 mL medication to patient
≈ 0.2 mL medication left in needle

Filter needles.

Clinical Insight 23-5 ▶ Mixing Two Kinds of Insulin in One Syringe

What You Should Know
Various combinations of rapid-acting, intermediate-acting, and long-acting insulin may be prescribed. Some can be mixed; some cannot. ✚ Insulins may come premixed from the pharmacy to minimize the possibility of error. If your agency requires you to mix insulins, carefully follow each step as outlined.

- Lente insulins (Lente and Lantus) can be mixed with each other, but not with neutral protamine Hagedorn (NPH).
- Even though they are compatible, do not mix Lente with regular insulin, except for patients who are already controlled on this mixture. Lente will bind with regular insulin, delaying the onset of action.
- A general rule is "clear before cloudy." Regular insulin is clear; all other types are cloudy. Therefore, you would draw up regular insulin into the syringe before Lente or NPH insulin, which are modified. If you draw up a modified type first, the needle may transfer it into the unmodified (regular) vial.

What You Should Do
Follow these steps when drawing up insulin from two vials into one syringe. The procedure assumes you are mixing regular (unmodified) insulin with a modified (e.g., NPH) insulin. NOTE: If regular insulin is cloudy, do not use it. Return it to the pharmacy.

1. **Maintain sterile technique throughout.**
2. **Before preparing the insulin**—Rotate the vials between the palms of your hands for at least 1 minute, and invert them to ensure an adequate concentration. Do not shake the vials because this can create bubbles, which take up space and make it difficult to measure the dose precisely.
3. **Scrub vial stoppers** with alcohol or other antiseptic (they are usually multidose vials).

(Continued)

Clinical Insight 23-5 ▸ Mixing Two Kinds of Insulin in One Syringe—cont'd

4. **Inject air into "cloudy" vial**—Using an insulin syringe and needle, inject an amount of air equal to the amount of insulin to be withdrawn from the vial of modified insulin (cloudy vial). Do not allow the needle tip to touch the insulin.
5. **Inject air into "clear" vial**—Using the same syringe, inject the appropriate amount of air into the vial of regular insulin (clear vial).
6. **Withdraw insulin from "clear" vial**—Do not withdraw the needle; withdraw the correct dose of regular insulin.
7. **Measure the dose of "clear"**—Remove the syringe from the regular insulin. Eject air and remove all air bubbles to measure the correct dose.
8. **Calculate combined dose**—Calculate the total amount on the syringe that the combined types of insulin should measure.
9. **Withdraw insulin from "cloudy" vial.**
   a. Return to the (first) vial of modified insulin (cloudy) and draw the correct dose into the syringe. (For example, if you have 5 units of regular insulin in the syringe and you need 10 units of NPH, the plunger should be at the 15-unit mark when you have drawn up the NPH.)
   b. Recall that you have already added air to this vial in a previous step. Draw up the medication slowly and exactly to the total dose, being very careful not to create bubbles and to withdraw only the amount needed. You cannot return any excess to the vial because it is now a mixture of two medications.

10. **Administer the insulin mixture** within 5 minutes after preparation. Even NPH insulin will bind with regular insulin and delay the onset of its action. ▼

Step 4 Inject air (cloudy insulin vial).
Step 5 Inject air (clear insulin vial).
Step 6 Withdraw dose (clear vial).
Step 9 Withdraw dose (cloudy vial).

Total dose is mixture of clear and cloudy insulins.

Total dose is a mixture of clear and cloudy insulins.

Clinical Insight 23-6 ▸ Administering Anticoagulant Medication Subcutaneously

Because of the anticoagulant properties of heparin and enoxaparin (Lovenox), you will need to adapt your technique for subcutaneous injections in the following ways:
- Enoxaparin-prefilled syringes and graduated prefilled syringes are available with a system that shields the needle after injection.
- Use a ⅜-inch 25- or 26-gauge needle.
- After drawing up the correct dose, add 0.2 mL of air to the syringe.
  To ensure that all of the medication is injected into the subcutaneous (subQ) tissue and is not tracked into the superficial tissue.
- Do not expel the air bubble from the syringe before the injection.
  To avoid the loss of drug when using prefilled syringes.
- With your nondominant hand, pinch or spread the skin; insert the needle at a 90° angle, using your dominant hand.
  - If the patient has very little subcutaneous tissue, use a ⅝-inch needle and insert it at a 45° angle.
- Introduce the whole length of the needle into a skinfold held between the thumb and forefinger; hold the skinfold throughout the injection.
- Alternate administration among sites on the abdomen. Give the injection subQ deep on the abdomen, at least 2 inches away from the umbilicus.
- Do not aspirate before injecting.
  This can traumatize tissue and cause bruising.
- Do not massage the site after injecting.
  This can cause bleeding and bruising. It may also cause the heparin to be absorbed more rapidly than desired.
- Keep a record of the sites used. Most agencies have a chart of the body on which to record the sites injected.
- ✚ Several mix-ups between heparin and insulin have been reported. To help avoid this, in addition to observing the three checks and six rights:
  1. Do not store heparin and insulin vials beside each other.
  2. Have another RN check your preparation before administering IV heparin or insulin.
  3. Think critically (e.g., ask yourself if giving heparin or insulin makes sense given the patient's diagnosis).
  4. Remember that heparin and insulin syringes are different.

TABLES: ABBREVIATIONS

Common Medication-Related Abbreviations

ABBREVIATION	EXPLANATION	ABBREVIATION	EXPLANATION
Ac	before meals: example 0700, 1100, 1700 hours	p.m.	evening
		po or PO	by mouth
ad lib	as desired	prn	as needed
a.m.	morning	qh, (q1h, q1hr)	every hour
bid	twice a day: example 0900, 2100 hours	q2h, q2hr	every 2 hours: example 0800, 1000, 1200 hours, etc.
c̄	with	q3h, q3hr	every 3 hours: example 0900, 1200, 1500 hours, etc.
fl oz	fluid ounce		
g, gm, or GM	gram	q4h, q4hr	every 4 hours: example 0200, 0600, 1000, 1400, 1800, 2200 hours
gtt	drop		
h, hr	hour	q6h, q6hr	every 6 hours: example 0600, 1200, 1800, 2400 hours
IM	intramuscular		
IV	intravenous	qid or QID	four times a day: example 1000, 1400, 1800, 2200
IVPB	intravenous piggyback	qs	sufficient quantity
Kg or kg	kilogram	s̄	without
KVO	keep vein open	stat or STAT	at once
L or l	liter	sup or supp	suppository
mEq	milliequivalent	susp	suspension
mL or mL	milliliter	tab	tablet
OTC	over the counter	Tbsp	tablespoon
oz	ounce	tid or tid	three times a day: example 1000, 1400, 1800 hours
pc	after meals: example 0900, 1300, 1900 hours		
		T or tsp	teaspoon

Table Institute for Safe Medication Practices (ISMP) List of Error-Prone Abbreviations, Symbols, and Dose Designations

Abbreviations for Doses/Measurement Units

ABBREVIATIONS	INTENDED MEANING	MISINTERPRETATION	CORRECTION
Cc	Cubic centimeter	Mistaken as u (units).	Use "mL."
IU**	International unit(s)	Mistaken as IV (intravenous) or the number 10.	Use "unit(s)." IU can be expressed as "units."
L	Liter	Mistaken as the number 1.	Use "L" (uppercase) for liter.
Ml	Milliliter	Lowercase l mistaken as the number 1.	Use "mL" for milliliter.
MM or M	Million	Mistaken as thousand. M is the roman number for thousand.	Use "million."
M or K	Thousand	M has been used to abbreviate million and thousand.	Use "thousand."
Ng or ng	Nonagram	Mistaken as mg. Mistaken as nasogastric.	Use "nanogram" or "nanog."
U or u	Unit(s)	Mistaken as the number 0 or 4, causing a 10-fold overdose or greater (e.g., 4U seen as "40" or 4u seen as "44"); mistaken as "cc" so dose given in volume instead of units (e.g., 4u seen as 4cc).	Use "unit."
mcg	Microgram	Mistaken as "mg."	Use "mcg."

Abbreviations for Routes of Administration

ABBREVIATIONS	INTENDED MEANING	MISINTERPRETATION	CORRECTION
AD, AS, AU	Right ear, left ear, each ear	Mistaken as OD, OS, OU (right eye, left eye, each eye).	Use "right ear," "left ear," or "each ear."
IN	Intranasal	Mistaken as "IM" or "IV."	Use "intranasal" or "NAS."
IT	Intrathecal	Mistaken as intratracheal, intratumor, intratympanic, or inhalation therapy.	Use "intrathecal."
OD, OS, OU	Right eye, left eye, each eye	Mistaken as AD, AS, AU (right ear, left ear, each ear).	Use "right eye," "left eye," or "each eye."
per os	By mouth, orally	The "os" can be mistaken as "left eye" (OS-oculus sinister).	Use "PO," "by mouth," or "orally."
SC, SQ, subQ, or sub q	Subcutaneous(ly)	SC and sc mistaken as SL (sublingual); SQ mistaken as "5 every"; the "q" in "sub q" has been mistaken as "every" (e.g., a heparin dose prescribed sub q 2 hours before surgery), misunderstood as "every 2 hours."	Use "SUBQ" or spell out "subcutaneous(ly)."

Table Institute for Safe Medication Practices (ISMP) List of Error-Prone Abbreviations, Symbols, and Dose Designations—cont'd

Abbreviations for Frequency/Instructions for Use

ABBREVIATIONS	INTENDED MEANING	MISINTERPRETATION	CORRECTION
BT	Bedtime	Mistaken as "bid" (twice daily).	Use "bedtime."
HS	Half-strength	Mistaken as bedtime.	Use "half-strength."
hs	At bedtime, hours of sleep	Mistaken as half-strength.	Use "bedtime" or "HS" (ALL UPPERCASE letters).
i/d	One daily	Mistaken as "tid."	Use "1 daily."
o.d. or OD	Once daily	Mistaken as "right eye" (OD-oculus dexter), leading to oral liquid medications administered in the eye.	Use "daily."
*Q.D., QD, q.d., or qd	Every day	Mistaken as q.i.d., especially if the period after the "q" or the tail of the "q" is misunderstood as an "i."	Use "daily."
Qhs, qhs	Nightly at bedtime	Mistaken as "qhr" or every hour.	Use "nightly" or "HS."
Qn, Qn	Nightly or at bedtime	Mistaken as "qh" (every hour).	Use "nightly" or "at bedtime" or "HS."
*Q.O.D., q.o.d. or qod, QOD	Every other day	Mistaken as "q.d." (daily) or "q.i.d." (4 times daily) if the "o" is poorly written.	Use "every other day."
q1d	Daily	Mistaken as q.i.d. (4 times daily).	Use "daily."
q6PM, etc.	Every evening at 6 PM	Mistaken as every 6 hours.	Use "6 PM nightly" or "6 PM daily."
Ss	Sliding-scale (insulin)	Mistaken as "55."	Spell out "sliding scale"; use "one-half."
SSRI	Sliding-scale regular insulin	Mistaken as selective-serotonin reuptake inhibitor.	Spell out "sliding scale (insulin)."
SSI	Sliding-scale insulin	Mistaken as strong solution of iodine (Lugol's).	Spell out "sliding scale (insulin)."
TIW or tiw	3 times a week	Mistaken as "3 times a day" or "twice in a week."	Use "3 times weekly."
BIW or biw	2 times a week	Mistaken as 2 times a day.	Use "2 times weekly."
UD	As directed ("ut dictum")	Mistaken as unit dose (e.g., diltiazem 125 mg IV infusion "UD" misinterpreted as meaning to give the entire infusion as a unit [bolus] dose).	Write out "Use as directed."

Miscellaneous Abbreviations Associated With Medications

ABBREVIATIONS	INTENDED MEANING	MISINTERPRETATION	CORRECTION
D/C	Discharge or discontinue	Premature discontinuation of medications if D/C (intended to mean "discharge") has been misinterpreted as "discontinued" when followed by a list of discharge medications.	Use "discharge" and "discontinue."
IJ	Injection	Mistaken as "IV" or "intrajugular."	Use "injection."
OJ	Orange juice	Mistaken as OD or OS (right or left eye); drugs meant to be diluted in orange juice may be given in the eye.	Use "orange juice."

(Continued)

Table Institute for Safe Medication Practices (ISMP) List of Error-Prone Abbreviations, Symbols, and Dose Designations—cont'd

Apothecary or Household Abbreviations

ABBREVIATIONS	INTENDED MEANING	MISINTERPRETATION	CORRECTION
gr	Grain(s)	Mistaken as gram.	Use the metric system (e.g., mcg, g).
dr	Dram(s)	Mistaken as doctor.	Use the metric system (e.g., mL).
min	Minim(s)	Mistaken as minutes.	Use the metric system (e.g., mL).
oz	Ounce(s)	Mistaken as zero or O_2.	Use the metric system (e.g., mL).
tsp	Teaspoon(s)	Mistaken as tablespoon(s).	Use the metric system (e.g., mL).
Tbsp or tbsp	Tablespoon(s)	Mistaken as teaspoon(s).	Use the metric system (e.g., mL).

Dose Designation or Other Information

DOSE DESIGNATIONS OR OTHER INFORMATION	INTENDED MEANING	MISINTERPRETATION	CORRECTION
½ tablet	Half tablet	1 or 2 tablets.	Use text ("half tablet") or reduced font-size fractions ("½ tablet").
Roman numerals used for doses (e.g., V)	5	Mistaken as a designated letter V or the wrong numeral (e.g., 10 instead of 5).	Use only Arabic numerals (e.g., "1," "5") to write doses.
*Trailing zero after decimal point (e.g., 1.0 mg)	1 mg	Mistaken as 10 mg if the decimal point is not seen expressed in whole numbers.	Do not use trailing zeros for doses.
*No leading zero before a decimal dose (e.g., .5 mg)	0.5 mg	Mistaken as 5 mg if the decimal point is not seen.	Use zero before a decimal point when the dose is less than a whole unit.
Drug name and drug dose run together (especially problematic for drug names that end in "l" e.g., Inderal 40 mg)	Inderal 40 mg Tegretol 300 mg	Mistaken as Inderal 140 mg. Mistaken as Tegretol 1300 mg.	Place adequate space between the drug name, dose, and unit of measurement.
Ratio expression of a strength of a single-entity injectable drug product (e.g., Epinephrine 1:1,000; 1:10,000; 1:100,000)	1:1,000—contains 1 mg/mL 1:10,000—contains 0.1 mg/mL 1:100,000—contains 0.01 mg/mL	Mistaken as wrong strength.	Write out the strength using quantity per total volume (e.g., 0.5 mg/mL)
Numeric dose and unit of measurement run together (e.g., 10 mg)	10 mg	The "m" can be mistaken for a zero, leading to a 10-fold dosing error.	Place adequate space between the drug name, dose, and unit of measurement.

Table Institute for Safe Medication Practices (ISMP) List of Error-Prone Abbreviations, Symbols, and Dose Designations—cont'd

DOSE DESIGNATIONS OR OTHER INFORMATION	INTENDED MEANING	MISINTERPRETATION	CORRECTION
Abbreviations such as mg. or mL. with a period after the abbreviation	mg or mL	The period is unnecessary and could be mistaken as the number 1 if written poorly.	Use mg, mL, etc. without a period.
Large doses without properly placed commas (e.g., 100000 units or 1000000 units)	100,000 or 1,000,000 units	100000 has been mistaken for 10,000 or 1,000,000; 1,000,000 has been mistaken for 100,000.	Use commas for dosing units at or above 1,000 or use such words as 100 "thousand" or 1 "million" to improve readability.

Drug Name Abbreviations

DRUG NAME ABBREVIATIONS	INTENDED MEANING	MISINTERPRETATION	CORRECTION

✚ **Note:** Pharmacists do not accept prescriptions for abbreviated medications. To prevent errors, do not abbreviate drug names when communicating medical information.

Antiretroviral medications	DOR: doravirine TAF: tenofovir alafenamide TDF: tenofovir disoproxil fumarate	DOR: Dovato (dolutegravir and lamivudine). TAF: tenofovir disoproxil fumarate. TDF: tenofovir alafenamide.	Use complete drug names.
APAP	acetaminophen	Not recognized as acetaminophen.	Use complete drug name.
ARA A	vidarabine	Mistaken as cytarabine (ARA C).	Use complete drug name.
AT II and AT III	AT II: angiotensin II (Giapreza) AT III: antithrombin III (Thrombate III)	AT II (angiotensin II) mistaken as AT III (antithrombin III). AT III (antithrombin III) mistaken as AT II (angiotensin II).	Use complete drug name.
AZT	zidovudine (Retrovir)	Mistaken as azathioprine or aztreonam.	Use the complete drug name.
CPZ	prochlorperazine (Compazine)	Mistaken as chlorpromazine.	Use complete drug name.
DPT	Demerol-Phenergan-Thorazine	Mistaken as diphtheria-pertussis-tetanus.	Use complete drug name.
DTO	Diluted tincture of opium, or deodorized tincture of opium (Paregoric)	Mistaken as tincture of opium.	Use complete drug name.
HCl	hydrochloric acid or hydrochloride	Mistaken as potassium chloride (the "H" is misinterpreted as "K").	Use complete drug name unless expressed as a salt of a drug.
HCT	hydrocortisone	Mistaken as hydrochlorothiazide.	Use complete drug name.
HCTZ	hydrochlorothiazide	Mistaken as hydrocortisone (seen as HCT 250 mg).	Use complete drug name.
*MgSO$_4$	magnesium sulfate	Mistaken as morphine sulfate.	Use complete drug name.
*MS, MSO$_4$	morphine sulfate	Mistaken as magnesium sulfate.	Use complete drug name.
MTX	methotrexate	Mistaken as mitoxantrone.	Use complete drug name.

(Continued)

Table Institute for Safe Medication Practices (ISMP) List of Error-Prone Abbreviations, Symbols, and Dose Designations—cont'd

DRUG NAME ABBREVIATIONS	INTENDED MEANING	MISINTERPRETATION	CORRECTION
Na at the beginning of a drug name (e.g., Na bicarbonate)	Sodium bicarbonate	Mistaken as no bicarbonate.	Use complete drug name.
NoAC	Novel/new oral anticoagulant	No anticoagulant.	Use complete drug name.
OXY	Oxytocin	Mistaken as oxycodone, oxycontin.	Use complete drug name.
PNV	Prenatal vitamins	Mistaken as penicillin VK.	Use complete drug name.
PCA	procainamide	Mistaken as patient-controlled analgesia.	Use complete drug name.
PTU	propylthiouracil	Mistaken as mercaptopurine.	Use complete drug name.
T3	Tylenol with codeine No. 3	Mistaken as liothyronine.	Use complete drug name.
TAC	triamcinolone	Mistaken as tetracaine, adrenaline, cocaine.	Use complete drug name.
TNK	TNKase	Mistaken as "TPA."	Use complete drug name.
TPA of tPA	Tissue plasminogen activator, Activase (alteplase)	Mistaken as TNKase (tenecteplase), or less often as another tissue plasminogen activator, Retavase (retaplase).	Use complete drug name.
$ZnSO_4$	zinc sulfate	Mistaken as morphine sulfate.	Use complete drug name.

Stemmed/Coined Drug Names

STEMMED DRUG NAMES	INTENDED MEANING	MISINTERPRETATION	CORRECTION
Levo	Levofloxacin	Mistaken as Levophed (norepinephrine).	Use complete drug name.
"nitro drip"	nitroglycerine infusion	Mistaken as sodium nitroprusside infusion.	Use complete drug name.
"Norflox"	norfloxacin	Mistaken as Norflex.	Use complete drug name.
"IV Vanc"	Intravenous vancomycin	Mistaken as Invanz.	Use complete drug name.

Symbols Used With Medication Administration

SYMBOLS	INTENDED MEANING	MISINTERPRETATION	CORRECTION
ℨ	Dram	Symbol for dram mistaken as "3."	Use the metric system.
ℳ	Minim	Mistaken as "mL."	Use the metric system.
x3d	For 3 days	Mistaken as "3 doses."	Use "for 3 days."
> and <	More than and less than	Mistaken as opposite of intended; mistakenly using incorrect symbols; "<10" mistaken as "40."	Use "more than" or "less than."

Table Institute for Safe Medication Practices (ISMP) List of Error-Prone Abbreviations, Symbols, and Dose Designations—cont'd

SYMBOLS	INTENDED MEANING	MISINTERPRETATION	CORRECTION
↑ and ↓	Increase and decrease	Mistaken as opposite of intended; mistakenly have used the incorrect symbol; ↑ mistaken as the letter T, leading to misinterpretation as the start of a drug name, or mistaken as 4 or 7.	Use increase and decrease.
/ (slash mark)	Separates two doses or indicates "per"	Mistaken as the number 1 (e.g., "25 units/10 units" misread as "25 units and 110" units).	Use "per" rather than a slash mark to separate doses.
@	At	Mistaken as "2."	Use "at."
&	And	Mistaken as "2."	Use "and."
+	Plus or and	Mistaken as "4."	Use "and."
°	Hour	Mistaken as zero (e.g., q2° seen as q 20).	Use "hr," "h," or "hour."
Φ or ⊘	zero, null sign	Mistaken as numerals 4, 6, 8, 9.	Use) or zero, or describe intent using whole words.
#	Pounds	Mistaken as number sign.	Use the metric system (kg or g) rather than pounds. Use lb if referring to pounds.

Sources
Institute for Safe Medication Practices. (2021). *List of error-prone abbreviations, symbols, and dose designations*. https://www.ismp.org/recommendations/error-prone-abbreviations-list
Institute for Safe Medication Practices. (2019). *List of confused drug names*. https://www.ismp.org/recommendations/confused-drug-names-list
Report medication errors and near misses to the ISMP Medication Errors Reporting Program (MERP) at https://www.ismp.org/report-error/merp.
*Listed on The Joint Commission's "Do Not Use" List, effective January 1, 2004.

MEASURING AND CALCULATING DOSAGE

Medications are not always available in the exact dosage the patient needs. Therefore, you must be proficient in calculating drug dosages to be sure your patients receive the correct amount of medication.

Drugs in solid form (e.g., tablets, powders) are measured by weight (e.g., milligrams [mg], grains). Drugs used for irrigation, infusion, and injection are liquids (usually solutions), measured by volume, generally milliliters (mL).

- A *solution* can be either a solid dissolved in a fluid or a given volume of one liquid dissolved in a given volume of another liquid.
- Solution concentrations may be expressed as a proportion. A 1/100 solution is a solution of 1 gram of solid dissolved in 100 mL of fluid, or 1 mL of fluid mixed with 100 mL of another fluid.
- Think of solutions as a quantity of solid drug dissolved in a quantity of liquid diluent. The diluent merely carries the medication. When you see a vial marked "50 mg/mL," for example, you will know this means that in each milliliter (mL) of diluent there are 50 mg (in weight) of the solid, active medication.
- Your task is to determine how many milliliters of liquid you need to give the patient to receive the prescribed milligrams of active drug.

Medication Measurement Systems

Medications are usually prescribed and measured using the metric system; however, a few are still dispensed using the apothecary and household systems. You will sometimes need to make conversions from one measurement system to another.

Metric System. The metric system is the preferred system to measure drug dosage because it promotes accuracy by allowing for calculation of small drug dosages. A disadvantage of this system in the United States is that many people outside the healthcare system are not familiar with it. It contains the following:

- *Meter,* the unit for linear measurement, is a little longer than a yard.
- *Liter,* used for capacity or volume, is a little larger than a quart.
- *Gram,* the unit for weight, is a little more than the weight of a steel paper clip. The following are the metric units you will use in preparing medications.

Weights
  1 mg (milligram) = 1000 mcg or (micrograms)
  1 gm (gram)   = 1000 mg (milligrams)
  1 kg (kilogram)   = 1000 g or gm (grams)

Volume
  1000 mL (milliliters)   = 1 L (liter)
  1000 (cubic centimeters)   = 1 L (liter)

The following are examples of medication prescriptions using the metric system:

- Milk of Magnesia 30 mL orally daily at bedtime
- Cefazolin 1 gm IV q8hr

Apothecary System. The British apothecary system of measurement (Roman or Arabic numerals) has been used in the United States since colonial times. This system uses grains, fractions (e.g., gr ¼) instead of decimals (e.g., 0.25). Only a few medications (e.g., aspirin, phenobarbital) are measured using this system because it is less convenient and less precise. For example, *5 grains* might be written as *grains V* or *gr V*.

➕ To avoid a dosage error, write out the intended unit of measurement (The Joint Commission, 2019a). For example, write grains so gr (grains) is not mistaken for gm (grams).

Key Point: *Keep in mind the apothecary abbreviations are prone to misinterpretation and error because they are not often used.* The following are the units used in preparing medications:

Volume
  1 minim (m)   = 1 drop (gtt)
  1 fluid dram (dr) = 60 minims
  1 fluid ounce (oz) = 8 fluid drams

Weight
  1 dram (dr) = 27.34 grains (gr)
  1 grain   = 60 milligrams (mg)

The following are Roman numerals you will use most often:

  M = 1000   X = 10
  D = 500   V = 5
  C = 100   I = 1
  L = 50   II = 2

The following are examples of medication prescribed using the apothecary system:

Aspirin grains V orally q4hr prn for fever greater than 101°F
Chloramphenicol otic 2 gtts in each ear tid daily

➕ With the exception of drops (gtts), many institutions no longer use the apothecary system of measurement. If it is used, verify the intended dose with the prescriber and pharmacist.

Household System. Although it is easier to teach a patient about home medications using this system (e.g., teaspoons, ounces, cups), nurses do not often use it because drug dosages are less precise and can lead to medication dosing errors. The following are household units of measurement with metric conversion:

Volume
  1 tsp (t)   = 5 mL
  1 tablespoon (tbsp or T)   = 3 teaspoons (tsp) = 15 mL

6 tsp or 2 T	=	1 ounce (oz)	=	30 mL
16 T or 8 oz	=	1 cup (c)	=	240 mL
16 T or 8 oz	=	1 glass	=	240 mL
2 C	=	1 pint (pt)	=	480 mL
2 pt	=	1 quart (qt)	=	946.4 mL
4 qt	=	1 gallon (gal)		

Weight

1 oz	=		=	28.35 gm
16 oz	=	1 pound (lb)	=	0.45 kg

Length

12 inches (in.)	=	1 foot (ft)	=	30.5 cm
3 feet (ft)	=	1 yard (yd)	=	91.4 cm

The following is an example of a medication prescribed using the household system:

Amoxicillin 250 mg per 5 mL; give 1 tsp PO tid

Special Measurements: Units and Milliequivalents

Key Point: *Note that units and mEq cannot be directly converted to the apothecary, metric, or household system.*

Units are used to measure insulin, a drug used by people with diabetes to help control their blood sugar (glucose). The standard strength preparation of insulin is 100 international units (U100). In this strength, 1 mL of the fluid medication contains 100 units of insulin.

Heparin (an anticoagulant) and penicillin (an antibiotic) are also prescribed in units. The following are medications prescribed using units:

NPH insulin 14 units subcutaneous every morning
Heparin 4000 units subcutaneous bid (twice daily)

Key Point: *Be aware that not all units are the same.* For example, 1 mL of heparin does not contain 100 units of heparin. You must always read the container label to know the number of units per milliliter.

Milliequivalents (mEq) indicate the strength of the ion concentration in a drug. A milliequivalent is the number of grams of a solid contained in 1 mL of a solution. Electrolytes, such as potassium chloride (KCl), are measured in mEq. The following are medications prescribed using *mEq*:

KCl 20 mEq orally bid (twice daily)
D_5W 1000 mL with KCl 40 mEq q8hr

Calculating Dosages

You should be able to calculate accurately using several methods and formulas. Inaccurate calculations result in incorrect dosages and could harm the patient.
One easy formula to remember is the following:

$$\frac{\text{Dose on hand}}{\text{Quantity (or volume) on hand}} = \frac{\text{Desired dose}}{\text{Quantity (or volume) desired}}$$

Or

$$\frac{DH}{QH} = \frac{DD}{X}$$

Remember: You must pay attention to *both* the milligrams (weight of the drug) marked on the medication container *and* the milliliters (amount of liquid in which the medication is dissolved). For example, the provider prescribes meperidine (Demerol) 25 mg IM now. You have a prefilled syringe containing meperidine (Demerol) 50 mg in 1 mL volume. How much of the liquid (how many mL) would you administer to the patient?

$$\frac{DH}{QH} = \frac{DD}{X} \text{ or } \frac{50 \text{ mg}}{1 \text{ mL}} = \frac{25 \text{ mg}}{X}$$

Therefore (recalling your algebra),

$$50X = 25 \text{ mL},$$
so X = 25 divided by 50,
so X = 0.5 mL

Here is an alternative formula you can use for calculating dosages:

$$\frac{\text{Dose desired (DD)}}{\text{Dose on hand (DH)}} \times \text{quantity on hand (QH)} = \text{desired quantity}$$

$$\frac{\text{Dose desired (25 mg)}}{\text{Dose on hand (50 mg)}} \times \text{quantity on hand (1 mL)} \times \text{desired quantity}$$

Think Like a Nurse: Clinical Judgment in Action 23-1A

Mr. Pearson (Meet Your Patients, in Volume 1) has been prescribed nifedipine (Procardia XL) 60 mg orally daily. You have available Procardia XL (extended-release nifedipine) 30-mg tablets. Calculate the number of tablets you will need for one dose. Calculate how many tablets you will need in a 24-hour period.

Conversions Within One System

When a drug prescription is written in the same system as the preparation you have on hand, you can easily make conversions. For example, in the metric system, if you want to **convert grams to milligrams,** you simply *multiply* by 1,000 (because 1 g = 1,000 mg). So, if you have 2.5 grams,

$$2.5 \text{ gm} \times 1,000 = 2,500 \text{ mg}$$

To change milligrams to grams, *divide* by 1,000—move the decimal three places to the left. For example, if you wanted to know the equivalent of 250 mg in grams:

You know that 1,000 mg = 1 gm
By dividing: 250 mg ÷ 1,000 mg = 0.25 gm
Or by moving the decimal point three places to the left: 250.0 mg = 0.250 gm

Use exactly the same procedures to convert liters (L) and milliliters (mL). For example, if you wanted to know how many milliliters are the equivalent of 0.25 L:

You know that 1 L = 1,000 mL
By multiplying: 0.25 L × 1,000 = 250 mL
By moving the decimal point three places to the right, 0.250 L = 250 mL (Note that you must add a zero to *have* three places to the right.)

Within the apothecary system or the household system, use the equivalents and follow a similar process of multiplying and dividing. *Note: You cannot just move the decimal in these systems.* For example, suppose you have a dram ii (2-dram) tablet and you need to know how many grains you have (apothecary system). You know that 1 dram = 27.3 grains, so multiply:

2 drams (dr) × 27.3 grains (gr) = 54.6 grain, rounded to 55 grain

In the household system, suppose you have 4 tbsp of a liquid and you need to know what part of a cup that represents. You know that 1 cup = 16 tablespoons, so substitute the equivalent and divide:

16 tbsp = 1 cup

So,

4 tbsp = 16 ÷ 4 = ¼ cup

KnowledgeCheck 23-1A

Lanoxin 0.25 mg orally daily is prescribed for a patient with congestive heart failure. The label on the package you have reads "Lanoxin 0.125 mg" How many tablets will you give? Use the "dose on hand (DOH)" formula.

Conversions Between Systems

You will sometimes need to make conversions from one measurement system to another. For example, you may need to convert pounds to kilograms because many medications are prescribed as "milligrams per kilograms" (e.g., "Give 2 mg per kg of body weight"). The following are the basic methods for converting between systems.

- **Metric and Apothecary—Weights**

Grams and grains
(Memorize: 1 gm = 15 gr)
To convert grams to grains—*multiply* the grams by 15.
To convert grains to grams—*divide* the grains by 15.

Grains and milligrams
(Memorize: 1 gr = 60 mg)
To convert grains to milligrams—*multiply* the grains by 60.
To convert milligrams to grains—*divide* the milligrams by 60.

- **Metric and Apothecary and Household—Liquid Volume**

Liters and ounces
(Memorize: 1 L = 34.4 oz)
To convert liters to ounces—*multiply* the liters by 34.4.
To convert ounces to liters—*divide* the ounces by 34.4.

Ounces and milliliters
(Memorize: 1 ounce = 30 mL)
To convert ounces to milliliters—*multiply* the ounces by 30.
To convert milliliters to ounces—*divide* the milliliters by 30.

Milliliters and drops
(Memorize: 1 mL = 15 drops or 15 minims)
To convert milliliters to minims or drops—*multiply* milliliters by 15.
To convert minims and drops to milliliters—*divide* the minims or drops by 15.

KnowledgeCheck 23-2A

Work the following conversions:

- How many drops are in 4 mL?
- How many milliliters are in 2 oz?
- Convert 16 oz to liters.
- You have 3 gm. How many grains is this?
- You have 10 mg. How many grains is this?

How Should I Calculate Dosage for a Child?

You must be very careful when calculating medication dosages for children and infants. Confusion between pounds and kilograms is a source of dosing error in pediatrics. Most drug references list normal pediatric ranges, which can serve as additional verification.

Key Point: *The standard measurement for pediatric patients is kilograms, and prescriptions for pediatric dosages are usually either calculated by the prescriber or stated in terms of "milligrams per kilogram of body weight."* For example, you might have a prescription for "Erythromycin 30 mg/kg of body weight." You know that 1 kg equals 2.2 lb. and that the child weighs 44 lb.

- Convert the weight to kilograms by dividing 44 by 2.2. The child thus weighs 20 kg.
- Multiply the prescribed dose (30 mg) by body weight (20 kg): 30 mg × 20 kg = 600 mg.
- 600 mg is the dosage for a 20-kg child.

You should rarely need to calculate a child's dosage on the basis of an adult dose, because medication prescriptions should specify the exact dosage for the individual child, and the medication is dispensed using pediatric-specific medication formulations and concentrations. However, if you must calculate a child's dosage, use either the body surface area (BSA) formula by using a Nomogram for children, or Clark's rule for children to verify the safety of pediatric prescriptions.

Nomograms. To find a child's BSA using the nomogram, you must know the child's height and weight. To use a nomogram, you draw a straight line between the child's height (on the left scale) and weight (on the right scale) and note where the lines cross midline.

▶ To see a nomogram example, go to https://www.manuelsweb.com/ped_dose_nomo.htm

Clark's Rule Another formula used in pediatrics to determine safe dosage range is Clark's rule. This rule is mostly used for children ages 2 and younger. The dosing for the drug erythromycin is a good example of how to use this rule. The usual adult dose for erythromycin is 250 to 500 mg. To determine the safe dosage range of erythromycin for a child 2 years and younger, use Clark's rule.

1. Using this formula, you assume that an average adult weighs 150 lb (68 kg) (this is the standard for the rule).

$$\text{Adult dose} \times \frac{\text{child's weight in lb}}{150} = \text{child's dose}$$

2. According to Clark's rule, if the maximum adult dose of erythromycin is 500 mg, then the maximum dose for an infant weighing 15 lb is:

$$500 \times 0.1 = 50 \text{ mg}$$

▶ If you need a Web-based dosage calculator, go to https://www.easycalculation.com/medical/pediatric-dosage-clark-rule.php.

CLINICAL REASONING
Applying the Full-Spectrum Nursing Model

Because these are clinical judgment questions, they usually do not have a single answer. Discuss the questions with your peers—discussion can stimulate critical thinking.

PATIENT SITUATION

Leonard LeMonte is a 57-year-old African American man who has come to his primary care provider because of persistent headaches that increase in intensity over the course of the day. His overall health has been good, although he is approximately 50 to 60 pounds overweight. His medical history is significant for borderline primary hypertension and noninsulin-dependent diabetes, type 2 (diet-controlled). Mr. LeMonte tells you he works in a high-stress environment. He shares with you that he fears losing his job and not being able to pay his bills and meet other financial commitments for his family. He also states that he has little time for hobbies or recreational outlets because he works so many hours.

THINKING

1. *Theoretical Knowledge (Facts and Principles):* You see in the medical records that the provider prescribed repaglinide (Prandin) to treat Mr. LeMonte's diabetes. By what route is this medication given?

2. *Critical Thinking (Inquiry):* If you did not know the answer to the first question, specifically how did you get that information? State your source.

DOING

3. *Nursing Process (Assessment):* To evaluate Mr. LeMonte's response to his diabetes medication, what questions do you need to ask him?

4. *Practical Knowledge (Skills):* Mr. LeMonte tells you that he forgot to take his Prandin this morning and also at lunchtime. What should you do?

CARING

5. *Self-Knowledge:* In what areas do you feel compassion for Mr. LeMonte, on which you might build a caring relationship?

6. *Self-Knowledge:* What do you identify as your strength in dealing with Mr. LeMonte's healthcare needs?

7. *Ethical Knowledge:* Mr. LeMonte tells you that he frequently skips doses of his Prandin because he can't afford the expense. He asks you not to tell his wife because he doesn't want her to worry. What will you do?

Critical Thinking & Clinical Judgment

Because these are clinical judgment questions, they usually do not have a single answer. Discuss the questions with your peers—discussion can stimulate critical thinking.

1. Your patient is prescribed Humulin R insulin 30 units subcutaneously. You have available in a multidose vial Humulin R insulin; the label reads "100 units per mL."

   a. What equipment and supplies do you need to administer this medication? Be specific.

   b. What practical knowledge (psychomotor skills) will you need?

   c. Regarding the psychomotor skills, what are the two aspects that require the most careful attention? Explain your thinking.

   d. What will you do to ensure that you have the correct dosage?

   e. What specific technique steps will you take to decrease the risk for infection?

   f. Suppose that after drawing the insulin into the syringe, you see that instead of the 30 units prescribed, you have only 20 units in the syringe. What will you do?

2. A provider prescribes heparin 4,000 units subcutaneous q12hr for Mr. Dale. You have on hand heparin 10,000 units/mL. How many milliliters should you draw up?

The following is patient information for questions 3 through 6 and 8:
Recall the patients from Chapter 23, Meet Your Patients, in Volume 1. Questions 3 through 6 and 8 refer to those patients. They are listed here for your convenience.

- Margaret Marks, an 82-year-old woman who has a fractured hip and has periods of confusion.
- Cary Pearson, a 70-year-old man with feeding and swallowing difficulties who receives his medications through a gastrostomy tube.
- Cyndi Early, a 32-year-old woman with diabetes who is scheduled for surgery at 1000 today.
- James Bigler, a 44-year-old man who has had a repair of a compound fracture of the right arm and is receiving intravenous fluids and medications.
- Rebecca Jones, an 84-year-old woman with compression fractures of two lumbar vertebrae resulting from a fall.

---

3. It is 0800, and you have begun organizing your medication pass for this shift by verifying the MAR entries against the provider's prescriptions. You notice that Mr. Bigler has been prescribed Toradol 30 mg IM q6hr. His last dose was supposed to have been given at 0600, but there is no documentation that the medication was administered.

   a. What should you do?

   b. Should you assume the night shift nurse administered the medication but forgot to document that they had given it, and give the 0600 dose late? Why, or why not?

   c. When should the next dose be administered?

   d. If the night nurse did *not* administer the medication as prescribed, what type of medication error did they make? What factors could have caused this error?

   e. Assuming that the nurse *did* administer the medication as prescribed at 0600, what error did the night nurse make? Which of the rights of medication was violated?

4. You receive the laboratory results for Cary Pearson's potassium level and find it to be 3.1 mEq/L. You notify the provider and receive a verbal prescription to add 20 mEq of KCl to his IV of D$_5$½ NS; 5% dextrose in half-strength NS [0.45% saline] to infuse at 125 mL/hr. The IV infusing is a new 1,000-mL bag that is almost full.

   a. Write the prescription as you would write it on the order sheet.

   b. What information must you put on the additive label for this bag?

   c. Suppose the situation were slightly different. There is only 100 mL of IV fluid left in Mr. Pearson's IV bag when you call the provider, who prescribes, "Add 10 mEq to the IV, and infuse it at 125 mL/hr." Would you ask for clarification of this prescription? Why or why not?

   d. Change the situation again. You have taken the prescription in this way: "Add 20 mEq of KCl to 1,000 mL of D$_5$½ NS and infuse at 125 mL/hr." You are preparing this medication and find that Mr. Pearson currently has 500 mL remaining in his IV infusion. Should you add the KCl to this IV infusion or wait until you hang a new 1,000-mL bag? If you do add it, how much KCl will you add? What is your rationale for your decision?

   e. You begin preparing the infusion with the 20 mEq of KCl to be added and find you have available a vial containing KCl 40 mEq in a 10-mL vial. How many milliliters of KCl will you add to the bag of fluids?

5. Dr. Xi has prescribed heparin 8,000 units subcutaneous q12hr for Mrs. Marks.

   a. You have vials of heparin containing 10,000 units/mL. How many mL of heparin will you administer?

   b. To prevent tissue trauma and hematoma and to help ensure adequate absorption, what precautions should you take while administering heparin?

   c. What syringe and needle will you select for administration, and why?

6. You are checking Mrs. Early's medical records and find that the provider has prescribed a medication the patient lists as having an allergy. What steps should you take?

7. A patient has been taking warfarin sodium (Coumadin) 3 mg daily for the past 3 years. They have tolerated the medication well, but recently they have noticed more bleeding tendencies, such as nosebleeds and hematuria (blood in urine). You assess the patient and find that they have gross hematuria today and numerous bruises over their body. To answer the following questions, what theoretical knowledge do you need, and where can you find it? (*Note:* After you get the information you need, answer the following questions.)

   a. What could be causing these bleeding episodes?

   b. What laboratory test is indicated in this situation, and what result do you expect?

   c. What actions should you take in this situation?

8. James Bigler (Meet Your Patients, in Volume 1) has had a postoperative repair of a compound fracture of the right arm and is receiving IV fluids and medications, including opioid analgesics and antibiotics. He also has a herniated intervertebral disk and severe muscle spasms. He received his first dose of an oral muscle relaxant, cyclobenzaprine (Flexeril) 10 mg, at midnight. At 0800, he received another dose. At 0900, he received an IV antibiotic, and while awake, he has been self-administering his opioid analgesic using his patient-controlled analgesia (PCA) IV pump about every 4 hours in a low dose. Consider these facts:

   - The most common side effect of Flexeril is drowsiness. It has a half-life of 24 to 72 hours.

   - Common side effects of opioids are drowsiness, decreased respiratory rate and depth, decreased blood pressure, and constipation (if taken long term).

   - Besides allergies, the most common adverse effect of Mr. Bigler's antibiotic is diarrhea.

Mr. Bigler's muscle relaxant (Flexeril) is to be administered every 8 hours. When you enter his room to administer his 1600 dose, you find that he is extremely sleepy. He will awaken when you shake him or speak to him, but he falls right back to sleep and is slurring his words. These are new symptoms for him.

   a. Is there anything obvious about his medical diagnosis that might be producing these symptoms? If so, what?

   b. Which of his medications could cause these symptoms, and why?

   c. What would you do? Would you give the 1,600 dose of cyclobenzaprine (Flexeril)?

9. Mrs. Thomas lives alone and until a few months ago was able to take care of herself. When her eyesight began to deteriorate, she had difficulty self-administering her medications.

   a. Discuss the assessment required to determine whether she is at risk for ineffective management of her medication regimen.

   b. Mrs. Thomas was prescribed lorazepam (Ativan) 1 mg orally. Is this prescription complete? If not, what is missing? What actions should you take?

   c. Mrs. Thomas has a prescription for digoxin (Lanoxin) 1.25 mg orally every morning. You have available Lanoxin 0.25 mg, and you calculate that five tablets should be administered. You check a drug guide and find that the usual dose is 0.125 mg to 0.25 mg orally daily. What actions should you take?

10. Calculate dosages for the following medications that you will be administering during your medication pass today. Are there any prescriptions you would question? If so, why?

    a. Cephalexin (Keflex) 500 mg IV q6hr. You have on hand Keflex 1 gm in 1 mL of solution.

    b. Furosemide (Lasix) 280 mg orally daily. You have 40-mg tablets of Lasix available.

    c. Meperidine (Demerol) 10 mg intramuscularly to a child. You have Demerol 25 mg/mL available in a prefilled syringe. In addition to calculating the dosage, describe the equipment you would use to administer the Demerol to a child.

11. Describe the procedure for giving atropine sulfate 0.4 mg IM along with morphine 10 mg IM using the same syringe. The atropine is in a single-dose vial containing 0.4 mg of atropine in 0.5 mL of fluid. The morphine is in a prefilled 10 mg injectable cartridge containing 10 mg in 1 mL of fluid.

12. You have a prescription to administer injectable phenytoin (Dilantin) and furosemide (Lasix). You would like to administer them in the same syringe. What theoretical and practical knowledge do you need to decide whether you can do this?

13. For each of the following patient problems, (1) state what you think might be the cause and (2) state one thing you might have done to prevent the problem.

    a. When you give Mrs. King an intramuscular injection in her ventrogluteal muscle, she complains of pain.

    b. Several weeks after receiving an intramuscular injection in the dorsogluteal site, Mr. Aguilar begins having pain in his left lower back and hip; the pain proceeds down his leg. He is beginning to limp when he walks.

    c. Several days after receiving a subcutaneous injection, Patti Deal's upper arm is red, hot, painful, and swollen. There is pus oozing from the injection site.

    d. Immediately after an intramuscular injection, a patient starts showing severe, unexpected symptoms.

14. For each of the following concepts, use critical thinking to describe how or why it is important to nursing, patient care, or administering medications. Note that these are *not* to be merely definitions.

Pharmacology

Drug classification systems (e.g., according to use or chemical traits)

The United States Pharmacopeia–National Formulary (USP-NF)

Drug excretion

Therapeutic levels

Side effects and adverse reactions

The apothecary system

Household measurements

Units and milliequivalents

Standing prescriptions

Rights of medication administration

Ventrogluteal site for intramuscular injection

Medication errors

What Are the Main Points in This Chapter?

▸ Drugs are classified according to their use, body systems, and chemical or pharmacological traits. Learning the classifications helps you to remember the characteristics of individual drugs.

▸ The form (preparation) of a drug affects its speed of onset, intensity of action, and route of administration.

▸ In the United States, the Food and Drug Administration (FDA) regulates the manufacturing, sale, and effectiveness of all medications. Various state and federal agencies and legislation also regulate the administration of medications.

▸ Controlled substances must be stored, handled, disposed of, and administered according to regulations established by the U.S. Drug Enforcement Agency (DEA).

▸ In general, intravenous (IV) medications are absorbed most rapidly, followed by intramuscular, subcutaneous, buccal, and oral medications.

▸ Metabolism is the chemical inactivation of a drug into a form that the body can excrete; drug metabolism takes place mainly in the liver.

▸ The primary route of drug excretion is from the kidneys; other routes are the liver, gastrointestinal tract, lungs, and exocrine glands.

▸ The therapeutic level of a drug is the concentration in the blood serum that produces the desired effect without toxicity.

▸ Medication effects can be primary (therapeutic and intended) or secondary (nontherapeutic and unintended). Secondary effects include side effects, adverse reactions, toxic reactions, allergic reactions, and idiosyncratic reactions.

▸ The metric system is preferred for medications; however, for a few medications, the apothecary and household systems are still used.

▸ You are legally responsible for the medications you administer. You must question prescriptions you believe to be incorrect.

▸ To help prevent medication errors, observe the three checks (before and after pouring or drawing up a medication, and at the bedside) and the six rights of medication (right drug, right dose, right time, right route, and right patient, as well as right documentation immediately after giving the medication).

▸ If you make a medication error, it is essential that you immediately assess the patient's vital signs and physical status, report findings to the primary care provider, and notify the nurse manager of your unit.

▸ The oral route is the one most commonly used; it is convenient and safe.

▸ Buccal and sublingual medications are held in the mouth so that they will be absorbed through the mucous membrane.

▸ For patients who cannot swallow or who have feeding tubes, you can give oral medications through enteric (e.g., nasogastric [NG] and gastrostomy) tubes. The medications are given one at a time and the tube must be flushed before and after each medication.

▸ Topical medications may have local and systemic effects; transdermal patches are applied for their systemic effect.

▸ Nebulization is the production of a fine spray, fog, powder, or mist from a liquid drug.

▸ Parenteral medications require the use of sterile technique to prevent infection.

▸ Needle length and gauge are chosen based on the type of medication, the route of administration, and the amount of adipose and muscle tissue the patient has.

- Needleless systems and safety syringes reduce the likelihood of needlestick injury.
- Always dispose of needles in special sharps containers. If you must recap a needle, use a one-handed technique.
- The ventrogluteal site is the preferred intramuscular injection site for adults. Other sites are the vastus lateralis and the deltoid. Use the rectus femoris site only if no other sites are available, and never in infants and children. Do not use the dorsogluteal site.
- Experts agree the anterolateral thigh (vastus lateralis) is preferred for infants who are not walking, and some recommend using it throughout childhood. Others recommend using the ventrogluteal site when the child starts walking and the gluteal muscle increase in mass. The deltoid can be used for older children if the muscle mass is adequate.
- Medications may be given intravenously by adding the medication to a large-volume (primary infusion), by the IV push technique, or by intermittent (piggyback setup) infusion.
- You should report medication errors immediately after they occur; a risk management process for monitoring causative factors should be in place.
- The most common reasons for a patient to have a central venous access device (CVAD) are to:
  - Give long-term IV therapy.
  - Provide total parenteral nutrition when the patient cannot eat normally.
  - Have blood drawn without the trauma and complications of repeated venipuncture.
  - Be used when peripheral IV line placement is difficult.

Knowledge Map

MEDICATION ADMINISTRATION

DRUGS
- Prescription
- Non-prescription (OTC)

DRUG NAMES:
- Chemical name
- Generic (official) name
- Brand name (trade)

DRUG CLASSIFICATIONS:
- By their use
- By body systems
- By pharmacological traits

EFFICACY INFLUENCED BY:
- Pharmacokinetics
  - absorption
  - distribution
  - metabolism
  - excretion
- Pharmacodynamics
  - interaction with target cells
  - how biological response occurs

FACTORS CONTRIBUTING TO DRUG SAFETY:
- Reliable drug info
  - USP; national formulary; PDR; drug reference books
- State/Federal Regulation
  - Nurse Practice Act
  - U.S. drug laws
  - regulation of controlled substances
- Improved storage/distribution systems

MEDICATION ORDERS

TYPES:
- Standard written
- Verbal
- Telephone
- Standing
- One-time

CORRECT COMPONENTS:
- Patient name
- Date/time
- Drug name
- Dose and frequency
- Route
- Signature of prescriber

ADMINISTRATION SAFEGUARDS

PREPARING: THREE CHECKS →
- Label against MAR prior to pouring
- Label against MAR AFTER preparing med at the bedside

ADMINISTRATION: SIX RIGHTS →
- Drug
- Dose = accurate calculations
- Time → know "window"
- Route
- The Joint Commission two patient identifiers
- Documentation

ROUTES OF ADMINISTRATION

NON-PARENTERAL:
- Oral
  - buccal
  - sublingual
- Topical
  - cream/ointment
  - transdermal
- Ophthalmic
- Otic
- Nasal
- Vaginal/rectal
- Inhaled

PARENTERAL:
- Intradermal
- Subcutaneous
- Intramuscular
- Intravenous

ERROR PREVENTION
- 3 checks/6 rights
- Check calculations w/second person
- Watch look-alike, sound-alike drugs
- Check decimals; use correctly
- Question multiple vials/tabs if single dose
- Question abrupt increase in doses

NURSING SKILLS:
- Appropriate needle/syringe
- Withdrawal from amp/vial
- Correct site
- Correct administration technique

UNIT 4

Supporting Physiological Functioning

24 Nutrition
25 Urinary Elimination
26 Bowel Elimination
27 Sensation, Perception, & Response
28 Pain
29 Physical Activity & Immobility
30 Sexual Health
31 Sleep & Rest
32 Skin Integrity & Wound Healing
33 Oxygenation
34 Circulation & Perfusion
35 Hydration & Homeostasis
36 Caring for the Surgical Patient

CHAPTER 24

Nutrition

STUDENT RESOURCES

The questions and exercises in this book allow you to practice the kind of thinking you will use as a full-spectrum nurse. Critical-thinking questions usually have more than one right answer, so we do not provide "correct" answers for these features. Try to answer these questions yourself. It is more important to develop your nursing judgment than to just cover content. You will learn more by discussing the questions with your peers. If you are still unsure, see the Davis Advantage chapter resources for suggested responses.

To explore learning resources for this chapter,

Go to www.DavisAdvantage.com and find:

Answers and Suggested Responses for all questions in this chapter
Concept Map
Knowledge Map
References and Bibliography

Key Concepts

Energy
Metabolism
Nutrition

Related Concepts

See the Concept Map on Davis Advantage.

Example Problems

Overweight and Obesity
Undernutrition and Malnutrition

Caring for the Williams Family

Stanley Williams has been diagnosed with hypertension, type 2 diabetes mellitus, obesity, osteoarthritis, and tobacco abuse. Assad Johnson, FNP-BC, has advised an 1800-kcal diabetic diet with no added salt and a daily brisk 30-minute walk. Mr. Williams discusses these challenges with his daughter Jayden Robinson.

A. Why might Assad have selected this diet plan? Discuss the rationale for each component (i.e., 1800-kcal, diabetic diet, no added salt).

B. Mr. Williams' diet is complex. He tells you he is overwhelmed by the many changes asked of him. How might Assad streamline his instructions about Mr. Williams' diet?

C. Mr. Williams asks what the best way is for him to monitor his weight loss progress at home and how Assad will monitor his progress. How would you respond?

D. Identify teaching tools that might help Mr. Williams understand his diet.

Practical Knowledge clinical application

480 UNIT 4 Supporting Physiological Functioning

To apply concepts that support patient nutrition, you will need to master techniques for assessing nutrition status, feeding patients, administering supplemental feedings, and working with nasogastric (NG) and nasoenteric (NE) tubes.

PROCEDURES

Procedure 24-1 ■ Checking Fingerstick (Capillary) Blood Glucose Levels

▶ For steps to follow in *all* procedures, refer to the Universal Steps for All Procedures on the page facing the inside back cover.

Equipment
- Blood glucose meter
- Test strip
- Sterile lancet (and injector, if available)
- Alcohol (or other antiseptic) pad, if required by policy
- 2 in. × 2 in. gauze pad or cotton ball
- Procedure gloves

Glucometers should be assigned to individual patients. If this is not possible, you must clean and disinfect the device between patients. Do not use insulin pens for more than one person. Injectors, too, should be assigned to individual patients; if possible, use single-use lancets that permanently retract upon puncture. Keep trays or carts with these supplies outside patient rooms. If there are unused supplies, do not use them for another patient. Do not carry supplies in your pocket. Change gloves and perform hand hygiene between fingerstick procedures.
These measures help prevent needlestick injury and transmission of bloodborne pathogens (American Diabetes Association, n.d.; Centers for Disease Control and Prevention, 2005).

Delegation
You can delegate this procedure to a licensed practical nurse (LPN) or unlicensed assistive personnel (UAP) who have been adequately trained in performing the skill if the patient's condition allows. Most patients perform this procedure independently at home.

Preprocedure Assessments
- **Assess the patient's comprehension of the procedure.**
  Understanding reduces anxiety and promotes cooperation.
- **Assess potential puncture sites for bruising, inflammation, open lesions, poor circulation, or edema.**
  Avoid such sites because of risk for infection and inaccurate results.
- **Check for factors such as anticoagulant therapy, bleeding disorders, or low platelet count.**
  These place the patient at risk for bleeding after skin puncture.

▶ When performing the procedure, always identify your patient according to agency policy, using two identifiers, and be attentive to standard precautions, hand hygiene, patient safety and privacy, body mechanics, and documentation.

▶ *Note:* The steps of this procedure will vary depending on the type of glucose meter used.

Procedure Steps

1. **Verify the medical prescription** for frequency and timing of testing.
   Timing and frequency of testing are crucial for accurate insulin dosing and managing optimal blood glucose.

2. **Ask the patient to wash their hands** with soap and warm water and to dry completely using a clean towel; or disinfect with alcohol-based hand sanitizer.
   Reduces the risk for infection and dilates capillaries at the puncture site. Also ensures that the testing site is free of any sugar residue.

3. **Turn on the blood glucose meter.** Calibrate it according to the manufacturer's instructions.
   Calibration readies the meter for testing and checks it for accuracy.

4. **Check that the strip is the correct type** for the monitor. Check the expiration date on the container of reagent strips. If the strips are expired, replace them.
   Expired strips may alter test results. Each brand of monitor uses a unique type of reagent strip.

5. **Don procedure gloves.**
   Gloving protects against exposure to blood.

6. **Remove the reagent strip** from the container and place it into the blood glucose meter. Then tightly seal the container.
   A tight seal protects reagent strips from exposure to air and light.

CHAPTER 24 Nutrition 481

7. **Select and clean a fingerstick site** with soap and warm water or an alcohol-based (or other antiseptic) pad, according to facility policy. Allow the site to dry thoroughly.
   Helps protect the patient from infection by removing some surface microorganisms. Allowing the alcohol to dry thoroughly will decrease pain of the skin puncture. Using alcohol is controversial, however, because it may interfere with the reagent on the strip, giving a false low reading; it also dries the skin. Follow agency policy and consult practice guidelines periodically.

8. **Use a different site each time** you check the glucose.
   Adult and child: the lateral aspect of a finger (palmar surface, distal phalanx)
   Infant: heel or great toe
   The lateral aspect of the finger contains fewer nerve endings than does the central fingertip, so it hurts less.

9. **Position the finger** (or heel or great toe for an infant) in a dependent position and massage from the base toward the tip of the finger.
   A dependent position promotes blood flow to the site via gravity and pressure, ensuring an adequate specimen. The massaging action increases blood flow to the tip of the finger, which may prevent the need for repuncture.

10. **Prick the finger** (or another site) with the lancet semiautomatic injector:
    a. Engage the sterile injector and remove the cover.
    b. Place the disposable lancet firmly in the end of the injector.
    c. Place the back of the patient's hand on the table, or otherwise secure the finger (e.g., hold the finger and hand firmly).
    d. Position the end of the injector firmly against the skin, perpendicular (at a 90° angle) to the chosen puncture site.
    e. Push the release switch, allowing the needle to pierce the skin.
    Proper positioning and stabilization of the site ensure that the lancet pierces to the correct depth. This prevents patient injury and allows for adequate blood sampling. Patients tend to pull away as you perform the puncture. ▼

11. **Allow the drops of blood to release naturally** or apply light pressure above the puncture site, if necessary, until a drop of blood is collected.
    Light pressure promotes a better blood sample for testing without causing injury to the puncture site. Firm or excessive pressure may lead to unreliable readings (Hortensius et al., 2011).

12. **Place the reagent strip test** patch close to the drop of blood. Allow contact between the drop of blood and the test strip. Do not smear the blood over the reagent strip.
    This ensures adequate blood sample for testing. ▼

13. **Insert the strip into the glucometer,** if it is not already inserted (follow the manufacturer's instructions); allow the blood sample to remain in contact with the test strip for time specified by the manufacturer.
    For some glucometers you insert the test strip before pricking the finger; with others you put the blood on the reagent strip and then insert the strip into the meter. The blood sample must be on the reagent strip for the specified time to ensure accurate test results.

14. **Using a gauze pad,** gently apply pressure to the puncture site.
    Pressure stops the bleeding by promoting coagulation.

15. **After the glucometer signals, read** the blood glucose level indicated on the digital display. ▼

16. **Turn off the meter** and dispose of the reagent strip, gauze pad, alcohol pad, and lancet in the safe collection containers (e.g., a sharps container for the lancet).
    Proper disposal prevents sharps injury and the spread of infection via bloodborne pathogens.

17. **Remove the procedure gloves** and dispose of them in the proper container. Perform hand hygiene.
    Hand hygiene and gloving reduce the transmission of microbes.

? What if . . .

- **The patient has poor circulation or is a child or older adult?**

Place a heel warmer or warm cloth on the site for about 10 minutes before obtaining the blood sample. Alternatively, position the patient's hand below the waist for 1 minute.
Capillaries in infants are very small; older adults may have poor peripheral circulation. The warmth may dilate the capillaries, helping you obtain an adequate amount of blood; the dangling of extremities allows blood to pool in the extremity, making it easier for you to obtain the quantity of blood needed.

(continued on next page)

Procedure 24-1 ■ Checking Fingerstick (Capillary) Blood Glucose Levels (continued)

- **The patient is taking an anticoagulant?**

  After the procedure, hold pressure for 2 minutes and then apply a pressure bandage if needed. Recheck the site after 5 minutes to make sure bleeding has stopped.

- **The monitor shows an extremely unusual result or an error message?**

  Repeat the process using a different finger or site.

- **The patient uses a noninvasive method to measure blood glucose?**

  A continuous glucose monitor (CGM) is used to track blood sugar more closely. One type of CGM is worn like a wristwatch. Using an electrical current, it pulls fluid from the skin to give a blood glucose reading. Another style uses a small sensor just below the skin of the abdomen and measures glucose in the interstitial fluid.
  - The CGM will take readings automatically every 5 to 30 minutes and will download data to a computer, tablet, or smartphone.
  - Advise the patient to shave their arm if it is very hairy, or the reading may not be accurate.
  - The patient should wear the device for a 2-hour warm-up before taking a reading and should not bathe or swim during that time.

  This does not replace the patient's fingerstick method. Its purpose is to track trends in blood glucose. It also benefits patients whose blood sugar goes dangerously low overnight, which could go undetected.

Evaluation

- Assess the puncture site for bleeding or bruising.
- Evaluate the patient's understanding of the procedure and the test results.
- Promptly notify the provider of abnormal test results, or administer insulin based on test results, if prescribed.

Patient Teaching

- Explain the procedure, test results, and treatment to the patient.

  Information allows the patient to participate in his plan of care and typically increases adherence to the therapeutic regimen.
- If the patient will be performing fingerstick blood glucose testing at home, teach the patient how to perform the procedure. Ask the patient to perform a return demonstration.
- Discuss the importance of maintaining glycemic control.
- If the patient will be performing fingerstick blood glucose testing at home, teach the patient to do the following:

  Read the manufacturer's instructions carefully and contact the company if you have any questions.

  Always use the test strips that are recommended for the meter.

  Take your meter to your health provider's office so the provider can make sure you are measuring your blood sugar correctly.

  Perform quality control checks (read the instructions) to make sure the glucometer is measuring accurately.

  Clean the meter according to the manufacturer's directions. Some meters will give you an electronic alert telling you when to clean them.

Home Care

- Assess the client's ability to perform fingerstick blood glucose monitoring independently.

  A change in the patient's condition may not allow the patient to perform testing. Certain conditions, such as arthritis and limited vision, may limit dexterity.
- Advise the patient about purchasing home glucose monitoring equipment.
- Explain how to dispose of lancets in a labeled, puncture-proof container with a secure lid.
- Instruct caregivers to wear gloves when obtaining a blood sample for glucose monitoring.
- At home, patients do not need to cleanse their fingers with an alcohol wipe before puncturing it. However, they should wash their hands with soap and water and dry well.

Documentation

- Record the fingerstick blood glucose result in the progress notes or special flow sheet, including the date and time the test was performed.

- Note whether the provider was notified and record any treatment given.
- Document patient teaching.
- If the fingerstick is performed in response to patient symptoms, you may need to write a narrative note.

Practice Resources
American Diabetes Association (n.d.); CDC (2005); Hortensius, Slingerland, Kleefstra, et al. (2011); Mayo Clinic Staff (2022, February 1); U.S. Food and Drug Administration (USFDA, 2021, November 1, updated).

Thinking About the Procedure

The video **Checking Fingerstick (Capillary) Blood Glucose Levels,** along with questions and suggested responses, is available on the **Davis's *Nursing Skills Videos*** Web site at www.fadavis.com.

Procedure 24-2 ■ Inserting Nasogastric and Nasoenteric Tubes

➤ For steps to follow in *all* procedures, refer to the Universal Steps for All Procedures on the page facing the inside back cover.

Equipment
- Nasogastric tube (commonly 16 or 18 Fr for adults, but sometimes smaller) or nasoenteric (small bowel) tube (8 Fr, 10 Fr, or 12 Fr)
- Stylet or guidewire (for small-bore tubes), according to agency policy
- Procedure gloves
- Linen-saver pad or towel
- Water-soluble lubricant
- 50- to 60-mL catheter-tip syringe or bulb syringe for Salem sump tubes; 30-mL luer-lock syringe for small-bore feeding tubes
- Hypoallergenic tape (about 2.5 cm [1 in.] wide) or tube fixation device
- Indelible marker
- Skin adhesive
- Stethoscope
- Emesis basin
- Basin with warm water
- Glass of water with a straw
- Penlight
- Tongue blade
- pH test strip
- Tissues
- Safety pin
- Gauze square or small plastic bag
- Rubber band
- Suction equipment (if tube is being connected to suction)

Delegation
This procedure should not be delegated because it requires knowledge of anatomy and physiology and the ability to adapt the procedure based on patient responses. You can, however, delegate associated oral hygiene needs.

(continued on next page)

Procedure 24-2 ■ Inserting Nasogastric and Nasoenteric Tubes (continued)

Preprocedure Assessment

- Verify the medical prescription for type of tube to be placed and whether it is to be attached to suction or drainage.
- Verify the patient's need for NG or NE intubation (e.g., surgery involving the gastrointestinal [GI] tract, impaired swallowing, or decreased level of consciousness).
  NG or NE intubation decreases the risk for aspiration in these patients. In many institutions, only specially trained nurses are allowed to place small-bowel feeding tubes.
- Assess each naris for patency, deviated septum, and skin breakdown. Ask the patient to close each nostril alternately and breathe. Select the nostril with the greatest air flow. Ask the patient to blow the nose, if not contraindicated.
  A septal defect or facial fracture may cause obstruction, placing the patient at risk for nasal membrane trauma if insertion is attempted through the affected naris.
- Check health history for anticoagulant therapy, coagulopathy, nasal trauma, nasal surgery, epistaxis, deviated septum, and other conditions that may indicate the need for tube insertion via endoscope or fluoroscope.
  The medical provider should be notified if patient history or status places the patient at risk for injury during NG or NE insertion.
- Assess the level of consciousness and ability to follow instructions.
- Assess for a gag reflex, using a tongue blade.
  Diminished or absent gag reflex places the patient at risk for aspiration.

➤ When performing the procedure, always identify your patient according to agency policy, using two identifiers, and be attentive to standard precautions, hand hygiene, patient safety and privacy, body mechanics, and documentation.

Procedure Steps

1. **Prepare the tube.**

   Plastic Tube
   Wrap the tube around your index finger and then unwrap it and proceed or place in a basin of warm water for 10 minutes and proceed.

   Small-Bore Tube
   Insert a stylet or guidewire and secure into position, according to agency policy. (Small-bore tubes may come with the guidewire in them. If so, flush the tube with sterile water to lubricate the wire for easy removal. Leave the wire in place until the tube is positioned and its placement has been checked on x-ray film. Once the guidewire is removed, do not reinsert it.) Agency policy determines which nurses are authorized to place small-bore tubes.
   Warm water softens a plastic tube to make it easier to insert. (Most tubes are polyurethane or silicone based.) Wrapping a plastic tube around your index finger helps the tube flex into a curve and aids in insertion. A guidewire facilitates passage of small-bore tube but can cause trauma if not secured in a proper position.

2. **Assist the patient into a high Fowler's position** with pillow behind the head and shoulders. Raise the bed to a comfortable working level.
   This position facilitates tube insertion and prevents aspiration should the patient vomit during tube insertion. Gravity facilitates passage of the tube. Raising the bed reduces strain on the nurse's back.

3. **Measure the tube for placement.**

   Nasogastric Tube
   Measure the length of the tube to be inserted by measuring from the tip of the nose to the earlobe and from the earlobe to the xiphoid process. Mark the length with tape or indelible ink.
   This measurement indicates the distance the tube must be inserted to reach the stomach. ▼

   Nasoenteric Tube
   Add 8 to 10 cm (3 to 4 in.) to the NG tube measurement, as directed, and mark the tube.

4. **If you are right-handed,** stand on the patient's right side; if you are left-handed, stand on the patient's left side. **Drape** a linen saver pad over the patient's chest, and hand the patient an emesis basin and facial tissues.
   Draping protects the patient's gown from becoming soiled during tube insertion.

5. **Prepare the fixation device.** Cut a 10-cm (4-in.) piece of hypoallergenic tape if securing tube with tape; split the bottom end lengthwise 2.5 cm (2 in.). If using a commercial feeding tube attachment device, have it ready at this time.
   To secure the tube after insertion.

6. **Arrange a signal** by which the patient can communicate if they want to stop (e.g., raising a hand).
   Relieves anxiety by giving the patient some control over the procedure.

7. **Don procedure gloves** if you have not already done so.
   Reduces the spread of microorganisms.

8. **Wrap 10 to 15 cm (5 to 6 in.) of the end of the tube** tightly around your index finger, then release.
   Forms the tube into a curve that helps it conform more easily to the shape of the nasopharynx.

9. **Lubricate the distal 10 cm (4 in.) of the tube** with a water-soluble jelly.
   Lubrication eases the passage of the tube and prevents injury to the nasal mucosa. Water-soluble lubricant will dissolve if it is aspirated, whereas oil-based lubricants do not dissolve in the respiratory tract and would cause inflammation and blockage of airways if they enter the lungs. Some nurses prefer water as a lubricant because aqueous jelly dries and can block nasal passages, which is irritating to the patient. Some tubes have a surface lubricant and require only that you dip them in room-temperature water.

10. **Hand the patient** a glass of water with a straw, if they are awake, alert, and able to swallow.
    Instructing the client to swallow water during insertion eases passage.

11. **Instruct the patient** to hold the head straight up and extend the neck back against the pillow (slightly hyperextended).
    a. Grasp the end of the tube above the lubricant with the curved end pointing downward.
    b. Carefully insert the tube along the floor of the nasal passage, on the lateral side, aiming toward the ear.
    c. You will feel slight resistance when the tube reaches the nasopharynx; use gentle pressure, but do not force the tube to advance. The patient's eyes may tear; if so, provide tissues.
    d. Continue inserting the tube until just past the nasopharynx by gently rotating the tube toward the client's opposite naris.
    Hyperextending the neck straightens the curve where the nasal passage meets the pharynx (nasopharyngeal junction). Gentle insertion prevents trauma to the nasal mucosa. Forcing against resistance can traumatize the mucosa. Tears are normal.

12. **Pause for a moment** to allow the patient to relax and perhaps use tissues. Explain that the next step requires them to swallow.
    Stopping to relax can give the patient a feeling of control. The rest can also reduce gagging.

13. **Instruct the patient to flex** the head toward the chest, take a small sip of water, and swallow.
    This maneuver closes the trachea and opens the esophagus. ▼

14. **Rotate the tube 180°.**
    Rotation helps to redirect the tube so that it will not enter the patient's mouth.

15. **Direct the patient to sip** and swallow the water as you slowly advance the tube. (If the patient is not allowed water, instruct them to dry swallow or suck air through the straw.) Advance the tube 5 to 10 cm (2 to 4 in.) with each swallow.
    Moving the tube with each swallow uses normal peristaltic movement to help advance the tube into the stomach. Swallowing closes the epiglottis so that the tube cannot advance into the trachea.

16. **Continue advancing the tube** to the desired distance.

17. **Temporarily secure the tube** with one piece of tape. Then verify tube placement.

    ✚ Never rely on a single bedside method. You can use a combination of the following methods to verify placement at the bedside; however, radiographic verification is the only reliable method and should be done before medications or fluids are given through the tube for the first time (Metheny & American Association of Critical-Care Nursing, 2016, updated 2020, January 29).

    ▶ Go to Box 24-5: Comparison of Methods for Checking Nasogastric Tube (NGT) Feeding Tube Placement, in Volume 1.

    If you do not secure the tube, at least temporarily, it may move out of position—especially if you are waiting for placement to be confirmed by x-ray film.

    a. Inspect the posterior pharynx for presence of coiled tube.
       Visualization confirms that the tube has gone beyond the oropharynx.
    b. Aspirate gently to withdraw stomach contents and measure aspirate pH. Aspirate gently over a period of up to 5 minutes, if necessary, to obtain gastric fluid.
       The pH of stomach contents is normally 1 to 5.5; however, many situations commonly alter the pH of gastric contents, so the usefulness of this method is limited. pH testing is helpful only if the fluid is acidic; if it is alkaline, the gastric contents may have been altered (e.g., by enteral feedings or antacids and other medications), or the tube may be in the lung. This procedure does not reliably confirm gastric placement and should be used in combination with other methods.
    c. Take note of the amount, color, and consistency of the aspirate.
       Gastric aspirates are often white or greenish and may be curdled. Intestinal aspirates will be smaller in quantity, yellowish due to the presence of bile, and not curdled.
    d. Ask the patient to speak.
       If they can do so, the tube is probably in the stomach. Use this only to confirm other methods; it is not reliable enough to use as the primary method of verification.

(continued on next page)

Procedure 24-2 ■ Inserting Nasogastric and Nasoenteric Tubes (continued)

18. **If the tube is not in the stomach,** advance it another 2.5 to 5 cm (2 to 4 in.) and repeat steps 17a through 17e.

19. **After you confirm proper placement,** clamp the end of the tube or connect it to the drainage bag, infusion pump, or suction machine.

20. **Secure the tube using one of the following methods:**

Securing the Tube With 1-Inch (2.5-cm) Tape

   a. Apply skin adhesive to the patient's nose; allow it to dry.
   A skin adhesive helps the tape to adhere and protects skin from breakdown.

   b. Use the 5-cm (2-in.) piece of hypoallergenic tape, split lengthwise for 2.5 cm (1 in.) at one end.
   A split tape can be wrapped around the tube in opposite directions to hold the tube in place more securely.

   c. Apply the intact end of tape to the patient's nose.

   d. Wrap the split strips around the tube where it exits the nose.

Securing the Tube With Tape

   e. Use 0.5-inch (1.3-cm) tape, 4 inches (10 cm) long. Apply one end of tape to the patient's nose and wrap the other end downward around the tube and then back up to secure on the opposite side of the nose. ▼

Securing the Tube With a Tube Fixation Device

   f. Peel the backing off the pad and place the wide end of the pad over the bridge of the nose.

   g. Position the connector around the NG or NE tube where it exits the nose.

21. **Curve and tape the tube to the patient's cheek** (not necessary with some commercial tube fixation devices).
    Securing the tube to the cheek reduces the tension on the naris.

22. **Fasten the tube to the patient's gown:** Tie a slipknot around the tube with a rubber band. Loop a rubber band in a slipknot near the connection. (Alternatively, wrap a short piece of tape around the tube to form a tab.) Then fasten the rubber band or the tab to the gown with a safety pin (or tape).
    Reduces discomfort produced by the weight of the tube and prevents movement that may cause dislocation of the tube and irritation of the nose.

23. **Elevate the head of the bed** 30° unless contraindicated.

24. **Mark the tube** where it enters the naris with tape, or measure the length from the naris to the connector.
    a. In the medical record, record either the incremental marking on the tube or the external length of the tube.
    b. Evaluate whether the incremental marking or external tube length changes, and, if a change is observed, use other bedside tests such as visualization and pH testing of tube aspirate to help determine whether the tube has become dislocated. If in doubt, obtain a radiograph to determine tube location.
    c. Document tube type, tip location, and external markings in the health record and in follow-up assessments.
    A marked tube allows you to easily notice whether tube placement has changed.

? What if...

- **The patient is confused, combative, or comatose?**

   a. If the patient is comatose, place them into a semi-Fowler's position. Have a coworker use a pillow to help position the patient's head forward for insertion.

   b. If the patient is confused and combative, ask a coworker to assist you with insertion.

- **The patient gags, coughs, or chokes (at steps 11 and 15)?**

   a. Stop advancing the tube. Ask the patient to take deep breaths and drink a few sips of water.
   Helps suppress the gag reflex.

   b. Instruct the patient to breathe easily and take some sips of water.

   c. If coughing continues, pull the tube back slightly.

   d. If gagging continues, use a tongue blade and penlight to check the tube position in the back of the throat.
   The tube may be coiled in the back of the throat.

   e. Continue to advance the tube to the desired distance.

   f. If the tube is coiled in the back of the throat, the patient coughs excessively during insertion, the tube does not advance with each swallow, or the patient develops respiratory distress (e.g., gasping, coughing, or cyanosis), withdraw the tube completely and allow the patient to rest before reinserting.
   The tube may be in the patient's trachea.

- **I am unable to obtain an aspirate (at step 17b) when confirming tube placement?**

   a. Use a 50-mL syringe and aspirate very slowly over at least 5 minutes.
   b. Flush the tube with air, then aspirate.
   c. Turn the patient to the left side, wait 20 minutes, then aspirate again.

- **The prescription states the tube needs to be in the jejunum?**
  a. To advance the tube into the jejunum after the tube has been placed in the stomach, position the patient on the right side.
  Positioning on the right side allows gravity to assist tube passage through the pyloric sphincter.
  b. Advance the tube 5 to 7.5 cm (2 to 3 in.) hourly over several hours (up to 24 hours) until x-ray confirms placement.
  Weighted tubes will advance by gravity and peristalsis if a loop of the designated length is made at the entrance to the naris. After reading the initial x-ray, the radiologist or primary physician can provide the measurement needed to advance the tube to the desired position. Note that specially trained nurses usually place these tubes at the bedside.

- **The procedure is anticipated to cause pain or discomfort?**
  Commercial viscous lidocaine is sometimes used to aid in patient comfort. Some practitioners use them for all NG insertions.
  a. You may insert 2% viscous lidocaine into the nasal passage with a syringe before tube placement.
  b. Alternatively, you can apply an anesthetic spray to the nasal and oropharyngeal mucosa.

- **The patient is a child?**
  a. Children usually require a tube of a smaller diameter.
  b. Encourage parents to comfort infants and children and participate in their care.
  c. You may need to apply restraints during insertion.
  To prevent dislodging of the tube.
  d. Monitor more frequently for complications.
  Small children are not able to communicate problems with the tube.

Evaluation
- Assess how well the patient tolerated the procedure (e.g., discomfort, gagging, coughing?).
- Note the color, consistency, and pH of NG or NE aspirate.
- Ask the patient whether she feels comfortable.
- Assess respiratory status.

Patient Teaching
- Explain that the sensation of the tube should decrease with time.
- Explain the importance of immediately reporting tension on the tube or displacement of the tape or fixation device.
- Discuss the need for frequent mouth care while the tube is in place.

Home Care
- Assess the client or caregiver's ability to maintain an NG or NE tube at home.
- Assess the home environment to determine the client's risk for infection.
- Instruct the client or caregiver about aspirating stomach contents and measuring pH.
- Teach the client or caregiver how to verify tube placement.
- Explain to the client or caregiver how to properly secure the NG or NE tube.
- Reinforce the need for frequent mouth care.

Documentation
- Chart the date and time of insertion, size and type of the NG or NE tube and insertion site (which naris), length of tube from the tip of the nose to the end of the tube, tolerance of the procedure, any abnormal findings, and methods for confirming NG or NE tube placement.
- Document the volume and description of gastric contents.
- Document respiratory status, including any sign of distress.
- Document the date and time of x-ray confirmation of the tube with report of tube position.
- NG or NE tube insertion is documented in the progress notes and flow sheets in most agencies.

Practice Resources
American Association of Critical-Care Nurses (2016, April); American Association of Critical-Care Nurses, Wiegand, (ed.) (2016); Emergency Nurses Association Clinical Practice Guideline Committee & Kilian, Reeve, Delao, et al. (2019, May); Institute for Safe Medication Practices (2010, 2014); Metheny & American Association of Critical-Care Nurses (2016, updated 2020, January 29); National Institutes of Health (2020, November 3, reviewed); Shlamovitz & Shah (2022, May 3, updated); Simons & Abdallah (2012).

Thinking About the Procedure

The video **Inserting Nasogastric and Nasoenteric Tubes,** along with questions and suggested responses, is available on the **Davis's *Nursing Skills Videos*** Web site at www.fadavis.com.

Procedure 24-3 ■ Administering Feedings Through Gastric and Enteric Tubes

> For steps to follow in *all* procedures, refer to the Universal Steps for All Procedures on the page facing the inside back cover.

Equipment

- Prescribed feeding formula at room temperature
- Filtered water or prescribed diluent, if ordered
- Tube feeding administration set and bag
- 60-mL luer-lock or catheter-tip syringe (two needed for syringe feeding)
- Connector to connect administration set to the feeding tube
- Stethoscope
- Enteral feeding infusion pump, recommended for continuous and cyclic feedings
- IV pole
- Linen-saver pad
- Graduated container
- pH strip
- For gastrostomy and jejunostomy tubes: a small precut gauze dressing

Delegation

You can delegate the procedure to the UAP or LPN if the patient's condition is stable and the UAP's skills allow. You must verify peristalsis, tube placement, and feeding tube patency before the feeding is started. Remind the UAP to position the patient upright and to report patient discomfort and any difficulty with the infusion.

Preprocedure Assessment

- **Verify the feeding tube is in proper placement** before starting the procedure.

Tube placement after insertion must be verified by radiography before the first feeding. For subsequent feedings, use more than one bedside method for verifying correct tube placement. One method is to aspirate and measure gastric residual volume. *(NOTE: For patients with a jejunostomy tube, do not measure the residual volume.)*

- You can also estimate tube placement by checking the length of the exposed tube: (1) Compare the length from the naris with the connector recorded after x-ray confirmation of placement, or (2) observe the mark that was made on it where it entered the nostril after insertion.

These methods help confirm that the tube has not become displaced since radiography. If there is significant change in length, tube position must again be confirmed by radiography.

- Assess fluid status by checking breath sounds, mucous membranes, skin turgor, edema, and intake and output.

These signs indicate fluid volume excess or insufficiency.

- Obtain baseline weight and laboratory studies.

Weight change is a sensitive measure reflecting fluid and nutrition status.

- Monitor vital signs before and after feedings.

Vital signs may vary from baseline because of pain, impaction, or dehydration.

- Auscultate for bowel sounds before each feeding or every 4 to 8 hours for continuous feedings. Also check for distention, nausea, vomiting, and diarrhea.

These symptoms may indicate intolerance of tube feedings. If GI motility is impaired, feedings accumulate in the stomach along with gastric secretions, predisposing the patient to reflux and aspiration. Some medications (e.g., opioids) also slow gastric emptying.

- Assess frequency of bowel movements.

Diarrhea may indicate intolerance of the formula, excessive feeding, or gastrointestinal disease.

- Check patient history for food allergies.

Helps prevent allergic reaction to ingredients in the feeding formula.

- **For gastrostomy and jejunostomy tubes:** Assess the exit site at every shift. Report redness or drainage to the physician.

Leaking of gastric or intestinal contents may cause skin breakdown.

Procedure 24-3A ■ Administering Feedings Through Gastric and Enteric Tubes Using a Closed System: Infusion Pump

➤ When performing the procedure, always identify your patient according to agency policy, using two identifiers, and be attentive to standard precautions, hand hygiene, patient safety and privacy, body mechanics, and documentation.

Procedure Steps

1. **Check the medical prescription** for the type of feeding, rate of infusion, and frequency of feeding.
   A medical prescription is required for enteral feedings. Rate and frequency of feeding are crucial for providing adequate nutrition.

2. **Elevate the head of the bed** 30° to 45° unless contraindicated.

3. **Check the expiration date** of the tube feeding formula.
   Expired formula should be discarded.

4. **Prepare the formula.**
   a. ✚ Inspect the container of feeding solution. If the bag, bottle, or can has been opened or damaged in any way, don't use it.
   b. Shake the feeding formula thoroughly. Examine the solution. It should be uniform in color and consistency. Most often the formula is room temperature. Follow the manufacturer's instructions for safe storage.
   Because the formula goes directly into the stomach and is not warmed by the mouth and esophagus, cold formula may cause abdominal cramping and increase the risk for diarrhea.

5. **Prepare the equipment** for administration.
   a. Don procedure gloves. Fill a disposable tube feeding container with a 4- to 6-hour supply of feeding formula. Or use a prefilled bottle with feeding formula. Follow similar procedure for flush bag if using a two-bag system.
   Limit hang time to help prevent bacterial growth and prevent air from entering the GI tract.

   b. ✚ Label the container with the patient's name, room number, date, start time, formula type, feeding rate, and your initials. Write a warning using large, bold letters—for instance, "WARNING! For Enteral Use Only—NOT for IV Use."
   Labeling identifies the formula and prevents misconnection of the feeding tube into an IV line. Labeling also helps avoid administering formula past the expiration date.

   c. ✚ Be sure adapters and connectors used in the enteral system are incompatible with female luer-lock rigid connectors used for IV infusion.
   Prevents tube feeding misconnection with an IV line.

   d. Hang the tube feeding container on an IV pole with the label facing forward. A prefilled container can safely hang for 24 to 36 hours (some agencies allow for 48 hours).
   Closed systems decrease the risk of contamination and prevent air from entering the GI tract.

   e. Open the administration set package. Make sure the tubing does not touch the floor.
   f. Close the clamp on the tubing before attaching the set to the container.
   g. Remove the cap from the end of safety connector. This adapter must *not* be compatible with IV tubing. Do not touch the end of the connector or let it touch another surface.
   h. Insert the proximal end of the tubing (with the safety adapter) into the cross-shaped opening of the port on the feeding tube bag.

   Twist the collar in a clockwise direction until it is securely fastened. ▼

6. **Prime the tubing with the feeding solution.**

7. **Thread the administration set** tubing through the infusion pump according to the manufacturer's instructions. Be sure to close the roller clamp. Be sure to move the clamp on your feeding tube to different sections of the tube.
   Clamping the tube prevents air from entering the stomach or gastric contents from leaking out. Moving the clamp prevents permanent kinking of the tube. ▼

(continued on next page)

Procedure 24-3 ■ Administering Feedings Through Gastric and Enteric Tubes (continued)

8. **Connect the distal end of the tubing** primed with feeding solution to the connector or directly to the NG or NE tube.

9. **Turn on the infusion pump.** Set the correct infusion rate and volume to be infused. Follow the pump manufacturer's instructions. Trace the tubing from the bag back to the patient before starting the feeding to ensure that you have not inadvertently hooked the feeding bag or bottle to the IV line.

10. **Unclamp the tube** and begin the infusion.

11. **When the feeding volume is complete,** stop the flow, flush the tube, and disconnect the feeding by turning off the pump and closing the roller clamp.

12. **Disconnect the feeding tube** from the administration tubing.

13. **Flush feeding tube** with the prescribed amount of water—typically 15 to 50 mL if there is no fluid restriction.

14. **Cap the proximal end of the feeding tube.**
    Prevents leaking of gastric contents and stops air from entering the stomach.

15. **Keep the head of the bed elevated** at 30° to 45° for 1 hour after administering the tube feeding.
    Reduces the risk for aspiration of gastric contents.

16. **Provide or assist with regular oral hygiene** and encourage frequent gargling.
    Reduces oropharyngeal discomfort from the tube.

17. **When you finish the procedure,** remember the universal steps that apply after all procedures. For example, leave the patient in a safe, comfortable position with the call device in easy reach.

Procedure 24-3B ■ Administering Feedings Through Gastric and Enteric Tubes Using an Open System: Syringe

Procedure Steps

First follow the previous steps 1 through 4. Then proceed as follows:

1. **Prepare the equipment for administration.**
   a. Don procedure gloves.
   b. Label the syringe with the patient's name, room number, date, time, formula type, feeding rate, start time, and your initials. Write a warning using large, bold letters—for instance, "WARNING! For Enteral Use Only—NOT for IV Use."
   Labeling identifies the formula, prevents misconnection of the feeding tube into an IV line, and helps avoid administering formula past the expiration date.

2. **Remove the plunger from the syringe.**

3. **Clamp or pinch off** the end of the feeding tube to begin the feeding.
   Prevents air from entering the feeding tube.

4. **Attach the syringe to** the proximal end of the feeding tube.

5. **Fill the syringe** with the prescribed amount of formula.

6. **Unclamp the feeding tube;** elevate the syringe. Do not elevate the syringe more than 18 inches (45 cm) above the insertion site. Allow the feeding to flow slowly.
   Gravity facilitates the flow of formula through the feeding tube. Rate of flow is determined by the height of the syringe. Feeding slowly prevents sudden stomach distention, which can lead to diarrhea, cramping, nausea, and vomiting. ▼

7. **When the syringe is nearly empty,** refill the syringe until the prescribed amount of feeding has been administered.
   If the tubing runs dry, air may enter the stomach and cause discomfort associated with gas.

8. **When the feeding volume** is infused, clamp or pinch the end of the feeding tube.

9. **Disconnect the syringe** from the feeding tube.

10. **Flush feeding tube** with the prescribed amount of water—typically 15 to 50 mL if there is no fluid restriction.

11. **Cap the proximal end** of the feeding tube.
    Prevents spillage of gastric contents and stops air from entering the stomach.

12. **Keep the head of the bed elevated** at 30° to 45° for 1 hour after administering the tube feeding.
    Elevation reduces the risk for aspiration of gastric contents.

13. **Provide or assist with** regular oral hygiene and encourage frequent gargling.
    Oral care reduces oropharyngeal discomfort from the tube.

? What if . . .

- **When checking for residual, the volume is more than the formula flow rate for 1 hour?**

  Reinstill the gastric residual volume. Residual gastric contents should be reinfused in the absence of pain or abdominal distention.
  If the residual is greater than 250 mL and if there is no abdominal pain or distention, elevate the head of the bed and continue the infusion. Recheck in 1 hour. If the residual is still greater than 250 mL, stop the infusion for 4 hours and recheck. If still greater than 250 mL, call healthcare provider (Boullata, Carrera, Harvey, et al., 2017).
  If residual is less than 250 mL, restart the infusion at 50% original rate and monitor.
  If the gastric residual volume is greater than or equal to 250 mL after a second gastric residual check, a promotility agent may be considered in adult clients (Boullata, Carrera, Harvey, et al., 2017).
  High residual volumes indicate delayed gastric emptying.

- **When checking for residual, none is obtained?**

  Use a large syringe (e.g., 60 mL) and inflate 20 mL of air into the tube, if agency policy permits; this may move the tube away from the gastric wall or clear the tube of any residual formula, medication, or water.

- **When irrigating the feeding tube (at step 10), resistance is met? Or when instilling the feeding, the fluid does not flow?**

  Do not force the solution.
  Do not use any fluid other than water for flushing.
  Check for kinks in tubing and that the pump is working correctly.
  Turn the client onto their left side.
  Remove any enteral feeding solution remaining in the tube. Try instilling 5 mL of warm water into the tube and clamping the tube for 5 minutes. Then apply gentle negative pressure to the tube with a syringe.
  Try flushing with a smaller (e.g., 10 or 20 mL) syringe.
  If these measures fail, the tube may need to be removed and a new one inserted; contact the primary care provider. (*Note:* There are other methods, such as the alkalinized enzyme method; they require a medical prescription.)
  Forcing the solution may damage the tube. However, you can use a smaller syringe to exert slightly more pressure.

- **The patient has a cuffed tracheostomy tube?**

  Inflate the cuff before administering the feeding, and keep the cuff inflated for least 15 minutes afterward.
  Cuffing helps to prevent aspiration.

- **During the feeding, the patient vomits or complains of nausea or feeling too full?**

  Stop the feeding and assess the patient's condition. Flush the tube, wait an hour, then measure gastric contents and restart the feeding at a slower rate. You may need to obtain a medical order to decrease the volume of the feedings.

- **The patient has a jejunostomy tube?**

  Do not instill air into the tube or check for residual before feeding.
  The tube is in the jejunum rather than the stomach, and the jejunum isn't normally a reservoir; therefore, no residual volume is present in the jejunum. Gastrostomy and jejunostomy tubes are often placed through the upper abdominal wall; such tubes, of course, cannot inadvertently migrate into the airway. Injecting air into the tube is not necessary and introduces air into the GI tract, causing the patient discomfort from gas.

  Clean the insertion site daily with soap and water. You may apply a small, precut gauze dressing to the site.
  Helps prevent bacterial growth; prevents infection.

  Be aware that the delivery rate will likely be slower for jejunostomy tubes because of the unavailability of the stomach as a reservoir.

(continued on next page)

Procedure 24-3 ■ Administering Feedings Through Gastric and Enteric Tubes (continued)

Evaluation
- Evaluate the patient's tolerance to the tube feeding; did the patient have any abdominal discomfort, nausea, vomiting, or diarrhea?
- Auscultate bowel sounds and vital signs every 4 hours.
- Check gastric residual volume every 4 hours.
- Monitor intake and output every 8 hours.
- Weigh patient at least 3 times per week.
- Assess the exit site for signs of skin breakdown.
- Assess frequency of bowel movements.
- Check laboratory values to evaluate nutrition status.

Patient Teaching
- Demonstrate the procedure to the patient and caregiver if the patient will be continuing tube feedings at home.
- Explain the importance of flushing the feeding tube with sterile water every 4 hours while the patient is awake to maintain tube patency and fluid and electrolyte balance.
- Discuss the importance of remaining upright for at least 1 hour after the feeding.

Home Care
- Provide written instructions.
- Be sure the client has a 7-day supply of enteral feedings.
- Identify with the client the person who will be responsible for care of the enteral tube and administration of feedings at home.
- Explain to the client and caregiver how to measure the prescribed amount of tube feeding formula and water for flushes by using household measuring equipment.
- Explain the importance of washing reusable equipment thoroughly with soap and water to prevent the spread of infection.
- Discuss how and where to purchase and store the formula.
- If home feedings are to be delivered by pump:
  - Facilitate a home care visit to provide training about the feeding pump.
  - Arrange for delivery of the feeding pump before discharge (or refer to the appropriate professional for this).
  - Ensure that the client has a 7-day supply of disposable feeding sets and 50-mL syringes upon discharge.

Documentation
- Chart the type of tube feeding, rate and volume of infusion, amount of gastric residual volume (if any), and tolerance of procedure.
- Tube feeding intake is documented on the intake and output portion of the flow sheet in most agencies.
- Record all flushes as intake. Subtract any liquids that you aspirate and do not reinstill (e.g., when gastric residual is too high).

Practice Resources
Bloom & Seckel (2022); Boullata, Carrera, Harvey, et al. (2017); Dietitians Association of Australia (2018); Durfee, Adams, Arthur, et al.; Home and Alternate Site Task Force; American Society for Parenteral and Enteral Nutrition (2014); Hodin & Bordeianou (2018); Institute for Safe Medication Practices (ISMP) (2010, July 15); The Joint Commission (2007); McClave, Taylor, Martindale, et al. (2016); Metheny & American Association of Critical-Care Nurses (2016, updated 2020, January 29); Memorial Sloan Kettering Cancer Center (2020); National Institutes of Health (NIH) (2020, November 3 updated); Powers, J. (2019).

Thinking About the Procedure

The videos **Administering Feedings Through Gastric and Enteric Tubes With Infusion Pump** and **Administering Feedings Through Gastric and Enteric Tubes Using an Open-System Syringe,** along with questions and suggested responses, are available on the **Davis's** *Nursing Skills Videos* Web site at www.fadavis.com.

Procedure 24-4 ■ Removing a Nasogastric or Nasoenteric Tube

▶ For steps to follow in *all* procedures, refer to the Universal Steps for All Procedures on the page facing the inside back cover.

Equipment
- Linen-saver pad
- 60-mL luer-lock or catheter-tip syringe
- Procedure gloves
- Stethoscope
- Disposable plastic bag
- Emesis basin
- Gauze square

Preprocedure Assessments
- Auscultate the abdomen for the presence of bowel sounds.
  Bowel sounds and flatus confirm peristalsis, which indicates bowel function is present.
- Assess the patient's ability to consume an oral diet.
  Confirms readiness for discontinuing the NG or NE tube.
- Determine how long it has been since the patient's last enteral feeding.

Delegation
This procedure should not be delegated to the LPN or UAP.

▶ When performing the procedure, always identify your patient according to agency policy, using two identifiers, and be attentive to standard precautions, hand hygiene, patient safety and privacy, body mechanics, and documentation.

Procedure Steps

1. **Check the patient's health record** to confirm removal of the tube. For feeding tubes, make sure tube feeding has been stopped at least 30 minutes before removal.

2. **Assist the patient to a sitting** or high Fowler's position.
   Proper body alignment facilitates tube removal.

3. **Place the plastic bag and emesis basin** on the bed or within reach. Hand the patient facial tissue. Explain that the procedure may cause some gagging or nasal discomfort, but it will be brief.
   Patients often need to blow their noses after this procedure.

4. **Drape a linen-saver pad or towel** across the patient's chest, and don procedure gloves.
   Draping protects the gown and linens from soiling. Maintains universal precautions.

5. **If you have not already done so,** perform hand hygiene and don procedure gloves.

6. **If the NG tube is connected** to suction, turn off suction and disconnect the tube.

7. **Stand on the patient's right side** if you are right-handed and left side if left-handed.

8. **Attach the syringe** to the proximal end of the NG or NE tube and flush the tube with 15 mL of water, normal saline, or air.
   Flushing clears the tube of feeding formula or gastric secretions that could cause irritation or be aspirated during tube removal.

9. **Unfasten the tube** from the patient's gown and then remove the tape from the patient's nose. Use an adhesive-remover pad to help loosen the tape as necessary.

10. **Clamp or pinch the end** of the tube in your hand. Hold gauze up to the patient's nose and be ready to grab the tube with the towel in the opposite hand upon removal.
    Prevents gastric fluids from leaking out the end of the tube onto the nurse or patient.

11. **Ask the patient to take a deep breath** and hold it.
    Breath holding closes the epiglottis to prevent aspiration.

12. **Quickly, steadily, and smoothly** withdraw the tube and place it in the plastic bag.
    Rapid removal in one steady motion prevents tissue trauma. The plastic bag acts as a barrier to gastric fluids until the tube can be placed in the trash. Seeing and smelling the tube may cause the patient to become nauseated.

13. **If the patient cannot do so,** clean the patient's nares and provide mouth care. Remove the tape residue from the nose with adhesive remover.
    Promotes patient comfort and prevents infection.

14. **If the NG tube was connected** to suction, measure the drainage and note the character of the content. Dispose of the tube and drainage equipment according to facility policy.
    For patients receiving enteral feedings or gastric suction, record their intake and output. Proper equipment disposal prevents the spread of infection.

15. **Remove and dispose of gloves** in the nearest receptacle.

(continued on next page)

Procedure 24-4 ■ Removing a Nasogastric or Nasoenteric Tube (continued)

Evaluation

- Assess the nares for signs of skin breakdown or bleeding.
- Monitor the patient for signs of GI dysfunction, such as food intolerance, nausea, vomiting, and abdominal distention. Auscultate for bowel sounds.
  GI dysfunction could necessitate reinsertion of the tube.
- Monitor intake and output every 8 hours.
- Weigh the patient regularly.
- Check laboratory values to evaluate nutrition status.

Patient Teaching

- Instruct the patient or caregiver on how to remove the feeding tube.
- Explain the importance of reporting nausea, vomiting, food intolerance, or abdominal distention to the physician.
- Explain the importance of and procedure for drinking fluids, if not contraindicated.

Home Care

The procedure does not require special adaptation for home care, except that you might want to place the tube in a plastic zippered storage bag before discarding it in the trash receptacle.

Documentation

- Chart the date and time of removal as well as the patient's tolerance of the procedure.
- Document the amount of drainage if the tube was connected to suction.
- Note any complications after NG or NE tube removal, such as food intolerance, nausea, vomiting, and abdominal distention.

Thinking About the Procedure

The video **Removing Nasogastric or Nasoenteric Tube,** along with questions and suggested responses, is available on the **Davis's *Nursing Skills Videos*** Web site at www.fadavis.com.

Procedure 24-5 ■ Administering Parenteral Nutrition

▶ For steps to follow in *all* procedures, refer to the Universal Steps for All Procedures on the page facing the inside back cover.

Equipment

- Parenteral nutrition solution
  - Keep the PN refrigerated until 60 minutes before use; do not give cold. Do not hasten warming by placing in a microwave oven or hot-water bath.
    Cold solution can cause pain, hypothermia, and venous spasm. Nutrients in PN solution are stable only for this short time. Nutrients could precipitate, causing catheter blockage or emboli.
  - Some pharmacies deliver the solution before infusion. Be sure the PN has not been mixed more than 24 hours beforehand. However, in home care you may find that solutions are mixed and delivered weekly.
- Procedure gloves
- Sterile gloves

- Intravenous administration set, extension set if indicated (free of plasticizers, such as DEHP, when fat emulsion is to be infused)

Permission for use granted by Cook Medical Incorporated, Bloomington, Indiana.

- 0.22-micron filter (1.2-micron filter if solution contains albumin or lipids)
  A 0.22-micron filter will remove most particulates and microorganisms that might have been introduced during mixing, but it is too fine for larger-molecule lipids to infuse properly.
- Time tape
  Even though the PN is delivered by infusion pump, there have been numerous recalls of infusion pumps because of malfunction. This

simple tape provides valuable information quickly and is an additional safety measure.

- 70% alcohol pads or chlorhexidine gluconate (CHG)-based pads (e.g., 2% CHG in 70% isopropyl alcohol)
- Infusion pump
- 10-mL syringe and saline
  To check for catheter patency
- Blood glucose testing monitor
- Intake and output record
- Transparent dressing or sterile gauze and tape (if dressing is to be changed)
- Catheter stabilization device (e.g., StatLock)
  These are recommended for all catheters and must be changed with each dressing change.
- If the dressing is to be changed, you also need a transparent dressing or sterile gauze, tape, and a mask.

Delegation

Do not delegate this skill to the LPN or UAP because administration of parenteral nutrition requires advanced assessment and critical-thinking skills. The LPN or UAP can assist by monitoring vital signs and verifying patient identity with you. Instruct them about complications associated with PN and ask them to inform you of any signs or symptoms or change in the patient's condition.

Preprocedure Assessments

- Assess nutrition status and nutrition needs (e.g., daily weights, intake and output [I&O], laboratory results). Patients requiring PN have complex nutrition needs, and actual nutrition status is assessed by a nurse or dietitian specializing in nutrition support.
- Check the prescriber's orders for type and concentration of additives in each container and for rate of infusion. Standardized order forms are recommended by the American Society for Parenteral and Enteral Nutrition (ASPEN).
- Check the patient's record to confirm that proper CVC tip placement has been established before the initial PN administration.
- Check agency policy.
  Some agencies may require tubing and filter change with every bottle or bag. The CDC recommends changing the PN set every 72 hours and a fat emulsion set at least every 24 hours.
- Check the blood glucose level.
- Assess for apparent patency of the IV site.
  If PN is being administered continuously by pump, the infusion is running, and there is no leakage from the insertion, you can begin the first few steps of the procedure. Actual patency is confirmed at step 14.

➤ When performing the procedure, always identify your patient according to agency policy, using two identifiers, and be attentive to standard precautions, hand hygiene, patient safety and privacy, body mechanics, and documentation.

Procedure Steps

1. **Gather equipment and place** at the bedside.
   Promotes efficient use of time.

2. **Identify the patient,** using two identifiers, according to agency policy. As an extra precaution, some institutions require that two people identify the patient.
   Multiple patient identifiers help to avoid "wrong-patient" errors. PN solutions are mixed to meet individual needs.

3. **Explain to the patient** the procedure and the rationale for it.
   Respects the patient's right to be informed.

4. **Perform hand hygiene** and don procedure gloves.
   Reduces transmission of infectious microorganisms.

5. **Position the patient supine** in bed.

6. **Obtain and examine the PN** container. Check for leaks, cloudiness, or floating particles. Do not use if any of these are present. Some agencies require that two people examine the solution.

Solutions Containing Lipids (3-in-1 Admixture)
Do not administer the admixture if it has a brown layer, oil droplets, or oil on the surface. This indicates that the emulsion has "broken," and the large lipid droplets can cause fat emboli if administered.
   Key Point: *Note that this solution requires a 1.2-micron filter.*
   To reduce the risk of adverse events such as fat emboli.

7. **Compare the bag with the patient's identification band;** check for correct bag number, expiration date, and additives and their concentration. Compare with the original prescription. Have a coworker verify with you.
   Ensures that the correct solution is administered. Check the expiration date to ensure that the solution will be discarded after that date and time. PN solutions are calculated and prepared using the recommendations for sterile compounding of solutions. The nurse should not add anything to the bag, either before it is hung or while it is infusing.

8. **Connect the IV tubing to the PN** solution; prime the tubing. Note that priming may be done manually now or later (on the pump after the tubing is loaded into the pump), depending on the design of the pump. Be sure to identify the correct port and IV line. Trace the PN tubing from the bag to the patient.
   Priming tubing removes air bubbles and prevents air from entering the patient's bloodstream, possibly causing air embolism. If there is PN already infusing, the old tubing must be removed from the pump and the rate regulated manually for the short time it takes to prime the new administration set.

(continued on next page)

Procedure 24-5 ■ Administering Parenteral Nutrition (continued)

When Using IV Tubing Without an Inline Filter

If the IV tubing does not have an inline filter, attach the filter and the extension tubing before priming. Attach the filter as close to the catheter site as possible.

9. **Place the IV tubing in the infusion pump.** (Prime the tubing if not previously done.) Set the pump to the prescribed rate.
   Administration via pump (preferably volumetric) helps prevent complications associated with too-rapid infusion. PN solutions must be administered by infusion pump with reliable, audible alarms. Catheter tip placement must be confirmed before initial PN administration.

10. **Identify the correct IV catheter** and lumen for the PN. This is usually a peripherally inserted central catheter (PICC line) or a centrally inserted venous line designated solely for PN.
    PN must be administered via a central venous catheter (e.g., subclavian catheter, internal jugular, or PICC), the tip of which is positioned in the superior vena cava/right atrial juncture. Most guidelines state that a specific intravenous line be reserved for parenteral nutrition and not used for any other purpose. If a single-lumen catheter is used, it is used only for PN. If a multilumen catheter is used, one lumen will be dedicated for the PN, and blood and other fluids should not be given through that lumen.

11. **Clamp the catheter and the old PN administration set,** if still connected, before disconnecting the tubing.
    a. A clamp should be present on the central line catheters with valves built into the catheter itself.
       The central line for the PN should already be clamped if no PN is running. If a previous bag is running, always clamp the PN line near the patient before disconnecting. Clamping prevents air from entering the catheter when you open the connection.
    b. As an additional safety measure, instruct the patient to perform the Valsalva maneuver just as you change the tubing.
    c. If Valsalva is contraindicated for a patient, instruct the patient to exhale at a specific time when the lumen is open.
       The Valsalva maneuver increases intrathoracic pressure and creates positive pressure in the central vessels, also helping prevent air embolism.

12. **Remove and discard gloves.** Perform hand hygiene.
    In steps 1 through 11, you were observing universal precautions. From this step forward, the emphasis is on preventing the introduction of microorganisms into the catheter lumen or the catheter insertion site.

13. **Don clean gloves (or sterile gloves if** your agency policy requires them). Disconnect the old administration set. Using a chlorhexidine gluconate (CHG)–alcohol pad or a 70% alcohol pad, thoroughly scrub all surfaces of the central line injection cap and extension leg (in a needleless system) or the luer-lock, including threads.
    Because PN solutions are a good medium for growth of pathogens, and because the IV line enters the central circulation, the risk for sepsis is relatively high.

14. **Determine patency of the line.** Use a 10-mL syringe to aspirate for blood, looking for a brisk return; then flush with saline. If the PN is running continuously on a pump, there are no occlusion alarms, and the dressing is dry and intact, these are also signs—but not proof—of patency.
    When PN is running continuously on a pump, the pump creates a constant fluid flow through the lumen to help keep it patent. There is some controversy about this step. Some experts prefer to aspirate for blood only for the first bag of a continuous infusion, and thereafter to flush without aspirating. As always, follow agency policy.

15. **Attach the infusion tubing** to the designated PN port and then turn the luer lock to secure the connection. "Luer-slip" connections should not be used. Do not use tape.
    Securing the connection with a luer-lock connection prevents separation of the connection and decreases the risk for sepsis or embolism. Tape, even sterile tape, has been found to be a medium for bacterial colonization.

If the Previous Infusion Is Still Connected

Be sure the access line and the line to the old infusion bag are clamped (step 11). Quickly disconnect from the central line, thoroughly cleanse the port, and connect the new infusion.

16. **Trace the tubing from the patient back to the bag.** Then start the infusion. Check again to make sure the catheter–tubing connection is secure. Infuse at the rate prescribed (depending on the patient's tolerance). PN is usually started at a rate of 40 to 50 mL/hr and then advanced 25 mL/hr every 6 hours.
    PN solutions may contain as much as 70% dextrose. A gradual rate increase allows the patient's pancreatic beta cells time to increase their insulin output to handle the increased glucose load. For lower concentrations of dextrose, you can usually run the same rate for the complete 24-hour volume. Tracing the tubing back to the bag is a double-check against misconnections.

17. **Label the tubing** with the date and time of change (if it is new tubing or if you have changed the tubing).
    Labeling allows other nurses to know when tubing is due to be changed and a new solution must be hung.

18. **Remove and discard gloves.** Perform hand hygiene.

? What if...

- **When I flush the catheter (at step 14), I meet resistance?**

  Examine the insertion site for leaking fluid or inflammation. Aspirate and try again to flush *gently*. Never forcibly flush against resistance. Reposition the patient and ask them to cough. Roll the patient's shoulder or raise the arm on the same side the catheter is on. If these measures fail, notify the primary care provider.

  Occlusion may be caused by a clot; drug precipitation; or catheter migration, kinking, or compression. Forceful flushing may discharge a clot into circulation. Other measures to clear a catheter require a medical order.

- **The rate falls behind or the pump gives occlusion alarms?**

  First check to be sure the pump is turned on, the bag is not empty, and all clamps are fully open. Change the filter if it is clogged. Perform the steps in the preceding item. If those measures do not work, change the pump and send it to biomedical engineering to be checked. Do not attempt to catch up by increasing the rate.

  A slow rate may indicate a clogged filter or injection cap, a kinked catheter, or a malfunctioning pump. A clogged filter must be changed; you cannot run the PN without a filter.

- **The 24-hour total deviates from the prescribed infusion rate by 10% or more?**

  Notify the primary care provider or nutrition support team.

- **A PN solution must be discontinued abruptly for any reason?**

  Notify the primary care provider or nutrition support team. Another solution of 5% or 10% dextrose may be started.

  The dextrose solution is started to prevent rebound hypoglycemia. Note that if it is a catheter complication that requires this discontinuation, 10% dextrose is the highest concentration that can be infused through a peripheral vein because infiltrated hyperosmolar fluid causes tissue injury.

- **The patient no longer needs parenteral nutrition?**

  You may need to decrease the rate gradually, perhaps over 48 hours, before discontinuing the infusion completely. Be sure the patient either receives enteral nutrition or consumes food during the next few hours after stopping PN.

  To prevent rebound hypoglycemia.

Evaluation

These are postprocedure evaluations. For ongoing monitoring, see Clinical Insight 24-3.

- Assess vital signs, I&O, and weight.
- Observe that the solution is infusing at the prescribed rate.
- Assess patient's tolerance to the infusion (e.g., observe for pulmonary edema; check laboratory results).
- Observe for skin rashes, flushing, color changes, or other signs of allergic reactions; notify the primary care provider. NOTE: These are not common.
- Monitor blood glucose and do not increase the infusion rate until glycemic control is established.

Patient Teaching

- Inform the patient and family of the purpose and duration of the nutritional support.
- Teach them to recognize and report to the nurse symptoms of complications associated with PN.
- Teach the patient that the dressing must remain occlusive and to notify nurse if it comes loose or gets wet.
- Teach the patient the importance of measures to prevent blood infections.

Home Care

- The home environment must provide dry storage space for supplies, a refrigerator for storing admixtures, a clean low-traffic area for procedure preparation, and electronic outlets for any electronic equipment.
- Teach safe disposal of supplies.
- Provide verbal and written instructions of the procedures; demonstrate and ask for a return demonstration. Role play "what would you do if...?" situations with the patient.
- Clients at home often administer their daily 24-hour total over 12 to 16 hours during the night. This allows them to disconnect from the infusion in the morning, flush the central line, and be free to pursue their usual activities during the day.
- Instruct about solution hang time and management of the access device.

  Depending on the anticipated length of therapy, patients may be sent home with a permanent venous access device.

- Provide 24-hour phone numbers for the primary care provider and home care agency.
- Home PN is less expensive than treatment in the hospital and in many cases is associated with a lower risk of infection.
- Home nutritional support is usually under the direction of specialized nutrition support teams.

(continued on next page)

Procedure 24-5 ■ Administering Parenteral Nutrition (continued)

Documentation

- A special form may be used for documenting PN administration.
- Bag number, date and time hung, volume, type of fluid, rate of delivery, additives
- Date and time of dressing or tubing change (if performed)
- Patient's tolerance of procedure
- Pre- and postadministration assessment data, including complications and response to therapy
- Results of fingerstick blood glucose checks
- If insulin is required, type, amount, and route/site administered
- Weight
- I&O

Practice Resources

A.S.P.E.N. Board of Directors and Task Force on Parenteral Nutrition Standardization; Kochevar, Guenter, Holcombe, et al. (2007); Ayers, Boullata, Gervasio, et al. (2014); Boitano, Bojak, McCloskey, et al. (2010); Boullata, Carrera, Harvey, et al. (2017); Boullata, Holcombe, Sacks, et al. (2016); Infusion Nurses Society (2016); McClave, Taylor, Martindale, et al. (2016); Mehta, Skillman, Irving, et al. (2017); Mueller, Compher, Druyan, et al. (2011).

Procedure 24-6 ■ Administering Lipids

➤ For steps to follow in *all* procedures, refer to the Universal Steps for All Procedures found on the page facing the inside back cover.
➤ *Note:* If administering through a central line, refer to Procedure 24-5 for precautions associated with central lines.
➤ *Note:* This procedure is for administering fat emulsions. If you are administering an admixture with the parenteral nutrition solution, use Procedure 24-5.

Equipment

- Intravenous lipid solution (not refrigerated)
- Special tubing (infusion set) for lipids
  Must be without plasticizers (DEHP). Set should be labeled to that effect.
- Needleless cannula (if using a split septum needleless connector that requires it)
- 70% isopropyl alcohol pads or chlorhexidine gluconate
- Procedure gloves
- Time tape
- Infusion pump
- Intake and output record
- If a filter is used, it must be a 1.2-micron filter.
  Lipid particles are large and will clog a smaller size.

Delegation

Do not delegate this skill to the LPN or UAP because administration of lipids requires advanced assessment and critical-thinking skills. The LPN or UAP can assist by monitoring vital signs and verifying patient identity with you. Instruct them about complications associated with lipids and ask them to inform you of any signs or symptoms or change in the patient's condition.

Pre-Procedure Assessments

- Assess for rash; eczema; dry, scaly skin; poor wound healing; and sparse hair.
  These are signs of essential fatty acid deficits.
- Check the history for anemia; coagulation disorders; and abnormal liver, pancreatic, or respiratory function.
  These factors predispose to fat emboli. Your role as a staff nurse is to be certain the PN prescriber is aware of these factors; they do not necessarily contraindicate giving the PN.
- Check peripheral IV site for erythema, infiltration, and patency. Check the central venous access site for erythema or other signs of infection.
- Take baseline vital signs just before infusing the lipids.
  An immediate reaction can occur upon starting the infusion. Note that not all guidelines require this action.
- Check patient's blood glucose level before infusing.
  Lipid infusion can raise the patient's blood glucose.

➤ When performing the procedure, always identify your patient according to agency policy, using two identifiers, and be attentive to standard precautions, hand hygiene, patient safety and privacy, body mechanics, and documentation.

Procedure Steps

1. **Review the prescriber's orders,** including rate of infusion; identify the patient; and explain the purpose of the procedure.
   Verifying helps to prevent dosage and wrong-patient errors. Explaining respects the patient's right to be informed and encourages cooperation.

2. **Gather supplies** and place at bedside. Adjust lighting as needed.
   Organization promotes efficient use of time.

3. **Perform hand hygiene** and don procedure gloves.
   To reduce transmission of infectious microorganisms.

4. **Position the patient supine** in bed.

5. **Be certain lipids are not cold.**
   Cold infusion can cause discomfort.

6. **Examine the bottle** for a layer of froth (indicates leakage) or for separation into fat globules or layers, or cloudiness.
   Do not use the lipids if these occur.

7. **Label the bottle** with the patient's name and identifier, room number, date, time, rate, and start and stop times. Label the tubing with date and time. Note: When lipids are infused with parenteral nutrition, the lipid infusion must be completed within 12 hours.
   Labeling helps ensure that the patient receives the correct infusion.

8. **Compare the lipids bottle** with the patient's wrist band; compare with the prescription (bag number, expiration date). Have a colleague verify.

9. **Determine patency of the IV line** (see Procedure 24-5).

10. **Cleanse the stopper** on the IV bottle with an antiseptic swab; allow to dry.

11. **Connect the special DEHP-free** lipids-infusion tubing to the bottle, twisting the spike as you insert it. **Key Point:** *You must use new tubing for each bottle.*
    Twisting the spike helps ensure that particles from the stopper do not fall into the bottle. New tubing reduces the growth of microorganisms (the feeding provides a medium for fungal growth).

12. **Place the primed tubing** in the pump and attach the tubing to the IV catheter lumen.
    Identify the correct IV line and port for the infusion. Trace the tubing from the bag back to the patient.
    a. Thoroughly scrub the catheter injection port or hub and the luer-lock threads with an antiseptic wipe.
    b. If you are infusing lipids simultaneously with PN, attach the primed lipid tubing to the injection port/hub closest to the patient, below the tubing filter, or through a Y-connection at the catheter hub.
    c. Turn the luer-lock to secure the connection.
    d. NOTE: If a previous infusion has been running, clamp the catheter lumen and the old administration set tubing before disconnecting and changing the tubing.
    Prevents blood backup in the line.

13. **Begin the infusion.** Ideally, infuse slowly at first: 1.0 mL/min for adults and 0.1 mL/min for children (or as prescribed by the physician). Check again to be sure the catheter-tubing connection is secure.
    Slow infusion allows time to assess if the patient will have an adverse reaction to the lipids. Nausea, vomiting, and elevated temperature have been reported when lipids are infused quickly.

14. **Take the vital signs now,** then every 10 minutes for 30 minutes, and according to agency protocol. Observe for side effects (e.g., chills, fever, flushing, dyspnea, nausea, vomiting, headache, back pain).

15. **If no reactions occur,** adjust to the prescribed infusion rate and continue monitoring according to your agency's protocol.

16. **Remove gloves and perform hand hygiene.**

17. **When the infusion is finished,** discard the bottle or bag and IV administration set.
    Formula contains sugars that are a medium for growth of pathogens.

? What if...

- **The entire bottle of lipids is not used?**
  Discard partially used bottles.
  Prevents contamination.

Evaluation

- If ordered, monitor serum lipids 4 hours after discontinuing the infusion.
- Monitor the IV site for infection, inflammation, and infiltration.
- Monitor for symptoms of fat emboli.
- Monitor the IV line for patency.
- Monitor for allergic reactions (nausea, vomiting, headache, chest pain, back pain, fever).
- Monitor for lipid intolerance (triglyceride levels, liver function tests, hepatosplenomegaly, decreased coagulation, cyanosis, dyspnea).

Patient Teaching

- Inform the patient and family of the purpose and duration of the nutritional support.
- Teach the patient to recognize and report symptoms of complications associated with lipid infusion.

Home Care

- The home environment must provide dry storage space for supplies, a refrigerator for storing solutions, a clean low-traffic area for procedure preparation, and outlets for any electronic equipment.

(continued on next page)

Procedure 24-6 ■ Administering Lipids (continued)

- Teach safe disposal of supplies.
- Provide verbal and written instructions for the procedures; demonstrate and ask for a return demonstration.
- Instruct about solution hang time and management of the access device.
- Provide 24-hour phone numbers for the primary care provider and home care agency.

Documentation

- A special form may be used for documenting lipids and PN administration.
- Bottle number, date and time hung, volume, type of fluid, and rate of delivery
- Status of dressing and date and time of dressing or tubing change (if performed)
- Patient's tolerance of the procedure and any problems encountered
- Pre- and postadministration assessment data and blood tests, if any
- Condition of the IV site
- Weight
- I&O

Practice Resources

Infusion Nurses Society (2021, revised); McClave, Taylor, Martindale, et al. (2016); Sepulveda & Pak (2022).

CLINICAL INSIGHTS

Clinical Insight 24-1 ➤ Measurements to Evaluate Body Composition

Measuring Skinfold Measurements

- Take measurements directly on the skin, not through clothing.
- Take each reading as soon as the jaws of the caliper contact the skin and the reading has stabilized.
- In each site, take three readings in quick succession and average the results to the nearest 0.1 mm. *Accuracy of this method varies with the technique.*
- Add the averages of all skinfold sites to arrive at a total skinfold measurement. The combined measurements of triceps skinfold and midupper arm circumference yield a better estimate of muscle and fat areas than does a single measurement.
- To determine the percentage body fat, compare the final calculated measurement with the values in the appropriate body fat and skinfolds table for the age and sex of the patient. *The most reliable location is the triceps for children and female individuals and the subscapular area in male individuals.*

Triceps Skinfold

- Locate the midpoint on the posterior side of the dominant upper arm.
- With the client's arm hanging loosely at the side, palpate the measurement site at the midpoint to become familiar with distinguishing muscle from adipose soft tissue.
- From 1 cm above the midpoint, grasp a vertical pinch of skin and only the subcutaneous fat layer between the thumb and index finger. Gently pull the skinfold away from the underlying muscle.
- Place the skinfold caliper at the midpoint, and slowly release the jaw of the caliper while maintaining a grasp of the skinfold.

Clinical Insight 24-1 ➤ Measurements to Evaluate Body Composition—cont'd

Subscapular Skinfold
- Follow the same procedure, except measure on the back, just under the shoulder blade. Grasp below the tip of the inferior angle of the scapula 45° to vertical.

Biceps Skinfold
- Follow the same procedure, except measure the muscle belly of the biceps. With the patient's arm hanging loosely at the side, grasp the skin and subcutaneous fat layer on the front of the upper arm, over the biceps, about level with the nipple.

Suprailiac Skinfold
- Follow the same procedure, except measure approximately 1 inch above the hipbone, above the iliac crest in the midaxillary line.

Midupper Arm Circumference
- Keeping the client's dominant arm parallel to the body, bend the elbow 90°.
- Using a tape measure, measure the distance between the **acromion** (the bony protrusion of the back of the upper shoulder) and the **olecranon process** (tip of the elbow).
- Mark the midpoint between these two landmarks.
- Ask the client to relax the arm so that it hangs loose and parallel to the body.
- Position the tape around the upper arm at the marked midpoint. Make sure the tape is snug but not so tight as to indent or pinch the skin.
- Record the circumference to the nearest 0.1 cm.

Calculating Waist-to-Hip Ratio (WHR)
- Use a tape measure to measure the circumference of the waist (at the umbilicus with abdominal muscles relaxed). Position the tape snugly but not constricting.
- Use a tape measure to measure the circumference of the hips at their widest point, keeping tape parallel to the floor.
- Calculate the waist-to-hip ratio using the following formula:

$$\text{waist circumference (cm)} \div \text{hip circumference (cm)} = \text{WHR}$$

Example: Robert's waist measurement is 106 cm, and his hip measurement is 114 cm. WHR is 106 ÷ 114 = 0.93.

Clinical Insight 24-2 ▸ Assisting Patients With Meals

General Guidelines
- Recommend having one feeding assistant for every two or three patients who need assistance, allowing about 20 to 30 minutes to feed a patient. Prolonged mealtimes do not promote appetite; nor does hurrying.
- Feeding assistants should be supervised by an RN or LPN.
- Do not interrupt meals with medications.
- Encourage family members to share mealtimes.
- If the patient's condition allows, encourage them to get out of bed for meals or go to the dining room for social time while eating.

Preparation
- Assess for rituals used before meals (e.g., blessings of food).
- Provide an opportunity for toileting, oral hygiene, and handwashing before meals.
- Assist the patient to eat and drink only as necessary; encourage independence.
- Provide privacy during meals if the patient is embarrassed; to further maintain dignity, use a napkin, not a bib, over the patient's clothes.
- Check for proper fit of dentures.
- Provide music during the meal if the patient wishes.
- Demonstrate the use of assistive devices and alternative methods for eating and drinking.

Assisting the Patient
- If the patient must eat in bed, place the head of the bed at the highest tolerable level, and adjust the overbed table to be in easy reach.
- If the patient can feed themselves, prepare the food on the tray (e.g., open food containers, cut the meat, peel an orange, open the dairy and butter containers, mash food if needed).
- If the patient is visually impaired, identify the locations of the meal on the tray based on a clock face (e.g., "The coffee is at 1 o'clock above the plate on the right").

Feeding the Patient
- Feed the patient if they are unable to feed themselves.
- Sit down while feeding the patient; do not rush.
- Position yourself so you can make eye contact.
- Be sure to provide adequate time for the patient to chew and swallow.
- If possible, ask the patient what food they would like next.
- Serve one food at a time; serve small amounts.
- Serve finger foods (e.g., fruit, bread) to promote independence.
  - Cue older adults whenever possible with words or gestures.
- Have casual conversation with the patient while feeding to make mealtime more pleasant and relaxed.

After the Meal
- Help the patient to wash hands or use the rest room.
- Record the amount of food and fluid the patient consumes.
- Document feeding behaviors.
- Document changes in nutrition status.
- Document staffing and staff education and availability of a supportive interdisciplinary team.

Assisting Older Adults With Dementia

As do all people, older adults with dementia differ in their abilities to eat and communicate. The following are general tips, but you should tailor interventions to each person's specific abilities to achieve the best results. In addition to many of the preceding interventions, try some of the following measures.
- Assess the patient's self-feeding abilities.
- Assess the patient's cognitive limitations and communication abilities.
- Assess for and treat pain.
- Minimize distractions: turn off the TV; discourage people from entering the room.
- Help the patient to a comfortable chair if possible.
- Assist with oral hygiene and hand hygiene.
- Remove any unnecessary eating utensils; serve only one food at a time.
- Remove items that should not be eaten (e.g., packets of salt or pepper) and hot items that could be spilled.
- Cue the patient verbally to help with self-feeding (e.g., "take a bite," "chew," "swallow").
- Pantomime eating motions so the patient can imitate them.
- Place your hand over the patient's hand to begin and guide self-feeding (hand-over-hand).
- When assisting, sit at eye level and interact socially with the patient.
- Involve family members if they have assisted with feeding at home.
- Train and supervise UAPs in interacting with and feeding patients with dementia.
- Do not assist too soon—give the patient time to eat independently.
- Do not feed too fast. Feed at a rate that is safe and comfortable for the patient.

Practice Resources
Ebersole, Hess, Touhy, et al. (2019); Liu, Cheon, & Thomas (2014); Porter Starr, Borack, Rincker, et al. (2022).

Clinical Insight 24-3 ▶ Monitoring Patients Receiving Enteral Nutrition

Monitor the following:
- **Position of the feeding tube.** Periodically check the placement of the tube. As a rule, check on each shift or at each intermittent feeding. For double-lumen tubes, keep the air vent above the level of the patient's stomach *so it will not act as a siphon and leak stomach contents.*
- **NG or NE tube insertion site.** An NG or NE tube is secured by adhesive to the nose. Regularly check the skin, gently cleanse the area (with soap and water as for normal washing; avoid harsh skin cleansers), and retape the tube as needed. Report tissue breakdown, epistaxis (nosebleed), or sinusitis, *as they may signal a need for insertion of a percutaneous endoscopy gastrostomy (PEG) tube.*
- **Gastrostomy tube, PEG/PEJ insertion site.** Inspect the insertion site for erythema or drainage, *which are signs of infection.* Clean it daily with soap and water.
- **Fluid balance.** Measure all intake and output.
- **Weight.** To assess the adequacy of the feeding, regularly weigh the patient—same time of day, same type of clothing. There is usually a medical prescription for frequency of weighing. *Frequent weight checks allow adjustment of the feeding orders to achieve the desired goal.*
- **Tube feeding residual volume.** To assess residual volume, aspirate the feeding tube to determine the amount of feeding remaining in the stomach. If the aspirate quantity is equal to or greater than the formula flow rate for 1 hour (or, alternatively, a total of 250 mL), the patient may be receiving too much fluid or may have delayed gastric emptying. However, you should not automatically stop the feeding in the absence of other feeding intolerance; if you obtain a single sample of an increased residual volume, recheck it in 1 hour (Metheny et al., 2016, updated 2020, January 29).
  Because gastric residual volume is not a consistent and reliable indicator of feeding intolerance, the American Society for Parental and Enteral Nutrition (ASPEN) more recently recommends moving away from checking gastric residual volume as part of the routine care to monitor ICU patients receiving enteral nutrition. Instead, a more accurate way to determine enteral digestion is to assess for GI intolerance defined by vomiting, diarrhea, abdominal distention and discomfort, reduced passage of flatus or stool, and abnormal abdominal radiographs (McClave et al., 2016).
- **Frequency of bowel movements.** Bowel movements should occur regularly.
  Constipation is usually due to inadequate water or fiber. Some commercial feedings contain fiber. You may add free water and perhaps fiber to other formulas.
  Diarrhea may indicate intolerance of the formula, excessive feeding, or gastrointestinal disease.
- **Bowel sounds.** Check before each feeding, or every 4 to 8 hours for continuous feedings. *Peristalsis must be present. Flatus is a better indication of complete bowel function than bowel sounds.*
- **Abdominal distention.** Measure abdominal girth daily, at the umbilicus.
- **Serum electrolyte levels.** Monitor regularly (per protocol or prescription).
- **Urine for sugar and acetone.** This is sometimes done as a bedside screening for hyperglycemia. *However, treatment is based on blood sugar levels.*
- **Skin turgor, hematocrit, and urine specific gravity.** *These are indicators of dehydration and overhydration, although skin turgor alone is not a reliable sign.*
- **Serum blood urea nitrogen (BUN) and sodium levels.** *This is especially important for high-protein formulas. Insufficient fluid intake combined with high protein intake may overload the kidneys so that nitrogenous wastes are not excreted adequately.*

Clinical Insight 24-4 ▶ Monitoring and Maintenance Interventions for Patients Receiving Parenteral Nutrition

Monitoring

For patients receiving PN, you will need to monitor the following:

Catheter Insertion Site
- Assess catheter insertion site for swelling, redness, drainage, or tenderness (signs of infection and/or phlebitis in PICC lines).
  The hypertonic PN creates a risk for phlebitis.
- Observe for swelling in the extremity on the same side of catheter insertion (sign of infiltration or phlebitis).
- Observe for catheter retraction from the vein; observe the length of the catheter from the insertion site to the hub at insertion and periodically.

Supplies and Equipment
- Monitor tubing connections to see that they are secure.
- Monitor to see that the dressing is secure and dry.
- Check the rate and amount infused at least hourly to ensure the line is patent, the PN is flowing freely, and the pump is functioning properly.

Weight
- Regularly weigh the patient (according to medical order or agency policy, but commonly daily or 3 times per week). (1) Frequent weight checks allow for assessing the adequacy of the formula and making adjustments as needed to achieve the desired goal. (2) Because of the hypertonicity of the solutions, fluid overload can occur. Rapid weight increase is an indicator.

Glucose
Check blood glucose every 4 to 6 hours until stable, and then at least daily.
The high proportion of glucose in the formulas can cause hyperglycemia, the most common complication of PN. You may need to administer regular insulin according to a sliding scale (or the pharmacist may add it directly to the PN solution). The risk for hyperglycemia is lower with 3:1 PN solutions.

Fluids
Monitor intake and output. Diuresis and dehydration can occur if hypertonic dextrose is infused too rapidly.

Laboratory Values
Patients receiving PN require regular laboratory studies (the following are examples and not a comprehensive list). The frequency of the studies depends on the patient's condition.
- Electrolytes, blood sugar, albumin, BUN, and creatinine (used for formula adjustment and to evaluate electrolyte balance and glucose metabolism)
- Albumin, transferrin, transthyretin (prealbumin), or retinol-binding protein (used to assess visceral protein status)
- 24-hour urine for urine urea nitrogen (weekly) to evaluate nitrogen balance
- Complete blood count (CBC) and differential (to monitor changes in immune function)
- Liver function studies
- Serum zinc
- Plasma urea
- Plasma and urine osmolality
- Blood gases

Symptoms of Complications
- *Electrolyte imbalances.* Symptoms depend on the electrolytes affected. Monitor laboratory values.
- *Sepsis.* Temperature greater than 100°F (37.8°C) orally, rapid pulse from baseline, chills, hypothermia, edema or erythema of skin, exudate from catheter insertion site, malaise, leukocytosis (increased white blood cell count), altered level of consciousness.
- *Air embolus.* Cyanosis, tachypnea, hypotension, heart murmur
- *Catheter dislodgement or thrombosis.* Swelling of arm or neck, pain, difficulty flushing catheter, difficulty infusing PN

Nutrition Status
- Calculate the daily calorie intake.
- Perform nutrition assessment at 2-week intervals.
- Possibly measure arm circumference and triceps skinfold thickness.
- Monitor serum albumin levels.
- Most agencies have specialized nutrition teams who will monitor these parameters.

Maintenance
- Change the dressing over the catheter every 24 hours or according to agency policy or when it becomes wet, soiled, or nonocclusive. Use sterile technique.
- Secure connections with luer-lock connectors; do not use tape.
- Place filter as close to the patient's administration system and change the filter every 24 hours (Ayers et al., 2014).
- Do not hang PN bottles for more than 12 hours (some guidelines and agency policies specify 24 hours).
  Its high nutrient concentration makes PN solution ideal for bacterial growth.
- Use sterile aseptic technique when changing the dressing for a central line as well as when changing the solution and tubing.
- Do not use the PN infusion line for administering any other medicines or solutions.
  To decrease the risk of contamination and infection.
- Infuse PN by pump with a reliable, audible alarm to protect against "free flow."
- If an infusion falls behind schedule, do not increase the rate in an attempt to catch up. This can cause osmotic diuresis and dehydration.
- When PN is discontinued, it may be done gradually (perhaps over as many as 48 hours).
  To prevent a sudden drop in blood sugar.

ASSESSMENT GUIDELINES AND TOOLS
Screening for Nutrition Problems

Patients who have risk factors for nutrition problems should be evaluated using one of the methods in this section: subjective global assessment, Nutrition Screening Initiative (NSI) for Older Adults, and Mini-Nutritional Assessment (MNA).

Focused Assessment

Subjective Global Assessment

Using the subjective global assessment (SGA) method, an experienced clinician examines the general medical history and physical examination to evaluate a client's nutrition status. There are six components pertinent to nutrition status:

1. *Weight history*—over previous 6 months
2. *Dietary history*—including a comparison of usual, recommended, and current intake as well as changes in eating patterns over the past weeks or months
3. *Gastrointestinal symptoms history*—anorexia, nausea, vomiting, and diarrhea
4. *Energy level*—including activity level and functional abilities
5. *Existing disease*—evaluation of the metabolic demands of any disease states along with acute stressors that may alter those demands
6. *Physical examination data*—regarding loss of fat stores, muscle wasting, and the presence of edema and ascites

As a clinician, you would analyze these components to rate the client's nutrition status as normal, mild, moderate, or severe. The effectiveness of this method depends largely on the experience of the clinician (Detsky, McLaughlin, Baker, et al., 1987).

Focused Assessment

Nutrition Screening Initiative (NSI) for Older Adults: Indications of Impaired Nutrition Status

The NSI requires collection and evaluation of data in four areas: clinical, dietary, body composition, and biochemical. In addition, it identifies indicators of impaired nutrition status.

Major indicators	Minor indicators	Symptoms	Physical signs	Laboratory values
➤ Significant weight loss over time	➤ Concurrent syndromes	➤ Anorexia, nausea, or dysphagia	➤ Poor oral or dental status	➤ Reduced levels of serum albumin, transferrin, or prealbumin
➤ Significantly high or low weight for height	➤ Alcoholism	➤ Early satiety	➤ Dehydration	
➤ Significant change in functional status	➤ Cognitive impairment	➤ Changed bowel habits	➤ Poorly healing wounds	➤ Folate deficiency
➤ Significant and inappropriate food intake	➤ Chronic renal insufficiency	➤ Fatigue or apathy	➤ Loss of subcutaneous fat or muscle mass	➤ Iron deficiency
➤ Significant reduction in midarm circumference	➤ Multiple concurrent medications	➤ Memory loss	➤ Fluid retention	➤ Zinc deficiency
➤ Significant decrease in skinfold	➤ Malabsorption syndromes			➤ Reduced levels of ascorbic acid
➤ Osteoporosis or osteomalacia				
➤ Folate or vitamin B deficiency				

Mini-Nutritional Assessment

The Mini-Nutritional Assessment (MNA) is a quick and easy method of identifying individuals with nutrition risk or with malnutrition. This tool was developed primarily for use in older clients. It consists of two parts. The first part screens for nutrition risk: loss of appetite, altered sense of taste and smell, frailty, depression. The second part is completed only if the individual is identified to be at risk: anthropometric measurements (body weight and body mass index, skinfold measurements), nutrition habits, general condition, and self-evaluation for dietary intake (Reber, Gomes, Vasiloglou, et al., 2019). The final score, which tallies the scores of both parts, is the malnutrition indicator score. Indications of malnutrition require interprofessional follow-up. To see and use the MNA,

➡ Go to the Web site **www.mna-elderly.com.**

References

Guigoz (2006); Rubenstein, Harker, Salva, et al. (2001); Vellas, Villars, Abellan, et al. (2006).

Focused Assessment

If you identify nutrition problems or risks using the screening tools, you should perform a more in-depth nutrition assessment, such as the following. The nutrition component of a focused nutrition assessment includes both subjective (history) and objective (physical examination) data.

Focused Nutrition Assessment

Nutrition History

Item	Components
Demographic data	Name, date, age, sex, gender, date of birth, address, occupation, workplace
Chief complaint	Client's subjective statement of health problem, including onset and duration
Present illness and current health	Detailed data about chief complaint as it relates to nutrition status
	Recent diet changes and reasons
	Recent weight loss or gain and over what period
	Usual body weight: 20% above or below desirable weight?
	Change in appetite
	Unusual stress/trauma (surgery, job, family)
	Medications, prescriptions
	Alcohol, nicotine, caffeine consumption
Health history	Previous illnesses, trauma, major dental problems, or issues that could interfere with ability to shop, prepare food, chew, or swallow
	Allergies (i.e., environmental, foods, drugs)
	Eating disorders
	Chronic disease or surgery that affects gastrointestinal (GI) tract
	Substance abuse
	Nutrition programs
	Depression

Focused Nutrition Assessment—cont'd

Item	Components
Family health history	Genetic/familial disorders that could affect nutrition status: cardiovascular or GI disorders, Crohn's disease, diabetes, cancer, sickle cell anemia, allergies, celiac disease, other food intolerances, obesity
Dietary history	Current food intake pattern using one of the following methods: 24-hour–7-day recall, as appropriate; food frequency questionnaire; food record; and comparison to dietary guidelines and Dietary Reference Intakes (DRIs)
	Special dietary considerations, restrictions
	Fad diets
	Vitamin and mineral supplements
	Commercial dietary supplements
	Nonconventional dietary supplements
	Food preferences, dislikes
	Dietary influences from ethnic, cultural, or religious practices
	Counseling needs (based on food knowledge)
Medication history	Recent use of steroids, immunosuppressants, chemotherapy, anticonvulsants, or oral contraceptives
Socioeconomic factors	Adequate food storage, refrigeration, food preparation, payments:
	Supplemental Security Income (SSI); Supplemental Nutrition Assistance Program (SNAP); Women, Infants, and Children (WIC) program
	Who shops for, prepares, and cooks food?
	Location/availability of retail food/grocery store or availability of transportation
Personal factors	Stress/coping mechanisms, self-concept, social supports
	Daily activity level and exercise regimen

Nutrition-Focused Physical Examination

Correlate the following physical examination findings with the dietary history, screening methods, anthropometric measurements, and laboratory results.

I. The General Survey

Assess vital signs, height, weight, and overall impressions.

- **Overall appearance.** Does the client look ill? Do they appear adequately nourished? You will want to investigate any concerns you have as you move through the physical examination.
- **Temperature.** An increase in temperature raises the client's metabolic rate and need for fluid, is a sign of infection, and may decrease the client's appetite.
- **Blood pressure (BP) and heart rate** are affected by fluid status. An elevated BP may be related to fluid volume excess; a low BP may be a sign of dehydration. Heart rate usually increases when fluid volume is low.
- **Height and weight.** Calculate the body mass index (BMI) based on these measures:

$$\text{BMI} = \text{weight in kilograms} \div (\text{height in meters})^2$$

(Continued)

Focused Nutrition Assessment—cont'd

Classification of Body Mass Index Values

Classification	BMI (kg/m^2)	Risk of comorbidities
Underweight*	<18.5	Low
Normal weight	18.5–24.9	Average
Preobese	25.0–29.9	Mildly increased
Class I obesity	30.0–34.9	Moderate
class II obesity	35.0–39.9	Severe
class III obesity	>40.0	Very severe

*NOTE: In adults in long-term care settings or with serious illness, nutrition support should be implemented for those with a BMI of less than 21. In this population, a BMI of less than 21 is associated with increased mortality (Centers for Disease Control and Prevention, 2022, June 3 last reviewed).

II. Integumentary System

- **Skin turgor** is an indicator of fluid status. Poor skin turgor may result from dehydration. Swelling may result from overhydration.
- **Skin integrity** reflects overall nutrition status. Poor wound healing may suggest inadequate intake of protein, vitamin C, or zinc. Patients with uncontrolled diabetes or severely restricted diets often have slow-healing wounds, especially in the feet and legs.
- **Areas of warmth or erythema.** These are signs of inflammation or infection.
- **Other nutrition-related skin changes** include red, swollen skin lesions (caused by niacin deficiency); excessive bleeding seen as petechiae or ecchymosis (caused by vitamin K or C deficiency); and xerosis (dry skin).
- **Abnormal nail findings** include spoon-shaped, brittle nails (caused by iron deficiency); dull nails with transverse ridge (caused by protein deficiency); pale, poor-blanching, or mottled nails (caused by vitamin A or C deficiency); bruising or bleeding beneath nails (caused by protein or caloric deficiency); and splinter hemorrhages (caused by vitamin C deficiency).
- **Hair** will grow slowly, thin, or break easily if protein is deficient.

III. The Head and Neck

The condition of the mouth, teeth, and gums has a major effect on a client's choice of food, ability to chew, and ability to swallow.

- **Facial paralysis or drooping** of one side of the face may be a result of stroke, injury, or nerve irritation, which also affects the ability to chew and swallow (dysphagia).
- **Enlarged thyroid gland.** Look for swelling of the thyroid, which may be related to hypothyroid or hyperthyroid states. Both disorders affect metabolic rate and energy requirements.
- **Eyes.** Nutrition deficits may cause the eyes to be red and dry and the conjunctiva pale.
- **Lips and tongue.** The lips may be chapped, red, or swollen. The tongue may be bright red, purple, or swollen or may have longitudinal furrows.
- **Teeth and gums.** Look for cavities; mottled or missing teeth; and spongy, bleeding, or receding gums.
- **Lymph nodes.** Palpate for enlarged or tender lymph nodes under the chin and along the neck. Nodes that are swollen can signal infection, such as a sore throat.

IV. Cardiovascular System

You will have gained initial information about the cardiovascular system by taking the vital signs. As you follow up and listen to the heart and check pulses, you should explore any abnormal vital signs.

- **Bounding pulses** are associated with fluid overload, fever, and hypertension.
- **Weak, thready pulse** may indicate dehydration, shock, or hypotension.
- **Edema in the extremities** may be a sign of fluid overload, inadequate protein stores, or electrolyte imbalance.

V. Abdominal Examination

- **A scaphoid or concave abdomen** indicates loss of subcutaneous fat, possibly caused by malnutrition.
- **A round or protuberant abdomen** points to obesity caused by excess caloric and/or high fat intake.

Focused Nutrition Assessment—cont'd

> - ***A generalized enlarged abdomen*** may signify *ascites* (fluid in the abdominal cavity) caused by liver malfunction. Ascites results from three mechanisms: abnormal movement of protein and water into the abdomen, sodium and fluid retention, and decreased albumin production in the liver.
> - ***Hyperactive bowel sounds*** are heard with gastrointestinal (GI) infection, laxative use, and malabsorption disorders.
> - ***Hypoactive bowel sounds*** suggest sluggish motility in the GI tract.

VI. Musculoskeletal System

> - ***Thin extremities with excess skinfolds*** may indicate muscle atrophy and fat loss related to malnutrition, especially protein and calories. This may also occur because of prolonged bedrest and inadequate food intake. Skinfold measurement is also useful in assessing muscle and fat stores.
> - Look for any obvious **swelling, deformities, or limitation in range of motion** of the joints.
> - ***Kyphosis*** of the spine may indicate osteoporosis and possible insufficient calcium intake.
> - ***Joint pain*** on palpation or with movement is a sign of arthritis or gout. Arthritis may affect ability to shop for groceries, prepare food to eat, and use utensils for eating and drinking. Gout is often induced by diets high in *purines* (food substances that break down into uric acid), obesity, and excess alcohol intake.

VII. Neurological System

The neurological examination will provide insight into the client's ability to perform independent tasks.

> - Look for **altered level of consciousness or signs of behavioral disturbances and dementia** through general conversation and appropriateness of answers to specific questions.
> - Assess **coordination and reflexes.**
> - Assess for **cognitive deficits or severe psychiatric disorders.** A client with cognitive deficits or severe psychiatric disorders may have difficulty preparing food or judging appropriate nutrient choices.
> - Assess for **motor or sensory deficits.** Clients with motor or sensory deficits may be unable to purchase, prepare, or eat a variety of foods.
> - ***Confusion, weakness, diminished reflexes, paresthesia, and sensory loss*** may be clues to vitamin B deficiencies.
> - ***Tetany or severe and generalized muscle spasm*** may indicate calcium or magnesium deficits.

VIII. Signs of Severe Malnutrition

Malnutrition is a condition of impaired development or function caused by a long-term deficiency, excess, or imbalance in energy and/or nutrient intake.

> - Symptoms of undernutrition caused by insufficient food include reduced physical activity, weight loss, and reduced height.
> - Children, older adults, and people with chronic illnesses such as cancer, HIV infection, and chronic obstructive pulmonary disease (COPD) are most likely to experience malnutrition. Malnutrition can occur with obesity.
> - To assess for malnutrition in children, compare weight, height, and head circumference to the standards (norms) for the child's age.
> - Other indicators in children include the presence of iron-deficiency anemia.
> - In adolescents, look for a delay of stages of sexual maturation.

DIAGNOSTIC TESTING

Tests Reflecting Nutrition Status: Norms

Note: Norms are for adults (aged 19 to 65) unless otherwise noted.

Blood glucose	70 mg/dL to 100 mg/dL
	▸ Capillary blood sugar is frequently assessed at the bedside with a simple fingerstick.
	▸ Serum blood glucose is assessed by drawing a venous blood sample. The level is measured in the laboratory.
	The American Diabetes Association (n.d.) recommends preprandial (before a meal) plasma glucose level of 80 to 130 mg/dL for patients with diabetes. For patients with diabetes, postprandial (1–2 hours after eating) plasma glucose should be less than 180 mg/dL.
Serum albumin	3.4–4.8 g/dL
Prealbumin	12–42 mg/dL (aged 6 yr–adult)
Globulin	2.3–3.4 g/dL
Blood urea nitrogen (BUN)	5–18 mg/dL (children)
	8–21 mg/dL (aged 14–adult); 10–31 mg/dL (adult older than 90)
Creatinine	0.5–1 mg/dL (female)
	0.6–1.2 mg/dL (male)
Hemoglobin	13.2–17.3 g/dL (male)
	11.7–15.5 g/dL (female)
	12.6–17.4 g/dL (male, older adult)
	11.7–16.1 g/dL (female, older adult)
Hemoglobin A1c (HbA1c)	For patients without diabetes:
	Normal: 4.0–5.6%
	Prediabetes: 5.7–6.4%
	Diabetes: 6.5% and above

CLINICAL REASONING
Applying the Full-Spectrum Nursing Model

PATIENT SITUATION

Mrs. Ong is a 75-year-old retired schoolteacher who suffered a stroke 8 months ago. Since leaving the hospital, she has been living in a nursing home. Mrs. Ong has residual weakness on the right side—her dominant side—and has not mastered the use of tableware with her left hand. On admission to the nursing home 7 months ago, she weighed 150 pounds. Today she weighs only 125 pounds. Mrs. Ong refuses to go to the dining room for meals. The UAPs report that she eats a few bites of most foods but never eats more than half of anything.

THINKING

1. *Theoretical Knowledge:*

    a. Based on Mrs. Ong's sex, age, and activity level, make a rough estimate of the number of kcal/day she needs.

    b. What are two other more precise ways you could determine Mrs. Ong's ideal body weight?

2. *Critical Thinking (Considering Alternatives):* What are some possible explanations for why Mrs. Ong is not eating all her food?

DOING

3. *Practical Knowledge:*

    a. Suppose you have decided to use the general ideal weight guide to determine Mrs. Ong's ideal weight. What, specifically, would you need to do? You do not need to calculate; just list the action steps.

    b. Suppose you have decided to determine Mrs. Ong's body mass index (BMI). What equipment would you need?

    c. What is the formula for calculating BMI from the height and weight?

4. *Nursing Process (Nursing Diagnosis/Analyzing Cues):* Write a nursing diagnosis for Mrs. Ong. Use just the data provided in the situation. Assume her BMI is 20.

CARING

5. *Self-Knowledge:* What would you be feeling if you were in Mrs. Ong's situation?

6. *Ethical Knowledge:* What are one or two things you would do to help Mrs. Ong feel cared for and cared about?

Critical Thinking and Clinical Judgment

1. Recall the employees (Isaac Schwartz and Sujing Lee) interviewed in the Meet Your Patient scenario in Volume 1. In addition, you now have two more patients, Wakenda Pierre and Luceno Jarin. Their information is in the following paragraphs:

    - Isaac Schwartz, a 65-year-old accountant, works long hours. He describes a sedentary lifestyle, no tobacco use, infrequent alcohol use, no medical problems, and a nutrition history of skipping meals and daily consumption of restaurant food. You measure his height as 69 in. and weight as 245 lb.

    - Sujing Lee, a 29-year-old project manager, regularly works 65 hours per week. Sujing is 30 weeks pregnant. She does not smoke or drink and has never been hospitalized or had surgery. She has gained a total of 25 lb since becoming pregnant. Her diet consists mainly of traditional Chinese food. She eats three meals a day and always brings lunch from home. Lately, she has been feeling "tired all the time." At the screening, she weighs 126 lb and is 63 in. tall.

    - Wakenda Pierre is a 38-year-old administrative assistant. She exercises at the gym 4 or 5 days per week, smokes an occasional cigarette, has 2 or 3 drinks every night before dinner, struggles with keeping her blood pressure under control, and eats fast food for breakfast and lunch every day. She is 72 in. tall and weighs 165 lb.

    - Luceno Jarin is a 65-year-old business executive. He tells you he was diagnosed with type 2 diabetes mellitus 5 years ago. He is struggling to follow his prescribed diet. He drinks alcohol sporadically and walks briskly 30 minutes every day of the week. He is 67 in. tall and weighs 205 lb.

    a. Determine each client's BMI. Based on these results, what conclusions can you make about their weight status?

    b. What are the likely causes of each person's weight status?

    c. What additional work-up would be recommended for each person?

    d. What indications would lead you to believe that each client has adopted a healthier lifestyle?

2. The following are three clients admitted to the medical-surgical unit of your local hospital. On their admission, the primary nurse collected the following information:

	CLIENT 1	CLIENT 2	CLIENT 3
Weight	175 lb	100 lb	250 lb
Height	70 in.	59 in.	65 in.
Sex/age	Male/40 years old	Female/18 years old	Male/65 years old
Usual daily caloric intake	2,500 kcal	1,000 kcal	2,500 kcal
Usual activity level	Moderate	High	Light
Serum albumin	Normal	Low	Normal
Serum glucose	Normal	Low	High

a. Identify which client(s) is/are at risk for nutrition imbalance.

b. Which client is at risk for developing malnutrition?

c. What additional information would support this conclusion?

d. What nursing interventions would you initiate at this time?

3. After 3 days, you examine how well each of these clients is doing using the same parameters as admission day.

	CLIENT 1	CLIENT 2	CLIENT 3
Weight	170 lb	103 lb	250 lb
Current daily caloric intake	2,500 kcal	1,500 kcal	1,500 kcal
Intake (mL)	2,000	2,000	1,000
Output (mL)	1,800	1,900	500
Current activity level	Up as tolerated	Up as tolerated	Bedrest
Serum albumin	Normal	Low	Normal
Serum glucose	Normal	Low	High

a. In comparison with the admission data, there are some changes. Which client's health status is a priority now, and why?

b. What is/are the most likely cause(s) of this concern?

c. Which nursing interventions should be initiated for this client while hospitalized? Focus on nutrition needs.

d. Identify appropriate education that should begin during hospitalization for this client.

4. For each of the following concepts, use critical thinking to describe how or why it is important to nursing, patient care, or nutrition. Note that these are *not* to be merely definitions.

Energy balance	Basal metabolic rate
Body mass index	Nutrients
Weight management	Nutrition history
Body weight standards	Enteral feedings
Parenteral nutrition	Special diets
Nutrition screening	

What Are the Main Points in This Chapter?

- Reliable guidelines for designing a nutritious diet include the Dietary Reference Intakes (DRIs), the USDA Dietary Guidelines, and the nutrition facts panel found on packaged foods in the United States.
- ChooseMyPlate is a food guide that illustrates healthful dietary choices. It stresses six concepts for healthy eating: activity, moderation, personalization, proportionality, variety, and gradual improvement.
- Energy nutrients are carbohydrates, proteins, and fats (lipids). Other important nutrients are water and the micronutrients: fat-soluble vitamins, water-soluble vitamins, and minerals.
- Carbohydrates include simple sugars called monosaccharides and disaccharides and complex carbohydrates called *polysaccharides*.
- Glucose, a monosaccharide, is the primary source of energy for the brain as well as for the body during moderate-to-intense physical activity.
- Proteins are made up of amino acids and are required for cell and tissue growth, maintenance, and repair. They also act as buffers in acid–base balance. Proteins are an energy source.
- Lipids, including fats and oils, are classified as glycerides, sterols, and phospholipids. They are essential components of cells, fuel the body at rest and during light activity, aid in absorption of fat-soluble vitamins, and promote a sense of satiety when eaten. Low-density lipoproteins (LDLs) are the "bad" cholesterol. High-density lipoproteins (HDLs) are the "good" cholesterol.
- Saturated fats and trans fats are less healthful lipid choices than mono- and polyunsaturated fats. Saturated fats and trans fats raise LDL cholesterol levels in the blood.
- The essential fatty acids omega-6 and omega-3 help protect against heart disease when they replace trans fats in the diet. They are found mainly in vegetable oils, nuts, seeds, and fatty fish.
- Nutrients must be consumed at least at a minimal level to meet the body's physiological needs. This level is called Dietary Reference Intake (DRI).
- The fat-soluble vitamins are A, D, E, and K. Water-soluble vitamins are C- and B-complex vitamins.
- Minerals (e.g., calcium, iron, magnesium) are important for transmitting nerve impulses, regulating fluid balance, strengthening bones, and producing energy.
- The basal metabolic rate (BMR) is a measure of the energy required by resting tissue to maintain basic function.
- Factors influencing a client's nutrition status include developmental stage, pregnancy and lactation, education, lifestyle choices, vegetarianism, dieting for weight loss, culture, religion, disease processes, functional limitations, economic factors, and modified or special diets.
- Many people must follow a modified diet to assist in managing illnesses. In addition, all inpatients must have a diet prescribed by their primary healthcare provider.
- When examining an individual's nutrition balance, it is important to screen for nutrition problems. When risk factors are present, thoroughly assess nutrition history, physical findings, anthropometric measurements, imaging techniques, and biochemical values.
- A food record is the most accurate method of obtaining data about a client's actual food intake.
- The body mass index (BMI), skinfold measurements, and body part circumferences are estimates of body composition.
- Laboratory or biochemical indicators of nutrition status include blood glucose and serum protein levels or indices such as albumin, urea, and hemoglobin.
- Vitamin and mineral supplementation may be appropriate for some people, but supplementation does not replace the need for a balanced diet.

- Government programs provide some assistance for clients who cannot afford to buy food.
- Nutrition requirements of older adults are similar to those for all adults, with a slight reduction in the need for calories, and the more likely need for nutrient supplementation. Nutrition problems are also similar, but the incidence is higher among older adults.
- Nurses can help support nutrition for patients who have deficits in self-care or impairment of swallowing by assisting patients with meals and providing swallowing therapy.
- Nutrition imbalance can range from inadequate to excessive amounts of a single nutrient relative to overall caloric intake.
- Obesity is a major problem in the United States, both in children and in adults.
- Interventions for underweight/undernutrition include measures to improve the patient's appetite, assisting with meals, and providing enteral and parenteral nutrition.
- Nasogastric tubes are inserted to lavage the stomach; collect a specimen of the stomach contents; or prevent nausea, vomiting, and gastric distention. They are also placed to facilitate enteral feeding.
- The most accurate way to check enteral tube placement is by radiographic (x-ray) verification. To check enteral tube placement at the bedside, you could also use a combination of techniques: aspirate stomach contents to observe color and measure the pH (normally 1 to 5.5 for stomach contents); serial observations for respiratory distress, residual volume, length of tube extending outside the body; and capnometry. Do not rely on a single technique.
- Potential complications associated with enteral feedings include aspiration, infection, diarrhea, and electrolyte imbalance.
- Meticulous sterile technique when administering parenteral nutrition is critical because the solution is delivered into a large central vein; if infection occurs, sepsis is almost immediate.

Knowledge Map

TYPES
MACRONUTRIENTS
- Carbohydrates
- Proteins
- Lipids (fats)

MICRONUTRIENTS
- Vitamins
- Minerals

SOURCE OF INFORMATION
- DRIs
- USDA guidelines
- USDA Food Pyramid
- Nutrition facts panels

FACTORS AFFECTING BMR
- Body composition
- Body and environmental temp
- Disease states
- Physical exertion

NUTRIENTS
- Underweight / Malnutrition
- Obesity

- Potential obesity
- Healthy / Potential underweight

- BMR
- Physical Activity

NUTRITION: TOTAL ENERGY NEEDS

Factors affecting:
- Developmental stage
- Lifestyle choices
- Culture; ethnicity
- Religious beliefs
- Disease processes
- Functional limitations

MEETING NUTRITIONAL NEEDS

ASSESSING NUTRITIONAL STATUS
- Body composition
  - Skin fold
  - Circumferences
  - BMI
  - Imaging
- Laboratory values
  - Blood glucose
  - Pre-albumin; albumin
  - Urea/creatinine
  - WBC; hemoglobin

SUPPORTING SPECIAL NEEDS
- Impaired swallowing
- Patients who are NPO
- Older adults
- Assisting with meals
- Improving patient's appetite

PROVIDING SPECIAL DIETS
- Clear liquid
- Full liquid
- Mechanical soft
- Pureed
- Calorie restricted
- Sodium or fat restricted
- Diabetic
- Renal
- Protein controlled
- Calorie protein push
- Antigen avoidance

ALTERNATIVE FEEDING METHODS
- Enteral: NG, NE, PEG tube, G-button
- Parenteral

CHAPTER 25

Urinary Elimination

STUDENT RESOURCES

The questions and exercises in this book allow you to practice the kind of thinking you will use as a full-spectrum nurse. Critical-thinking questions usually have more than one right answer, so we do not provide "correct" answers for these features. Try to answer these questions yourself. It is more important to develop your nursing judgment than to just cover content. You will learn more by discussing the questions with your peers. If you are still unsure, see the Davis Advantage chapter resources for suggested responses.

To explore learning resources for this chapter,

Go to www.DavisAdvantage.com and find:

Answers and Suggested Responses for all questions in this chapter
Concept Map
Knowledge Map
References and Bibliography

Key Concepts
Urinary elimination

Related Concepts
See the Concept Map on Davis Advantage.

Example Client Conditions
Urinary incontinence
Urinary retention
Urinary tract infection (UTI)

Caring for the Williams Family

At a recent visit to the Family Health Center, Stanley and Nadine Williams confide that Stanley's mother, Charlene Williams, has had several "accidents." She has denied the problem, but Nadine tells you that she helped her mother-in-law with laundry recently and found that many of the clothes smelled of urine. They ask you how to approach Charlene about this problem.

A. How would you respond?

B. What suggestions, if any, could you make to Stanley and Nadine about treatment for Charlene?

C. Nadine says that she has been told that surgery is the best form of treatment. She asks you whether this is true. How would you answer her question?

PracticalKnowledge clinical application

This section provides procedures and clinical insights you will need to support your patients' urinary function. You will also find assessment guidelines and information about diagnostic tests of urinary function.

PROCEDURES

Procedure 25-1 ■ Measuring Postvoid Residual Urine Volume With a Portable Bladder Scanner

➤ For steps to follow in *all* procedures, refer to the Universal Steps for All Procedures on the inside back cover of volume 2.

Equipment
- Portable bladder scanning device
- Ultrasound gel
- Clean gloves
- Tissues
- Antiseptic swabs or wipes

Delegation
Measuring urine, including postvoid residual volume (PVR) with the use of a portable bladder scanner, may be delegated to specially trained unlicensed assistive personnel (UAP) in some facilities. However, you must be sure that the UAP knows how to perform the procedure correctly, including proper cleansing of the bedpan/urinal and the graduated container according to the facility's policies. Also, complete the following assessments, and instruct the UAP when to stop the procedure and seek assistance from the nurse and to report the results immediately. In some instances, you may choose to perform the bladder scan to ensure accuracy and expedite any necessary treatment.

Preprocedure Assessments
- *Cognitive status.* Determine whether the patient can be instructed to complete this procedure on their own and/or whether they can follow directions.
- *Mobility status.* Determine whether the patient can be permitted to get out of the bed to use the toilet.
- *Urinary status.* Determine the patient's ability to control bladder function.
- *Postvoid residual urine volume,* if needed. Determine the timing and amount of the last voiding.

  Note: A bladder scan should be done as soon as possible after voiding and within no more than 15 minutes.
- *Palpate the bladder* to assess for distention.

➤ When performing the procedure, always identify your patient according to agency policy, using two identifiers, and be attentive to standard precautions, hand hygiene, patient safety and privacy, body mechanics, and documentation.

Procedure Steps

1. **Perform hand hygiene,** and don clean gloves.
   Prevents transmission of bacteria.

2. **Assist the patient to the supine** position. Uncover only the patient's lower abdomen and suprapubic area.

3. **Clean the scanner head** with antiseptic wipes.
   Prevents transmission of microorganisms between patients.

4. **Turn the device on.**

5. **Select the patient sex by touching the icon on the device.** If a patient has had a hysterectomy, follow the manufacturer's directions for sex selection. In some cases, you will select the MALE icon for a patient who has undergone hysterectomy.
   The device is calibrated to adjust for uterus and bladder anatomy.

6. **Palpate the symphysis pubis,** and apply an ample quantity of warmed ultrasound gel midline on the abdomen, approximately 2.5 to 4 cm (1 to 1.5 inches) above the symphysis pubis.
   The gel ensures proper transmission of the ultrasound. Warm gel is more comfortable for the patient.

7. **Position the scanner head** in the gel, and aim it toward the bladder, pointing slightly downward toward the patient's coccyx.

Proper placement allows for an accurate reading. ▼

(continued on next page)

Procedure 25-1 ■ Measuring Postvoid Residual Urine Volume With a Portable Bladder Scanner (continued)

8. **Press and release the SCAN** button. Hold the scanner head steady until the scan is finished.
   An audible tone indicates the scan is complete.

9. **Read the bladder volume measurement.** Repeat the scan to ensure accuracy.
   Note: Some scanners will also display an image of the bladder. The bladder image should be centered on the crossbars. If it is not, reposition the scanner head, and repeat the scan. ▼

10. **Press DONE when finished.** Print the results by pressing PRINT.
    A printout provides for accurate documentation and may, in some facilities, be added to the patient record.

11. **Wipe the gel from** the patient's skin with tissue, cover the patient, and return the patient to a comfortable position.

12. **Clean the scanner head** with antiseptic. Remove gloves and perform hand hygiene.

? What if...

- **The healthcare provider prescribes hourly monitoring of the patient's urine output?**

Obtain a special collection bag with a small measuring chamber; document urine output on the I&O record every hour. Be sure that the cylinder does not overflow in the hour. Check the collection bag more frequently if the input is increased or if the patient has a diuretic.

Taking several readings ensures maximum accuracy.

Evaluation

- Note any unusual characteristics of the urine (e.g., color, odor, presence of sediment or mucus).
- Note any difficulties with urination (e.g., pain, dribbling, difficulty beginning urination).
- Continue to monitor that urine is flowing freely from the indwelling catheter and that the drainage bag is below the level of the bladder.
- Assess for bladder distention.
  Bladder distention indicates poor bladder emptying.

  NOTE: If the facility has a bladder-scanning device, scan to determine whether there is residual urine.

Patient Teaching

Instruct the patient and/or primary caregiver to document fluid intake and urine output on the I&O record.

Home Care

Teach the client and/or the primary caregiver how to collect and measure urine and how to document fluid intake and urine output on the I&O record.

Documentation

- Record urine volume and record the time and date the specimen was collected, per agency policy (e.g., in the nurse's notes or a patient graphic flow sheet, depending on the agency).
- Document the characteristics of the urine, including color, odor, particulate matter, blood, and clarity.
- Document any difficulty with voiding, including pain or burning with urination, frequency, or difficulty starting the urine flow.
- For PVR, document the time and amount of the last void before the scan and the amount of residual urine. Follow agency policy related to attaching a printout of the bladder scan to the patient record.

Sample documentation

00/00/00   1500   Voided 75 mL of clear, yellow urine with no odor, blood, or mucus. Pt states that he still feels full. Bladder palpated just above level of symphysis pubis. Bladder scan performed—350 mL of residual urine in bladder. Dr. Roy contacted and straight catheterization prescribed.─────────────────────S. Tran, RN

Practice Resources
Agency for Healthcare Research and Quality (2017, March); Appendix C Sample Bladder Scan Policy (2020, October); Ballstaedt & Woodbury (2020); Boyer, Steltzer, & Larrabee (2009).

Thinking About the Procedures

The videos **Measuring Postvoid Residual Urine Volume With a Portable Bladder Scanner,** along with questions and suggested responses, are available on the **Davis's *Nursing Skills Videos*** Web site at www.fadavis.com.

Procedure 25-2 ■ Obtaining a Urine Specimen for Testing

➤ For steps to follow in *all* procedures, refer to the Universal Steps for All Procedures on the inside back cover of Volume 2.

Equipment

Collecting a Clean-Catch Urine Specimen

- Prepackaged collection kit
- If no kit is available:
  - Sterile specimen container
  - Antiseptic solution
  - Sterile cotton balls or 2 × 2 inch gauze pads
- Washcloth and towel, or perineal wipes
- Perineal wash solution
- Two pairs of clean procedure gloves
- Patient identification labels
- Bedpan or bedside commode for an immobile patient

Obtaining a Sterile Urine Specimen From a Catheter

- Clean gloves
- Antiseptic swab or wipe
- Sterile specimen container with a lid
- Patient identification label
- Sterile 5- to 10-mL syringe with a sterile 21- to 25-gauge needleless access device

Collecting a 24-Hour Urine Specimen

Note: Some tests require using a double-storage container. Be sure to find out if you need a double-storage container and preservative, and if there are special instructions for collection of the sample.

- Basin and ice, possibly (check with the laboratory to determine whether the specimen needs to be kept cold during the 24-hour collection)
- Large collection container

Delegation

You may delegate this procedure to the UAP, but you must be sure that he or she knows how to perform the procedure correctly, including proper cleansing and maintaining sterility of the container. You must complete the following assessments and instruct the UAP to report any abnormalities seen in the urine (e.g., blood, foul odor, mucus) or any patient complaints of dysuria. The UAP should bring the specimen to you for inspection.

Preprocedure Assessments

- **Cognitive status:** Determine whether the patient can follow directions and complete this procedure on their own.
- **Mobility status:** Assess the patient's ability to ambulate to the bathroom or bedside commode.
  To determine where the specimen will be collected.
- **Urinary status:** Assess the patient's ability to control urinary flow.
  To plan how to best collect a urine specimen.

(continued on next page)

Procedure 25-2 ■ Obtaining a Urine Specimen for Testing (continued)

Procedure 25-2A ■ Collecting a Clean-Catch Urine Specimen

> When performing the procedure, always identify your patient according to agency policy, using two identifiers, and be attentive to standard precautions, hand hygiene, patient safety and privacy, body mechanics, and documentation.

Procedure Steps

1. **Perform hand hygiene. Don procedure gloves.**

2. **Open the prepackaged kit.** Remove the contents.
   - Open the sterile specimen cup, being careful not to touch the inside of the lid or container. Place it within easy reach.
   - Make sure to place the lid with the inside surface facing upward. Do not touch the inside of the lid.
   - Open the packages of towelettes or cotton balls.

3. **Cleanse the perineum and urethra.**

For Female Patients
   a. Open the antiseptic towelette provided in the prepackaged kit. If there is no towelette, pour the antiseptic solution over the cotton balls.
   b. To cleanse the perineum, separate the folds of the urinary opening (labia) with fingers. Wipe down one side of the meatus using one pad and discard the towelette or cotton ball. Then wipe the other side with a second towelette or cotton ball. Wipe down the center over the urinary meatus with the third towelette and discard it. Use each towelette or cotton ball only once.
   Following the "clean to dirty" principle decreases the likelihood of contamination of the specimen and the urethra with feces. ▼

   c. Continue to hold the labia apart until the specimen is obtained.
   To help keep bacteria from the labia from contaminating the urine specimen.

For Male Patients
   a. If the penis is uncircumcised, retract the foreskin back from the end of the penis.
   Allows for better access when cleansing the area around the meatus.
   b. Use the towelette provided in the prepackaged kit or pour antiseptic solution over cotton balls. You might also use 2 × 2-inch gauze pad soaked with povidone–iodine to cleanse the periurethral area.

   ✚ Before using an iodine-based solution, be sure to check the patient's health history for allergy to iodine.

   c. With one hand, grasp the penis. With the other hand, use the towelette or soaked cotton balls to cleanse the entire head of the penis in a circular motion from the meatus outward away from the urethral opening. Use each towelette or cotton ball only once.
   Prevents contamination of the specimen.
   d. Keep one hand in place to retract the foreskin (if uncircumcised) or to hold the penis (for a patient who is unable to assist).

4. **Pick up the sterile specimen container** and hold it near the meatus. Instruct the patient to begin voiding into the toilet.

5. **Allow a small stream of urine to pass;** then, without stopping the urine stream, place the specimen container into the stream, collecting approximately 30 to 60 mL. Check with the agency laboratory to determine how much urine to collect.
   Midstream urine collection prevents specimen contamination.

6. **Remove the container from the stream,** and allow the patient to finish emptying the bladder into the toilet. Note: For men, if the penis is uncircumcised, replace the foreskin over the glans when the procedure is finished.

7. **Carefully replace the container lid,** touching only the outside of the cap and container. Avoid touching the rim of the cup to the genital area. Ensure there is no toilet paper, feces, pubic hair, menstrual blood, or anything else in the urine sample.
   Maintains sterility of specimen and prevents cross-contamination.

8. **Label the container** with the correct patient information (in many institutions, labels are pre-printed or barcoded). Place the container in a facility-specific carrier (usually a plastic bag) for transport to the laboratory.

9. **Remove your gloves and perform hand hygiene.** If the specimen has been obtained in a bedpan, leave your gloves on until you have removed, emptied, and stored the bedpan properly.
   Hand hygiene and gloving prevent transmission of bacteria.

10. **Assist the patient back to bed,** or remove the bedpan or urinal, if applicable. (See Procedure 26-2 for instructions on removing a bedpan.) Raise the side rails and place the call bell in a convenient location.

11. **Transport the specimen** to the laboratory in a timely manner.
    Delayed testing can cause inaccurate results (e.g., casts in urine will break up if urine is allowed to sit for an extended period).

Procedure 25-2B ■ Obtaining a Sterile Urine Specimen From a Catheter

▶ When performing the procedure, always identify your patient according to agency policy, using two identifiers, and be attentive to standard precautions, hand hygiene, patient safety and privacy, body mechanics, and documentation.

Procedure Steps

1. **Don procedure gloves** and empty the drainage tube of urine.

2. **Clamp the drainage tube** below the level of the specimen port for 15 to 30 minutes to allow a fresh sample to collect. If the client's urine is flowing briskly, you may not need to clamp the catheter.

3. **Remove your contaminated gloves and perform hand hygiene.** Then don a sterile pair before scrubbing the specimen port with an antiseptic swab or wipe.
   Aseptic technique is used to obtain a catheter sample of urine (Loveday, Pratt, Wilson, et al., 2014).

4. **Insert the needleless access device** with a 10-mL syringe into the specimen port, and aspirate to withdraw the amount of urine you need. ▼

5. **Once you have the sample,** transfer the specimen into a sterile specimen container.

6. **Discard the needleless access device** and syringe in a safe container.

7. **Tightly cap** the specimen container.

8. **Remove the clamp** from the catheter. Remove gloves and perform hand hygiene.

   ✚ Be sure to unclamp the tubing of the urinary collection bag after you obtain the sample.
   Urine backflow can cause bladder distention and lead to stasis-induced urinary tract infection (UTI).

9. **Label and package the specimen** with the correct patient identification, according to agency policy. *To avoid "wrong patient" error.*

10. **Transport the specimen to the laboratory.** If immediate transport is not possible, refrigerate the sample, per agency policy.

    ✚ Never disconnect the catheter from the drainage tube to obtain a sample. Interrupting the system creates a portal of entry for pathogens, thereby increasing the risk of contamination.

Procedure 25-2C ■ Collecting a 24-Hour Urine Specimen

▶ When performing the procedure, always identify your patient according to agency policy, using two identifiers, and be attentive to standard precautions, hand hygiene, patient safety and privacy, body mechanics, and documentation.

Procedure Steps

1. **Use a large collection container** (usually supplied by the laboratory) to collect all urine voided in the 24-hour period. If you need to use more than one container during the 24-hour period, use one container at a time. When it is full, collect the urine in the next container. Label it with the patient's name and the date and time of the first voiding (labels may be preprinted or bar coded).

2. **To begin collection,** have the patient empty the bladder and discard the urine. Record the time. This is the start time of the 24-hour collection.
   This urine was produced before the start of the collection period and should not be part of the specimen collection.

3. **Collect all urine voided** during the next 24 hours. Just before the collection period ends, ask the patient to void again, and add this last specimen to the collection container. Store the collection container in a designated refrigerator or surrounded by ice.
   If the laboratory does not receive the entire collection, the results will be inaccurate.

4. **Inform the patient and all staff** about the collection.
   Communication can help prevent accidental discarding of urine.

5. **Post signs in prominent** locations, such as the patient's bathroom or entry door, to remind staff of the ongoing collection.
   Key Point: *It is essential that none of the urine voided during the 24-hour period be accidentally discarded.*

6. **Check to be sure the container is properly labeled** with the correct patient information (name, date, and time the test ended). Place the container in a facility-specific carrier (usually a plastic bag), and transport it to the laboratory in a timely manner, following agency protocol.

? What if . . .

■ **A urine culture is prescribed?**
Be sure to list current antibiotic therapy on the laboratory request form.
This information is important to accurately determine sensitivity of the microorganisms.

■ **A clean-catch urine sample is needed from an immobile patient?**
For the patient using a bedpan, raise the head of the bed to semi-Fowler's position.

(continued on next page)

Procedure 25-2 ■ Obtaining a Urine Specimen for Testing (continued)

Facilitates correct direction of urine flow down into the specimen container you are holding. In addition, this is the anatomical position for voiding.

- **I need to collect a urine sample from an infant?**
    1. Remove the paper covering adhesive patches on the back side of the specimen bag before applying it to the clean and dry perineal area. Start at the narrow area between the anus and the vaginal or scrotal area. Press the adhesive sides firmly against the skin while avoiding wrinkles in the skin against the patch.
    2. It is easier to apply the lower portion of the bag first. The area must also be dry for the adhesive to stick to the skin. Because infants urinate frequently, it is best to work quickly to catch the specimen. Work upward to secure the bag around the entire genital area.
    3. After the specimen bag has been applied, put a diaper on the infant/child. Remember to check the collection bag every 15 to 30 minutes to see if there is a specimen. If the infant has not urinated in 2 to 3 hours, discard the bag, recleanse the area, and apply a new bag.
    It is possible there was a leak in the seal between the skin and the adhesive sides of the specimen collection bag.
    4. Once a specimen is obtained in the bag, remove it gently, and pour the urine into a sterile specimen cup. Label it with the patient-identifying information. ▼

- **The female patient is menstruating?**

    Instruct the patient to insert a clean tampon for starting the stream of urine. *A tampon will prevent contamination of the sample with menstrual fluid.*

Evaluation

- Note any unusual characteristics of the urine (e.g., color, odor, clarity, crystals, blood, mucus).
- Note any difficulties with urination (e.g., pain, burning, dribbling, difficulty beginning).

Patient Teaching

- **For a clean-catch specimen,** teach the patient how to collect the specimen, focusing on how to maintain sterility of the specimen.
- **For the 24-hour urine specimen,** emphasize the need to collect all urine during the 24-hour period. If the procedure is to be completed at home, tell the patient to refrigerate the urine specimen for up to 24 hours until it can be transported to the laboratory. Instruct the patient to place the specimen in a plastic bag, separate it from food items, and label it appropriately.
- **For clean-catch and 24-hour urine specimens,** instruct a menstruating patient that perineal cleansing is especially important. The patient may use a tampon to prevent leakage during specimen collection. Instruct the patient to notify the laboratory that they are menstruating.
- Explain that prepackaged antiseptic wipes cannot be flushed down the toilet.

Documentation

- Urine volume in the patient record, per agency protocol, and the time and date that the specimen was collected.

Some facilities use a desktop card filing system or flow sheets; others require documentation in nursing notes or on electronic health records.

- Characteristics of the urine—color, odor, particulate matter, blood, clarity, or other qualities.
- Any difficulty with voiding, including pain or burning with urination, frequency, or difficulty starting the urine flow.

Sample documentation

> mm/dd/yyyy 0800 Order noted for clean-catch urine specimen. Explained to client the procedure for cleaning and obtaining urine specimen. Client stated "I must clean my bottom from front to back using the toilet in here. Then begin to void and stop voiding. Then void directly into this container." Assisted client to bedside commode. 100 mL of clear yellow urine without foul odor, blood, or particles collected. Pt. denies difficulty voiding, pain, and burning. Urine container labeled per protocol and sent to laboratory.
> ———— L. Schaaf, RN

> mm/dd/yyyy 1000 Order noted for sterile urine specimen. Foley catheter clamped for 15 minutes. Port on Foley cleansed with antiseptic agent. 30 mL of pink tinged-urine without foul odor or sediment removed. Specimen labeled per protocol and sent to laboratory.
> ——— L. Schaaf, RN
>
> mm/dd/yyyy 1200 Order noted for 24-hour urine collection. Explained procedure to client. Client stated, "I will call you when I void. This first void will be flushed and the test will begin. During the test, I will void in the white hat that is in the commode. Then every time that I void, I will call you to empty the urine into the big container. The big container for the urine must be kept cold with ice." ——— L. Schaaf, RN

Practice Resources

Cleveland Clinic (n.d.); Dolan & Cornish (2013); Jones, Sibai, & Fakih (2016, February); Siegel et al. (2007); Skobe (n.d.); Van Leeuwen & Bladh (2017); Wound, Ostomy, and Continence Nurses Society (2016).

Thinking About the Procedure

The video **Obtaining a Sterile Urine Specimen From a Catheter,** along with questions and suggested responses, is available on the **Davis's *Nursing Skills Videos*** Web site at www.fadavis.com.

Procedure 25-3 ■ Inserting an Intermittent Urinary Catheter (Straight Catheter)

▶ For steps to follow in *all* procedures, refer to the Universal Steps for All Procedures on the inside back cover of Volume 2.

Equipment

- Washcloth and towel
- Periwash solution
- Procedure gloves, at least two pairs
- Catheter insertion kit containing:
  - Sterile gloves
  - Urinary catheter
  - Antiseptic cleansing agent, forceps, and cotton balls or a packet of sterile antiseptic swabs or wipes
  - Sterile waterproof drapes
  - Sterile lubricant
  - Urine receptacle
  - Specimen container
- Extra pair of sterile gloves and extra sterile catheter
  Obtaining extra supplies prevents the need to leave the bedside to obtain additional supplies should the gloves or catheter become contaminated.
- Bath blanket
- Procedure lamp or flashlight
- Topical anesthetic gel (e.g., 2% lidocaine, [Xylocaine]), according to agency policy and patient need ▼

Straight catheter kit

(continued on next page)

Procedure 25-3 ■ Inserting an Intermittent Urinary Catheter (Straight Catheter) (continued)

Delegation

In some institutions, UAPs receive special training to practice this skill. In such instances, you may delegate this task to the UAP. However, you must complete the following assessments and instruct the UAP when to stop the procedure and what abnormal findings to report. You must, from time to time, supervise to ensure that the procedure is being performed correctly.

Preprocedure Assessments

- Assess the patient's cognitive level.
  To determine whether the patient will be able to follow instructions.
- Assess for the presence of conditions that may impair the patient's ability to assume the necessary position.
  To determine whether you will need assistance to help the patient maintain the correct position.
- Assess the presence and degree of bladder distention.
  To establish baseline values against which to evaluate future data.
- Determine time of last voiding or last catheterization.
  To interpret the significance of the amount of urine obtained in this catheterization.
- Assess the general body size of the patient and size of the urinary meatus.
  To determine whether you need to choose a different-sized catheter.
- ✚ Determine whether the patient is allergic to iodine (if that is the antiseptic solution in the kit). If so, use a different solution or sterile, normal saline.
- ✚ Determine whether the patient is allergic to latex.
  Many catheters are made of latex.
- Note any signs and symptoms of bladder infection (e.g., elevated temperature, urinary frequency, dysuria).
- Note any conditions (e.g., enlarged prostate in men) that may make it difficult to pass the catheter.
- Assess the need for additional lighting.
  It is sometimes difficult to visualize a woman's urinary meatus. Supplemental, direct lighting helps.

▶ When performing the procedure, always identify your patient according to agency policy, using two identifiers, and be attentive to standard precautions, hand hygiene, patient safety and privacy, body mechanics, and documentation.

▶ Note: Before starting the procedure, gather the appropriate supplies and prepare the patient. Explain to the patient the reason for the catheter insertion, the expected length of time catheterization will be needed, and the sensations she is likely to have.

Procedure Steps

Note: The following steps are described for a female patient. If your patient is a male, refer to the procedure variation for Intermittent Urinary Catheterization (Straight Catheter) for a Male Patient, immediately after the Procedure Steps for females.

1. **If you are right-handed,** stand and work on the patient's right side; if you are left-handed, stand and work on the patient's left side.

2. **Position the patient supine** (dorsal recumbent) to allow you to see the urinary meatus:
   a. Flex the patient's knees and place their feet flat on the bed.
   b. Instruct the patient to relax their thighs and allow them to rotate externally. Obtain help with positioning the patient if the patient is confused, unable to cooperate or follow directions, or unable to hold her legs in position.
   The urinary meatus is sometimes difficult to visualize on women because it may resemble skinfolds or other anatomical landmarks in the area.

3. **Don clean procedure gloves.**

4. ♥ **iCare** **Drape the patient.** Fold the blanket in a diamond shape, over the perineum.
   Providing privacy promotes comfort.

5. **Lift the corner of the privacy drape** to expose the perineum; position the procedure light to allow optimal visualization of the perineum, and locate the urinary meatus.
   Locating the meatus during this step helps prevent delays at subsequent steps when it is important to maintain sterile technique.

6. **Cleanse the perineal area** with periwash solution; let dry.
   Cleansing the perineum before inserting the catheter reduces the number of skin bacteria, thus preventing transmission of microorganisms into the bladder.

7. **Remove and discard gloves.** Perform hand hygiene.
   To prevent the transmission of microbes.

8. **Organize your work area.**
   a. Arrange the bedside table or overbed table within your reach.
   b. Open the sterile catheter kit, according to manufacturer's instructions, and place it on the bedside or overbed table.
   c. Position a biohazard bag or other trash receptacle so that you will not have to reach across the sterile field (between the patient's legs) to dispose of soiled cotton (e.g., a trashcan on the floor beside the bed; a trash bag on the bed near, but not between, the patient's feet; or the outer wrapping of the catheter kit).
   Carrying contaminated objects above a sterile field can contaminate the field.

CHAPTER 25 Urinary Elimination 525

9. **Place the sterile underpad and drape.**

   NOTE: *This step assumes the waterproof drape is packed as the top item in the kit. If your kit is different, see the What If... section.*
   The drapes provide sterile work surfaces and help prevent contamination of your gloves and sterile supplies.

   a. Remove the underpad from the kit carefully, allowing it to fall open as you remove it. Do not touch other kit items. Place it flat on the bed, shiny side down, and tuck the top edge under the buttocks, taking care to touch only the corners of the drape.
   b. Remove the sterile glove package, and don sterile gloves (see Procedure 20-7: Sterile Gloves [Open Method]). *Note: Once you are wearing the sterile gloves, you may touch items inside the catheter kit, arranging the supplies as needed.*
   c. Place the fenestrated drape, which has a hole in the center. Pick up the drape, allowing it to unfold as you remove it, without touching any other objects from the kit. Place the drape over the perineum with the hole over the labia. See the photos below and in Step 11. ▼

10. **Organize kit supplies on the sterile field,** and prepare the supplies in the kit.

    a. Open the antiseptic package and pour the solution over the cotton balls; or use sterile, normal saline to moisten the cotton balls.

    Note: Some kits contain a packet of sterile antiseptic swabs or wipes. Open the end of the packet where you feel the "sticks," leaving the swabs covered by the packet.
    b. Place the forceps near the cotton balls. Omit this step if using swabs.
    c. Open the specimen container if you need to collect a specimen.
    d. Remove any unneeded supplies, such as the urine specimen container, from the urine collection basin.
    e. Remove the plastic wrapper from the catheter if it is covered.
    f. Open the packet or uncap the syringe filled with sterile lubricant.
    g. Squeeze sterile lubricant into the kit tray; roll the catheter slowly in the lubricant to generously lubricate the first 2.5 to 5 cm (1 to 2 inches). Leave the catheter tip in the lubricant or on the sterile field until ready to use.
    Lubrication allows for ease of insertion of the catheter. Prevents trauma to the mucosa.
    h. Touching only the box or sterile side of the wrapping, place the sterile catheter kit down onto the sterile field between the patient's legs or the side of the bed.
    This approach allows you to reach supplies during catheter insertion. It also extends the sterile field created by the sterile underpad.

11. **Cleanse the urinary meatus.**

    a. Place your nondominant hand above the labia, and with your thumb and forefinger, spread the patient's labia, pulling upward (or anteriorly) at the same time, to expose the urinary meatus. Hold this position throughout the procedure—firm pressure is necessary. If the labia slip back over the urinary meatus, they are considered contaminated, and you will need to change gloves and repeat the cleansing procedure.
    When a female patient is supine, gravity may cause tissues above the meatus to fall downward and obscure the meatus from sight. Once placed on the patient's perineal area, your hand is considered contaminated.
    b. With your dominant hand, pick up a moistened cotton ball with the forceps (or swab) and cleanse the perineal area, taking care not to contaminate your sterile glove.

    ▪ Use one stroke and a new cotton ball or swab for each area.
    ▪ Wipe from front to back (clitoris to anus).
    ▪ **If there are five cotton balls or swabs:** Wipe in this order: far labium majora, near labium majora, inside far labium minora, inside near labium minora, and directly down the center over the urinary meatus.
    ▪ **If there are only three cotton balls or swabs:** Cleanse only the inside far labium minora, inside near labium minora, and down the center of the urethral meatus.
    ▪ Discard the used cotton balls or swabs as you use them. Be careful not to move them across the open and sterile kit.
    Because the urethra is close to the anus in female patients, thorough cleansing of the perineum is very important to reduce contamination of the catheter and prevent bacteria from being introduced into the urethra. Following the "clean to dirty" principle prevents recontamination of the cleansed area. ▼

(continued on next page)

Procedure 25-3 ■ Inserting an Intermittent Urinary Catheter (Straight Catheter) (continued)

12. **Prepare the urine receptacle.** Place it 10 cm (4 inches) from the meatus (for women).
    The end of the catheter will need to reach into the container to catch the draining urine.

13. **Insert the catheter.** ▼

    a. Grasp the catheter with your dominant hand, no more than 7.5 cm (3 inches) from the tip. Keep the rest of the catheter coiled in the palm of your hand. Slowly insert the end of the catheter into the meatus. Ask the patient to take slow, deep breaths until the initial discomfort has passed.
    Bearing down helps relax the external sphincter and makes insertion easier and more comfortable. Holding the catheter close to the distal end will help to keep the tip stable and prevent it from being inserted into the vaginal opening. Deep breathing by the patient helps relax the sphincters. Coiling the catheter in your hand keeps you from contaminating the catheter.

    b. Ask the patient to bear down as though they are trying to void.

    c. Continue inserting the catheter gently until urine flows, for 5 to 7.5 cm (2 to 3 inches). After you see urine, insert the catheter another 2.5 to 5 cm (1 to 2 inches).

    d. ✚ If there is slight resistance as the catheter goes through the sphincters, twist the catheter slightly, or apply gentle pressure, but do not force the catheter while inserting it. You might need to remove it and cautiously attempt the insertion action again using a new catheter.
    Forcing may damage mucosa. Insert the catheter more deeply after urine flow to be sure the catheter is well into the bladder so that the bladder can be emptied completely. The catheter might not advance while being inserted when it is misplaced in the vagina or if there is a stricture within the urethra or sphincter spasm.

    e. If the catheter touches the labia or unsterile linens or if you inadvertently place it in the vagina, it is contaminated; you must insert a new, sterile catheter. Leave the contaminated catheter in the vagina while you are inserting the new one into the meatus.
    Leaving the catheter in the incorrect location serves as a visual landmark and helps avoid making the same mistake again.

14. **Manage the catheter** and/or urine collection device.

    a. Continue to hold the catheter securely with your nondominant hand while urine drains from the bladder.
    Holding the catheter like this prevents the catheter from being expelled by the bladder or because of urethral contractions.

    b. If you are to collect a urine specimen, use your dominant hand to take the specimen container, and put it into the flow of urine until you obtain the correct amount of urine. Cap the container, maintaining sterile technique. See Procedure 25-2B.

    c. When the flow of urine stops and the bladder has been emptied, pinch the catheter, and slowly withdraw it from the meatus. Discard the catheter in an appropriate receptacle.
    Withdrawing slowly promotes adequate urinary drainage, preventing urinary stasis. Pinching prevents urine from dribbling out of the end of the catheter.

    d. Remove the urine-filled receptacle; set it aside outside the patient care area to be emptied when the procedure is finished.
    Keeps the urine from spilling on the bed.

15. **Cleanse the patient's perineal** area, as needed; let dry.
    This removes residual antiseptic solution from the area, an especially important step if you used povidone–iodine (Betadine). Betadine left on intact healthy skin can cause irritation.

16. **Remove and discard** disposable supplies (e.g., drapes).

17. **Remove your gloves** and perform hand hygiene.
    Prevents transmission of bacteria.

18. **Return the patient** to a comfortable position, with the call device within reach.

Intermittent Urinary Catheterization (Straight Catheter) for a Male Patient

Procedure Steps	Nursing Action
1. Position the patient.	Position the patient supine, legs straight and slightly apart.
2. Drape the patient.	Cover the patient's upper body with a blanket; fold bed sheets down to expose the penis.
3. Don procedure gloves and cleanse the perineum.	After donning procedure gloves, wash the penis and perineal area with perineal wash solution; let dry. If you are using a topical anesthetic gel (e.g., Xylocaine), use a syringe (no needle) to insert it into the urethra now. ■ Remove and discard gloves. ■ Perform hand hygiene.
4. Organize the work area.	■ Open the sterile catheter kit and place on overhead table without contaminating the inside of the wrap. ■ Position a trash receptacle nearby.
5. Place the sterile underpad and sterile drape.	■ Remove underpad from the kit before donning sterile gloves. ■ Place the drape shiny side down between or across the patient's thighs.
6. Don sterile gloves.	Remove the sterile glove package, and don sterile gloves (see Procedure 23-7: Sterile Gloves [Open Method]). *Note: Once you are wearing the sterile gloves, you may touch items inside the catheter kit to arrange the supplies, as needed.*
7. Place the fenestrated drape.	Allow the fenestrated drape to fall open while removing it from the kit and without touching other kit items. Place the drape with the center hole over the penis.
8. Organize kit supplies on the sterile drape.	■ Open the antiseptic package and pour over cotton balls or use antiseptic swabs or wipes. Sterile, normal saline is also acceptable for cleansing the urethral opening (follow agency guidelines). ■ Open the sterile specimen container. ■ Remove any unneeded supplies. ■ Remove the wrapper from the catheter. ■ Touching only the kit or inside of the wrapping, place the sterile catheter kit down onto the sterile field between the patient's legs.
9. Lubricate the catheter.	■ Do not lubricate the catheter if you have already inserted a lubricant (lidocaine-based product) directly into the urethra. ■ If the lubricant comes in a packet, squeeze it into the kit tray, and roll the catheter slowly in it to generously lubricate 12.5 to 17.5 cm (5 to 7 inches) of the catheter. Leave the catheter tip in sterile lubricant or on the sterile field until ready to use. ■ If your kit contains a prefilled syringe of lubricant, gently insert the tip of the syringe into the urethra and instill the lubricant.
10. Expose the urinary meatus.	■ With your nondominant hand, grasp the penis, taking care not to contaminate the surrounding drape. This glove is no longer sterile. ■ Hold the penis gently, but firmly, at a 90-degree angle to the body, exerting gentle traction. ■ If the penis is uncircumcised, retract the foreskin to fully expose the meatus. If the foreskin accidentally falls over meatus and does not remain retracted, or if you release the penis during cleansing, you must change gloves and repeat the cleansing procedure.
11. Cleanse the urinary meatus.	■ Continuing to hold the penis with your nondominant hand, hold the forceps in your dominant hand and pick up a cotton ball. Cleanse the glans in a series of circular motions, starting at the meatus and working partially down the shaft of the penis. ■ Repeat with at least two more cotton balls or swabs. Discard the cotton balls or swabs as they are used. Do not move them across the open sterile kit and field.

(continued on next page)

Procedure 25-3 ■ Inserting an Intermittent Urinary Catheter (Straight Catheter) (continued)

Procedure Steps	Nursing Action
12. Prepare the urine receptacle.	■ Maintaining sterile technique, with your dominant hand place the plastic urine receptacle between the patient's thighs, close enough to the urinary meatus for the end of the catheter to rest inside the container as the urine drains. ■ With the dominant hand, hold the catheter 5 to 7.5 cm (2 to 3 inches) from the tip with remainder coiled in the palm of the hand and the distal end of the catheter is in the plastic container.
13. Insert the catheter into the urinary meatus.	■ Ask the patient to bear down as though trying to void; slowly insert the end of the catheter into the meatus. Instruct the patient to take slow, deep breaths until the initial discomfort has passed. ✚ If you feel resistance, withdraw the catheter. Do not force against resistance. ■ Continue inserting the catheter to about 17.5 to 22.5 cm (7 to 9 inches) or until urine flows. After you see urine, insert the catheter another 2.5 to 5 cm (1 to 2 inches).
14. Collect a specimen, if needed.	If a urine specimen is to be collected, continue to grasp the penis, and use your dominant hand to place the specimen container into the flow of urine; cap container using sterile technique.
15. Manage the catheter.	■ When the flow of urine stops and the bladder has been emptied, pinch the catheter, and slowly withdraw it from the meatus. ■ Replace the foreskin if the penis is uncircumcised. ■ Discard the catheter in a biohazardous waste receptacle.
16. Finish the procedure.	Remove gloves and perform hand hygiene. Return patient to a comfortable position with the call device within reach.

? What if...

- **The sterile gloves are packed as the top item in the catheter kit?**
- **A woman is unable to maintain a dorsal recumbent position?**
- **The patient is having a menstrual period?**
- **The patient has an erection during the procedure?**

You will find instructions for these situations at the end of Procedure 25-4.

Evaluation

- Note any difficulty with catheter insertion.
  This can indicate structural problems, especially in an older male patient with an enlarged prostate gland.
- Note the characteristics of the urine obtained (e.g., amount, color, odor, presence of sediment or mucus).
- Assess and palpate for absence of bladder distention.
  Note: Some facilities have a portable bladder-scanning device that will allow you to determine whether residual urine remains. Palpating the bladder helps you to determine whether it has been emptied.

Documentation

- Document the reason for the catheter and/or clinical indication for continuing catheterization.
- Document the time and date of the procedure.
- Document the size of catheter used.
- Record the amount of urine obtained on the I&O portion of the graphics sheet. Record the color of urine, odor, presence of mucus, blood, and so on, in the nursing notes.
- Record the patient's subjective statements.
- If you collected a specimen, document it, and note the time it was sent to the laboratory.
- Some facilities require that you record the amount of saline used to inflate the balloon.

Practice Resources

Agency for Healthcare Research and Quality (2017, March last reviewed); Beauchemin et al. (2018, September); Goetz et al. (2018); Gould et al. (2019, updated); Newman et al. (2017); Shlamovitz & Kim (2021, November, updated); Thangavelu-Veluswamy (2020, October 8, reviewed); Vahr et al. (2013, March); Wound, Ostomy, and Continence Nurses Society (WOCN) (2016).

Thinking About the Procedure

The video **Intermittent Urinary Catheterization,** along with questions and suggested responses, is available on the **Davis's Nursing Skills Videos** Web site at www.fadavis.com.

Procedure 25-4 ■ Inserting an Indwelling Urinary Catheter

▶ For steps to follow in *all* procedures, refer to the Universal Steps for All Procedures on the inside back cover of Volume 2.

Equipment
- Washcloth and towel
- Periwash solution
- Procedure gloves, at least two pairs
- Catheter insertion kit containing:
  - Sterile gloves
  - A double-lumen or triple-lumen catheter with a balloon tip for inflation
  - Antiseptic cleansing agent, povidone-iodine, or sterile saline
  - Forceps
  - Cotton balls
  - Sterile waterproof drapes
  - Sterile lubricant
  - Prefilled syringe with sterile water (to inflate the catheter balloon)
  - Urine collection bag with drainage tubing (often the tubing is preconnected to the catheter)
  - Specimen container
- Extra pair of sterile gloves and extra sterile catheter
  Obtaining extra supplies prevents the need to leave the bedside to obtain additional supplies should the gloves or catheter become contaminated.
- Bath blanket
- Procedure lamp or flashlight
- Topical anesthetic gel (e.g., 2% lidocaine [Xylocaine]), according to agency policy and patient need
- Commercial or hydrocolloid securement
- Safety pin and elastic band (if needed to secure tubing to the bed; you can usually use the clamp that is on the drainage tubing)

Indwelling catheter kit

Delegation
In some institutions, UAPs undergo special training to learn this skill. In such instances, you may delegate this task to the UAP. However, you must complete the following assessments and instruct the UAP when to stop the procedure and what abnormal findings to report. You must from time to time supervise to ensure that the procedure is being performed correctly.

Preprocedure Assessments
- Assess the patient's cognitive level.
  To determine whether the patient will be able to follow instructions.
- Assess for conditions that may impair the patient's ability to assume the necessary position.
  To determine whether you will need assistance to help the patient maintain the correct position for catheter insertion.
- Assess the presence and degree of bladder distention.
  To establish a baseline against which to evaluate future data.
- Determine time of last voiding or last catheterization.
  To interpret the significance of the amount of urine obtained in this catheterization.
- Assess the general body size of the patient and size of the urinary meatus.
  To determine whether you need to choose a different-sized catheter.
- ✚ Determine whether the patient is allergic to iodine (if that is the antiseptic solution in the kit). If so, use a different solution or sterile, normal saline.
- Determine whether the patient is allergic to latex.
  Many catheters are made of latex.
- Note signs and symptoms of bladder infection (e.g., elevated temperature, urinary frequency, dysuria).
- Note any conditions (e.g., enlarged prostate in men) that may make it difficult to pass the catheter.
- Assess the need for extra lighting.
  It is sometimes difficult to visualize a woman's urinary meatus. Supplemental, direct lighting helps.

(continued on next page)

Procedure 25-4 ■ Inserting an Indwelling Urinary Catheter (continued)

➤ When performing the procedure, always identify your patient according to agency policy, using two identifiers, and be attentive to standard precautions, hand hygiene, patient safety and privacy, body mechanics, and documentation.

➤ *Note:* **The following steps are described for a male patient.** If your patient is female, refer to the Procedure Variations for Female Patients, immediately after the procedure steps.

Procedure Steps

1. **If you are right-handed,** stand and work on the patient's right side; if you are left-handed, stand and work on the patient's left side.

2. **Place the patient supine,** with the legs straight and slightly apart (frog-leg position). If the patient is confused, unable to follow directions, or unable to hold their legs in the correct position, obtain help with the procedure.

♥ **iCare 3. Drape the patient.** Cover the patient's upper body with a blanket; fold the bedsheets down to expose the penis.
Covering the patient preserves modesty and enhances a feeling of security, while ensuring that you can visualize the urinary meatus.

4. **Don clean procedure gloves.** Cleanse the penis and perineal area with antiseptic solution; let dry.
Cleansing the area of skin bacteria reduces the risk of transmitting microbes into the bladder.

5. **If you are using topical anesthetic** gel, use a syringe (no needle) to insert it into the urethra.
This is frequently used for men to provide local anesthesia. You insert it now because it takes 5 minutes for the gel to take effect at the time you are ready to insert the catheter.

6. **Remove and discard gloves.** Perform hand hygiene.
To prevent the transmission of microbes.

7. **Organize your work area:**
   a. Arrange the bedside table or overbed table within your reach.
   b. Open the sterile catheter kit, according to the manufacturer's instructions, and place it on the bedside or overbed table.
   c. Position a plastic bag or other trash receptacle so that you will not have to reach across the sterile field to dispose of soiled cotton balls and so forth (e.g., a trash can on the floor beside the bed; a trash bag or the kit outer wrapper on the bed near, but not between, the patient's feet).
   Carrying contaminated objects above a sterile field can contaminate the field.

8. **Place the sterile underpad** and drape.
   NOTE: This step assumes the waterproof drape is packed as the top item in the kit. If your kit is different, see the What If... section.
   These drapes provide sterile work surfaces and help prevent contaminating your gloves and sterile supplies.
   a. Remove the underpad from the kit carefully. Drop the underpad shiny side down between or across the patient's thighs, touching only the corners.
   b. Remove the sterile glove package and don sterile gloves (see Procedure 23-7: Sterile Glove [Open Method]).
   Note: Once you are wearing the sterile gloves, you may touch any items inside the catheter kit to arrange the supplies, as needed.
   c. Place the fenestrated drape, which has a hole in the center. Pick up the drape, allowing it to unfold as you remove it, without touching any other objects. Place it with the center hole over the penis.

9. **Organize the kit supplies** on the sterile field and prepare the supplies in the kit.
   a. Open the antiseptic packet. Pour antiseptic solution or sterile, normal saline over the cotton balls.
   Note: Some kits contain a packet of sterile antiseptic swabs or wipes. Open the end of the packet where you can feel the "sticks," leaving the swabs covered by the remainder of the packet.
   b. Place the forceps near the cotton balls.
   c. Open the specimen container if you are to collect a specimen.
   d. Remove any unneeded supplies, such as the specimen container, from the kit. Remove the plastic wrapper from the catheter if it is covered.
   e. Do not lubricate the catheter if you have already inserted a lubricant (2% lidocaine topical gel) directly into the urethra.

Variation: Lubricant in a Syringe
If the sterile lubricant in the kit is packaged in a syringe, you will insert the lubricant into the urethra at Step 11.

Variation: Lubricant in a Packet
If the lubricant comes in a packet, squeeze the lubricant into the kit tray and roll the catheter slowly in the lubricant. Generously lubricate 12.5 to 17.5 cm (5 to 7 inches) of the catheter. Leave the catheter tip in sterile lubricant or on the sterile field until ready to use.
   f. Attach the sterile water-filled syringe to the balloon port of the catheter.
   g. Touching only the box or sterile side of the wrapping, place the sterile catheter kit down onto the sterile field on top of the man's thighs. You may, alternatively, set up the sterile field between his legs.
   Placement of supplies in this manner allows you to reach supplies during catheter insertion.
   h. If the bedside bag is preconnected to the catheter itself, leave the bag on or near the sterile field until after the catheter is inserted.

10. **Cleanse the urinary meatus.** ▼

   a. With your nondominant hand, reach through the opening in the fenestrated drape and grasp the penis, taking care not to contaminate the surrounding drape. This glove is no longer sterile.
   b. Hold the penis gently, but firmly, at a 90-degree angle to the body, exerting gentle traction.
      Supporting the shaft with the fingers straightens the urethra, easing insertion of the catheter.
   c. If the penis is uncircumcised, retract the foreskin to fully expose the meatus. If the foreskin unintentionally falls over the meatus or if you drop the penis during cleansing, you must change gloves and repeat the cleansing procedure.
      Retracting the foreskin allows for full cleansing of the area.
   d. Continuing to hold the penis with your nondominant hand, hold the forceps in your dominant hand and pick up a cotton ball. Cleanse the glans in a series of circular motions, starting at the meatus and working partially down the shaft of the penis.
   e. Repeat with at least two more cotton balls or swabs. Discard the cotton balls or swabs as you use them. Do not move them across the open sterile kit and field.
      Following the "clean to dirty" principle prevents recontamination of the cleansed area.
   f. Continue to grasp the penis with your nondominant hand during the next steps. This glove is no longer sterile.

11. **Instill lubricant** (if not done previously).

   Variation: Lubricant Packaged in a Syringe
   Before beginning the procedure, you should have made sure that the catheter kit contains a prefilled syringe of lubricant rather than a packet. Gently insert the tip of the prefilled syringe into the urethra and instill the lubricant (unless you have already inserted 2% lidocaine topical gel).

   Variation: Lubricant in a Packet
   If the kit contains a single packet of lubricant, make sure you have already generously lubricated 12.5 to 17.5 cm (5 to 7 inches) of the catheter. This is not the technique of choice.

12. **Insert the catheter.** ▼

   a. With your dominant hand, stabilize the catheter before inserting it by holding the catheter approximately 5 to 7.5 cm (2 to 3 inches) from the tip. Keep the rest of the catheter coiled in the palm of your hand if the catheter is not already preconnected to the drainage tube.
      Coiling the catheter in your hand prevents contamination of the catheter. When you preconnect the drainage bag before you insert the catheter, you keep the urine from draining onto the bed. Frequently, the catheter and the drainage bag are connected by the manufacturer.
   b. With your nondominant hand, continue to hold the penis gently, but firmly, at a 90-degree angle to the body, exerting gentle traction.
      Supporting the shaft with the fingers straightens the urethra, easing insertion of the catheter.
   c. Ask the patient to bear down as though trying to void; slowly insert the end of the catheter into the meatus. Ask the patient to take slow, deep breaths until the initial discomfort has passed.
      These strategies help the patient to relax the external sphincter and make insertion easier and more comfortable.
   d. Continue inserting the catheter to about 17.5 to 22.5 cm (7 to 9 inches) or until urine flows. You will feel slight resistance at the level of the internal sphincter. Continue to advance almost to the bifurcation (Y-connector).

   ✚ You will commonly feel resistance at the prostatic sphincter. Hold the catheter firmly against the sphincter until the resistance eases. Then advance the catheter, but do not force it.
   This prevents compromised circulation and painful swelling.

   e. Lower the penis and replace the foreskin.

13. **Manage the catheter.**
   a. Continue to hold the catheter securely with your nondominant hand to stabilize the catheter's position in the urethra. Use your other hand to pick up the water-filled syringe and inflate the catheter balloon.
      Holding the catheter until the balloon is inflated decreases the chance that

(continued on next page)

Procedure 25-4 ■ Inserting an Indwelling Urinary Catheter (continued)

the catheter will be expelled by bladder or urethral contractions. The inflated balloon prevents the catheter from slipping out of the bladder. ▼

A Catheter placement, male.

B Catheter placement, female.

b. If the patient complains of pain on inflation of the balloon, withdraw the water from the balloon, and reposition the catheter by advancing it 2.5 cm (1 inch).
Pain usually indicates that the balloon was in the urethra instead of in the bladder.

c. After the balloon is inflated, pull back gently on the catheter until you feel resistance. Lower the penis and replace the foreskin.
This indicates that the balloon is correctly positioned at the neck of the bladder.

14. **Connect the drainage bag** to the end of the catheter if it is not already preconnected. Hang the drainage bag on the side of the bed, below the level of the bladder.
Hanging the drainage bag below the bladder promotes adequate urinary drainage by gravity, preventing urinary stasis.

15. **Using a commercial catheter securement,** secure the catheter to the thigh or the abdomen. If you must use tape, use hypoallergenic tape.
Securing the catheter prevents urethral irritation related to tugging or pulling of the catheter. Commercial catheter securement devices are preferable to tape for catheter securement.

16. **Cleanse the patient's perineal area,** as needed; let dry. Cover the patient.
Removes residual antiseptic solution from the area, an especially important step if you used povidone–iodine (Betadine). Betadine left on intact healthy skin can cause irritation.

17. **Remove and discard disposable** supplies (e.g., drapes).

18. **Remove gloves** and discard them into biohazard receptacle. Perform hand hygiene.

19. **Return the patient** to a comfortable position, with the call device placed within reach.

Indwelling Catheter Insertion for a Female Patient

Procedure Steps	Nursing Action
1. Position the patient.	Flex the patient's knees; place her feet flat on the bed (dorsal recumbent position). Instruct the patient to relax her thighs and allow them to rotate externally. *Note: Obtain help if the patient is confused, unable to follow directions, or unable to hold her legs in the correct position.*
2. Drape the patient.	Fold the blanket in a diamond shape, wrapping the corners around the patient's legs and folding the upper corner down over the perineum. See Procedure 25-3, Step 4.
3. Cleanse the perineal area.	■ Don clean procedure gloves. ■ Lift the corner of the privacy drape to expose the perineum. ■ Position the procedure light to allow optimal visualization of the perineum, and locate the urinary meatus. ■ Cleanse the perineal area with antiseptic solution or sterile normal saline (per agency policy); let dry. ■ Remove and discard gloves. Perform hand hygiene.
4. Organize the work area.	■ Arrange the bedside table or overbed table within your reach. ■ Open the sterile catheter kit, according to the manufacturer's directions, and place it on the table. ■ Position a plastic bag or other trash receptacle so that you will not have to reach across the sterile field to dispose of soiled cotton balls and other items.

Procedure Steps	Nursing Action
5. Apply the sterile underpad and fenestrated drape.	▪ Remove the sterile underpad from the kit before donning sterile gloves. Be sure not to touch other kit items with bare hands. Touching only the corners, place the drape shiny side down under the patient's buttocks. ▪ Carefully remove the sterile glove package from the kit, and don sterile gloves. ▪ Pick up the fenestrated drape; allow it to unfold without touching other objects; place over the perineum with the opening over the labia.
6. Organize the kit supplies on the sterile field.	▪ Open the antiseptic packet and pour solution over the cotton balls, and position forceps nearby. Or if the kit comes with antiseptic swabs, open the packet so the sticks are convenient to grasp. You may also use sterile, normal saline for cleansing the urethral opening (follow agency policy). ▪ Open the specimen container if a specimen is to be collected. Remove any unneeded supplies. ▪ Remove the plastic wrapper from the catheter if it is covered. Squeeze the sterile lubricant into the kit tray. Roll the catheter slowly in the lubricant, being sure to generously lubricate the first 2.5 to 5 cm (1 to 2 inches) of the catheter. Leave the catheter tip in the sterile lubricant or on the sterile field until ready to use. ▪ Attach the sterile water-filled syringe to the balloon port of the catheter. Leave the syringe attached to the catheter. ▪ Touching only the box or sterile side of the wrapping, place the sterile catheter kit down onto the sterile field. You may, as an alternative, set up the sterile field between the patient's legs.
7. Spread the labia and cleanse the urinary meatus.	▪ Place your nondominant hand above the labia, and, with thumb and forefinger, spread the patient's labia, pulling up at the same time to expose the urinary meatus. Use firm pressure to hold this position throughout the procedure. If the labia accidentally slip back over the meatus during cleansing, change your gloves and repeat this step. ▪ Wipe from the clitoris to the anus, wiping in the order of the far labium majora, near labium majora, inside far labium, inside near labium, and directly down the center over the urinary meatus. ▪ Discard cotton balls or swabs as they are used; do not move them across the open, sterile kit and field. Use only one stroke and a new cotton ball or swab for each area.
8. Insert the catheter.	▪ Ask the patient to bear down as though they are trying to void. ▪ Grasp the catheter with your dominant hand, no more than 7.5 cm (3 inches) from the tip. Slowly insert the end of the catheter into the meatus. ▪ Ask the patient to take slow, deep breaths until the initial discomfort has passed.
9. Manage the catheter.	▪ If the catheter touches the labia or unsterile linens, or if you inadvertently place it in the vagina, it is contaminated; you must insert a new, sterile catheter. Leave the contaminated catheter in the vagina while you are inserting the new one into the meatus; this keeps you from making the same mistake again. ▪ Continue inserting the catheter gently until urine flows, for a distance of 5 to 7.5 cm (2 to 3 inches). After you see urine, insert the catheter another 2.5 to 5 cm (1 to 2 inches). ▪ After urine flows, stabilize the catheter in the urethra with your nondominant hand; use the dominant hand to pick up the sterile water-filled syringe and inflate the catheter balloon. ▪ If the patient complains of pain when inflating the balloon, withdraw the water out of the balloon. Then reposition the catheter by advancing it 2.5 cm (1 inch).
10. Secure the catheter.	▪ Hang the drainage bag on the side of the bed below the level of the bladder. ▪ Using a commercial catheter securement device, if available, secure the catheter to the thigh.
11. Finish up.	▪ Remove and discard disposable supplies in a biohazard receptacle. ▪ Remove and discard gloves. Perform hand hygiene. ▪ Return the patient to a comfortable position, with the call device within reach.

(continued on next page)

Procedure 25-4 ■ Inserting an Indwelling Urinary Catheter (continued)

? What if...

- **The sterile gloves are packed as the top item in the catheter kit?**

  - Grasp the corner and remove the sterile glove package, taking care not to touch anything else in the package. Don the sterile gloves. Once you have donned the sterile gloves, you may touch any item inside the catheter kit to arrange the supplies, as needed.
  - Place the sterile underpad: Grasp the edges of the sterile drape. Fold the entire edge down 5 to 7.5 cm (2 to 3 inches) and toward you, making a "cuff" to protect your gloves. Be careful not to touch unsterile objects with your gloves or the drape.

  For female patients: Carefully slide the drape under the patient's buttocks without contaminating your gloves. Ask the patient to raise her hips slightly if she can.

  For male patients: Drop the sterile underpad across thighs.
  - Continue with the fenestrated drape, as described in the standard procedures.

- **The patient is having a menstrual period?**

  Before sending a specimen for diagnostic testing, note on the laboratory form that the patient is having a menstrual period.
  Blood from a menstrual period in the urine specimen might lead to misinterpretation of the result.

- **A patient is unable to maintain a dorsal recumbent position?**

  Use Sims' position (side-lying with the upper leg flexed at the hip). Cover the rectal area.
  Prevents contamination from the rectal area to the urethra.

- **A patient has an erection during the procedure?**

  Treat the situation professionally. Take a break until the erection goes away. Never force the catheter.
  Forcing the catheter can cause urethral trauma.

Evaluation

- Note any difficulty with catheter insertion.
  This can indicate structural problems, especially in an older male patient with an enlarged prostate gland.
- Note the characteristics of the urine obtained (e.g., amount, color, odor, presence of sediment or mucus).
- Assess and palpate for absence of bladder distention.

  Note: Some facilities have a portable bladder-scanning device that will allow you to determine whether residual urine remains. Palpating the bladder helps you to determine whether it has been emptied. A portable bladder scanner may also be used to determine whether residual urine remains.
- For indwelling catheters, continue to monitor that drainage is not obstructed and that the drainage bag is below the level of the bladder.

Home Care

For inserting indwelling catheters in the home, teach clients:
- When to change the catheter.
  Changing indwelling catheters at routine, fixed intervals is generally not recommended (Gould, Umscheid, Agarwal, et al., 2019, updated). Clients should be taught to change catheters based on clinical indications, such as impaired urine drainage or encrustation.
- How to prevent catheter blockage (e.g., increase fluid intake).
  Fluids increase the urine volume, helping to reduce the deposit of sediment or other particles in the tubing.
- To empty the drainage bag frequently and to keep the bag below the level of the bladder.
- How to prevent UTIs (e.g., maintain a closed system, hand washing before handling catheter equipment, prevent blockage of urine outflow, adequate fluid intake, taking a shower rather than a bath).
- How to prevent discomfort at the urethra.
- Use of a leg bag.
- To eat foods that help acidify urine: meat, eggs, cheese, prunes, cranberries, and whole grains.
- How to obtain additional supplies suitable for individual needs.

Documentation

- Document the reason for indwelling urinary catheterization.
- Time and date of the procedure.
- The size of catheter used.
- Amount of urine obtained (on the I&O portion of the graphics sheet).
- Color of urine, odor, presence of mucus, blood, and so on (in the nursing notes).
- The patient's subjective statements.
- Any specimen collected; note the time it was sent to the laboratory.
- For an indwelling catheter: In addition, some facilities require that you record the amount of sterile water used to inflate the balloon.
- Include a date for removal or review for continued need.

Sample documentation

00/00/00   1010   Order noted for insertion of indwelling catheter. Explained the procedure to Pt and reason for insertion. Pt verbalized understanding of the procedure and need for catheter. Placed Pt in a dorsal recumbent position with blankets to keep Pt warm and provide privacy. Perineal care completed. 14 Fr. Foley catheter inserted using sterile technique per protocol. Foley draining dark yellow urine with sediment and foul odor. No mucus or blood noted in urine. Bladder is not distended. Client returned to semi-Fowler's position. No needs noted at this time. Reminded Pt to call nurse if there is any discomfort associated with urinary catheterization. Call light placed in Pt's dominant hand. ——————C. Chin, RN

Practice Resources

Agency for Healthcare Research and Quality (2017, March last reviewed); Beauchemin (2017, April); Goetz et al. (2018); Gould et al. (2019, updated); Lachance & Grobeina (2019, May 4); Newman et al. (2017); Shlamovitz & Kim (2021, November, updated); Society of Urological Nurses (2021a, 2021b, March-April); Thangavelu-Veluswamy (2020, October 8, reviewed); Wound, Ostomy, and Continence Nurses Society (2016).

Thinking About the Procedure

The video **Indwelling Urinary Catheterization,** along with questions and suggested responses, is available on the **Davis's** *Nursing Skills Videos* Web site at www.fadavis.com.

Procedure 25-5 ■ Applying an External (Condom) Urinary Catheter

➤ For steps to follow in *all* procedures, refer to the Universal Steps for All Procedures on the inside back cover of Volume 2.

Equipment
- Condom catheter
- Two pairs of clean procedure gloves
- Washcloth and towel
- Disposable basin of soap and purified water or antiseptic wash or sterile, normal saline
- Bath blanket, if available
- Urine collection bag (e.g., bedside drainage bag or leg bag)
- Disposable tape measure
- Skin prep (per agency policy)
- Scissors
- Commercial leg strap

Delegation

You may delegate the application of a condom catheter to the UAP once you have assessed the UAP's skill level and completed the preprocedure assessments. Instruct the UAP to report any alterations in the skin integrity along the shaft of the penis.

Preprocedure Assessments
- Assess the patient's cognitive status.
  Knowing whether the patient can follow directions helps determine how to approach the procedure. Find out if the patient may be prone to pulling on the catheter.
- Assess pattern of voiding (e.g., degree and time of incontinence).
  Helps determine when the condom catheter should be applied.
- Assess the skin along the shaft of the penis, the glans, and the meatus (for swelling or excoriation).
  The condom catheter cannot be used on excoriated, irritated skin or over areas of impaired skin integrity.
- Note whether and how much the penis is retracted toward the body.
  There is an increased risk of nonadherence and leakage of urine in a patient with a retracted penis.
- Assess for the presence of neuropathy.
  Patients with neuropathies that affect sensation in the penis may not feel skin irritation from the condom catheter and will need to be assessed more frequently.

➤ When performing the procedure, always identify your patient according to agency policy, using two identifiers, and be attentive to standard precautions, hand hygiene, patient safety and privacy, body mechanics, and documentation.

Procedure Steps

1. **Determine appropriate size** of the external catheter by measuring the circumference of the penis using a disposable paper tape. Obtain a correctly sized catheter.
   A catheter that is too small impairs circulation. A catheter that is too large allows leakage of urine.

2. **Perform hand hygiene,** and don clean procedure gloves.
   Hand hygiene and gloving prevent the transmission of bacteria.

3. **Organize the supplies** and prepare the leg bag or bedside drainage bag for attachment to the condom catheter by removing it from the packaging and placing the end of the connecting tubing near the perineal area.

4. **Position the patient supine.** If the patient has difficulty breathing, raise the head of the bed to 30 degrees.

5. **Fold down the bed covers** to expose the penis and drape the patient by using the bath blanket.
   Covering the patient reduces patient embarrassment.

(continued on next page)

Procedure 25-5 ■ Applying an External (Condom) Urinary Catheter (continued)

6. **Gently cleanse the penis** with soap and filtered water or antiseptic perineal wipes. Rinse and dry it thoroughly. If the patient is uncircumcised, gently retract the foreskin, cleanse the glans, and return the foreskin to its natural resting position. Excess hair along the shaft of the penis may be carefully clipped off with the scissors.
   Cleansing the penis not only helps to prevent infection but it also helps the condom catheter to adhere better to the shaft.

7. **Perform hand hygiene;** change procedure gloves.

8. **Apply skin prep, adhesive solution** (if used by your agency) to the shaft of the penis, and allow it to dry. *Note:* Some external condom catheters require the placement of the special adhesive strip onto the penis before the application of the condom. Follow the manufacturer's directions.

9. **Grasp the penis** in your nondominant hand. With your dominant hand, place the condom catheter at the end of the penis, and slowly unroll it along the shaft toward the patient's body. Leave 2.5 to 5 cm (1 to 2 inches) between the end of the penis and the drainage tube on the catheter.
   Careful unrolling in this manner helps prevent irritation of the glans caused by rubbing and allows for expansion of the penis if an erection were to occur. ▼

10. **Secure the external urinary catheter** in place on the penis.
    a. Ensure that the condom is not twisted.
       Twisting can obstruct urine flow.
    b. Do not use regular bandage or surgical dressing tape to hold an external condom catheter in place.
       Regular tape does not expand and could lead to decreased blood flow to the penis.

    Variation: Catheter With Internal Adhesive
    c. Gently grasp the penis and compress so that the entire shaft comes in contact with the condom.

    Variation: Catheter With External Adhesive Strip
    d. Wrap the strip around the outside of the condom in a spiral direction, taking care not to overlap the ends.
       Prevents constriction of blood flow to the penis.

11. **Assess the proximal end** of the condom catheter. If a large portion of the condom is still rolled above the adhesive strip, you may need to clip the roll.
    Clipping the roll prevents constriction of blood flow.

12. **Attach the tube end** of the condom catheter to a drainage system (e.g., a leg bag). Make sure there are no kinks in the tubing.
    Kinks impede the flow of urine. Urine that does not drain away from the meatus can cause irritation and skin breakdown and possibly cause the condom catheter to fall off.

13. **Secure the catheter tubing** to the patient's thigh by using a commercial leg strap or hydrocolloid stabilization securement device.
    A leg strap controls movement of the tubing and accidental pulling on the condom catheter. ▼

14. **Cover the patient,** and return him to a comfortable position, with the call bell within reach. Raise the side rails and lower the bed.

15. **Remove your gloves** and perform hand hygiene.

16. **Change the condom daily** or more often, if needed.
    This helps to prevent urinary tract infection and allows for inspection of the skin.

? What if...

- **The urine flow becomes obstructed?**

  Check the catheter and collecting tube for kinking; readjust, if needed, and make certain that the tubing is secured properly to the patient's thigh. Replace the catheter and tubing, if necessary.

Evaluation

Within 30 minutes of condom application, assess for the following:
- Urine flow (should not be obstructed)
- Swelling or discoloration of the penis
  Swelling or discoloration might indicate that the condom is too tight.

Monitor

- Penis for circulatory changes
- Position and patency of the drainage tubing
- Characteristics of the urine (e.g., amount, color, odor, bleeding)
- Patient comfort
- Leakage of urine

Home Care

- Clients and caregivers should wash their hands before and after any manipulation of the penis or apparatus.
- Daily bag decontamination with a diluted (1:10) bleach solution has been found effective in reducing bacteria.
- Teach the client and the caregiver to recognize the signs and symptoms of skin irritation and excoriation as well as the symptoms of UTI.
- Teach the client or the caregiver to notify the care provider and discontinue use of the condom catheter if skin irritation or swelling occurs; if urine becomes thick and cloudy, pink, or red; if urine has mucus in it; or if no urine has drained from the catheter in 6 to 8 hours.
- Change the external condom catheter every 24 hours.
- Keep the collecting bag below the level of the bladder.
- Regularly empty the collection bag before it becomes completely full.
- Never allow the draining spigot to come in contact with the nonsterile collecting container.
- Disinfect the catheter–tubing junction before disconnecting them (if they must be disconnected).
- Avoid disconnecting the catheter and drainage tube unless the catheter must be irrigated.

Documentation

- Document the date and time of application of the external catheter in the nursing notes.
- Note any unusual findings related to the condition of the skin on the penis.
- Document characteristics of urine (e.g., color, odor, consistency, blood).

Practice Resources
Gray, Skinner, & Kaler (2016); Newman & Wein (2018); Wound, Ostomy, and Continence Nurses Society (n.d.).

Thinking About the Procedure

The video **Applying an External Condom Urinary Catheter,** along with questions and suggested responses, is available on the **Davis's** *Nursing Skills Videos* Web site at www.fadavis.com.

Procedure 25-6 ■ Removing an Indwelling Catheter

> For steps to follow in *all* procedures, refer to the Universal Steps for All Procedures on the inside back cover of Volume 2.

Equipment
- Syringe (5 to 30 mL, depending on balloon size)
- Clean procedure gloves
- Towel or drape
- Receptacle for the catheter, such as an emesis basin
- Hygiene supplies (washcloth, warm filtered water or perineal wash solution, towel)

Delegation
In some institutions, unlicensed UAPs undergo special training to learn this skill. In such instances, you may delegate this task to the UAP. However, you must complete the following assessments and instruct the UAP about what abnormal findings to report.

Preprocedure Assessments
- Assess the patient's cognitive level.
  Knowing whether the patient can follow directions helps determine how to approach the procedure and also to know if the patient may be prone to pulling on the catheter or your hands when you are removing the catheter.
- Assess the condition of bladder (e.g., distention), perineum, and meatus (e.g., color, swelling, crusting, drainage, lesions).
  This information helps establish a baseline for later assessment.

(continued on next page)

Procedure 25-6 ■ Removing an Indwelling Catheter (continued)

> When performing the procedure, always identify your patient according to agency policy, using two identifiers, and be attentive to standard precautions, hand hygiene, patient safety and privacy, body mechanics, and documentation.

Procedure Steps

1. **Gather the necessary supplies.**

2. **Explain to the patient what you are about to do,** what they will feel, and that you will need to monitor her urination after removal.

3. **Perform hand hygiene** before and after removing the catheter.

4. **Wear clean procedure gloves** during the removal.
   Gloving prevents transmission of bacteria.

♥ **iCare 5. Explain that this procedure** is nearly always pain-free, but patients may feel a little pressure as the balloon deflates and the catheter is removed.

6. **Instruct** the patient to assume the supine position.

7. **Place the catheter receptacle** near the patient (e.g., on the bed).

8. **Place a waterproof drape** or towel.

   Variation: Female Patient: Place the drape between the patient's legs and up by the urethral meatus.

   Variation: Male Patient: Place the drape on his thighs.
   These methods preserve modesty and a feeling of security and prevent soiling of the bed.

9. **Obtain a sterile specimen** (see Procedure 25-2B), if needed. Some agencies require a culture and sensitivity test of urine when an indwelling catheter is removed.

10. **Wash the perineum** with soapy water or periwash before removal of the catheter.
    The perineum and catheter surfaces are colonized with bacteria. Cleansing this area reduces the risk for urinary catheter-associated infection.

11. **Remove the device securing** the catheter to the patient.

12. **Deflate the balloon completely** by inserting a syringe into the balloon valve and allowing the balloon to self-deflate. Allow at least 30 seconds for the balloon to deflate. *Note:* Follow the manufacturer's directions for balloon deflation. If the direction is to attempt aspiration, it should be done slowly and gently.
    Aspiration of the balloon may collapse the lumen and cause the formation of creases and ridges that may make removal of the catheter difficult.

13. **Verify that the total fluid** volume has been removed by checking the balloon size printed on the balloon port.
    If water remains in the balloon, removal of the catheter may cause urethral trauma.

14. **Ask the patient to relax** and take a few deep breaths as you slowly withdraw the catheter from the urethra. Pinch the catheter while removing it.
    Deep breathing helps the patient to relax the sphincters.

15. **Wrap the catheter in the towel** or drape or place in the catheter receptacle.

16. **Again, cleanse the perineal area** with warm filtered water or perineal wash solution on gauze pads or perineal disposable wipes. A mild soap may also be used.
    Cleansing the perineum prevents transmission of bacteria.

17. **Measure the urine** and empty it in the toilet; discard the catheter, drainage tube, and collection bag in the biohazard waste.

18. **Explain to the patient** the need to monitor the first few voidings after catheter removal. If the patient toilets independently, place a receptacle in the toilet or use a bedside commode. Ask the patient to notify the nurse when they void and to save the urine.

19. **Remove and discard gloves;** perform hand hygiene.

20. **Record the procedure** (see Documentation, as follows).

21. **Return the patient to** a position of comfort with the call device within reach.

? What if...

- **The balloon does not empty completely when I aspirate?**

  Do not pull on the catheter. Report to the charge nurse or the primary healthcare provider before continuing the procedure.
  Pulling on the catheter could cause injury to the urethra.

Evaluation

- Observe for signs and symptoms of infection.
  Signs of a catheter-associated urinary tract infection include the presence of significant bacteriuria in a patient with signs or symptoms of UTI, such as fever, malaise, flank pain, dysuria, altered mental status, or hematuria.
- Observe the condition of the meatus.
- Monitor the next few voidings. Place a collection container in the commode if the patient is ambulatory.
- Assess the characteristics of the urine at the time the catheter is removed. Then note the time of the first voiding and the amount voided, and observe the urine for color, amount, odor, and presence of blood.
- Compare voidings over the next 8 to 10 hours to the patient's intake.
- Monitor for bladder distention. A portable bladder-scanning device may be used to quantify any residual urine.

Patient Teaching

- Explain to the patient that you need to monitor the first few voidings after catheter removal to ensure that they do not have difficulty reestablishing bladder control.
- Teach the patient to notify you when they void and to save the urine (if the patient toilets independently).

Home Care

For patients who will have catheters at home, teach the patient and family the following:

- Steps for removing the catheter that you learned in this procedure
- To notify a healthcare provider if the patient is unable to urinate within 8 hours after catheter removal, or if the abdomen becomes distended and painful
- The signs and symptoms of UTI
  Signs and symptoms of UTI develop rapidly and can include a strong, persistent urge to urinate; a burning sensation when urinating; passing frequent, small amounts of urine; blood in the urine (hematuria); fever; flank pain; or an alteration in mental status.
- Increase fluid intake if not contraindicated by other health conditions.
- ❖ The patient should never remove a catheter unless trained by a healthcare provider. Remove the catheter only when prescribed by the provider.

Documentation

- Date and time the catheter was removed
- Amount of urine (on the I&O portion of the graphics sheet)
- Characteristics of urine (e.g., color, odor, cloudiness, turbidity, or blood)
- Time the specimen was sent to the laboratory
- Amount of fluid returned from balloon by self-deflation, amount of urine in drainage bag, and notification of first void
- Any unusual findings in your assessment of the perineum
- How the patient tolerated the procedure
- Patient teaching

Sample documentation

00/00/00   1010   Order noted for removal of indwelling catheter. Explained the procedure to patient. Pt stated, "I'm finally getting this thing out." Placed Pt in a dorsal recumbent position with blanket to provide privacy. Perineal care completed. Allowed retention balloon to self-deflate, obtaining 10 mL of liquid. Removed catheter, using gentle pulling motion. Pt expressed no discomfort during removal. Perineal care again given. 250 mL of clear, yellow, strong-smelling urine noted in drainage bag. Instructed client to increase fluid intake, especially water, and to notify a nurse when voiding for the first time. ——————————————————————D. Drumpf, RN

Practice Resources

Agency for Healthcare Research and Quality (2020, June, reviewed); Brown (2015); Clayton (2017, April); Cooper et al. (2016, July); Griffiths & Fernandez (2009); Newman, Cumbee, & Rovner (2017); Rimmer et al. (2020); Thangavelu-Veluswamy (2020, October 8, reviewed); Okrainec (2017); Wound, Ostomy, and Continence Nurses Society (2016); Yates (2008).

Thinking About the Procedure

▶ The video **Removing an Indwelling Urinary Catheter,** along with questions and suggested responses, is available on the **Davis's Nursing Skills Videos** Web site at www.fadavis.com.

Procedure 25-7 ■ Irrigating the Bladder or Catheter

➤ For steps to follow in *all* procedures, refer to the Universal Steps for All Procedures on the inside back cover of Volume 2.

Equipment

Intermittent Irrigation Through a Three-Way Catheter
- Bag of sterile irrigation solution
- Connecting tubing (to connect the bag to the irrigation port)
- IV pole
- Antiseptic swabs or wipes
- Bath blanket

Intermittent Irrigation via the Specimen Port Using a Syringe
- Sterile container
- Sterile 60-mL syringe with large-gauge needleless access device
- Sterile irrigation solution
- Two pairs of clean procedure gloves
- Antiseptic swabs or wipes

Continuous Bladder Irrigation
- Three-way (or triple-lumen) indwelling catheter in place
- Sterile irrigation solution at room temperature
- Connecting tubing
- Antiseptic swabs or wipes
- IV pole
- Bath blanket
- Measuring container
- Pair of clean procedure gloves

Delegation

Irrigation of an indwelling catheter requires nursing assessment and clinical decision-making. Because of the high potential for urinary tract infection, you should not delegate this procedure to the UAP. Bladder/catheter irrigation may be delegated with supervision to qualified LPNs who are trained in the procedure.

Preprocedure Assessments

- Note the characteristics of the urine (e.g., amount, color, odor, presence of clots or mucus).
- Assess for the presence and degree of bladder distention.
  This information helps establish a baseline for assessment.
- Note patient complaints of discomfort.
- Assess the patient's cognitive status.
  To determine whether the patient will remain still during the procedure.
- Check the chart for the amount and type of sterile solution to use.
- Determine whether the irrigant is to remain in the bladder for any length of time.

Procedure 25-7A ■ Intermittent Bladder or Catheter Irrigation

➤ When performing the procedure, always identify your patient according to agency policy, using two identifiers, and be attentive to standard precautions, hand hygiene, patient safety and privacy, body mechanics, and documentation.

➤ *Note:* This is the procedure for the closed methods of irrigation. ✚ The open method is no longer recommended. Because of the risk for infection, you should never disconnect the drainage tubing from the catheter.

Procedure Steps

Procedure Variation: Three-Way (Triple-Lumen) Indwelling Catheter

1. **Before starting irrigation,** prepare the connection tubing and the irrigation solution warmed to room temperature.
   a. Close the clamp on the connection tubing.
   b. Spike the tubing into the appropriate portal on the irrigation solution bag, using aseptic technique.
   c. Invert the solution and hang it on an IV pole.
   d. Remove the protective cap from the distal end of the connection tubing. Hold the end of the tubing over the sink or trash receptacle.
   e. Open the roller clamp and allow the solution to fill the tubing. Be sure to keep the end sterile.
   e. Reclamp the roller on the tubing to stop the flow of the irrigation solution.
   f. Recap the tubing.

2. **Perform hand hygiene,** and don procedure gloves.
   To reduce the transmission of microbes.

3. **Place the patient in the supine position.**

4. ♥ **iCare** **Drape the patient** so only the connection port on the indwelling catheter is visible.
   Protects patient privacy.

5. **Before initiating the flow** of the irrigation solution, empty any urine that is in the drainage bag, and perform hand hygiene. Then document the volume on the I&O record.
   Starting the procedure with an empty drainage bag gives you a baseline for correct calculation of true urine output during irrigation.

6. **Scrub the catheter port** with antiseptic swabs or wipe or sterile, normal saline.
   To remove microorganisms and help prevent UTI.

7. **Connect the irrigation tubing** to the catheter port.

8. **Slowly open the roller clamp** on the irrigation tubing to the desired flow rate.
   Slow instillation prevents patient discomfort.

9. **Instill or irrigate** with the prescribed amount of irrigant. If the irrigant is to remain in the bladder for a certain period, clamp the drainage tubing for that time.

10. **When the correct amount** of irrigant has been used and/or the goals of the irrigation have been met, close the roller clamp on the irrigation tubing, leaving the tubing connected to the catheter for use during the next irrigation.
    You can assess whether the goals of irrigation have been met by inspecting the color of the urine and assessing for presence of clots, mucus, or blood. Clamping the drainage tubing prevents immediate outflow.

11. **Remove gloves,** perform hand hygiene, and return the patient to a position of comfort.

Procedure Variation: Two-Way Indwelling Catheter

12. **Don clean procedure gloves.** Empty any urine in the bedside drainage bag.
    Emptying the bag will ensure accurate output results.

13. **Perform hand hygiene,** and don clean gloves.
    Gloving prevents the transmission of microorganisms.

♥ **iCare 14. Drape the patient** so that only the specimen removal port on the drainage tubing is exposed. Place a waterproof drape beneath the exposed port.
Draping ensures patient privacy and prevents soiling of the bed linens.

15. **Open the sterile irrigation** supplies. Pour approximately 100 mL of the irrigating solution, warmed to room temperature, into the sterile container, using aseptic technique.
    Warm solution is more comfortable to the patient.

16. **Scrub all surfaces** of the specimen removal port with an antiseptic swab or wipe.
    Cleaning the port reduces the risk of transmission of pathogens into the bladder.

17. **Draw up the irrigation solution** into the syringe. Connect the syringe to the specimen port. For catheter irrigation, use a total of 30 to 40 mL; for bladder irrigation the amount is usually 100 to 200 mL, unless irrigation is prescribed postoperatively (in which case more irrigation might be needed).

18. **Clamp or pinch the drainage** tubing distal to the specimen port.
    Clamping prevents irrigant from going down into the drainage bag and not into the catheter and/or bladder.

19. **Inject the solution into the port.** Hold the specimen port slightly above the level of the bladder. If you meet resistance, have the patient turn slightly, and attempt a second time. If resistance continues, stop the procedure, and notify the primary healthcare provider.
    Holding the port above the level of the bladder enhances gravitational flow of irrigant into the bladder. ➤

20. **When the irrigant has been injected,** remove the syringe. Refill the syringe, if necessary.

21. **Unclamp or release** the drainage tubing, and allow the irrigant and urine to flow into the bedside drainage bag by gravity. (If the solution is to remain in the bladder for a prescribed time, leave the tubing clamped for that period.)

22. **Repeat the procedure, as necessary,** until the prescribed amount has been instilled or until the goal of the irrigation is met (e.g., removal of clots and mucus, free flowing of urine).

23. **Remove gloves,** perform hand hygiene, and return the patient to a position of comfort with the call device within reach.

(continued on next page)

Procedure 25-7 ■ Irrigating the Bladder or Catheter (continued)

Procedure 25-7B ■ Continuous Bladder Irrigation

▶ When performing the procedure, always identify your patient according to agency policy, using two identifiers, and be attentive to standard precautions, hand hygiene, patient safety and privacy, body mechanics, and documentation.

Procedure Steps

1. **If one is not already present,** insert a three-way (triple-lumen) indwelling catheter.
   A triple-lumen catheter provides an access for the irrigation solution without disrupting the sterile drainage unit.

2. **Prepare the tubing and the irrigation fluid** warmed to room temperature:
   a. Close the clamp on the connecting tubing.
   b. Spike the tubing into the portal on the irrigation solution container, using aseptic technique.
      This prevents the introduction of microorganisms into the solution.
   c. Invert the container and hang it on the IV pole.
      The elevated bag allows the solution to flow by gravity.
   d. Remove the protective cap from the distal end of the connecting tubing. Hold the end of the tubing over a sink or other receptacle. Open the roll clamp slowly and allow the solution to fill the tubing completely. Reclamp the tubing. Recap the tubing.
      Priming the tubing flushes air from tubing, preventing bladder distention.

3. **Perform hand hygiene,** and don clean procedure gloves.
   To prevent the spread of microorganisms.

   ♥ **iCare 4. Place the patient supine** and drape the patient so that only the connection port on the indwelling catheter is visible.
   Draping prevents exposure of the genital area and protects patient privacy.

5. **Place a waterproof barrier** drape under the irrigation port. Scrub the irrigation port with antiseptic swabs or wipes. Pinching the tubing and using aseptic technique, connect the end of the irrigation infusion tubing to the irrigation port of the catheter.

6. **Before initiating the flow** of the irrigation solution, empty any urine that may be in the bedside drainage bag, and document the volume on the I&O record.
   Starting the procedure with an empty bag gives you a baseline for correct calculation of true urine output during irrigation. The I&O record provides data for evaluating urinary status.

7. **Remove your gloves** and perform hand hygiene.
   Gloving and hand hygiene prevent the transmission of microorganisms.

8. **Cover the patient** and return him or her to a position of comfort, with the call device within reach.

9. **Open the roller clamp** on the tubing and regulate the flow of the irrigation solution to meet the desired outcome for the irrigation.
   The goal of continuous bladder irrigation for patients who have had transurethral resection of the prostate is to keep urine light pink to clear. ▶

10. **Monitor the flow rate** for 1 to 2 minutes to ensure accuracy.
    Monitoring the irrigation fluid for a minute or two prevents rapid introduction of solution into the bladder, which would cause patient discomfort.

? What if...

- **The draining irrigant solution and/or urine looks like it has red blood cells (RBCs) in it?**

Stop the irrigation and report to the primary healthcare provider.
Increased RBCs in urine may indicate bladder irritation and possible trauma to the inner mucosal lining of the bladder.

- **I meet resistance when irrigating?**

Ask the patient to turn slightly, and attempt a second time. If resistance continues, stop the procedure, and notify the primary healthcare provider.

Evaluation

- Note the flow rate of irrigant and/or inability to instill irrigant into the catheter.
- Note the characteristics of urine output (e.g., presence of output, color, amount, clots, mucus).
- Note patient report of discomfort (e.g., pain, spasms).
- Assess for development of bladder distention accompanied by lack of urine outflow. A portable bladder scanner may be used to quantify the amount of fluid retained in the bladder.

Home Care

For clients who will have continuous bladder irrigation at home, you will need to teach the family the necessary steps of the procedure. Also teach them to:

- Empty the urine collection device before beginning the procedure.
- Use strict aseptic technique when irrigating the bladder or catheter.
- Irrigate the catheter using the closed method, which carries the least risk for introducing bacteria into the bladder. The catheter and drainage tubing should never be disconnected.
- Identify signs and symptoms of urinary retention and UTI.
- Wash their hands before and after any manipulation of the catheter site or apparatus.
- Be certain to maintain unobstructed flow.
- For the syringe method, the client will need access to syringes and needleless access devices and a process to dispose of them properly.

Documentation

- Date and time of procedure, the type of irrigant, and the total volume infused
- Characteristics of the urine (e.g., color, odor, clarity, sediment, presence of clots or mucus)
- Evidence of catheter patency (e.g., flow of urine, absence of distention)

Sample documentation

mm/dd/yyyy 1415 Bladder irrigation per orders with 1 liter sterile saline solution. Urine with frank blood visible. Cleared to pale, straw-color at the completion of bladder irrigation. Mucous shreds and clots cleared. Pt. tolerated procedure without complaints of pain, discomfort, or burning. Catheter patency evidenced by free flow of urine and absence of distention.............................M.M.Baker, RN

Practice Resources

Agency for Clinical Innovation (ACI) Urology Network (2019, June, amended); Agency for Healthcare Research and Quality (2017, March, reviewed); Appendix C Sample Bladder Scan Policy (2020, October); Harmon & Hassoun (2017, Fall); Shepherd, Mackay, & Hagan (2017); Weber, Purvis, VanDenBergh, et al. (2017).

Thinking About the Procedure

The videos **Intermittent Bladder Irrigation: Three-Way (Triple-Lumen) Indwelling Catheter, Intermittent Bladder Irrigation: Two-Way Indwelling Catheter,** and **Continuous Bladder Irrigation,** along with questions and suggested responses, are available on the **Davis's *Nursing Skills Videos*** Web site at www.fadavis.com.

CLINICAL INSIGHT

Clinical Insight 25-1 ▸ Teaching Clients About Clean, Intermittent Self-Catheterization

In the home setting, this is a clean procedure rather than a sterile one. It is referred to as clean, intermittent self-catheterization (CISC).

Clean, Intermittent Self-Catheterization for Male Patients

1. **Try to void before catheterization.** If you are unable to void or if the amount is less than 3 ounces (or the amount specified by your healthcare provider), then insert the catheter.
2. **Assemble the catheter, lubricant, and drainage receptacle.**
3. **Thoroughly wash** your hands with soap and water; cleanse the penis and the urethral opening.
4. **Lubricate** the catheter to 15 cm (6 inches).
5. **Stand over the toilet,** or assume a comfortable position (e.g., sitting on the toilet).
6. **Hold the penis** perpendicular (at a right angle) to your body.
7. **Gently insert** and advance the catheter.
8. **When you meet resistance,** at the level of the prostate, take deep breaths to try to relax, and advance the catheter.
9. **When the urine flow starts,** advance the catheter 2.5 cm (1 inch) more; return the penis to its natural position; hold the catheter in place until the urine flow stops and the bladder is empty.
10. **Withdraw the catheter** slowly in small increments to be sure that the entire bladder has been emptied.
11. **Wash the catheter** with soap and water, if it is reusable (or follow the manufacturer's instructions for cleaning). Rinse and dry it well. If it is disposable, discard it immediately.
12. **Store catheters** in a clean, dry, secure place.
13. **Record the amount** of urine obtained.

Clean, Intermittent Self-Catheterization for Female Patients

1. **Try to void before catheterization.** If you are unable to void or if the urine amount is less than 3 ounces (or less than the amount specified by your healthcare provider), then insert the catheter.
2. **Assemble the catheter, lubricant, and drainage receptacle;** a good light is important.
3. **Thoroughly wash your hands** with soap and water.
4. **Cleanse your labia and urethra** with soap and water or with a moist towelette; rinse well. Cleanse and rinse from front to back.
5. **Lubricate the catheter** to about 2.5 cm (1 inch).
6. **Assume a comfortable position** for urinating. Some patients perform CISC standing up with one foot on the toilet.
7. **Use a hand mirror** to locate the urethral opening, which is between the clitoris and the vagina.
8. **Spread your labia** with the second and fourth fingers; use the middle finger to feel for the urethral opening.
9. **Gently insert the catheter** into the opening, guiding it upward toward your umbilicus (belly button) until urine flows. This is usually 5 to 8 cm (2 to 3 inches) past the urethral opening.
10. **When urine flows,** advance the catheter another 2.5 cm (1 inch). Hold it in place until the urine flow stops and your bladder is empty.
11. **Withdraw the catheter slowly** in small increments to be sure the entire bladder has been emptied.
12. **If the catheter is reusable,** wash it with soap and water; rinse and dry it well (or follow the manufacturer's instructions for cleaning). If it is disposable, discard it immediately.
13. **Store catheters** in a clean, dry, secure place.
14. **Record the amount** of urine obtained.

Practice Resources

Beauchemin et al. (2018, September); Goetz et al. (2018); Yates (2015); Zhang et al. (2018).

ASSESSMENT GUIDELINES AND TOOLS

Focused Assessment

Urinary Elimination History Questions

Usual Urination Pattern
- How often do you urinate?
- Do you get up in the middle of the night to urinate?
- Do you have difficulty getting to the bathroom in time to urinate?
- Does urine ever leak when you cough, laugh, or exercise?
- Does urine ever leak on the way to the bathroom?
- Do you need to use pads or tissue in your underwear to catch urine?
- Do you have any difficulty starting voiding?

Appearance of Urine
- How would you describe your urine?
- Have you noticed unusual odor with urination?

Changes in Urination Habits or Urine Appearance
- Have you had any changes in your voiding pattern recently?
- Have you had any changes in the appearance or odor of your urine?

History of Urination Problems
- Have you had any problems with urinary tract infections or kidney and bladder problems?
- Have you ever lost control of urination?
- Have you ever had urinary tract surgery or diagnostic procedures?

Use of Urination Aids
- What aids, if any, do you use to help with urination?
- What is your usual fluid intake over the course of a day?
- What medications are you taking? Have they had any effect on your urination pattern?

Lifestyle Questions
- Where is your bathroom located? Can you get to it easily?
- Can you manage your clothing when you go to the bathroom?
- How much fluid do you drink each day?
- How many caffeinated beverages do you drink?
- Do you smoke?
- Are you bothered by constipation?
- Do you do high-impact exercise (e.g., jogging)?

Presence of Urinary Diversions
- Have you ever had urinary tract surgery?
- If so, what and when?
- Gather data on the client's usual care of the stoma, use of appliances, and adjustment to the ostomy.

For Infants and Young Children
- Has the child been toilet-trained?
- What elimination routines have been established?

Guidelines for Physical Assessment for Urinary Elimination

Physical assessment for urinary elimination includes examination of the kidneys, bladder, urethra, and skin surrounding the genitals, as appropriate. For a complete discussion of physical examination of the genitourinary system, see Chapter 19, Procedures 19-17 and 19-18, in this volume.

The Kidneys

Technique	Rationale
The **costovertebral (CV) angle** is formed by the junction of the 12th rib and the spine on both sides of the back. Place one palm flat on the CV angle and lightly strike it with the closed fist of the other hand (see the accompanying figure).	You cannot usually palpate the kidneys. Instead, examine them by assessing for costovertebral angle tenderness (CVAT). If kidney inflammation is present, percussion of this angle produces pain.

The Bladder

Inspect, palpate, and percuss the lower abdomen. Correlate your findings with data about the client's fluid intake and voiding.

▸ Inspect the lower abdomen.	▸ An empty bladder, or one with limited urine, is small and sits below the symphysis pubis.
	▸ In contrast, a distended bladder rises above the symphysis pubis. If it is very distended, you may be able to see a rounded swelling above the symphysis pubis.
▸ Lightly palpate the lower abdomen to define the bladder margin. Observe the patient's response to palpation, noting signs of tenderness or discomfort.	An empty bladder, or one with limited urine, will not be palpable.
▸ Percuss the area.	A distended bladder produces a dull sound as opposed to the normal tympanic sound of intestinal air.

The Urethra

▸ Inspect the urethral orifice. Look for erythema, discharge, swelling, or odor.	These are all signs of infection, trauma, or inflammation.

The Perineal Area

▸ Frequently inspect skin color, condition, texture, turgor, and presence of urine or stool.	Clients who have urine leakage or a urinary catheter are at risk for perineal skin problems. Ammonia in urine may cause skin excoriation, skin breakdown, and subsequent infection. If both urine and stool are present on the skin, the likelihood of skin breakdown increases.

DIAGNOSTIC TESTING

Urinalysis

Characteristic Findings	Expected	Variations
Color	A freshly voided sample is pale yellow to deep amber.	▸ Color is lighter, or even clear, if fluid intake is high or urine output is excessive. ▸ Color is darker as it becomes more concentrated (e.g., with decreased fluid intake or excessive fluid loss). ▸ Color is affected by certain foods (e.g., beets, carrots, asparagus) and medications (e.g., antacids, phenazopyridine). ▸ Dark, tea-colored urine can indicate liver disease or vasculitis. ▸ Color is affected by some medications.
Clarity	A freshly voided sample should be translucent. If urine sits for some time, it will become cloudy.	▸ Cloudiness in a freshly voided sample indicates the presence of other constituents in the urine (e.g., bacteria, RBCs, WBCs, sperm, prostatic fluid, or vaginal discharge).
Odor	Fresh urine is mildly odorous.	▸ Certain foods, such as garlic, onions, and asparagus, may give urine a distinctive odor. ▸ Vitamins (e.g., B_6) and medication can change the odor of urine. ▸ Bacteria with a bladder or kidney infection give urine an ammonia-like odor. ▸ A sweet odor may indicate an inborn metabolic disorder (maple syrup urine disease). ▸ Diabetes and liver failure can cause a different odor.
pH	5.0–9.0	▸ Indicates the kidneys' ability to help maintain balanced hydrogen ion concentration (acid–base balance) in blood. ▸ The pH increases (more alkaline) if the client eats dairy products or citrus fruits or has a vegetarian diet. ▸ The pH decreases (urine becomes more acidic) if the client eats a high-protein diet or consumes cranberry juice.
Specific gravity	1.002–1.030	▸ Reflects the kidneys' ability to concentrate urine. ▸ Rises with dehydration or kidney disease. ▸ Decreases as fluid intake increases.
Protein	<20 mg/dL	▸ Most common indicator of renal disease (e.g., diabetic nephropathy, glomerulonephritis, nephrosis, or toxemia of pregnancy). ▸ May be increased in benign proteinuria secondary to stress or physical exercise. ▸ Foamy urine can mean higher protein level than normal.
Glucose	Negative	▸ Indicates elevated blood sugar (as in diabetes).
Ketones	Negative	▸ Indicates impaired carbohydrate metabolism. ▸ May be detected with diabetes, fever, fasting, high-protein or low-carbohydrate diet, or vomiting and in the postanesthesia period.
Hemoglobin	▸ Negative on dipstick ▸ If RBCs are assessed via microscopic examination: less than 5/hpf (high-power field)	▸ Detected with UTI, bladder or kidney disease or cancer, enlarged prostate, trauma, lupus, or sickle cell anemia. It also may be present in samples obtained during menstruation.

(Continued)

Urinalysis—cont'd

Characteristic Findings	Expected	Variations
Bilirubin	Negative	▸ Increased bilirubin occurs with liver disease, cancer, gallstones, or hepatitis.
Urobilinogen	Up to 1 mg/dL	▸ Increased in cirrhosis, heart failure, liver disease, infectious mononucleosis, malaria, and pernicious anemia.
Nitrite	Negative	▸ Increased in bacteriuria, presence of nitrite-forming bacteria, such as *Escherichia coli*.
Leukocyte esterase	▸ Negative ▸ If WBCs are assessed via microscopic examination: less than 5/hpf	▸ Increased in bacterial infection, calculus formation, fungal or parasitic infection, glomerulonephritis, interstitial nephritis, or tumor.
Renal cells	None seen	▸ Indicates damage to the tubular network. (Renal cells come from the lining of the collecting ducts.)
Transitional cells	None seen	▸ Occurs with infection, trauma, and malignancy. (Transitional cells line the renal pelvis, ureter, bladder, and proximal urethra.)
Squamous cells	Rare	▸ Typically insignificant. (Squamous cells line the vagina and distal portion of the urethra.)
Casts	Rare hyaline; negative	▸ Large numbers of *hyaline casts* are seen in renal disease and hypertension, with diuretic use, and in fever. ▸ *Granular casts* occur in renal disease, viral infection, or lead intoxication.
Crystals	Absent in freshly voided sample	▸ May indicate an old sample, stone formation in the urinary tract, gout, high dietary intake of oxalates, liver disease, or side effect of chemotherapy.
Bacteria, yeast, parasites	None seen	▸ Microbes in urine indicate urinary tract infection (UTI).

Source: Adapted from Van Leeuwen & Bladh (2021). *Davis's comprehensive handbook of laboratory & diagnostic tests with nursing implications* (9th ed.). Philadelphia, PA: F.A. Davis.

Blood Studies: BUN and Creatinine

Normal Ranges		Levels May Be Increased in:	Levels May Be Decreased in:
Blood urea nitrogen (BUN)	8–21 mg/dL	▸ Renal failure	▸ Inadequate protein intake
Creatinine	0.5–1.2 mg/dL	▸ Impaired renal perfusion	▸ Malabsorption syndromes
		▸ Kidney inflammation	▸ Liver disease
		▸ Kidney obstruction	
		▸ Dehydration	
		▸ Excessive protein intake	
		▸ Use of total parenteral nutrition (TPN)	

Adapted from Van Leeuwen & Bladh (2021). *Davis's comprehensive handbook of laboratory & diagnostic tests with nursing implications* (9th ed.). Philadelphia, PA: F.A. Davis.

Studies of the Urinary System

Direct Visualization Studies

Cystoscopy
Direct visualization of the urethra, bladder, and ureteral orifices by insertion of a scope. May be used to obtain biopsies and treat any pathology of visualized areas.
PREPARATION
- Instruct the patient that the procedure is performed under anesthesia. This anesthesia may be general, spinal, or local.
- Ensure that a signed consent form is included with the chart.
- Restrict food and fluids for 8 hours if the patient is receiving general anesthesia. For local anesthesia, allow intake of only clear liquids for 8 hours before the procedure.

POSTPROCEDURE CARE
- Monitor vital signs and intake and output (I&O).
- Observe the characteristics of urine after the procedure.
- Encourage increased fluid intake.
- Report suprapubic or flank pain, chills, or difficulty urinating.

Cystometry
Done to determine whether a muscle or nerve problem is causing problems with how well the bladder holds or releases urine. A catheter is inserted into the bladder and a pressure probe into the rectum. Warm fluid is injected and connected to the *cystometer,* which measures how much the bladder can hold and the pressure in the bladder. A gas or contrast material is sometimes used.
PREPARATION
- Ensure a signed consent form is included with the chart.
- Explain that patient cooperation with positioning and activity is crucial during the test.
- There are no food or fluid restrictions before the test.

POSTPROCEDURE CARE
- Monitor vital signs and I&O.
- Encourage increased fluid intake.
- Report suprapubic or flank pain, chills, or difficulty urinating.

Indirect Visualization Studies

Intravenous Pyelography (IVP) and Retrograde Pyelography

IVP uses IV radiopaque contrast medium to visualize the kidneys, ureters, bladder, and renal pelvis. It evaluates renal function by analyzing flow of contrast over time.

Retrograde pyelography uses radiopaque contrast medium to visualize the renal collecting system. Contrast media is injected via a ureteral catheter inserted through a cystoscope.
PREPARATION
- Assess for history of allergies. Radiopaque dyes can be highly allergenic for some patients; therefore, this test is contraindicated for patients with allergies to shellfish or iodinated dye.
- Ensure baseline BUN and creatinine results are available. This test is contraindicated for patients with renal failure.
- Ensure that a signed consent form is included with the chart.
- Restrict food and fluids for 8 hours before the procedure. Check agency protocols for specific guidelines, especially related to fluid intake.
- Some patients may require a laxative the evening before the surgery to clear the gastrointestinal tract and improve visualization.
- Check to be sure patients with diabetes who take insulin make an adjustment to the insulin dose when fasting for this examination.
- Determine the patient is not pregnant, breastfeeding, or with an intrauterine device (IUD) in place.
- Ask whether the patient has had an x-ray test using barium contrast material (e.g., barium enema) or have taken a medication containing bismuth (e. g., Pepto-Bismol) in the 4 days before the test. These can affect the test results.
- Check for a history of bleeding disorders or if the patient is taking any anticoagulant, aspirin, or other medications that affect blood clotting. It may be necessary to hold these medications before the procedure.

POSTPROCEDURE CARE
- Encourage increased fluid intake.
- Monitor vital signs and I&O.
- Observe for reactions to the contrast media: rash, nausea, hives.

Ultrasonography
Using contrast media, computed tomography (CT) examines body sections from different angles by using a narrow x-ray beam to produce a three-dimensional image of the area of the body being scanned.
PREPARATION
- Ensure a signed consent form is included with the chart.
- There are no food or fluid restrictions with renal ultrasonography. A patient undergoing bladder ultrasonography may be required to drink five to six glasses of fluid 90 minutes before the procedure to ensure a full bladder.

POSTPROCEDURE CARE
- No special care is required.

Computed Tomography
Using contrast media, CT examines body sections from different angles by using a narrow x-ray beam to produce a three-dimensional image of the area of the body being scanned.
PREPARATION
- Obtain history of allergies. This test is contraindicated in patients with allergies to shellfish or iodinated dye.

(Continued)

Diagnostic Testing

Studies of the Urinary System—cont'd

- Ensure a signed consent form is included with the chart.
- For renal CT, food and fluids are usually restricted for 2 to 4 hours before the procedure.
- Remove all metal objects from the patient's body (e.g., eyeglasses, rings, safety pins).

POSTPROCEDURE CARE
- Monitor vital signs and I&O.
- Observe for reactions to the contrast media: rash, nausea, hives.

Renal Biopsy

Removal of a piece of kidney tissue for microscopic evaluation, usually done with ultrasound guidance.

PREPARATION
- Ensure baseline coagulation studies and hemoglobin results are available.
- Ensure a signed consent form is on the chart.
- Nothing by mouth (NPO) 6 to 8 hours before an open biopsy procedure and at least 4 hours before a needle biopsy procedure. Protocols may vary among facilities.
- Instruct the patient that sedation and/or pain medication may be given.

POSTPROCEDURE CARE
- Monitor vital signs and I&O.
- The patient will be on bedrest for 6 to 24 hours, as prescribed.
- Monitor biopsy site for bleeding.
- Monitor urine for presence of blood.

Source: Adapted from Van Leeuwen & Bladh (2021). *Davis's comprehensive handbook of laboratory & diagnostic tests with nursing implications* (9th ed.). Philadelphia, PA: F.A. Davis.

Nursing Care Plan

Client Data

Desmond Washington, a 69-year-old man, comes to the clinic 4 weeks after having a prostatectomy for prostate cancer. He was discharged from the hospital on postoperative day 4 and went home with an indwelling urinary catheter. The catheter was removed at his last visit, 9 days after surgery.

Mr. Washington is friendly, greeting other patients in the clinic and chatting with the clinic personnel. When his nurse brings him to an examination room and asks how he feels, he says, "I saw the sun come up today. I appreciate that more now. The good Lord has given me a new lease on life, and I intend to use it!" His nurse continues, "That's great, Mr. Washington. How have you been doing since the catheter was removed?" Mr. Washington's smile fades. He lowers his voice and says, "You know, I think that's the worst part of this whole thing. I hate wearing these diapers—they make me feel, well, like an old man. I'm certainly not ready for this."

The nurse continues, "Do you have *any* control of your urine?" Mr. Washington explains, "I may go for hours and stay dry, and then it seems for no reason, I wet myself. Take yesterday, for example. I was sitting on the sofa watching the ball game when someone came to the door. I got up to answer the door, and suddenly, I felt wet. I didn't even have anything to drink so I could make it through the afternoon and stay dry. And if I cough? Forget it. Can something be done so I can hold my urine again?"

Nursing Diagnosis

Stress urinary incontinence related to disruption of the urinary sphincter and related pelvic muscles by surgery as evidenced by client report of involuntary loss of urine with increased intra-abdominal pressure.

NOC Outcomes	Individualized Goals/Expected Outcomes
Urinary continence (0502) Urinary elimination (0503)	*By the next visit, Mr. Washington will:* 1. Describe three things he can do that will help regain urinary continence. 2. Explain three interventions to cope with leaked urine. 3. Report that he is drinking adequate amounts of fluids during the day.

NIC Interventions

Urinary elimination management (NIC 0590)
Urinary incontinence care (NIC 0610)

Nursing Interventions/Activities	Rationale
1. Obtain midstream voided urine specimen for urinalysis.	Urinary tract infection (UTI) can cause or worsen urinary incontinence (UI) (Mayo Clinic Staff, 2021; Nambiar, Bosch, Cruz, et al., 2018). Dipstick urinalysis is a rapid, convenient, inexpensive, and easy-to-perform test to detect UTI (Skobe, n.d.), although not always reliable for ruling out UTI (Chu & Lowder, 2018).
2. Identify factors that contribute to Mr. Washington's incontinence by using an incontinence journal for a minimum of 3 days, including variations in his usual activities.	Identifying activities or other factors that cause loss of urine control can guide specific interventions. Becoming aware of activities or other factors that cause loss of urine control can guide specific interventions. A journal may help people identify patterns that could otherwise be missed (NIDDKD, 2021a; Nambiar et al., 2018; Trowbridge & Hoover, 2022).
3. Use portable bladder scanner to confirm pelvic floor muscle strength.	Pilates exercise program is also effective for improving strength of pelvic floor muscles in recovering continence in men after prostatectomy (Appendix C Sample Bladder Scan Policy, 2020, October; Chmielewska, 2019; Pedriali et al., 2016).

(continued)

Nursing Care Plan (continued)

Nursing Interventions/ Activities	Rationale
4. Teach urgency suppression techniques to delay voiding.	Gradually lengthening the time between urination can help stretch the bladder so it can hold more urine (NDDKD, 2021a, July; NIDDKD, 2021c, July; Roscow & Borello-France, 2017).
5. Teach pelvic floor muscle physiotherapy using a resistance band to strengthen and improve urinary control.	PFMEs strengthen pelvic muscles and enhance sphincter control. Some studies have shown that PFMEs increase UI without side effects in men who have undergone prostatectomy (Campbell et al., 2012; Chmielewska, 2019, December 2; Glazener et al., 2011; Nambiar et al., 2018; Pan et al., 2019, May; Roscow & Borello-France, 2017; Van Kampen et al., 2000; Appendix C Sample Bladder Scan Policy, 2020, October, last reviewed).
6. Use surface electromyography (sEMG) biofeedback when needed in conjunction with abdominal training to help Mr. Washington isolate pelvic floor muscles.	Biofeedback allows clients to receive auditory or visual (or both) cues when the proper muscles are contracted to learn how to improve strength of pelvic floor muscles (Chmielewska, 2019, December 2; Hill & Alappattu, 2017, May; McIntosh, 2015, July August; Pan et al., 2019; Roscow & Borello-France, 2017; Starr, Drobnes, & Cornelius, 2016).
7. Teach timed voiding. Have Mr. Washington void on a schedule of every 2 hours.	Bladder training with voiding on a schedule can reduce the amount of urine in the bladder, thus reducing the likelihood of leakage with activities of daily living (Davis & Wyman, 2020, February; Bedretdinova et al., 2016).
8. Administer prescribed medications.	A variety of medications can increase bladder capacity and decrease frequency of urination (e.g, antimuscarinics, beta-3 agonists, beta-3 adrenergic receptor stimulators, tricyclic antidepressants) (NIDDKD, 2021a, July). Other medication may be prescribed to reduce urinary leakage.
9. Instruct Mr. Washington to use neuromuscular electrical stimulation.	This treatment is used to retrain and strengthen weak urinary muscles and improve bladder control. A probe is inserted into the anus, and a current is passed through the probe at a level below the pain threshold, causing a contraction. The patient is instructed to squeeze the muscles when the current is on. After the contraction, the current is switched off (Anderson et al., 2015; Roscow & Borello-France, 2017).
10. Explain the need to drink adequate fluids and not limit fluids to prevent UI. Also avoid drinking fluids at bedtime. Help Mr. Washington identify ways to drink a minimum of 1,500 mL/day.	Adequate fluid intake is important to maintain dilute urine, which is less irritating to the bladder; to maintain systemic hydration; and to reduce the risk for constipation, which can contribute to UI.
11. Advise patient to avoid caffeine; salty, spicy, and acidic foods; and alcohol. Encourage a high-fiber diet.	Caffeine and spicy foods increase bladder irritability. Alcohol interferes with signals for urination (Goode, 2011; Nambiar et al., 2018). Salty foods can cause the body to retain water, which eventually goes to the bladder. They also increase thirst. Dietary fiber can prevent constipation, a cause of UI (Mayo Clinic Staff, 2021, December 17).
12. Advise the client to keep a healthy weight.	As body mass index (BMI) increases, so does the likelihood of urinary leakage (Gordon, 2017; NIDDKD, 2021a, July).
13. Assist the client in selecting absorbent products that collect urine temporarily while continence management is ongoing.	Incontinence products (e.g., male incontinence guards, underpads, adult incontinence briefs) contain urine, keep skin clean and dry, reduce odor and embarrassment, and reduce the risk for skin breakdown (Davis & Wyman, 2020, February; Nambiar et al., 2018; Vasavada, 2021, July 12).

Nursing Care Plan (continued)

Nursing Interventions/ Activities	Rationale
14. Help Mr. Washington develop a personal hygiene routine that will maintain skin integrity and control odor.	Conscientious skin care and good hygiene will reduce the risk of skin irritation and infection. Use warm (not hot) water, and pat (don't scrub) the perineal area. A barrier cream repels fluid and reduces skin excoriation. Controlling odor is important in reducing embarrassment and preventing social isolation (Davis & Wyman, 2020, February).
15. Offer referral to a support group. Encourage the client to speak to family and friends about UI.	Support groups provide a sense of community and enhance problem-solving skills of members. In sharing their struggle, the patient may find that other people in their life have bladder problems as well (NIDDKD, 2021a, July).
16. Explain that urinary incontinence is common after prostatectomy but that it may be only temporary.	UI can be a troubling complication of prostatectomy for many male patients. Fortunately, it often resolves within 6 to 12 months after surgery (McIntosh, Andersen, & Reekie, 2015, July–August; Yu Ko & Sawatzky, 2008; Roscow & Borello-France, 2017).

It is important for nurses to understand the pathophysiology of urinary incontinence differs between male and female patients and that interventions that are successful in female patients may or may not be equally successful in male patients.

Evaluation

Mr. Washington currently has a positive attitude and is focused on surviving his cancer first and on managing complications of surgery second. Although he previously had been placing folded paper towels in his underwear to collect urine because he thought absorbent products were too expensive, now, with guidance from his nurse, he identified products he could afford to manage his UI. He liked that they would not be visible through his clothing.

At Mr. Washington's next visit, the nurse will review the initial collaborative goals and stated outcomes and perform a client assessment to determine whether the goals were reached in the stated time.

As time passes, incontinence may persist and may become more frustrating for him once he is fully recovered from surgery. Mr. Washington initially declined referral to a support group, but he may be more interested in joining one in the future for help dealing with long-term consequences of prostatectomy.

References

Anderson, C. A., Omar, M. I., Campbell, S. E., et al. (2015). Conservative management for postprostatectomy urinary incontinence. *Cochrane Database of Systematic Reviews, 1*, CD001843. doi:10.1002/14651858.CD001843.pub5

Appendix C Sample Bladder Scan Policy. (2020, October, last reviewed). Toolkit for reducing catheter-associated urinary tract infections in hospital units: Implementation guide. Agency for Healthcare Research and Quality, Rockville, MD. Retrieved July 1, 2020, from http://www.ahrq.gov/professionals/quality-patient-safety/hais/cauti-tools/impl-guide/implementation-guide-appendix-c.html

Campbell, S. E., Glazener, C. M., Hunter, K. F., et al. (2012). Conservative management for postprostatectomy urinary incontinence (Review). *Cochrane Database of Systematic Reviews, 1*. https://doi.org/10.1002/14651858.CD001843.pub5

Chmielewska, D., Stania, M., Kucab-Klich, et al. (2019, December 2). Electromyographic characteristics of pelvic floor muscles in women with stress urinary incontinence following sEMG-assisted biofeedback training and Pilates exercises. PLoS ONE, 14(12), e0225647. https://doi.org/10.1371/journal.pone.0225647

Davis, N. J. & Wyman, J. F. (2020, February). Managing urinary incontinence. *American Journal of Nursing, 120*(2), 55-60.

Dowling-Castronovo, A. (2018, revised). Urinary incontinence assessment in older adults, part 1—transient urinary incontinence. *Try This: Best Practices in Nursing Care to Older Adults, 11*(1). https://hign.org/sites/default/files/2020-06/Try_This_General_Assessment_11_Part_1.pdf

Glazener, C., Boachie, C., Buckley, B., et al. (2011). Urinary incontinence in men after formal one-to-one pelvic-floor muscle training following radical prostatectomy or transurethral resection of the prostate (MAPS): Two parallel randomised controlled trials. *Lancet, 378*, 328–337. http://dx.doi.org/10.1016/S0140-6736(11)60751-4

Goode, P. S., Burgio, K. L., Johnson, T. M., et al. (2011). Conservative treatment of postprostatectomy incontinence. *JAMA, 305*, 151–159. doi:https://doi.org/10.1007/978-3-319-55829-5_4

(continued)

Nursing Care Plan (continued)

Gordon, B., Shorter, B., Isoldi, K. K., et al. (2017). Obesity with comorbid stress urinary incontinence in women: a narrative review to inform dietetics practice. *Journal of the Academy of Nutrition and Dietetics, 117*(6), 889–907.

Hill, A., & Alappattu, M. (2017, May). Quality-of-life outcomes following surface electromyography biofeedback as an adjunct to pelvic floor muscle training for urinary continence: A case report. *Journal of Women's Health Physical Therapy, 41*(2), 73-82. doi: 10.1097/JWH.0000000000000065

Mayo Clinic Staff. (2021, December 17). *Urinary incontinence.* https://www.mayoclinic.org/diseases-conditions/urinary-incontinence/symptoms-causes/syc-20352808

McIntosh, L., Andersen, E., & Reekie, M. (2015, July–August). Conservative treatment of stress urinary incontinence in women: A 10-year (2004–2013) scoping review of the literature. *Urological Nursing, 35,* 179–186, 203. DOI:10.7257/1053-816X.2015.35.4.179

Nambiar, A. K., Bosch, R., Cruz, F., et al. (2018). EUA guidelines on assessment and nonsurgical management of urinary incontinence. *European Urology, 73,* 596–609. doi:https://doi.org/10.1016/j.eururo.2017.12.031

National Institutes of Diabetes and Digestive and Kidney Diseases (NIDDKD). (2021c July, reviewed). *Treatments for bladder control problems (urinary incontinence).* https://www.niddk.nih.gov/health-information/urologic-diseases/bladder-control-problems/treatment

Pan, L.-H., Lin, M.-H., Pang, S.-T., et al. (2019, May). Improvement of urinary incontinence, life impact, and depression and anxiety with modified pelvic floor muscle training after radical prostatectomy. *Journal of Men's Health,* 1-10. https://doi.org/10.1177/1557988319851618

Pedriali, F. R., Gomese, C. S., Soares, L., et al. (2016, March 21). Is Pilates as effective as conventional pelvic floor muscle exercises in the conservative treatment of postprostatectomy urinary incontinence? A randomised controlled trial. *Neurology and Urodynamics, 35*(5). https://doi.org/10.1002/nau.22761

Roscow, A. S., & Borello-France, D. (2017). Treatment of male urinary incontinence postradical prostatectomy using physical therapy interventions. *Journal of Women's Health Physical Therapy, 40*(3), 129–138. doi: 10.1097/JWH.0000000000000064

Skobe, K. (n.d.). *The basics of specimen collection and handling of urine testing.* https://www.bd.com/en-ca/offerings/capabilities/specimen-collection/educational-services-and-materials/labnotes/labnotes-14-2-2004

Starr, J. A., Drobnis, E. Z., & Cornelius, C. (2016, March–April). Pelvic floor biofeedback via a smart T phone app for treatment of stress urinary incontinence. *Urological Nursing, 36*(2), 88–97.

Trowbridge, E. R., & Hoover, E. F. (2022, March). Evaluation and treatment of urinary incontinence in women. *Gastroenterology Clinics of North America, 51*(1), 157-175. https://doi.org/10.1016/j.gtc.2021.10.010

Van Kampen, M., De Weerdt, W., Van Poppel, H., et al. (2000). Effect of pelvic-floor reeducation on duration and degree of incontinence after radical prostatectomy: A randomised controlled trial. *Lancet, 355,* 98–102.

Vasavada, S. P. (2021, July 12). *Urinary incontinence.* http://emedicine.medscape.com/article/452289-overview

WebMD. (2022, January 27, reviewed). *Food and drink to tame an overactive bladder.* https://www.webmd.com/urinary-incontinence-oab/food-drink

Yu Ko, W. F., & Sawatzky, J. V. (2008). Understanding urinary incontinence after radical prostatectomy: A nursing framework. *Clinical Journal of Oncology Nursing, 12*(4), 647–654. http://dx.doi.org/10.1188/08.CJON.647-654

CLINICAL REASONING
Applying the Full-Spectrum Nursing Model

PATIENT SITUATION

An older woman, Mrs. Patel, has several health concerns, including diabetes and obesity. She seeks healthcare because she feels burning with urination, frequency, and urgency. You explain to her these are signs of a urinary tract infection (UTI). You discover while taking the nursing history that she also has urinary incontinence (UI). When asked about toileting habits, she tells you she often does not make it to the bathroom, even at home. This has been going on for about 3 years now. She has trouble getting up and walking upstairs to the bathroom because of a foot ulcer that is not healing well. Mrs. Patel's affect is flat, with little expression. During your time with her, she seems to have little interest in talking about her health concerns. When you ask her about what she does to get out or socialize, she is hesitant to go far because she is afraid of "accidents" and carrying an embarrassing odor.

THINKING

1. *Theoretical Knowledge (Recall of Facts and Principles):*

    a. What kind(s) of UI is this patient likely to have?

    b. What are this patient's risk factors for UI?

2. *Critical Thinking (Contextual Awareness):*

    a. What aspects of this situation have you experienced or observed previously in your role as a healthcare provider?

    b. How might those past experiences affect your perception in this situation?

DOING

3. *Practical Knowledge (Patient Teaching):*

    a. How could you encourage Mrs. Patel to seek healthcare for managing her UI?

    b. What might you ask your patient to do to get a better idea of her bladder history and toileting habits?

    c. By looking at Mrs. Patel's bladder diary, you see a pattern suggestive of UI. What other behavioral strategies might you suggest for improving her ability to have control of her bladder?

CARING

4. *Self-Knowledge:*

    a. Have you ever personally experienced urinary urgency, when you had trouble getting to the bathroom in time? Reflect on this experience and examine how you might feel if you were incontinent much of the time.

    b. In what way(s) can you show compassion for the patient who has UI?

Critical Thinking and Clinical Judgment

1. You receive a report from the UAP that a patient with no history of urinary elimination problems has had 150 mL of oral liquids in 6 hours and has voided 100 mL of clear, dark amber urine. His vital signs at the start of the shift were as follows: blood pressure 108/76 mm Hg; pulse 72 beats/min; respirations 18 breaths/min; and temperature 98.6°F (37.0°C). The most recent check revealed blood pressure 112/80 mm Hg; pulse 88 beats/min; respirations 22 breaths/min; and temperature 100.4°F (38.0°C).

   a. What conclusion might you draw about what has caused these symptoms?

   b. What actions should you take?

2. As you make patient rounds, you discover a collection bag for an indwelling catheter placed on the bed above the level of the patient's bladder.

   a. What should you do first? What assessments should you make?

   b. What teaching would be important in this situation?

3. The UAPs complain that Mr. Jones, a patient with dementia, keeps urinating in his trashcan and in the hallway.

   a. What special measures could be taken to assist Mr. Jones in finding the bathroom?

   b. What data could be helpful in developing a plan for Mr. Jones?

4. For each of the following concepts, use critical thinking to describe how or why it is important to nursing, patient care, or urinary elimination. Note that these are *not* to be merely definitions.

   Blood pressure   Hydration

   Kidney tubules   Specific gravity

   Developmental stage   Urinary incontinence

   Privacy

What Are the Main Points in This Chapter?

- The urinary system consists of two kidneys, two ureters, the urinary bladder, and the urethra.
- The kidneys filter nitrogen and other metabolic wastes, toxins, excess ions, and water from the bloodstream and excrete them as urine.
- The bladder has a normal average storage capacity of 500 mL (1 pint), but it may distend, when needed, to a capacity twice that amount.
- Voiding occurs when contraction of the detrusor muscle pushes stored urine through the relaxed internal urethral sphincter into the urethra.
- The kidneys produce urine at a rate of approximately 60 mL per hour, or 1500 mL per day. Most people urinate about five or six times per day.
- Voiding and control of urination require normal functioning of the bladder and the urethra, as well as an intact brain, spinal cord, and nerves supplying the bladder and the urethra.
- As adults age, the number of functional nephrons gradually decreases, along with the ability to dilute and concentrate urine. The potential volume of the bladder also decreases as the bladder wall loses elasticity; thus, older adults need to urinate more frequently.
- Substances that contain caffeine act as diuretics and increase urine production.
- A diet high in salt causes water retention and decreases urine production.
- Medications with anticholinergic effects inhibit the free flow of urine and may contribute to urinary retention.
- An adequately hydrated adult produces clear yellow urine. Concentrated urine is darker in color, but dilute urine can appear colorless.
- A clean-catch urine specimen is preferred for many diagnostic tests. To collect this specimen, the client must cleanse the genitalia before voiding and collect the sample in midstream.
- Sterile urine specimens may be obtained by inserting a catheter into the bladder or withdrawing a sample from an indwelling catheter.
- A 24-hour urine collection requires collection of all urine voided in that period. The start time of the 24-hour collection begins when the first voided urine is discarded.
- A routine urinalysis is one of the most commonly prescribed laboratory tests. It is used as an overall screening test as well as an aid to diagnose renal, hepatic, and other diseases.
- Normal urine is free of bacteria, viruses, and fungi. Urinary tract infections are often caused by the introduction of *Escherichia coli,* which normally live in the colon, into the urethra and bladder.
- Urinary retention is an inability to empty the bladder. It may occur because of obstruction, neurological problems, infection, surgery, medications, or anxiety.
- Urinary catheterization is the introduction of a pliable tube (catheter) into the bladder to allow drainage of urine.
- Urinary incontinence (UI) is a lack of voluntary control over urination. Nurses can independently perform the primary interventions to manage UI.
- A urinary diversion is required when the bladder must be removed or bypassed. There are three options: a conventional urostomy or ileal conduit, a continent urinary reservoir, or a neobladder.
- A patient with a urinary diversion requires physical and psychological care. The goal is to have the patient become comfortable with their changed body and assume self-care.

Knowledge Map

STRUCTURES:
- Kidneys – filter; regulate
- Nephrons – urine formation
- Ureters – urine transport
- Bladder – urine storage
- Urethra – urine transport
- Sphincters – flow control

URINATION

FACTORS AFFECTING:
- Developmental stage: infants, elders
- Personal; sociocultural; environmental
  - time; privacy; loss of dignity
- Nutrition; hydration
- Activity
- Medications
- Surgery/anesthesia

PATHOLOGICAL CONDITIONS AFFECTING URINATION:
- UTI
- Calculi
- BPH
- Cardiovascular & metabolic diseases
- Neurogenic bladder
- Impairments: mobility, communication, cognition

ASSESSING URINE:
- Intake and output
- Urine studies
  - analysis
  - specific gravity
  - dipstick
- Specimens from:
  - fresh-voided
  - clean-catch
  - sterile specimen
  - 24-hour collection

PROMOTING NORMAL URINATION:
- Provide privacy
- Position properly
- Establish toileting routines
- Provide adequate fluids/nutrition
- Assist with voiding

URINARY CATHETERIZATION
- Straight catheter
- Indwelling catheter
- Suprapubic catheter

- Skin care
- Lifestyle changes
- Bladder training
- Scheduled voiding
- Kegels
- Biofeedback
- Anti-incontinent devices

COMMON URINARY PROBLEMS:
- Urinary tract infections
  - urethritis; cystitis; pyelonephritis
- Urinary retention
- Urinary incontinence:
  - urge
  - stress
  - overflow
  - functional
  - transient
  - reflex
  - enuresis
- Urinary diversions
  - cutaneous ureterostomy
  - ileal conduit
  - Kock pouch (continent urostomy)

CHAPTER 26

Bowel Elimination

STUDENT RESOURCES

The questions and exercises in this book allow you to practice the kind of thinking you will use as a full-spectrum nurse. Critical-thinking questions usually have more than one right answer, so we do not provide "correct" answers for these features. Try to answer these questions yourself. It is more important to develop your nursing judgment than to just cover content. You will learn more by discussing the questions with your peers. If you are still unsure, see the Davis Advantage chapter resources for suggested responses.

To explore learning resources for this chapter,

Go to www.DavisAdvantage.com and find:

Answers and Suggested Responses for all questions in this chapter
Concept Map
Knowledge Map
References and Bibliography

Key Concepts

Bowel elimination
Motility

Related Concepts

See the Concept Map on Davis Advantage.

Example Problems

Bowel incontinence
Constipation and impaction
Diarrhea

Caring for the Williams Family

Nadine Williams arrives at the family health center for a scheduled appointment, accompanied by her granddaughter, Kayla Robinson. Recently, Nadine has been constipated and has had several episodes of bleeding with bowel movements (BMs). She has read that a change in bowel habits is a sign of colon cancer and is worried about that. She brought her granddaughter along because she is also having bowel problems. Kayla's bowel habits are erratic. At times she has a soft BM daily. However, she has also had bouts of constipation and diarrhea. Nadine would like advice on her granddaughter's elimination status. As a critical thinker, you will begin by obtaining accurate, credible information.

A. What history questions would be appropriate to ask Nadine regarding her bowel concerns? What data do you need? How can you get the data? Are the data accurate? What information is important; what is not? Write some specific questions, just as you would ask them in an interview.

B. What physical assessments would you conduct for Nadine to add to, and possibly to validate, your subjective data?

C. Now you must consider the context. What factors must you consider when gathering a history on Kayla?

(Continued)

Caring for the Williams Family (continued)

D. The family nurse practitioner (FNP) examines Nadine and determines that she has external hemorrhoids that have been bleeding because of recent straining at stool. The FNP prescribes rectal suppositories to decrease the swelling of the hemorrhoids and asks you to teach Nadine about necessary lifestyle changes. What additional information will you need to gather to provide this teaching? Recall that you have already obtained a significant amount of information from the history questions. Again, think about context: Whatever the content of your teaching, Nadine will be using that information to care for herself and her granddaughter in her home.

E. The FNP examines Kayla and tells you that the examination is normal. Use your theoretical knowledge of bowel elimination and Kayla's developmental stage to think of possible reasons for her erratic bowel pattern.

Practical Knowledge
clinical application

To help you promote normal bowel elimination and support patients who have bowel elimination problems, this section applies concepts from Volume 1 to provide practical knowledge of procedures and clinical insights. You will also find assessment guidelines for assisting patients who are having diagnostic studies of the gastrointestinal system.

PROCEDURES

The procedures in this chapter will help you provide care to patients who have problems with bowel elimination.

Procedure 26-1 ■ Testing Stool for Occult Blood

➤ For steps to follow in *all* procedures, refer to the Universal Steps for All Procedures on the inside back cover.

Equipment
- Clean gloves
- Tongue blade or other wooden applicator
- Clean, dry collection container to place in the commode; or a clean, dry bedpan
- Facility-specific fecal occult blood test (FOBT) slide or test paper
- Developing solution

Delegation
You can delegate the collection and testing of a stool sample for occult blood to the unlicensed assistive personnel (UAP) if the UAP has the necessary skills and the patient's condition is stable. Inform the UAP of any special considerations (e.g., the need to assist the patient with ambulation or the need for a bedpan). Instruct the UAP to inform you if there is visible blood in the stool and to show you the FOBT slide for evaluation of results when the test is complete.

Preprocedure Assessment
- Assess the patient's mobility status.
  Determines the patient's ability to participate in stool collection, the need for a bedpan or commode, and so forth.
- Assess the patient's dietary history for the past 24 to 48 hours.
  Some foods, such as red meat, chicken, fish, horseradish, turnips, or raw vegetables, may lead to a false-positive reading. Vitamin C in excess of 250 mg per day can produce a false-negative result (MEDLINE Plus, 2020).
- Assess medication history.
  If the patient is taking medications, such as salicylates, NSAIDs, iron, oxidizing drugs (e.g., iodine salts, boric acid), reserpine, corticosteroids, anticoagulants, colchicine, and high doses of vitamin C, consult with a physician. These medications may cause a false-positive reading. If possible, they will be discontinued for 7 days before the test. If the patient must have them, then the results must be interpreted by taking them into consideration.

CHAPTER 26 Bowel Elimination   561

- Assess for the presence of hemorrhoids.
  Any source of blood may cause a false-positive result for intestinal bleeding.
- If the patient is female, ask whether she is menstruating.
- Check the expiration date on the developing solution for the FOBT test slide.
- Assess the patient's or family's understanding of the need for the stool test.
  Provides a baseline for health teaching.

➤ When performing the procedure, always identify your patient according to agency policy, using two identifiers, and be attentive to standard precautions, hand hygiene, patient safety and privacy, body mechanics, and documentation.

Procedure Steps

1. **Determine whether the test** will be done by the nurse at the point of care (e.g., in the home or at the bedside) or by laboratory personnel.
   Because of the regulatory and billing practices in some settings, this test may be completed by laboratory personnel.

2. **Gather the necessary testing supplies.** Be sure you understand the directions for the testing kit you are using.
   This procedure gives instructions for using the FOBT slide method.

3. **Ask the patient to void** before collecting the stool specimen.
   Helps prevent contaminating the stool with urine.

4. **Perform hand hygiene and don procedure gloves.**

5. **Place a clean, dry container** for the stool specimen into the toilet or bedside commode in such a manner that any urine falls into the toilet and the fecal specimen falls into the container. Obtain a clean, dry bedpan for a patient who is immobile.
   Using a sample of stool that comes in contact with either urine or water may produce an inaccurate test result.

6. **Instruct the patient to defecate** into the container, or place the patient on the bedpan. Do not contaminate the specimen with toilet tissue.

7. **Once the specimen has been obtained** and the bedpan removed or the patient assisted to bed as necessary, perform hand hygiene, and don clean procedure gloves.
   Prevents the spread of intestinal bacteria.

8. **Explain the purpose of the test.** Explain to the patient that serial specimens may be needed.
   Testing serial specimens decreases the chances of a false-negative finding.

9. **Open the specimen side** of the FOBT slide. With a tongue depressor or other applicator, collect a small sample of stool and spread it thinly onto one "window" of the FOBT slide.

10. **With a different applicator** or the opposite end of the tongue depressor, collect a second small sample of stool from a different location in the large sample. Spread the second sample thinly onto the second "window" of the slide.
    Reduces the possibility of a false-negative result. ▼

11. **Wrap the tongue depressor** in tissue and a paper towel; place it in a waste receptacle. Do not flush it.
    Prevents transfer of microorganisms. Flushing would likely clog the plumbing.

12. **Close the FOBT slide.**
    Prevents the transfer of microorganisms from the specimen smears on the slide.

13. **If the test is to be done by laboratory personnel,** transfer the specimen to a clean dry container, being careful not to contaminate the outside of the container with feces. Label the specimen in the presence of the patient according to agency policy, and place it into the proper receptacle for transportation to the laboratory.

14. **If you are to perform the test,** turn the slide over, and open the opposite side of the FOBT slide. Follow the directions on the package regarding the number of drops of the developing solution.
    Ensures an accurate reading. ▼

15. **Remove gloves and** perform hand hygiene.

(continued on next page)

Procedure 26-1 ■ Testing Stool for Occult Blood (continued)

Evaluation
- Observe the color of the paper inside the FOBT slide windows for 30 to 60 seconds.
- If the paper turns blue, consider the test for occult blood to be positive.

Patient Teaching
- Inform the patient of the reasons for performing the test.
- Explain the possible implications of a positive occult blood test, if one is obtained.

Home Care
- Determine the client's level of cognition and manual dexterity to assess ability to follow instructions and physically perform the test.
- Explain necessary dietary and medication restrictions (see the Preprocedure Assessment section of this procedure).
- Instruct the client to collect the specimen in a clean, dry container. If an appropriate container is not available, the client may use the toilet.
- If defecating in the toilet, the client should flush it immediately before obtaining the sample. If commercial toilet bowl cleaners are in use, remove them from the tank, and flush twice. Then lay rice paper (from the kit) directly on the water; it is okay to get it wet. When using the probe to take the stool sample, take the sample from any area of stool that is above the water line.
- Protect the slide from heat, light, and household chemicals.
- Home collection slides come in a kit, connected together as a set of three. Instruct the client not to tear them apart.
- Emphasize to the client that each sample should be from separate bowel movements on separate days.
- After all three specimens have been collected over the course of at least 3 days, store the slide in a paper envelope to air dry.
- The client must place the slides in the special mailing pouch that comes with the slides, if they are to be sent back to the laboratory. The slides should be returned to the care provider or laboratory no later than 14 days after the first sample was collected. For additional instructions,

▶ Go to the **Hemoccult Web site** at https://www.beckmancoulter.com/download/wsr-118305

Documentation
- Document the date and time of the specimen collection, both in the patient record and on the specimen container or FOBT kit.
- Note the appearance of the stool (e.g., color, odor) and the presence of blood, mucus, or other abnormal constituents.
- Note any rectal bleeding or discomfort during and after defecation.
- Document the test results on the appropriate agency form.
- Notify the appropriate care provider of the results.

Sample Documentation

06/14/xx   0915   Specimen taken from 2 separate sections of yellowish brown soft stool containing mucus. No rectal bleeding or discomfort with defecation. Specimen sent to laboratory; test results pending.   —S. Hoeszle, RN

Practice Resources
American Cancer Society (2019); Davidson et al. (2021); The Joint Commission Accreditation Program (2022); Lee et al. (2020); Siegel et al. (2007).

Procedure 26-2 ■ Placing and Removing a Bedpan

▶ For steps to follow in *all* procedures, refer to the Universal Steps for All Procedures on the inside back cover.

Equipment
- Bedpan
- Two pairs of clean gloves
- Toilet tissue
- Prepackaged disposable wipes
- Waterproof pad
- Bedpan cover
- Linen-saver pad

Delegation
You may delegate the placement and removal of a bedpan to the UAP after ensuring that the UAP has the necessary skills and that the patient's condition is stable. Complete the preprocedure assessments, and inform the UAP of any special considerations (e.g., medical or surgical conditions that will necessitate the use of a fracture pan, extra care with turning or required positioning based on medical condition).

Preprocedure Assessments
- Assess the patient's level of consciousness, ability to follow directions, mobility status, and physical status.
  Helps determine whether one or two persons are needed to complete the procedure
- Determine the patient's comfort level—note the presence of rectal or abdominal pain, hemorrhoids, or perianal irritation.
  Pain can cause difficulty with positioning and bearing down during defecation. Any unexplained pain should be evaluated by the primary care provider.

- Identify factors that will necessitate the use of a fracture pan. (Examples include a fractured pelvis; total hip replacement; lower back surgery; presence of casts, splints, or braces on lower limbs; or obesity.)
- Auscultate bowel sounds and palpate for distension if indicated.
  The colon, when full of fecal matter, is a rounded, firm mass. A smooth, round mass above the symphysis pubis is a distended bladder.
- Review the patient's chart to determine the need to obtain a stool specimen.
  Promotes efficiency by allowing you to obtain a specimen container before placing the patient on the bedpan.

Procedure 26-2A ■ Placing a Bedpan

➤ When performing the procedure, always identify your patient according to agency policy, using two identifiers, and be attentive to standard precautions, hand hygiene, patient safety and privacy, body mechanics, and documentation.

Procedure Steps

1. **Obtain the necessary supplies** and take them to the patient's room. Warm prepackaged disposable wipes and leave at the bedside for use during bedpan removal.
   The patient will need to wash hands after using the bedpan.

2. **If the bedpan is metal,** place it under warm, running water for a few seconds. Then dry it, making sure bedpan is not too hot.
   A warm bedpan allows the patient to be more comfortable and helps relax the anal sphincter. Most bedpans now are made of disposable plastic.

3. **Raise the siderail** on the opposite side from where you are working.
   Prevents patient from falling out of bed and gives the patient something to hold on to while moving around in bed.

4. **Raise the bed** to a comfortable working height.
   Allows you to use good body mechanics and prevents muscle strain.

5. **Prepare the patient** by folding down the covers to a point that will allow for placement of the bedpan, yet exposing only as much of the body as necessary.
   Privacy facilitates elimination by promoting relaxation.

6. **Perform hand hygiene** and don clean procedure gloves.
   Prevents the spread of microorganisms via contact with urine or feces.

7. **Observe for the presence of** dressings, drains, intravenous fluids, and traction; and be sure there is a linen-saver pad in place.
   These appliances may hinder the patient from assisting with the procedure and may create the need for assistance from another caregiver.

Procedure Variation: For the Patient Able to Move/Turn Independently in Bed

8. **Position the patient.**

Variation: Supine Position
   a. Lower the head of the bed, placing the patient in a supine position.
   b. Ask the patient to lift their hips. The patient may need to raise their knees to a flexed position, place their feet flat on the bed, and push up. You can also assist the patient to raise their hips by sliding a hand under the small of the patient's back.

Variation: Semi-Fowler's Position
   c. Place the bed in a semi-Fowler's position.
   d. Ask the patient to raise their hips by pushing up on raised side rails or by using an overhead trapeze.

9. **Place the bedpan.**

Variation: Regular Bedpan
   a. Place the bedpan under the patient's buttocks so that the wide, rounded end is toward the back.
   Sliding the pan against the patient's skin may cause damage to skin.

Variation: Fracture Pan
   b. Place the wide, rounded end of the pan toward the front.

10. **Instruct or assist the patient** to lower their hips onto the bedpan. Move to Step 16.

Procedure Variation for the Patient Unable to Move/Turn Independently

11. **Ask for help** from another healthcare worker if the patient's condition warrants.

12. **With the patient in the supine position,** lower the head of the bed.

13. **Assist the patient to** the side-lying position. Use a turn sheet, if necessary.

14. **Place the bedpan.**

Variation: Regular Bedpan
   a. Place the bedpan under the patient's buttocks so that the wide, rounded end is toward the back. Do not push the pan under the patient's buttocks. ▼

(continued on next page)

Procedure 26-2 ■ Placing and Removing a Bedpan (continued)

Variation: Fracture Pan
b. Place the wide, rounded end toward the front. ▼

15. **Holding the bedpan in place,** slowly roll the patient back and onto the bedpan.

16. **Replace the covers;** raise the head of the bed to a position of comfort for the patient. Place a rolled towel, blanket, or small pillow under the sacrum (lumbar curve of the back).

17. **Place the call device** and toilet tissue within the patient's reach. Return the bed to its lowest position if not already done, and raise the upper side rails.
Provides privacy, comfort, and safety.

18. **Remove your gloves** and perform hand hygiene.
Prevents the transmission of intestinal bacteria.

Procedure 26-2B ■ Removing a Bedpan

➤ When performing the procedure, always identify your patient according to agency policy, using two identifiers, and be attentive to standard precautions, hand hygiene, patient safety and privacy, body mechanics, and documentation.

Procedure Steps

1. **Don clean procedure gloves.** Open the warmed prepackaged disposable wipes and place them near the work area.

2. **If the patient is immobile,** lower the head of the patient's bed. Pull down the covers only as far as needed to remove the bedpan.
Lowering the head of the bed is necessary only if the patient is immobile.

3. **Offer the patient toilet paper.** Assist patients who are unable to complete this task independently.

4. **Ask the mobile patient to raise their hips.** Stabilize and remove the bedpan. If the patient is unable to raise their hips, stabilize the bedpan and assist them to the side-lying position.
Stabilizing the bedpan prevents spillage of contents.

5. **Cleanse the buttocks** with a warm, prepackaged disposable wipe. Allow to air dry.
Provides comfort and hygiene and decreases the risk of skin irritation and breakdown.

6. **Replace covers and position** the patient for comfort. Offer the patient the second wipe to cleanse their hands.
Encourages independence with personal hygiene and decreases transmission of bacteria.

7. **Empty the bedpan** into the patient's toilet. Measure the output if that is part of the treatment plan. Clean the bedpan, following facility-specific guidelines.
If there is no toilet in the patient's room, cover the bedpan and carry it to the nearest toilet or soiled utility room for emptying.

8. **Remove the soiled gloves** and perform hand hygiene.
Prevents transmission of infectious microorganisms.

? What if . . .

■ **My patient is an older adult?**

Offer a bedpan at set intervals, perhaps in conjunction with a turning schedule. For elderly clients with limited mobility, you may wish to keep the bedpan readily available.
To minimize episodes of incontinence and/or falls. Trying to get out of bed to use the toilet is a common cause of falls.

Evaluation

- Assess the amount and characteristics of any urine and/or stool.
- Observe the skin on the perineum and buttocks for redness and breakdown.

Home Care

Teach the patient's family the steps of this procedure.

Documentation

- Document the amount of urine voided if intake and output are being recorded.
- Note the presence of any unusual characteristics of either stool or urine, and include in the nursing notes. If there are no unusual characteristics, document the passage of stool or urine in the graphic records.

Practice Resources

Ayello et al. (2020); Balas et al. (2020); Gray-Micelli et al. (2020); Siegel, et al. (2007).

Thinking About the Procedure

The video **Placing a Bedpan and Removing a Bedpan,** along with questions and suggested responses, is available on the **Davis's** *Nursing Skills Videos* Web site at www.fadavis.com.

Procedure 26-3 ■ Administering an Enema

> For steps to follow in *all* procedures, refer to the Universal Steps for All Procedures on the inside back cover.

Equipment

- Enema administration container, correct enema solution, or prepackaged enema—depends on the type of enema ordered.
  - *Enema kit:* This may be a grouping of supplies that includes a small plastic bucket or a 1-liter plastic bag with attached tubing, disposable toweling, lubricant, and castile soap.
  - *Prepackaged enema solution:* If a prepackaged enema (e.g., Fleet) is ordered, you may need to obtain the preparation from the pharmacy or central supply department.
- Prepackaged disposable wipes and/or toilet tissue
- Bath blanket
- Waterproof pad
- Bedpan with cover or bedside commode, if needed
- Water-soluble lubricant
- Clean procedure gloves
- IV pole

Delegation

You may delegate this procedure to the UAP if the UAP is trained and the patient is stable. Complete the preprocedure assessments, and instruct the UAP about conditions under which the procedure should be stopped (e.g., severe abdominal pain occurs, bleeding is seen, or the patient is unable to retain the solution). Instruct the UAP to report the results of the enema and show you any stool that appears to be abnormal (e.g., containing blood or pus).

Preprocedure Assessments

- Assess for history of bowel disorders (e.g., diverticulitis, ulcerative colitis, recent bowel surgery, abdominal pain, abdominal distention, hemorrhoids).
  Some disorders put the patient at risk for complications, such as mucosal irritation or perforation. Abdominal pain along with hypoactive bowel sounds and distention could indicate a bowel obstruction.

- Inspect the abdomen for the presence of distention.
  Establishes baseline for effectiveness of the enema.

- Review the patient's chart for the presence of increased intracranial pressure, glaucoma, or recent rectal or prostate surgery.
  An enema may cause the patient to strain, therefore increasing the pressure on the brain or surgical incisions.

- Review laboratory results, paying particular attention to blood urea nitrogen (BUN), creatinine, and electrolytes.
  Hypertonic and hypotonic enemas have been linked to fluid and electrolyte changes. Phosphate enemas (Fleet brand) have been associated with hyperphosphatemia and hypocalcemia.

- Note the date and time of the patient's last bowel movement, recent bowel movement pattern, and bowel sounds.
  Establishes baseline for evaluating bowel function.

- Assess the patient's cognitive level and mobility.
  Determines the patient's ability to follow instructions and the need for placing them on a bedpan for the enema.

- Assess the patient's rectal sphincter control.
  Will determine whether you need to administer the enema with the patient on the bedpan. Also influences the amount of solution to instill.

- Assess for fecal impaction.
  May necessitate obtaining a prescription for a different type of enema.

(continued on next page)

Procedure 26-3 ■ Administering an Enema (continued)

Procedure 26-3A ■ Administering a Cleansing Enema

> When performing the procedure, always identify your patient according to agency policy, using two identifiers, and be attentive to standard precautions, hand hygiene, patient safety and privacy, body mechanics, and documentation.

Procedure Steps

1. **Before administering** a prescribed enema, explain the purpose of the enema and what the patient can expect (e.g., the patient will probably have some cramping with a large-volume enema). Reassure the patient that you will be immediately available to help them to the restroom or bedpan.

2. **Place the bedpan nearby** or the commode near the bed.
   So you can reach the bedpan during the procedure, or so the patient can easily get to the commode.

3. **Open the enema supplies or kit.** Attach the tubing to the enema pail, if you are using a pail.
   The 1-liter enema bag comes with preconnected tubing.

4. **Close the clamp on the tubing** and fill the container with 500 to 1,000 mL of warm solution. The water temperature should be lukewarm—105°F to 110°F (40°C to 43°C).

   ✚ Check the temperature with a bath thermometer. Never warm the enema solution in a microwave oven.

   a. For infants, use 50 to 150 mL of solution.
   b. For toddlers, use 250 to 350 mL of solution.
   c. For school-age children, use 300 to 500 mL of solution.
   Cold solution causes intestinal cramping. Very hot solution can damage the intestinal mucosa. Use the correct amount of solution to decrease the necessity of repeating the procedure.

5. **Add castile soap** (or the soap solution used by your facility) to the fluid at this time if a soapsuds enema has been prescribed.
   Soap causes mucosal irritation, which stimulates peristalsis and defecation.

6. **Hang the container** on the IV pole. Holding the end of the tubing over a sink or waste can, open the clamp, and slowly allow the tubing to prime (fill) with solution. Reclamp the tubing when the tubing is filled.
   Expresses air from the tubing. Air introduced into the bowel may cause intestinal distention and discomfort.

7. **Don clean procedure gloves.**
   Prevents the transmission of intestinal bacteria.

8. **Position the patient:** Ask or assist the patient to turn to a left side-lying position with the right knee flexed.
   Allows the enema solution to fill the rectum and lower intestine following the natural flow of gravity.

   a. If the patient has shortness of breath associated with a respiratory condition, elevate the head of the bed very slightly. Avoid the semi-Fowler's position.
   The semi-Fowler's position increases the likelihood that gravity will cause the solution to leak out.

   b. ✚ Do not administer the enema with the patient on the toilet. The curved rectal tubing can scrape the rectal wall.

   c. If the patient has poor sphincter control, position on the bedpan in a comfortable dorsal recumbent position.
   Patient will not be able to retain all of the enema solution.

9. **Place the waterproof pad** under the patient's buttocks or hips.
   Prevents soiling of bed linens.

♥ iCare 10. **Cover the patient** with the bath blanket, exposing only the buttocks and rectum.
Promotes patient privacy.

11. **Depending on the patient's** mobility status, place the bedpan flat on the bed, directly beneath the rectum, up against the patient's buttocks.

12. **Lubricate the tip of the enema** tubing generously.
   Allows for ease of insertion, decreases patient discomfort, and helps prevent mucosal irritation.

13. **If necessary, lift the superior buttock** to expose the anus. Slowly and gently insert the tip of the tubing approximately 7 to 10 cm (3 to 4 in.) into the rectum. Have the patient take slow, deep breaths as you complete this step. If the tube does not pass with ease, do not force it. Allow a small amount of fluid to infuse and then try again, inserting the tube slowly.
   Helps the patient to relax, provides additional lubrication, and decreases reflex tightening of the anal sphincter. ▼

14. **Remove the container from the IV pole,** and hold it at the level of the patient's hips. Unclamp to begin instilling the solution.
    Lowering the container slows the force of the instillation, decreasing pressure, cramping, discomfort, and reflex expulsion of the solution.

15. **Slowly raise the level** of the container so that it is 30 to 45 cm (12 to 18 in.) above the level of the hips. Adjust the pole and rehang the container. Continue a slow, steady instillation of the enema solution.
    The height of the container determines the speed of the flow. A slow, steady rate of infusion decreases cramping and increases the patient's ability to retain the solution.

16. **Continuously monitor the patient** for pain or discomfort and ability to retain the solution. If the patient has difficulty with retaining the solution, lower the container, stop the flow for 15 to 30 seconds, and then resume the procedure.

    ✚ If the patient feels pain or you meet with resistance at any time during the procedure, stop and consult with the primary care provider.

17. **When the correct amount** of solution has been instilled, clamp the tubing, and slowly remove it from the rectum. If there is stool on the tubing, wrap the end of the tubing in a disposable wipe or toilet tissue until it can be rinsed or disposed of.
    Prevents transmission of pathogens.

18. **Clean the rectal area,** cover the patient, and instruct the patient to hold the enema solution for approximately 5 to 15 minutes. Be certain the call device is within reach.
    - Retention of the enema solution will distend the bowel and increase the stimulus to defecate.
    - Leaving the solution in the bowel too long may result in fluid and electrolyte complications.
    - Retaining hypertonic solutions may result in dehydration related to large amounts of fluids moving from the capillary bed into the bowel. Excessive retention of hypotonic solutions may cause fluid overload.

19. **Dispose of the enema supplies** or, if they are reusable, clean and store them in an appropriate location in the patient's room.
    Maintains a pleasant environment and helps prevent transfer of pathogens.

20. **Remove your gloves and perform hand hygiene.**
    Prevents transmission of intestinal pathogens.

21. **Depending on the patient's mobility,** assist them onto the bedpan, to the bedside commode, or to the toilet when they feel the need to defecate. Perform hand hygiene and use clean procedure gloves as necessary.

22. **After the patient has defecated,** remove the bedpan or assist the patient to bed; inspect the stool for color, consistency, and quantity.

Procedure 26-3B ■ Administering a Prepackaged Enema

> When performing the procedure, always identify your patient according to agency policy, using two identifiers, and be attentive to standard precautions, hand hygiene, patient safety and privacy, body mechanics, and documentation.

Procedure Steps

1. **Open the prepackaged enema.** Remove the plastic cap from the container. Clip the tip of the container if it does not have a hole in it. The tip of the enema container comes prelubricated. However, you may need to add extra lubricant.
   Extra lubricant increases comfort and eases insertion of the tube into the rectum.

2. **Follow Steps 7 through 13 of Procedure 26-3A** (regarding gloving, positioning, draping, and inserting the enema tip).

3. **Tilt the container slightly** and slowly roll and squeeze the container until all of the solution is instilled.
   Ensures that the container empties completely and that an adequate amount of solution is instilled. ▼

4. **Withdraw the container tip** from the rectum. Wipe the area with a disposable wipe or toilet tissue.
   Prevents transmission of pathogens.

5. **Cover the patient and instruct** them to hold the enema solution for approximately 5 to 10 minutes. Be certain the call light is within reach.
   Retention of the enema solution will distend the bowel and increase the stimulus to defecate. Retaining the solution for longer than the prescribed time has been associated with dehydration and electrolyte imbalances.

6. **Dispose of the empty container.**
   Maintains a pleasant environment.

7. **Follow Steps 19 through 22 of Procedure 26-3A** (regarding equipment disposal, assisting the patient, and observations of stool).

(continued on next page)

Procedure 26-3 ■ Administering an Enema (continued)

Procedure 26-3C ■ Administering an Oil-Retention Enema

▶ When performing the procedure, always identify your patient according to agency policy, using two identifiers, and be attentive to standard precautions, hand hygiene, patient safety and privacy, body mechanics, and documentation.

▶ Note: An oil-retention enema may be administered to help a client pass hard stool. It also may be administered before digital removal of stool, or it may be given at least 1 hour before a cleansing enema. See Procedure 26-4 for digital removal of stool.

Procedure Steps

1. **Obtain a commercial** oil-retention enema kit; these kits include a small rectal tube. If a commercial kit is not available, use a small tube and about 90 to 120 mL of the prescribed solution.
   A small tube allows for slower infusion, which minimizes cramping and thereby promotes retention.

2. **Warm the oil** to body temperature by running warm tap water over the container. Test a drop on your arm.
   If the oil is too cold, it will cause cramping and expulsion of the oil. If it is too warm, it may injure the patient.

3. **Follow Steps 7 through 13 of Procedure 26-3A** (regarding gloving, positioning, draping, and inserting the enema tip).

4. **Instill the oil into the rectum.**
   Softens stool and lubricates the rectum for easier passage of stool.

5. **Withdraw the container tip** from the rectum. Wipe the area with a disposable wipe or toilet tissue.

6. **Cover the patient and instruct** the patient to retain the oil for at least 30 minutes.

7. **Follow Steps 19 through 22 of Procedure 26-3A** (regarding equipment disposal, assisting the patient, and observations of stool).

Procedure 26-3D ■ Administering a Return-Flow Enema

▶ When performing the procedure, always identify your patient according to agency policy, using two identifiers, and be attentive to standard precautions, hand hygiene, patient safety and privacy, body mechanics, and documentation.

▶ Note: A return-flow enema (Harris flush) may be ordered to help a patient expel flatus and relieve abdominal distention.

Procedure Steps

1. **Obtain a rectal tube and solution** container (e.g., bag or pail).

2. **Prepare 100 to 200 mL** (for adults) of tap water or saline. The temperature should be lukewarm: 105°F to 110°F (40°C to 43°C).

3. **Follow Steps 7 through 13 of Procedure 26-3A** (regarding gloving, positioning, draping, and inserting the enema tip).

4. **Instill all the solution** into the patient's rectum.

5. **Lower the tube and container** below the level of the rectum, and allow the solution to flow back into the container.

6. **Repeat this process several times,** or until the distention is relieved.

7. **Follow Steps 19 through 22 of Procedure 26-3A** (regarding equipment disposal, assisting the patient, and observations of stool).

? What if...

- The solution for a return-flow enema becomes thick with fecal matter?

  Discard it and begin again with new solution.

Evaluation

- Observe the amount, color, and consistency of the stool.
- Evaluate the patient's tolerance of the procedure (e.g., amount of cramping, discomfort).
- Determine whether the prescriber's orders require subsequent enema administration.
- Some bowel examinations require repeated enemas or enemas administered until the returns are "clear." For the latter, you will need to examine the return and determine whether stool particles are still present. "Clear" does not mean absence of color but rather absence of stool particles and transparency of the liquid.

Patient Teaching

- Teach the patient that dependence on enemas can disrupt the normal process that stimulates defecation.
- Teach dietary and lifestyle changes that promote regular elimination (e.g., increased fluid intake, high-fiber diet, increased exercise).

Home Care

- Show the patient the box for a prepackaged enema, and instruct them to purchase this type of enema at a local grocery or pharmacy.
- Assess the patient's ability to administer their own enema. If you determine that they will be unable to do so, encourage them to seek assistance and instruct the caregiver in the task.
- Teach the patient or caregiver proper handwashing. Encourage them to purchase nonsterile procedure gloves.
  Patients and caregivers may not be aware of the serious infections that can be caused by gram-negative intestinal bacteria.
- If the patient will be attempting to self-administer a cleansing enema, help them determine how and where to hang the container so that it is at the proper height.
- If a soapsuds enema is to be administered in the home setting, teach the patient which household soaps may be substituted for castile soap.
  Some soaps used in the home for cleaning purposes may be too harsh and irritating to the intestinal mucosa.

Documentation

- Document on the nursing notes type of enema given and, if applicable, the amount of the solution instilled; patient's tolerance of the procedure; and characteristics and amount of stool.
- If the prescription is to administer enemas until the returns are clear, document the color of the return solution and the amount of stool seen.
- For prepackaged enemas, some facilities require documentation on the medication administration record (MAR) of the time given and the nurse's initials.

Sample Documentation

06/04/xx   0825   Fleet enema administered (see MAR). Patient had no cramping; retained enema for 5 minutes. Passed moderate amount of solid, formed, brown stool with no mucus, but with streaks of bright red blood on the surface. ——————— R. Cline, RN

Thinking About the Procedure

The video **Administering a Cleansing Enema**, along with questions and suggested responses, is available on the **Davis's** *Nursing Skills Videos* Web site at www.fadavis.com.

Procedure 26-4 ■ Removing Stool Digitally

> For steps to follow in *all* procedures, refer to the Universal Steps for All Procedures on the inside back cover.

Equipment

- Two pairs of clean procedure gloves
- Water-soluble lubricant (containing lidocaine, if agency policy permits)
- Bedpan and cover
- Prepackaged disposable wipes (or moistened towelettes)
- Bath blanket
- Waterproof pad

Delegation

This procedure should not be delegated to a UAP. Ongoing assessment of the patient by the professional nurse is required when stool is manually removed from the rectum. The nurse must monitor the patient for complications, such as bleeding and vagal stimulation. Nursing judgment is necessary in determining the need to halt the procedure.

Preprocedure Assessments

- ✦ Assess the patient's baseline vital signs and history of heart disease. Be sure to monitor the patient's pulse before and during the procedure.
  Digital removal of stool can stimulate the vagus nerve, causing bradycardia. Patients who have a history of heart disease or dysrhythmia are at greater risk. You should check the physician order before administering.
- Assess the patient's white blood cell (WBC) count.
  If the patient has a compromised immune status, evidenced by a low WBC count, you should discuss this procedure with the primary care provider to evaluate the risks and benefits of the procedure.
- Assess the patient's cognitive level and mobility.
  Determines the patient's ability to follow directions and turn in bed.
- Determine the time of the patient's last bowel movement.
  The longer stool remains in the lower bowel, the more water can be absorbed and the more likely it is that hard stool may form in the rectum.
- Assess the patient for history of fecal impaction.
  Can be a recurrent problem for immobile, disabled, or institutionalized patients.
- Assess stool consistency.
  Patients who are immobilized may become incontinent of watery stool. They may be able to pass small sections of hard stool or small quantities of watery stool. The latter, which may be intermittent or continuous, is a symptom of high colon impaction.
- Ask whether the patient has pain on defecation.
  Pain can cause the patient to suppress defecation.
- Assess the patient's pattern of bowel movements, diet, exercise, mobility, and medications (e.g., iron supplements or opioid analgesics).
  Determine whether any of these factors contribute to the problem, and add this information to the nursing care plan to help prevent recurrence.

(continued on next page)

Procedure 26-4 ■ Removing Stool Digitally (continued)

- Assess bowel sounds and any abdominal distention.
  Peristalsis may be present without gastrointestinal patency. This creates abdominal distention, which can aggravate constipation.

Guidelines

- Prevention of fecal impaction is the best treatment, but if impaction has occurred, the stool must be removed. The procedure is both painful and embarrassing to your patient.
- An order from the healthcare practitioner may be necessary to perform digital disimpaction. Check your facility policy.
- Some practitioners may prescribe an oil-retention enema before the procedure to soften and moisten the stool, making removal easier.
- Many also advise that you follow digital removal of stool with either an oil-retention and/or a tap water enema to ensure evacuation of stool that may not have been reached by digital removal.
- Trim and file your fingernails if they extend past the end of your fingertips.
- **CAUTION:** Some resources suggest that this procedure should be done in small steps (no more than four finger insertions in one session), giving a series of suppositories between stool removal episodes. This is thought to prevent patient fatigue and pain, reduce the risk of injury to the rectal tissue, and minimize vagal stimulation.

> When performing the procedure, always identify your patient according to agency policy, using two identifiers, and be attentive to standard precautions, hand hygiene, patient safety and privacy, body mechanics, and documentation.

Procedure Steps

1. **Determine whether lubricant** containing lidocaine is to be used, and obtain the correct lubricant.
   May decrease rectal discomfort for the patient.

2. **Cover the patient** with the bath blanket. Assist the patient to turn on the left side, with right knee flexed toward the head. Place the waterproof pad halfway beneath the left hip.
   Provides privacy and exposes the anus for visualization. The pad protects the bed from being soiled.

3. **Don clean procedure gloves.** Some sources recommend double-gloving.
   Prevents the transmission of intestinal bacteria.

4. **Expose the buttocks.** Place a clean, dry bedpan on the waterproof pad next to the buttocks in line with the rectum.

5. **Open the packet of prepackaged disposable** wipes, or have toilet tissue ready to cleanse the rectal area when you complete the procedure.

6. **Generously lubricate either** the gloved forefinger and/or middle finger on your dominant hand.

   Helps prevent discomfort, pain, and mucosal injury.

7. **Slowly slide one lubricated** finger into the rectum. Observe for perianal irritation.
   The patient may need skin care to reduce pain during additional bowel evacuation. ▼

8. **Gently rotate your finger** around the mass and/or into the mass.
   Assists in determining the amount and texture of the fecal bulk.

9. **Begin to break the stool** into smaller pieces. At this point, you may insert a second finger and gently "slice" apart the stool, using a scissoring motion. Remove pieces of stool via the rectum as they become separated, and place them in the bedpan. ▶

10. **As you proceed, instruct** the patient to take slow, deep breaths.
    Helps the patient to relax the anal sphincter.

11. **Continue to manipulate** and remove pieces of stool, allowing the patient to rest at intervals. Reapply lubricant (containing lidocaine, if permitted) each time you reinsert your fingers.
    Rest periods allow for assessment of and attention to the patient's comfort level and tolerance for the procedure.

12. **Assess the patient's heart rate** at regular intervals.
    Bradycardia is a sign of vagal stimulation. Stop the procedure if the patient's heart rate falls or the rhythm changes from your initial assessment.

13. **When removal of stool** is complete, cover the bedpan and set it aside. Use a prepackaged disposable wipe and/or toilet tissue to cleanse the rectal area.
Provides personal hygiene and decreases transmission of pathogens.

14. **Assist the patient to return** to a position of comfort. Note the color, amount, and consistency of the stool, and dispose of it properly.

15. **Remove your gloves and** perform hand hygiene.
Prevents transmission of intestinal pathogens.

? What if...

- **The patient is an infant?**
When treating infants with fecal impactions, avoid enemas and mineral oils. Glycerin suppositories may be used to soften the stool before removal.

Evaluation

- Determine whether evacuation of the retained stool was complete. Perform a rectal examination to assess for presence of stool.
- Reassess vital signs and compare the results to the initial assessment. Continue to monitor for 1 hour for bradycardia.
- Assess bowel sounds.
- Palpate the abdomen for tenderness and firmness.
- Ask the patient whether they feel relief from rectal pressure or abdominal discomfort.

Patient Teaching

Retained stool is most often the result of poor dietary habits, lack of fluid intake, lack of exercise, inattentiveness to the urge to defecate, and laxative abuse. Focus patient teaching on lifestyle changes that will facilitate a regular bowel elimination pattern.

Home Care

Home care should focus on preventing constipation that would require the digital removal of stool. Teach clients about high-fiber foods, adequate water intake, and the importance of exercise. Digital removal of stool may be necessary for some clients as part of a bowel-training program, (e.g., patients who are paraplegic or quadriplegic). You can teach this procedure to the caregiver in the home.

Documentation

Document the following:
- Bowel movement on the graphic record
- Procedure and the patient's tolerance for the procedure in the nursing notes
- Patient's pulse rate on the vital signs record
- Any unusual characteristics of the stool (e.g., black or green color, blood, or mucus)

Sample Documentation

07/11/XX   1815   Impacted stool removed digitally. No perianal irritation noted. Removed moderate amount (approximately 6 oz [170g]) dry, hard, gray-colored stool. Pulse 78 before removal; 84 after. Encouraged 8 oz of fluid every hour. ——————————————— C. Bryan, RNC

Practice Resources

Daniali et al. (2020); Hayat et al. (2017); Nazarko (2017); Siegel et al. (2007).

Procedure 26-5 ■ Inserting a Rectal Tube

> For steps to follow in *all* procedures, refer to the Universal Steps for All Procedures on the inside back cover.

Equipment

- 22- to 34-French rectal tube for adults. Choose the size according to the size of the client. For children or petite adults, a smaller tube (12- to 18-Fr) may be required.
- Water-soluble lubricant
- Procedure gloves
- Toilet paper
- Skin care items (e.g., soap, skin cleanser, disposable wipes)
- Collecting device (waterproof pad, graduated cylinder partially filled with water, a urine collection bag nicked at the top to vent)
- Paper tape
- Stool specimen container if needed

Preprocedure Assessments

- Obtain baseline vital signs.
- Auscultate bowel sounds; percuss for tympany.
- Observe and palpate the degree of abdominal distention.
- Ask whether the patient is passing any flatus.
- Assess discomfort caused by flatulence.
- Assess the condition of perianal tissues.
- Assess the history of cardiac disease.
Insertion of a rectal tube can stimulate the vagus nerve, causing bradycardia.

(continued on next page)

Procedure 26-5 ■ Inserting a Rectal Tube (continued)

> When performing the procedure, always identify your patient according to agency policy, using two identifiers, and be attentive to standard precautions, hand hygiene, patient safety and privacy, body mechanics, and documentation.

Procedure Steps

1. **Wear procedure gloves.**
   Follows standard precautions.

2. **Ask the patient to lift their hips** or roll from side to side to place a waterproof pad.
   Protects against soiling of linens.

3. **Attach a collecting device** to the end of the rectal tube: Tape a plastic bag or urine collection bag around the distal end of the rectal tube and vent the upper side of the bag. Alternatively, use one of these variations:

   Alternatively, use one of these variations:
   - Insert the tube into the specimen container.
   - Place the end of the tube in a graduated container partially filled with water.
   Collects small pieces of stool expelled with flatus. Venting the plastic bag prevents overinflation and bursting the bag. An advantage of using water in the container is that gas generates bubbles, and you will be able to assess the effectiveness of the rectal tube based on the amount of bubbling in the container.

4. **Place patient in left side-lying** position. Cover for privacy.
   Allows the tube to follow the normal curve of the rectum and sigmoid colon when inserted.

5. **Lubricate the tip** of the rectal tube.
   Prevents trauma to the rectal mucosa.

6. **Separate the buttocks** and ask the patient to take a deep breath. Gently insert the tube into the rectum.
   Adults: 10 to 12.5 cm (4 to 5 in.)
   Children: 5 to 10 cm (2 to 4 in.).
   Deep breaths relax the anal sphincter and ease tube insertion.

7. **For adults, tape the tube** in place; for children, hold it manually.

8. **Leave the rectal tube in** place for 15 to 20 minutes. If distention persists, you may reinsert the tube every 2 to 3 hours.
   Leaving the tube in place for more than 20 minutes may cause pressure necrosis of the mucosa; prolonged stimulation of the anal sphincter may result in loss of the neuromuscular response.

9. **Assist the patient to move** about in bed to promote gas expulsion. A knee–chest position is ideal.
   Because gas is lighter than fluid or solid, the position promotes passage of flatus. Unfortunately, many patients cannot tolerate this position.

10. **Remove the tube,** wipe the patient's buttocks with tissue, and assist to clean the rectal area as needed.
    Prevents transmission of microorganisms from feces; promotes patient comfort and skin integrity.

11. **Dispose of used equipment,** or clean it if it is to be reused. Follow agency procedures for cleaning.

Evaluation
- Evaluate the patient's response to the procedure (e.g., vital signs, fatigue).
- Assess abdominal distention and abdominal comfort.

Patient Teaching
- Teach the patient that chewing gum, sucking on hard candy, using a straw, smoking, and drinking carbonated beverages increase air swallowing and abdominal distention.
- Teach factors that promote normal elimination (e.g., exercise, increased fluid intake, adequate dietary fiber).

Documentation
Record the following:
- Date and time tube was inserted
- Size of tube and characteristics of feces collected
- Abdominal distention before and after the procedure
- Pulse and respiratory rates before and after the procedure
- Tolerance of procedure and any complications
- Patient and family teaching

Procedure 26-6 ■ Changing an Ostomy Appliance

▶ For steps to follow in *all* procedures, refer to the Universal Steps for All Procedures on the inside back cover.

▶ *Note:* Some pouches come with the wafer attached, some without. These instructions assume that the wafer is attached.

▶ *Note:* Also see Clinical Insight 26-2: Guidelines for Ostomy Care.

Equipment
- Ostomy pouch
  - One-piece pouch with the wafer attached, or a two-piece system with a separate wafer and pouch
  - Clamp for pouches with an opening at the bottom (a new clamp is not used each time; usually one clamp is packaged with each box of pouches)
- Skin care items per agency protocol or recommended by the enterostomal therapist (e.g., pH-balanced skin cleanser, skin prep, skin barrier wipe, adhesive remover, adhesive paste, and stoma paste if needed to fill and smooth skin surface)
- Stoma measuring guide (or precut template)
- Scissors
- Pen or pencil
- Two pairs of clean procedure gloves
- Prepackaged disposable wipes
- Toilet tissue
- 4 in. × 4 in. gauze pad
- Bedpan or container for **effluent** (fecal material)
- Plastic bag (for disposal of used pouch)
- Plastic bag for disposal of other contaminated articles
- Waterproof pad
- Ostomy deodorant
- Hypoallergenic paper tape (optional) or ostomy belt
- Bath blanket

Delegation
During the immediate postoperative period, the professional nurse must assess the newly created stoma and peristomal skin area and use clinical judgment when changing a pouch. You may delegate to a UAP if it is a preexisting, stable stoma and if you are sure the UAP is qualified to perform the task. If you do delegate this task, instruct the UAP to report any changes or unusual findings (e.g., changes in stoma color, swelling, peristomal redness, excoriation, deviations from expected amount) and color and consistency of drainage from the stoma.

Preprocedure Assessments
- Assess the type of stoma (e.g., ileostomy, colostomy, urostomy), number of stomas, and location on the abdomen (e.g., is the stoma near structures that will affect care?).
  Determines the type of pouch or system to use.

- Assess stoma color, shape, size, and/or length of protrusion or retraction; stoma construction (end, loop, double barrel); direction of stoma lumen; and discharge. Does the stoma lie flat or does it protrude?
  The stoma should be moist and red or pink. Alterations in stoma color (purple, black, or blue) may indicate poor circulation and possible necrosis and should be reported to the primary provider. Protruding or retracted stomas will need special adjustments in wafer measurement and placement. It is normal for a new stoma to have yellow or blood-tinged mucus or dried blood on it.

- Assess peristomal skin for redness, rash, irritation, or excoriation. Observe the existing skin barrier and pouch for leakage and length of time in place. You may have to remove the pouch to observe the stoma fully, depending on the type of pouch (i.e., if the pouch is opaque). Notify the provider or an ostomy specialist immediately if you note peristomal skin abnormalities.
  Preserving peristomal skin is critical because skin excoriation may cause an ineffective seal between the wafer and the skin and leakage of effluent. This in turn causes more skin and tissue damage. Leakage may indicate the need for a different type of pouch system or sealant.

- Determine the changing schedule for the pouch.
  Pouches are usually changed every 3 to 5 days, preferably before leakage occurs. Frequency also depends on the type of stoma, the equipment used (e.g., one- or two-piece pouch), the effluent, the patient's preference, and the climate (i.e., pouches are changed more frequently during the summer). To decrease skin irritation, avoid changing the entire system. In a one-piece or two-piece pouching system, change the skin barrier only every 3 to 7 days, never daily.

(continued on next page)

Procedure 26-6 ■ Changing an Ostomy Appliance (continued)

- Observe abdominal shape and incision, if present.
  Abdominal shape determines the proper placement of the pouch. Because of stomal and abdominal characteristics, some patients may need convexity in their ostomy pouching system to avoid leakage.
- Assess the patient's willingness to look at the stoma, touch the appliance, and discuss or participate in the task.
  May indicate a readiness or desire to learn.
- Assess the patient's condition and self-care ability. Consider vision, dexterity or mobility, and cognitive ability.
  Helps determine best type of appliance to use.
- Auscultate for bowel sounds.
  Determines the presence of peristalsis.
- Observe for effluent from the stoma, and document your findings.
  Change the skin barrier pouch at times of lower effluent output. Avoid changing after meals, when the gastrocolic reflux increases chance of fecal effluent output. Mucous secretion is normal.
- Assess whether a new clamp will be needed or the one on the pouch can be used again.
- Consult a peristomal nurse or the primary care provider to determine whether an ostomy should be irrigated.
  Many patients with left-end colostomies may be safely irrigated as a method of continence management. An ileostomy, however, drains liquid containing high concentrations of sodium, chloride, potassium, magnesium, and bicarbonate.

> ✚ Ileostomies should never be irrigated, except in cases of food blockage near the stomal outlet. Only a qualified person, such as an enterostomal therapy nurse, may perform a gentle lavage.

> ▶ When performing the procedure, always identify your patient according to agency policy, using two identifiers, and be attentive to standard precautions, hand hygiene, patient safety and privacy, body mechanics, and documentation.

Procedure Steps

1. **Perform hand hygiene** and don clean procedure gloves.
   Prevents transmission of pathogens.

2. **Fold down the bed covers** to expose the ostomy site. Place a clean towel across the patient's abdomen under the existing pouch.
   Helps prevent spilling effluent onto the patient.

3. **Position the patient** so that no skinfolds occur along the line of the stoma.
   Ensures an adequate seal between the wafer and the skin, preventing leakage.

4. **If the present ostomy pouch** is drainable, empty it into the bedpan.
   Pouches should be drained when they are one-third to one-half full because the weight of the contents may dislodge the skin seal; ostomy drainage is irritating to the skin. The pouch also collects flatus, which needs to be expelled because it can disrupt the skin seal.

   a. To calculate the amount of output in milliliters for an ostomy with a liquid effluent (e.g., ileostomy or urostomy), use a graduated measuring container.

   b. For pouches that you open by unrolling them at the bottom, you must remove a clamp to empty the pouch. Save this clamp for reuse.

   Note: Some pouches cannot be drained.

5. **Remove the appliance** by applying a silicone-based (hexamethyldisiloxane) adhesive remover with one hand as you press the skin away from the wafer barrier with your other hand. Avoid pulling the appliance straight off. Begin at the top and work downward. ▼

   Silicone-based adhesive removers are preferred over alcohol- or oil-based products. Pulling the appliance from the skin tends to strip the loosely bound epidermal skin layers, making the skin more susceptible to moisture loss and irritation from effluent. Silicone-based products reduce the bind strength, whereas alcohol dissolves the adhesives; alcohol may cause dryness and irritation. It also causes pain if the skin is not intact. If you use an oil-based solvent, the new pouch will not adhere to the oily skin.

6. **Place the old pouch and wafer** in the plastic bag for disposal. If the pouch is not a drainable one, dispose of it according to agency protocol.
   Prevents transmission of infections caused by fecal bacteria.

7. **Inspect the stoma** and peristomal skin area for redness, rash, irritation, or excoriation (see Preprocedure Assessments).

8. **Remove your gloves and** perform hand hygiene.
   Decreases the spread of intestinal bacteria.

9. **Don clean procedure gloves.**

10. **Cleanse the stoma** and surrounding skin using a skin cleansing agent with a pH of 5.5 that is designed to both cleanse and moisturize the skin.
    Removes old adhesive and any effluent that has leaked. Helps prevent skin irritation and/or breakdown and maintain skin moisture. Select cleansing agents that protect the stratum corneum lipids and proteins.

11. **Remove gloves and perform hand hygiene.**

12. **Measure the size of the stoma.** You can accomplish this in several ways.
    a. Place a standard stoma measuring guide over the stoma.
    b. Reuse a previously cut template.
    c. Measure the stoma from side to side (approximating the circumference).

    The stoma may need to be remeasured frequently during the initial postoperative period because the size of the stoma may change as edema subsides. ▼

13. **Place a clean 4 in. × 4 in. gauze pad** over the stoma.
    Gauze will absorb any leaking effluent, keeping the skin clean and dry during application of the new pouch.

14. **Trace the size of the opening** (obtained in Step 12) onto the paper on the back of the new wafer. Cut the opening. The opening in the wafer should be approximately 1/16 to 1/8 in. (1.5 to 3 mm) larger than the circumference of the stoma. Hold the wafer between the palms of your hands to warm the adhesive ring.
    Allows for skin movement with activity and prevents impaired circulation to the stoma. Warming the adhesive ring enhances the integrity of the seal by making the ring more sticky so that it will bond better with the skin.

15. **Don clean procedure gloves.**

16. **Apply ostomy skin care products** at this time using your clinical judgment, hospital protocol, or the recommendations of the enterostomal therapist (e.g., wipe around stoma with skin prep, apply skin barrier powder or paste, or apply extra adhesive paste).
    These products prevent or treat excoriated skin and/or ensure a tight seal between the wafer and the skin.

17. **Remove the gauze** from the stoma. Center the wafer opening around the stoma, and gently press it down. Make sure the bag is pointed toward the patient's feet. Press your hand firmly against the newly applied wafer and hold for 30 to 60 seconds.

18. **Peel the paper off the wafer.** Center the wafer opening around the stoma and gently press it down. Make sure the bag is pointed toward the patient's feet. Press your hand firmly against the newly applied wafer and hold for 30 to 60 seconds.
    Heat from the hand activates the adhesive ring, making it adhere better, thus promoting optimal wear time. Some sources also suggest taping down the edges of the wafer.

19. **Remove your gloves** and perform hand hygiene.

20. **Return the patient** to a comfortable position.

21. **Dispose of the used ostomy** pouch following your facility's policy for biohazardous waste.

❓ What if...

- **My patient has a two-piece pouch?**

  After applying the wafer around the stoma with a good seal (Step 18), attach the bag following manufacturer's instructions.

- **My patient's ostomy uses an open-ended pouch?**

  After applying the wafer securely around the stoma, fold the end of the pouch over the clamp and close the clamp, listening for a click to ensure that it is secure.

- **When cleansing the stoma (Step 10), I notice that the stoma is bleeding?**

  Slight bleeding of the stoma is normal; report excessive bleeding to the primary care provider.

Evaluation

Make the following observations:
- Characteristics of stoma: color, size, presence of edema, and shape
- Presence of blisters, redness, or excoriation on peristomal skin
- Amount and characteristics of effluent: color, odor, consistency
- Whether the patient expressed a desire to participate in the task
- Whether the patient demonstrated nonverbal cues that they are ready to learn about the task (e.g., looking at the stoma)

Patient Teaching

Patient teaching is aimed at preparing the patient to complete this skill at home. The patient (or a caregiver) will need to be instructed on completing all the steps of the procedure.

Home Care

- Assess the patient's self-care ability and assist the client to establish a routine for changing the stoma wafer/pouch (see Clinical Insight 26-2). The client may need to stand in front of a mirror or sit to change the ostomy appliance if they are unable to view the stoma easily.

(continued on next page)

Procedure 26-6 ■ Changing an Ostomy Appliance (continued)

- Teach the client that slight bleeding is normal when the stoma is washed.
- The client should not use soaps and lotions containing oils. They decrease the adhesiveness of the wafer.
- The appliance and wafer cannot be flushed down the toilet.
- Teach the client to report to the primary care provider changes in the color or size of the stoma and/or the presence of peristomal irritation or skin breakdown.
- Provide information about ostomy supply vendors and community support groups, such as Ostomates (https://www.ostomy.org/support-group-finder/).

Documentation

Document the following:
- Your assessment of the stoma and peristomal skin area
- Patient's tolerance of the procedure
- Type of appliance used, including the manufacturer and part number
- Use of any special ostomy skin care products
- Amount of liquid effluent (on the intake and output [I&O] portion of the graphics record)
- Patient teaching and the degree to which the patient participated in the procedure

Sample EHR documentation

Practice Resources

Contrada (2019); John et al. (2019); Nagano et al. (2019); Siegel et al. (2007); Tielemans et al. (2019).

Thinking About the Procedure

The video **Changing an Ostomy Appliance,** along with questions and suggested responses, is available on the **Davis's *Nursing Skills Videos*** Web site at www.fadavis.com.

Procedure 26-7 ■ Irrigating a Colostomy

▶ For steps to follow in *all* procedures, refer to the Universal Steps for All Procedures on the inside back cover.

Equipment

- Irrigation equipment
  - One-piece system with a fluid container connected to tubing with cone or two-piece system with a container separate from tubing with cone
  - Irrigation sleeve (a sleeve without adhesive backing requires a belt to hold it in place)
  - Clamp for a sleeve with an opening at the top
  - Prescribed irrigating solution (usually 500 to 1,000 mL warm tap water, 40°C to 43°C [100°F to 105°F])
- IV pole or other equipment to hang the irrigation container
- Chair
- Water-soluble lubricant
- Silicone-based adhesive remover
- Skin cleansers and barriers as recommended by your agency
- Toilet tissue
- Prepackaged disposable wipes
- Waterproof pad
- Two pairs of clean procedure gloves
- Toilet facilities that include a flushable toilet and a hook or some other device to hold the irrigation container; or bedpan or bedside commode (for patients with impaired mobility)
- New ostomy appliance and skin barrier or stoma cap cover
- Ostomy deodorant (optional)
- Plastic bag for disposal of the used pouch

Delegation

The initial irrigation of a newly created colostomy requires nursing judgment and clinical decision making. Initially, this procedure should not be delegated to the UAP, although in some situations it may be delegated to an LPN, depending on agency policy.

Preprocedure Assessments

- Evaluate the defecation pattern (or absence) nature of stool, placement of stoma, abdominal distention, and nutrition pattern.
  Findings may indicate the need to irrigate to stimulate elimination function; consistency of stool varies along the length of the gastrointestinal (GI) tract.

- Identify the type of ostomy.
  Many patients with left-end colostomies may be safely irrigated as a method of continence management. However, do not irrigate an ileostomy.

- Assess the patient's usual bowel pattern.
  The purpose of irrigating a colostomy is to promote a regular pattern for bowel elimination.

- Assess for abdominal distention.
  Report distention to the primary care provider, because it may indicate excess gas or inflammation.

- Assess hydration.
  The colon may absorb some of the irrigation fluid if the patient is very dehydrated.

- Assess cognitive level and mobility.
  Determines the necessity for a bedpan or bedside commode. Also determines whether patient teaching will be effective.

- Assess the patient's ability to maintain a sitting position.

▶ When performing the procedure, always identify your patient according to agency policy, using two identifiers, and be attentive to standard precautions, hand hygiene, patient safety and privacy, body mechanics, and documentation.

Procedure Steps

1. **Place an IV pole near** the location of the procedure (e.g., in the bathroom, next to the bedside commode, or next to the bed).
   Allows you to work efficiently.

2. **Assist the patient to the bathroom** or commode, if possible. Ask the patient whether they prefer to sit directly on the toilet or on a chair in front of it. If the patient must remain in bed, elevate the head of the bed.
   Patients with impaired mobility can sit directly on or in front of the bedside commode, or they may remain in bed in the side-lying position.

3. **Prepare the irrigation container.**
   a. For two-piece systems, connect the tubing to the container. Clamp the tubing. Fill the container with 500 to 1,000 mL of warm tap water.

   ✚ Water that is too cold will cause cramping, nausea, and discomfort. Water that is too hot will damage the intestinal mucosa.

   Note: Some ostomy resources suggest that using 1,000 mL of water will promote a more effective irrigation of the entire colon and decrease the necessity to irrigate more than once a day.

4. **Hang the solution container** on the IV pole. Adjust the pole so that it reaches the height of the patient's shoulder (approximately 45 cm [18 in.] above the stoma).
   The height of the container regulates the force of the flow.

5. **Unclamp the tubing to prime it** and allow it to fill.
   Removes air from the tubing, preventing gas pains.

6. **Perform hand hygiene** and don clean procedure gloves.
   Prevents the transmission of pathogens.

7. **Remove the existing colostomy** appliance (if the patient is wearing one) following the steps in Procedure 26-6.
   Use of ostomy skin care preparations may be needed when you replace the pouch.

(continued on next page)

Procedure 26-7 ■ Irrigating a Colostomy (continued)

8. **Dispose of the used colostomy appliance** properly. Empty the contents into the bedpan or toilet, and discard the pouch in a moisture-proof (e.g., plastic) bag.
   Prevents transmission of intestinal bacteria.

9. **Assess the characteristics** of the stoma and the surrounding skin (see Clinical Insight 26-2).

10. **Apply the colostomy irrigation sleeve,** following the manufacturer's directions.
    - *If your patient is sitting on a toilet* or bedside commode, then the end of the sleeve should hang down past the patient's pubic area but not down into the water. Place a waterproof pad under the sleeve over the patient's thighs.
    - *If your patient is in bed,* place the end of the sleeve into the bedpan.
    Prevents leakage and spilling of irrigation fluid and effluent.

11. **Generously lubricate the cone** at the end of the irrigation tubing with water-soluble lubricant.
    Prevents irritation and damage to the stoma and intestinal lumen.

12. **Open the top of the irrigation** sleeve; insert the cone gently into the colostomy stoma, and hold it solidly in place.
    Gentle insertion prevents damage to the mucosa. ▼

13. **Open the clamp on the tubing,** and slowly begin the flow of water. The fluid should flow for about 10 to 15 minutes or as the patient can tolerate.
    Proceeding slowly allows the patient to adjust to the distention of the bowel.

14. **If the patient complains** of discomfort, stop the flow for 15 to 30 seconds, and ask the patient to take deep breaths.
    Allows the patient to rest and adjust to the pressure of solution. Cramping may indicate that the bowel is ready to empty, the water is too cold, the flow is too fast, or the tube contains air.

15. **When the correct amount** of solution has instilled, clamp the tubing, and remove the cone from the stoma.

16. **Wrap the end of the cone** in tissue or paper towel until you can clean or dispose of it properly.
    Prevents transmission of intestinal bacteria.

17. **Close the top of the irrigation** sleeve with a clamp.
    Prevents spillage of irrigation fluid and feces.

18. **Wait for evacuation to occur:**
    - *If the patient is sitting,* ask the patient to remain sitting until most of the irrigation fluid and bowel contents have evacuated. Alternatively, you can clamp the end of the sleeve and ask the patient to ambulate to stimulate complete evacuation of stool.
    - *If the patient is in bed,* massaging the abdomen may also help stimulate return.
    This should take about 30 minutes on average. You might wait for about an hour to be certain all the fecal material has been returned.

19. **When evacuation is complete,** open the top clamp, and rinse and remove the irrigation sleeve. Set it aside.
    The irrigation sleeve is reusable, but it should be rinsed promptly to make thorough cleansing easier in the following steps.

20. **Change gloves.**

21. **Cleanse the stoma** and peristomal skin area with a warm prepackaged disposable wipe. Prep the skin and apply a new colostomy appliance, if the patient is wearing one, following the steps in Procedure 26-6. Otherwise, cover the stoma with a small gauze bandage.

22. **Clean the irrigation sleeve** with mild soap and water. Allow it to dry. Place the irrigation supplies in the proper place (e.g., in a plastic container or plastic bag).
    The irrigation sleeve must be cleaned well to avoid odors and transmission of pathogens.

23. **Remove your gloves** and perform hand hygiene.
    Prevents healthcare-associated infections.

24. **Assist the patient back to** a position of comfort.

? What if...

- **My patient has a colostomy sleeve without an adhesive backing?**

  Place the belt around the patient's waist, and attach the ends to the pouch flange on either side.

Irrigation solution

Irrigation cone inserted into stoma

Evaluation

Observe the following:
- Characteristics of the stool: color, amount, consistency
- Signs of bleeding from stoma or bowel
- Presence or absence of abdominal distention
- Patient's tolerance of procedure (e.g., cramps, fatigue)
- Patient's ability to participate in the irrigation

Patient Teaching

- Explain to the patient the purpose for the procedure.
- Explain that using sufficient fluid will decrease the need for multiple irrigations during the day.
- Teach the steps of the irrigation procedure to prepare the patient to complete the task at home.
- Explain that it takes approximately 6 to 8 weeks to achieve bowel regulation with irrigations.

Home Care

- Help the client determine where this procedure will be completed in the home setting.
- Make sure the client has resources for purchasing the supplies for the irrigation. Provide resources and contact information.
- Help the client locate a place to hang the irrigation container. There may be a hook on the bathroom wall, for instance.
- If the irrigating solution does not flow well, the client should:
  Check the tubing for kinks.
  Change the position of the cone.
  Put the container at a slightly higher level.

- Explain and demonstrate how to care for the irrigation supplies (e.g., how to rinse and clean the sleeve and/or belt, if used).

Documentation

Document the following:
- Your assessment of the stoma and peristomal area
- The amount of irrigation solution used
- The date and time that you performed the irrigation
- Characteristics of the stool returned in the irrigation fluid
- Patient teaching

Sample Documentation

06/14/xx   0830 AM   Ostomy irrigated with 750 mL warm tap water. Small amount of loose, formed, flaky stool returned in the fluid, with some undigested food apparent. No blood; very small amount of mucus. Stoma pink, peristomal area without redness. Explained procedure steps to patient as it was performed. Patient stated he will do some of the steps tomorrow. —————————————— C. Hiam, RNC

Practice Resources

Bauer et al. (2016); Berti-Hearn et al. (2019a, 2019b); Cobb et al. (2015); Farahani et al. (2020); Siegel et al. (2007).

Thinking About the Procedure

The video **Irrigating a Colostomy,** along with questions and suggested responses, is available on the **Davis's Nursing Skills Videos** Web site at www.fadavis.com.

Procedure 26-8 ■ Placing Fecal Drainage Devices

➤ For steps to follow in *all* procedures, refer to the Universal Steps for All Procedures on the inside back cover.

Equipment

External Fecal Collection Device

- pH-balanced soap and water or recommended skin cleanser
- Skin protection wipes (e.g., peristomal wipes to protect skin and improve adherence)
- Self-adhesive fecal containment device
- Procedure gloves
- Linen-saver pad
- Scissors

Internal Fecal Collection System

- Fecal device kit: Contains soft silicone catheter tube assembly, a syringe, and a collection bag
- Water-soluble lubricant
- Approximately 100-mL container of tap water or saline (follow the manufacturer's directions for amount and type of solution)
- 500 mL of lukewarm irrigant (water or saline)
- 60-mL luer-tip syringe and a catheter tip syringe (if not contained in the kit)
- Protective skin care dressing (e.g., Stomahesive, DuoDerm)
- Tape
- Procedure gloves, mask, and goggles or face shield
- pH-balanced soap and water or recommended skin cleanser

(continued on next page)

Procedure 26-8 ■ Placing Fecal Drainage Devices (continued)

- Scissors
- Linen-saver pad

Delegation

Application of an external fecal collection system may be delegated to the UAP. Insertion of a internal fecal collection device is usually performed by a professional nurse but may be delegated to an LPN depending on agency policy.

Preprocedure Assessments

- Assess the patient's bowel patterns.
  Fecal diversion is indicated when the patient is incontinent of liquid or semiliquid stools (flowing).

- Assess for allergies to silicone. If the patient is sensitive or allergic to any of the materials in the device, it cannot be used.

- Inspect perirectal skin.
  External devices should not be used in patients with impaired skin integrity.

For Indwelling Devices

- Assess whether the patient has had a recent bowel movement (BM).
  Patients who have not had a BM for two or more days should be considered as having firm stool and will likely be given a bowel prep or enema before insertion of the indwelling device.

- Check for the presence of any indwelling anal or rectal device (e.g., thermometer for continuous temperature monitoring).
  The treatment plan may need to be changed. If suppositories or enemas are a part of the current treatment plan, collaborate with the prescriber, because these medication delivery mechanisms will need to be changed.

- ✚ Identify factors that increase your patient's risk for bleeding, including medications (anticoagulant and/or antiplatelet therapy) and laboratory results (PT, PTT, platelets).
  Patients with an increased risk of bleeding should be monitored carefully.

- ✚ Check the chart for contraindications to an indwelling fecal management system (e.g., proctitis, lacerations, rectal surgery in the past year, large or painful hemorrhoids).
  If your patient has a history of any of these problems, contact the primary care provider immediately. You may elect to use an external device, but an internal fecal catheter is contraindicated.

- ✚ Internal fecal catheters should not be used for children.

Procedure 26-8A ■ Applying an External Fecal Collection System

▶ When performing the procedure, always identify your patient according to agency policy, using two identifiers, and be attentive to standard precautions, hand hygiene, patient safety and privacy, body mechanics, and documentation.

Procedure Steps

1. **Recruit another nurse** or UAP to help you. Assist the patient to a side-lying position and drape to expose the buttocks.
   For successful application (without leakage) it is best to have one caregiver position the patient and a second person apply the device.

2. **Don procedure gloves.**
   Observes standard precautions.

3. **Cleanse the perineal area** and dry well. If perianal hair is present, trim it away.

4. **Wipe the area with** skin protectant wipes.
   To obtain a leak-proof seal, the device should be attached to clean, dry skin. The wipes protect the skin and improve adherence.

5. **Spread the buttocks apart** to expose the anus.

6. **Remove the backing from the adhesive** on the fecal bag, then apply it, being careful to place the opening in the bag over the anus and to avoid gaps and creases.
   Careful application helps to obtain a leak-proof seal.

7. **Release the buttocks.** Connect the fecal incontinence pouch to a drainage bag.

8. **Hang drainage bag below the patient.**
   To collect and promote gravity drainage of fecal material.

Procedure 26-8B ■ Inserting an Indwelling Fecal Drainage Device

▶ When performing the procedure, always identify your patient according to agency policy, using two identifiers, and be attentive to standard precautions, hand hygiene, patient safety and privacy, body mechanics, and documentation.

▶ *Note:* Because devices differ markedly, it is best to follow the manufacturer's instructions for placing the device. The following are generic instructions.

▶ *Note:* Also see Clinical Insight 26-1: Caring for a Patient With an Indwelling Fecal Drainage Device.

Procedure Steps

1. **Ensure that a primary care** provider has performed a digital rectal examination.
   To assess for contraindications and to check sphincter tone. When sphincter tone is compromised, the patient may not be able to retain the device.

2. **Don procedure gloves,** mask, and goggles or face shield.
   To protect from splatters when irrigating or disconnecting the device. Usually the devices are used for incontinence of loose, if not liquid, stool.

3. **Position the patient** in the left side-lying position.
   Allows access to the rectum.

4. **Remove any indwelling device.**
   The presence of a foreign body between the inflated balloon and rectum may damage rectal mucosa, and a seal cannot be maintained.

5. **Depending on the type** of device, verify proper inflation and deflation of the intraluminal balloon. Attach the syringe, inflate with the recommended amount of air, deflate, and remove the syringe.

6. **Again, depending on the device,** fill the retention cuff with 35 to 40 mL of water; disconnect syringe and check for leaks. After verifying function, slowly and completely aspirate all fluid from cuff and balloon and disconnect the syringe.

7. **Connect the indwelling tube** to the collection bag. Clamp and hang the bag lower than the level of the patient.

8. **Some systems have an** "introducer," which you must inflate with about 25 mL of air through a connector on the tube. Disconnect the syringe. ▼

9. **Insert your lubricated, gloved** index finger into the balloon cuff finger pocket (located above the position indicator line) and coat the balloon generously with lubricant.
   This allows for digital guidance during insertion.

10. **Gently insert the balloon end** of the catheter through the anal sphincter until the balloon is beyond the anus and well inside the rectal vault.
    This helps prevent accidental expulsion of the device.

11. **Inflate the retention cuff** with water or saline per the manufacturer's guidelines. Do not overfill. If the catheter will not accept the recommended amount of fluid, see the What If… section at the end of this procedure. ▶

12. **Remove the syringe** from the inflation port and put gentle traction on the catheter.
    To determine whether the balloon is securely in the rectum and appropriately positioned against the rectal floor.

13. **If you inflated an intraluminal** balloon or introducer in Step 8, you

(continued on next page)

Procedure 26-8 ■ Placing Fecal Drainage Devices (continued)

must now completely aspirate the air from it.

■ **Do not leave an air-inflated intraluminal balloon in an unattended patient.**

An inflated balloon can cause tissue necrosis after a period of time.

14. **If the device has anchoring** straps, apply protective skin care dressing and tape one strap to each of the patient's buttocks.
Prevents internal migration of the tube and occlusion by twisting of the tube.

15. **Position the tubing along** the patient's leg, avoiding kinks and obstruction, and position the collection bag lower than the patient.
Promotes flow of stool from the rectum to the collection bag.

? What if...

■ **When irrigating, the catheter will not accept the recommended amount of fluid?**

Deflate the balloon and reposition the catheter.
The catheter is probably not positioned correctly. Do not use more than the recommended amount of fluid, because it would result in excessive pressure on the rectal vault and may cause mucosal or sphincter damage.

■ **Rectal bleeding occurs with an internal fecal management device?**

Discontinue the device and notify the physician.
Bleeding may indicate pressure necrosis from the device.

Evaluation

- Confirm catheter/bowel lumen patency by irrigating the bowel according to manufacturer's instructions and physician's order. Regular irrigation is required to facilitate evacuation through most devices.
Stool needs to be of loose consistency to pass through the indwelling tube.
- Assess how well the patient tolerated the procedure.
- Note the color, consistency, and odor of stool.
- Monitor the amount of stool in the collection bag. Change the fecal pouch at least every 72 hours (per protocol) and whenever there is evidence of leakage.
- When the collection bag is approximately two-thirds full, change it.
- Monitor for abdominal distention and pain.
- Regularly assess that connections are secure and that the device is not leaking.
- In addition, for indwelling devices, monitor
  - Length of time the device is in place.
  Not intended for use longer than 26 days.
  - Rectal bleeding
  May indicate tissue necrosis, bowel perforation, or fistula formation; device must be removed.

Documentation

Document the following:
- Date, time, and type of collection device used
- Your assessment of the perineal skin
- Patient's tolerance of the procedure
- Characteristics and amount of stool in the collection bag (output)
- Patient/family teaching

Sample Documentation

09/15/xx   1435   After prepping skin, an external fecal collection device was applied. Patient tolerated procedure well. Rationale for device was explained. Pt and family verbalized they will report leaking, pain, or discomfort. Device is draining large amounts of brown liquid stool, with no visible mucus or blood. ———————— J. Smiley, RN

Practice Resources

Ayello et al. (2020); Robson et al. (2019) Siegel et al. (2007); Wound, Ostomy and Continence Nurses Society (2017).

Thinking About the Procedure

The video **Applying an External Fecal Collection System**, along with questions and suggested responses, is available on the **Davis's Nursing Skills Videos** Web site at www.fadavis.com.

CLINICAL INSIGHTS

Clinical Insight 26-1 ▸ Caring for a Patient With an Indwelling Fecal Drainage Device

With an indwelling fecal drainage device, a catheter is present in the rectum and connected to a drainage tube and collection bag.

Nursing Goal 1: Prevent injury to rectal sphincter and/or rectal mucosa.

- Do not add air or fluid to the balloon port of the catheter.
- Check the catheter frequently for kinks or obstructions.
- Monitor for signs of complications and notify the healthcare provider immediately if patient has rectal pain, rectal bleeding, abdominal distention, or abdominal pain.
- Monitor stool for change in consistency (solid or soft-formed stool cannot pass through the catheter and will cause an obstruction).
- How to discontinue the catheter:
  1. Attach a 60-mL syringe to the balloon inflation port and deflate the retention balloon by pulling back on the plunger.
  2. Grasp the catheter as close to the patient as possible and slowly slide it out of the anus.
  3. Dispose of the device according to agency policy for disposal of medical waste.

Nursing Goal 2: Maintain free flow of liquid stool.

- Monitor the patient for changes in stool consistency. If the stool is no longer liquid and flowing, the device must be discontinued.
- Make sure the tubing and bag remain below the level of the patient.
- Irrigate the tube as often as necessary to maintain patency:
  1. Fill a 60-mL syringe with room-temperature tap water.
  2. Attach it to the irrigation port of the catheter and flush by depressing the plunger.
  Be sure you are using the irrigation port, NOT the balloon inflation port.
  3. Be sure to subtract the irrigation fluid from the stool volume to maintain an accurate record of intake and output.
- Change the collection bag when it is three-fourths full.
  1. Remove the collection bag from the tubing. Snap the cap onto the used bag and dispose of according to agency policy for medical waste.
  2. Snap new collection bag securely onto the device.

Nursing Goal 3: Prevent transmission of pathogens to others.

- Follow the agency protocol for hand hygiene. Always wear clean procedure gloves when handling the fecal management device.
- Monitor stool cultures and implement isolation protocols as indicated. If a stool sample is ordered, you may obtain it from the collection bag:
  1. If the collection bag is more than 24 hours old, place a new collection bag before obtaining a sample.
  2. Cut the collection bag at the bottom and transfer stool to an appropriate container for transport to the laboratory.
  3. Apply a new collection bag to the connector at the end of the catheter.

Nursing Goal 4: Maintain perineal skin integrity or prevent wounds from being contaminated by stool.

- Monitor insertion site for leakage and signs of infection.
- If perineal wounds are present, keep clean and dry; notify the primary provider if signs of infection are present.
- Perform perineal care according to agency policy.

Clinical Insight 26-2 ▸ Guidelines for Ostomy Care

Assess stoma appearance.
- The stoma should be moist and red or pink.
- ⊕ Immediately report to the surgeon a stoma that is pale, dusky, or black in color; dry; or with sloughing tissues. These are signs of inadequate blood supply to, and possible necrosis of, the portion of intestine that has been externalized.
- Protruding or retracted stomas will need special adjustments in wafer measurement and placement. It is normal for a new stoma to have yellow or blood-tinged mucus or dried blood on it.

Preserve peristomal skin.
- Preserving peristomal skin is critical because skin excoriation may cause an ineffective seal between the wafer and the skin and leakage of effluent. This, in turn, causes more skin and tissue damage. Leakage may indicate the need for a different type of pouch system or sealant.
- Use recommended moisture-proof barrier creams and skin care products.

Plan for and change the pouch as scheduled.
- Change the skin barrier pouch at times of lower effluent.
- Avoid changing after meals, when the gastrocolic reflux increases chance of fecal effluent. Mucous secretion is normal.
- Pouches are usually changed every 3 to 5 days, preferably before leakage occurs. Frequency also depends on the type of stoma, the type of equipment used (e.g., one- or two-piece pouch), the effluent, the patient's preference, and the climate (e.g., pouches are changed more frequently during the summer).
- To decrease skin irritation, avoid changing the entire system. In a one-piece or two-piece pouching system, change the skin barrier only every 3 to 7 days, never daily.

Assess the patient's self-care ability.
- Patients with poor vision may need to use magnification mirrors and yellow-tinted sunglasses to help reduce glare and improve contrast when they perform stoma care.
- Patients with immobility or spinal cord injury may need equipment that has a longer pouch that the patient can empty independently when sitting.
- Impaired dexterity or vision may warrant the use of a one-piece system or precut pouch and skin barrier, whereas a two-piece system may be better for patients who need to keep the skin barrier in place for several days and change just the pouch.
- Patients who are blind can be taught to change their own equipment.

Determine whether the ostomy should be irrigated.
- Consult a peristomal nurse or the primary care provider to determine whether an ostomy should be irrigated.
- Many patients with left-end colostomies may be safely irrigated as a method of continence management. An ileostomy, however, drains liquid containing high concentrations of sodium, chloride, potassium, magnesium, and bicarbonate.
- ⊕ Ileostomies should never be irrigated, except in cases of food blockage near the stomal outlet. Only a qualified person, such as an enterostomal therapy nurse, may perform a gentle lavage. For lavage, normal saline is preferred because excessive lavage could lead to a serious fluid and electrolyte imbalance.

Promote psychological adaptation.
- Be available to discuss the patient's reaction to the stoma. Your attitude and willingness to discuss the patient's body changes will help your patient begin adapting.
- Show acceptance when working with the patient and the stoma.
- Provide adequate ventilation and odor control when assessing the stoma or ostomy appliance.
- Provide ample time to explain stoma care and use of ostomy appliances. For most patients, this is a lifelong task; therefore, patient teaching is essential.
- Teach the client about diet modifications.
- Encourage patients to return to their usual activities as much as possible.
- Encourage patients to discuss intimacy issues associated with the ostomy. Use the PLISSIT model (in Chapter 30) if necessary, and convey to them that sexual functioning is an appropriate topic to discuss. You may wish to use the United Ostomy Associations of America's *Intimacy After Ostomy Surgery Guide* (https://www.ostomy.org/wp-content/uploads/2018/03/Intimacy-After-Ostomy-Surgery-Guide.pdf), or give it to the patient.
- Refer the patient to the local ostomy association, if one is available. Most of the counselors are skillful because they also have ostomies. They can share practical information based on their own experience with similar challenges. To find the local chapter, consult your phone book, or

▶ Go to the **United Ostomy Associations of America** Web site at https://www.ostomy.org/

ASSESSMENT GUIDELINES AND TOOLS

Focused Assessment

Bowel Elimination

Nursing History

Ask questions such as the following:
1. **Normal bowel pattern**
   - How often do you have a bowel movement (BM)?
   - What time of day do you usually have a BM?
   - Do you follow any routines to help you have a BM?
2. **Appearance of stool**
   - How would you describe your stool?
   - What color is your stool?
   - How would you describe the texture of your stool—hard, soft, or watery?
   - What shape is the stool?
   - Have you noticed unusual odor with your stool?
3. **Changes in bowel habits or stool appearance**
   - Have you had any recent changes in your bowel pattern?
   - Have you noticed any changes in the appearance, texture, or odor of your stool?
4. **For clients with a bowel diversion,** also gather data on the client's usual care of the stoma, use of appliances, and adjustment to the ostomy.
5. **History of elimination problems**
   - What has been your experience with bowel elimination problems?
   - Have you had any problems with constipation, diarrhea, or severe bloating or gas?
   - Have you ever lost control of your bowels?
   - Have you ever had bowel surgery or diagnostic procedures of the digestive tract?
6. **Use of bowel elimination aids,** including diet, exercise, medications, and remedies
   - What aids, if any, do you use to help you have a BM?
   - What foods help you maintain your bowel pattern?
   - What foods do you avoid? What effect do these foods have on you?
   - What is your usual fluid intake over the course of a day?
   - What is your usual exercise pattern?
   - What medications are you taking? Have they had any effect on your bowel elimination pattern?
   - What is your current stress level? What effect does stress have on your bowel elimination pattern?

Physical Assessment

Examine the abdomen, rectum, and anus.
- Recall that in abdominal assessment, the order of the examination is inspection, auscultation, percussion, and palpation.
- Observe the size, shape, and contour of the abdomen.
- Percuss and palpate the abdomen for tenderness, presence of air or solid, and presence of masses.
- Inspect the anus for signs of hemorrhoids.
- Depending on the policies of your institution as well as your skill with assessment, you might also palpate the anus and rectum for the presence of stool or masses.
- When listening to bowel sounds, note the presence and timing of the sounds and the presence of any bruits. Note whether the sounds are normal, hyperactive, hypoactive, or absent. (If you need to review, see Focused Nursing History in Volume 1.)
- If, after listening for 3 to 5 minutes, you hear no bowel sounds, you should listen in several areas before describing them as absent.

For a complete discussion of physical examination of the abdomen, rectum, and anus,

> Go to Chapter 19, **Procedure 19-14: Assessing the Abdomen,** and **Procedure 19-19: Assessing the Anus and Rectum,** in Volume 2.

DIAGNOSTIC TESTING

Direct Visualization Studies of the Gastrointestinal Tract

- These studies are invasive procedures; ensure that the patient has signed an informed consent.
- All of the procedures require some degree of advance preparation, such as fasting. Check agency policy, as preparation may vary.
- Preparing the patient includes explaining what they will experience and feel during the procedure.
- When the patient is sedated (e.g., with midazolam or diazepam), a crash cart must be in the room during the procedure and the patient monitored with pulse oximetry.
- All of the procedures require teaching for aftercare.
- For all tests, explain that rectal bleeding is normal for a few days if polyps were removed or a biopsy was taken.

Esophagogastroduodenoscopy (EGD)

A *fiberoptic endoscope*, a long, flexible tube with a light and lens, is introduced through the mouth and advanced for visualization of the esophagus, stomach, and duodenum. The physician may also perform tissue biopsies or coagulate bleeding sites through the endoscope.

Preparation
- Instruct the patient to fast for 6 to 12 hours before the test (instructions usually are "NPO after midnight").
- Remove the patient's dentures and eyewear before the test.
- Because the tube is introduced through the mouth, patients often require sedation to limit gagging.

During the Test
- The patient will be sedated but awake.
- A local anesthetic will be sprayed into the patient's mouth and throat to lessen the gag reflex.

Posttest Care
- Check vital signs and gag reflex (per agency protocol).
- Keep the patient NPO until the gag reflex returns; then instruct the patient to eat lightly during the next 12 to 24 hours.
- Instruct the patient to resume normal activity, medications, and diet in 24 hours.
- Observe, and teach patient to observe, for potential complication: esophageal or bowel perforation—cyanosis, substernal or abdominal pain, vomiting blood, continuing difficulty swallowing, or black and tarry stools.
- Explain to the patient that they will have a sore throat and hoarseness for a few days. Suggest gargling with saltwater and using throat lozenges.
- Caution the patient to notify the physician immediately if they have severe pain, fever, difficulty breathing, or expectoration of blood.
- Inform the patient that belching, bloating, or flatulence is a result of introducing air into the intestine and will be temporary.

Sigmoidoscopy

A rigid metal scope or a flexible fiberoptic scope is used to visualize the anal canal, rectum, and sigmoid colon. The patient is usually not sedated. During the examination, the physician may perform a biopsy, remove polyps (small growths), or coagulate sources of bleeding in the area. This procedure is also used as screening for colon cancer.

Preparation
- A light meal before the test may be allowed. For flexible sigmoidoscopy, the patient may be asked to follow a clear liquid diet for a day before the examination.
- Administer two commercially prepared, small-volume enemas before the test.
- For a flexible sigmoidoscopy, a strong laxative solution may also be prescribed.
- Have the patient void before the procedure.

During the Test
- Drape the patient for modesty.
- The patient may feel pressure, cramping, or the urge to defecate; encourage slow, deep breathing through the mouth to help alleviate the feeling.

Posttest Care
- Observe for potential complication: bowel perforation (see discussion of EGD).
- The patient may resume normal activity.
- Explain that air was introduced into the intestines to distend them for better visibility and that this may cause gas pains or flatulence for a few hours.
- A small amount of blood in the first bowel movement is normal. Notify the physician of significant bleeding.

Fiberoptic Colonoscopy

Provides direct visualization of the rectum, colon, entire large intestine, and distal small bowel. A flexible scope is inserted through the rectum and advanced to the cecum. Colonoscopy is useful in detecting lower GI disease. It is also often used for cancer screening instead of a sigmoidoscopy, because colonoscopy provides greater visualization of the colon. This is the preferred test for clients with suspected problems above the level of the sigmoid colon.

Preparation
- The colon and rectum must be empty and clean so the physician can view the linings during the examination. Practitioners have different colon-cleansing routines to achieve this, such as the following:
  - Instruct the patient:
    Three days before the colonoscopy, eat only low-fiber foods.
    Two days before, continue eating only low-fiber foods.
    One day before, consume a clear liquid diet (nothing purple or red).

Direct Visualization Studies of the Gastrointestinal Tract—cont'd

> The evening before, drink a strong laxative drink (OTC or as prescribed) to clean out the colon for the procedure.

> Remain NPO after midnight the night before the examination.

> The patient will be sedated before the test, so they will need someone to drive them home.

During the Test

> Position the patient on their side with knees flexed. Drape for modesty.

> Monitor vital signs.

Posttest Care

> Monitor vital signs (per agency protocol).

> Observe for potential complication: bowel perforation (see discussion of EGD).

> Explain that air was introduced into the intestines to distend them for better visibility and that, as a result, the patient may have gas pains or flatulence for a few hours.

> Instruct the patient to resume a normal diet when they have recovered from sedation.

Source: American Cancer Society. (2022). Colorectal cancer. https://www.cancer.org/cancer/colon-rectal-cancer.html; Van Leeuwen, A., Poelhuis-Leth, D., & Bladh, M. (2019). *Davis's comprehensive handbook of laboratory and diagnostic tests with nursing implications* (7th ed.). Philadelphia: F.A. Davis.

Indirect Visualization Studies of the Gastrointestinal Tract

Abdominal Flat Plate

An anterior-to-posterior (AP) x-ray view of the abdomen is used to detect gallstones, fecal impaction, and distended bowel. This test requires no preparation and no special posttest care.

Barium Enema (BE)

Radiological examination of the rectum, colon, and distal small bowel. A rectal tube is inserted into the rectum or an existing ostomy. Barium (a contrast medium) is instilled. The patient must retain the barium through several position changes while air is instilled and radiographs are obtained. The test is especially useful for visualizing polyps, diverticula, and tumors. In addition, it may be used to reduce certain obstructions. As a rule, patients are not sedated.

Preparation

> The test is invasive, so a signed informed consent is necessary.

> Patient instructions: Low-residue diet for several days before the procedure; consume only clear liquids the evening before the procedure; NPO for 8 hours before the test; possibly avoid dairy products that day.

> Administer a laxative, suppository, or cleansing enema the day before the test and cleansing enemas on the morning of the procedure (check agency policy). Enema administration is discussed in this chapter. For complete instructions on inserting a suppository, see Chapter 26, Procedure 26-6, Inserting a Rectal Suppository.

Posttest Care

> The patient may have bloating and cramping after the test and will probably feel the need to empty their bowels as soon as the test is finished.

> Instruct the client to resume food, fluids, and medications withheld before the procedure.

> Instruct the client to take a mild laxative and increase fluid intake (four glasses) to aid in elimination of barium (unless contraindicated). Barium can cause constipation for a few days.

> Explain that stools will be white or light colored for 2 to 3 days; if patient is unable to eliminate barium, they should call the physician.

Ultrasonography (Ultrasound)

Detects tissue abnormalities such as masses, cysts, edema, or stones. An ultrasound probe, called a transducer, is moved over the skin surface of the abdomen. The probe emits a sound wave that abdominal tissue and organs reflect back based on their density. The sound waves may be transformed into images visible on a computer screen.

Computed Tomography (CT) Scan

Useful in diagnosis of many abdominal disorders. Examines body sections from various angles using a narrow x-ray beam and produces a three-dimensional picture of the area of the body being scanned. The patient needs to lie very still during the procedure. A CT scan may be enhanced by injecting contrast dye that allows for improved visualization of circulatory function.

Preparation
If contrast dye is to be used:

> Determine that the patient is not allergic to contrast medium, iodine, or shellfish.

> Check blood urea nitrogen and creatinine levels to ensure adequate kidney function.

(Continued)

Indirect Visualization Studies of the Gastrointestinal Tract—cont'd

- Patients taking metformin (Glucophage) should discontinue it on the day of the test and withhold it for 48 hours after to prevent lactic acidosis.
- Restrict food and fluids for 6 to 8 hours if contrast medium is to be given.
- Sometimes the patient is asked to drink about 450 mL of a dilute barium solution 1 hour before the CT scan to distinguish GI from other abdominal organs.

During the Test
- Explain that the patient may feel nausea or warmth or have a metallic taste or a transient headache after injection of contrast medium. Instruct the patient to take slow, deep breaths if this occurs.

Posttest Care
- Patient may resume normal diet, activity, and medication.
- Renal function should be assessed before metformin (Glucophage) is restarted.
- The patient should increase fluid intake to help eliminate contrast medium.
- Diarrhea may occur after ingestion of oral contrast medium.
- Observe for delayed allergic reactions (e.g., hives, headache, nausea, vomiting) if contrast medium was used.

Magnetic Resonance Imaging (MRI)
Produces cross-sectional images of the body. MRI uses a strong magnetic field and radio waves. This type of diagnostic test does not use ionizing radiation, so it is free of the hazards of x-rays. MRIs are very sensitive and may be used to detect edema, hemorrhage, blood flow, infarcts, tumors, and infections in organ structures. When used, the contrast medium is noniodinated, and it is administered intravenously to enhance contrast between normal and abnormal tissues. The patient must lie still in a narrow tube, sometimes for up to an hour.

Preparation
- Determine the presence of metal in the body, such as shrapnel or flecks of ferrous metal in the eye.
- Instruct the patient to remove all external metallic objects before entering the scanning room (e.g., jewelry, body piercing rings, eyeglasses, hairpins, credit cards).
- Food and fluids are not always restricted. The patient may be NPO for 4 to 6 hours before the examination.
- Have the patient void before the procedure.

Posttest Care
- The patient can resume normal activity, medication, and diet.
- If a contrast medium was used, observe for delayed allergic reactions.

Source: Van Leeuwen, A., Poelhuis-Leth, D., & Bladh, M. (2019). *Davis's comprehensive handbook of laboratory and diagnostic tests with nursing implications* (7th ed.). Philadelphia: F. A. Davis.

Nursing Care Plan

Client Data

Olivia Grimaldi, 59 years old, is admitted to the orthopedic unit after having a total knee replacement. She is receiving intravenous opioid analgesics for pain. Mrs. Grimaldi's nurse sits down to talk and complete the nursing admission assessment. The conversation turns to a discussion of bowel habits.

Nurse: Mrs. Grimaldi, we pay special attention to bowel elimination because many people on this unit have problems. How often do you have a bowel movement?

Mrs. G: Not as often as I'd like. I used to be very regular, but lately everything is all mixed up.

Nurse: What has changed? Tell me what's going on.

Mrs. G: Oh, it's so embarrassing. I haven't told anyone about this.

Nurse: When did this problem start?

Mrs. G: Everything started going bad when I fell and landed on this knee a few months ago. Nothing was broken, but the pain has been just awful. I knew I had arthritis, but I never felt anything like this. I couldn't sleep, the pain was so bad. The doctor put me on some pain pills—narcotics—and they helped, but I got so constipated. I started using laxatives to go to the bathroom, but I kept needing to use more and more. Sometimes I would take a laxative and then I would have to get to the bathroom quickly. I had a couple of accidents because I couldn't get to the toilet quickly enough.

Nurse: I think this is something we'll be able to help you with, Mrs. Grimaldi.

The nurse discovers that Mrs. Grimaldi drinks about 32 to 40 ounces of fluid each day and has used several stimulant laxatives and enemas to relieve her constipation. Her mobility has been significantly impaired for the past 2 months.

Nursing Diagnosis

Bowel incontinence related to overdistention of the rectum secondary to chronic constipation, as evidenced by client report of constipation when taking opioids and subsequent fecal incontinence with the use of laxatives.

NOC Outcomes

Bowel continence (0500)
Bowel elimination (0501)

Individualized Goals/Expected Outcomes

By discharge, Mrs. Grimaldi will:
1. Be free from fecal impaction.
2. Begin to establish a regular pattern of stool evacuation.
3. Describe four actions she can take to reduce the risk of constipation.

Within 1 month, Mrs. Grimaldi will:
1. Control stool passage without any episodes of fecal incontinence.

NIC Interventions

Bowel management (0430)
Bowel training (0440)

Nursing Activities

1. Conduct a comprehensive assessment of all factors related to fecal incontinence and impaired bowel elimination.

Rationale

Fecal incontinence has multiple possible causes. The best nursing actions are those based on client assessment/recognizing cues (Deb et al., 2020). Constipation is attributed to immobility, weak straining ability, use of constipating drugs, neurological disorders, lack of dietary fiber, and poor fluid intake (Menees et al., 2022).

(continued)

Nursing Care Plan (continued)

Nursing Activities	Rationale
2. During physical examination, inspect the perianal skin for possible causes of fecal incontinence or skin irritation resulting from exposure to liquid stool.	Congenital abnormalities and hemorrhoids can lead to incontinence (Menees et al., 2022). Skin tags can make cleansing difficult and lead to minor soiling that is difficult to distinguish from actual fecal incontinence.
3. Inquire about Mrs. Grimaldi's access to the bathroom and toileting facilities at home and work. Provide regular toileting assistance as long as she needs it during her hospitalization.	A lack of convenient access to the toilet can precipitate fecal incontinence (Nazarko, 2017).
4. Work with Mrs. Grimaldi to establish a bowel reeducation program, starting with bowel cleansing.	Cleansing is indicated for rectal impaction or palpable stool in the descending or sigmoid colon. Cleansing with manual disimpaction, laxatives, and/or enema removes any potential blockages to stool elimination (Menees et al., 2022).
5. Ensure that Mrs. Grimaldi drinks 30 mL/kg of fluids per day and gradually increases dietary fiber with bran or with bulking agents. Mrs. Grimaldi is drinking only about 1,200 mL of fluid per day. If she weighs 125 lb (56.7 kg), she would need to drink at least 1,700 mL of fluid per day.	Increasing fluid intake may help to normalize stool consistency in clients with constipation who do not have adequate fluid intake (Menees et al., 2022). Increasing dietary fiber improves stool consistency and reduces fecal incontinence (O'Donnell, 2020); however, unless the diet is deficient in fiber, adding fiber does not necessarily alleviate constipation. Bulk should be added to the diet slowly to reduce the risk of bloating, gas, or diarrhea. Dosing of bulking agents can be increased weekly until desired results are achieved; the results are more important than the amount of fiber ingested.
6. Teach Mrs. Grimaldi about how her body works to produce stool; ways to gently signal the body to defecate; the importance of responding to the urge to defecate; and how immobility, medications, and dehydration can cause constipation.	Gaining knowledge about body functions allows clients to be active participants in their care. Addressing causes of constipation can reduce the risk of recurrence (O'Donnell, 2020).

Evaluation

Review initial outcomes and goals. Reassess daily progress toward stated discharge goals.

The day before Mrs. Grimaldi's discharge she had no palpable stool on physical examination, and she no longer needed the intravenous analgesics; her patient-controlled analgesia (PCA) pump was discontinued. She was drinking approximately 20 mL/kg per day of fluids, she had begun taking 2 tablespoons of psyllium dissolved in water every morning, and she had a bowel movement each of the previous 2 days with stool of normal consistency for the first time in more than a month. She was able to state the actions she would take at home: Continue the bulk supplements, try to increase her fluid intake to 30 mL/kg per day, use nonconstipating analgesics, and increase her mobility each day. The nurse charted that the goals were met.

References

Butcher, H., Bulechek, G., Dochterman, J., et al. (2018). *Nursing interventions classification (NIC)*. (7th ed.). St. Louis, MO: Elsevier.

Deb, B., Prichard, D. O., & Bharucha, A. E. (2020). Constipation and fecal incontinence in the elderly. *Current Gastroenterology Reports, 22*(11), 1-16.

Menees, S., & Chey, W. D. (2022). Fecal incontinence: Pathogenesis, diagnosis, and updated treatment strategies. *Gastroenterology Clinics, 51*(1), 71-91.

Moorhead, S., Swanson, E., Johnson, M., et al. (Eds.). (2018). *Nursing outcomes classification (NOC)* (6th ed.). St. Louis, MO: Elsevier.

Nazarko, L. (2017). Understanding and managing constipation in older adults. *Practice Nursing, 28*(12), 517-526.

O'Donnell, K. F. (2020). Fecal incontinence: A stepwise approach to primary care management. *The Journal for Nurse Practitioners, 16*(8), 586-589.

CLINICAL REASONING
Applying the Full-Spectrum Nursing Model

PATIENT SITUATION

Lucy Franklin is a frail, older woman, a long-time resident in a long-term care facility. She can no longer communicate and lies in whatever position the UAPs place her in bed, seldom moving. She is very thin, does not eat or drink, and is being fed entirely through a gastrostomy tube. She is incontinent of both stool and urine and has recently started having copious diarrhea, probably from the tube feedings, but that has not been established definitively. The skin on Lucy's back, buttocks, and perineum is still intact, but it is quite red now. The healthcare team is considering various measures for controlling the diarrhea, but until that can be achieved, nurses want to protect her skin integrity.

THINKING

1. *Theoretical Knowledge:*

    a. Other than tube feedings, what else could be causing Lucy's diarrhea?

    b. In addition to skin integrity impairment, what are some other risks associated with diarrhea?

    c. Why is fecal incontinence, especially with diarrhea, a risk factor for skin integrity impairment?

2. *Critical Thinking:*

    a. *(Contextual Awareness):* What other factors in Lucy's situation do you think might make her even more vulnerable to skin integrity impairment? If you do not yet have the theoretical knowledge you need, draw on your own experiences—and think carefully about everything you know about Lucy.

    b. *(Considering Alternatives):* A fecal incontinence pouch is being discussed as an intervention to preserve Lucy's skin integrity. Do you think it should be an external system or an internal system? Why?

DOING

3. *Practical Knowledge:*

    It has been decided that an external fecal collection system will be used. Describe the steps you will take to apply this system after you have made the necessary assessments.

4. *Nursing Process (Assessment/Recognizing Cues):*

    What ongoing assessments will you need to make after the fecal collection system is applied?

CARING

5. *Self-Knowledge:*

    How comfortable would you be with applying Lucy's fecal collection system? What aspects of the situation make you most uncomfortable?

Critical Thinking and Clinical Judgment

1. Your neighbor is aware that you are a nursing student and calls you for advice. She has a 12-year-old daughter with diarrhea. "Everything runs through her," states the mother. There are also two other children in the house, ages 6 years and 18 months. Both have had watery stools this morning. Your neighbor explains that her husband has an ileostomy and has been hospitalized since yesterday. Your neighbor has no symptoms but is very worried. She asks, "Do we all need to go to the hospital?"

    a. Consider alternatives. What are the most likely explanations for the diarrhea?

    b. Based on your theoretical knowledge, how would you explain why her husband was hospitalized, while the rest of the family members, who have the same symptoms, remain at home?

    c. After reassuring her, what advice should you offer your neighbor about self-care for her and the children's elimination problem?

2. Consider the following patients:

    - A 54-year-old man diagnosed with colon cancer who now has a new sigmoid colostomy

    - A 21-year-old woman with Crohn disease (an inflammatory bowel disorder) who has just had an ileostomy

    - A 36-year-old trauma victim who has a new double-barreled transverse colostomy

    a. How are these patients similar?

    b. Regarding their surgery, what nursing care priorities do these patients share?

    c. How do the major concerns for these patients differ? (Consider the context. How are their surgical and self-care situations different?)

3. For each of the following concepts, use critical thinking to describe how or why it is important to nursing, patient care, or bowel elimination. Note that these are *not* to be merely definitions.

    Digestion (in the mouth, esophagus, stomach, and small intestine)

    Large intestine (colon)

    Rectum and anus

    Fluid intake

    Location of a bowel diversion

    Bowel sounds

    Providing privacy

    Diarrhea

What Are the Main Points in This Chapter?

- Bowel elimination is a normal process by which waste products are eliminated from the body.
- Feces are a mixture of insoluble fiber and other indigestible material, bacteria, and water.
- During defecation, the internal and external anal sphincters relax; the rectum contracts; and peristalsis increases in the sigmoid colon, propelling feces through the anus.
- The frequency of bowel movements (BMs) varies. As long as stools are passed without excessive urgency, with minimal effort and no straining, and without the use of laxatives, bowel function is regarded as normal.
- The bowel pattern set in childhood normally continues into adulthood. Adequate fiber, fluid, and exercise are required to maintain this pattern.
- Factors affecting bowel function include developmental stage, personal and sociocultural factors, nutrition, hydration, activity level, stress, anesthesia, medications, pregnancy, surgery and other procedures, and pathological conditions.
- To promote regular defecation, provide privacy for the patient and allow time to use the toilet.
- Constipation is a decrease in frequency of BMs and the passage of dry, hard stool that requires more effort to pass.
- Bulking agents are the preferred medication for treating constipation.
- Habitual use of laxatives, with the exception of bulking agents, may cause reliance on medication for bowel elimination.
- Fecal impaction is detected by digital examination of the rectum. To treat a fecal impaction, an enema or digital removal of stool is required.
- An enema is the introduction of solution into the rectum to soften feces, distend the colon, and stimulate peristalsis and evacuation of feces.
- Monitor patients with diarrhea for intake and output, body weight, and vital signs to assess for fluid losses; provide hygiene measures to protect the skin.
- Bowel incontinence may be managed by providing assistance to the bathroom at regular intervals and at the times BMs are most likely to occur and by beginning a bowel training program.
- External or internal fecal collection devices can be used to protect perianal skin or to collect large stool samples. They minimize odor, allow for accurate measurement of output, and improve patient comfort.
- A bowel diversion is a surgically created opening for elimination of digestive waste products.
- The **effluent** (fecal matter) of an ostomy ranges from liquid to solid, depending on the part of the bowel that is being diverted.
- A healthy stoma ranges in color from deep pink to brick red and is shiny and moist at all times.
- A client with a bowel diversion must adapt to the stoma for elimination and learn to care for the stoma.

UNIT 4 Supporting Physiological Functioning

Knowledge Map

BOWEL ELIMINATION

FACTORS AFFECTING:
- Developmental stage
- Personal/cultural
  - Time
  - Privacy
- Nutrition/hydration
- Activity level
- Medications
- Procedures
- Pregnancy

PATHOLOGICAL CONDITIONS:
- Pain
- Immobility
- Neurological
- Cognitive changes
- Food allergies
- Diverticulosis/itis

BOWEL DIVERSIONS:
- Ileostomy/Kock pouch
- Colostomy:
  - Permanent
  - Temp → loop

STRUCTURES:
- Mouth: Digestion begins
- Esophagus: Transit of food to stomach
- Stomach: Mechanical digestion
- Small intestine: Digestion/absorption; passage to large intestine
- Large intestine: Absorption of vitamins/minerals
- Rectum/anus: Waste elimination

ASSESSMENT:
- Bowel sounds
- Elimination pattern
- Appearance of stool
- Change in bowel habits/patterns
- Use of elimination aids

DIAGNOSTIC TESTING:
- Visualization:
  - Direct
  - Indirect
- Labs:
  - Occult blood
  - Parasites

PROMOTING NORMAL/REGULAR DEFECATION:
- Provide privacy
- Position properly
- Timing related to meals
- Promote adequate fluids and balanced diet
- Encourage exercise

MANAGE DIARRHEA:
- Assess stools
- Attend to fluid needs
- Provide hygiene/skin care
- Antidiarrheals

MANAGE CONSTIPATION:
- Increase dietary fiber
- Increase fluid intake
- Increase activity

MANAGE IMPACTIONS:
- Enemas: Cleansing; retention; return flow
- Digital removal of stool

MANAGE BOWEL INCONTINENCE:
- Fecal collection pouch
- Bowel training
- Promote hygiene; skin care
- Review diet/fluid intake

MANAGE BOWEL DIVERSION:
- Assessing effluent → amount, consistency
- Stoma assessment/care → size, color
- Peristomal skin care
- Patient teaching: Diet, appliance management
- Supporting patient self-concept

CHAPTER 27

Sensation, Perception, & Response

STUDENT RESOURCES

The questions and exercises in this book allow you to practice the kind of thinking you will use as a full-spectrum nurse. Critical-thinking questions usually have more than one right answer, so we do not provide "correct" answers for these features. Try to answer these questions yourself. It is more important to develop your nursing judgment than to just cover content. You will learn more by discussing the questions with your peers. If you are still unsure, see the Davis Advantage chapter resources for suggested responses.

To explore learning resources for this chapter,

Go to www.DavisAdvantage.com and find:

Answers and Suggested Responses for all questions in this chapter
Concept Map
Knowledge Map
References and Bibliography

Key Concepts

Perception
Reception
Sensation

Related Concepts

See the Concept Map on Davis*Advantage*.

Caring for the Williams Family

Charlene Williams, Stanley Williams' mother, has been having blurred vision. At a recent ophthalmology appointment, she was told she has bilateral cataracts that will require surgical removal. She reports to the primary care clinic today, accompanied by Stanley. Charlene tells you, "I don't know what happened. I was pulling into a parking space at the grocery store, and the next thing you know, I hear this loud crash. I don't know how I did it, but I hit the car next to me. I just didn't see it."

Stanley is very concerned and questions whether his mother should be allowed to drive. Charlene is visibly upset. "I don't want to hurt anyone, but I don't want to lose all my freedom." Stanley insisted on this appointment to discuss his concerns.

A. What data will you need to gather from Charlene and Stanley?

B. What assessments will you need to perform?

C. How will cataract surgery most likely affect Charlene? You will need to learn about the surgery and recovery to answer this question.

D. What information would you offer to Charlene and Stanley?

Practical Knowledge clinical application

To provide support for patients with sensorineural alterations, you will need practical knowledge about assessing and diagnosing sensorineural functions. You will find those in Assessment Guidelines and Tools.

Nursing interventions involve caring for patients who have vision and hearing deficits. This section includes a procedure for otic irrigations, which may be used to correct hearing loss resulting from a cerumen-blocked ear canal. Some procedures to support sensory function, such as instilling medications and irrigating the eye, are presented in the procedures in Chapter 23 of this volume. For other interventions, see Volume 1 of this chapter.

PROCEDURE

Procedure 27-1 ■ Performing Otic Irrigation

➤ For steps to follow in *all* procedures, refer to the Universal Steps for All Procedures on the inside back cover.

Equipment

- An ear irrigation system, such as the Welch Allyn ear wash system or an electronic jet ear irrigator

  ✚ Using a metal syringe is no longer recommended and is considered dangerous. An ear irrigation system is also preferred over an Asepto or bulb syringe because of the better ability to control pressure and remove cerumen (Harkin, n.d.).

- Asepto syringe, or rubber bulb syringe (if an ear irrigation system is not available)
- Irrigating solution (usually normal saline solution or sterile water, but may be an antiseptic solution), warmed to body temperature
- Cerumenolytic (optional)
- Bath towel and moisture-resistant towel
- A headlight or bright, external light if one is available
- Emesis basin
- Otoscope
- Cotton balls
- Procedure gloves

Delegation

You must assess the patient before performing this procedure and evaluate patient responses during and after the procedure. The procedure requires knowledge of anatomy and physiology, use of an otoscope, and sometimes use of sterile technique. Therefore, you should not delegate otic irrigation to unlicensed assistive personnel (UAP).

Preprocedure Assessments

- Determine whether there are contraindications for ear irrigation.
  Contraindications include ruptured tympanic membrane, present or recent middle ear infection, prior surgery on the ear, cleft palate, or acute inflammation of the ear canal.
- Assess the external ear for drainage.
  Do not irrigate the ears if drainage is present. Drainage from the ear may be a sign of rupture of the tympanic membrane.
- Assess the external ear for cerumen.
  Impacted cerumen is the most common reason for performing an ear irrigation.
- Assess the external ear canal for redness, swelling, or foreign objects; visualize the tympanic membrane. If a foreign object is present, attempt to remove it before irrigation.
  Establishes the baseline. If you irrigate with a foreign object in the ear, it may cause the object to swell and become more difficult to remove. Also, if you cannot visualize the tympanic membrane, it may be perforated; if so, otic irrigation is contraindicated.
- Assess for pain or hearing loss.
  Establishes the baseline. Cerumen blockage in the ear canal may result in a conductive hearing loss.

➤ When performing the procedure, always identify your patient according to agency policy, using two identifiers, and be attentive to standard precautions, hand hygiene, patient safety and privacy, documentation, and body mechanics.

Procedure Steps

1. **Assist the patient into a** sitting or lying position, with the head tilted slightly toward the affected ear. Explain what you are going to do.
   Positioning facilitates administering the solution and allows fluid to run along the roof of the ear canal. Knowing what to expect may decrease patient anxiety and improve their ability to cooperate during the procedure.

2. **Place a cerumenolytic of choice** in the external auditory canal and leave it in the ear for 15 to 30 minutes before initiating irrigation.
   Softens the earwax before irrigation for easier removal.

3. **Warm the irrigating solution** to body temperature; fill the reservoir of the irrigator.

CHAPTER 27 Sensation, Perception, & Response 597

Placing cool solutions in the ear can cause dizziness.

4. **Assemble the irrigator** if necessary; place a clean disposable tip on it.

5. **Don gloves, face mask, and eye protection;** put on the headlight.
   The gloves are needed because of the risk of exposure to body fluids. The headlight facilitates direct vision.

6. **Drape the patient** with a plastic drape; place a towel on the patient's shoulder on the side being irrigated. Ask the patient to hold an emesis basin under the ear to collect the irrigating fluid that drains out of the ear.

   Note: An emesis basin is not necessary if a comprehensive ear wash system is used. Drape and towel protect the client's clothing.

7. **Set the irrigator pressure** to the minimum level. Let it run for 20 to 30 seconds to prime the tubing or nozzle before irrigation. (If you must use an Asepto or rubber bulb syringe, fill the syringe with about 50 mL of the irrigating solution, and expel any remaining air.)

8. **Straighten the ear canal.**
   a. For a child younger than 3 years old, pull the pinna down and back.
   b. For older children and adults, pull the pinna upward and outward.
   Straightens the ear canal so that the solution can flow through the length of the canal.

9. **Instruct the patient to notify** you if they have any pain or dizziness during the irrigation. Explain to the patient that they may feel warmth, fullness, or pressure when the fluid reaches the tympanic membrane.
   Pain or dizziness may indicate a contraindication to the procedure.

10. **Place the tip of the nozzle** (or syringe) about 1 cm (½ in.) above the entrance of the ear canal; direct the stream of irrigating solution gently along the top of the ear canal toward the back of the patient's head.

    ✚ Do not direct the water stream directly at the tympanic membrane.
    Direct pressure can cause bleeding, pain, or perforation of the tympanic membrane.

    a. Do not occlude the ear canal with the nozzle.
    b. Instill the solution slowly.
    c. Allow the solution to flow out as it is instilled.
    d. Repeat these steps for 5 minutes or until you can see cerumen in the return solution.

11. **Inspect the ear with** an otoscope to evaluate cerumen removal. See Procedure 19-7: Assessing the Ears and Hearing if you need to review otoscopic examination.
    Allows visualization of the canal.

12. **Continue irrigating until** the examination indicates the canal is cleaned of cerumen and debris.
    The irrigating solution will soften the cerumen, easing removal. Blocking the canal prevents the outward flow of the solution.

13. **Place a cotton ball loosely** in the ear canal; ask the patient to lie on the side of the affected ear.
    The cotton ball will absorb excess fluid that drains by gravity.

14. **Clean and disinfect the irrigator,** according to the manufacturer's instructions or agency protocols. Dispose of the disposable tips.

? What if . . .

- **The cerumen is very hard or I have difficulty removing it?**

  The irrigating solution will help soften it, so you may attempt again after 15 minutes.

- **The patient is an infant or young child?**

  Ask another caregiver to immobilize the child during the irrigation.

Evaluation
- Observe the quantity and quality of ear cerumen you removed.
- Observe the appearance of the ear canal.
- Assess for complaints of pain or dizziness.
- Assess for improvement in hearing acuity.
- Reassess for drainage on the cotton ball.

Patient Teaching
- Avoid use of cotton-tipped swabs.
  They simply push cerumen deeper into the ear.
- Keep the ear dry for a few days. Use cotton balls coated with petroleum jelly when bathing.
  Exposure to a wet environment, such as a swimming pool, may increase the risk of bacterial or fungal infection. Petroleum jelly serves as a barrier to keep water from entering the ear.
- Clean ears daily with washcloth, soap, and water. If wax buildup is a problem, over-the-counter preparations (oils) can be used.
- Notify the primary care provider if you have ear pain, vertigo, or ringing in the ears.
  Ear irrigation is an invasive procedure and may result in otitis media, trauma to the external meatus, vertigo, tinnitus, and perforation of the tympanic membrane, although this is not common.

Home Care
- Provide the caregiver with instructions on ear care as stated previously.
- Teach parents to avoid irrigation in young children unless absolutely necessary. Oil- or water-based ear drops may be used to treat a wax problem in a child, applying the oil when the child is asleep.

(continued on next page)

Procedure 27-1 ■ Performing Otic Irrigation (continued)

■ ✚ Teach patients that ear candling is a not advisable. Candling consists of putting a hollow cone soaked in beeswax or paraffin in the ear and lighting the other end. The heat is supposed to draw out wax, but there is no evidence that it is effective. People using ear candles have burned themselves, blocked their ear canals with candle wax, and punctured their tympanic membranes (eardrums).

Documentation
- Document the ear solution used, the quantity, character, and odor of cerumen or drainage.
- Chart the condition of the ear canal and tympanic membrane after the irrigation.

Sample Documentation

00/00/0000   1220   Pt reported bilateral decreased hearing acuity. External ear canals occluded with dried cerumen. Irrigated with warm water using electronic ear irrigation system. Large amount of dry, brown cerumen removed with irrigation. External cannula and tympanic membrane intact after procedure with no report of pain, no bleeding, and no drainage. ————————N. Ephrain, RN

Practice Resources

Harkin (n.d.); Schumann Toscano, & Phleghaar (2022, April 30, updated); Schwartz, Magit, Rosenfeld, et al. (2017, January); Van Wyk (2018, May 9, updated).

CLINICAL INSIGHTS

Clinical Insight 27-1 ▶ Communicating With Clients Who Are Visually Impaired

- ♥ **iCare** ■ Introduce yourself when you enter the room.
- Address the client by the preferred name so that they can be certain you are addressing them.
- When you enter a room with a client who is visually impaired, describe the room, room layout, and activities that are occurring.
- Explain unfamiliar sounds, such as the paging system and monitor and pump alarms.
- If the client has limited vision, be sure to position yourself in the client's field of vision.
- Speak to the client before you touch them so that they are prepared for your touch.
- Do not speak loudly unless the client has a hearing impairment.
- Let the client know when you are leaving the room.
- Use the words "see" and "look" as you would with a sighted person.
- Avoid expressions, such as "over there" or "right here." Guide the client to the location or place her hand on the object.

Clinical Insight 27-2 ▶ Communicating With Clients Who Are Hearing Impaired

♥ **iCare** Difficulty communicating can be anxiety provoking for patients and frustrating for both patients and caregivers, especially in a healthcare setting. A caring nurse will:

Assess the patient's method of receiving speech.
- If the patient wears a hearing aid, check to see that it is turned on.
- If not, does the patient read lips or use sign language? (Only about one-third of spoken words can be understood by speech reading.)
- If possible, arrange a hearing evaluation for the client and construction of any required hearing aids.

Position yourself and minimize noise.
- Don't chew gum or eat while talking. Many clients use lip reading to interpret speech.
- Make sure you are clearly visible to the client before you start speaking.
- Face the client directly; keep your hands away from your mouth.
- If the hearing deficit is predominantly in one ear, move closer to the less affected ear.
- Minimize environmental noise (e.g., turn off the TV).

Communicate the message.
- Speak slowly and articulate clearly, in a natural way. Don't shout. Shouting distorts your words.
- Don't drop your voice at the end of a sentence.
- Use simple, plain language, but longer phrases (e.g., "Would you like me to get you a drink of water?" instead of "Do you want a drink?")
- Use gestures to provide visual cues (e.g., act out what you want the patient to do).
- Use paper, pencil, or computer communication when necessary. Consider literacy skills.

Clinical Insight 27-2 ▶ Communicating With Clients Who Are Hearing Impaired—cont'd

Interpret the client's responses.
- Observe the client's verbal responses, facial expressions, and body language for clues to understanding. An inappropriate response is a sign of misunderstanding.
- Be aware the client may nod agreement or say "yes" even when they do not understand what is being said.
- Confirm that the client understood you by asking them to repeat what you said, especially if you are giving specific information, such as a time or place. Many numbers and words sound alike (e.g., "fifteen" and "fifty"; or "Prozac" and "Prograf").
- If the person does not understand what you've said, rephrase your statement. Don't repeat the same words.
- **For older adults:** Use a low-pitched voice. The ability to hear high-pitched tones is lost first with aging.

ASSESSMENT GUIDELINES AND TOOLS

Always consider your patient's sensory–perceptual status. Sensory deficits, deprivation, and overload have a significant influence on quality of life and may be especially troublesome for institutionalized patients.

Hearing Screening in Older Adults

For adults 50 years and older who have not noticed hearing loss, the USPSTF found insufficient evidence to recommend for or against routine screening. However, adults with conductive hearing loss, congenital hearing loss, or sudden hearing loss caused by recent noise exposure should consult a provider for hearing testing (USPSTF, 2021, March).

Nurses may administer the *Hearing Handicap Inventory for the Elderly Screening Version (HHIE-S)* to assess the emotional and social effects of hearing impairment in older adults (Ventry & Weinstein, 1983). The HHIE-S is an easily administered 10-question reliable tool that has been used worldwide since the 1980s. It is designed for older adults in clinical and community settings. This tool does not determine the extent of hearing loss as audiometric testing in a sound-protected environment does but rather assesses the effect on the hearing impairment in everyday life. The goal of the HHIE-S is to identify individuals who would likely benefit from intervention.

Other Sensory Assessment Tools

Nursing History: Overall Sensory–Perceptual Status

Usual Sensory Function

Ask questions such as the following:
- How would you rate your vision?
- How would you evaluate your ability to see objects up close or at a distance?
- Do you have any difficulty hearing conversations or listening to the radio or television?
- Have you had any difficulty locating sounds?
- Do you have ringing or buzzing in your ears?
- Do you enjoy the taste of food?
- Do you notice any difficulty with your ability to smell?
- Do you have any pain or discomfort?
- Do you have any areas of numbness or tingling on your body?
- Do you have any difficulty with sensing hot or cold?
- Describe your level of coordination.
- What medications are you taking? Have they had any effect on your vision, hearing, sense of taste, smell, touch, or balance?
- What is your current stress level?
- What is your usual activity level?
- What is your preferred activity level?

Assess for Risk Factors for Impaired Sensory Function
- Developmental level (e.g., older adults)
- Health status (usual and current state of health, current health concerns such as Ménière's disease, history of hospitalizations and surgeries)
- Medications (i.e., look up adverse effects to determine what, if any, effect the medications have on sensory function)
- Stress (current and usual stress level, major sources of stressors, usual coping mechanisms)

(Continued)

Nursing History: Overall Sensory–Perceptual Status—cont'd

- Lifestyle (normal activity, noise, interaction levels, hobbies, and usual lifestyle)

History of Sensory Problems

Ask about the following:

- Have you had any problems with blurred vision, double vision, sensitivity to light, blind spots, objects moving in front of your eyes, or eye pain?
- Have you ever felt unable to follow a conversation because of difficulty hearing?
- Have you ever had problems with your ability to taste or smell?
- Have you ever had areas of numbness or tingling?
- Has anyone in your family ever been diagnosed with a stroke or circulation problem?
- Have you ever had episodes of confusion or disorientation?

Use of Sensory Aids, Including Diet, Exercise, Medications, and Remedies

- Does the patient wear glasses or contact lenses at any time? If so, determine the following:
  When was the patient's last eye examination?
  Are the glasses clean and in good repair? Are the glasses within easy reach?
  Are contact lenses in good condition? Is the patient able to care for them?
- Does the patient wear a hearing aid? If so, determine the following:
  Can the patient hear adequately with the hearing aid in place?
  Are the batteries working?
  Is the hearing aid clean?
  How much help does the patient need to place the aid in the ear?
- Does the patient use a cane or walker? If so:
  Has the cane or walker been properly fitted to the patient?
  How often does the patient use the device when walking?
- What factors determine when the device will be used?

Assess Mental Status

- Assess behavior, appearance, response to stimuli, speech, memory, and judgment. If you need more specific instructions, see Chapter 19, Procedure 19-16, Steps 1–10 and Questions for Evaluating Cognitive Status, at the end of the procedure.

- **For older adults,** the Mini-Cog is a rapid screening for Alzheimer's and dementia (Borson et al., 2000) and for assessing memory. It consists of three memory questions for memory recall using instructions to draw a clock face.

- Assess level of orientation: Have the patient tell you their name, the date, and their current location. If they can answer these questions correctly, describe them as "awake, alert, and oriented to person, place, and time" (AA&O×3).

Assess Level of Consciousness

Alert	Is the patient awake and aware of the environment and themselves, speaking clearly, making eye contact?
Confused	Are actions and speech inappropriate?
Lethargic	Is speech slow or sluggish? Are mental processes and movements sluggish?
Obtunded	This is a low level of awareness and response to environment. Document it if it occurs.
Stuporous	This occurs when the patient can be aroused by vigorous stimulation but seems confused during periods of arousal.
Comatose	In this state, there is no spontaneous movement, no verbalization, and only nonpurposeful movement with stimulation (Huntley, 2008).

- Also see Chapter 19, Procedure 19-16: Assessing the Sensory-Neurological System, Glasgow Coma Scale, and Full Outline of Unresponsiveness Scale.

Assess Support Network for Clients With Sensory Deficit

- Are there support persons to help the patient by assuming chores they can no longer perform?
- Are there people who provide comfort to ease the patient's distress about sensory losses?
- Who can provide sensory stimulation?
- Who can help reorient and calm the patient?
- Does the patient need help with transportation to maintain social contact?

Focused Assessment

Bedside Assessment of Sensory Function

Sense	Assessment process
Vision	Use the Snellen chart, or have the patient read a newspaper.
	Observe for squinting.
Hearing	Perform the whisper test.
	Inspect the ear canals for hardened cerumen.
	Observe patient conversations. Are there frequent requests for repeating information or misunderstandings?
	How loud is the patient's radio or television?
	To screen hearing in older adults, you will find a useful tool if you go to http://consultgerirn.org/uploads/File/trythis/try_this_12.pdf.
Smell	Ask the patient to close their eyes and identify common smells (e.g., coffee, vanilla, cloves, tobacco).
Taste	Ask the patient to close their eyes and identify common tastes (e.g., salt, lemon, and sugar). Give water between tastes.
Tactile	With their eyes closed, touch the patient with a wisp of cotton. Have the patient identify when you have touched them. Repeat this process with a sharp object, such as a needle.
	With their eyes closed, ask the patient to identify where you are touching their body.
Kinesthesia	Have the patient perform the Romberg test. See Chapter 19, Procedure 19–7.
	Have the patient perform alternating rapid motions, such as tapping heels or clapping.
	Observe the patient's gait and movement.

CLINICAL REASONING
Applying the Full-Spectrum Nursing Model

PATIENT SITUATION

Clint Gossage is an 85-year-old man who lives at home alone. His wife moved to a nursing home a year ago. Although Mr. Gossage has many self-care deficits, he is still able to live at home, with regular visits from a home health nurse and community services to help with some meals and bathing. When you visit him, you notice that he shouts when talking to you, looks at you intently when you speak, and constantly asks you to repeat what you say. You examine his external ear canal and note that there is some hardened cerumen in the canal. He is not wearing a hearing aid. The patient record reveals tympanic membrane scarring and a diagnosis of conductive hearing loss.

THINKING

1. *Theoretical Knowledge:* Describe the pathophysiology of conductive hearing loss.

2. *Critical Thinking (Considering Alternatives):* Based on your knowledge of conductive hearing loss and your assessment of Mr. Gossage, what is the first follow-up question you would ask him about his hearing?

DOING

3. *Practical Knowledge:* At a subsequent visit, you discover that Mr. Gossage has impacted cerumen in his left ear. After obtaining a medical prescription, you prepare to perform an otic irrigation.

    a. To what temperature will you warm the solution?

    b. What position would you use for Mr. Gossage?

    c. Describe how you would place the tip of the syringe (or ear wash system) for irrigating.

    d. After the ear is cleared of cerumen and you have finished irrigating, what should you do next? And what position will you have Mr. Gossage assume when you do it?

4. *Nursing Process (Diagnosis):*

    a. Write a nursing diagnosis that focuses on Mr. Gossage's safety and relates to hearing.

    b. Based on your nursing diagnosis, what safety measures would you recommend for Mr. Gossage's home? (Do not address the hearing aid issue here.)

CARING

5. *Ethical Knowledge:* Now think back to the first visit with Mr. Gossage. What are some reasons that he might not have been wearing a hearing aid? Consider physical changes associated with aging.

Critical Thinking & Clinical Judgment

1. Review the following patient scenarios.

    - **Margaret** is 84 years old. She is a retired schoolteacher who loves to read, work in her garden, and volunteer at the local children's hospital. She is a light-eyed, older adult with a long history of smoking. She lived in the southern region of the United States most of her life, reporting that she rarely used sunglasses most of her life. She has developed macular degeneration and is progressively losing her sight.

    - **Rocky** is 55 years old. He is a former guitar player in a heavy-metal band. He now works in music production. He has significant hearing loss related to chronic exposure to loud music. Most recently he has developed tinnitus, which has exacerbated his hearing loss.

    - **Abdul** is 31 years old. He is a chef at a local four-star restaurant. He suffered a head injury in a motor vehicle accident. A few days after his injury, he noticed that he had difficulty smelling and tasting food, and there was a change in his appetite. In addition to tiring easily and failing to remember the events after his injury, Abdul has sensitivity to light and noise. He is cranky and has isolated himself from others.

    - **Vitoria** is 66 years old. She is a licensed architect working for a firm in the downtown area. Recently she has been under a lot of stress. She began drinking lots of coffee, smoking cigarettes, and working long hours. She was admitted to the hospital with right-sided weakness and slurred speech. She is being evaluated for a cerebrovascular accident.

    a. For each client, write a nursing diagnosis to reflect their sensory–perception problem. Write one other nursing diagnosis that might result from the sensory–perceptual problem. Explain your thinking.

    b. Each of the patients is experiencing a sensory deficit. What interventions would be most appropriate to address each patient's concerns?

c. Which patient(s) is/are most likely to have difficulty adapting to the sensory deficit? How would you determine how each patient is adapting?

d. Which patient, if any, is most likely to have sensory overload?

2. Examine the clinical unit that you are visiting for your current clinical rotation. What unit factors contribute to the development of sensory overload?

3. What factors in the clinical unit contribute to the development of sensory deprivation?

4. For each of the following concepts, use critical thinking to describe how or why it is important to nursing, patient care, or sensory perception. Note that these are *not* to be merely definitions.

   Sensory stimulation   Sensory deficits

   Sensory overload   Sensory aids

   Sensory deprivation

What Are the Main Points in This Chapter?

- The purpose of sensation is to allow the body to respond to changing situations and maintain homeostasis.
- A sensory experience involves four components: stimulus, reception, perception, and an arousal mechanism.
- Reception is the process of receiving stimuli from nerve endings in the skin and body.
- Perception is the ability to interpret the impulses transmitted from the receptors and give meaning to the stimuli.
- Humans respond to sensations when they are alert and receptive to stimulation. The response to a stimulus is based on intensity, contrast, adaptation, previous experience, illness, or injury.
- Sensory deprivation is caused by a deficiency of meaningful stimuli.
- Sensory deprivation can be due to environmental conditions or to interference with the reception or perception of stimuli.
- Sensory overload develops when either environmental or internal stimuli—or a combination of both—exceed a level that the client's sensory system can effectively process. It can also occur in clients with neurological or mental health disorders who are unable to adapt to continuing, nonmeaningful stimuli.
- The patient with impaired vision, hearing, tactile sensation, olfactory sensation, or kinesthesia is at risk for injury.
- Visual and hearing changes may diminish the ability to communicate and may hamper social interaction.
- Developmental issues, culture, health status, medications, stress level, and individual preferences affect sensory perception.
- To assess sensory–perceptual function, assess factors affecting sensory perception, mental status, recent changes in sensory stimulation, use of sensory aids, the patient's environment, and the support network.
- Nursing strategies to address impaired sensory perception include activities to promote sensory function, prevent and treat sensory overload and deprivation, assist patients with sensory deficits, and communicate with patients with altered mental status.

Knowledge Map

SENSORY PERCEPTION

COMPONENTS OF

RECEPTION:
- Receiving, converting, and transmission of stimuli by receptors
- Examples:
  - mechanoreceptors
  - thermoreceptors
  - proprioceptors

PERCEPTION:
- Brain gives meaning to stimuli received

RESPONSE:
- To any given stimuli

Factors affecting (Reception/Perception):
- Receptor location
- Number of receptors
- Intensity of stimuli
- Past experience
- Knowledge & attitude
- Intact RAS

Factors affecting (Response):
- Intensity
- Contrast between stimuli
- Adaptation to stimuli
- Prior experience with stimuli

FACTORS AFFECTING Sensory function
- Developmental level
- Culture
- Illness and medications
- Stress level
- Personality
- Lifestyle

NURSING ASSESSMENT
- Mental status
- Changes in sensory function
- Use of sensory aids → glasses, hearing aid, canes
- Stimuli in the environment/pt's response
- Support network

SENSORY ALTERATIONS

SENSORY DEPRIVATION: RAS depression due to lack of meaningful stimuli

SENSORY OVERLOAD: Environmental/internal stimuli at a level higher than the sensory system can effectively process

SENSORY DEFICITS: Impairments in vision; hearing; taste; smell; touch; proprioception

PROMOTING OPTIMAL SENSORY FUNCTION

Preventing Sensory Deprivation:
- Help with sensory aids
- Make regular contact with patient; ensure continuity of care
- Include touch; avoid isolation
- Provide orientation cues: message board; calendar; TV
- Encourage social interaction
- Monitor sedating medications
- Stimulate senses: smells; pet therapy

Preventing Sensory Overload:
- Minimize unnecessary stimuli: pain, nausea, noxious odors
- Establish a schedule for care including uninterrupted sleep
- Promote calm, low stress environment
  - teach relaxation techniques
  - limit visitors

VISION:
- Clean glasses in reach
- Sufficient light
- Magnification/large print

HEARING:
- Functioning hearing aid
- Clean ear canal
- Closed caption: TTY phone
- Written communication

- Care of the confused patient
- Care of the unconscious patient

CHAPTER 28

Pain

STUDENT RESOURCES

The questions and exercises in this book allow you to practice the kind of thinking you will use as a full-spectrum nurse. Critical-thinking questions usually have more than one right answer, so we do not provide "correct" answers for these features. Try to answer these questions yourself. It is more important to develop your nursing judgment than to just cover content. You will learn more by discussing the questions with your peers. If you are still unsure, see the Davis Advantage chapter resources for suggested responses.

To explore learning resources for this chapter,

Go to www.DavisAdvantage.com and find:

Answers and Suggested Responses for all questions in this chapter
Concept Map
Knowledge Map
References and Bibliography

Key Concepts
Pain
Pain management

Related Concepts
See the Concept Map on Davis Advantage.

Caring for the Williams Family

Review the introduction to the Williams family at the front of this volume. Stanley Williams has bilateral knee pain secondary to osteoarthritis.

A. To develop a pain management plan, what patient data do you need to know?

B. How will you get the data you need? What sources should you use?

C. What types of nursing knowledge (theoretical, practical, ethical, or self-knowledge) are needed to develop a pain management plan?

Practical Knowledge knowing how

When caring for patients with pain, you will need to be skilled in medication administration, including use of patient-controlled analgesia (PCA) pumps, and caring for patients who have an epidural catheter.

PROCEDURE

Procedure 28-1 ■ Setting Up and Managing Patient-Controlled Analgesia by Pump

➤ For steps to follow in *all* procedures, refer to the Universal Steps for All Procedures on the inside back cover.

Equipment
- PCA pump (infuser and central unit)
- Manufacturer's instructions for the pump
- Cartridge, syringe, or other type of sealed unit containing the medication
- Connecting tubing (to connect the PCA device to the patient's IV line)
- Maintenance IV supplies, as needed
- IV pole
- Antiseptic swab
- Flowsheet (electronic or paper)
- 1 pair of clean procedure gloves (if venipuncture is necessary)

Delegation
Because an opioid medication is delivered intravenously to the patient, this procedure is outside the scope of the practice of unlicensed assistive personnel (UAP) and should never be delegated. Furthermore, the UAP should not administer a dose for the patient, even if they ask the UAP to do so. You can inform the UAP of expected side effects and ask them to report their observations to you.

Preprocedure Assessment
- Assess physical conditions that can affect respirations. Respiratory assessment should include evaluation of respiratory rate, depth, pattern, effort, breath sounds, oxygen saturation, and capnography.
  Respiratory diseases (e.g., chronic obstructive pulmonary disease [COPD] and asthma) and conditions such as head injury and sleep apnea increase the risk for respiratory depression with opioid use.
- Assess level of consciousness and cognitive level.
  Determines whether the patient will be able to follow directions for self-dosing.
- Review laboratory values reflecting liver and kidney function, such as blood urea nitrogen (BUN), creatinine, and liver enzymes.
  Opioid analgesics are typically metabolized through the liver or kidneys.
- Assess the respiratory rate, pulse, blood pressure, and oxygen saturation at baseline, at initiation of PCA, or with a change in drug. Check vital signs every 15 minutes for 1 hour, every hour for 4 hours, and then every 2 hours while infusing. Also, check patient's vital signs at any handoffs or shift changes (San Diego Patient Safety Council, 2014, updated; McGinley, 2013, July/August).
  A change in vital signs (e.g., hypotension, respiratory rate below 8) may indicate adverse responses to opioid administration.
- Be aware of the patient's age and weight.
  Age is a factor when you are verifying the dose. Older patients and very young children are at increased risk for respiratory suppression so may require lower doses.
- Assess the patient's baseline pain level using a standardized pain assessment tool or numeric scale ranging from 0 to 10.
  A quantified self-report is one of the most accurate measures of pain (Contrada, 2019).
- Assess the patient's manual dexterity.
  Patients with impaired fine motor control or upper extremity injury may not be able to operate the self-dosing mechanism.
- Review medications currently in use.
  The risk of respiratory depression increases when a PCA pump is used in conjunction with other CNS depressants, such as diazepam (Valium).
- Assess the extent of family involvement. Identify any family anxiety over the patient's pain. Reinforce that only the patient should use the PCA button.
  Only the patient should administer the medication. PCA by proxy (someone other than the patient pushing the dosing button) is a major factor contributing to adverse patient outcomes (Wuhrman et al., 2007).

➤ When performing the procedure, always identify your patient according to agency policy, using two identifiers, and be attentive to standard precautions, hand hygiene, patient safety and privacy, body mechanics, and documentation.

Procedure Steps

1. **Don clean procedure gloves;** initiate IV therapy if the patient does not currently have an IV solution infusing. Refer to Procedure 35-1 as needed.

2. **Obtain the medication** and double-check it with the original prescription. You may need to remove air from the vial by pushing the injector into the vial. Connect the PCA tubing to the vial (or cartridge).

   ✚ Some PCA systems use a key to open the PCA module.
   Some vials may not be filled with medication. Ejecting the air makes it faster to prime the connecting tubing.

3. **Double-check your dose** calculation with another nurse before starting the infusion or wasting medication.

   ✚ Some systems are loaded with a drug library already programmed to the needs of the facility and with features in place to ensure proper delivery of medication to patients.
   To prevent medication errors in dosing:

   a. On-demand dose (the amount of drug to be delivered with each push of the button).
   b. The "lockout" interval (the number of minutes allowed between each administration of an on-demand dose [e.g., q10min]). Even if the patient pushes the button more frequently, the PCA pump will not administer a dose until the preset time between doses has been met.
   c. Basal rate or continuous infusion (the amount of medication to be delivered automatically by the pump over 1 hour) should be used with caution. Giving the medication continuously without the patient having to push a button takes away some of the inherent safety of a PCA.
   d. One-time bolus (or *loading*) dose, which you administer after setting up the pump.
   e. The 1-hour or 4-hour lockout interval (the maximum dose allowed in that time frame). For example, if the patient has a 4-mg on-demand dose with a 10-minute lockout interval, the patient can receive a maximum of six 4-mg doses per hour for a total of 24 mg/hr and a maximum dose of 96 mg in 4 hours.

   NOTE: PCA prescriptions are usually written in milligrams; however, pump settings may be in milliliters. In such cases, you must verify the concentration (milligrams per milliliter) to set the pump correctly.

4. **Prime the tubing; then clamp** the tubing above the connector.
   Priming prevents air from entering the pump and causing malfunction. Clamping prevents an accidental bolus of medication getting to the patient.

5. **Insert the cartridge or vial** into the pump; lock the pump. Follow the manufacturer's instruction manual (e.g., some pumps can be set only if the door is closed and locked).
   Depending on the pump, it may be a syringe, a cartridge, or other sealed container that can be "locked" into the pump. Locking the pump prevents unauthorized access to the opioid and dosing features.

6. **Turn the pump on; set** the parameters according to the prescriptions and your calculations. The settings may include:
   a. On demand
   b. Lockout interval
   c. Basal rate or continuous infusion—if applicable
   d. The 1-hour or 4-hour lockout dosage limit
   e. The one-time loading dose—if applicable

7. **Scrub the port on the IV** tubing closest to the patient, using alcohol or a chlorhexidine gluconate (CHG)–alcohol product; then connect the PCA pump tubing.
   Removes gross contamination and discourages growth of pathogens.

8. **Open the clamp and** administer the bolus (loading) dose if prescribed. Remain with the patient as the dose is delivered.
   A loading dose is usually larger than the basal and on-demand doses because pain is likely to be more severe before the pump is initiated. Remaining with the patient allows you to observe for adverse effects.

9. **Close the pump door;** lock the machine with the key.

10. **Check for flashing lights** or alarms that may indicate the need to correct settings.

11. **Be sure to release tubing clamps** if you previously clamped the tubing; press the start button to begin pump operation.

12. **Ensure that the battery life** is sufficient or, preferably, that the pump is plugged into an appropriate electrical outlet.
    To avoid battery failure.

13. **Place the control button** for on-demand doses within the patient's reach. Be sure the PCA cord is placed away from the call bell.
    To avoid error in self dosing with PCA. ▼

(continued on next page)

Procedure 28-1 ■ Setting Up and Managing Patient-Controlled Analgesia by Pump (continued)

? What if...

- **The patient cannot verbally communicate pain status?**

  Use an alternative standardized pain tool, such as the FACES pain scale or a behavioral measure, to determine pain level.

  Pain assessment in patients who are uncommunicative may include behavioral or physiological indicators to assess and monitor the effectiveness of pain medication.

- **The infusion infiltrates?**

  Discontinue the IV and establish another IV site. Follow facility policy for application of cold or warm compresses to the infiltrated area. Assess pain level. You may need to contact the prescriber for a bolus dose if the IV has been interrupted for an extended period or the patient has insufficient pain relief.

Evaluation

- Monitor the patient's pain level, sedation level, and respiratory rate at least every hour for the first 24 hours or according to facility policy after initiating PCA.
  Promotes the early detection of respiratory depression, oversedation, or inadequate pain control.
- Perform routine assessment of number and frequency of doses and pump settings per facility protocol.
- Check the IV site for redness, infiltration, or phlebitis.
- Check the IV tubing for patency (e.g., for kinks) to be sure the medication is infusing.

Patient Teaching

Patients who are candidates for use of PCA should be trained before surgery rather than in the immediate postoperative period, when the effects of anesthesia impair learning. Reinforce or teach the patient and family the following:

- Safe and correct use of the PCA pump.
- The benefits of PCA for controlling pain.
- The pump will deliver only the amount of medication prescribed. Pushing the button too many times will not result in overdosing.
- The patient cannot accidentally roll over on the button and unintentionally give additional medication.
- If pain is not being relieved, the patient should tell the nurse so adjustments can be made to the PCA.
- The pump will alarm when nearly empty, alerting nurses to change the syringe.
- The PCA button is to relieve pain, not to help the patient sleep.
- Signs and symptoms of allergic reaction and which ones to report.
- How to rate pain using a standard pain scale.
- The patient is the only one who may push the pain-dosing button. Explain why family members should not give doses by proxy.

Documentation

You will usually document PCA initiation on a specialized checklist or flowsheet. Items charted include:

- Time the infusion was begun, including the drug, the patient demand dose, the loading dose, the basal dose if applicable, lockout interval, and hourly limit
- Patient's baseline pain level and evaluation of subsequent pain level performed at intervals determined by facility policy
- Baseline respiratory rate, pulse, blood pressure, and oxygen saturation; routine evaluation of subsequent vital signs performed at intervals determined by facility policy
- Sedation level
- Continuous monitoring of vital signs, level of consciousness, and pain status, as well as the number and frequency of doses
- Unusual occurrences (e.g., oversedation, IV infiltration) in the nursing notes

Thinking About the Procedure

➤ To practice applying clinical reasoning to this procedure,

➤ Go to the **Davis's** *Nursing Skills Video* **Setting Up and Managing Patient-Controlled Analgesia by Pump**

For questions and suggested responses,

Practice Resources

d'Arcy, 2008a; Pastino & Lakra, 2019; San Diego Patient Safety Council, 2014, updated.

CLINICAL INSIGHT

Clinical Insight 28-1 ➤ Caring for the Patient With an Epidural Catheter

Nursing care of the patient with epidural analgesia focuses on:
- Safely administering analgesia
- Assessing pain while achieving maximum pain control
- Preventing or identifying adverse reactions

Contraindications

Epidural analgesia is contraindicated in patients who have:
- Increased risk for bleeding: anticoagulant therapy, other bleeding problems
- Infection at the insertion site or in the bloodstream
- Increased intracranial pressure.
- Allergy to local anesthetic or opioid
- Spinal defects, previous spinal surgery, or certain neurological conditions (e.g., multiple sclerosis).

Monitoring

- **Monitor vital signs,** especially for respiratory depression and hypotension (every hour for the first 24 hours, then every 4 hours if the patient is stable).
- **Assess pain intensity** using a pain rating scale (per institution's protocol) and degree of motor and sensory block.
- **Monitor the site** for leaking or drainage.
- **Check connections for leaks.** This can be fixed by carefully retightening connections. If the filter is cracked, replace with a new one using sterile technique.
- **Assess for urine retention.** Keep careful intake and output (I&O) records.
  Urinary retention is one side effect of epidural opioids.
- **Observe for verbal and nonverbal signs of headache** as a result of dural puncture. Treatment consists of bedrest, analgesics, and liberal hydration. Caffeine is also helpful and may be administered IV. If unresolved after 72 hours, patient might receive an epidural blood patch.
  An epidural blood patch is an injection of the patient's own blood into the epidural space to prevent headache.
- **Observe for signs of catheter migration:** nausea, a decrease in blood pressure, and a loss of motor function without a recognizable cause.
- **Observe for signs of local anesthesia toxicity** occurring when anesthesia is injected directly into the bloodstream instead of the epidural space. The patient might report numbness or tingling around the mouth or ringing in the ears (tinnitus); or you may assess irritability, tremors, seizures, or cardiac arrhythmias (Portenoy & McCaffery, 2011; Sawheney, 2012).

Prevention

- **Clearly label solutions with "For epidural use only"** using large font. Store IV and epidural medication in separate locations.
  Prevents errors in medication administration.
- **Mark all lines** *clearly:* Most epidural tubing is marked with a yellow stripe.
  Epidural lines must not be confused with IV solution for an arterial or venous catheter.
- **Ensure the tape is secure on the tubing** connected to the patient.
  To prevent catheter migration.
- **Use strict aseptic technique** when changing tubing, including mask and sterile gloves for access and maintenance procedures.

Discontinuing the Catheter

- **If you are specially trained to remove an epidural catheter:**
  1. Loosen the tape securing the catheter.
  2. While wearing clean gloves, apply slow, steady pressure to withdraw the catheter.
  3. Inspect the catheter on removal. You must be able to see the tip of the catheter. If not, a portion of the catheter may still be lodged in the patient's epidural space. Notify the anesthesia team immediately of this finding.
- If the catheter cannot be withdrawn with minimal force, try placing the patient in the same position for removal as the patient was in during insertion of the catheter.
- Cleanse the insertion site, and cover with a dry sterile dressing.

ASSESSMENT GUIDELINES AND TOOLS

Pain Assessment

Taking a Pain History

Taking a pain history is the most effective way to perform an assessment. Each agency has a different assessment form for this history, but the questions typically will include the following:

- Do you have pain now?
- When did the pain begin?
- Where is the pain located?
- How do you rate your pain? (Use a pain scale.)
- How would you describe your pain? Sharp? Dull? Achy? Burning?
- How often do you have pain? Is it constant or intermittent?
- Is there a rhythm or pattern to your pain? Is there anything you do that triggers the pain?
- What makes the pain better? What makes it worse?
- How many days this past week has pain interfered with your ability to do what you would like to do?
- Does pain interfere with your ability to take care of yourself?
- Does pain wake you up at night?
- Does pain interrupt your concentration and reduce your ability to think clearly?
- Does pain prevent you from participating in pleasurable activities, hobbies, and socializing with friends?
- Have you had this type of pain in the past?
- Do you have any other symptoms (such as nausea and vomiting) when you feel pain?
- Have you used any medications to treat the pain? If so, were they effective? How often do you need to take pain relievers?
- What, if any, alternative treatments have you used for pain?
- What past experiences or cultural factors, if any, influence the pain?

Observing for Nonverbal Indicators of Pain

Physiological (Involuntary) Responses
SYMPATHETIC RESPONSES (ACUTE PAIN)
- Increased systolic blood pressure
- Increased heart rate and force of contraction
- Increased respiratory rate
- Increased alertness (resulting from dilated blood vessels to the brain)
- Dilated pupils
- Rapid speech

PARASYMPATHETIC RESPONSES (DEEP OR PROLONGED PAIN)
- Decreased systolic blood pressure, possible syncope
- Decreased pulse rate
- Changeable breathing patterns
- Withdrawal
- Constricted pupils
- Slow, monotonous speech

Behavioral Responses (Voluntary)
- Withdrawing from painful stimuli
- Moaning
- Facial grimacing
- Crying
- Agitation
- Guarding the painful area

Psychological (Affective) Responses
- Anxiety
- Depression
- Anger
- Fear
- Exhaustion
- Hopelessness
- Irritability

Using Pain Scales

The most used pain scales are the Visual Analog Scale (VAS), the Numerical Rating Scale (NRS), the Simple Descriptor Scale (SDS), and the Wong-Baker FACES rating scale.

Visual Analog Scale
The Visual Analog Scale (VAS) is a 10-cm horizontal line in which "No pain" is written on the left side and "Worst pain imaginable" is written on the right. Patients point to a location on the line that reflects their current pain. Although this rating system is simple and quick, some patients have problems with the abstract nature of the scale.

No pain   Worst pain imaginable

Numerical Rating Scale
The Numerical Rating Scale (NRS) is a line numbered from 0 to 10. Zero indicates no pain at all, whereas a 10 indicates the worst possible pain. Patients choose a number from 0 to 10 to denote their level of pain. To use this scale, the patient must be able to count to 10. A scale of 0 to 5 may be more helpful for cognitively impaired patients.

0   1   2   3   4   5   6   7   8   9   10

Pain Assessment—cont'd

Simple Descriptor Scale
The Simple Descriptor Scale (SDS) is a list of adjectives that describe various levels of pain intensity. The simplest version of this scale uses the words *mild, moderate,* and *severe.* An SDS with many words is not recommended; it is time consuming to describe and may not be understood by many patients.

Wong-Baker FACES Pain Rating Scale
The FACES Scale uses simple illustrations of faces to depict various levels of pain. It requires no numerical or reading skill. Initially developed for use with children older than the age of 3, the scale has proved to be extremely useful for adults with communication and cognitive impairments as well.

Wong-Baker FACES Pain Rating Scale

0	1	2	3	4	5
No hurt	Hurts little bit	Hurts little more	Hurts even more	Hurts whole lot	Hurts worst

Explain to the person that each face is for a person who feels happy because he has no pain (hurt) or sad because he has some or a lot of pain. Face 0 is very happy because he doesn't hurt at all. Face 1 hurts a little bit. Face 2 hurts a little more. Face 3 hurts even more. Face 4 hurts a whole lot. Face 5 hurts as much as you can imagine, although you do not have to be crying to feel this bad. Ask the person to choose the face that best describes how he is feeling. Rating scale is recommended for persons age 3 and older.

From Wong-Baker FACES Foundation (2018). Wong-Baker FACES Pain Rating Scale. http://www.WongBakerFACES.org. Originally published in *Whaley & Wong's Nursing Care of Infants and Children.* © Elsevier Inc.

Revised Faces Pain Scales
The Faces Pain Scale—Revised (FPS-R) is a self-report measure of pain intensity developed for children. It was adapted from the Faces Pain Scale to make it possible to score pain levels using the widely accepted 0-to-10 metric. The use of grimacing can reflect the experience of pain more accurately than rating faces with smiles and tears.

Give direction for the person to score the chosen face 0, 2, 4, 6, 8, or 10 where 0 means *no pain* and 10 means *very much pain.* This scale is intended to measure how they feel inside, not how their face looks.

Hicks, C. L., von Baeyer, C. L., Spafford, P. van Korlaar, I., Goodenough, B. (2001). The Faces Pain Scale—Revised: Toward a common metric in pediatric pain measurement. *Pain, 93,* 173–183.

Bieri, D., Reeve, R., Champion, G. D., Addicoat, L., & Ziegler, J. (1990). The Faces Pain Scale for the self-assessment of the severity of pain experienced by children: Development, initial validation and preliminary investigation for ratio scale properties. *Pain, 41,* 139–150.

▶ To see FACES scales using photos of children of various ethnicities,

▶ Go to the **OUCHER! Web site** at www.oucher.org.

Pain Relief Diary

Client Pain Relief Diary

For pain relief I am using:

Medications _____

Alternative therapy (relaxation, distraction, etc.) _____

I will call my physician if _____ (filled in by nurse before discharge)

My goals are a pain rating of _____

Date	Time	Number of pills	Pain scale 0 1 2 3 4 5 6 7 8 9 10	Goal met? Yes No	Activity

Focused Assessment

Richmond Agitation–Sedation Scale

Score	Term	Description
+4	Combative	Overtly combative or violent; immediate danger to staff
+3	Very agitated	Pulls on or removes tube(s) or catheter(s) or has aggressive behavior toward staff
+2	Agitated	Frequent nonpurposeful movement or patient–ventilator dyssynchrony
+1	Restless	Anxious or apprehensive but movements not aggressive or vigorous
0	Alert and calm	
−1	Drowsy	Not fully alert but has sustained (more than 10 seconds) awakening, with eye contact, to voice
−2	Light sedation	Briefly (less than 10 seconds) awakens with eye contact to voice
−3	Moderate sedation	Any movement (but no eye contact) to voice
−4	Deep sedation	No response to voice, but any movement to physical stimulation
−5	Unarousable	No response to voice or physical stimulation

Sessler, C. N., Gosnell, M. S., Grap, M. J., et al. (2002). The Richmond Agitation–Sedation Scale: Validity and reliability in adult intensive care unit patients. *American Journal of Respiratory Critical Care Medicine, 166*, 1338–1344. DOI: 10.1164/rccm.2107138

Focused Assessment

Opioid Risk Tool—Revised (ORT-R)

This tool should be administered to patients upon an initial visit before beginning or continuing opioid therapy for pain management. A score of 2 or lower indicates low risk for future opioid use disorder; a score of >/=3 indicates high risk for opioid use disorder.

Mark each box that applies	Yes	No
Family history of substance abuse		
Alcohol	1	0
Illegal drugs	1	0
Prescription drugs	1	0
Personal history of substance abuse		
Alcohol	1	0
Illegal drugs	1	0
Prescription drugs	1	0
Age 16–45 years	1	0
Psychological disease		
Attention deficit disorder (ADD), obsessive compulsive disorder (OCD), bipolar, schizophrenia	1	0
Depression	1	0
Scoring total		

Source: Cheatle, M, Compton, P, Dhingra, L, Wasser, T, O'Brien, C. (2019, January 25). Development of the revised Opioid Risk Tool to predict opioid use disorder in patients with chronic nonmalignant pain. *The Journal of Pain, 0*(0) 1–10. DOI:https://doi.org/10.1016/j.jpain.2019.01.011

CLINICAL REASONING
Applying the Full-Spectrum Nursing Model

PATIENT SITUATION

Dieter Schmidt is a 48-year-old patient with a 2-year history of cervical spine injury that began after a motor vehicle accident (MVA). Presenting symptoms were neck pain when turning his head, biceps weakness, and pain down the arm with tingling into the fingertips. He is unable to sit for extended periods or walk distances. Initially he received treatment with medication, TENS to the site, physical therapy, and cervical fusion. Despite trying all treatments available to him, including surgery, Dieter continues to suffer chronic pain and fatigue. After prolonged suffering with no relief, he develops a cynical attitude toward healthcare. He begins missing more and more scheduled appointments for physical therapy. He describes the stress he feels from the economic downturn affecting his land development business and fears bankruptcy. As a result, he has given up previous hobbies and most social activities. His relationships with his family and friends are increasingly strained as the pain persists over time.

THINKING

1. *Theoretical Knowledge:*
   What is the mechanism that explains how pain is transmitted in the spine?

2. *Critical Thinking (Considering Alternatives, Deciding What to Do):*
   a. When planning care for Mr. Schmidt, what approach would you take in helping him to set goals for his rehabilitation?

   b. Why do you think Mr. Schmidt displays a negative attitude and reduced compliance toward rehabilitative therapies?

DOING

3. *Practical Knowledge:*
   a. (*Nursing Process: Assessment*): What questions would you ask Mr. Schmidt to assess the impact of pain on his daily living and quality of life?

   b. (*Nursing Process: Interventions*): In addition to drug therapy, what other measures might you teach Mr. Schmidt to do to control his pain and increase his comfort?

CARING

4. *Self-Knowledge:*
   Have you ever had chronic pain, such as back pain, fibromyalgia, arthritis, migraines, sports injuries, or other types? If so, how has it affected your daily life? Has your pain affected your relationships? Has it interfered with your job or recreational activities? In what other ways would you say chronic pain has reduced the quality of your life?

Critical Thinking and Clinical Judgment

1. Mrs. Jennings is a 37-year-old woman with terminal metastatic breast cancer. Although she is suffering from intractable pain, she resists opioid use because she fears being heavily sedated. Her time is limited, and she wants to be as alert as possible for her husband and young children.

   a. What is it about the patient's situation that may intensify her pain?

   b. Would you suggest using alternative therapies? Why or why not?

2. Mr. Lopez is a 39-year-old construction worker who fell from a roof at a construction site 8 months ago and is still having back pain from the accident. To manage pain, he is prescribed an oral opioid every 4 hours on a prn basis. He is still out of work and has great difficulty walking, so he spends most of the day in a recliner watching TV and drinking beer. Mr. Lopez also sleeps most nights in the recliner. He states that the alcohol is the only thing that helps his pain. How would you alter his pain management plan to get better relief? What is your rationale for these changes?

3. If you were delegating vital signs to unlicensed assistive personnel (UAP), what instructions would you give?

4. For each of the following concepts, use critical thinking to describe how or why it is important to nursing, patient care, or pain management. Note that these are *not* to be merely definitions.

Nociceptive pain   Opioid pain medications

Neuropathic pain   Adjuvant therapies

Unrelieved pain   Fear of addiction

Pain scales   Nonpharmacological pain management

Pain flowsheets   Nonopioid pain medications

What Are the Main Points in This Chapter?

- Pain is whatever the person says it is and exists whenever the person says it does.
- Pain has a protective function, warning us of potential or actual tissue damage and prompting us to act.
- Pain can be classified by its origin, cause, duration, and quality.
- Nociceptive pain results from injury to body tissues. Pain begins when mechanical, thermal, or chemical stimuli activate nociceptors, which send pain impulses to the spinal cord.
- Neuropathic pain occurs with injury to one or more nerves. A pain signal is transmitted even in the absence of painful stimuli.
- Fast pain impulses are carried on large-diameter A-delta fibers, whereas slow pain impulses are carried on thinner C fibers.
- Perception of pain occurs in the frontal cortex of the brain.
- Pain can be modulated by the endogenous analgesic system or by the gate control mechanism.
- Some of the factors that influence pain are emotional factors, life span variations, past pain experiences, sociocultural factors, inability to communicate, and cognitive impairment.
- Serious physiological, emotional, and psychological problems can result from unrelieved pain.
- Nonpharmacological pain relief measures include cutaneous stimulation, immobilization, and cognitive–behavioral intervention.
- Pharmacological measures include nonopioid analgesics, opioid analgesics, and adjuvant analgesics.
- Local and regional anesthesia, nerve blocks, and ablation therapy can relieve short- and long-term pain.
- Surgical interruption of pain conduction pathways is an option for intractable pain. Options depend on the type and location of pain.
- Opioid addiction among individuals being treated for pain is rare.
- The nurse assesses the patient for pain thoroughly and often (e.g., when the patient is admitted to a healthcare facility and when checking vital signs, before and after an intervention, when there is a change in clinical condition, and when the patient reports pain).
- The patient's self-report is the most reliable indicator of pain, especially for those suffering chronic pain.
- Misconceptions about pain can interfere with pain management.
- Older adults are at risk for undertreatment of pain.
- Planning for the patient's pain management program includes discovering the patient's own goals, educating the patient and family, and developing a nursing plan of care.
- It is important to continually assess the effectiveness of pain management strategies.

Knowledge Map

CHAPTER 28 Pain

PAIN

Definitions
- **A.P.S.**—Unpleasant sensory emotional experience associated with actual/potential tissue damage
- **McCaffrey**—whatever the person says it is, and existing whenever the person says it does.

CLASSIFIED ACCORDING TO:

Origin
- Cutaneous
- Visceral
- Somatic
- Radiating
- Referred
- Phantom
- Psychological

Cause
- Nociceptive
- Neuropathic

Duration
- Acute
- Chronic
- Intractable

FACTORS INFLUENCING PAIN
(Also influence person's definition)
- Emotions
- Developmental stage
- Sociocultural factors
- Impaired communication/cognition

PAIN MANAGEMENT

PHARMACOLOGIC:
- Non-opioids/NSAIDS
- Opioids: mu agonists; agonist antagonists
- Adjuvants: anticonvulsives; antidepressants

NONPHARMACOLOGIC:
- TENS
- Acupressure/acupuncture; massage; therapeutic touch
- Heat and cold
- Immobilization
- Distraction/humor
- SMR
- Guided imagery
- Hypnosis

NURSING CONSIDERATIONS IN PAIN MANAGEMENT:
- ID misconceptions
- Tailor the plan to needs of the elderly; substance abusers
- Teaching patient/family
- Thorough documentation

NURSING ASSESSMENT: PAIN
- **When:**
  - As the 5th vital sign
  - On admission
  - Before and after procedures and pain management strategies
  - With rest and activity
- **How:**
  - Obtain pain history
  - For children: art and play: FACES
  - Adults: Pain scales
  - Assessing nonverbal cues

PHYSIOLOGY OF PAIN

TRANSDUCTION: Activation of nociceptors by stimuli

TRANSMISSION: Conduction of impulses to spinal cord/brain

PERCEPTION: Recognition of and response to stimulus

Responses
- **Sympathetic**
  - Elevated BP/HR/resp; pupil dilation
- **Parasympathetic**
  - Low BP/HR constricted pupils
- **Behavioral**
  - Moaning, crying, grimacing, withdrawing
- **Psychological**
  - Anxiety, depression, exhaustion, hopelessness

CHAPTER 29

Physical Activity & Immobility

STUDENT RESOURCES

The questions and exercises in this book allow you to practice the kind of thinking you will use as a full-spectrum nurse. Critical-thinking questions usually have more than one right answer, so we do not provide "correct" answers for these features. Try to answer these questions yourself. It is more important to develop your nursing judgment than to just cover content. You will learn more by discussing the questions with your peers. If you are still unsure, see the Davis Advantage chapter resources for suggested responses.

To explore learning resources for this chapter,

Go to www.DavisAdvantage.com and find:

Answers and Suggested Responses for all questions in this chapter
Concept Map
Knowledge Map
References and Bibliography

Key Concepts

Fitness
Mobility
Physical activity

Related Concepts

See the Concept Map on Davis Advantage.

Example Client Condition

Immobility

Caring for the Williams Family

As you may recall, Stanley Williams has been advised to diet and exercise as part of the treatment plan for hypertension, type 2 diabetes mellitus, obesity, and osteoarthritis. Assad Johnson's examination has revealed no other cardiovascular problems.

Caring for the Williams Family (continued)

A. Design a fitness program for Stanley. Describe the program in detail. Recall that Stanley has been relatively sedentary.

B. Compare the type of program you would recommend for Stanley with the type of program appropriate for his granddaughter, Kayla.

C. What type of fitness program would be most appropriate for Charlene Williams, Stanley's mother? What additional information do you need to know to answer this question?

Practical Knowledge clinical application

In the next sections you will learn about procedures and techniques for positioning, moving, turning, transferring, and ambulating patients safely. Although the American Nurses Association (ANA, 2021) recommends that you use assistive equipment for all patient lifting and transferring, you may encounter situations in which equipment is not available or you do not have time to get it (e.g., in an emergency). In such situations, using good body mechanics may help you decrease the risk of injury to you and the patient.

PROCEDURES

Procedure 29-1 ■ Moving and Turning Patients in Bed

> For steps to follow in *all* procedures, refer to the Universal Steps for All Procedures on the inside back cover.

Equipment
- Nonlatex gloves, if you may be exposed to body fluids
- Friction-reducing device, such as a transfer roller sheet or scoot sheet
- Pull or lift (draw) sheet
- Pillows, as needed

Delegation
You may ask unlicensed assistive personnel (UAP) to assist with moving a patient up in bed, turning a patient, or logrolling a patient after ensuring that the UAP has the necessary skills and that the patient's condition is stable. Complete the assessment; inform the UAP of any special considerations when moving the patient.

Preprocedure Assessment
Assess the following:
- Level of comfort
  If the patient is uncomfortable, you may need to administer an analgesic before moving.
- Level of consciousness, ability to follow directions, and ability to assist with the move
- Any restrictions in movement or position (ask the patient and check the provider's orders)
- Physical size of the patient and the assistive devices available
- The patient's health status. Identify problems that may affect positioning (e.g., respiratory or cardiac problems, pain).
- Presence of equipment such as IV setups, pumps, or casts and know what must be moved with the patient
  The preceding assessments all help determine how many assistants and equipment you need, the patient's ability to assist in the procedure, and how to proceed with the move safely.

(continued on next page)

Procedure 29-1 ■ Moving and Turning Patients in Bed (continued)

Procedure 29-1A ■ Moving a Patient Up in Bed

> When performing the procedure, always identify your patient according to agency policy, using two identifiers, and be attentive to standard precautions, hand hygiene, patient safety and privacy, body mechanics, and documentation.

Procedure Steps

Key Point: *Medicate the patient for pain, if needed, before moving the patient in bed.*

1. **Lock the bed wheels.** Lower the head of the bed; place the patient in a supine position. Position one nurse on each side of the bed. Lower the side rails on the "working" side of the bed. Raise the height of the bed to waist level.
   These actions allow you to work with gravity and move the patient more easily while maintaining good body mechanics.

2. **Ensure that a friction-reducing device,** such as a transfer roller sheet, is in place under the drawsheet. If it is not in place, turn the patient from side to side to place the device under the drawsheet. You can improvise this device by placing a clean, unused plastic bag or plastic film under the drawsheet.
   A transfer roller sheet facilitates movement by reducing friction. This also helps to reduce back injury to the nurse.

   NOTE: This procedure uses a transfer roller sheet. This device is inexpensive and readily available. Scoot sheets further reduce the risk of back and musculoskeletal injury; however, their availability varies. Having a second person to help move a patient up in bed is the safest approach for staff and patients. Also follow the guidelines in Clinical Insight 29-1.

3. **Remove the pillow** from under the patient's head. Place it at the head of the bed.
   A pillow prevents patient from hitting their head on the headboard.

4. **Instruct the patient to fold** their arms across their chest. If an overhead trapeze is in place, ask the patient to hold the trapeze with both hands if able. Have the patient bend their knees with feet flat on the bed.
   This position facilitates the patient's assistance with the move.

5. **Instruct the patient to flex** their neck.
   Protects the neck while moving.

6. **With a nurse positioned** on either side of the patient, grasp and roll the drawsheet close to the patient.

7. **Stand as close as possible** to the client without twisting your back.

8. **Position your feet with a wide** base of support. Point your feet toward the direction of the move. Flex your knees and hips.
   Allows you to maintain proper body mechanics and prevents injury while moving the patient. ▼

9. **Instruct the patient,** on the count of 3, to lift their trunk and push off with their heels toward the head of the bed. With your weight on your foot nearest to the foot of the bed, lean forward toward the head of the bed. Move along the patient's side instead of reaching. Use gentle rocking motions to reduce exertion.
   Shifting your weight allows you to use your momentum to move the patient, which helps protect your back from injury.

10. **Repeat until the patient** is positioned near the head of the bed. If you used a plastic sheet to reduce friction, remove it now.
    Plastic is water impermeable, so it allows moisture to pool under the patient and creates a risk for impaired skin integrity.

11. **Straighten the drawsheet;** tuck it in tightly at the sides of the bed.
    A wrinkle-free sheet prevents uneven pressure, discomfort, and skin irritation.

12. **Place a pillow under** the patient's head; assist them to a comfortable position.
    Provides comfort and good body alignment.

13. **Place the bed in low position;** raise the side rail.
    Helps prevent falls.

14. **Place the call device** in a position where the patient can easily reach it.
    Allows patient to call for help, if needed.

Procedure Variation: Use of an Approved Mechanical Lifting Device

15. **Lock the bed wheels.** Lower the head of the bed; place the patient in a supine position. Position at least one nurse on each side of the bed. Lower the side rails. Raise the height of the bed to waist level.

16. **Using the drawsheet, turn** the patient to one side of the bed. Position the midline of the full body sling at the patient's back. Tightly roll the remaining half of the sling; tuck the fabric under the drawsheet. ▼

17. **With a second nurse positioned** on either side of the patient, use the drawsheet to turn the patient to the opposite side of the bed. Unroll the full body sling; reposition the patient supine.

CHAPTER 29 Physical Activity & Immobility 619

18. **Attach the sling** to the overbed lifting device or mechanical lift. Be sure the fasteners are securely attached to the lifting device.

19. **Engage the lift** to raise the patient completely off the bed. Advance the lift toward the head of the bed until the patient is at the desired level. ▶

20. **Lower the lift;** turn the patient to the desired position. You may leave the sling in place for future movement, or you may remove it by turning the patient from side to side.

    NOTE: If a full body sling is not available, use a friction-reducing device, such as a transfer roller sheet, and at least three staff members.

Procedure 29-1B ■ Turning a Patient in Bed

➤ When performing the procedure, always identify your patient according to agency policy, using two identifiers, and be attentive to standard precautions, hand hygiene, patient safety and privacy, body mechanics, and documentation.

➤ *Note:* This procedure describes the use of a transfer roller sheet. This device is inexpensive and readily available.

➤ *Note:* This procedure describes turning the patient by two nurses. With one nurse, some details differ.

Procedure Steps

1. **Lock the bed wheels.** Lower the head of the bed; place the patient in a supine position. Position one nurse on each side of the bed. Lower the side rail. Raise the height of the bed to waist level.
   Lowering the side rails and raising the bed allow you to move the patient while maintaining good body mechanics and working with gravity to prevent injury.

2. **Position the patient for turning.**
   a. Remove the pillow from under the patient's head and place it at the head of the bed.
   b. Stand as close as possible to the patient without twisting your back.
   c. Roll the patient side to side and place a friction-reducing device under the drawsheet. Smooth any wrinkles as needed. Tuck the friction-reducing device snugly under the mattress.

   Note: You can improvise this device by placing a large, clean plastic bag or plastic film under the drawsheet.

   d. Move the patient to the side of the bed you are turning them away from by rolling up the drawsheet close to the patient's body and pulling it.
   e. Align the patient's legs and head with the trunk.
   This allows you to position the patient in the center of the bed after turning. ▶

3. **Place the patient's near leg** and foot across the far leg (e.g., when turning the patient to their right, place their left leg over their right leg).

4. **Place the patient's near arm** (e.g., left when turning right) across their chest. Position the patient's underneath arm up and away from their body.
   Positioning the patient's legs and their near arm facilitates turning. Abducting and rotating the other arm prevent it from being caught under the patient during the turn.

5. **Each nurse positions their feet** with a wide base of support with one foot forward of the other. Bend from the hips; grasp both ends of the drawsheet at the level of the patient's hip and the other at the level of the shoulder.
   A wide base of support allows you to maintain good body mechanics while performing the move.

6. **Instruct the patient** that the turn will occur on the count of 3.
   Counting coordinates and facilitates patient cooperation with the move.

7. **On the count of 3, flex** your knees and hips and shift your weight. The nurse positioned on the side toward which the patient will turn shifts their weight to the back foot. The nurse on the opposite side shifts their weight forward. Move along the patient's side instead of reaching. Use gentle rocking motions to reduce exertion.
   Provides the best leverage to turn the patient. ▼

(continued on next page)

Procedure 29-1 ■ Moving and Turning Patients in Bed (continued)

8. **If a plastic film is used,** remove it after you turn the patient.

9. **Position the dependent shoulder** forward. Place pillows behind the patient's back and between legs to maintain the patient in the lateral position. Replace the pillow under the patient's head.
Positioning ensures that patient is not putting excess pressure on the inferior shoulder. Pillows help maintain good body alignment.
Refer to **Table 29-3: Positioning a Bed-Bound Patient,** in Volume 1.

10. **Place the bed in low position;** raise the side rail.
Helps ensure patient safety.

11. **Place the call device** in a position where the patient can easily reach it.
Allows patient to call for help, if needed.

Procedure 29-1C ■ Logrolling a Patient

➤ When performing the procedure, always identify your patient according to agency policy, using two identifiers, and be attentive to standard precautions, hand hygiene, patient safety and privacy, body mechanics, and documentation.

Procedure Steps

1. **Lock the bed wheels.** Lower the head of the bed with the patient supine. Lower the side rail on the side where you are standing but keep the opposite rail in the up position. Raise the height of the bed to waist level.
Lowering the side rail and raising the bed allow you to move the patient while maintaining good body mechanics and working with gravity to prevent back injury.

2. **You should already have** a drawsheet with an underlying friction-reducing device, such as a transfer roller sheet, to move the patient to the side of the bed on which you are standing. (You can improvise this device by placing a clean, unused plastic bag or plastic film under the drawsheet.)

3. **Position one staff member** at the patient's head and shoulders; they are responsible for moving the head and neck as a unit. Position the other person at the patient's hips. If you need three staff members, position one at the shoulders, one at the waist, and the third at thigh level. One staff member must maintain the patient's head and neck in alignment. The other members assist with moving the rest of the body in alignment. ➤

4. **Each nurse should position their** feet with a wide base of support with one foot slightly more forward than the other.
Facilitates proper body mechanics and minimizes risk of injury to staff members.

5. **Use the drawsheet** or transfer sheet to move the patient to the side of the bed on which the nurses are standing. The move must be smooth so that the patient's head and hips are kept in alignment. Position the patient's head with a pillow.
A transfer sheet maintains straight alignment of the spine.

6. **Instruct the patient to fold** their arms across their chest.

7. **Place a pillow** between the patient's knees.
A pillow prevents internal rotation of the hip and spine with movement. Maintains straight alignment of the spine.

8. **Raise the side rail;** move to opposite side of the bed.
Side rails keep the patient from falling out of bed.

9. **Lower the side rail** on the "new" side of the bed; face the patient. All nurses should position their feet with a wide base of support, with one foot forward of the other. Place your weight on the forward foot. Bend from the hips; position your hands evenly along the length of the drawsheet.
Provides the best leverage to turn the patient while maintaining spine alignment. ▼

10. **All nurses flex their knees** and hips and shift their weight to the back foot on the count of 3. Be sure to support the head as the patient is rolled to their side.
Allows you to maintain straight alignment and body mechanics while performing the move.

11. **Place pillows to maintain** the patient in the lateral position.
Refer to **Table 29-3: Positioning a Bed-Bound Patient,** in Volume 1.
A pillow provides support and maintains proper alignment.

12. **Place the bed in low position;** raise the side rail.

13. **Place the call device** in a position where the patient can easily reach it.
Allows patient to call for help, if needed.

? What if...

- **My facility has instituted a no-lift policy and I have to pull the patient up in bed?**

  Use assistive equipment, such as friction-reducing devices, mechanical lifts, air-powered mattresses, and/or lateral transfer devices, to help prevent work-related injuries.

- **My patient is obese or unable to assist (totally dependent) and I need to lift them?**

  Minimize manual lifting in all cases and eliminate it where feasible. Therefore, follow facility recommendations/protocols and use approved devices. You should be familiar with the lift devices in your facility.

- **The patient has had a total hip replacement and I have to turn or logroll the patient?**

  Maintain the affected leg in abduction by using a pillow or abduction wedge between the legs.
  To ensure the hip will not become dislocated during turning.

- **The patient has a cast or is in traction, and I have to turn or logroll the patient?**

  Designate a person to assist in the turning by guiding the affected extremity.

- **The patient has an external fixation device, and I have to turn or logroll the patient?**

  Secure the device in place to keep it from moving when lifting or moving the limb as needed.
  By holding on to the device to secure it and keep it from moving, there is less movement of the healing bone and therefore less trauma and pain.

Evaluation

- Assess the patient's comfort level after the position change.
- Assess body position and alignment after position change.
- Assess skin for pressure areas.

Patient Teaching

- Explain to the patient the importance of maintaining spine alignment.
- Explain to the patient the importance of frequent position changes.
- Instruct the patient to ask the nurse when she needs to be turned sooner than scheduled.
- Teach the patient how they can assist with moving and turning.

Home Care

- Instruct the family member or caregiver in the techniques for moving, turning, or logrolling the patient.
- Discuss the shearing effects on the skin from sliding down in bed (see Chapter 35).
- Provide instruction on importance of changing position and maintaining proper body alignment.

Documentation

Repositioning and turning patients are considered routine aspects of care and are not usually charted every time they are done. However, document in the nursing notes any problems with positioning the patient or any areas of skin breakdown. You might also chart turning as an intervention when charting a specific problem. For example, if the patient has impaired skin integrity, you might describe the skin and chart, "Position changed hourly." Some facilities have flowsheets on which you indicate by a checkmark each time a patient is repositioned.

Practice Resources

Centers for Disease Control and Prevention (2012, February); Collins, Nelson, & Sublet, (2006); National Institute for Occupational Safety and Health (NIOSH) (2023, March); Nelson, & Baptiste, (2006, March); Occupational Safety and Health Administration, U.S. Department of Labor (n.d.); Waters, et al (2009, November).

Thinking About the Procedure

The videos **Moving a Patient Up in Bed, Moving a Patient Up in Bed Using a Mechanical Lifting Device, Turning a Patient in Bed,** and **Logrolling a Patient,** along with questions and suggested responses, are available on the **Davis's** *Nursing Skills Videos* Web site at www.fadavis.com.

Procedure 29-2 ■ Transferring Patients

➤ For steps to follow in *all* procedures, refer to the Universal Steps for All Procedures on the inside back cover.

Equipment
- Nonlatex gloves, if you may be exposed to body fluids
- Transfer board (for transferring from bed to stretcher, and sometimes bed to chair)
- Pull or lift (draw) sheet (for transfers)
- Gait transfer belt (for dangling and transferring from bed to chair)

Delegation
You may ask unlicensed assistive personnel (UAP) to dangle, transfer a patient from bed to stretcher, or transfer a patient from bed to chair. Ensure that the UAP has the necessary skills and that the patient's condition is stable. Inform the UAP of any special considerations when dangling or transferring the patient and evaluate the patient after transfer.

Preprocedure Assessment
- Assess for any restrictions in movement or position by asking the patient and checking the provider's orders.
- Observe for the presence of equipment such as IV lines, drains, or catheters.
- Assess possible side effects of medications (e.g., dizziness and sedation). Assess the patient's level of consciousness, ability to follow directions, and ability to assist with the move.
- Assess the physical size of the patient and your own strength and ability to move the patient.
- Before transferring a patient to a chair, assess the patient's tolerance of dangling.
  The preceding assessments inform you about activity tolerance, readiness to get out of bed, and ability to participate in the transfer. They help you determine how many assistants you need, the appropriate transfer device, and how to proceed with the move while preventing injury and dislodging of equipment.
- Assess vital signs; monitor for postural hypotension (light-headedness when sitting or standing up quickly from a recumbent position).
  If the patient is at risk for postural hypotension, you may need to allow additional time for the patient to change position.
- Assess the patient's level of comfort using a standardized pain scale.
  If the patient is in pain, you may need to administer an analgesic before moving.

Procedure 29-2A ■ Transferring a Patient From Bed to Stretcher

➤ When performing the procedure, always identify your patient according to agency policy, using two identifiers, and be attentive to standard precautions, hand hygiene, patient safety and privacy, body mechanics, and documentation.

Procedure Steps

1. ✚ **Lock the wheels on the bed.** Position the bed so that it is flat (if the patient can tolerate being supine) and at the height of the stretcher.
   Locking the wheels ensures client safety during the transfer. Having the bed flat helps prevent injury to staff because the patient is easier to move.

2. **Lower the side rails** and position at least one nurse on each side of the bed. Move the patient to the side of the bed where the stretcher will be placed by rolling up the drawsheet close to the patient's body and pulling it toward the designated side. Align the patient's legs and head with their trunk.
   Position patient to enable nurses to move them to the stretcher.

3. **Position the stretcher** next to the bed. Lock the stretcher wheels.
   Locking the wheels keeps the stretcher from moving during the transfer; prevents falls.

4. **Place the transfer board** against the patient's back.
   a. Place a friction-reducing device, such as a transfer roller sheet, over the transfer board. (You can improvise this device by placing a clean, unused plastic bag or plastic film under the drawsheet.)
   b. The nurse on the side opposite the stretcher uses the drawsheet to turn the patient away from the stretcher, while the other nurse places the transfer board against the patient's back halfway between bed and stretcher. Turn the patient to their back and onto the transfer board.

   Safely positions the transfer board under the patient, without friction. ▼

5. **Ensure the patient's feet** and shoulders are over the edge of the transfer board.
   To prevent injury to the patient from the edge of the board.

CHAPTER 29 Physical Activity & Immobility   623

6. **Ask the patient to raise their head** if able. Use the drawsheet to slide them across the transfer board onto the stretcher.
   Facilitates the move to the stretcher; prevents friction on patient's skin.

Procedure Variation: If Transferring a Patient From Bed to Stretcher With a Slipsheet

A slipsheet may be used instead of a transfer board. A slipsheet is a large, low-friction fabric that facilitates transfer. ▼

7. **With the drawsheet, turn** the patient away from the bed; remove the board and roller sheet.

8. **Position the midline of the slipsheet** under the patient. Roll the remaining half tightly and tuck it under the patient.

9. **Turn the patient back over to the** side near to the stretcher and pull the slipsheet through from under the patient.

10. **Place the patient supine;** lower the side rail on the side where the stretcher will be placed.

11. **Move the stretcher** next to the bed and lock the wheels on the stretcher.

12. **Position at least two nurses** on the far side of the stretcher.

Using the slipsheet, pull the patient onto the stretcher. ▼

13. ✚ **Be sure the stretcher** wheels are locked and the side rails raised for patient safety.

14. **Place the call device in reach** of the patient or position the patient where they can be seen by staff members at all times.

Procedure 29-2B ■ Dangling a Patient at the Side of the Bed

➤ When performing the procedure, always identify your patient according to agency policy, using two identifiers, and be attentive to standard precautions, hand hygiene, patient safety and privacy, body mechanics, and documentation.

Procedure Steps

1. ✚ **Lock the bed wheels.** Place the patient in a supine position; raise the head of the bed to 90°. Keep the side rail elevated on the side opposite where you are standing.
   Locking the wheels prevents the bed from moving as you move the patient. Raising the head of the bed prepares the patient to be dangled and requires less effort from you to help the patient sit erect.

2. **Apply a gait transfer belt** to the patient at waist level. Be sure the belt is snug but not uncomfortable.

3. **Place the bed in the low position.**
   Ensures patient safety and proper body mechanics.

4. **Instruct the patient to bend** their knees and turn the patient onto their side, if possible, keeping knees flexed.
   Prepares the patient to be able to dangle their legs over side of bed.

5. **Stand at the side of the bed,** facing the patient and using a wide base of support. Place your foot closest to the head of the bed forward of the other foot. Lean forward, bending at the hips, with your knees flexed. Instruct the patient to use their arm to push off the bed.
   Allows you to maintain proper body mechanics and prevents injury. ▼

6. **Position your hands** on each side of the gait transfer belt.

7. **Rock onto your back foot** as you assist the patient toward you with the gait transfer belt, thereby moving the patient into a sitting position at the side of the bed.
   Uses your body weight as leverage to reposition the patient preventing injury to your back. ▼

8. ✚ **Stay with the patient** as they dangle. Reassess comfort level and for dizziness.
   Helps prevent falls.

(continued on next page)

Procedure 29-2 ■ Transferring Patients (continued)

Procedure 29-2C ■ Transferring a Patient From Bed to Chair

▶ When performing the procedure, always identify your patient according to agency policy, using two identifiers, and be attentive to standard precautions, hand hygiene, patient safety and privacy, body mechanics, and documentation.

Procedure Steps

1. ✚ **Position the chair** next to the bed. If possible, lock the chair.
   Prevents the chair from moving during transfer. Ensures patient safety.

2. ✚ **Put nonskid footwear** on the patient.
   Prevents the patient from slipping during transfer.

3. ✚ **Place the bed in a low position;** lock the bed wheels.
   Prevents the bed from moving during the transfer. Low position allows the patient to place feet firmly on the floor.

4. **Apply a transfer belt.**
   Facilitates transfer of the patient to the chair and helps prevent back injury to the nurse.

5. **Assist the patient to dangle** at the side of the bed (see Procedure 29-2B). Be sure the patient doesn't need support before releasing them.

6. **Stand toward the bed,** facing the patient. Brace your feet and knees against the patient's legs. Pay particular attention to any known weakness. Bend your hips and knees, and, keeping your back straight, hold on to the transfer belt on both sides. If two nurses are available to assist with the transfer, one nurse should be on each side of the patient.
   Bracing provides stability. Bending the hips and knees allows you to use the major muscle groups and limit the risk of injury. Lifting the patient at waist level prevents injury to the arm or shoulder. ▶

7. **Instruct the patient** to place their hands by their sides and help to push off the bed.
   Having the patient help to push off the bed reduces the risk of injury to your back or neck.

8. **Ask the patient to stand** as you move to an upright position by straightening your legs and hips.
   Straightening your thighs and hips uses your large muscle groups and prevents injury to your back.

9. **Allow the patient to steady** themselves for a moment. Ask if they are feeling light-headed.
   Provides the patient an opportunity to rest before further movement. Allows you to evaluate their tolerance of activity and ability to maintain an upright posture before continuing.

10. **Instruct the patient to pivot** and turn with you toward the chair.
    Pivoting helps prevent twisting and straining the patient's back muscles.

11. **Assist the patient to position** themselves in front of the chair. Have the patient flex their hips and knees, and as they lower themselves to the chair, reach for arms of the chair. Guide their motion while maintaining a firm hold on them and keeping your back straight.
    Maintains good body mechanics and balance and ensures patient safety. ▼

12. **Assist the patient** to a comfortable position in the chair.

13. **Provide a blanket** if needed for warmth or privacy.

14. **Place the call device in reach** of the patient or position the patient where they can always be seen by staff members.

❓ What if...

■ **The patient is obese?**
   If the patient is obese or unable to assist, use a full body sling that allows the patient to assume a seated position. You may also use a powered standing assist lift, if one is available.

- **The patient has had hip surgery (replacement or fracture repair)?**
  When assisting the patient out of bed, raise the bed to a position that is high enough to allow the patient to exit the bed without acute hip flexion.
  To avoid hip injury or dislocation.

- **The patient becomes dizzy during the transfer?**
  Return the patient to sitting or recumbent position and assess their vital signs.

- **The patient has a weaker side, for example, from a cerebrovascular accident (CVA) or surgical procedure?**
  Instruct the patient to exit the bed from their unaffected side. Stand on the patient's weaker side.
  The stronger side should lead a transfer.

Evaluation
- Assess the level of patient participation in the transfer.
- Assess the patient's comfort level during the transfer and in the new position.
- Assess proper body position and alignment after the patient's position change.
- Assess the patient's vital signs for postural hypotension after dangling or transferring to a chair.

Patient Teaching
- Explain the importance of frequent position changes and getting out of bed to avoid complications of immobility.

Home Care
- Instruct the family member or caregiver in the proper technique for assisting the client to dangle at the bedside or transfer to a chair.
- Provide instruction in the importance of changing position and maintaining proper body alignment.

Documentation
Patients are usually moved to a stretcher for transport to a test or procedure. The movement is a routine aspect of care and is not documented. When dangling or transferring a patient to a chair, document in the nursing notes how much assistance was required, the use of assistive devices, any problems with positioning the patient, how long the patient was out of bed, and how the patient tolerated the activity.

Practice Resources
Centers for Disease Control and Prevention (CDC) (2012); Collins, Nelson, & Sublet, (2006); National Institute for Occupational Safety and Health (NIOSH) (2013); Nelson, & Baptiste, (2006); Occupational Safety and Health Administration, U.S. Department of Labor (n.d.); Waters, et al. (2009).

Thinking About the Procedure

> The videos **Transferring a Patient From Bed to Stretcher, Dangling a Patient at the Side of the Bed,** and **Transferring a Patient From Bed to Chair,** along with questions and suggested responses, are available on the Davis's *Nursing Skills Videos* Web site at www.fadavis.com.

Procedure 29-3 ■ Assisting With Ambulation

> For steps to follow in *all* procedures, refer to the Universal Steps for All Procedures on the inside back cover.

Equipment
- Nonlatex gloves if you may be exposed to body fluids
- Transfer belt
- Nonskid footwear

Delegation
You may ask unlicensed assistive personnel (UAP) to assist with ambulation. Ensure that the UAP has the necessary skills, and that the patient's condition is stable. Inform the UAP of any special considerations when assisting a patient with ambulation and evaluate the patient after the activity.

Pre-Procedure Assessment
- Assess for any restrictions in movement or position by asking the patient and checking the provider's orders.
- Observe for the presence of equipment such as IV lines, drains, or catheters.
- Assess possible side effects of medications (e.g., dizziness and sedation).
- Assess the patient's level of consciousness, ability to follow directions, and ability to assist with the move.
- Assess the physical size of the patient and your own strength and ability to move the patient.

(continued on next page)

Procedure 29-3 ■ Assisting With Ambulation (continued)

- Assess the patient's tolerance when dangling before beginning to ambulate.
  The preceding assessments inform you about activity tolerance, readiness to get out of bed, and ability to participate in the transfer. They help you determine how many assistants you need, the appropriate transfer device, and how to proceed with the move while preventing injury and dislodging of equipment.

- Assess vital signs; monitor for postural hypotension.
  If the patient is at risk for postural hypotension, you may need to allow additional time for the patient to change position and plan for adequate help.

- Assess the patient's level of comfort using a standardized pain scale.
  If the patient is uncomfortable, you may need to administer an analgesic before moving.

- Assess for factors that may increase the risk of falls (age, muscle weakness, chronic disease, gait disturbance).
  Identifies patients at risk.

Procedure 29-3A ■ Assisting With Ambulation (One Nurse)

▶ When performing the procedure, always identify your patient according to agency policy, using two identifiers, and be attentive to standard precautions, hand hygiene, patient safety and privacy, body mechanics, and documentation.

Procedure Steps

1. **Put nonskid footwear** on the patient.
   Prevents the patient from slipping while transferring and ambulating.

2. **Apply the transfer belt.**
   Allows you to safely support the patient during the transfer and ambulation.

3. **Place the bed in a low position;** lock the bed.
   Prevents the bed from moving during transfer. Makes it easier for the patient's feet to reach the floor.

4. **Assist the patient to dangle** at the side of the bed (see Procedure 29-2B if you need to review).

5. **Face the patient.** Brace your feet and knees against the patient's feet and knees. Pay particular attention to any known weakness. Bend your hips and knees; hold on to the transfer belt.
   Bracing provides stability of the patient's legs. Bending the hips and knees allows you to use the major muscle groups and limit injury. Lifting at the patient's waist level prevents injury to their arm or shoulder.

6. **Instruct the patient** to place their arms around you between the shoulders and waist (the location depends on your height and the height of the patient). Ask the patient to stand as you move to an upright position by straightening your legs and hips.
   Having the patient hold you on your trunk prevents injury to your neck. Straightening your thighs and hips uses your large muscle groups and promotes good body mechanics.

7. **Allow the patient to steady** themselves for a moment.
   Allows the patient an opportunity to rest before further movement and to regain equilibrium before walking.

8. **Stand at the patient's side,** placing both hands on the transfer belt. If the patient is weak on one side, position yourself on the weaker side.
   By standing on the weaker side, the patient is freer to reach with the stronger arm and grip wall or bed rails with their strong-side hand and use the stronger side for strength and balance. This position also keeps you clear of a cane or other assistive device, which would be used on the strong side, and allows you to support the weaker side to prevent the patient from falling. ▼

9. **Slowly guide the patient** forward. Observe for signs of fatigue or dizziness.
   Helps prevent falls.

10. **If the patient has an IV pole,** ask them to hold on to the pole on the side where you are standing. Assist the patient to advance the pole as you ambulate. Be sure the patient does not rely on the pole for support.
    Provides a grip for the patient and positions the IV pole near you so that you can assist the patient to move the pole. ▼

Procedure 29-3B ■ Assisting With Ambulation (Two Nurses)

➤ When performing the procedure, always identify your patient according to agency policy, using two identifiers, and be attentive to standard precautions, hand hygiene, patient safety and privacy, body mechanics, and documentation.

Procedure Steps

1. ✚ **Put nonskid footwear** on the patient.
   Prevents the patient from slipping during the transfer and ambulation.

2. ✚ **Apply the transfer belt.**
   Allows you to support the patient during transfer and ambulation.

3. ✚ **Place the bed in low position;** lock the bed.
   Prevents the bed from moving during transfer and prevents the patient from falling.

4. **Assist the patient to dangle** at the side of the bed (see Procedure 29-2B, as needed).

5. **Each nurse should stand facing** the patient on opposite sides of the patient. Brace your feet and knees against the patient, paying particular attention to any known weakness. Bend from the hips and knees and hold on to the transfer belt.
   Bracing provides stability. Bending the hips and knees allows you to use the major muscle groups and limit injury. Lifting at the patient's waist level prevents injury to their arm or shoulder.

6. **Instruct the patient to place** their arms around each of you between the shoulders and waist (the location depends on your height and the height of the patient). Ask the patient to stand as both of you move to an upright position by straightening your legs and hips.

7. **Allow the patient to steady** themselves for a moment.
   Allows the patient an opportunity to rest before further movement and to regain equilibrium. Allows you to evaluate the patient's tolerance for activity and ability to maintain an upright posture before ambulating.

8. **Both nurses stand at** the patient's sides, grasping hold of the transfer belt. If no belt is available, the nurses grasp each other's arms at the patient's waist.
   Helps patient maintain an erect posture. ▼

9. **Slowly guide the patient forward.** Observe for signs of fatigue or dizziness.
   Ensures client safety.

10. **If the patient has an IV pole,** one nurse advances the IV pole along the side of the patient by holding the pole with the outside hand. Remind the patient not to use the IV pole for support.
    Positions the IV pole out of the path of the patient. Because the IV pole is on rollers, it will not support the patient if he starts to fall.

? What if...

■ **The patient has a weaker side (e.g., from a stroke or musculoskeletal injury)?**

If the patient has weakness on one side, provide additional support but allow them to use that side as they are able.
This will force them to use their weaker side.

Evaluation
- Assess the level of patient participation in the transfer.
- Assess patient comfort with ambulation.
- Assess posture and base of support.
- Assess vital signs for postural hypotension.

Patient Teaching
- Instruct the patient to inform you if they feel dizzy or weak.
- Explain the importance of ambulation to prevent complications of immobility.

Home Care
- Teach family members or caregivers how to assist the patient with ambulation.
- Provide instruction on importance of ambulation.

Documentation
Document in the nursing notes how much assistance was required, any problems with ambulation, and the distance walked.

Sample Documentation
00/00/0000   0630   Pt assisted to ambulate to doorway in room. Required minimal assistance from one nurse. Placed in chair for 30 min and then assisted back to bed. Required maximum assist from two nurses to return to bed. ———————————————— B. Bowen, RN

Practice Resources
Centers for Disease Control and Prevention (2012, February); National Institute for Occupational Safety and Health (NIOSH) (2013); National Institute for Occupational Safety and Health (NIOSH), Centers for Disease

(continued on next page)

Procedure 29-3 ■ Assisting With Ambulation (continued)

Control and Prevention (CDC). (2018); Nelson, Baptiste, (2006, March); Occupational Safety and Health Administration, U.S. Department of Labor (n.d.); Waters, et al. (2009).

Thinking About the Procedure

The videos **Assisting With Ambulation (One Nurse)** and **Assisting With Ambulation (Two Nurses)**, along with questions and suggested responses, are available on the **Davis's Nursing Skills Videos** Web site at www.fadavis.com.

CLINICAL INSIGHTS

Clinical Insight 29-1 ▶ Applying Principles of Body Mechanics

Principles of body mechanics are the rules that enable you to move your body without causing injury. Use the following guidelines to decrease the risk of back and other injuries. Teach them to your patients as well.

The American Nurses Association (n. d.) states you should use mechanical equipment (e.g., lift, transfer sheet) or get assistance for lifting and transferring whenever possible. Do not rely on body mechanics alone to prevent injury.

Account for Patient Factors

Patient lifting, transfer, and movement is based on:
- **Patient dependency levels.** Select equipment after determining the patient's ability to assist in the transfer. Categories include total dependence, extensive dependence, partial assistance, supervision required, independence.
- **Weight and size of patients.** Ensure proper equipment and assistive staff are available.
- **Environmental constraints.** Low ceilings may not allow for installation of overhead lifts. Room configuration with an L-shape may prevent use of certain types of lifts. Structural support in the ceiling is necessary for installation of lift tracts. Width of doors and hallways may dictate equipment for safe maneuvering.
- **Type of patient handling and movement equipment available.** Sit-to-stand lifts, floor-based sling lifts, ceiling-lifts, inflatable devices, safety equipment for staff.
- **Tasks for patient handling, movement, and mobility.**
  - **Vertical and lateral transfers** to and from a bed, chair, stretcher, toilet/bedside commode, wheelchair).
  - **Weighing** patients on bed scales
  - **Showering** or bed bath
  - **Lifting** off the mattress for linen change or daily patient care
  - **Repositioning in bed** (side to side or up to the head of the bed) or in a chair

Make Use of Inanimate Objects and Get Help When Possible

- **Raise the height of the bed and over-the-bed table to waist level** when you are working with a patient.

- **Get help to move a heavy object** or patient. Assess the object or patient you are going to lift. If you have any doubt that you can do it by yourself, get help from a coworker.
- **Use assistive devices at all times** to limit the risk of back and musculoskeletal injury.
- **Maintain competency** in using all assistive and transfer devices.

Use Your Body Correctly

- **Use a wide base of support** (feet apart).
- **Minimize bending and twisting.** These movements increase the stress on the back. Instead, face the object or person, and bend at the hips or squat.
- **Squat to lift heavy objects** from the floor. (Squatting lowers your center of gravity.) Push against the strong hip and thigh muscles to raise yourself to a standing position. Avoid bending at the waist.
- **Use the muscles in your legs** as the power for lifting. Bend your knees, keep your back straight, and lift smoothly. Repeat the same movements for setting the object down.
- **Keep objects close to your body** when you lift, move, or carry them. The closer an object is to the center of gravity, the greater the stability and the less strain on the back.
- **Use both hands and arms** when you lift, move, or carry heavy objects.
- **Do not stand on tiptoes to reach** an object. If you must use a ladder or stepstool to reach for an object, make sure it is stable and adequate to position your body close to the object.
- **Push, slide, or pull heavy objects** whenever possible rather than lifting.
- **Maintain a good grip** on the patient or object you are moving before attempting to move it.
- **When possible, keep your elbows bent** when you carry an object.
- **Work with smooth and even movements.** Avoid sudden or jerky motions.

Clinical Insight 29-2 ➤ Performing Passive Range-of-Motion Exercises

Passive range of motion (PROM) is the movement of the joints through their full range of motion by another person. Nurses frequently perform PROM to maintain joint mobility. Refer to Table 29-1.

- **Explain the purpose of PROM.** You may teach family members and caregivers about the importance of ROM exercises and ask for their help in exercising the patient when they visit.
- **Observe the patient as you perform PROM.** You may need to perform the exercises in several short segments if the patient tires easily or has discomfort.
- **Support the patient's limb** above and below the joint that is to be exercised.
- **Move the joint in a slow, smooth, rhythmic manner.** Avoid fast movements; they may cause muscle spasm.
- **Never force a joint.** Some patients may have limited ROM. Move each joint to the point of resistance. This should not be painful.
- **Perform PROM** at least twice daily. Move each joint through ROM 3 to 5 times with each session. Consider incorporating PROM into care activities, for example, while bathing or turning the patient.
- **Return the joint to a neutral position** when exercise is complete.
- **Encourage active exercise** whenever possible.

Thinking About the Procedure

The video **Performing Passive Range-of-Motion Exercises,** along with questions and suggested responses, is available on the **Davis's *Nursing Skills Videos*** Web site at www.fadavis.com.

Clinical Insight 29-3 ➤ Assisting With Physical Conditioning Exercises to Prepare for Ambulation

Patients who have been confined to bed for more than a week or who have sustained major injury require conditioning before they are able to resume walking. Conditioning exercises include the following.

Quadriceps and Gluteal Drills

- Ask the patient to tighten their thigh muscles by pushing downward with their knees and flexing their feet. Each leg may be done separately if moving both is contraindicated.
- Ask the patient to hold the position for a count of 5 and then relax.
- Repeat this process 2 or 3 times per hour during the waking hours.
- To exercise the gluteal muscles, ask the patient to pinch their buttocks together.
- Do this exercise when the patient exercises their quadriceps muscles.
- Instruct the patient not to hold their breath as they exercise.

Arm Exercises

- Install a trapeze bar on the patient's bed. Ask the patient to do pull-ups on the bar from a lying position. This exercises the biceps muscles.
- To exercise the triceps muscles, ask the patient to lift their upper body off the mattress by firmly pressing down with the palms.
- The patient can also do push-ups from a seated position at the side of the bed or from a stationary chair or wheelchair.

Dangling

- Dangling is a seated position at the side of the bed, feet resting on the floor.
- Provide a footstool if the patient's feet do not reach the floor.
- Assess for light-headedness or postural hypotension.
- Do not progress to ambulation until the patient is comfortable and stable in the dangling position.

Daily Activities

- Encourage your patient to be active in bed by repositioning and turning themselves.
- Encourage the patient to get out of bed and into a chair before attempting to walk.
- Encourage the patient to perform as many of their activities of daily living (ADLs) as possible.
- ADLs exercise many of the muscle groups used in ambulation.

Clinical Insight 29-4 ➤ Teaching Patients to Use Walking Aids

Canes

Sizing Canes
- Ask the patient to stand erect; place the cane tip 20 cm (4 in.) to the side of the foot.
- The top of the cane should reach the top of the hip joint so that the patient can hold the cane with their elbow flexed 30°.

Teaching Patients to Use Canes Safely
- Hold the cane on the stronger side.
- Distribute weight evenly between the feet and cane.
- Advance the cane and weaker leg simultaneously, then bring the stronger leg through.
- Avoid leaning over or on the cane.
- Maintain the integrity of the rubber tip for traction.

Walkers

Sizing Walkers
- Ask the patient to stand erect, holding on to the walker.
- The walker should extend from the floor to the hip joint so that the patient can comfortably hold the walker with 30° flexion of the elbow.

Teaching Patients to Use Walkers Safely
- Stand between the back legs of the walker. Do not stand too far behind the walker.
- Pick up the walker and advance it as you step ahead. Do not advance it so far as to lose balance.
- If one leg is weaker, move it forward as the walker moves forward.
- Do not slide the walker (unless it has wheels).

Crutches

Sizing Crutches
- Ask the patient to lie down wearing the nonskid shoes that she will use when walking.
- Measure the distance between the heel and the anterior fold of the axilla, then add 2.5 cm (1 in.).
- Select a crutch that can be adjusted to this height.
- Have the patient stand; position the crutch tip 10 to 15 cm (4 to 6 in.) to the side of the heel. Adjust the axillary crutch pad three fingerbreadths below the axilla.
- Adjust the handgrips so that the patient can comfortably grasp the bar while the elbow is slightly flexed. The patient's axilla should not rest on the crutch pad.

Teaching Patients to Use Crutches Safely
- When first teaching crutch walking, instruct the patient to stand near a wall with a chair behind them. Help the patient to stand and grip the crutches. Ask the patient to sway from side to side on the crutches to become accustomed to weight bearing by the arms.
- *Tripod position* is the basic crutch gait standing position. Place crutches 15 cm (6 in.) in front of the feet, with the crutch point 15 cm from the patient's center. In this position, a triangle is formed by the crutches and the body.
- Five crutch gaits exist (see accompanying chart): 2-point gait, 3-point gait, 4-point gait, swing-to gait, and swing-through gait.

✜ To teach the patient how to go up and down stairs, instruct them to lead with the unaffected leg when going up the stairs and to lead with the affected leg when going down the stairs.

Navigating stairs with crutches can be dangerous. When possible, have the patient practice this technique before discharge. When having a patient practice, the nurse should always stand below the patient on the stairs to prevent falling.

Clinical Insight 29-4 ▶ Teaching Patients to Use Walking Aids—cont'd

NOTE: **Read this table from bottom to top.**

2-Point gait	3-Point gait	4-Point gait	Swing to	Swing through
• Partial weight bearing, both feet; faster, but less support than a 4-point gait	• Non-weight bearing; faster than a 4-point gait; can use with walker	• Partial weight bearing, both feet; patient must shift weight constantly	• Weight bearing, both feet; can use with walker	• Weight bearing; requires the most coordination and balance
4. Advance right foot and left crutch	4. Advance right foot	4. Advance right foot	4. Lift both feet; swing them forward, landing feet next to the crutches	4. Lift both feet; swing them forward, landing feet in front of the crutches
3. Advance left foot and right crutch	3. Advance left foot and both crutches	3. Advance left crutch	3. Advance both crutches	3. Advance both crutches
2. Advance right foot and left crutch	2. Advance right foot	2. Advance left foot	2. Lift both feet; swing them forward, landing feet next to the crutches	2. Lift both feet; swing them forward, landing feet in front of the crutches
1. Advance left foot and right crutch	1. Advance left foot and both crutches	1. Advance right crutch	1. Advance both crutches	1. Advance both crutches
Tripod position	Tripod position	Tripod position	Tripod position	Tripod position

Crutch gaits. The shaded area represents weight bearing. The arrow shows movement.

ASSESSMENT GUIDELINES AND TOOLS

Focused Assessment

Assessing Activity and Exercise

Suggested History Questions

Usual Activity

Describe your typical daily activity level.

If the patient has very restricted activity, ask the following questions:
- Are you able to care for yourself regarding hygiene, dressing, toileting, and getting out of bed?
- If the patient has ADL limitations: Who helps you with these daily activities?

If the patient does not indicate restricted activity, ask the following questions:
- What is your usual form of exercise?
- How often do you exercise?
- How long are your exercise sessions?
- How long have you been engaged in this type of activity?
- What types of exercise or sports have you participated in previously?
- Describe your activity level over the past 10 years.
- Are you exercising more or less than in the past?
- What factors have changed your activity level?

Fitness Goals

What aspects of exercise do you enjoy? What aspects of exercise do you dislike?

What do you think are the benefits of exercise?

How do you schedule your exercise?

What motivates you to exercise?

What are your current fitness goals?

Mobility Concerns

Do you have any pain or discomfort with activity?

Do you avoid any activities because of pain, discomfort, shortness of breath, or chest pain?

If the patient answered yes to either question, describe the following:
- Type of problem
- Onset of concern
- Frequency of problem
- Activities that trigger and relieve
- Severity and type of symptoms
- Effect of problem on day-to-day activities
- Treatments used to alleviate and how they worked

Underlying Health Concerns

Do you have any healthcare problem that affects your ability to engage in activity or exercise?

If so, describe the problem and the effect.

What medications do you take?

Have you ever been told you have a bone problem? If so, what was the nature of the problem?

Have you ever had a fracture, strain, or sprain? If so, where was the problem? When did it occur? How did it occur?

Have you ever had weakness of the muscles or problems coordinating movement?

Do you have any cardiac or respiratory problems that affect your ability to perform activities?

Have you ever had anxiety or depression that affected your ability to participate in activities?

Lifestyle

What kind of work do you do?

Describe your typical work activities.

How many hours per week do you work?

What other commitments do you have (school, family, other obligations)?

External Factors

Are there any restrictions in your home that limit your ability to be active?

Do you feel you need an assistive device?

Are you comfortable exercising outside your home or in your neighborhood?

Focused Physical Assessments for Activity and Body Alignment

With the patient standing, observe from the anterior, posterior, and lateral views. Check for the following:

Shoulders and hips are level.

Toes are pointed forward.

The spine is straight, with no abnormal curvatures noted.

The posture is not slumped.

Ask the patient to sit down; observe as they do so.

Do they have difficulty lowering their torso?

Can they control the movement?

Are they able to get into this position with ease?

When they sit, do they slump?

If the patient cannot stand or sit, assess their alignment in bed. Look for ability to move in bed, as well as the posture the patient maintains.

Assessing Activity and Exercise—cont'd

Joint Function

Assessing joint function includes inspection and palpation of the joints and assessment of range of motion.

Begin your assessment at the neck and systematically work your way through each of the joints.

At each joint observe for swelling, erythema, asymmetry, or obvious deformity.

Compare the size of the muscles above and below the joint and on each side of the body.

Palpate the joint for temperature and crepitus. Warmth over a joint indicates inflammation or infection. Be sure to compare body temperature over several joints and right to left. **Crepitus** is a grating sensation with movement of a joint. It can often be heard as well as felt. Crepitus is associated with degenerative joint disease or arthritic changes in the joint.

As you palpate the joint, move it through its range of motion.

Muscle Strength

Assess muscle strength by having the patient push and then pull against your hands.

Start at the neck; test the strength of all major joints' range of motion.

To see a nurse using a performing passive range-of-motion exercise,

> The video **Performing Passive Range-of-Motion Exercises,** along with questions and suggested responses, is available on the **Davis's** *Nursing Skills Videos* Web site at www.fadavis.com.

Gait

Gait is divided into two phases: stance and swing.

Stance—In the stance phase, the heel of one foot strikes the ground while the opposite foot pushes off and leaves the ground.

Swing—In the swing phase, the leg from behind moves in front of the body. When the right leg is in stance mode, the left leg is in swing mode.

You must observe the patient walking. Normal gait includes the following features:

- Head is erect, gaze forward.
- Heel strikes the ground before the toe.
- Opposite arm moves forward at the same time.
- Feet are dorsiflexed in the swing phase.
- Gait is coordinated and rhythmic.
- Weight is evenly distributed, with minimal swing from side to side.
- Movement starts and stops with ease.
- Movement is at a moderate pace.

If the patient uses an assistive device, such as a cane, crutch, or walker, pay attention to how they use it. Ask the patient to ambulate a short distance with and without the device to determine whether the device is providing stability.

Activity Tolerance

Assess and record vital signs before having the patient engage in 3 minutes of activity.

Select an activity appropriate for the patient. For example, if the patient uses a walker, ask the patient to walk down the hallway. For a patient without obvious health limitations, consider asking them to run in place for 3 minutes.

Observe the patient throughout the exercise. If they show any signs of distress, stop the exercise, immediately take a set of vital signs, and repeat the vital signs every minute until they have returned to baseline.

If the patient can exercise continuously for 3 minutes, assess the patient at the end of the 3-minute period and at 1-minute intervals. Note the change in heart rate, blood pressure, and respiratory rate.

This type of approach is not appropriate for patients who easily become short of breath, develop chest pain, or are very unsteady on their feet. Instead, for example, limit your assessment to determining the amount of assistance the patient needs to turn in bed or get out of bed.

Muscle Mass and Strength

As you observe the patient, compare muscle mass on the right and left sides. If you notice an obvious discrepancy in size, measure the circumference of the limbs and compare.

To assess strength, ask the patient to push against your hand with the hands and feet. Once again, compare both sides.

For guidelines for assessing mobility in the home,

> See the **Chapter 29, Home Care box, Home Assessment for a Patient With Mobility Concerns,** in Volume 1.

CLINICAL REASONING
Applying the Full-Spectrum Nursing Model

PATIENT SITUATION

Mr. Ronald Ornduff is a 72-year-old retired man who lives with his wife in a one-story home. He has excellent general health with no significant health problems. Ronald typically walks with a moderate to vigorous pace in his neighborhood or at the local mall in the winter. He belongs to a health club and works out two or three times a week, walking on the treadmill, using the weight machines, or taking a basic conditioning class. Ronald considers himself fit and of an acceptable weight for his age. When going outdoors to pick up the morning paper, he slipped on a patch of ice and fell. You are now caring for him 2 days after hip surgery. He has pain and seems fearful his injury could be the beginning of a decline in his health.

THINKING

1. *Theoretical Knowledge:*

   a. Based on Mr. Ornduff's age, physical condition, and activity level, make a rough estimate of the number of minutes per week of physical activity he should have after he recovers from surgery and resumes full mobility. What are the benefits of this physical activity?

   b. As a nurse planning the care for a patient after hip surgery, what complications of immobility should you assess for?

2. *Critical Thinking (Considering Alternatives):* What are some possible barriers for an older adult's participation in physical activity? What might you teach your patient to do to overcome those barriers?

DOING

3. *Practical Knowledge:*

   a. How might you position your patient after hip surgery?

   b. What equipment would you need to position your patient after surgery? Is there anything you can set up that will help your patient move around in bed when he can tolerate it?

   c. What type of physical activity would you recommend Mr. Ornduff incorporate into his exercise plan after he recovers fully from his surgery? What benefit will these exercises provide?

4. *Nursing Process (Diagnosis):* Write at least two nursing diagnoses for Mr. Ornduff. Use just the data provided in the situation. Assume he is 2 days postop.

CARING

5. *Self-Knowledge:* What would you be feeling if you were in Mr. Ornduff's situation of being physically fit one day and suffering pain and immobility the next?

6. *Ethical Knowledge:* What are one or two things you would do to help Mr. Ornduff feel cared for and cared about?

Critical Thinking and Clinical Judgment

1. In Volume 1, you were introduced (Meet Your Patient) to Helen Jillian, a 72-year-old woman with hypertension, high cholesterol levels, and chest pain. She is 5 ft 1 in. tall and weighs 340 pounds. Ms. Jillian is admitted to the hospital for another episode of chest pain. You are assigned to care for her. Her provider has ordered her to be out of bed in the chair at least twice daily and to ambulate every day. How will you safely move this patient from bed to chair and assist her with ambulation? Work through that decision by answering the following questions.

    a. What aspects of this situation require the most careful attention (what are the risks; what could go wrong)?

    b. What steps can you take to prevent those difficulties?

2. Ms. Jillian is refusing to get out of bed. "I'm sick," she tells you. "If you make me get out of bed, I'll probably have chest pain." How would you respond to this statement?

3. Vince Fulk is an 85-year-old man who sustained a massive cerebrovascular accident (stroke). He is unresponsive and immobile. What activity or mobility interventions should you incorporate into his plan of care? What is your rationale for these interventions?

4. For each of the following concepts, use critical thinking to describe how or why it is important to nursing, patient care, or activity and exercise. Note that these are *not* to be merely definitions.

    Body mechanics   Activity tolerance

    Exercise   Assistive devices

    Immobility

What Are the Main Points in This Chapter?

- The skeletal system includes bones, cartilage, ligaments, and tendons. The skeleton forms the framework of the body and protects the internal organs.
- Movement depends on the interaction between the skeleton and the muscles. The ligaments, tendons, and cartilage serve as the interface between these two systems.
- Contraction of skeletal muscles causes the muscles to shorten, thus causing the bones to move at the joints.
- There are four natural curves to the spine. Proper posture maintains these natural curves in good alignment.
- In the human body, the center of gravity is below the umbilicus at the top of the pelvis. The feet provide the base of support.
- Range of motion (ROM) is the degree of maximum movement at a joint. Active range of motion (AROM) is when the patient independently moves joints through flexion, extension, abduction, adduction, and circular rotation. Passive range of motion (PROM) is performed by another person when the patient is unable to do so for themselves.

- Principles of body mechanics are the rules that allow you to move your body with proper alignment, strength, and balance without causing injury.
- The U.S. Department of Health and Human Services recommends a minimum of 150 minutes per week of moderate-intensity, or 75 minutes per week of vigorous-intensity aerobic physical activity, or an equivalent combination of moderate- and vigorous-intensity aerobic physical activity.
- A well-rounded exercise program focuses on flexibility and balance, resistance training, and aerobic conditioning.
- Regular physical activity each week, sustained for months and years, can produce long-term health benefits. Strong evidence links regular physical activity with a lower risk for early death, heart disease, stroke, type 2 diabetes, hypertension, colon and breast cancers, and depression.
- Together with a healthy diet, regular physical activity aids in weight management, better heart and lung function and muscular fitness, fall prevention, and improved memory and mental clarity in older adults.

- People who are physically active tend to feel better and have more energy. Sleep quality is improved. And, overall, for many people, physical activity promotes a sense of optimism and positive self-esteem.
- Factors that influence activity and exercise level include developmental stage, health concerns, nutrition, lifestyle, attitudes, and external factors.
- Severe illness associated with prolonged immobilization causes physiological changes in almost every body system.
- A nursing history focused on activity and exercise assesses usual activity, commitment to fitness goals, mobility concerns, underlying health concerns and injuries, lifestyle, attitude of hardiness and persistence, and external factors.
- Physical assessment that is focused on activity and exercise examines the musculoskeletal system and activity tolerance. Important data include vital signs, height, weight, body mass index, body alignment, joint function, gait, and activity tolerance.
- Patients require a change of position at least every 2 hours to prevent pressure injury, muscle discomfort, damage to superficial nerves and blood vessels, or contractures.
- Range-of-motion exercises maintain joint mobility and limit the complications of immobility.
- Patients who have been confined to bed for more than a week or who have sustained major injury require ROM and muscle strength conditioning before they are able to resume walking.
- Canes, braces, walkers, and crutches promote stability for patients to walk independently and move safely.

Knowledge Map

CHAPTER 29 Physical Activity & Immobility

POSITIONING PATIENTS:
Why: prevents skin breakdown; contractions; discomfort
Ways to position:
- Fowler's
- Lateral
- Prone
- Sims
- Supine

Positioning devices:
- Adjustable beds; siderails
- Pillows
- Trapeze; footboard/foot cradle

MOVING PATIENTS:
In bed: Moving up in bed; turning; logrolling for spinal surgery/injury
Transfer out of bed: to stretcher or wheelchair
Assistive devices:
- Transfer board
- Mechanical lift
- Transfer roller or belt

PROMOTING ACTIVITY:
Performing range of motion:
- Active
- Passive

Assisting with ambulation:
- Assess readiness; patient condition
- Obtain assistance/equipment
- Physical conditioning prior to

Ambulation aids:
- Cane
- Walker
- Braces
- Crutches

PRINCIPLES GUIDING CARE
- Use lifting devices
- Get adequate help
- Use good body mechanics
- Assess pt size/restrictions
- Control pt pain; explain activity interventions
- Avoid friction

ACTIVITY AND EXERCISE

Eliminating → **HAZARDS OF IMMOBILITY:**
- Muscle atrophy; stiff joints
- Decreased respiration depth; pooling secretions; pneumonia/atelectasis
- Venous pooling; clotting; orthostatic hypotension
- Glucose intolerance; reduced muscle mass; stress response
- Constipation; flatus; ileus
- Urinary stasis; calculi
- Depression; anxiety; sleep disturbances; apathy

TYPES:
- Isometric
- Isokinetic
- Aerobic
- Anaerobic

PROGRAMS:
- Flexibility training
- Resistance training
- Aerobic conditioning

Promoting → ACTIVITY EXERCISE
Bones, Muscles, & Neurological Control

Diseases Affecting / *Factors Affecting* / *Body Mechanics* → **MOBILITY**

SPECIFIC DISEASES:
- M/S: hip dysplasia, scoliosis
- Bone formation: OI
- Joint mobility: arthritis
- Bone integrity: osteoporosis/osteomyelitis
- Trauma
- Neuro: SCI, MS

Factors Affecting:
- Developmental stage
- Nutritional status
- Lifestyle
- Stress
- Environmental/socioeconomic factors

COMPONENTS:
- Body alignment: posture; proper spinal curve position
- Balance: via alignment; line of gravity through center of gravity
- Coordination: neuromuscular pairing for smooth movement
- Joint mobility: ROM

CHAPTER 30

Sexual Health

STUDENT RESOURCES

The questions and exercises in Volume 2 allow you to practice the kind of thinking you will use as a full-spectrum nurse. Critical-thinking questions usually have more than one correct answer, so we do not provide "correct" answers for these features. Try to answer these questions yourself. It is more important to develop your nursing judgment than to just cover content. You will learn by discussing the questions with your peers. If you are still unsure, see the Davis Advantage chapter resources for suggested responses.

To explore learning resources for this chapter,

Go to www.DavisAdvantage.com and find:

Answers and Suggested Responses for all questions in this chapter
Concept Map
Knowledge Map
References and Bibliography

Key Concepts

Sexual dysfunction
Sexual health
Sexuality

Related Concepts

See the Concept Map on Davis Advantage.

Caring for the Williams Family

As you may recall, Stanley and Nadine Williams are raising their 3-year-old granddaughter, Kayla. Kayla has made friends with Kyrie, a little boy at preschool. Kayla has asked whether they can play together. Nadine works at the preschool and knows Kyrie and his family. She is unsure whether she should allow her granddaughter to play with Kyrie because Nadine is uncomfortable with the boy's family. Kyrie was conceived via artificial insemination and is being raised by a lesbian couple. His parents are open about the relationship and shared the conception information with Nadine voluntarily.

A. Nadine calls the clinic to speak with you. She explains the situation and asks you whether you think it would be a problem to allow the children to play together. She is concerned that being around this family may be a bad influence on Kayla. How would you respond?

B. Nadine remains concerned and presses you for more information. She is concerned that Kayla's knowledge that Kyrie is being raised by same-sex parents may "influence Kayla toward these types of relationships." How would you address her concerns?

C. Nadine admits that Stanley does not agree with her. "He told me that sexual orientation is genetic." How would you react to this statement?

Practical Knowledge
practical application

In this section you will find guidelines to assist you in assessing/recognizing cues and planning care/prioritizing hypotheses and generating solutions related to patients' sexual health.

CLINICAL INSIGHTS

Clinical Insight 30-1 ▸ Providing Care After Sexual Assault

- **Carefully collect information about the incident** and document findings in a fact-based manner, following your institution's protocol.
- **Be sensitive to the victim's fear, anxiety, and guilt** related to the event.
  Open discussion without communicating judgment or disapproval helps with fact finding for better care.
- **Assess the victim's emotional status**, including sexual identity, stress disorder, and risks for suicide and self-harm. Also discuss the potential for sexual and physical violence, including violence within relationships.
- **When collecting a nursing history on people from vulnerable populations (e.g., disabilities), be sure to screen for sexual violence.**
- **Administer prophylactic treatment** to patients who have been assaulted (vaginally, anally, or orally) to prevent sexually transmitted infections (STIs), such as chlamydia and gonorrhea. If there is a significant risk for HIV, prophylaxis may be prescribed within 72 hours of exposure.
- **Administer vaccines to prevent hepatitis B and human papillomavirus (HPV),** as prescribed and according to your agency's policy.
- **Administer emergency pregnancy prevention** (e.g., the "morning after" pill) to patients who have been vaginally assaulted even if penetration is uncertain, according to your agency's policy.
- **Document pregnancy status** with a urine or blood sample.
- **Teach follow-up care.** The victim should receive follow-up care within 1 week after the event to assess for healing of injuries and presence of STIs. If vaginal penetration occurred, advise the victim to obtain pregnancy testing again 2 weeks after the event.
- **Follow the current reporting requirements** for sexual assault in your state. Some states require reporting assault of children and adolescents, even if they do not consent to the reporting.
- **Know support services** available in your community for victims of abuse. Refer the victim to a sexual assault center for support, counseling, and additional information. Because of the long-term psychological and emotional consequences of sexual assault, most victims benefit from counseling.

Clinical Insight 30-2 ▸ Guidelines for Taking a Sexual History

- ♥ **iCare** ■ **Provide privacy.**
  - Usually it is not enough merely to pull the curtains around the bed. Ask others who may be able to overhear private conversation behind the curtain to leave the room.
  - Talk to the client alone.
  - In some situations, it is also beneficial to talk to the partners as a unit, with the consent of both.
- **Protect confidentiality.** Assure your client that information will not be shared with others, unless directly related to planning or delivering healthcare.
- **Be relaxed in your approach,** and allow the client time to fully answer your questions. Your manner and attitude are critical in putting the client at ease.
- **Make eye contact.** Do not act embarrassed or allow your body language to show your discomfort.
- **Avoid communication stoppers,** such as the following:
  - "I'm asking you these questions only because I have to."
  - "I know that you probably won't want to tell me, but …."
  - "You're not having any sexual problems, are you?"
- **Consider a more inviting opening:**
  - "Many people are embarrassed when asked questions about their sexuality, but whatever you tell me will remain confidential."
  - "Many people hesitate to talk about sexual problems. However, your sexual health is important to your overall health, and I would like to ask you a few questions about that."
- **Be aware of verbal and nonverbal cues** that indicate concerns. Many people will cloak their concerns in comments such as these: "I suppose that I won't need to worry about sexy lingerie any longer," or "Sex is for the young. I just have to accept that I'm sick and older now." Be careful that your response to such statements does not either negate or validate your patient's identity as a sexual being. Follow up with comments that encourage the client to provide more details (see Chapter 15 if you would like to review communication techniques).
- **Realize the client may be embarrassed.** If the client is uncomfortable discussing topics about their own sexual health, reassure them by letting them know that some information, because of its private nature, may be difficult to discuss but is important.
- **Encourage your client to use terminology that they are comfortable with.**
- **Help the client feel comfortable.** Consider statements such as the following:
  - "Most people wonder how this surgery [or illness] may affect their sexual functioning."
  - "Whenever these medications are suggested, there are questions about sexual side effects."
  - "Have you thought about the kinds of adaptations you may have to make in your sex life after this surgery/treatment/illness?"
- **Begin with a less sensitive topic** such as "When was your last menstrual period?" or "How is your relationship with your partner [spouse]?" Then you can move into more sensitive areas: "Many older female patients have some vaginal dryness that creates discomfort during intercourse. Do you have any concerns about this?"

Clinical Insight 30-3 ➤ Teaching Your Patient to Use a Condom

Using Male Condoms

The male condom is a sheath that covers the penis during sexual activity.
- Put the condom on before the penis touches the vagina, mouth, or anus.
- Inspect the package to ensure that the condom has not been damaged.
- Open the package without tearing the condom.
- Squeeze out the air at the tip of the condom, and unroll it over the erect penis, leaving some space at the tip to collect the ejaculate.
- After sex, to avoid breaking the condom, hold the condom at the rim as the penis is withdrawn. Discard the condom. Wash your hands.
- Use a new condom if you want to have sex again.

Using Female Condoms

The female condom is a plastic pouch that fits inside the vagina so that all vaginal tissue is protected from contact with the penis. The condom is inserted with the inner ring placed high in the vagina near the cervix and the outer ring on the labia.
- Insert the condom before the penis touches the vagina.
- Inspect the package to ensure that the condom has not been damaged.
- Open the package without tearing the condom.
- Put the inner ring and pouch inside the vagina.
- Push the inner ring as far into the vagina as it will go.
- Ensure that the outer ring stays outside the vagina.
- If needed, add lubricant to the inside of the condom.
- After sex, gently pull out the condom and discard.

Do
- Use latex condoms unless you or your partner are allergic to latex, or use polyurethane condoms.
- Treat condoms gently, and keep them out of the sun.
- Use only water-based lubricants to reduce friction and prevent tearing.
- Check the expiration date of the condom and packaging. Old condoms may be brittle and more likely to break.

Don't
- Don't store condoms in your wallet or other place where body heat can break down the latex.
- Don't use fingernails or teeth to open the condom wrapper; doing so can tear the condom.
- Don't reuse a condom.
- Don't use lotions or oils with condoms; these may cause breakage.

TABLES

Methods of Contraception

CONTRACEPTION METHOD	ADVANTAGES	DISADVANTAGES
Abstinence—No sexual intercourse	100% effective Cost free	Lack of sexual expression May create stress in relationship
Fertility awareness (natural family planning, rhythm method)—Intercourse only during the infertile phase of the menstrual cycle	Cost free May be consistent with religious teachings No physical side effect	Requires cooperation of both partners Menstrual cycle must be regular Relatively high failure rate; pregnancy may result No protection against STIs
Withdrawal (coitus interruptus)—Removal of the penis from the vagina before ejaculation	Cost free	Requires discipline and mutual cooperation Preejaculatory fluid may contain sperm Relatively high failure rate; pregnancy may result No protection against STIs
Male and female condoms	Obtained without a prescription Relatively inexpensive Protect against STIs	Must be put on before penetration; therefore, may diminish spontaneity of intercourse May decrease sensation for both partners Cannot use certain types of condoms if either partner has latex allergy
Spermicides—Jelly, creams, or foams placed in the vagina	Obtained without a prescription More effective when used with a barrier (condom)	Significant pregnancy rate when used without a barrier (condom) No protection against STIs
Contraceptive sponge	May offer some protection against STIs Can be inserted into the vagina up to 24 hours before intercourse Inexpensive	Not fully effective against pregnancy
Vaginal ring	Highly effective in preventing pregnancy Does not have to be inserted before each act of intercourse—can be left in place for weeks to months, depending on the type	Requires a prescription because it is a hormonal method Similar risks as oral contraceptives Costs similar to or greater than those for oral contraceptives Correct insertion is key factor in effectiveness of the method
Oral contraceptives (birth control pills)	Highly effective Do not interfere with intercourse Regulate menstrual flow Decrease menstrual cramps	Require a healthcare visit and prescription May be a significant cost Must be taken as prescribed to be effective Drug interactions No protection against STIs Carry some undesirable side effects Contraindicated for some patients (e.g., those who smoke, who have significant varicose veins)

Methods of Contraception—cont'd

CONTRACEPTION METHOD	ADVANTAGES	DISADVANTAGES
Depo-Provera injections	Duration of 3 months Highly effective Do not interfere with intercourse	Require a healthcare provider visit Amenorrhea (may be seen as an advantage) No protection against STIs
Intrauterine device (IUD)—A small piece of plastic that also may contain metal or a hormone; placed through the cervix into the uterus by a healthcare provider	Highly effective May remain in place for years Does not interfere with intercourse	Increased risk of pelvic inflammatory disease (PID) Must be inserted by a healthcare provider Increased menstrual flow and cramping No protection against STIs
Diaphragm—Latex dome-shaped cup with a flexible rim that is inserted in the vagina and fits over the cervix Note: Cervical (silicone) cups provide a better fit for women who have not been pregnant or had vaginal deliveries.	Few side effects Quite effective if used properly with spermicide	Requires an examination to provide the best fit Must be inserted before intercourse, thereby compromising spontaneity Must be removed about 6 hours after intercourse Must be used with a spermicide Increased risk of urinary tract infection (UTI) No protection against STIs
Hormonal implant—Small rod(s) containing hormones that are inserted under the skin, usually in the back of upper arm	One of the safest and most effective forms of birth control available (World Health Organization, 2020) Users do not have to think about their birth control every day or for every instance of intercourse. Menstrual periods are fewer and lighter for most women. Effective for 3 or more years Can be removed at any time Does not contain estrogen	No protection against STIs May be able to see the rod if the patient is very thin A small number of patients have longer and heavier periods with breakthrough bleeding. May be limited availability More expensive than some other birth control methods Surgical procedure
Female sterilization (tubal ligation)	Effective Long-term cost effectiveness	Usually not reversible No protection against STIs
Male sterilization (vasectomy)	Effective Long-term cost effectiveness Does not interfere with sexual performance May be reversible in some cases	Psychological effects No protection against STIs

ASSESSMENT GUIDELINES AND TOOLS

Guidelines and Questions for Taking a Sexual History

Topics to Include in a Sexual History

The topics to include in the sexual history depend on the nature of the patient's concern. The following topics are most commonly included:

- Reproductive history
- Sexual self-concept
- History of sexually transmitted infections
- History of sexual dysfunction
- Present sexual functioning
- Other factors that affect sexuality, such as medications and diseases
- Signs or symptoms of sexual abuse (see Procedure 6-1: Assessing for Abuse)
- Knowledge level about sex, reproduction, and contraception

Tailor your assessment to meet the client's needs. For example, Frank Thanee (Meet Your Patients) is concerned about his family's reaction to his partner and his sexual orientation. In his situation, you would focus your assessment on his sexual self-concept, family relationships, present sexual functioning, and specific concerns about his heart and the impending family visit.

Questions to Ask Female Patients

Menstrual Cycle
- How old were you when you started your menstrual periods?
- When was your last menstrual period?
- How often are your periods? How would you describe the flow? How long does your period last?
- Do you have any problems with your periods, such as cramping, breast pain, or heavy flow?
- Does your menstrual period ever prevent you from going to work or school or participating in the activities you enjoy?
- What products do you use during your period, such as tampons and pads? Do you ever use douches, either during your period or at other times?

Cancer Screening
- When was your last Pap smear?
- Have you ever had an abnormal Pap smear? If so, how was it treated?
- Have you received a vaccine for HPV?
- Do you examine your breasts? If so, how often?
- Have you noticed asymmetry, lumps, or masses in your breasts? If so, describe them and show me where they are.
- When was your last mammogram? What were the results?
- Is there any history of breast cancer in your family?

Childbearing History
- How many living children do you have?
- How many times have you been pregnant?
- Have you ever had a miscarriage? An abortion?
- How many of your births were preterm (before 37 weeks)? Term?

Sexual Activity
- How often do you typically have sexual intercourse per month?
- Are you satisfied with the frequency or quality of sexual activity?
- Is there anything in your life that prevents you from sexual activity?
- Do you have any difficulty achieving orgasm?
- Is sexual intercourse ever painful for you?

Questions to Ask Male Patients

Sexual Activity
- How many times a month do you typically have sexual intercourse?
- Do you have any difficulty achieving or maintaining an erection or orgasm?
- Are you satisfied with the firmness of your erection?
- Do you experience premature ejaculation or have difficulty achieving orgasm?

Cancer Screening
- Have you been taught to examine your testicles? Do you practice testicular self-examination?
- Is there a history of testicular cancer in your family?

Questions to Ask Both Male and Female Patients

Illnesses and Medications
- What types of illnesses have you been treated for in the past?
- Have you ever been hospitalized? Have you ever had surgery?
- What medications, herbal remedies, or over-the-counter medicines do you take?
- Has any medical treatment, surgery, or medication affected your sexual functioning?

Family Responsibilities
- Do you have children? If so, how many? How many are still at home? Dependent on you?

Focused Assessment

Guidelines and Questions for Taking a Sexual History—cont'd

- Are you responsible for other children or adults? (This question may reveal whether the person continues to care for an adult, disabled child, or grandchildren.)

Genitalia
- Have you noticed any redness, swelling, discharge, itching, or odor in your genital area?
- Have you noticed asymmetry, lumps, or masses in the genitals? If so, describe them and show me where they are.
- Have you ever been told you have a hernia?
- Have you ever had trauma to your genitals?
- Are you having any problems urinating?

Sexual Patterns
- Are you sexually active? If not, have you ever been?
- Can you provide information on the gender of your sexual partners?
- What types of sexual activity do you engage in? Oral, anal, or genital?
- How many partners do you currently have? How many partners have you had in the past 6 months?
- How would you describe your satisfaction with your current sexual relationship?
- What are your thoughts about how this procedure/illness may affect your sexual relationship?

- Have you had any recent changes in your sexual function—in your level of desire, your sexual activity, participation, or satisfaction?
- Do you have any concerns about your sexual function, including your level of desire, activity, participation, or satisfaction?

Contraception (as Appropriate)
- Do you use birth control? If so, what type and how often?
- How satisfied are you with your method of contraception?

Sexually Transmitted Infections
- Have you ever been treated for an STI? If so, what type?
- Are you concerned about STIs or HIV?
- What precautions do you take to avoid STIs?

Abuse
- Have you ever been forced to have sex against your will?
- Have you ever been threatened or abused by a partner?
- Do you ever feel threatened by your partner?
- For guidelines for your approach to taking a sexual history, see Clinical Insight 30-2.

CLINICAL REASONING
Applying the Full-Spectrum Nursing Model

PATIENT SITUATION

Debra is perimenopausal at age 52, and her husband Roberto is 59. At times, she has been feeling tired and moody in the afternoon. At her annual gynecological visit, Debra tells you that she feels a lower level of sexual desire than she used to. Debra says, "I chalk it up to being very busy at work and yet still having so many demands on my time and energy with care of our three kids and housework." Debra is physically active, exercising four times a week, and is in good general health. She takes no medication and is within 15 pounds of her normal weight. Debra still has her period, but the flow is very heavy and cramping is more uncomfortable than it ever had been.

Recently, Debra has noticed that Roberto has been taking longer to achieve an erection, and his erection is not as firm as it used to be. He is generally in good health except for high blood pressure and high blood cholesterol levels. He takes medication for both conditions.

THINKING

1. *Theoretical Knowledge (Factual Information):*

    a. What are the common physical and emotional manifestations occurring with perimenopause?

2. *Critical Thinking (Analyzing Alternatives, Deciding What to Do):*

    a. How would you respond to Debra when she asks for information and support regarding her husband's erectile dysfunction?

    b. Debra asks you whether her desire for sexual intimacy will continue to decline after she goes through "the change of life." Describe in detail what you would tell her.

DOING

3. *Practical Knowledge:*

   a. What general topics would you explore with Debra to assess her sexual history?

   b. What questions would you ask Roberto to assess his sexual history?

CARING

4. *Self-Knowledge:* What might you be feeling if you were in Debra's situation?

5. *Ethical Knowledge:* What are one or two things you would do to help Debra and Roberto feel cared for and cared about?

Critical Thinking and Clinical Judgment

1. A 34-year-old married woman was hospitalized yesterday after an alleged rape. You are assigned to provide her nursing care. She will remain hospitalized for several days because of a head injury she suffered during the rape.

   a. How can you best approach this woman to establish a positive rapport?

   b. What fears is this patient likely to express?

   c. The patient's spouse is coming to visit. What concerns do you think that they may have?

   d. You begin to feel overwhelmed by this couple's emotions and questions. What can you do to help provide this couple with optimal care?

2. You are assigned a 26-year-old male patient who recently had a spinal cord injury. The doctors have talked to him about the possibility of regaining motor function and perhaps being able to walk again after intense therapy. He now seems most concerned about his relationship with his 25-year-old fiancée.

   a. What aspects of their relationship do you think he is concerned about?

   b. Do you have enough theoretical and patient information regarding his injury to answer all his concerns?

   c. As you consider some of the changes in sexual functioning that may follow a spinal cord injury, what suggestions might you share with him?

   d. What clues would indicate that talking to the fiancée may be appropriate?

3. You are seeing Jessica, a 14-year-old girl, at the clinic. Her throat culture is positive for gonorrhea. The girl's mother has gone to the coffee shop. The doctor has left a prescription for antibiotics. You are left to take care of the discharge from the clinic.

   a. How would you explain the culture results to Jessica?

   b. Jessica tells you that she cannot possibly have a sexually transmitted infection because she has not had sexual intercourse. How would you respond?

   c. Jessica tells you that she has had oral sex with her boyfriend, but no one else. What education regarding STIs and antibiotics would be appropriate?

   d. What information would you give the mother when she returns?

4. A 45-year-old married man with young children has just been informed that he is HIV positive. He is shocked by the news. He admits he had an extramarital relationship 7 years ago.

   a. What concerns is he likely to have? As his nurse, what biases will you have to put aside to help him?

   b. What theoretical knowledge would you need at a later time to help him deal with questions about sexual activity?

   c. What patient information would you need to help him deal with questions about sexual activity?

5. Review the following scenarios from Meet Your Patients in Volume 1.

   - **Jocelyn Carter.** Two days after Jocelyn Carter underwent a fine-needle aspiration to evaluate a small breast mass, her surgeon informed her that the mass was malignant. He recommended a mastectomy (removal of the breast). Today, she arrives alone at the surgery registration area. You ask how she is feeling, and she tells you that the past week has been a whirlwind of activity. "I had to arrange childcare, cancel a business trip, and organize the house so that I could take a few days off to have the surgery. My husband is working overseas this fall, so he couldn't be here to help me. Honestly, I don't know how I'm feeling. I haven't had time to think about it." A few minutes later, as she waits in the surgery holding area, she begins to cry. You hold her hand and ask whether she would like to talk. She asks you, "Do you think my husband will still want me? I'm afraid he will be turned off when he looks at me."

   - **Gabriel Thomas.** This patient comes to the outpatient clinic complaining of a throbbing headache for the past 3 days. He explains that he has tried several over-the-counter medicines and has had no relief. You check his blood pressure, and measure the reading at 240/130 mm Hg. When you ask whether he has ever been treated for high blood pressure, he replies, "Are you another one of these people trying to get me to take drugs that will ruin my sex life?"

   - **Frank Thanee.** Frank has heart disease; he had a mitral valve replacement 3 days ago. He has been transferred to the cardiology floor for an additional day of hospitalization. His partner, Greg, has spent the past 3 days at the hospital and has just left to check on the apartment and feed their cat. Frank confides that he is worried about his parents' expected visit. "I've never been able to tell them about Greg. They wouldn't be able to understand our relationship, much less approve of it based on their religion. I don't know how to handle this. What do you think I should do?"

   a. Write etiologies for each of the patients. The nursing diagnosis label is provided for you in each case.

   Jocelyn Carter—sexuality patterns alterations

   Gabriel Thomas—sexuality patterns alterations

   Frank Thanee—sexual dysfunction

   b. For each of the patients, instead of the sexuality diagnosis, use the cues (assessment data) to identify another nursing diagnosis label that you should explore to see whether it fits the situation better. Consult a nursing diagnosis handbook, as needed.

   Jocelyn Carter:

   Gabriel Thomas:

   Frank Thanee:

6. An infant is born with ambiguous sex organs. The provider has informed the parents that they will need to make a decision regarding which sex they want to assign to the child. They also have the option of waiting and letting the child decide later.

    a. What do you think the parents need to consider in making this decision?

    b. What emotional factors may be involved in this decision?

7. For each of the following concepts, use critical thinking to describe how or why it is important to nursing, patient care, or sexual health. Note that these are *not* to be merely definitions.

Sexual health	Sexual expression
Gender	Sexually transmitted infections
Sexual orientation	Fertility control

What Are the Main Points in This Chapter?

- Sexuality is a broad and complex aspect of the self, with physical, emotional, social, and spiritual dimensions.
- Sexuality involves how we feel about ourselves as individuals and how we interact with others and our environment.
- Gender, gender roles, gender identity, and sexual orientation contribute to expression of our sexuality throughout the life cycle.
- There are both typical and atypical forms of sexual expression.
- Culture, religion, lifestyle, sexual knowledge, and physical health all influence our attitudes toward sexuality, sexual behaviors, and intimate relationships.
- Sexual victimization is a societal and healthcare concern.
- Physical and psychological health status affects sexuality and sexual functioning.
- Sexual health is challenged by high-risk sexual behaviors, STIs, negative interpersonal relationships, and sexual dysfunctions.
- Four phases of the sexual response cycle are excitement, plateau, orgasm, and resolution.
- A sexual history is a component of the nursing assessment.
- There are strategies you can use to help you gain comfort and competence in collecting sexual data.
- The PLISSIT model was developed as a guideline for counseling for sexual problems: permission, limited information, specific suggestions, and intensive therapy.
- Sexual well-being may be enhanced through nursing interventions such as counseling for sexual problems; dealing with inappropriate sexual behavior; and teaching about body function and reproduction, self-care, contraception, and prevention of STIs.

Knowledge Map

CHAPTER 30 Sexual Health

SEXUAL IDENTITY
Perception of

- Cisgender
- Transgender
- Nonbinary

- Heterosexual
- Homosexual
- Bisexual

SEXUAL EXPRESSION
- Fantasy
- Erotic dreams
- Masturbation
- Oral/genital/anal stimulation
- Intercourse
- Celibacy
- Paraphilias

GENDER ROLES

SEXUAL ORIENTATION

GENDER ID

REPRODUCTION

- Eroticism
- Pleasure
- Intimacy

SEXUALITY

Factors affecting

Optimum expression

- Culture
- Religion
- Lifestyle
- Sexual knowledge
- Medication
- Psychiatric disorders
- Physical disorders

DEVELOPMENTAL FACTORS
- Tactile stimulation
- Exploration of self
- Parental role models
- Development of sex characteristics
- Sexual exploration
- Development of intimate relationships
- Dealing with the physical changes of aging

SEXUAL HEALTH

NURSING SKILLS — identify and treat

SEXUAL PROBLEMS
- STIs
- Dysmenorrhea
- Premenstrual dysphoric disorder
- Negative intimacy
- Sexual exploration
- Sexual harassment
- Rape

THEORETICAL KNOWLEDGE
- Dispel myths
- Taboos

SELF-KNOWLEDGE
- Beliefs
- Attitudes
- Comfort level

COMMUNICATION
- Privacy
- Relaxed affect
- Non-verbal expression
- Comfortable terms

SEXUAL RESPONSE DISORDERS
- Low libido
- Arousal disorders
- Orgasmic disorders

CHAPTER 31

Sleep & Rest

STUDENT RESOURCES

The questions and exercises in this book allow you to practice the kind of thinking you will use as a full-spectrum nurse. Critical-thinking questions usually have more than one right answer, so we do not provide "correct" answers for these features. Try to answer these questions yourself. It is more important to develop your nursing judgment than to just cover content. You will learn more by discussing the questions with your peers. If you are still unsure, see the Davis Advantage chapter resources for suggested responses.

To explore learning resources for this chapter,

Go to www.DavisAdvantage.com and find:

Answers and Suggested Responses for all questions in this chapter
Concept Map
Knowledge Map
Care Plan
Care Map
References and Bibliography

Key Concepts

Sleep
Rest

Caring for the Williams Family

Nadine Williams arrives at the clinic accompanied by her husband, Stanley. She appears very tired. Stanley tells you that she has been sleeping poorly. "She worries so much. She worries about Kayla, our grandchild. She worries about our kids. Now she's worried about my mother. When we were going through that mammogram scare, she was even worse!"

Mrs. Williams shrugs her shoulders. "I can't help it. I'm like that. I've always been a worrier. But it's gotten worse lately. Now I worry and get so emotional. I lie in bed thinking about all this stuff and end up in tears. Then, when I finally get to sleep, I wake up covered with sweat. I've tried extra soy for hot flashes, melatonin from the health food store, herbal tea, and even Benadryl—but nothing seems to work. I'm so tired. But when I get up, I have to deal with all these little kids at work. They're bouncing all over the place and noisy. I just get so short-tempered with them. That's not like me. I can't take this anymore."

A. Patient data: Clearly Mrs. Williams has a sleep problem. Underline the data that are defining characteristics (symptoms) of a sleep problem.

B. Patient data: Which data suggest ideas about the etiologies (causes) of Mrs. Williams' sleep problem?

Caring for the Williams Family (continued)

C. *Nursing diagnosis:* Two NANDA-I sleep-related nursing diagnoses are sleep deprivation and disturbed sleep pattern. You have already identified the patient's defining characteristics. Now, what *knowledge* do you need to decide which of these NANDA-I labels to use?

D. How could you obtain this knowledge?

E. Sleep deprivation is defined as prolonged periods of time without sleep and disturbed sleep pattern is defined as time-limited disruption of sleep. Can you make the diagnoses based on this knowledge? Why or why not?

F. Following are some of the defining characteristics for these two nursing diagnoses. Certainly there is some overlap between the two sets of symptoms. Nevertheless, which set seems to be a better fit for Mrs. Williams? Why?

Disturbed Sleep Pattern
Verbal complaints of not feeling well rested
Dissatisfaction with sleep
Change in normal sleep pattern
Decreased ability to function
Reports being awakened
Reports difficulty falling asleep

Sleep Deprivation
Daytime drowsiness
Apathy
Decreased ability to function
Agitation
Irritability
Hallucinations
Anxiety
Inability to concentrate
Slowed reactions
Combativeness
Fatigue
Fleeting nystagmus
Hand tremors
Heightened sensitivity to pain
Lethargy, listlessness, malaise
Perceptual disorders (e.g., disturbed body sensation, delusions, feeling afloat)
Restlessness
Transient paranoia

G. Write a nursing diagnosis for Mrs. Williams.

Practical Knowledge clinical application

This section will help you learn to give a back massage, assist you in obtaining a sleep history, and provide standardized language to use in planning care for clients with sleep problems.

ASSESSMENT GUIDELINES AND TOOLS

This section will assist you in screening for sleep problems.

Focused Assessment

Questions for a Sleep History

A brief assessment for all patients should include questions about the following:

Usual Sleeping Pattern
- When do you go to sleep and wake up?
- How many hours do you sleep?
- Do you have a regular sleep schedule?
- How would you rate the quality of your sleep on a scale of 1 to 10, with 10 meaning "great"?
- Do you take a nap? If you do, for how long?
- How often do you wake up during sleep, for example, to go to the bathroom?
- Do you feel adequately rested when you wake up?

Sleeping Environment
- Would you like a night light?
- What room temperature do you prefer?
- What noise level do you prefer (for example, radio, television, absolute quiet)?

Bedtime Routines/Rituals
- What do you typically do in the hour before bedtime?
- What do you do to help you fall asleep?

Sleep Aids
- Do you need a special pillow or positioning aid?
- Do you take any sleep medications or other drugs, natural sleep aids, or homeopathic remedies that may affect sleep?

Sleep Changes or Problems
- Have your sleep patterns changed? If so, how?
- How often do you have trouble falling asleep? Staying asleep?
- Do you currently, or have you in the past, ever had a sleep disorder (e.g., narcolepsy, insomnia)?
- Do you remember your dreams after you wake? Do you ever have night terrors? Do you sleepwalk?
- Do you ever had an unpleasant creeping feeling, crawling, or tingling, relieved only by moving the legs at night?
- Do you snore? Does your own snoring or grunting ever wake you or anyone in the room?
- Do you wear a cap at night? Do you require oxygen at night? Or any other medical aid or therapy while you sleep?
- Do you grind your teeth while you sleep? Do you wear a dental appliance to prevent grinding?
- Do you have any kind of pain that makes it difficult for you to fall asleep or stay asleep?
- Is there anything that I have not asked that might help you sleep while you are in the hospital (having surgery, receiving home care)?

If the client reports having satisfactory sleep, that is an adequate assessment, and you merely need to support her usual sleep patterns and rituals. When you suspect a sleep problem, you will perform a more in-depth assessment, such as a detailed sleep history or sleep diary.

Focused Assessment

Sleep Log

A sleep log provides specific information on the patient's sleep–wakefulness patterns over a long period. The diary is usually kept for 14 days and may include the following.

Note: If you work a night shift, adjust the time for sleep and waking in these questions accordingly.

Completed in the Morning

1. Time you went to bed: _____
2. Approximate time you fell asleep: _____
3. Times you woke during the night: _____
4. Times you fell back to sleep: _____
5. Time you woke up in the morning: _____
6. Did you feel refreshed upon waking up? _____
7. What did you eat or drink just before bedtime? _____
8. What mental and physical activities did you engage in during the 2 to 3 hours before bedtime? _____
9. Were you worried or anxious about anything when you went to bed? _____
10. Sleep medications you have taken: _____ Any repeated doses? _____ Times: _____

Completed in the Evening

1. How sleepy did you feel during the day?
   ____ Sleepy; struggled to stay awake during the day
   ____ Somewhat tired
   ____ Fairly alert
   ____ Wide awake
2. Any naps during the day? _____ If so, for how long? _____
3. Frequency of pain medication taken and times: _____
4. Exercise during the day? _____ If so, for how long? _____ What time of the day? _____
5. Number of alcoholic drinks: _____ What time: _____
6. Number of caffeinated drinks: _____ What time: _____
7. Number of tobacco products: _____ What time: _____

CLINICAL REASONING
Applying the Full-Spectrum Nursing Model

PATIENT SITUATION

A 43-year-old healthy woman, Maria Lupe, is being seen for her annual gynecological health visit. She tells you she lies awake in bed for hours before falling asleep at night. Sometimes she falls asleep without problems but will wake up and then have trouble going back to sleep. After feeling as though she had been awake nearly all night, Maria wakes in the morning feeling exhausted. She tells you she feels tired all the time and can't seem to get things done during her time off because of her fatigue. Maria admits to feeling irritable with her coworkers and children. Because of her lack of rest, she doesn't have the desire to do things socially anymore.

THINKING

1. *Theoretical Knowledge:* The NANDA-I definition and defining characteristics of insomnia differ slightly from the medical diagnosis of insomnia.

    a. What is insomnia, as defined medically (e.g., by the National Sleep Foundation)?

    b. What other health conditions might a medical diagnosis of insomnia be confused with?

    c. What factors either lead to or aggravate insomnia, as described medically?

2. *Critical Thinking (Contextual Awareness):*

    a. Obviously Maria has trouble sleeping. Based on the data you have, do you consider her difficulty sleeping significant enough to require consultation with her primary healthcare provider? Explain your thinking.

DOING

3. *Nursing Process (Assessments):*

    a. When conducting a sleep history for Maria, what questions would you ask her to (1) describe more fully her sleeping problem and (2) identify the cause of her sleeping problem?

    b. What would you suggest Maria do to help you gain more information about her sleeping problem?

4. *Nursing Process (Nursing Diagnosis):* Based on the data in the Patient Situation, would you use a nursing diagnosis of sleep deprivation or insomnia for Maria? Explain your thinking. Use a nursing diagnosis handbook, as needed, to compare the defining characteristics of the two diagnoses.

5. *Nursing Process (Interventions):* How might you help your patient manage her insomnia other than using prescription medication? What might you suggest?

CARING

6. *Self-Knowledge:*

    a. Have you ever had trouble falling or staying asleep? How did you feel at the time and in the morning? Describe your experience.

    b. How might you provide better emotional care and support to your patient after recalling your own episodes of sleeping difficulty?

Critical Thinking and Clinical Judgment

1. You are assigned to the care of Dayana, a 23-year-old woman with anorexia nervosa, an eating disorder. Dayana attends therapy each day, seems to be taking her medications, and is eating the necessary amount of food at each meal. But she continues to lose weight. The nurse working the night shift reports that Dayana is unable to sleep at night, seems anxious, paces the hall, and cries. Dayana is unwilling to talk about her inability to sleep, but you read in her chart that she was sexually abused during the night while living in a foster home. While in her room, you find a stash of her sleep-inducing medication.

    a. What do you think may be contributing to Dayana's difficulty falling sleep? Explain your reasoning.

    b. Why might you want to tell other caregivers about the sleeping pills? What reasons can you think of for *not* telling?

    c. For you to deal effectively with Dayana's sleep problem, what theoretical knowledge would you need?

    d. Now assess your current theoretical knowledge. Do you need more knowledge about certain topics to help Dayana? If so, where can you find out what you need to know?

2. You are a home health nurse. One of your patients is a 75-year-old man named Alonso. He is struggling to walk because of complications of diabetes. He states that he sleeps during the day, taking several naps. His chief complaint today is a pain in his left foot. You observe numerous books about alternative medicine as well as various dietary supplements in his home. He states he can manage his diabetes using herbs and refuses to take insulin or other prescribed medication.

    a. Do you have enough information to conclude that Alonso has a sleep problem? Explain your answer.

    b. Examine the patient situation (context). What factors lead you to suspect that Alonso may not be sleeping enough at night?

    c. What would you do to find out whether Alonso is getting enough sleep?

    d. Imagine how you would feel about Alonso's decision to forgo his medication and use herbal treatments.

    e. What personal values and biases do you have that will affect the way you respond to Alonso?

3. Imagine that you are a registered nurse at a local nursing home. Gwen, an 84-year-old woman, has captured your heart. Gwen has severe rheumatoid arthritis with pain and joint deformities, so she cannot ambulate or perform activities of daily living independently. Gwen's family visits every weekend, and they always bring cookies or candy, usually chocolate. Gwen likes to eat these treats just before bedtime, right after her bedtime medications. She receives a stool softener, a sleeping pill, and a pain pill for her arthritis. Lately she has been waking up at least twice each night, seeming quite confused. She tells the day shift nurse that she needs another sleeping pill at bedtime because "I'm not sleeping as well as I used to, because I have to get up so many times to go to the bathroom." She also seems more sluggish than usual during the day. You will need to integrate all available information. Don't worry if you do not know much about arthritis or if there are other things you have not yet studied. Just try to reason out the questions based on the knowledge you *do* have.

   a. If you have not yet studied arthritis and urinary elimination, you may lack some theoretical knowledge you need to answer the following questions. What information do you need? Where would you go to get it?

   b. What are some reasons that Gwen might be waking up?

   c. What might be causing her confusion at night?

   d. Should you address the problem of having chocolate before bed? Why or why not?

   e. List as many interventions as you can that you might use to address the problem of eating sweets before bed.

   f. Consider the consequences. How might her family react if you suggest that they bring something besides sweets?

   g. What teaching might you do with the family?

4. For each of the following concepts, use critical thinking to describe how or why it is important to nursing, patient care, or sleep and rest. Note that these are *not* to be merely definitions.

   Sleep

   Rest

   Theoretical knowledge about the physiology of sleep

   Circadian rhythm

   Stages of sleep (e.g., REM sleep)

   Sleep apnea

   Sedatives

   Sleep diary

What Are the Main Points in This Chapter?

- Sleep is a basic physiological need for health and wellness.
- Sleep and rest promote physical, mental, and spiritual well-being by restoring energy and reducing body demands while the body repairs itself.
- Illness can interfere with the ability to sleep and rest; conversely, people who suffer from sleep disorders have an increased susceptibility to illnesses.
- The hypothalamus and various neurotransmitters are involved in the physiology of sleep.
- Circadian rhythm is a biorhythm that is influenced by both internal and external stimuli, especially the light–dark patterns of day and night.
- The brain waves produced during REM sleep are similar to those of alert wakefulness. REM is characterized by rapid eye movements and dreaming.
- Duration of sleep varies with age.
- Factors affecting sleep include developmental needs and stressors, work, exercise, foods, other lifestyle factors, use of medications, illness, pain, and the environment.
- Common sleep disorders include insomnia, sleep apnea, and narcolepsy.
- It is important in a health history to obtain information about the patient's typical sleep patterns and rituals; this may require use of a sleep diary.
- Nursing interventions to promote sleep include clustering nursing care, creating a restful environment, promoting comfort, and supporting bedtime rituals and routines.
- Pain is one of the most common deterrents to and interruption of sleep. Hormonal fluctuations and stress also contribute to sleep difficulties.
- Sleep-inducing medication, as a rule, should be used only as a temporary measure.
- Teaching patients and their families about the importance of rest and sleep and measures to aid improving sleep quality and duration is an important health promotion intervention.

Knowledge Map

CHAPTER 31 Sleep & Rest

SLEEP AND REST

Benefits of SLEEP
- Restores energy
- Time for restoration and repair
- Strengthens immune system
- Improves learning/adaptation
- Facilitates storage of long-term memory
- Decreases stress/enhances coping
- Enhances wellness/recovery from illness

Factors Affecting
- Age
- Lifestyle: Work, exercise, nutrition
- Illness; disease symptoms, anxiety
- Environment; temp, noise, bedclothes

SLEEP
Cyclically occurring state of decreased motor activity and perception

REST
Inactivity/mild activity after which a person feels refreshed

Essential for physical, mental, and spiritual well-being

PHYSIOLOGY/STAGES

BIORHYTHMS:
- Internal biological clock; synchronized with environmental factors
- Influence physical/mental functions

CIRCADIAN RHYTHM:
- Based on day/night pattern in 24-hour cycle
- Affects level of functioning
- Regulated by cells in hypothalamus
- Disrupted by night work, travel, hospitalization

NREM:
- Stage I: Light sleep; easily awakened
- Stage II: Slowing of body processes
- Stage III: Deeper; difficult to arouse; relaxed muscles

REM:
- Stage IV: 90 minutes after onset; increased brain wave activity; dreaming; essential for mental/emotional restoration

SLEEP DISORDERS
- Insomnia
- Sleep/wake schedule disorder
- Restless legs syndrome
- Sleep deprivation
- Snoring
- Narcolepsy
- Hypersomnia
- Sleep apnea
- Parasomnias
  - Sleepwalking
  - Sleep talking
  - Bruxism
  - Night terrors
  - REM disorders
  - Enuresis
- Secondary disorders
  - Depression
  - Hyper/hypothyroidism
  - Pain
  - Airway passage obstruction

To promote — NURSING INTERVENTIONS:
- Adjust healthcare routine to promote sleep
- Provide a restful environment
- Use comfort measures
- Support bedtime routines/rituals
  - Hygiene; snacks
- Promote relaxation
- Pharmacotherapy to promote sleep

DISORDERS EXACERBATED BY SLEEPLESSNESS
- CAD
- Asthma
- COPD
- Diabetes
- Duodenal ulcers
- Epilepsy

CHAPTER 32

Skin Integrity & Wound Healing

STUDENT RESOURCES

The questions and exercises in this book allow you to practice the kind of thinking you will use as a full-spectrum nurse. Critical-thinking questions usually have more than one right answer, so we do not provide "correct" answers for these features. Try to answer these questions yourself. It is more important to develop your nursing judgment than to just cover content. You will learn more by discussing the questions with your peers. If you are still unsure, see the Davis Advantage chapter resources for suggested responses.

To explore learning resources for this chapter,

Go to www.DavisAdvantage.com and find:

Answers and Suggested Responses for all questions in this chapter
Concept Map
Knowledge Map
References and Bibliography

Key Concepts

Skin integrity
Wound
Wound healing

Related Concepts

See the Concept Map on Davis Advantage.

Example Client Condition

Pressure injury

Caring for the Williams Family

Kayla Robinson, Stanley and Nadine Williams' 3-year-old grandchild, fell at the neighborhood playground. She has abrasions on her knees, a deep puncture wound on her left hand, and a laceration on her scalp. Mr. and Mrs. Williams bring her to the clinic for assessment. She is crying loudly and moving all extremities. No treatment has been given.

Caring for the Williams Family (continued)

A. What should be your first course of action?

B. What kind of care will Kayla need at the clinic?

C. You determine that the scalp laceration will need to be sutured. What actions should you take to prepare Kayla for the suturing?

D. One week later, Kayla arrives at the clinic with her grandmother to have the sutures removed. The scalp laceration is dried and healed. When you inspect her other wounds, you notice that her left knee is erythematous, warm, and painful to touch and that there is a moderate amount of purulent drainage. What assessment questions should you ask?

E. Nadine tells you that Kayla would not allow her to clean or dress the abraded knees. You cleanse Kayla's knee and remove several small pieces of gravel from the wound bed. The wound is yellow and malodorous. What kind of care will Nadine need to provide to Kayla to heal the left knee?

Practical Knowledge clinical application

As a nurse, you will care for many patients who have wounds or who are at risk for impaired skin integrity. To apply your theoretical knowledge of wound assessment and wound care, you will need practical knowledge found in the Procedures and Clinical Insights.

PROCEDURES

Specific nursing interventions directed at maintaining skin integrity or healing wounds make use of procedures for obtaining wound cultures, cleansing wounds, and dressing wounds; for placing and removing wound closures, caring for wound drains, and applying binders and bandages; and Clinical Insights for applying local heat and cold therapy.

Procedure 32-1 ■ Obtaining a Wound Culture by Swab

➤ For steps to follow in *all* procedures, refer to the Universal Steps for All Procedures on the inside back cover.

➤ *Note:* This procedure uses modified sterile technique because wound care is now usually performed using a clean approach rather than strict sterile technique.

Equipment
- Three pairs of clean nonsterile gloves
- Aerobic culturette tube with sterile calcium alginate or rayon swab
- Sterile 4 in. × 4 in. gauze in an impermeable tray or separate 4 × 4 packs and an impermeable barrier
- Sterile 0.9% (normal) saline solution for irrigation, warmed to body temperature when possible
  (cold solution lowers the temperature of the wound bed and slows the healing process)
- 35-mL syringe
- 19-gauge angiocatheter
- Gown and face shield
- Emesis basin
- Water-resistant disposable drapes

Delegation
This procedure requires knowledge of wound healing. It needs to be performed by a registered nurse (RN). Do not delegate this skill to unlicensed assistive personnel (UAP).

Preprocedure Assessments
NOTE: If the wound is covered when you begin, you will make these assessments once you remove the soiled dressing and after cleansing the wound.

- Assess for pain.
  Wounds may be painful, and wound irrigation may increase pain. Provide prescribed pain medication 30 minutes before performing the procedure, if indicated.

(continued on next page)

Procedure 32-1 ■ Obtaining a Wound Culture by Swab (continued)

- Determine whether the wound requires sterile, modified sterile, or clean technique.
  Sterile technique is used for acute surgical wounds and for wounds that have undergone recent sharp debridement, or when the healthcare provider prescribes it. Chronic wounds are colonized with bacteria and may be cared for using clean technique, as in this procedure. To perform sterile wound irrigation, see Procedure 32-2.
- Assess the amount and type of tissue present in the wound bed.
  Granulating tissue is beefy red with a velvety appearance. It appears with the growth of new blood vessels and connective tissue. Pale pink tissue may indicate compromised blood supply to the wound bed. Necrotic tissue, which is black, brown, or yellow in appearance, is nonviable and inhibits healing. **Only red granulating tissue should be swabbed for a culture.**
- Assess the type and amount of exudate.
  Exudate may be a sign of infection.
- Assess the wound for odor.
  A foul odor may indicate infection. Cleanse wounds before you assess for odor because some dressings interact with wound drainage to produce an odor.
- Assess the tissue surrounding the wound edge.
  Surrounding tissue that is red, warm, and/or edematous may indicate infection.

➤ When performing the procedure, always identify your patient according to agency policy, using two identifiers, and be attentive to standard precautions, hand hygiene, patient safety and privacy, body mechanics, and documentation.

Procedure Steps

NOTE: Steps are for aerobic culture, except as noted.

1. **Position the patient** for easy access to the wound and to allow the irrigation solution to flow freely from the wound with the assistance of gravity. Place a water-resistant disposable drape between the patient and the bed to protect the bedding from any possible runoff.

2. **After performing hand hygiene,** put on a gown, face shield, and clean nonsterile gloves.

3. **Remove the soiled dressing.** Dispose of gloves and soiled dressing in a biohazard bag.

4. **Perform hand hygiene** and again don clean nonsterile gloves. If splashing or excessive drainage is expected, don personal protective equipment, including goggles and a gown.
   Soiled gloves are a source of contamination.

5. **Fill a 35-mL syringe** with an attached 19-gauge angiocatheter with 0.9% (normal) saline solution. Distilled, sterile water can also be used but is not as common. Make sure to remove and dispose of metal stylet in sharps container. Commercial irrigation kits containing a piston-tip syringe may also be used. Their use is discussed in Procedure 32-2.
   A 19-gauge angiocatheter with a 35-mL syringe provides 8 to 12 pounds per square inch (psi) of pressure and is effective for removing bacteria, necrotic tissue, exudate, and/or metabolic wastes.

6. **Gently irrigate the wound** with a back-and-forth motion from the cleanest to most contaminated part of wound. Hold the angiocatheter tip generally 2 to 5 cm from the wound bed. Use volumes of 50 to 100 mL per cm of laceration length/diameter.
   Irrigating from the most contaminated part of the wound prevents flow of contaminated solution over the cleansed area. ▼

7. **Dispose of the irrigation supplies;** remove and dispose of gloves in the biohazardous waste receptacle. If a stylet is in the area, place it in a sharp collection container.
   Prevents contamination and needlestick injury.

8. **Obtain an aerobic culturette tube** with calcium alginate or rayon swap (not cotton tip); twist the top of the tube to loosen the swab.
   Swab specimens are not suitable for anaerobic culture. Culture for anaerobic organisms may be obtained via tissue biopsy or needle aspiration specimens only.

9. **Don clean gloves.**

10. **Locate an area of red granulation tissue** in the wound bed.

11. **Using Levine's technique, press the culture swab** against a 1 cm square area of red granulating tissue, and rotate the swab for 5 seconds using a rolling motion. Apply enough downward pressure to the swab to cause tissue fluid to be expressed.
    Fluid from deeper within the wound bed is more indicative of the microbial colonization than culturing the surface of the wound. Levine's technique is as accurate a tissue biopsy but is less invasive.
    a. Swab only the area of the wound with granulation tissue. Avoid wound edges.

CHAPTER 32 Skin Integrity & Wound Healing   661

b. Do not swab culture areas where slough or eschar is present.
Areas of avascular or necrotic tissue are considered contaminated.

c. Do not roll the swab in exudative material.
Pus is a collection of white blood cells that have already done their work as well as other wound debris. The culture specimen must be wound tissue or wound fluid, not surface fluid or exudate.

d. Do not swab multiple sites with the same culturette. Use more than one culturette if several areas need to be cultured. ▼

12. **Carefully reinsert the swab** back into the culturette tube (aerobic or anaerobic culture, depending on the type of wound and type of organism). Break the liquid capsule at the bottom of the culture tube. Be sure the culture medium surrounds the swab.

13. **Label the tube** with patient's name, patient identifier, birthdate, source of specimen, and date and time of collection.

14. **Apply a clean wound dressing** if needed.

15. **Arrange for the specimen** to be immediately transported to the laboratory.

? What if...

- **I see another nursing student performing a Z stroke method of wound culture swab?**

  Consult your nursing instructor regarding the need to recollect the specimen using the Levine technique.
  Since Levine technique is more accurate than the Z stroke method, it should be used to determine the type and number of bacteria in the wound (Angel et al., 2011; Copeland-Halperin, Kaminsky, Bluefield, & Miraliakbari, 2016).

- **I determined this wound requires sterile technique?**

  After removal of soiled dressing, apply sterile gloves for irrigating, obtaining culture, and applying new sterile dressing.
  Sterile technique is used for acute surgical wounds and for wounds that have undergone recent sharp debridement, or when the healthcare provider prescribes it.

- **The culture tube is not sent to the laboratory within 72 hours?**

  If the culture swab is not sent to the laboratory within 48 to 72 hours, it must be discarded. Be sure to check the policy within your institution.
  The swab culture needs to be exposed to ideal laboratory conditions to allow microbial growth. If the culture sits on the unit too long, the culture medium might not produce reliable results. Most swab transport systems are validated for 48 to 72 hours after collection. However, if bacteria are suspected, the quicker the specimen is sent to the laboratory, the better.

- **The wound care and culture supplies are kept on a common treatment cart?**

  Common treatment carts should be left in the hall and not taken into individual rooms.
  When a mobile cart is rolled into a room, it is a source for possible cross-contamination.

Evaluation

- Assess the patient's pain level. Medicate as prescribed.
- Monitor laboratory reports for results of the swab culture.

Documentation

Document the following information (some agencies use a wound/skin flow sheet):

- Appearance and location of the wound and surrounding tissue. Note type, consistency and amount of exudate, and odor, if present, after irrigation.
- Patient's pain level before you obtained the culture.
- If the patient has been medicated for pain, document the drug and dose used, time given, and patient response.
- Method by which the wound was cleansed before you obtained the swab culture.
- Description of the area where the culture was obtained.
- Dressing reapplied to wound, if applicable.
- Education provided to the patient.

Practice Resources

Angel et al. (2011, April); Baranoski & Ayello (2020); Copeland-Halperin et al. (2016); Gabriel & Schraga (2021, August 27, updated); Haalboom et al. (2018); Levine et al. (1976); Non & Kosmin (2021, May 21, updated); Stallard (2018).

Thinking About the Procedure

➡ The video **Obtaining a Wound by Swab,** along with questions and suggested responses, is available on the Davis's *Nursing Skills Videos* Web site at www.fadavis.com.

Procedure 32-2 ■ Performing a Sterile Wound Irrigation

➤ For steps to follow in *all* procedures, refer to the Universal Steps for All Procedures on the inside back cover.

Equipment
- Nonsterile gloves
- Sterile gloves
- Gown and face shield
- Water-resistant disposable drapes
- Tepid (body temperature) irrigation solution
- Sterile gauze
- Dressing supplies
- Biohazardous waste container
- Sterile impermeable barrier
- Sterile bowl

For Step 10A Variation:
- Sterile emesis basin
- 35-mL syringe
- 19-gauge angiocatheter (needle removed)

For Step 10B Variation:
- Sterile commercial irrigation kit containing a sterile basin and piston-tip syringe

Delegation
This is an invasive, sterile procedure that requires nursing assessment, judgment, evaluation, and teaching during the procedure. It requires knowledge of wound healing and should be performed by a registered nurse. Do not delegate this skill to nursing assistive personnel (UAP).

Preprocedure Assessments
NOTE: If the wound is covered when you begin, you will make these assessments when you remove the soiled dressing and after cleansing the wound.

- Assess the amount and type of tissue present in the wound bed.
  Granulating tissue is beefy red with a velvety appearance. It appears with the growth of new blood vessels and connective tissue. Pale pink tissue may indicate a delay in wound healing because of compromised blood supply to the wound bed or lack of proper nutrition. Necrotic tissue, which is black, brown, or yellow in appearance, is nonviable and inhibits healing and is a source of bacterial growth. Wound irrigation should not be performed if the wound is actively bleeding, as irrigation may dislodge any clots that are forming.

- Determine whether the wound requires sterile, modified sterile, or clean technique for irrigation.
  Irrigation helps wounds to heal because it removes bacteria, old drainage, and necrotic tissue from the wound bed. Sterile technique is used for acute surgical wounds, for wounds that have undergone recent sharp debridement, or when the healthcare provider has ordered it. Chronic wounds are colonized with bacteria and may be irrigated with clean technique. Irrigation using clean technique is presented in steps 1 through 8 of Procedure 32-1.

- Assess the wound for signs of infection (erythema, induration, amount and type of drainage).
  Exudate may be a sign of infection. Infected wounds require higher flow pressures for irrigation.

- Assess the wound for odor.
  A foul odor may indicate infection. Cleanse wounds before you assess for odor, because some dressings interact with wound drainage to produce an odor.

- Assess the tissue surrounding the wound edge.
  Surrounding tissue that is red, warm, and/or edematous may indicate infection. Tissue that is macerated (white and moist) indicates too much fluid is being held against the skin, usually from saturated dressings.

- Assess for pain and the need to premedicate.
  Wound irrigation may be painful.

➤ When performing the procedure, always identify your patient according to agency policy, using two identifiers, and be attentive to standard precautions, hand hygiene, patient safety and privacy, body mechanics, and documentation.

Procedure Steps

1. **Administer pain medication** 30 minutes before the treatment, if necessary.

2. **Place the patient** for easy access to the wound and in a position that will allow the irrigation solution to flow freely from the wound with the assistance of gravity.

3. **After performing hand hygiene,** apply a gown, face shield, and clean nonsterile gloves.
   Personal protective equipment provides a barrier against splattering that commonly occurs during wound irrigation. For splashing, a face shield, mask, and protection over scrubs are advised.

4. **Remove the soiled dressing.** Dispose of gloves and soiled dressing in a biohazard bag.
   Soiled dressings contain body fluids and other contaminants and should be treated as biohazardous waste.

5. **Set up a sterile field** on a clean, dry surface. Add the following supplies to the field depending on the type of solution and equipment to be used for irrigation:

   Sterile gauze

   Sterile bowl

   Dressing supplies

   A sterile commercial irrigation kit, or a 19-gauge angiocatheter, 35-mL syringe, and sterile emesis basin

   Setting up a sterile field at bedside provides easy access to equipment for irrigation and reduces the risk for contamination when retrieving supplies after getting started. ▼

6. **Select irrigation solution** based on the wound assessment and goals of therapy. Sterile saline or sterile water is the solution of choice for irrigation of most wounds. Although cleansers are commonly prescribed for irrigation of wounds with debris or in dirty, necrotic wounds, tap water has now been shown to yield the same results as sterile saline in both wound infection rate and wound healing (Chan et al., 2016). ✚ Do not use povidone-iodine (Betadine) if the patient has an iodine allergy.

   Normal saline is isotonic and the commonly used wound irrigation solution because it is not damaging to healing granulation tissue. It is also isotonic (similar to the body's natural lowest salt-to-water balance). Sterile water contains no antimicrobial or bacteriostatic agents or added buffers. Cleansers contain surfactant (soaplike substance) that removes bacteria and cellular debris with less force and slow growth of bacteria, molds, and fungi. However, some antiseptic solutions can be harmful to healing tissues (e.g., hydrogen peroxide, acetic acid, povidone-iodine, bleach solutions, and sodium hypochlorite solutions [Dakin's solution]).

7. **Pour the tepid (room-temperature)** irrigation solution into the sterile bowl.

   Local cooling of wound tissues impairs healing. This can occur if you irrigate with refrigerated solutions and change dressings frequently.

8. **Don sterile gloves.**

   Gloving maintains sterile technique.

9. **Place the sterile basin** at the bottom of the wound to collect irrigation runoff.

10. **Fill the irrigation syringe.**

    If Using an Angiocatheter
    a. Attach the 19-gauge angiocatheter (with needle removed) to the 35-mL syringe and fill with the irrigation solution.

    A 19-gauge angiocatheter (with needle removed) and 35-mL syringe provide 8 psi of pressure and are effective for removing bacteria, necrotic tissue, exudate, and/or metabolic wastes.

    If Using a Piston-Tip Syringe
    b. Fill a piston-tip syringe with irrigation solution.

11. **Gently irrigate the wound.** Hold the angiocatheter tip or syringe tip 2 to 5 cm from the wound bed and use a back-and-forth motion, moving from the cleanest to most contaminated part of the wound.

    Irrigating from clean to dirty prevents flow of contaminated solution over cleansed area. Irrigating a clean, noninfected wound with gentle low pressure (8 psi) reduces disruption of the healthy, healing tissue. Irrigating an infected wound with higher flow (but <15 psi) selectively debrides necrotic tissue while protecting healthy tissue. Consult the provider. ▶

    a. Ensure any undermining or tunneling is irrigated as well.
    b. Repeat the irrigation until the solution returns clear.

    Flushing removes exudate, debris, and some surface bacteria.

12. **Remove the basin** or sterile container from the base of the wound.

13. **Gently pat the skin surrounding** the wound dry with sterile gauze.

    Moisture on the surrounding tissue may lead to maceration and further breakdown of the wound margins.

14. **Dress the wound as prescribed.**

15. **Consider applying a waterproof** skin protectant around the wound if drainage is heavy.

    Wound drainage contains irritating chemicals that can damage healthy tissues, especially at the wound edge and surrounding skin. Solutions used to keep the wound bed moist can also macerate or damage healthy skin if allowed to remain on intact skin.

16. **Dispose of the contaminated** irrigation fluid in a biohazard receptacle.

    Contaminated fluid is biohazardous waste.

17. **Remove soiled drapes** from the patient area.

(continued on next page)

Procedure 32-2 ■ Performing a Sterile Wound Irrigation (continued)

18. **Remove your gloves, face shield, and gown.** Dispose of these items in a biohazard collection container. *Contaminants from the irrigation may be present on these items, and they should also be considered biohazardous.*

19. **Reposition the patient** to a comfortable position. Change any linen that may have become wet during the procedure.

20. **Perform hand hygiene.** *Hand hygiene prevents cross-contamination and transmission of infectious organisms.*

? What if...

- **The patient has a wound covering a large area of the body?**

A general rule is that the larger the wound, the more solution is needed to clean it.

The purpose of cleansing a wound is to remove bacteria and debris by flushing the wound.

- **Peroxide or another antiseptic solution is prescribed?**

First, identify the reason that the solution was ordered for the wound type. Then identify the length of time it is to be used. Weigh the benefit of using the solution with the potential risks to healing tissues. Finally, discuss any concerns with the healthcare provider.

Peroxide is indicated more for acute, traumatic wounds to remove dirt and other debris. Peroxide and other commercial antiseptics can damage fibroblasts and cause air embolism if used to forcefully irrigate or pack a tunneling wound. Fibroblasts produce collagen, the major structural protein of skin and healing tissues.

- **All I have available for irrigation fluid is tap water?**

Tap water has been proven to be as effective as sterile water irrigation. Make sure the source of tap water is clean (sink, tub, etc.).

Tap water has now been shown to have same results as sterile saline in both wound infection rate and wound healing (Burch & Köpke, 2018; Chan et al., 2016). With the cheaper cost and more availability, tap water will become more of a standard for irrigation fluid.

Evaluation

- Determine whether the patient remains comfortable. If not, medicate according to prescriptions.
- Reassess the wound at regular intervals.

Patient Teaching

- Answer any questions the patient may have.
- Teach the patient about the expected healing process.
- Inform the patient and caregiver about signs and symptoms of infection and the need to report these findings.

Home Care

- Wound irrigation is commonly done in the home. In most cases, clean technique is used in the home setting.
- Irrigation solutions, such as saline, can be made and stored up to 7 days if refrigerated.
- Review with the family proper disposal of contaminated supplies.

Documentation

Document the following information (many agencies use a wound/skin flow sheet):

- Appearance and location of the wound, size, tissue in wound base, periwound tissue, type and amount of exudate, and odor, if present, after irrigation.
- The patient's pain level. If the patient has been medicated for pain, document the drug and dose used, time given, and patient response.
- Method by which the wound was cleansed.
- Dressing reapplied to the wound, if applicable.
- Education provided to the patient.

Sample Documentation

00/00/0000   0800   Dressing change to sacral wound using modified sterile technique due to saturation of old dressing with serious drainage. Patient premedicated with Lortab 5 mg PO 30 minutes before dressing change. Wound irrigated with normal saline using 19-gauge needleless angiocatheter and 35-cc syringe. Wound repacked with saline-moistened fluffed gauze and ABD pad to cover. Healing stage 4 pressure injury with 100% granulation tissue to the wound bed; 4 × 3.5 cm, with 1 cm of undermining at 6:00; copious serous drainage though no odor was noted. Periwound is slightly macerated; therefore, zinc-based barrier cream applied for protection. Patient reported no pain with procedure. Will continue to monitor and change dressing as needed. —————— L. Syzmanski, RN

Practice Resources

Burch & Köpke (2018); Chan et al. (2016); Lewis & Pay (2022, July 25, updated); Gabriel & Schraga (2021, August 27, updated); WOCN (2010, updated 2017, May/June).

Procedure 32-3 ■ Taping a Dressing

➤ For steps to follow in *all* procedures, refer to the Universal Steps for All Procedures on the inside back cover.

Equipment
- Nonsterile gloves
- Tape (cloth, plastic, foam, silklike, etc.)

Delegation
As a nurse, you are responsible for assessing the wound and evaluating interventions. However, this procedure may be delegated to unlicensed assistive personnel (UAP).

Preprocedure Assessments
- Assess the degree of importance of the dressing.
  The more critical the dressing, the more adhesion will be required.
- Assess the characteristics of the dressing material, weight and conformability, and the device or tubing to be held.
  Heavier dressings require higher adhesion. Bulky dressings may need high conformability or greater adhesion.
- Assess the skin surface (i.e., dry, damp, diaphoretic, oily, hairy, edematous, fragile, or impaired skin integrity).
  Fragile skin may require less adhesion, whereas damp or oily skin may require higher adhesion.
- Assess the anticipated wear time.
  Tape adhesion gets stronger over time. Breathable tapes can be used longer. Occlusive plastic tapes build up moisture and are used when adhesion is intended for a shorter time.
- Assess the patient's history and current medical conditions.
  Review allergies or sensitivities to tapes. Review medical conditions that may be affected by adhesives.
- Assess for activity level of the patient and the anticipated length of time the dressing will be needed.
  The more active the patient is, the more adhesion will be required.

➤ When performing the procedure, always identify your patient according to agency policy, using two identifiers, and be attentive to standard precautions, hand hygiene, patient safety and privacy, body mechanics, and documentation.

Procedure Steps

1. **Perform hand hygiene.** Don gloves.

2. **Place the patient in a comfortable position** that provides easy access to the wound.

3. **Ensure the skin surrounding the dressing is clean and dry.**

4. **Choose the type of tape** based on wound size, location, amount of drainage or edema, frequency of dressing changes, patient's activity level, and type of dressings used.
   Tapes come in many adhesive types and backings. Select the tape based on individual characteristics.
   a. Choose tape of the width that is appropriate for the dressing. The larger the dressing, the wider the tape needed for securing.
      For example, a large abdominal dressing may require 3-inch tape, whereas a small incision on an extremity may need only 0.5-inch tape.
   b. Choose a tape that stretches if the area is at risk for distention, edema, hematoma formation, or movement.
      Skin distention under tape may cause blistering or skin tears.

5. **Tear or cut strips that extend** approximately 1 to 1.5 inches (2.5 to 4.0 cm) beyond the dressing, depending on the size of the dressing.
   To anchor the dressing to the skin.

6. **Place the tape perpendicular** to the incision and without pulling or stretching the tape.
   Fewer skin tension injuries occur with perpendicular taping.

   a. When taping over joints, apply the tape at a right angle to the direction of joint movement, or at a right angle to a body crease. For example, tape a shoulder or knee horizontally, not lengthwise.
   b. Apply tape with an even amount of tension on both sides, being careful not to pull at the edges.
      This reduces the risk of skin damage. ▼

A   Correct   B   Incorrect — Too short / Too long, narrow / Too wide

C   Correct

(continued on next page)

Procedure 32-3 ■ Taping a Dressing (continued)

7. **Smooth tape in place** with your fingertips.
   To maximize the tape's adhesion to the skin surface.

8. **Replace tape if site becomes** edematous or the skin is not intact.

? What if...

- **The tape will not adhere to the patient's skin because of excess hair?**
  Remove the hair with clippers or scissors. Do not shave the site with a razor. *Shaving can cause nicks or abrasions to the skin that could become a portal of entry for bacteria.*

- **The patient's skin is diaphoretic or excessively oily?**
  Cleanse the skin with soap and water before the dressing change. Allow the skin to dry before applying the dressing and tape. You may also use polymer skin barriers to place a seal over the skin and allow the tape adhesive to adhere.

- **The patient has fragile skin (e.g., is an older adult)?**
  Use skin sealant preparations under adhesives. Use the least adhesive product possible. *The junction between the epidermis and dermis on an older adult is not as strong as it is in a younger person.*

- **The patient is allergic to tape adhesives?**
  Use hypoallergenic products. *Circular wraps, ace bandages, or other such products may be used to secure dressings.*

Evaluation

- Verify type of tape that is appropriate for the patient and dressing.
- Note whether the tape adheres comfortably to the skin.
- Ensure that the patient verbalized understanding of the treatment.
- Inspect the dressing daily for intactness, edema, or hematoma.

Patient Teaching

- Teach the patient about the expected healing process.
- Educate the patient about the purpose of the procedure.
- Instruct the patient to keep the dressing dry.

Documentation

Document the following information (many agencies use a wound/skin flow sheet):

- Type of dressing and tape applied
- Location and characteristics of wound
- Education given to patient

Sample Documentation

00/00/0000   0815   Dressing applied to left hip incision using conformable cloth tape. Wound edges are well approximated with no drainage noted. Periwound skin is dry and intact without erythema, induration, or odor. Wound cleaned with normal saline using sterile technique. Educated patient about the purpose of the dressing and expected course for wound healing. Will continue to monitor. ———————————— B. Hopkins, RN

Procedure 32-4 ■ Removing and Applying Dry Dressings

► For steps to follow in *all* procedures, refer to the Universal Steps for All Procedures on the inside back cover.

► *Note:* This procedure uses clean technique because wound care is now usually performed using clean rather than sterile technique.

Equipment

- Three pairs of clean nonsterile gloves
- Normal saline solution for irrigation, warmed to body temperature when possible
  Cold solution lowers the temperature of wound bed and slows the healing process.
- Tray of sterile 4 in. × 4 in. gauze
- Sterile gauze for dressings
- Tape
- Adhesive removal pads

Delegation

This procedure requires knowledge of wound healing. It should be performed by a registered nurse. Do not delegate this skill.

Preprocedure Assessments

NOTE: When you begin, the wound will likely be covered with a dressing. You will make these assessments when you remove the soiled dressing and after cleansing the wound.

- **Assess for pain at least 30 minutes before performing the procedure.**
  Wounds may be painful. Provide pain medication 30 minutes before performing the procedure, if needed, to allow the medication time to be distributed in target tissues. Changes in the quality or severity of pain are some symptoms linked with infection.

- **Assess the type and amount of exudate.**
  Exudate may be a sign of infection.

- **Assess the wound for odor.**
  A foul odor may indicate infection. Clean wounds before you assess for odor, because some dressings interact with wound drainage to produce an odor.

CHAPTER 32 Skin Integrity & Wound Healing   667

- Assess the tissue surrounding the wound edge.
  Surrounding tissue that is red, warm, and/or edematous may indicate infection.
- Determine the type of dressing needed.
  The type of dressing depends on the characteristics of the wound and the goal of treatment. Dry dressings are appropriate when there is no need to keep the wound bed moist, such as a wound healing by primary intention or a wound covered by eschar.

⊕ *Removing a dry dressing can also interfere with wound healing by disrupting granulation tissue and can cause pain to the patient.*

➤ When performing the procedure, always identify your patient according to agency policy, using two identifiers, and be attentive to standard precautions, hand hygiene, patient safety and privacy, body mechanics, and documentation.

Removing the Dressing

1. **Place the patient in a** comfortable position that provides easy access to the wound.
   Provides for patient comfort and proper nurse body mechanics during dressing change.

2. **Perform hand hygiene** and don nonsterile procedure gloves.
   Hand washing is one of the most important measures for preventing infection transmission.

3. **Gently loosen the edges of the tape** of the old dressing at an angle parallel to the skin.
   a. Hold that edge with one hand and gently raise the edge until it is taut but not pulling on the skin.
   b. Using your other hand, push down on the exposed skin at the point where the tape and skin meet. Push the skin from the tape. Adhesive remover pads are advised to help prevent tearing of fragile skin.
   The pull–push method will help prevent skin stripping from the adhesive and reduce discomfort and skin trauma as you remove the tape.

4. **Beginning at the edges** of the dressing, lift the dressing toward the center of the wound. If the dressing sticks, moisten it with normal saline before removing it completely.
   Moistening the dressing decreases the risk of bleeding and/or removal of granulating tissue.

5. **Assess the type and amount** of drainage on the soiled dressing.
   Allows for evaluation of wound healing. Purulent drainage is an indication of infection.

6. **Dispose of the soiled** dressing and gloves in a biohazard receptacle.
   Soiled dressings contain body fluids and other contaminants and should be disposed of as biohazardous waste.

7. **Remove the cover of a tray** of sterile 4 in. × 4 in. gauze. Moisten the gauze with sterile saline.
   The sterile container tray is impermeable and allows you to moisten the gauze while maintaining sterility. Gauze will not shed fibers into the wound (as do cotton balls). Fibers and any other foreign bodies in a wound promote inflammation and delay healing.

8. **Don clean nonsterile gloves.**

9. **Gather a gauze pad** by pulling the four corners up toward the middle. Use the center ball of the gauze to cleanse the wound.
   Forming a ball with the gauze pads prevents contamination of gloved hands during cleansing.

10. **Gently cleanse the wound** with the saline-moistened gauze by lightly wiping a section of the wound from the center toward the wound edge. Discard the gauze in a biohazard receptacle and repeat in the next section using a new piece of gauze with each wiping pass.
    Removes surface bacteria and exudate.

11. **Discard the gloves** and soiled gauze in a biohazard bag.

12. **Reassess wound** for size, color of tissue present, amount and type of exudate, and odor.

Applying Dry Dressing

13. **Perform hand hygiene.**

14. **Open sterile gauze packages** on a clean, dry surface.
    Maintains sterility of gauze. ▼

15. **Don nonsterile procedure gloves.**

16. **Apply a layer of dry dressings** over the wound. If drainage is expected, use an additional layer of dressings.
    The first layer serves as a wick for drainage. A second layer is needed if increased absorption is required.

17. **Place strips of tape at the ends** of the dressing and evenly spaced over the remainder of the dressing. Use strips that are sufficiently long to secure the dressing in place. Tape the dressing around all edges, "window-paning," if appropriate.
    Edges remain taped down and dressing stays intact.

18. **Remove gloves** and discard them in a biohazard receptacle.

19. **Assist the patient** to a comfortable position.

(continued on next page)

Procedure 32-4 ■ Removing and Applying Dry Dressings (continued)

? What if...

- **Signs of infection are noted with wound assessment?**

  Notify the healthcare provider. Cultures, wound care interventions, and potentially even antibiotics may be required.

- **The wound is not approximated?**

  Place the patient in a supine position, apply adhesive skin closures, and cover with sterile saline dressings. Notify primary healthcare provider.
  This could indicate wound dehiscence.

- **The skin surrounding the incision is not intact?**

  Clean the area with sterile saline, dry thoroughly, and apply protective moisture barrier dressing. Consider using Montgomery straps.
  Montgomery straps are useful when dressings must be changed frequently because they do not cause trauma to the skin.

- **A drain or drainage tube is present?**

  Always clean the drain site after cleaning the primary incision site.
  Reduces the risk of cross-contamination.

Evaluation

- Determine whether the dressing is clean, dry, and intact.
- Verify that the patient had minimal discomfort during the procedure.

Patient Teaching

- Teach the patient about the expected healing process.
- Inform the patient and caregiver about the signs and symptoms of infection and the need to report these findings.

Home Care

- Help the patient to store dressings appropriately to keep them clean, for example, in a plastic container with a lid.
- Teach the patient or caregivers to dispose of contaminated dressings and gloves by double-bagging them in moisture-proof bags (e.g., plastic grocery bags).
- Advise the patient and family whether they can get the wound wet (e.g., during bathing). If it must be kept dry, demonstrate how to cover it with a waterproof barrier (e.g., a plastic bag).

Documentation

Sample Documentation

00/00/0000   1420   Pt with no report of pain. Gauze dressing removed from lateral aspect of right forearm without difficulty. No drainage noted on gauze. Surrounding skin intact. Abrasion on right, lateral forearm cleansed with normal saline. Sterile gauze dressing reapplied to wound and anchored with cloth tape. Pt instructed to report any change at wound site, such as bleeding, drainage, or increase in pain. ———————————— D. Enferma, RN

Practice Resources

Armstrong & Meyer (2022, July 9, updated); Baranoski & Ayello (2020); Dabri & Phillips (2016).

Thinking About the Procedure

➤ The video **Removing and Applying Dry Dressings,** along with questions and suggested responses, is available on the **Davis's *Nursing Skills Videos*** Web site at www.fadavis.com.

Procedure 32-5 ■ Removing and Applying Wet-to-Damp Dressings

➤ For steps to follow in *all* procedures, refer to the Universal Steps for All Procedures on the inside back cover.

➤ *Note:* This procedure uses clean technique, because wound care is now usually done using a clean or modified sterile approach rather than sterile technique. However, sterile technique is recommended for wounds that have recently had sharp debridement, have a drain, or are fresh surgical wounds; also used for patients with immunodeficiency.

Equipment

- Three pairs of clean nonsterile gloves
- Sterile or clean solution, typically normal saline or water, warmed to body temperature when possible
  Cold solution reduces the temperature of the wound bed and slows the healing process.
- Water-resistant disposable drapes
- Sterile fine-mesh gauze in a tray for dressing
- Thick surgical pad
- Tape or Montgomery straps
- Adhesive removal pads

Delegation

This is an invasive procedure that requires knowledge of wound healing. It should be performed by a registered nurse. Do not delegate this skill to unlicensed assistive personnel (UAP).

Preprocedure Assessment

NOTE: When you begin, the wound will likely be covered with a dressing. You will make these assessments when you remove the soiled dressing and after cleansing the wound.

- **Assess the amount and type of tissue present in the wound bed.**
  Granulating tissue is beefy red with a velvety appearance. It appears with the growth of new blood vessels and connective tissue. Pale pink tissue may indicate compromised blood supply to the wound bed. Necrotic tissue, which is black, brown, or yellow in appearance, is nonviable and inhibits healing.

- **Assess the type and amount of exudate.**
  Exudate may be a sign of infection.

- **Assess the wound for odor.**
  A foul odor may indicate infection. Clean wounds before you assess for odor, because some dressings interact with wound drainage to produce an odor.

- **Assess the tissue surrounding the wound edge.**
  Surrounding tissue that is red, warm, and/or edematous may indicate infection.

- **Assess for pain.**
  Wounds may be painful. Assess for pain and provide prescribed pain medication 30 minutes before performing procedure, if needed. A change in the quality or intensity of pain may be a sign of infection.

> When performing the procedure, always identify your patient according to agency policy, using two identifiers, and be attentive to standard precautions, hand hygiene, patient safety and privacy, body mechanics, and documentation.

Removing the Wet-to-Damp Dressing

1. **Place the patient in a comfortable position** that provides easy access to the wound.
   Provides for patient comfort during dressing change.

2. **Perform hand hygiene** and don clean, nonsterile gloves.
   Hand washing complies with standard precautions, helping to prevent transfer of pathogens.

3. **Gently loosen the edges** of the tape of the old dressing. Hold that edge with one hand and gently raise the edge until it is taut but not pulling on the skin. Using your other hand, push down on the exposed skin at the point where the tape and skin meet. Push the skin from the tape. Use adhesive remover pads to avoid tearing fragile skin.
   The pull–push method will help prevent skin stripping from the adhesive and reduce discomfort and skin trauma as you remove the tape.

4. **Beginning with the top layer,** lift the dressing from the corner toward the center of the wound. If the dressing sticks, moisten it with normal saline or sterile water before completely removing it. Remove first from one side of the wound toward the wound, and then from the other side. Continue to remove layers until you have removed the entire dressing.
   Moistening the dressing decreases the risk of bleeding and/or removal of granulating tissue. ▼

5. **Assess the type and amount** of drainage present on the soiled dressing.
   Type of drainage is an indication of the stage of healing. Purulent drainage is an indication of infection.

6. **Dispose of the soiled dressing** and gloves in a biohazard container. Wash your hands.
   Soiled dressings contain body fluid contaminants and should be disposed of as biohazardous waste.

7. **Remove the cover of a tray** of sterile 4 in. × 4 in. gauze. Moisten the gauze with sterile saline or water.
   The sterile container tray is impermeable and allows you to moisten the gauze while maintaining sterility. Gauze will not shed fibers into the wound (as do cotton balls). Fibers and any other foreign bodies in a wound promote inflammation and delay healing.

8. **Don clean procedure gloves.**
   Avoids introducing microorganisms into the wound.

9. **Gather a gauze pad** by pulling the four corners up toward the middle. Use the center of the gauze to cleanse the wound.
   Prevents contamination of your gloves during wound cleansing.

10. **Using gauze moistened** with saline or filtered water, gently wipe a section of the wound from the center toward the wound edge. Discard the gauze in a biohazard receptacle and repeat in the next section using a new piece of gauze with each wiping pass.
    Removes surface bacteria and exudate. Prevents transfer of microorganisms from the skin to the wound.

11. **Reassess the wound** for location, amount of tissue present, exudate, and odor.
    Allows for determination of most effective treatment and type of dressing.

12. **Discard the gloves** and soiled gauze into a biohazard bag. Perform hand hygiene.
    Soiled gauze contains contaminants and should be disposed of as biohazardous waste.

Applying a Wet-to-Damp Dressing

13. **After establishing a sterile field** using a sterile impermeable barrier, open a sterile gauze pack tray and a thick surgical pad. The amount of

(continued on next page)

Procedure 32-5 ■ Removing and Applying Wet-to-Damp Dressings (continued)

gauze you use depends on the size of the wound.
Maintains sterile field and supplies.

14. **Moisten sterile gauze** with saline solution or sterile water for irrigation.

15. **Don clean nonsterile** gloves.

16. **Squeeze out excess moisture** from the gauze. Apply a single layer of moist, fine-mesh gauze to the wound. Be sure to place gauze in all depressions or crevices of the wound. You may need to use forceps or a cotton applicator to ensure that you fill deep depressions or sinus tracts with gauze. "Fluff" the mesh gauze before placing in the wound so as it dries it acts as a wick for any drainage.
Maintains a moist environment for the wound bed. ▼

17. **Apply a secondary moist layer** over the first layer. Repeat this process until the wound is filled with moistened sterile gauze—but do not tightly pack the gauze into the wound. Do not extend the moist dressing onto the surrounding skin.
Packing the gauze tightly can restrict blood flow to the area. Moist dressings on the surrounding skin can cause maceration.

18. **Cover the moistened gauze** with a thick surgical pad.
Protects the wound from external contaminants. ▼

19. **Secure the dressing** with tape or Montgomery straps (see Fig. 32-16). *Montgomery straps are useful when dressings must be frequently changed because they do not cause trauma to the skin.*

20. **Dispose of gloves** and materials in the biohazard waste receptacle.

21. **Perform hand hygiene.** Notes the date and time of the dressing.

22. **Assist the patient** to a comfortable position.

❓ What if . . .

- **Gauze becomes dry between dressing changes?**

  Moisten dressings with sterile saline before removing them; change dressing more frequently; consider using a semiocclusive dressing.
  A moistened dressing prevents debridement of granulating tissue, maintains a moist environment, and prevents tissue injury. Dressings that become too dry will injure healthy tissue and impair healing.

- **The patient has multiple wounds?**

  The most infected wound should be treated last. Remember to always change your gloves in between wound dressing changes.
  The risk of cross-contamination is reduced when moving from clean to dirty and with fresh gloves.

Evaluation

- Evaluate whether the patient feels pain with the procedure and afterward.
- Note whether the patient verbalizes understanding of the procedure.

Patient Teaching

- Teach the patient about the expected healing process.
- Inform the patient and caregiver about signs and symptoms of infection and the need to report these findings.

Home Care

- Help the patient store dressings appropriately to keep them clean, such as in a plastic container with a lid.
- Teach the patient or caregivers to dispose of contaminated dressings and gloves by double-bagging them in moisture-proof bags (e.g., plastic grocery bags).
- Advise the patient and family whether they can get the wound wet (e.g., during bathing). If it must be kept dry, demonstrate how to cover it with a waterproof barrier (e.g., a plastic bag).

Documentation

Document the following information (many agencies use a wound/skin flow sheet):

- Appearance and location of the wound, type and amount of exudate, and odor, if present, after cleansing
- The patient's pain level before and after the procedure
- Pain medication given including the dose, time, your name, and the patient's response
- Method of cleansing the wound
- Type of dressing applied to the wound
- Education provided to the patient
- Pressure relief measures, as applicable

Practice Resources

Baranoski & Ayello (2020); Bhimji (2021, March 15, reviewed); Bryant & Nix (2023, April); Wechter (2021, March); WOCN (2017, May/June).

Thinking About the Procedure

The video **Removing and Applying Wet-to-Damp Dressings,** along with questions and suggested responses, is available on the **Davis's *Nursing Skills Videos*** Web site at www.fadavis.com.

Procedure 32-6 ■ Applying a Negative Pressure Wound Therapy (NPWT) Device

▶ For steps to follow in *all* procedures, refer to the Universal Steps for All Procedures on the inside back cover.

Equipment
- Suction unit (pump)
- Collection canister with connecting tubing
- Open-pore reticulated polyurethane foam dressing
- Semipermeable transparent adhesive dressing
- Skin preparation product or sealant (skin prep)
- Sterile 4 in. × 4 in. gauze
- Clean nonsterile gloves
- Two pairs of sterile gloves (if using sterile technique)
- Sterile scissors (if using sterile technique)
- Waterproof pad
- Bath blanket
- Goggles or safety glasses, mask, and protective gown
- 10- to 20-mL irrigation syringe
- Normal saline for irrigation
- Emesis basis
- Biohazard bag for contaminated materials

Procedure 32-6A Open-Pore Reticulated Polyurethane Foam Therapy
- GranuFoam (black), white, or silver foam dressing
- Therapeutic regulated accurate care (TRAC) pad

Procedure 32-6B Gauze Dressing Application (i.e., Chariker-Jeter Dressing Method)
- Fenestrated drain
- Ostomy paste

Delegation
As a nurse, you are responsible for assessing the wound and evaluating interventions. You should not delegate application of a negative pressure wound therapy device to a UAP. However, you may ask the UAP to report to you any changes in the wound dressing, pressure in the unit, or alarms.

Preprocedure Assessments
- Assess the type of wound to be treated with negative pressure.
  Negative pressure wound therapy (NPWT) is used to promote wound healing by secondary or tertiary intention in acute, chronic, traumatic, and dehisced wounds; partial-thickness burns; or flaps and grafts. NPWT will prepare the wound bed for closure, reduce edema, promote granulation formation, and remove exudate and infective material.

- Determine whether there is any contraindication to use of a NPWT: nonenteric or unexplored fistulas; necrotic tissue with eschar; untreated osteomyelitis; malignancy in the wound or in exposed blood vessels, anastamosis sites, organs, or nerves.

- Assess patients for active or prolonged bleeding; patients who are on anticoagulant therapy or platelet aggregation inhibitors; or patients with infected, damaged, irradiated, or sutured blood vessels.
  Patients who are at increased risk for bleeding should be closely monitored. These conditions could be fatal if negative pressure is applied and bleeding is uncontrolled (exsanguination could occur). Notify the healthcare provider of these conditions.

- Assess the wound for bone fragments or sharp edges.
  When NPWT is activated, mechanical stress is placed on the wound. Sharp edges or bone may puncture protective barriers, vessels, or organs, causing injury; bleeding, if uncontrolled, could be fatal.

- Assess the wound for infection.
  Monitor infected wounds closely because they may require more frequent dressing changes than noninfected wounds.

- Assess the wound for size (length, width, and depth in centimeters); location and depth of undermining or tunneling; amount, character, and odor of drainage; type and percentage of tissue present in wound bed (granulation, slough, fibrin, necrotic); and periwound condition (i.e., intact, denuded, erythema, induration, or maceration).
  If no response or improvement in the wound condition occurs within 2 weeks, use of NPWT should be reevaluated.

- Assess the patient's nutrition status.
  Adequate protein stores are needed for wounds to heal. Evaluate the patient's albumin or prealbumin level before initiating therapy, as NPWT may deplete these levels and prevent healing.

- Assess for pain.
  Wound care is painful. Wound pain that is inadequately treated can lead to wound bed hypoxia that impairs wound healing and increases infection rates. Wound pain also negatively affects the patient's quality of life.

▶ When performing the procedure, always identify your patient according to agency policy, using two identifiers, and be attentive to standard precautions, hand hygiene, patient safety and privacy, body mechanics, and documentation.

▶ *Note:* The success of NPWT partially depends on the training and expertise of the clinician. Allow adequate time for this procedure. Experienced nurses need at least 15 minutes. You will need more time if problems arise, and even more if you are a novice.

▶ *Note:* This procedure assumes you are performing the initial application of vacuum-assisted closure (VAC) therapy. If you are changing the dressing, first read the "What If..." section near the end of this procedure.

(continued on next page)

Procedure 32-6 ■ Applying a Negative Pressure Wound Therapy (NPWT) Device (continued)

Procedure Steps

1. **Consider administering pain** medication before initiating negative pressure wound therapy.
   Allow sufficient time for the medication to take effect.

2. **Select the appropriate dressing** (per NPWT system used) to fill the entire wound cavity.
   Dressings should be placed directly against the wound surface to allow for equal suction/pressure throughout the wound bed.

3. **Obtain suction pump** unit as prescribed.
   Negative pressure wound therapy is provided by several manufacturers. Use the unit and dressing method that is approved by your facility.
   a. Place the suction unit upright on a level surface.
   b. Remove the canister from the sterile package and insert it into the pump.
   c. Connect the tubing to the canister.
   d. Ensure the opposite end of the tubing remains clean before connecting with the tubing from the dressing.
   e. You may place the suction unit at the end of the bed or hang it on an IV pole.
   f. Do not place the unit on the floor. Ensure the unit is not knocked over, as drainage from the canister can back up and contaminate the pump's filter, blocking suction.

4. **Place the waterproof bag** or trash receptacle so you can reach it easily during the procedure.
   Convenient placement facilitates access to safe disposal of the dressing into a trash receptacle for biohazardous waste.

5. **Assist the patient to a comfortable position** that allows for easy access to the wound.
   Facilitates access to the wound site with less contamination and promotes good body mechanics for the nurse.

♥ **iCare** 6. **Drape the patient** (use a bath blanket if needed) to expose only the wound area.
   Draping provides privacy and emotional comfort.

7. **Place a waterproof pad** as needed.
   An underpad protects the linens from moisture and drainage.

8. **Prepare a sterile or clean field** and add all supplies: gloves, scissors, irrigation supplies, gauze pad, selected wound dressings, tubing, and/or connectors.

9. **Don sterile or clean procedure gloves.** Use a gown and protective eyewear.
   Using sterile/aseptic versus clean technique is based on the wound type, physician preference, or facility protocol. A safe rule to follow is to use sterile gloves for a fresh noninfected wound and clean gloves for other wounds.

10. **Irrigate the wound** with 10 to 30 mL of sterile saline or other prescribed solution before all dressing changes. Use a 35-mL syringe and a 19-gauge angiocatheter (needle removed) to direct the flow of the irrigation fluid from the clean end toward the dirty end of the wound.
    Irrigation facilitates loosening of adherent tissue and removes debris and exudate while adhering to infection control principles of clean to dirty.

11. **Remove the excess solution** from the wound. Clean and dry the periwound skin with sterile gauze sponges, as needed. Consider a skin protectant around the wound edges.
    Excess moisture predisposes skin to maceration and possible damage. Applying a skin protectant can assist the drape in sticking to the skin and protecting the skin when the drape is removed (i.e., from stripping of skin by the adhesive).

12. **Remove soiled gloves** and don new, sterile ones for the procedure.
    Change gloves during patient care if the hands will move from a contaminated body site (e.g., perineal area or wound) to a clean body site.

13. **To apply appropriate dressing** per preferred negative pressure wound therapy unit, follow Procedure 32-6 A or 32-6B.

Procedure 32-6A ■ Open-Pore Reticulated Polyurethane Foam Therapy (i.e., Vacuum-Assisted Closure [VAC])

▶ When performing the procedure, always identify your patient according to agency policy, using two identifiers, and be attentive to standard precautions, hand hygiene, patient safety and privacy, body mechanics, and documentation.

Begin with steps 1 through 13 at the beginning of Procedure 32-6. Then proceed as follows:

1. **Select the appropriate foam dressing:** black, white, or silver.
   Black foam is sufficient for most wounds unless individual patient circumstances require white or silver. White foam is denser and will limit granulation formation. It may be used for painful or superficial wounds, tunneling/sinus tracts/undermining, or where granulation tissue growth needs to be limited. Silver dressings may act as a barrier to bacterial penetration in the wound bed. Silver may eradicate biofilms of colonized bacteria.

2. **Cut the foam dressing** to the appropriate size to fill the wound cavity. Do not cut the foam dressing over the wound. Rub the cut edges to remove any loose pieces.

If you cut the foam over the wound, particles may fall into the wound and create irritation. ▼

3. **Gently place the foam dressing** into the cavity without overlapping onto intact skin. Do not overfill the cavity or pack into deep crevices.
   a. Do not place foam into blind/unexplored tunnels.
      Forcing foam dressings into any area may damage tissue, alter the delivery of negative pressure, or hinder exudates or foam removal.
   b. Do not allow foam dressing to overlap onto healthy skin.
      Foam dressing becomes very wet during therapy and will macerate and damage intact skin.
   c. If you use more than one piece, note the total number of pieces that were placed into the wound so you can document them on the transparent dressing and in the patient record.
      An accurate record of the number of foam pieces is necessary to prevent retained material within the wound.

4. **Apply a liquid skin preparation** product to periwound, if needed.
   Skin preps can protect the periwound skin from excess fluid, adhesive stripping, or other damage.

5. **Apply transparent film/drape** 3 to 5 cm (1 to 2 in.) from wound margins without pulling, stretching, or wrinkling the drape. Do not push down or compress foam while placing drape.
   The occlusive dressing creates a seal to help create negative pressure within the wound. Tension from pulling, stretching, or wrinkling the dressing may lead to tissue injury. More pressure will be placed on the wound bed than necessary if you have flattened the foam before turning on the suction unit.

6. **Avoid placing dressings that wrap** all the way around an extremity. If necessary, place several smaller pieces of drape rather than one continuous piece.
   When pressure is applied, a circumferential dressing may interfere with circulation if wrapped too tightly.

7. **Identify a site over the dressing** for the suction track tubing apparatus.

8. **Pinch up a piece of drape** and cut at least a 2-cm round hole. Do not make a slit or X, as this may close off under pressure. ▼

9. **Place the track adhesive** and suction device directly over the hole in the drape and apply gentle pressure to secure.
   Negative pressure removes excess wound exudate from the wound bed. ▼

10. **Connect suction track tubing** to the canister tubing and open clamps. The canister is attached to a vacuum pump that provides either continuous or intermittent negative pressure, adjusted for the type of wound. Set suction to the prescribed pressure, which is typically in the range of −5 to −125 mm Hg (adjustable pressures, depending on the device used).
    Suction draws excess exudate away from the wound and into an evacuation container.

11. **Connect tubing from the dressing** to the suction track tubing going to the collection canister.
    Allows for collection and measurement of drainage.

12. **Position the tubing** and connector away from bony prominences and skin creases.
    Prevents pressure injury to the skin.

13. **Ensure clamps are open** on all tubing.

14. **Turn on power to the pump** and set to the prescribed therapy settings to initiate therapy.
    Therapy should be maintained for at least 22 out of 24 hours daily. Alternative wound care should be considered if the vacuum cannot be tolerated for this length of time.

15. **Listen for audible leaks** and observe dressing collapse or wrinkling as pressure is applied to the wound bed.
    With an adequate seal, the dressing will collapse almost immediately. Any leak (i.e., between the dressing and drape, around tubing, at skin crevices, or at tubing connection sites) will prevent collapse. ▼

16. **Change the canister** at least once a week or when filled. Write the date on the canister.
    This will help to know when it was changed last as well as how often it is being changed for fluid loss.

(continued on next page)

Procedure 32-6 ■ Applying a Negative Pressure Wound Therapy (NPWT) Device (continued)

Procedure 32-6B ■ Gauze Dressing Application (i.e., Chariker-Jeter Method)

▶ When performing the procedure, always identify your patient according to agency policy, using two identifiers, and be attentive to standard precautions, hand hygiene, patient safety and privacy, body mechanics, and documentation.

Begin with steps 1 through 13, at the beginning of Procedure 32-6. Then proceed as follows:

1. **Measure the length of drain** from wound margin, starting with the first hole perforation and pull back 1 cm.

2. **Moisten gauze** with normal saline.

3. **Wrap or "sandwich" the drain** in the moistened gauze and place in the wound base. Tuck gauze into any undermining areas to ensure contact with the wound bed.

4. **Apply a strip or small amount** of ostomy paste 1 cm from the wound edge and secure the drain as needed.
   Paste is occlusive and will help maintain a seal between the drain and the transparent film dressing. Paste that is too close to the wound edge can get sucked into the drain and occlude pressure.

5. **Apply liquid skin preparation** product to periwound, if needed. Extra drape, hydrocolloid, or transparent dressing may be used to protect fragile skin.
   Skin preps can protect the periwound skin from excess fluid, adhesive stripping, or other damage.

6. **Apply transparent film** approximately 1.0 to 2.5 cm (½ to 1 in.) beyond the wound margin to intact skin. Pinch the film around the drain tubing to ensure a tight seal.

7. **Avoid wrapping dressings** around an extremity. If necessary, place several smaller pieces of drape rather than one continuous piece.
   When pressure is applied, a circumferential dressing may interfere with circulation.

8. **Attach filter tubing** to the canister spout.

9. **Connect tubing** from the dressing to the evacuation tubing going to the collection canister.
   Allows for collection and measurement of drainage. ▼

10. **Position the tubing** and connector away from bony prominences and skin creases.
    Prevents pressure injury to the skin.

11. **Ensure clamps are open** on all tubing.

12. **Turn on power to pump** and set to the prescribed therapy settings to initiate therapy.
    Therapy should be maintained for at least 22 out of 24 hours daily. Alternative wound care should be considered if suction cannot be tolerated for this length of time.

13. **Listen for audible leaks** and observe dressing collapse as pressure is applied to the wound bed.
    With an adequate seal, the dressing will collapse almost immediately. Any leak (i.e., between the dressing and drape, around tubing, at skin crevices, or at tubing connection sites) will prevent collapse.

14. **Change the canister** at least once a week or when filled. Write the date on the canister.
    This will help to know when it was changed last as well as how often it is being changed for fluid loss.

? What if...

■ **I am changing the dressing instead of applying it for the first time?**

Use the following procedure steps. *NOTE: Dressings should be changed every 48 to 72 hours.*

Dressings left in the wound longer than the recommended time can become difficult to remove if tissue grows into the foam, or they can lead to infection or other adverse events.

a. Evaluate the need for analgesia.
b. Turn the suction pump unit off during the procedure.
c. Place a waterproof biohazard pad under the body part requiring the dressing change.
d. Perform hand hygiene and don sterile or clean gloves as appropriate.
e. Remove the transparent dressing using a push–pull method to gently pull up drape while pushing it slowly from the skin.
   Separating the drape from the skin in this manner will decrease the risk of tape stripping.
f. Gently remove gauze or foam dressing. If dressing is difficult to remove, instill normal saline onto the dressing for 15 to 30 minutes.
   Dressing removal can damage new granulation tissue if tissue has grown into the dressing.
g. Count all pieces of gauze or foam dressing that were removed to ensure none remains in the wound bed. Ensure no dressing is left in tunneled or undermined areas.
   Dressings are not bioabsorbable and can abscess if left in the wound.
h. Discard soiled dressings in a biohazard container.
i. Start at the beginning of Procedure 32-6 and perform steps 1 through 13. Then, as instructed in step 13, follow either Procedure 32-6A or 32-6B.

- **After 2 weeks, I see that the wound is not improving?**

  Consult with the healthcare provider or a wound care specialist. Average length of therapy is usually 4 to 6 weeks. Therapy should be discontinued if the wound shows no improvement in 1 to 2 consecutive weeks, the patient is unwilling or unable to follow the medical plan, or the goal of therapy has been met.

  The longer a wound is open, the longer it takes to heal and places the patient at risk for complications. A steady decrease in wound size should be seen every week. If NPWT is not effective, alternative wound care should be evaluated.

- **I cannot find or remove a piece of foam?**

  Notify the healthcare provider, as this may necessitate surgery.

  The retained material in the wound could likely create an inflammatory response.

- **There is a foul odor when the dressing is removed?**

  Clean the wound with normal saline to ensure odor is not emanating from the soiled dressing. If other signs of infection are present (i.e., fever, tenderness, redness, swelling, purulent drainage), notify the healthcare provider.

- **Suction cannot be maintained?**

  Identify why the seal cannot be maintained. If the wound is near the coccyx and gluteal fold, use a dollop of paste to help fill in the crack and maintain a seal. If the skin around the wound is moist, adhesive drape will not adhere to skin. Use a skin prep product or drape to protect the skin. If the tube is pulling away from the dressing or tension is being placed on the tube, anchor it with additional drape or tape several centimeters from the dressing or wound.

- **The canister is filling with blood?**

  Immediately discontinue negative pressure therapy. The gauze or foam dressing will not stop the bleeding, so take measures to control bleeding (i.e., hold pressure on wound). Do not remove dressing until the treating healthcare provider is consulted.

- **Dressing does not collapse or the alarm sounds?**

  a. Press firmly around the transparent dressing to seal.
  b. Verify the machine is turned on, all clamps are open, and tubing is not kinked.
  c. Check tubing and drape for leaks. Listen for leaks with a stethoscope or by moving your hand around the wound margins while applying slight pressure.
  d. Additional small pieces of transparent dressing may be used to seal around hardware, skinfold, or creases.
  e. Do not place multiple layers of drape or adhesive dressing.

     Several layers may decrease the dressing's moisture vapor transmission rate, increasing the risk of maceration.

  f. Never leave foam in place without an adequate seal for more than 2 hours. If an adequate seal cannot be achieved in that time, remove the foam, and apply a saline-moistened gauze dressing.

Evaluation

- Note the patient's response to the procedure.
- Continue to monitor wound healing and changes in periwound tissues.
- Monitor dressing every 2 hours to ensure it is firm and collapsed in the wound bed while therapy is on.
- Monitor the seal of the dressing and pressure settings.
- Monitor for brisk or bright bleeding, evisceration or dehiscence, and symptoms of infection. These must be reported to the healthcare provider.

Home Care

- Refer the patient to a home health agency for wound care.
- In limited circumstances, some patients or caregivers may be able to perform dressing changes. Determine their ability to perform dressing changes; teach and demonstrate as needed.
- Instruct the patient or family to visually check the dressing every 2 hours to ensure it is firm and collapsed in the wound bed.
- Review safety labeling, alarms, and pump instructions.
- Review conditions in which to seek medical care: bleeding, infection, unresolved alarms, or loss of suction.
- Review proper disposal of contaminated supplies.

Documentation

Document the following information:

- Date and time of dressing change
- Wound assessment: location of the wound, size (length, width, diameter), undermining or tunneling, amount and character of drainage, odor, wound bed including type and percentage of tissue seen, and periwound appearance
- Evaluation of therapy with evidence of healing
- Treatment selected: type of NPWT, type of gauze or foam, number of pieces placed in the wound
- Treatment settings: pressures, intermittent vs. continuous, or variable pressures
- Patient response to dressing change

(continued on next page)

Procedure 32-6 ■ Applying a Negative Pressure Wound Therapy (NPWT) Device (continued)

Sample documentation for Procedure 32-6B: Chariker-Jeter Dressing Application

00/00/0000.   1010   Patient reported pain rating 5 on a scale of 1 to 10. Administered hydrocodone 5.0 mg PO for pain at 0815 before initiation of negative wound pressure therapy. See eMAR. Stage 4 pressure injury to coccyx surgically debrided. Wound is 4 × 6 × 2 with no appreciable undermining. Wound bed is now clean of necrotic tissue with 100% pink tissue noted. Periwound has 2 cm of erythema to wound edges. Scant malodorous serosanguineous drainage. Using sterile technique, moistened saline gauze applied to wound bed with fenestrated drain. Ostomy paste applied at wound edge to assist in seal. Pump activated to 80 mm Hg continuous pressure. Patient rated pain in wound area as a 2 postprocedure. Plan: Begin dressing changes every 48 hours. —————— L. Opperta, RN

Practice Resources

Bukovcan et al. (2016); Bayer (2018); European Pressure Ulcer Advisory Pane (EPUAP), National Pressure Injury Advisory Panel (NPIAP), and Pan Pacific Pressure Injury Alliance (PPPIA) (2019); Gabriel & Schraga (2021, August 27 updated).

Thinking About the Procedure

The video **Open-Pore Reticulated Polyurethane Foam Therapy,** along with questions and suggested responses, is available on the **Davis's *Nursing Skills Videos*** Web site at www.fadavis.com.

Procedure 32-7 ■ Applying and Removing a Transparent Film Dressing

▶ For steps to follow in *all* procedures, refer to the Universal Steps for All Procedures on the inside back cover.

Equipment

- Clean nonsterile gloves
- Sterile gauze
- Normal saline solution or specified cleansing agent, warmed to body temperature when possible
  Cold solution lowers the temperature of the wound bed and slows the healing process.
- Scissors (if needed)
- Liquid skin preparation (if needed)
- Transparent film dressing

Delegation

Because assessment of the wound and knowledge of clean technique are important, you should not delegate this procedure to a UAP.

Preprocedure Assessment

- Assess the area to determine whether a transparent film dressing is appropriate.
  Transparent film dressings are indicated as primary dressings (dressings that touch the wound or area to be treated) to protect high-risk intact skin; for superficial or partial-thickness wounds that have little to no drainage (i.e., stage 1 or 2 pressure injury); and to assist in debriding eschar by autolysis. Films may be used as a secondary dressing to protect other types of dressings from bodily fluids (i.e., wounds near the perineum).

- Assess the wound to determine whether use of a transparent film is contraindicated.
  Films are contraindicated in third-degree burns, arterial ulcers, and infected wounds. Films should not be used to fill dead space.

- Determine the size of the wound.
  Film dressings are available in many sizes. Select the appropriate size based on wound measurements, allowing for a 2.5-cm (1-in.) perimeter of intact skin around the wound for the adhesive to stick.

- Assess the periwound area.
  Film dressings should be attached to intact skin. The adhesive is not waterproof and will not adhere to wet or moist skin.

▶ When performing the procedure, always identify your patient according to agency policy, using two identifiers, and be attentive to standard precautions, hand hygiene, patient safety and privacy, body mechanics, and documentation.

Procedure Steps

1. **Place the patient in a** comfortable position that provides easy access to the wound.

Applying the Dressing

2. **If a dressing is present, perform hand hygiene,** don clean nonsterile gloves, and remove the old dressing.

3. **Dispose of the soiled dressing** and gloves in the biohazard waste container.
   Observe universal precautions, preventing transfer of pathogens.

4. **Don clean nonsterile gloves** and cleanse the skin surrounding the wound with normal saline or a mild cleansing agent. Be sure to rinse the skin well if you use a cleanser. Allow the skin to dry.
   Cleansing prepares the skin for application of the dressing. Skin must be dry for the dressing to adhere.

5. **Cleanse the wound** with saline or wound cleanser as prescribed or according to agency procedure.
   Cleansing of wounds removes bacteria and necrotic debris from wound beds.

6. **Consider placing a skin barrier** around the wound before transparent film dressing application.
   Skin sealants may be applied to skin before tape to protect fragile skin from tears or epidermal stripping.

7. **Remove the center backing liner** from the transparent film dressing. ▼

8. **Holding the dressing by the edges,** apply the transparent film to the wound without stretching or pulling the dressing or the skin.
   This reduces the risk of skin damage.

9. **Remove the edging liner** from the dressing.

10. **Gently smooth and secure** the dressing to skin.
    Allows the dressing to adhere fully to the patient's skin.

11. **Dispose of soiled equipment** and remove your gloves.

Removing the Dressing

Transparent film dressings are typically changed every 3 days. Change dressing sooner if drainage extends beyond the edges of the wound onto periwound skin. To remove the dressing, do the following:

12. **Grasp one edge of the film** dressing.

13. **Gently lift the edge.**

14. **Stabilize the skin underneath** the elevated edge with your finger.
    Stabilizing the skin as the adhesive is taken off will prevent epidermal stripping.

15. **With the other hand, slowly peel** the dressing back over itself, "low and slow," in the direction of hair growth. Use of an adhesive removal pad is recommended especially for sensitive skin.
    Removing the dressing at an angle will increase the risk of pulling on the epidermis and causing mechanical trauma.

16. **As dressing is removed,** keep moving your finger as necessary to avoid newly exposed skin.

? What if . . .

- **The adhesive will not adhere to the patient's skin because of excess hair?**

   Hair may be removed with clippers/scissors. Do not shave the site with a razor.
   Shaving can cause nicks or abrasions to the skin that could become a portal of entry for bacteria.

- **The patient's skin is diaphoretic or excessively oily?**

   Cleanse the skin with soap and water before the dressing change. Allow the skin to dry before continuing with the dressing. Also, polymer skin barriers may be used to place a seal over the skin and allow the tape adhesive to adhere.

- **The patient has fragile skin (older adults)?**

   Skin sealant preparations may be used under adhesives.
   The junction between the epidermis and dermis on the older adult is not as strong as with a younger person. Less pressure or tension is needed to break those bonds and cause skin damage.

- **The dressing sticks to itself before it can be applied?**

   If a small portion of the dressing is stuck to itself, gently stretch, or pull the edges in opposite directions. If a large portion is involved, throw the dressing away and start over.
   Transparent dressings can be difficult to apply because they are polyurethane sheets coated on one side with an acrylic, hypoallergenic adhesive and are flimsy, making them clumsy to work with at times.

- **Purulent-appearing fluid has collected underneath the film dressing?**

   This does not necessarily mean the wound is infected. Remove the dressing and clean the wound per policy. Select an alternative dressing that will be more absorbent.
   Because films do not have absorptive capabilities, any drainage produced by the wound will pool underneath.

(continued on next page)

Procedure 32-7 ■ Applying and Removing a Transparent Film Dressing (continued)

Evaluation
- Verify the transparent film dressing is appropriate for the wound.
- Determine whether the dressing adheres comfortably to skin.
- Ensure that the patient verbalizes understanding of treatment.

Patient Teaching
- Educate the patient about the expected healing process.
- Teach the patient about the use of transparent film dressings.
- Inform the patient and caregiver about signs and symptoms of infection and the need to report these findings.

Documentation
Document the following information (many agencies use a wound/skin flow sheet):
- Wound assessment: location of the wound, size (length × width × diameter), undermining or tunneling, amount and character of drainage, odor, wound bed including type and percentage of tissue seen, and periwound appearance.
- Appearance and location of the wound, type and amount of exudate, and odor, if present, after cleansing.
- The patient's pain level before the procedure. If the patient has been medicated for pain, document the drug and dose used, time given, and the patient's response to analgesia.
- Method of cleansing the wound and surrounding skin.
- Type of dressing applied to the wound.
- Education provided to the patient.
- Preventive measures taken.

Practice Resources

Association of periOperative Registered Nurses (2022); Bryant & Nix (2023, April).

Procedure 32-8 ■ Applying a Hydrating Dressing (Hydrocolloid or Hydrogel)

▶ For steps to follow in *all* procedures, refer to the Universal Steps for All Procedures on the inside back cover.

Equipment
- Clean nonsterile gloves
- Hydrating dressing 3 to 4 cm (1.5 in.) larger than the wound
- Moisture-proof bag

Obtain the following items, only if needed:
- Normal saline solution warmed to body temperature when possible
  Cold solution lowers the temperature of wound bed and slows the healing process.
- Emesis basin
- Sterile gauze for cleansing
- Disposable clippers or scissors (to trim hair or dressing)
- Skin prep
- Measuring device
- Tape

Preprocedure Assessments
- Assess the area to determine whether a hydrating dressing is appropriate.
  Hydrating dressings are appropriate for wounds with small amounts of drainage. These dressings autolytically debride necrotic tissue from the wound bed. They may also be used to protect skin at risk for breakdown.
- Determine the size of the wound.
  Allows you to select a dressing of the appropriate size. Choosing a dressing size that extends beyond the ulcer ensures complete coverage.

Delegation
This procedure requires knowledge of wound healing, dressings, and infection control and prevention. You should not delegate this procedure to a UAP.

▶ When performing the procedure, always identify your patient according to agency policy, using two identifiers, and be attentive to standard precautions, hand hygiene, patient safety and privacy, body mechanics, and documentation.

Procedure Steps

1. **Place the patient in a comfortable position** that provides easy access to the wound.
   Provides for patient comfort and proper nurse body mechanics during dressing change.

2. **If a dressing is present, perform hand hygiene,** don clean nonsterile gloves, and remove the old dressing.
   Prevents transfer of pathogens.

3. **Dispose of the soiled dressing** and gloves in the biohazard waste container.
   Dressings may contain body fluids and other contaminants, so they must be disposed of in moisture-proof containers.

4. **Perform hand hygiene.** Don nonsterile gloves and cleanse the skin surrounding the wound with normal saline or a mild cleansing agent. Be sure to rinse the skin well if you use a cleanser. Allow the skin to dry or pat wound dry with sterile gauze. Do not attempt to remove residue that is left on the skin from the old dressing.
   Cleansing and drying prepare the skin for application of the dressing. Removing residue irritates the surrounding skin.

5. **Apply skin prep** to the area covered by tape.
   Skin prep protects intact skin from breakdown from tape removal.

6. **Cleanse the wound as directed.** Wound cleansing may be performed with clean or sterile technique, depending on the type of wound.
   Cleansing the wound removes microbes and necrotic debris from wound bed. Studies show using either saline or tap water is similarly effective for cleansing.

7. **Remove soiled gloves** and assess the condition of the wound. Note the size, location, type of tissue present, amount of exudate, and odor.
   Granulating tissue is beefy red with a velvety appearance. It appears with the growth of new blood vessels and connective tissue. Pale pink tissue may indicate compromised blood supply to the wound bed. Necrotic tissue, which is black, brown, or yellow in appearance, is nonviable and inhibits healing. A hydrocolloid dressing will interact with wound drainage to produce a thick, yellow gel that may have a foul odor. Clean the wound before assessing for exudate and odor.

8. **With the backing still intact,** cut the hydrating dressing, if necessary, to the desired shape and size. Size the hydrocolloid dressing so it will extend 3 to 4 cm (1.5 in.) beyond the wound margin on all sides and cover all areas of nonintact skin.
   Provides complete coverage of the wound.

9. **Don clean nonsterile gloves.** Hold hydrocolloid dressing between hands to warm it so that it adheres better. Then remove the backing of the hydrocolloid dressing, starting at one edge. Place the exposed adhesive portion on the patient's skin. Position the dressing to cover the wound. ▼

10. **Gradually peel away** the remaining liner; smooth the hydrocolloid dressing onto the skin by placing your hand on top of dressing and holding in place for 1 minute.
    Warmth helps the dressing adhere to the skin. ▼

11. **Assist the patient to** a comfortable position.

12. **Remove your gloves.** Perform hand hygiene.

? What if...

- **Signs of infection are noted?**

  Notify healthcare provider. Cultures may be prescribed. A different type of dressing may be prescribed, as well.

- **The surrounding skin is not intact?**

  Choose a larger size of hydrocolloid dressing to cover the nonintact area. Document your observations and report new findings to the healthcare provider.

Evaluation

- Verify that a hydrocolloid dressing is still appropriate for the wound.
- Note whether the dressing adheres comfortably to the skin.
- Ensure the patient verbalizes understanding of treatment.
- Inspect the dressing daily. Change it if it becomes dislodged, leaks, or wrinkles or if it develops an odor.

Patient Teaching

- Teach the patient about the expected healing process.
- Inform the patient and caregiver about signs and symptoms of infection and the need to report these findings.

Home Care

- Hydrating dressings may be required in the home setting. Teach caregivers to use the appropriate size and change the

(continued on next page)

Procedure 32-8 ■ Applying a Hydrating Dressing (Hydrocolloid or Hydrogel) (continued)

dressing if it begins to leak, develops an odor, or begins to separate from the skin.

Documentation

Document the following information (many agencies use wound care flow sheets):

- Appearance and location of the wound, type and amount of exudate, and odor, if present, after cleansing. Include wound measurements, if taken, and condition of surrounding skin.
- The patient's pain level before the procedure. If the patient has been medicated for pain, document the drug and dose used, time given, and patient response.
- Method of cleansing the wound and surrounding skin.
- Type of dressing applied to the wound.
- Use of skin prep.
- Education provided to the patient.

Sample Documentation

Practice Resources

Aderibigbe & Buyanna (2018); Armstrong & Meyr (2022, June 9, updated); Bryant & Nix (2023, April); Ghomi et al. (2019); WOCN (2010, updated 2017, May/June).

Thinking About the Procedure

The video **Applying a Hydrating Dressing (Hydrocolloid or Hydrogel),** along with questions and suggested responses, is available on the **Davis's** *Nursing Skills Videos* Web site at www.fadavis.com.

Procedure 32-9 ■ Placing Skin Closures

➤ For steps to follow in *all* procedures, refer to the Universal Steps for All Procedures on the inside back cover.

Equipment

- Adhesive skin closures
- Tincture of benzoin or skin protectant pads
- Forceps
- Normal saline
- Gauze
- Gloves (sterile if indicated)

Delegation

This procedure may be delegated to a UAP with the required training unless it is a new wound requiring sterile technique or has developed complications (e.g., dehiscence). Assessment of the incision line or wound is a licensed professional's responsibility and cannot be delegated.

Preprocedure Assessments

- Assess the type of wound to be closed.
  Adhesive closures are frequently used to keep surgical incisions well approximated. They may be used in conjunction with staples or sutures or after early staple/suture removal. Closures may be used to approximate the edges of lacerations or skin tears.

- Assess the wound for skin edge approximation.
  Wounds that are gaping or appear to have undermining should not be closed using adhesive closures.

- Assess the wound for drainage, amount, type, and odor.
  Wounds that are draining heavily might not be suitable for adhesive skin closures because the adhesive would not stick to the skin.

- Assess the periwound area or surrounding skin. Assessment should include skin color, texture, temperature, and integrity of the surrounding skin. Look for maceration (caused by heavy drainage), excoriation (from caustic effluent), stripping (from inappropriate adhesive removal), pustules, papules, or lesions.
  Adhesive closures should be placed only on intact skin.

- Assess the length of the wound, the location (over a joint), or whether edema may occur to determine the size of the skin closure used. Consider elastic skin closures if distention or movement is anticipated.
  Closures come in several lengths, widths, and flexibility capabilities to meet elasticity and conformability needs.

➤ When performing the procedure, always identify your patient according to agency policy, using two identifiers, and be attentive to standard precautions, hand hygiene, patient safety and privacy, body mechanics, and documentation.

Procedure Steps

1. **Perform hand hygiene** and don clean nonsterile gloves.
   Gloving prevents cross-contamination.

2. **Cleanse the skin** at least 5 cm (2 in.) around the wound with saline-moistened gauze. Pat the skin dry, allowing it to dry thoroughly.
   The skin surrounding the wound must be clean and dry for the strips to adhere.

3. **Apply a skin preparation product** and allow it to dry (or follow agency procedures). Avoid benzoin on fragile skin.
   Because the strips are prone to peeling off with moisture, benzoin enhances adhesion of the strips.

4. **Do not allow skin preparation** product to come into contact with the wound.
   It may impair healing.

5. **Peel back package tabs** to access the adhesive closures.

6. **Remove the card** from the package using modified sterile technique as necessary.
   Careful technique should be followed when applying to a surgical wound to minimize contamination and promote healing.

7. **Grasp end of the skin closure** with forceps or gloved hand and peel strip from the card at a 90° angle.
   Closures lifted at a lesser angle or directly back on themselves may "curl," complicating handling.

8. **Starting at the middle** of the wound, apply strips perpendicular to the wound, drawing the wound edges together. Apply closures without tension; do not stretch or strap closures.
   a. Apply half of the closure to the wound margin and press firmly in place.
   b. Using fingers or forceps, ensure skin edges are approximated.
   c. Press the free half firmly on the other side of the wound in a ladder fashion.
   d. Place the strips so that they extend at least 2 to 3 cm (¾ to 1 in.) on either side of the wound to ensure closure.
   e. Place the wound closure strips 3 mm (⅛ in.) apart along the wound. ▼

? What if . . .

- **A flap of skin rolls up on the edges?**

  Cleanse the wound with normal saline and reapproximate the edges of the skin flap with the intact epidermis. Apply skin closures across the flap.

- **The skin around the wound is swollen?**

  Apply skin closures without tension and reapply as swelling increases.
  This prevents pulling on the skin that can delay healing or disrupt the approximated borders of the wound, which is more likely to lead to scarring.

- **Edges are not accurately approximated or tension has been placed on the skin?**

  Remove the closure over the affected area, peeling each side toward the wound, and reapply.
  Use of adhesive products can cause superficial skin damage if the skin is stretched during application or with edema formation. Tension blisters are the most common problem associated with taping.

Evaluation

- Verify that skin closures are appropriate for the wound.
- Note whether the closures adhere comfortably to the skin.
- Ensure the patient verbalized understanding of the treatment.
- Inspect the wound daily. Lifted closure edges may be trimmed or closures replaced if less than half of the strip remains.

Patient Teaching

- Teach the patient about the expected healing process.
- Inform the patient or caregiver about signs and symptoms of infection and the need to report these findings.
- Instruct patient not to pull or tug on the strips.
  Improper removal may damage the underlying skin or the wound itself.
- Instruct the patient that they do not need to keep the strips dry. They can bathe and shower as directed by the healthcare provider.
- Instruct the patient that adhesive strips are often kept in place until they begin to separate from the skin on their own.

Documentation

Sample Documentation

00/00/0000 2040 Skin closures applied to surgical incision along right forearm. Wound edges are well approximated with slight erythema noted 4 mm from incisional site. Periwound skin is dry and intact with no drainage, induration, or odor noted. Wound cleansed with normal saline using sterile technique. Patient educated on the purpose of the closures and expected time and course of healing. Will continue to monitor. ——— S. Wong, RN

Practice Resource
Takayama et al. (2016).

Thinking About the Procedure

The video **Placing Skin Closures,** along with questions and suggested responses, is available on the **Davis's Nursing Skills Videos** Web site at www.fadavis.com.

Procedure 32-10 ■ Applying Binders

> For steps to follow in *all* procedures, refer to the Universal Steps for All Procedures on the inside back cover.

Equipment
- Abdominal binder, triangular arm binder, or T-binder
- Clean nonsterile gloves
- Measuring tape

Delegation
This procedure may be delegated to a UAP. Assessment of the incision line or wound is a licensed professional's responsibility and cannot be delegated.

Preprocedure Assessments
- Assess the condition of the wound (if one is present). Note the amount and type of drainage. A wound must be dressed before it is bandaged; if there is a significant amount of exudate, you will need to apply a secondary dressing.
- Assess for pain and check the circulation of the underlying body parts before and after applying the binder. Look for cool, pale, or cyanotic skin; tingling; and numbness.
- Determine whether the patient or family has the skills to reapply the binder when necessary.

> When performing the procedure, always identify your patient according to agency policy, using two identifiers, and be attentive to standard precautions, hand hygiene, patient safety and privacy, body mechanics, and documentation.

> Observe steps 1 through 7, regardless of the type of binder you use.

Procedure Steps

1. **Choose a binder** of the proper size.

2. **Perform hand hygiene** and don nonsterile gloves.

3. **Thoroughly clean and dry** the part to be covered.
   Moisture contributes to skin breakdown.

4. **Place the body part** in a comfortable position (e.g., with the joint slightly flexed) whenever possible.
   Prevents strain on ligaments and muscles.

5. **Pad between skin surfaces** (e.g., under the axilla) and over bony prominences.
   Prevents pressure and abrasion of the skin.

6. **Fasten from the bottom up,** especially for abdominal binders.
   Make sure the binder is secured with enough pressure to provide the needed support and control bleeding, but not so tightly that circulation is compromised or breathing impaired.
   Fastening from the bottom up gives upward support.

7. **Change binders** whenever they become soiled or wet.

Proceed to step 8, 14, or 20, depending on the type of binder you are using.

Procedure Variation: Applying an Abdominal Binder

8. **Measure the patient** for the abdominal binder.
   a. Place the patient in supine position.
   b. With a measuring tape, encircle the abdomen at the level of the umbilicus. Note the measurement. This is the length of the binder. ▼
   c. Measure the distance from the costal margin to the top of the iliac crests. This is the width of the binder.
   d. Dispose of gloves and measuring tape and perform hand hygiene.
   e. Based on the measurements, obtain an abdominal binder.

9. **Assist the patient to roll** to one side. Roll one end of the binder to the center mark. Place the rolled section of the abdominal binder underneath the patient. Position the binder appropriately between the costal margin and iliac crest.

10. **Make sure the binder** does not slip upward or downward.
    If the binder is positioned too high, it could impair lung expansion and gas exchange. If it is positioned too low, the binder will not provide adequate support.

11. **Assist the patient to turn** to the other side as you unroll the binder from underneath him. Pad any pressure areas or skin abrasions to avoid pressure injury.

12. **With your dominant hand, grasp the end of the binder** on the side farthest from you and steadily pull toward the center of the patient's abdomen. With your nondominant hand, grasp the end of binder closest to you and pull toward the center. Overlap the ends of the binder so that the hook-and-loop fasteners (e.g., Velcro) meet. ▼

CHAPTER 32 Skin Integrity & Wound Healing 683

13. **Assess the abdominal binder** every 2 to 3 hours. Observe that the binder has not shifted up or down or compromised the patient's breathing. Remove it to assess the underlying skin and dressings. Change wound dressings if they are soiled, or as prescribed.

Applying a Triangular Arm Binder

A triangular arm binder or sling is used to support the upper extremities. Obtain a commercial sling (consisting of a sleeve for the arm and a strap to go around the neck) or a triangular piece of fabric. To form a splint from a triangular cloth, follow these steps:

14. **Ask the patient to place** the affected arm in a natural position across the chest, elbow flexed slightly.
    Slight flexion prevents swelling of the hand and relieves pressure on the shoulder.

15. **Place one end of the triangle** over the shoulder of the uninjured arm and allow the triangle to fall open so that the elbow of the injured arm is at the apex of the triangle.

16. **Move the sling** behind the injured arm.

17. **Pull up the lower corner** of the triangle over the injured arm to the shoulder of the injured arm.

18. **Tie the sling with a square knot** at the neck on the side of the arm requiring support.
    A square knot will not slip and is easy to untie.

19. **Adjust the injured arm** within the sling.
    To ensure patient comfort. ▶

Applying a T-Binder

A T-binder is used to secure dressings or pads in the perineal area. A single T-binder is often used for women. A double T-binder is commonly used for men. To apply a T-binder, follow these steps:

20. **Position the waist tails** under the patient at the natural waistline. Bring the right and left tails together and secure them at the waist with pins or clips.

21. **For a single T-binder,** bring the center tail up between the legs of the patient. Secure the tail at the waist with pins or clips. ▶

22. **For a double T-binder,** bring the tails up on either side of the penis. Secure the tail at the waist with pins or clips. ▼

23. **Fasten the ties** at the waist using pins or clips.

? What if...

- **The patient is obese?**

  Obtain the appropriate size binder before applying. Do not try to position a binder that is too small for the patient.
  A poorly fitting binder can constrict circulation, cause pressure points that can injure the skin, and can restrict movement of the chest for adequate breathing. A binder that is too tight is uncomfortable and will not provide the proper support of an incision or wound needed for healing.

Evaluation

- Evaluate whether the patient's physical condition has changed since using the binder.
- Assess circulation to be sure the binder is not secured too tightly. Check color, warmth, tingling, sensation, and capillary refill.
- Assess the depth of breathing to be sure the binder is not restricting ventilation.
- Check the skin under the binder to be sure there are no areas of irritation, pressure, or skin abrasion.
- Assess incisions or wounds under the binder to be sure they are not bleeding and are healing properly.
- Monitor comfort regularly.
- Assess the patient's ability to perform activities of daily living while wearing the binder.

(continued on next page)

Procedure 32-10 ■ Applying Binders (continued)

Home Care
- Teach the patient and/or caregiver how to apply the binder in the proper position, snugly but not too tightly.
- Teach the family to inspect the site under the binder to be sure the skin is not pinched or with other points of pressure. This is especially crucial for older adults.
- Clean binders in warm, soapy water when soiled. Use a mesh laundry bag to keep the Velcro straps from catching other clothing in the washer. Air-dry thoroughly. Patients should have two binders at home—a clean one to wear while the other is laundered.
- Apply and remove binder to promote comfort and ensure good circulation. This also allows the patient and caregiver to inspect any incision or wound underneath.
- Binders for children at home could be decorated with permanent marking pens.
- Allow children to help with applying and removing the binder.

Documentation
Document the following information (many agencies use specialized wound care flow sheets):
- Appearance and location of the wound or incision under the binder, type and amount of exudates, and odor, if present, after cleansing
- Pain level before and after the procedure. If the patient has been medicated for pain, document the drug and dose used, time given, and patient response.
- Type of binder applied
- Date and time the binder was applied and removed
- Any change in the appearance of the wound or skin in contact with the binder
- Education provided to the patient

Procedure 32-11 ■ Applying Bandages

➤ For steps to follow in *all* procedures, refer to the Universal Steps for All Procedures on the inside back cover.

Equipment
- Appropriate bandage dressing
- Clean nonsterile gloves (2 pairs)
- Gauze sponges
- Normal saline
- Primary dressing (as prescribed)
- Scissors
- Tape or metal closures

Delegation
This procedure may be delegated to a UAP who has the appropriate training. Assessment of the incision line or wound is a licensed professional's responsibility and cannot be delegated.

Preprocedure Assessment
- Determine the body part or area to be bandaged.
  This allows you to choose the correct width of gauze or elastic bandage to use.
- Assess the condition of the wound (if one is present). Assess the wound for size (length, width, and depth in centimeters); location and depth of undermining or tunneling; amount, character, and odor of drainage; type and percentage of tissue present in wound bed (granulation, slough, fibrin, necrotic); and periwound condition (intact, denuded, erythema, induration, or maceration).
  Wound dressings should be chosen based on the characteristics of the wound.
- Assess for pain and check the circulation of the underlying body parts before and after applying the bandage. Look for cool, pale, or cyanotic skin; tingling; and numbness.
  Circulation to an extremity can be compromised if the bandage is too tight or the extremity swells after application.
- Determine whether the patient or family has the skills to reapply the bandage when necessary.
  Teaching might be needed for home care.

➤ When performing the procedure, always identify your patient according to agency policy, using two identifiers, and be attentive to standard precautions, hand hygiene, patient safety and privacy, body mechanics, and documentation.

Procedure Steps

Observe the following steps, regardless of the type of bandage you use:

1. **Choose a bandage of the proper width.** For example, use a 2.5-cm (1-in.) wide bandage for a finger, a 5-cm (2-in.) wide bandage for an arm, and a wider bandage for a leg.
   Prevents pressure and abrasion of the skin.

2. **Thoroughly clean and dry the part** to be covered. Use a nontoxic cleansing solution, such as normal saline.
   Cleaning the wound removes debris, exudates, and bacteria. Drainage and moisture on the skin contribute to irritation.

3. **Remove excess moisture** by gently patting the wound and surrounding skin with gauze sponge.
   Drainage and moisture contribute to skin breakdown.

4. **Stand facing the patient.**
   In this position you can wrap the bandage evenly in the proper direction.

5. **Bandage the body part** in a comfortable position (e.g., with the joint slightly flexed) whenever possible.
   This prevents strain on ligaments and muscles. Movement of the extremity (extension) may cause skin damage if the bandage is too tight, or the extremity is not properly positioned.

6. **Always work from distal** to proximal (or peripheral to central).
   This improves venous return and helps to prevent edema.

7. **If a wound is present,** apply a primary dressing, as prescribed, over the wound.
   A primary dressing is any dressing that is placed first in the wound bed. It provides exudate absorption, holds medications in place, provides antimicrobial coverage, or maintains a moist wound bed.

8. **Apply the bandage** with enough pressure to provide the needed support, but do not bandage too tightly. Make sure circulation to the area is not compromised.

9. **If possible, leave the fingers** (if you are bandaging an arm) or toes (if you are bandaging a leg or foot) exposed so that you can assess the circulation to the extremity. Begin the wrap along the pad of the foot or hand, just under the first bend of the toes or fingers (metatarsal or metacarpal joints).

10. **Begin the wrap** with the bandage against the skin. Unwind the bandage as if rolling it over the extremity.
    This helps to keep the bandage snug against the skin.

11. **Pad bony prominences** before bandaging if there are pressure concerns.

12. **Change bandages** whenever they become soiled or wet from external sources (stool, urine, etc.) and internal sources (drainage that has wicked on the outer surface of the bandage).
    Wound drainage contains chemicals, enzymes, and bacteria that can damage fragile healing tissues.

13. **After bandaging, assess** circulation and comfort regularly.

Proceed to step 14, 16, 19, 25, or 28, depending on the type of bandaging you are using.

Circular Turns

Use this technique to wrap a finger or toe, or as an anchor at the beginning and end of another wrapping technique.

14. **With one hand, hold one end** of the bandage in place. With the other hand, encircle the body part two times with the bandage—the second wrap should partially cover the first wrap. Continue to wrap the body part by overlapping two-thirds of the width of the bandage.

15. **Secure the bandage** with tape or metal clips when you are finished if circular turns are not being combined with another technique. ▼

Spiral Turns

Spiral turns are a variation of the circular turn technique. Spiral turns are often used to wrap an extremity.

16. **Anchor the bandage** by making two circular turns—the second wrap completely covering the first one.

17. **Continue to wrap** the extremity by encircling the body part with each turn angled at approximately 30° so that you are overlapping the preceding wrap by two-thirds of the width of the bandage.

18. **Complete the wrap** by making two circular turns and securing the bandage with tape or metal clips. ▼

Spiral Reverse Turns

Spiral reverse turns are used to bandage cylindrical body parts that are not uniform in size.

19. **Anchor the bandage** by making two circular turns.

20. **Bring the next wrap up** at a 30° angle.

21. **Place the thumb** of your nondominant hand on the wrap to hold the bandage. ▼

22. **Fold the bandage back on itself** and continue to wrap at a 30° angle in the opposite direction. ▼

Circular turns

Bandage folds over to make spiral reverse turn

(continued on next page)

Procedure 32-11 ■ Applying Bandages (continued)

23. **Continue to wrap the bandage,** overlapping each turn by two-thirds. Align each bandage turn at the same position on the extremity. ▼

24. **Complete the wrap** by making two circular turns and securing the bandage with tape or metal clips.

Figure-Eight Turns
The figure-eight wrap is used on joints (e.g., ankle, elbow).

25. **Anchor the bandage** by making two circular turns.

26. **Wrap the bandage** by ascending above the joint and descending below the joint to form a figure-eight. Continue to wrap the bandage, overlapping each turn by two-thirds. Align each bandage turn at the same position on the extremity. ▼

27. **Complete the wrap** by making two circular turns and securing the bandage with tape or metal clips.

Recurrent Turns
The recurrent turns wrap is usually used on amputation stump or head.

28. **Anchor the bandage** by making two circular turns.

29. **Fold the bandage back on itself;** hold it against the body part with one hand. With the other hand, make a half turn perpendicular to the circle turns and central to the distal end being bandaged. ▼

30. **Hold the central turn** with one hand and fold the bandage back on itself; bring it over the distal end of the body part to the right of the center, overlapping the center turn by two-thirds of the width of the bandage.

31. **Next, hold the bandage** at the center with one hand as you bring the bandage back over the end to the left of center. Continue holding and folding the bandage back on itself, alternating right and left until the body part is covered. Overlap by two-thirds of the bandage width with each turn.

32. **Start and return each turn** to the midline or center of the body part and angle it slightly more each time to continue covering the body part.

33. **Complete the bandage** by making two circular turns and securing the bandage with tape or metal clips.

34. **Assess circulation** and comfort of the body part.

❓ What if . . .

■ **Drainage breaks through the outer bandage more frequently than expected?**

Determine the cause of the drainage if possible (i.e., is it blood or serum?). Increased drainage may be a sign of infection and should be evaluated. You might need to change the dressing more often or an alternate, more absorbent type of dressing may be needed.

Wound exudates can harm healing tissues. Dressings that are saturated should be changed as soon as possible to prevent prolonged moisture exposure or maceration.

Evaluation

- Be sure the bandage is firmly wrapped without being too tight.
- Check the circulation is not compromised to the area distal of the bandage.
- Evaluate for numbness or pain around or distal to the bandaged area.

Patient Teaching

- Teach the patient about the expected healing process.
- Inform the patient and caregiver about signs and symptoms of infection and the need to report these findings.
- Instruct the patient and family about signs of circulation problems and how to remove the bandage if needed.

Home Care

- Refer the patient to a home health agency for wound care.
- Some patients or caregivers may be able to perform dressing changes. Determine the patient and/or caregiver's ability to perform dressing changes; teach and demonstrate as needed.

Documentation

Many agencies use wound care flow sheets.

Sample EHR Documentation

6 Lateral Aspect, Left Posterior Forearm, proximal end — Cancel
☐ Wound Healed

Wound Category:
☐ Surgical
☐ Lesions
☐ Decubitus
☑ Burns
☐ Body Modifications

Wound Type:
1st Degree - (Superficial) Skin red in color; Area turns white when touched; No blisters; Painful.
Second Degree - (Partial Thickness) Skin bright red in color; Area turns white when touched; Mottling;
Third Degree - (Full Thickness): Skin bright red in color; Area may or may not turn white when touched
Fourth Degree - (Full Thickness, Deep): Skin has charred patches; Charring may be black, brown or w

Length 4.8 cm
Width 2.4 cm
Depth __ cm

Wound Area:
☐ Skin is mottled (red/pink/white)
☐ Skin bright red in color
☐ Skin red in color
☑ Skin pink in color
☐ Fluid-filled blisters
☐ Wound edges are attached
☑ Undermining at wound edges

Wound Drainage/Exudate:
☐ Scant drainage/exudates
☐ Minimal drainage/exudates
☐ Draining serous fluid
☑ Draining serosanguinous fluid
☐ Draining blood-tinged fluid
☑ No odor
☐ Foul odor

Peri-Wound Area:

Dressing and Wound Care:
☐ No dressing, open to air
☑ Gauze dressing wraps
☐ Occlusive dressing
☐ Hydrocolloidal dressing
☐ Dressing clean, dry and intact
☐ Dressing reinforced, MD to perform 1st drsg change
☐ Wound cleansing & dressing change per MD orders

Solutions Used:
☐ None
☐ Neosporin
☐ Bacitracin
☑ Silvadene

Interventions:
☑ Increasing nutrition and hydration
☑ Burn recovery diet
☑ Keeping skin clean and dry
☐ Using paper tape
☐ Tape removal done slowly
☑ Pressure garments in use
☐ Face mask in use

Patient Response:
☐ No complaints at this time
☐ Tolerated procedure well
☑ Reports procedural pain
☐ Refused dressing change
☐ Refused Hydrotherapy
☑ Compliant with nursing regimen
☐ Non-compliant with nursing regimen

Notes:
mm/dd/yyyy 1200 Dressing change to left wrist burn site completed. Wound cleaned with normal saline. Wound bed with 50% epithelial tissue and 50% fibrin. No signs of infection noted. Silvadene re-applied. Dry gauze dressing placed with gauze circular wrap bandage to cover. Patient reported no pain during procedure.

Practice Resources

Bryant & Nix (2023, April); Le Badour et al. (2019).

Thinking About the Procedure

The video **Applying Bandages**, along with questions and suggested responses, is available on the **Davis's Nursing Skills Videos** Web site at www.fadavis.com.

Procedure 32-12 ■ Removing Sutures and Staples

> For steps to follow in *all* procedures, refer to the Universal Steps for All Procedures on the inside back cover.

Equipment
- Nonsterile gloves
- Suture removal kit or sterile scissors and forceps (Procedure 32-12A)
- Staple remover (Procedure 32-12B)
- Gauze

Delegation
This procedure cannot be delegated to a UAP. Assessment of the incision line or wound is a registered nurse's responsibility and cannot be delegated. The procedure requires assessment and judgment during removal and may require stopping the procedure if complications occur.

Preprocedure Assessment
- Assess staples to ensure none have rotated or turned instead of lying flat along the incision.

Procedure 32-12A ■ Removing Sutures

> When performing the procedure, always identify your patient according to agency policy, using two identifiers, and be attentive to standard precautions, hand hygiene, patient safety and privacy, body mechanics, and documentation.

Procedure Steps

1. **Obtain a suture removal kit.**
2. **Perform hand hygiene.** Don nonsterile gloves.
3. **Cleanse the wound** or suture line.
4. **Use the forceps** to pick up one end of the suture. ▼

   Suture types
   - Plain interrupted
   - Mattress interrupted
   - Plain continuous
   - Mattress continuous
   - Blanket continuous
   - Retention

5. **Slide the small scissors** around the suture and cut near the skin.
   This helps you avoid pulling the exposed portion of the suture through the underlying tissue.

6. **With the forceps, gently pull** the suture in the direction of the knotted side to remove it. ▼

   Removing interrupted sutures

7. **Apply a dressing** or adhesive skin closures if needed.
8. **Remove gloves** and dispose in proper biohazardous waste receptacle. Perform hand hygiene.

Procedure 32-12B ■ Removing Staples

1. **Perform hand hygiene.** Don nonsterile gloves.
2. **After cleansing the wound** or incision, position the staple remover so that the lower jaw is on the bottom.
3. **Place both tips of the lower jaw** of the remover under the staple. ▼

Removing staples

4. **Ensure the staple is** perpendicular to the plane of the skin. If not, reposition the staple with the tips of the lower jaw and apply gentle pressure, causing it to straighten the ends for easier removal.
5. **Lift slightly on the staple,** ensuring that it stays perpendicular to the skin.
6. **Continue to lift slightly** as you gently squeeze the handles together to close.
   Spreads the ends of the staples apart, freeing them from the skin.
7. **Lift the reshaped staple** straight up from the skin.
8. **Remove alternate staples** and check the tension on the wound.
9. **If there is no significant pull** on the wound, remove the remaining staples.
   Where there are many staples over an area of stress (abdomen, legs), the remaining staples are often removed a day or two later after ensuring the incision remains intact.
10. **Place the removed staples** on a piece of gauze.
    Staples are small and can be easily lost. Keeping them in one place prevents this.
11. **Apply a dressing** or adhesive closures, if needed.
12. **Dispose of the removed staples** in the sharp container.
    Ends of the staples are sharp and should be handled with care.
13. **Remove gloves and perform hand hygiene.**

? What if...

- **A staple gets stuck?**
  Gently manipulate the staple with the remover until it is perpendicular to the skin.
  When the skin is stapled, the edges of the staple are crimped to hold the incision together. For the staple to be removed, those edges must be reshaped and straightened. If one edge of the staple is reshaped and the other is not, continuing to remove it can cause pain and tissue trauma.

- **The incision needs a dressing once the staples or sutures have been removed?**
  New surgical incisions should be covered with a sterile dressing the first 24 to 48 hours, but not necessarily after that time. Apply a dressing if you are concerned about soiling or per your institution's policy.
  In a healing incision, epithelial resurfacing is complete in 24 to 48 hours. Though only a few cells thick, this epithelium is enough to keep the wound closed and provide a bacterial barrier.

Evaluation

- Note whether the incision is well approximated after the procedure.
- Ensure that the patient verbalized understanding of the treatment.
- Inspect the wound daily.

Patient Teaching

- Instruct the patient of signs and symptoms of wound infections (i.e., redness, drainage) and the need to report these findings.
- Instruct the patient that he may be able to shower once sutures or staples are removed, if approved by the healthcare provider.

Documentation

The following is an example (many agencies use wound care flow sheets):

Sample Documentation

00/00/0000   1815   Staples removed from abdominal midline incision. Incision edges well approximated without erythema, drainage, or swelling. Dry dressing applied. Patient tolerated the procedure without discomfort. Discussed purpose of staple removal with patient. Will continue to monitor wound daily. ———————— M. Dali, RN

Practice Resources

Sanja & Ramesh (2017).

Procedure 32-13 ■ Shortening a Wound Drain

➤ For steps to follow in *all* procedures, refer to the Universal Steps for All Procedures on the inside back cover.

Equipment
- Nonsterile gloves
- Sterile gloves
- Sterile scissors
- Two safety pins or other clips (sterile)
- Sterile gauze

Delegation
Assessment of the incision line or wound and the drain is a registered nurse's responsibility and cannot be delegated. This procedure should not be delegated to a UAP. The risk for accidently losing the drain into the body or pulling it out of the wound is too high.

Preprocedure Assessment
- Inspect the site around the drain, noting skin excoriation, tenderness, erythema, warmth to the touch, and drainage seeping from the wound.
  Could indicate a wound infection or irritation of the drain at the skin site. Excoriation can be the result of seeping drainage around the tube (e.g., if the tube diameter is not sufficient size to handle drainage output) or, more likely, an obstruction within the tubing.
- Assess the characteristics of the drainage, including color, volume of drainage, presence of blood, odor, pus, and any change in the type or amount of drainage through the tubing.
  A sudden decrease in drainage might indicate a blocked drain. Presence of fresh blood might be a sign of irritation within the wound. Pus and odor in the drainage could indicate wound infection.
- Check the suction apparatus to be sure it is functioning properly.
  A self-suction apparatus might need to be recompressed from time to time to maintain effective vacuum. Electric suction units can fail, delivering too much suction, which can lead to injury. Too little suction can contribute to insufficient drainage, which can lead to pressure on sutures if present, or cause the wound to become infected or heal more slowly.

➤ When performing the procedure, always identify your patient according to agency policy, using two identifiers, and be attentive to standard precautions, hand hygiene, patient safety and privacy, body mechanics, and documentation.

Procedure Steps

1. **Perform hand hygiene** and don nonsterile gloves. Remove wound dressings.
2. **Remove soiled gloves** and discard in a moisture-proof biohazard collection container. Perform hand hygiene.
3. **Open sterile supplies** (scissors, etc.).
4. **Don sterile gloves**; use sterile scissors to cut halfway through a sterile gauze dressing (for later use) or use a sterile precut drain dressing.
5. **If the drain is sutured in place,** use sterile scissors to cut the suture.
6. **Firmly grasp the full width** of the drain at the level of the skin and pull it out by the prescribed amount (e.g., 5 cm [2 in.]).
7. **Insert a sterile safety pin or clamp** through the drain at the level of the skin. Hold the drain tightly between your fingers and insert another pin above your fingers.
   The pin or clamp keeps the drain from disappearing into the wound. ▼
8. **Using sterile scissors, cut** the drain about 2.5 cm (1 in.) above the skin and pin. ▼
9. **Cleanse the wound,** using sterile gauze swabs and the prescribed cleaning solution. In some situations, you may use sterile forceps to manipulate the swabs.
10. **Apply precut sterile gauze** around the drain; then redress the wound. ▼
11. **Remove gloves** and discard in a biohazard container. Perform hand hygiene.
12. **Leave the patient** in a safe and comfortable position.

? What if...

I shorten the drain too much?

Immediately notify the surgeon who placed the drain.

The drain will need to be evaluated to be sure it remains intact, which it mostly likely will. Drainage tubing is secured under the skin surface and will probably not be dislodged with shortening.

Evaluation
- Assess the local area of skin around the drain after manipulating it.
- Note the patency of the drain after shortening it.
- Be sure the drain is secure after shortening.
- Evaluate for complications occurring related to shortening procedure.

Patient Teaching
- Patients should not shorten their own drains. Consult a healthcare provider if concerned about the length of tubing or drains.

Documentation
- Record the intervention.
- Note the amount and characteristics of the drainage.
- Document the appearance of the wound.
- Note any complications that occur with shortening a drain (e.g., manipulation of tubing causes bleeding or drainage at the site).

Sample Documentation

mm/dd/00/00/0000   0930   Penrose shortened 2.0 cm by postop orders. Drain intact. Pt tolerated procedure without complication. —— M. Garcia, RN

Thinking About the Procedure

The video **Shortening a Wound Drain,** along with questions and suggested responses, is available on the **Davis's *Nursing Skills Videos*** Web site at www.fadavis.com.

Procedure 32-14 ■ Emptying a Closed-Wound Drainage System

➤ For steps to follow in *all* procedures, refer to the Universal Steps for All Procedures on the inside back cover.

Equipment
- Drainage container with graduated markings
- Nonsterile gloves
- Disposal sink for biomedical material
- Biohazard disposal receptacle

Delegation
This procedure may be delegated to a UAP who is trained in the skill. Assessment of the wound and drainage characteristics is a licensed professional's responsibility and cannot be delegated.

Preprocedure Assessment
- Assess the appearance of the drainage tube site and sutures, if in place.
- Inspect for warmth, edema, redness, or pus where tubing penetrates the skin.
- Check to be sure the closed-wound drainage system is securely fastened at the connections and within the wound.
- Determine whether suction (electric, portable, or manual) is working properly.

➤ When performing the procedure, always identify your patient according to agency policy, using two identifiers, and be attentive to standard precautions, hand hygiene, patient safety and privacy, body mechanics, and documentation.

(continued on next page)

Procedure 32-14 ■ Emptying a Closed-Wound Drainage System (continued)

Procedure Steps

1. **Read the instructions** about the drainage device.
   Procedures vary among manufacturers and different systems.

2. **Perform hand hygiene.** Don nonsterile gloves and goggles or mask.

3. **Unfasten the drainage device** from the patient's gown.
   The drainage device is often pinned to the patient's gown to prevent it from dislodging.

4. **Open the drainage port** and empty the drainage into a small, graduated container. ▼

5. **With the port still open,** place the collection device on a firm, flat surface (e.g., the overbed table).

6. **Use the palm of one hand** to press down on the device and eject air from it. Do not stand directly over the air vent. Do not touch the drainage port.
   It can splash or bubble.

7. **Use your other hand to scrub** the port and plug with an alcohol-based antiseptic or povidone-iodine swab (Betadine) if the patient is not allergic to iodine. ▼

8. **Continuing to press down** on the device, replace the plug in the port. Do not touch the open port or the part of the plug that goes into the port.
   Creates a constant, negative pressure vacuum to facilitate suction.

9. **Attach the drainage device** to the patient's gown.
   Keeps it secure and prevents it from accidentally dislodging.

10. **Measure the drainage** in the graduated container. Discard drainage in the container for biohazardous material. Wash the graduated container. Do not stand in front of an air vent while doing so.
    Forced air in the room can cause the drainage to splash or bubble, introducing biohazardous material into the environmental air.

11. **Remove your gloves.** Perform hand hygiene.

12. **Document** in the patient's record.

? What if . . .

- **The wound drainage spills?**

  Don nonsterile gloves and protective clothing. Keep people away from the spill area. If sharps are present, remove with forceps. Contain the spill with absorbent pads and place all used materials in a red biohazard bag. Use an approved disinfectant. When finished, place all materials including gloves and gowns in the bag and dispose in the biohazard area.
  Proper handling of contaminated biomedical materials is important to prevent transmission of infectious organisms.

Home Care

- Teach family members who are emptying drainage systems at home to wear gloves and avoid touching the drainage port.

Documentation

- Note the date and time the drainage system is emptied.
- Record the volume lost. Report excess fluid loss to the healthcare provider.
- Describe the appearance of drainage, including presence of blood or purulent material.

Sample Documentation

00/00/0000   0750   Hemovac drained 18 mL serosanguineous fluid over 12 hours. No odor or purulent material noted at drainage site. ——— R. Ferretti, RN

Practice Resource
Wechter, D.G. (2020, February 28).

Thinking About the Procedure

The video **Emptying a Closed-Wound Drainage System,** along with questions and suggested responses, is available on the **Davis's *Nursing Skills Videos*** Web site at www.fadavis.com.

CLINICAL INSIGHTS

Clinical Insight 32-1 ▸ Applying Local Heat Therapy

Preparation
- Determine whether there are any contraindications to heat therapy, such as impaired circulation, bleeding, wound complications, or inability to tolerate the treatment.
- Explain the application and rationale to the patient.

Moist Heat (Irrigations, Compresses, Hot Soaks)

If skin is intact and heat is being applied for relaxation:
- Soak a washcloth or towel in warm water (105°F to 115°F [40°C to 46°C]) and wring out the excess before applying to the skin. Reapply and change water frequently to maintain a constant temperature.

For open areas, use a sterile gauze compress, a soak, or a bath:
- **To make a compress,** soak gauze in the heated solution (105°F to 115°F [40°C to 46°C]) and then apply it to the wound. Usually, you will use sterile gloves, gauze, and solution. Reapply compresses or towels and change the water frequently to maintain a constant temperature.
- **For a soak,** you will need to immerse the affected area. Sterilized tubs are often used for this procedure. *Soaking helps cleanse a wound and remove encrusted material.*
- **A bath** is a modification of a soak. The most used bath is a **sitz bath** (see Fig. 32-17), which soaks the patient's perineal area. A special tub or chair may be used. Because of infection control concerns, disposable sitz baths are preferred. Check that the water temperature is from 105°F to 110°F (40°C to 43°C). Instruct the patient to soak for 15 minutes.

Dry Heat (Aquathermia Pads)

Aquathermia pads (also called K-pads) are plastic or vinyl pads that circulate water in the interior to create a constant temperature.
- Connect the pad via tubing to the electric heating unit, which constantly exchanges water that has been heated to the specified temperature.
- Fill the reservoir about two-thirds full of distilled water.
- Set the temperature control to 98°F to 105°F (37°F to 40.5°C).
- Cover the pad with a protective case and apply it to the body part.
  To prevent tissue injury.

Dry Heat: Disposable Hot Packs and Hot Water Bags or Bottles

Hot water bags are common in the home use but not in healthcare agencies because of the danger of burns from improper use.
- Use water that is 115°F to 125°F (46°C to 52°C).
- Fill the bag about two-thirds full of warm tap water, expel the air from the bag, and close the top.
- Tip the bag upside down to test for leaking.
- Wrap the bag in a towel; place it on the patient.
- Never place a heat source directly on the patient's skin. Burns can occur.

Dry Heat: Electric Heating Pads
- Be sure that the body part is dry or that the pad has a waterproof cover.

✚ Safety Precautions for Electric Heating Pads
- Do not use pins (e.g., to hold a cover in place) or other sharp objects on the pad.
  The pin could go through a wire and cause an electric shock.
- Tell the patient to report any discomfort during the treatment.
- For home use, warn the patient about the danger of skin injury, especially from microwavable bags. *These can get too hot and lead to a burn.*
- Avoid direct contact with the heating device. Cover the heat source with a washcloth, towel, or fitted sleeve.
- Do not place the heating device (pad, bag) under the patient; place it over the body part.
  Helps prevent burns.
- Apply heat intermittently, leaving it on for no more than 15 minutes at a time in an area.
  This helps prevent tissue injury (e.g., burns, impaired circulation). It also makes the therapy more effective by preventing the rebound phenomenon.
- Check the skin frequently for redness or blistering.
- Caution patients to place the heating pad or device over the body area and never to lie on it.

Clinical Insight 32-2 ▸ Applying Local Cold Therapy

Preparation
- Determine whether there are any contraindications to the treatment, such as impaired circulation, bleeding, wound complications, or inability to tolerate the treatment.
- Explain the application and rationale to the patient.
- Assess for indications for cold application. Measure the patient's temperature.

Cooling Baths
A cooling bath is often used to treat a high fever (above 104°F [40°C]). It promotes heat loss through conduction and vaporization.
- Prepare a pan of water with a temperature from 65°F to 90°F (18°C to 32°C).
- You may add a fan to increase heat loss if the temperature is markedly elevated.
- Slowly sponge the face, arms, legs, back, and buttocks with the cool water. Do not dry the area; cover with a damp towel.
- Take about 30 minutes to complete the bath.
  Cooling the body too rapidly will cause shivering, which will increase heat production.
- You may also place ice bags or cold packs on the forehead in the axillae and the groin.
- Assess the patient constantly during a cooling bath.
  If the patient begins to shiver, the temperature may begin to rise.

Cold Compresses
- Apply a cool, damp cloth or towel to the body part.
- Renew the compress or cloth frequently.
  The temperature of the compress or cloth will rapidly rise toward body temperature.

Collars, Ice Bags, Commercially Prepared Cold Packs, Aquapads
- You can make an ice bag out of a nonsterile glove or small plastic bag by filling it with ice chips and tying a knot in the top.
- Fill the ice bag with ice chips or an alcohol-based solution.
- Cover ice bags or packs with a towel or soft cover.
- Apply to the skin for a maximum of 15 minutes and then remove. You may reapply the cold pack in 1 hour.

✚ Safety Precautions for Cooling Devices
- Measure water temperature with a bath thermometer.
- Tell the patient to report any discomfort during the treatment.
- Avoid direct contact with the cooling device. Cover the cold pack with a washcloth, towel, or fitted sleeve.
- Apply cold intermittently, leaving it on for no more than 15 minutes at a time in an area.
  Helps to prevent tissue injury (e.g., impaired circulation). It also makes the therapy more effective by preventing the rebound phenomenon: At the time the cold reaches maximum therapeutic effect, the opposite effect (vasodilation) begins.
- Observe for tissue damage: bluish purple, mottled appearance of the skin, numbness, and sometimes blisters and pain.
- Monitor for elevated blood pressure.

ASSESSMENT GUIDELINES AND TOOLS

Focused Assessment

History Questions for Skin and Wound Assessment
- What is your typical activity level?
- Do you ever use a wheelchair or mobile device to get around? Do you require assistance to get out of bed or a chair?
- Tell me about your usual diet.
- How much liquid do you drink each day?
- Do you have any areas of numbness and tingling?
- Have you had any recent changes in your skin?
- Do you have any sores or open areas? If so, how long have you had the wound?
- Have you ever had difficulty with wound healing?
- What kinds of healthcare problems have you been having?
- What medications—prescribed, herbal, or over the counter—are you taking?
- What is your typical hygiene routine?
- Do you ever lose control of your bladder or bowels?
- Do you use tobacco?
- How much time do you spend outdoors?
- Do you have diabetes? If so, how often do you check your feet? How often do you see a podiatrist? What is your average blood sugar?

Focused Assessment

Physical Examination: Wound Assessment

All Wounds

Assess all wounds for the following:

Location
Describe the location of the wound in anatomical terms. For example, you would describe an incision from cardiac surgery as a midsternal incision extending from the manubrium to the xiphoid process.

Size
- Measure the length and width of the wound in centimeters.
- To measure wound depth, gently insert a sterile cotton-tipped applicator into the deepest part of the wound. Measure the applicator from the skin level to the tip.
- If possible, use photo documentation, indicating the dimensions on the photo. This is especially useful in the case of a wound with an irregular border.

Appearance
Your description of the appearance of the wound should be detailed. You must describe the following:
- **Type of wound** (open or closed)
- **If the wound is sutured,** examine the closure. Are the wound edges approximated? Is there tension on any aspect of the wound? Are the stitches intact?
- **The color of the wound.** Redness and inflammation for the first 2 to 3 days is normal, but erythema or swelling beyond that time may indicate infection.
- **Condition of the wound bed (in an open wound).** A beefy red, moist appearance is evidence of healing. A pale color or dry texture indicates a delay in healing.
- **Examine for necrosis, slough, and eschar.** Examine for a tunnel or sinus tract in the wound bed; if there is one, inspect and probe it for depth and characteristics.
- **The skin surrounding the wound.** Observe for skin discoloration, hematoma, or additional injury to the surrounding tissue. Observe for maceration, tunnelling, crepitus, blistering, or erythema. Examine the edges of the wound for epithelial tissue and contraction. Look for undermining beneath the wound margins.

Drainage
- **Presence of drainage or exudate.** Describe the color, consistency, amount, and odor.
- **Assess the quantity of wound drainage** by weighing dressings before they are applied and again when they have been removed. The change in weight reflects the amount of drainage that they have absorbed.
- **If a drain is present,** measure the amount of fluid in the collection container.
- **Odor** may indicate fistula formation or contamination with bacteria. If a new odor develops, assess carefully for presence of a fistula.

Patient Responses
Ask your patients about pain, discomfort, or itching related to the wound or wound care.

Assessing an Untreated Wound

Your assessment should determine what, if any, additional professional support is necessary. Assess the following same aspects as for treated wounds: location, size, appearance, description of drainage, condition of wound margins, condition of surrounding skin, and effect of the wound on the patient. In addition, assess the following:

- **Bleeding.** If bleeding is profuse, apply direct pressure to the site. If bleeding continues after you apply pressure for 5 minutes or if blood is spurting from the wound, call the physician immediately.
- **Severity of the wound.** A gaping wound or a deep wound with fat, fascia, or muscle exposed will need additional care.
- **Last tetanus immunization.** Immunization should be given if (1) the last immunization was 10 years ago or longer, (2) the wound is contaminated with dirt or debris and the tetanus injection was given more than 5 years ago, or (3) it is uncertain when the patient last received an immunization.
- **Whether the wound was caused by a bite.** Determine whether the wound was caused by any type of bite, animal or human. A deep bite wound usually requires additional observation and/or antibiotics.
- **Pain.** Assess for pain. Any wound causing severe pain requires a comprehensive evaluation.
- **Numbness or loss of movement.** If any deficit is detected, the patient will need immediate evaluation.
- **Presence of chronic medical conditions.** Examples include diabetes, malnutrition, immunocompromise, a bleeding disorder. Patients with conditions that affect wound healing will need ongoing evaluation.

Braden Scale for Predicting Pressure Sore Risk

BRADEN SCALE FOR PREDICTING PRESSURE SORE RISK

Patient's Name _____ Evaluator's Name _____ Date of Assessment _____

Category	1	2	3	4
SENSORY PERCEPTION — ability to respond meaningfully to pressure-related discomfort	**1. Completely Limited** — Unresponsive (does not moan, flinch, or grasp) to painful stimuli, due to diminished level of consciousness or sedation. OR limited ability to feel pain over most of body.	**2. Very Limited** — Responds only to painful stimuli. Cannot communicate discomfort except by moaning or restlessness. OR has a sensory impairment which limits the ability to feel pain or discomfort over 1/2 of body.	**3. Slightly Limited** — Responds to verbal commands, but cannot always communicate discomfort or the need to be turned. OR has some sensory impairment which limits ability to feel pain or discomfort in 1 or 2 extremities.	**4. No Impairment** — Responds to verbal commands. Has no sensory deficit which would limit ability to feel or voice pain or discomfort.
MOISTURE — degree to which skin is exposed to moisture	**1. Constantly Moist** — Skin is kept moist almost constantly by perspiration, urine, etc. Dampness is detected every time patient is moved or turned.	**2. Very Moist** — Skin is often, but not always moist. Linen must be changed at least once a shift.	**3. Occasionally Moist** — Skin is occasionally moist, requiring an extra linen change approximately once a day.	**4. Rarely Moist** — Skin is usually dry, linen only requires changing at routine intervals.
ACTIVITY — degree of physical activity	**1. Bedfast** — Confined to bed.	**2. Chairfast** — Ability to walk severely limited or non-existent. Cannot bear own weight and/or must be assisted into chair or wheelchair.	**3. Walks Occasionally** — Walks occasionally during day, but for very short distances, with or without assistance. Spends majority of each shift in bed or chair.	**4. Walks Frequently** — Walks outside room at least twice a day and inside room at least once every two hours during waking hours.
MOBILITY — ability to change and control body position	**1. Completely Immobile** — Does not make even slight changes in body or extremity position without assistance.	**2. Very Limited** — Makes occasional slight changes in body or extremity position but unable to make frequent or significant changes independently.	**3. Slightly Limited** — Makes frequent though slight changes in body or extremity position independently.	**4. No Limitation** — Makes major and frequent changes in position without assistance.
NUTRITION — usual food intake pattern	**1. Very Poor** — Never eats a complete meal. Rarely eats more than 1/2 of any food offered. Eats 2 servings or less of protein (meat or dairy products) per day. Takes fluids poorly. Does not take a liquid dietary supplement. OR is NPO and/or maintained on clear liquids or IVs for more than 5 days.	**2. Probably Inadequate** — Rarely eats a complete meal and generally eats only about 1/2 of any food offered. Protein intake includes only 3 servings of meat or dairy products per day. Occasionally will take a dietary supplement. OR receives less than optimum amount of liquid diet or tube feeding.	**3. Adequate** — Eats over half of most meals. Eats a total of 4 servings of protein (meat, dairy products) per day. Occasionally will refuse a meal, but will usually take a supplement when offered. OR is on a tube feeding or TPN regimen which probably meets most of nutritional needs.	**4. Excellent** — Eats most of every meal. Never refuses a meal. Usually eats a total of 4 or more servings of meat and dairy products. Occasionally eats between meals. Does not require supplementation.
FRICTION & SHEAR	**1. Problem** — Requires moderate to maximum assistance in moving. Complete lifting without sliding against sheets is impossible. Frequently slides down in bed or chair, requiring frequent repositioning with maximum assistance. Spasticity, contractures or agitation leads to almost constant friction.	**2. Potential Problem** — Moves feebly or requires minimum assistance. During a move skin probably slides to some extent against sheets, chair, restraints or other devices. Maintains relatively good position in chair or bed most of the time but occasionally slides down.	**3. No Apparent Problem** — Moves in bed and in chair independently and has sufficient muscle strength to lift up completely during move. Maintains good position in bed or chair.	

Total Score _____

© Copyright Barbara Braden and Nancy Bergstrom, 1988 All rights reserved

Source: U.S. Department of Health and Human Services. (1992). *Clinical practice guideline. Pressure ulcers in adults: Prediction and prevention* (pp. 16–17). PPPPUA Publication No. 92-0047. Rockville, MD: Public Health Service. Copyright © Barbara Braden and Nancy Bergstrom, 1988. Reprinted with permission.

Norton Pressure Sore Risk Assessment Scale

Norton Scale for Assessing Risk of Pressure Ulcers

	Physical Condition	Mental Condition	Activity	Mobility	Incontinent	
	Good 4 Fair 3 Poor 2 Very bad 1	Alert 4 Apathetic 3 Confused 2 Stupor 1	Ambulant 4 Walk/help 3 Chair-bound 2 Bed 1	Full 4 Slightly limited 3 Very limited 2 Immobile 1	Not 4 Occasional 3 Usually/urine 2 Doubly 1	Total Score
Name/Date						

The Norton Scale uses five criteria to assess patients' risk for pressure ulcers. Scores of 14 or less indicate liability to ulcers; scores of <12 indicate very high risk.

Source: Norton, D., McLaren, R., & Exton-Smith, A. N. (1975). *An investigation of geriatric nursing problems in hospitals.* Churchill Livingstone. Used with permission.

PUSH Tool for Evaluation of Pressure Ulcers

PUSH Tool - Version 3.0

Patient Name:_____   Patient ID#:_____

Ulcer Location: _____   Date:_____

DIRECTIONS:
Observe and measure the pressure ulcer. Categorize the ulcer with respect to surface area, exudate, and type of wound tissue. Record a sub-score for each of these ulcer characteristics. Add the sub-scores to obtain the total score. A comparison of total scores measured over time provides an indication of the improvement or deterioration in pressure ulcer healing.

Length x Width	0 0 cm²	1 <0.3 cm²	2 0.3 - 0.6 cm²	3 0.7 - 1.0 cm²	4 1.1 - 2.0 cm²	5 2.1 - 3.0 cm²	Subscore
		6 3.1 - 4.0 cm²	7 4.1 - 8.0 cm²	8 8.1 - 12.0 cm²	9 12.1 - 24.0 cm²	10 > 24 cm²	
Exudate Amount	0 None	1 Light	2 Moderate	3 Heavy			Subscore
Tissue Type	0 Closed	1 Epithelial Tissue	2 Granulation Tissue	3 Slough	4 Necrotic Tissue		Subscore
							Total Score

Length x Width: Measure the greatest length (head to toe) and the greatest width (side to side) using a centimeter ruler. Multiply these two measurements (length • width) to obtain an estimate of surface area in square centimeters (cm²). **Caveat:** Do not guess! Always use a centimeter ruler and always use the same method each time the ulcer is measured.

Exudate Amount: Estimate the amount of exudate (drainage) present after removal of the dressing and before applying any topical agent to the ulcer. Estimate the exudate (drainage) as none, light, moderate, or heavy.

Tissue Type: This refers to the types of tissue that are present in the wound (ulcer) bed. Score as a "4" if there is any necrotic tissue present. Score as a "3" if there is any amount of slough present and necrotic tissue is absent. Score as a "2" if the wound is clean and contains granulation tissue. A superficial wound that is reepithelializing is scored as a "1". When the wound is closed, score as a "0".

- **4 - Necrotic Tissue (Eschar):** black, brown, or tan tissue that adheres firmly to the wound bed or ulcer edges and may be either firmer or softer than surrounding skin.
- **3 - Slough:** yellow or white tissue that adheres to the ulcer bed in strings or thick clumps, or is mucinous.
- **2 - Granulation Tissue:** pink or beefy red tissue with a shiny, moist, granular appearance.
- **1 - Epithelial Tissue:** for superficial ulcers, new pink or shiny tissue (skin) that grows in from the edges or as islands on the ulcer surface.
- **0 - Closed/Resurfaced:** the wound is completely covered with epithelium (new skin).

Note: Refer to the NPUAP Website (www.npuap.org) for further information regarding development and use of the PUSH Tool.

Version 3.0: 9/15/98
© National Pressure Ulcer Advisory Panel

PRESSURE ULCER HEALING CHART
(use a separate page for each pressure ulcer)

Patient Name:_____   Patient ID#:_____
Ulcer Location: _____   Date:_____

Directions: Observe and measure pressure ulcers at regular intervals using the PUSH Tool. Date and record PUSH Sub-scale and Total Scores on the Pressure Ulcer Healing Record below.

PRESSURE ULCER HEALING RECORD

DATE												
Length × Width												
Exudate Amount												
Tissue Type												
Total Score												

Graph the PUSH Total Score on the Pressure Ulcer Healing Graph below.

PRESSURE ULCER HEALING GRAPH

PUSH Total Score: 17, 16, 15, 14, 13, 12, 11, 10, 9, 8, 7, 6, 5, 4, 3, 2, 1, Healed 0

DATE:

Version 3.0: 9/15/98
© National Pressure Ulcer Advisory Panel

Source: National Pressure Ulcer Advisory Panel (NPUAP). (1998). Pressure ulcer scale for healing (PUSH) Tool, version 3.0. https://www.sralab.org/sites/default/files/2017-06/push3.pdf

DIAGNOSTIC TESTING

Tests for Assessing Wounds

Test	Normal Range	Comments
Leukocyte (WBC) count	5,000–10,000/mm^3	Usually done as a part of a complete blood count (CBC) but may be ordered as an independent test. White blood cells (WBCs) may increase when a wound develops; continued elevation may signal infection. A low WBC count may delay wound healing. Leukocytes are responsible for an inflammatory reaction at the wound site, phagocytosis of bacteria and cellular debris, and the creation of antibodies.
Serum protein **Serum albumin** **Serum prealbumin**	6.0–8.0 g/dL 3.4–4.8 g/dL 12–42 mg/dL	Low serum levels indicate limited nutritional stores that delay wound healing or place the patient at high risk for pressure injury. Serum protein may be monitored as an indicator of the ability to heal a wound or prevent a pressure injury. Serum protein and albumin levels are closely related. However, both fluctuate slowly. A more accurate measure of a patient's immediate protein stores is reflected in the prealbumin level.
Erythrocyte sedimentation rate (ESR)	<50 years old: 0–15 mm/hr; >50 years old: 0–20 mm/hr	In the presence of an inflammatory and necrotic process, blood proteins are altered. This test indicates whether the RBCs stick together, become heavier, and settle at the bottom of a laboratory tube when held vertically.
Coagulation studies: Partial thromboplastin time, activated (aPTT)	Varies with respect to equipment and reagents used. Critical values: >70 seconds or <53 seconds	Prolonged coagulation times may result in excessive blood loss or ongoing bleeding in the wound bed. Shortened coagulation times increase the risk for blood clot formation problems, such as deep vein thrombosis, pulmonary embolus, or stroke.
Prothrombin time (clotting time)	Critical values: >20 seconds (uncoagulated) or 3 times normal control (anticoagulated)	Altered coagulation may result from anticoagulant medications, a concurrent illness, trauma, or reaction to transfusions.
International normalized ratio (INR)	<2.0 for patients not receiving anticoagulation therapy; 2.0–3.0 for those receiving coagulation therapy	A standardized test to evaluate clotting times, considered the gold standard.
Wound cultures	Negative; no growth of pathogens	Wound cultures may be prescribed to determine the types of bacteria present in the wound. Cultures may be obtained by swab, aspiration, or tissue biopsy. A positive culture may not indicate an infection as chronic wounds are colonized with bacteria.
Tissue biopsy	Negative; no growth of pathogens	Wounds are not considered infected unless the bacteria count exceeds 100,000 organisms per gram of tissue. Exception: The presence of beta-hemolytic streptococci in any number indicates infection.

CLINICAL REASONING
Applying the Full-Spectrum Nursing Model

PATIENT SITUATION

Tio Santos is a 66-year-old man with obesity, diabetes, and hypertension. He is being seen for a wound on his right foot that doesn't seem to be healing. He injured his foot when repairing drywall at home. He is otherwise relatively sedentary at home. The wound is oozing, swollen, tender, and warm to the touch. Mr. Santos is now running a low-grade fever of 100.4°F (38°C) at home. He tells you his foot is very painful, especially with any weight bearing, and throbs when he is sitting or lying still. You measure the wound bed to be 6 cm x 4 cm and note purulent exudate at the distal edge. He is referred to an outpatient wound care center for treatment.

THINKING

1. *Theoretical Knowledge:*

   a. What is the Braden scale and why might it be used for Mr. Santos?

   b. What risk factors for delayed wound healing does Mr. Santos have?

2. *Critical Thinking (Considering Alternatives, Deciding What to Do):*

   a. To care for Mr. Santos' wound, should you use sterile gloves, clean nonsterile gloves, or no gloves? Explain your thinking.

DOING

3. *Practical Knowledge (Assessment):*

   a. What symptoms of infection does Mr. Santos have?

   b. To be certain the wound is infected, what would you need to know or do?

CARING

4. *Self-Knowledge:* Imagine you are Mr. Santos and have had a wound on your foot for 6 weeks. What would be the most troublesome symptom in your daily life? What would concern you the most?

Critical Thinking and Clinical Judgment

1. You are caring for a 22-year-old man with paralysis from the waist down secondary to a motor vehicle accident. He has been admitted to the hospital with a urinary tract infection manifested by a fever of 102°F (39°C) and lethargy. His family reports he has been withdrawn and sits in his wheelchair looking at his phone all day.

   a. What risk factors does this patient have for skin breakdown?

   b. What locations of his body should you be most concerned for the formation of pressure injury?

   c. What actions should you take to decrease the risk of pressure injury for your patient? What further information do you need?

2. A 63-year-old male patient is admitted to your unit after an emergency appendectomy. His appendix was ruptured, and the surgeon has left the wound open to heal by secondary intention. A Jackson–Pratt drain is in place in the wound bed. A moderate amount of purosanguineous drainage is visible in the drain. The surgeon has ordered saline-moistened gauze packing every 4 hours.

   a. What actions should you take as you prepare to do the first dressing change?

   b. How will you secure the dressing?

3. For the following patients, write a nursing diagnosis related to skin integrity. Include problem, etiology, and defining characteristics. If you do not have enough data for one of those components, state what additional data you need.

   a. Mrs. Whitefeather is 95 years old. She has cancer, and she has stopped eating and has become emaciated. Recently she has become too weak to move about in bed without help. However, her skin is intact with no redness, even over her bony prominences. She has a low score on the Braden Scale for Predicting Pressure Sore Risk.

   b. Mason Allen is 4 years old. He has a severe case of poison ivy and has blisters on his skin. He has been scratching and has bleeding, excoriated areas over his limbs, face, and trunk.

   c. Sabreen Hassen has a stage 2 pressure injury on her left heel.

4. For each of the following concepts, use critical thinking to describe how or why it is important to nursing, patient care, or skin integrity and wound healing. Note that these are *not* to be merely definitions.

   Shearing

   Friction

   Pressure

   Wound healing process

   Preventing pressure injury

   Wound assessment

   Dressing changes

What Are the Main Points in This Chapter?

- The layers of the skin are the epidermis (outermost), the dermis, and the subcutaneous layer (innermost).
- The major functions of the skin are protection of the internal organs, unique identification of an individual, thermoregulation, metabolism of nutrients and metabolic waste products, and sensation.
- Age, mobility, nutrition, hydration, moisture underlying conditions, medications, contamination or infection, diminished sensation, cognitive impairment, hygiene, and lifestyle are factors that influence the ability to maintain intact skin and heal wounds.
- If there are no breaks in the skin, a wound is described as **closed**. A wound is considered **open** if there is a break in the skin or mucous membranes.
- Acute wounds may be intentional (e.g., surgical incisions) or unintentional (e.g., trauma) and are expected to heal without complications.
- Wounds that exceed the anticipated length of recovery are classified as chronic wounds. Chronic wounds include pressure, arterial, and venous wounds and diabetic ulcers. A chronic wound may linger for months or years.
- **Clean wounds** are uninfected wounds with minimal inflammation. **Clean-contaminated wounds** are surgical incisions that enter the gastrointestinal, respiratory, or genitourinary tracts. **Contaminated wounds** include open, traumatic wounds or surgical incisions in which a major break in asepsis occurred. **Infected wounds** are wounds with evidence of infection, such as presence of microorganisms.
- A wound that involves minimal or no tissue loss and has wound edges that are approximated are said to heal by primary intention.
- A wound that involves extensive tissue loss and has margins that cannot be approximated, or is infected, heals by secondary intention.
- Tertiary intention healing, or delayed primary closure, occurs when two surfaces of granulation tissue are brought together. Initially the wound is allowed to heal by secondary intention.
- Healing occurs in three stages. The **inflammatory phase** lasts from 1 to 5 days and consists of two major processes: hemostasis and inflammation. The **proliferative phase** occurs from days 5 to 21. It is characterized by cell development aimed at filling the wound defect and resurfacing the skin. The **maturation phase** begins in the second or third week and continues until the wound is completely healed.
- Wound closure methods include adhesive strips (Steri-Strips), absorbent sutures, surgical staples, and surgical glue.
- Drainage is the flow of fluids from a wound or cavity. It is often referred to as exudate (fluid that oozes as a result of inflammation).
- Complications of wound healing include hemorrhage, infection, dehiscence, evisceration, and fistula formation.
- Pressure injury is caused by unrelieved pressure over time that compromises blood flow to tissue, resulting in ischemia in the underlying tissue.

- **A stage 1 pressure injury** is an area of persistent redness and does not blanch.
- **A stage 2 pressure injury** involves partial-thickness skin loss of the epidermis, dermis, or both.
- **A stage 3 pressure injury** is characterized by full-thickness skin loss involving damage or necrosis of subcutaneous tissue, which may extend down to, but not through, the underlying fascia. The ulcer appears as a deep crater.
- **A stage 4 pressure injury** involves full-thickness skin loss with extensive destruction; tissue necrosis; or damage to muscle, bone, or support structures. Undermining and sinus tracts (blind tracts underneath the epidermis) are common.
- Extrinsic factors leading to pressure injuries are those that alter the skin and tissue integrity and blood supply (e.g., aging, low blood pressure, neurological injury, poor nutrition, edema, and fever).
- Extrinsic factors include friction and shearing and exposure to moisture and pressure.
- Not all lower extremity ulcers are related to pressure. Some are caused by poor perfusion, such as venous stasis ulcers, diabetic foot ulcers, and arterial ulcers.
- An eschar is a black leathery covering of necrotic tissue. An ulcer covered by an eschar cannot be classified because it is impossible to determine the depth.
- The Braden, Norton, and PUSH scales evaluate risk for problems with skin integrity.
- When assessing a wound, note the following: the type of wound, the color of the wound and surrounding skin, the condition of the wound bed, drainage and odor, and the level of pain associated with the wound or wound care.
- Prevention of pressure injury includes skin care, nutrition, turning and positioning, using therapeutic mattresses and cushions, and patient/family teaching.
- Five types of debridement are used: sharp, mechanical, enzymatic, autolytic, and biotherapy (maggot debridement).
- Wound care therapies to promote healing might include negative pressure wound therapy, electrical stimulation, tissue growth factors, ultrasound, bioengineered skin substitutes, and surgical options.
- **Primary dressings** are ones that are placed in the wound bed and have contact with the wound. A **secondary dressing** covers or holds a primary dressing in place. Many dressings can act as both.
- Types of wound dressings are absorption, alginate, antimicrobial, collagen, gauze, foam dressings, hydrocolloid, hydrogel, skin sealants, and moisture barriers.
- Ideal wound irrigation pressures range from 4 psi to 15 psi. Current recommendations are to use a 35-mL syringe attached to a 19-gauge angiocatheter. This will deliver the solution at approximately 8 psi.
- Heat application promotes vasodilation, increases tissue metabolism, increases capillary permeability, reduces blood viscosity, and reduces muscle tension.
- The application of cold causes vasoconstriction, local anesthesia, reduced cell metabolism, increased blood viscosity, and decreased muscle tension.

Knowledge Map

NURSING INTERVENTIONS:
- Wound assessment
  - ID risk: Braden score
  - Wound culture
- Prevention strategies
  - skin care
  - nutrition
  - positioning
  - therapeutic mattress
  - patient/family teaching

PROCESSES:
- Regeneration
- Primary intention
- Secondary intention
- Tertiary intention

PHASES:
- Inflammatory
- Proliferative
- Maturation

WOUND HEALING

WOUND CLOSURES:
- Adhesive strips
- Sutures
- Surgical staples
- Surgical glue
- Negative pressure wound therapy

TYPES:
- Skin integrity
  - closed or open
- Healing time
  - acute or chronic
- Contamination
  - clean or infected
- Depth
  - Superficial
  - Partial-thickness
  - Full-thickness (penetrating)

CLEANSING:
- Removes exudate; slough, foreign material, microorganisms
- NS; dilute antimicrobial; wound cleanser
- Gentle technique; hydrotherapy

DEBRIDING:
- Sharp
- Mechanical
  - wet to dry
  - hydrotherapy
- Enzymatic
- Autolysis
- Biotherapy (maggot therapy)

WOUND CARE

DRESSINGS:
- Gauze
- Transparent films
- Hydrocolloids
- Hydrogels
- Absorptive → beads/ribbon/alginate
- FOAM
- Skin sealants and moisture barriers
- Antimicrobial

TYPES OF DRAINAGE:
- Serous
- Sanguinous
- Serosanguinous
- Purulent
- Purosanguinous

DRAINAGE DEVICES:
- Penrose drain
- Hemovac
- Jackson-Pratt
- Davol

Caused by unrelieved pressure that leads to tissue ischemia

PRESSURE INJURY

FACTORS INVOLVED:
- Intrinsic: immobility, impaired sensation, malnutrition
- Extrinsic: friction, shearing, moisture, pressure

Stages I–IV + unstageable + suspected deep tissue injury: increasing degree of tissue damage/loss/necrosis/death

WOUND: Disruption in the normal integrity of the skin

Special consideration

SKIN
- Epidermis
- Dermis
- Subcutaneous

FACTORS INFLUENCING INTEGRITY:
- Age
- Mobility
- Nutrition/hydration
- Decreased sensation/circulation
- Medications
- Moisture
- Fever
- Lifestyle
- Infection

CHAPTER 33

Oxygenation

STUDENT RESOURCES

The questions and exercises in this book allow you to practice the kind of thinking you will use as a full-spectrum nurse. Critical-thinking questions usually have more than one right answer, so we do not provide "correct" answers for these features. Try to answer these questions yourself. It is more important to develop your nursing judgment than to just cover content. You will learn more by discussing the questions with your peers. If you are still unsure, see the Davis Advantage chapter resources for suggested responses.

To explore learning resources for this chapter,

Go to www.DavisAdvantage.com and find:

Answers and Suggested Responses for all questions in this chapter
Concept Map
Knowledge Map
References and Bibliography

Key Concepts

Oxygenation
Respiration
Ventilation

Related Concepts

See the Concept Map on Davis Advantage.

Example Client Conditions

Pneumonia
URI and influenza

Caring for the Williams Family

Charlene Williams, Stanley's mother, has been complaining of fatigue and a persistent cough for approximately 2 weeks. Stanley has brought his mother to the family clinic where you are a nurse. Mrs. Williams appears disheveled. Her clothes are rumpled and her hair is tousled. Normally she is dressed neatly and wearing makeup. She has a hard time signing in at the desk and tells the receptionist she has a 1:00 p.m. appointment, but it is 9:00 a.m. Mrs. Williams' vital signs are as follows: BP, 142/90 mm Hg; pulse, 94 beats/min and regular; respirations, 24 breaths/min and labored; temperature, 99.6°F (37.5°C) oral.

(Continued)

Caring for the Williams Family (continued)

A. What additional assessment data would be useful to gather at this time?

B. During her visit at the clinic, you notice that Mrs. Williams is very confused. Her weight has dropped 7 pounds since her visit last month, her mucous membranes are dry, and she is dyspneic with any activity. She is diagnosed with pneumonia. Because of her rapid decline, Mrs. Williams is admitted to the hospital to receive intravenous antibiotics. At the hospital, her initial pulse oximetry reading is 90%, and she is unable to cough up secretions. Write the most appropriate nursing diagnosis to focus interventions for Mrs. Williams.

C. What actions should you anticipate taking?

D. The hospitalist (hospital-based physician) writes prescriptions for IV fluids, antibiotics, suction prn, and continuous pulse oximetry. What additional prescriptions will you need to provide care for Mrs. Williams? What therapy would you suggest?

E. Mrs. Williams requires suctioning to help remove secretions. She has a weak cough and crackles and rhonchi throughout all lung fields. There are few secretions in her oropharynx, and she bites down on the catheter. What technique would you use to suction her? Explain your choice.

F. After 4 days in the hospital, Mrs. Williams is discharged to home. She asks the hospital nurse, "What can I do to make sure I never get that sick again?" How would you answer this question?

Practical Knowledge clinical application

As you perform the procedures, apply the concepts and other theoretical knowledge you learned in Volume 1. This section will help you acquire the skills to safely provide for clients' oxygenation needs.

PROCEDURES

In this section you will find procedures necessary for supporting oxygenation. Some, but not all, of the procedures in this section can be delegated to qualified unlicensed assistive personnel (UAPs). Refer to the delegation notes in each procedure and to agency policies.

Procedure 33-1 ■ Collecting a Sputum Specimen

➤ For steps to follow in *all* procedures, refer to the Universal Steps for All Procedures on the inside back cover.

Equipment

For all sputum specimens, you will need a patient identification label, a completed laboratory requisition form, and a small plastic bag with a biohazard label (or container designated by the agency) for delivering the specimen to the laboratory. Depending on how you obtain the specimen, you also need the following:

Procedure 33-1A: Collecting an Expectorated Sputum Specimen

- Sterile specimen container with lid
- Personal protective equipment (PPE), as needed and based on precaution type
- Procedure gloves
- Glass of water
- Emesis basin
- Tissues
- Pillow (if abdominal or chest incision is present)

Procedure 33-1B: Collecting a Suctioned Sputum Specimen

- Sterile suction catheter or sterile suction kit
- Suction device (portable or wall)
- Sterile gloves
- PPE, as needed and based on precaution type
- Inline sputum specimen with trap (DeLee catheter)
- Sterile saline solution
- Oxygen therapy equipment, if indicated
- Linen-saver pad or towel

Delegation

You can delegate collection of an expectorated sputum specimen to a UAP who has been adequately trained in performing the skill. Assess the patient's respiratory status first; if the patient's condition is unstable, do not delegate the procedure. Do not delegate obtaining a specimen by tracheal suctioning.

Preprocedure Assessment

- Assess the patient's comprehension of the procedure.
  Understanding allays anxiety and promotes cooperation.
- Assess breath sounds; respiratory rate, depth, and pattern; skin and nailbed color; and tissue perfusion.
  You may need to delay sputum collection if the patient is in respiratory distress.
- Assess ability to deep-breathe, cough, and expectorate.
  If the patient is unable to deep-breathe, cough, and expectorate, suctioning may be necessary to obtain an adequate sputum specimen.
- Determine when the patient last ate or had a tube feeding, especially for a specimen obtained by suction.
  Specimen collection should be delayed for 1 to 2 hours after eating because the procedure may cause vomiting, which creates a risk for aspiration of stomach contents.
- If suctioning is required to obtain the specimen, check for factors such as anticoagulant therapy, bleeding disorders, or low platelet count.
  These factors place the patient at risk for bleeding when the suction catheter is introduced.

➤ When performing the procedure, always identify your patient according to agency policy, using two identifiers, and be attentive to standard precautions, hand hygiene, patient safety and privacy, body mechanics, and documentation.

Procedure Steps

1. **Verify the medical prescription** for type of sputum analysis.
   The type of sputum specimen determines the number of specimens required and the time of day the specimen should be collected. For example, specimens to confirm tuberculosis typically require three consecutive morning samples.

2. **Position the patient** according to the required specimen collection technique.
   a. *For an expectorated specimen,* assist the patient to high or semi-Fowler's position or to a sitting position at the edge of the bed.
   b. *For a suctioned specimen,* position the patient in high or semi-Fowler's position.
   These positions facilitate insertion of the suction catheter and the ability to cough. They also promote lung expansion and prevent aspiration should the patient vomit during the procedure.

3. **Drape a towel or linen-saver pad** over the patient's chest. Ask the patient to rinse their mouth and gargle with water.
   A towel or pad prevents soiling of the patient's gown during specimen collection.
   Rinsing the mouth removes flora that may contaminate the specimen; however, evidence is not conclusive on this point.

4. **If the patient has an abdominal** or chest incision, have the patient splint the incision with a pillow.
   Splinting the incision decreases discomfort when the patient coughs.

Procedure 33-1A ■ Collecting an Expectorated Sputum Specimen

Procedure Steps

Follow Steps 1 through 4, previously.

5. **Provide the patient with** the specimen container. Advise the patient to avoid touching the inside of the container. If you must hold the container, first don procedure gloves.
   The inside of the container should remain sterile. Wear gloves because you may come in contact with secretions or airborne bacteria when the patient coughs and expectorates. ➤

6. **Ask the patient to breathe** deeply for three or four breaths, and then ask the patient, after a full inhalation, to hold their breath and then cough.
   Deep breathing opens airways and stimulates the cough reflex. Coughing after a full inhalation creates enough force to mobilize secretions through the airways and into the pharynx.

7. **Instruct the patient to expectorate** the secretions directly into the specimen container.
   Prevents specimen contamination from outside organisms.

(continued on next page)

Procedure 33-1 ■ Collecting a Sputum Specimen (continued)

8. **Tell the patient to repeat deep breathing** and coughing until an adequate sample is obtained.
   Typically 5 to 10 mL of sputum is required to ensure adequate sputum analysis.

9. **Don procedure gloves** if you are not already wearing them; cover the specimen container with the lid immediately after the specimen is collected.
   Gloves protect you in the event the patient's coughing has contaminated the outside of the container. Covering the container immediately prevents spread of microorganisms.

10. **After the patient expectorates,** offer tissues and provide mouth care.
    Promotes patient comfort.

11. **Label the specimen container** with patient identification label that contains the name of the test and collection date and time.
    Correctly identifying the specimen ensures accurate diagnosis and treatment.

12. **Place the specimen in** a plastic bag with a biohazard label. Attach a completed laboratory requisition form.
    The plastic bag protects healthcare workers from exposure to microorganisms. The laboratory requisition form ensures proper processing of the specimen.

13. **Send the specimen** to the laboratory immediately, or refrigerate it if transport might be delayed.
    If bacterial cultures are delayed, contaminating organisms may grow, producing false culture results and possibly inappropriate treatment.

Procedure 33-1B ■ Collecting a Suctioned Sputum Specimen

Procedure Steps

Follow Steps 1 through 4, previously.

5. **Administer oxygen** to the patient, if indicated.
   Suctioning may cause hypoxemia.

6. **Prepare the suction device,** and make sure it is functioning properly.

7. **Don personal protective equipment (PPE).**
   Protects your eyes, nose, and mouth from splattering of secretions during suctioning. Minimizes exposure to body fluids and airborne diseases such as COVID-19 and prevents the spread of infection.

8. **Turn on the suction machine and open the suction catheter with a trap** (*DeLee* catheter) packaging. ▼

9. **Don sterile gloves.**
   Protects the patient's sterile airways from contamination by outside organisms.

10. **Attach the sterile suction** to the male adapter of the suction catheter with trap. The hand that touches the specimen trap tubing is no longer sterile.
    Ensures that the sputum specimen goes directly into the specimen trap instead of the suction tubing. ▼

11. **Lubricate the suction catheter** with sterile saline solution.
    Lubrication eases insertion and prevents trauma to mucosa.

12. **Insert the tip of the suction** catheter gently through the nasopharynx, endotracheal tube, or tracheostomy tube. Advance the tip into the trachea (see Procedure 33-6 or Procedure 33-8).
    Gentle insertion prevents airway trauma.

13. **When the patient begins** coughing, apply suction by placing your finger over the suction control port for 5 to 10 seconds to collect the specimen.
    Applying suction for longer than 10 seconds can cause hypoxia.

14. **If an adequate specimen** (5 to 10 mL) is not obtained, allow the patient to rest for 1 or 2 minutes, and then repeat the procedure. Administer oxygen to the patient at this time, if indicated.
    Allowing the patient to rest and administering oxygen prevent hypoxia. You must assess your patient continually during this procedure to ensure patient safety and respiratory status.

15. **When you have collected** an adequate specimen, discontinue suction, then gently remove the suction catheter.
    Applying suction during catheter removal can damage the airway mucosa.

16. **Remove the suction catheter** from the specimen trap by removing the top cap on the trap, and dispose of the catheter in the appropriate container.
    Disposal of contaminated supplies prevents the spread of infection.

CHAPTER 33 Oxygenation 709

17. **Remove the white cap** from the bottom of the trap and place on top of the trap to seal it. ▼

18. **If sputum comes in contact** with the outside of the specimen trap, clean the outside with a disinfectant, according to agency policy.
Prevents spread of infection to staff members who must handle the specimen.

19. **Label the specimen trap** with patient identification, name of the test, and collection date and time.
Correctly identifying the specimen ensures accurate diagnosis and treatment.

20. **Place the specimen** in a plastic bag with a biohazard label. Attach a completed laboratory requisition form.
Placing the specimen in a plastic bag protects healthcare workers from exposure to microorganisms. Completing the laboratory requisition form ensures proper processing of the specimen.

21. **Send the specimen to the laboratory** immediately, or refrigerate it if transport might be delayed.
If bacterial cultures are delayed, contaminating organisms may grow, producing false culture results and possibly inappropriate treatment.

Evaluation

- Evaluate the patient's respiratory status during and after the procedure, especially if suctioning was necessary.
- Examine the color, consistency, and odor of the sputum specimen.
- Promptly report laboratory results to the primary care provider.
- Evaluate the patient's understanding of the procedure and test results.

Patient Teaching

- Explain proper collection techniques to avoid specimen contamination.
- Show the patient proper coughing techniques to ensure an adequate specimen.
- Explain the importance of avoiding mouthwash before the procedure, as it may alter laboratory results.
- If the patient has an incision, show them how to splint his incision to avoid discomfort during coughing and expectoration.

Home Care

Explain how to collect an expectorated sputum specimen and the importance of sending the specimen to the laboratory immediately after collection.

Documentation

- Record the date and time the specimen was collected, the method of collection, and the type of specimen ordered.
- Note the amount, color, consistency, and odor of the specimen.
- Document the patient's tolerance of the procedure.

Sample Documentation

00/00/0000   0700   Patient suctioned via tracheostomy. Sputum specimen obtained and sent for acid-fast bacillus (AFB) analysis. Specimen contained 15 mL of yellow, tenacious, odorless sputum. Patient became short of breath with suctioning. 100% O_2 administered via tracheostomy hood for 10 minutes after suctioning. Shortness of breath abated with treatment. O_2 returned to 40%. ———— S. Ryan, RN

Practice Resources

Centers for Disease Control and Prevention (CDC) (n.d.a.), Texas Department of State Health Services, Laboratory Services Section Home (2009, updated May 2018).

Procedure 33-2 ■ Monitoring Pulse Oximetry (Arterial Oxygen Saturation)

▶ For steps to follow in *all* procedures, refer to the Universal Steps for All Procedures on the inside back cover.

Equipment

- Nail polish remover, if necessary
- Oximeter and probe sensor appropriate for patient age, size, and weight and for the desired location.

Delegation

Because it is noninvasive and simple to perform, the registered nurse (RN) can delegate application of the pulse oximeter probe and measurement of arterial oxygen saturation

(continued on next page)

Procedure 33-2 ■ Monitoring Pulse Oximetry (Arterial Oxygen Saturation) (continued)

(SaO$_2$) to a UAP or licensed practical nurse (LPN) who is adequately trained to perform the skill. Inform the UAP or LPN how often to take measurements, and instruct them to notify you immediately if SaO$_2$ falls below 95%. Although this procedure can be delegated, it is the responsibility of the RN to interpret the results, assess the patient, and notify the primary care provider.

Preprocedure Assessment

- Assess/recognize cues for the need for SaO$_2$ monitoring: low hemoglobin level; confusion, decreased level of consciousness, or respiratory distress; or risk factors, such as heart or pulmonary disease, recovering from anesthesia, or ventilator-dependent.
  SaO$_2$ monitoring helps detect oxygenation problems early. Monitoring is especially important in patients with risk factors. Patients with underlying pulmonary disease may have adapted to low oxygen saturation levels, so you may need to adjust the lower limit alarm and, if you have delegated the procedure, the level for notification for these patients.

- Assess the patient's respiratory status, including breath sounds; respiratory rate, depth, and pattern; tissue perfusion; SaO$_2$; and skin and nailbed color.
  Cues may suggest a decrease in oxygen saturation and validate oximetry readings.

- Determine the optimal location for the oximeter probe sensor, such as the fingertip, earlobe, forehead, or bridge of the nose. Check the capillary refill and pulse at the pulse closest to the site.
  To ensure accurate monitoring, choose a site that has adequate circulation, is free of artificial nails, and contains no moisture. Clinical Insight 33-1 offers suggestions on site placement based on patient factors.

- Assess for factors that may interfere with pulse oximetry measurement, such as hypotension, hypothermia, and tremors.
  The sensor requires adequate circulation to recognize hemoglobin molecules that absorb the emitted light. Tremors may produce artifact that may be misinterpreted by the oximeter, causing false readings.

- Check patient history for allergy to adhesives.
  An allergic reaction may occur if an adhesive-backed disposable probe sensor is used in a patient with a history of allergy to adhesives.

▶ When performing the procedure, always identify your patient according to agency policy, using two identifiers, and be attentive to standard precautions, hand hygiene, patient safety and privacy, body mechanics, and documentation.

▶ Note: This procedure explains how to apply a pulse oximeter. Refer to Clinical Insight 33-1 for tips for obtaining accurate pulse oximetry readings.

Procedure Steps

1. **Choose a sensor appropriate** for the patient's age, size, and weight and for the desired location.
   - If the patient is allergic to adhesive, use a clip-on probe sensor.
   - If the patient's peripheral circulation is compromised, use a nasal sensor.
   An appropriate type of sensor is more comfortable for the patient and ensures accurate readings.

2. **Prepare the site by cleansing** and drying it. If the finger is the site, remove nail polish or an acrylic nail, if present.
   Dirt and skin oils on the site can interfere with passage of light waves. Nail polish or acrylic nails may interfere with signal transmission, causing inaccurate SaO$_2$ measurement. However, a recent study found that nail polish did not cause a clinically significant change in readings in healthy people (Balaraman et al., 2020).

3. **Remove the protective backing** if you are using a disposable probe sensor that contains adhesive.

4. **Attach the probe sensor** to the chosen site. Make sure the photodetector and light-emitting diodes (LED) on the probe sensor face each other. Most probe sensors contain markings to facilitate correct placement.

When Using a Clip-on Probe Sensor

If you are using a clip-on probe sensor, warn the patient that they may feel a pinching sensation. Choose the site based on the status of circulation to the extremity and patient movement.
Inadequate circulation to the site and artifact caused by motion may alter SaO$_2$ results. The photodetector diodes and LED must be properly placed to ensure accurate readings.

5. **Connect the sensor probe** to the oximeter and turn it on. Check the pulse rate displayed on the oximeter to see whether it correlates with the patient's radial pulse. (Be sure the pulse oximeter is plugged in to an electrical socket.)
   Correlation between the oximeter pulse display and the patient's radial pulse confirms accurate readings.

6. **Read the SaO$_2$** measurement on the digital display when it reaches a constant value, usually in 10 to 30 seconds, but may take up to 2 minutes.
   The oximeter requires time to detect the pulse, calculate oxygen saturation, and register an accurate reading. ▶

7. **Set and turn on the alarm** limits for SaO₂ and pulse rate, according to the manufacturer's instructions, patient condition, and agency policy if continuous monitoring is necessary.
   Alarms must be set at appropriate levels to signify when SaO₂ or pulse rate falls below predetermined levels. Alarms help ensure prompt recognition and treatment of hypoxia.

8. **Obtain readings as prescribed** or indicated by the patient's respiratory status.
   Some agencies require a prescription for pulse oximetry to ensure reimbursement.

9. **Rotate the site** if continuous monitoring is indicated.

   For an Adhesive Probe Sensor
   Rotate the site every 4 hours.

   For a Clip-on Probe Sensor
   Rotate the site every 2 hours.
   Probe sensors and prolonged pressure may irritate the skin; rotating the site prevents skin breakdown.

10. **Remove the probe sensor,** and turn off the oximeter when monitoring is no longer necessary.
    Some oximeters are battery powered; leaving them on after use depletes the battery.

Evaluation
- Evaluate the patient's understanding of the procedure and the obtained values.
- Compare pulse oximetry results with the patient's clinical presentation.
- Evaluate the effectiveness of therapy by comparing SaO₂ results before, during, and after treatment.
- Assess the site every 4 hours if you are using an adhesive probe sensor or every 2 hours if you are using a clip-on probe sensor.

Patient Teaching
- Demonstrate the procedure to the patient and caregiver, especially if the patient will be continuing pulse oximetry at home.
- Explain to the patient and caregiver the significance of SaO₂ results.
- Discuss the signs and symptoms of hypoxia (confusion, restlessness, shortness of breath, dyspnea, cyanosis, and somnolence) with the patient and caregiver.

Home Care
- Explain where to obtain a pulse oximeter.
- Tell the client and caregiver when to notify the primary provider of abnormal results or signs and symptoms of hypoxia.
- Help the client identify risk factors that decrease SaO₂ levels.

Documentation
- Record the date and time of each pulse oximetry reading obtained. Most agencies use a flowsheet if frequent monitoring is necessary.
- Document whether readings are intermittent or continuous.
- If readings are continuous, record alarm parameters.
- Chart the patient's vital signs and SaO₂ results, and indicate whether the patient is breathing room air or receiving oxygen therapy. For oxygen therapy, note the oxygen concentration and the mode of delivery.
- Document acute decreases in SaO₂, any precipitating factors, treatment interventions, and the patient's response.

Sample Documentation
00/00/0000   0300   Pt stated "short of breath." Crackles throughout lung fields. BP 140/92, apical pulse 110 beats/min, resp rate 32 breaths/min. Pulse oximetry applied to left index finger, and SaO₂ 88% on room air. Places on O₂ at 4 L/min via nasal cannula. Dr. Jones notified. ─────────────── Kate Jackson, RNC

Practice Resources
American Association of Critical-Care Nurses (AACN) (2016); Balaraman et al. (2020); Bunker et al. (2014); Jones et al. (2015).

Thinking About the Procedure
To practice applying clinical reasoning to this procedure,

The video **Administering Oxygen,** along with questions and suggested responses, is available on the **Davis's Nursing Skills Videos** Web site at www.fadavis.com.

Procedure 33-3 ■ Performing Percussion, Vibration, and Postural Drainage

➤ For steps to follow in *all* procedures, refer to the Universal Steps for All Procedures on the inside back cover.

Equipment
- Bed capable of being placed in the Trendelenburg position
- Pillows
- Patient gown
- Facial tissues
- Emesis basin
- Sputum specimen container, if needed
- Suction equipment, if needed
- Stethoscope

Delegation
You should assess the patient to determine the need for the procedure and to evaluate whether the patient can tolerate the procedure. You should perform the initial procedure, but you can delegate subsequent treatments to a respiratory therapist or UAP who is adequately trained. Instruct the respiratory therapist or UAP to report any changes in the patient's condition immediately. The RN is responsible for ongoing assessment and monitoring of airway clearance and respiratory status.

Preprocedure Assessment
- Check the patient's chest x-ray results.
  Identifies which lung fields require treatment.
- Assess the patient's respiratory status, including respiratory rate, depth, and rhythm; breath sounds; color; and pulse oximetry results.
  Determines the need for and effectiveness of percussion, vibration, and postural drainage.
- Determine when the patient last ate.
  Postural drainage should not be performed for at least 2 hours after meals to prevent nausea, vomiting, and aspiration.
- Assess the patient for dysrhythmias, coagulopathy (a defect in blood clotting), hypertension, and pain or tenderness in the chest area being treated.
  If any of these are present, the procedure should be avoided because it might worsen these conditions.

➤ When performing the procedure, always identify your patient according to agency policy, using two identifiers, and be attentive to standard precautions, hand hygiene, patient safety and privacy, body mechanics, and documentation.

Procedure Steps

1. **Help the patient assume the appropriate** position, based on the lung field that requires drainage.
   Helps mobilize secretions in the affected lung field by gravity.

   a. **Apical areas of the upper lobes.** Ask the patient to sit at the edge of the bed, if possible. If needed, place a pillow at the base of the spine for support. If the patient is not able to sit at the edge of the bed, place them in high-Fowler's position. ▼

   b. **Posterior section of the upper lobes.** Position supine with a pillow under the hips and knees flexed. Have the patient rotate slightly away from the side that requires drainage. ➤

   c. **Middle or lower lobes.** Place the bed in the Trendelenburg position. Position the patient in Sims' position. To drain the left lung, position the patient on the right side. For the right lung, position the patient on the left side. ▼

   d. **Posterior lower lobes.** Keeping the bed flat, position the patient prone with a pillow under the abdomen. ▼

2. **Have the patient remain** in the desired position for 10 to 15 minutes, if tolerated.
   Allows adequate drainage of secretions by gravity from the desired lung field.

3. **Perform percussion** over the affected lung area while the patient is in the desired drainage position.
   Loosens and mobilizes secretions.

   a. Instruct the patient to breathe deeply and slowly.
      Relaxation helps the patient tolerate the procedure.

   b. Place a towel over the patient's skin or use the patient's gown to cover the area to be percussed.
      Protects the skin and promotes patient privacy and comfort.

   c. ✚ Avoid clapping over bony prominences, female breasts, or tender areas of the chest.
      Percussing over these areas may cause discomfort and compromise tissue integrity.

   d. Cup your hands, keeping your fingers flexed and your thumbs pressed against your index fingers.
      Cupping your hands promotes patient comfort during percussion.

   e. Place your cupped hands over the lung area that requires drainage.

f. Percuss the lung area for 1 to 3 minutes by alternately striking your cupped hands rhythmically against the patient. ▼

4. **Perform vibrations** while the patient remains in the desired drainage position. ▼

a. Place the flat surface of one hand over the lung area that requires vibration. Place your other hand on top of that hand at a right angle.
Using the flat surfaces of the hands provides a large surface area to transmit vibrations through the chest. Placing one hand on top of the other provides better leverage for vibrating.

b. Instruct the patient to inhale slowly and deeply.
Promotes relaxation and lung expansion.

c. Instruct the patient to make a "fff" or "sss" sound while exhaling.

d. As the patient exhales, press your fingers and palms firmly against the chest wall.
Vibrating during exhalation enhances the downward movement of the rib cage that occurs during exhalation.

e. Push down, and gently vibrate with your hands over the lung area.
Vibration helps mobilize secretions.

f. Continue performing vibrations for three exhalations.

5. **After performing postural** drainage, percussion, and vibration, allow the patient to sit up. Ask the patient to cough at the end of a deep inspiration. Suction the patient if they are unable to expectorate secretions. If a sputum specimen is needed, collect it in a specimen container.
Coughing helps clear the airway of secretions.

6. **Repeat Steps 1 through 5** for each lung field that requires treatment. The entire treatment should not exceed 60 minutes.
Treating for longer than 60 minutes fatigues the patient.

7. **Provide mouth care.**
Cleanses the mouth of secretions and promotes patient comfort.

Evaluation
- Evaluate the effectiveness of percussion, vibration, and postural drainage.
- Auscultate breath sounds every 2 to 4 hours, as indicated.
- Monitor pulse oximetry and arterial blood gas (ABG) results.
- Evaluate the need for further treatment.

Patient Teaching
- Demonstrate percussion, vibration, and postural drainage if the patient will be continuing it at home.
- Reinforce the importance of immediately reporting shortness of breath or any difficulty breathing.
- Explain the importance of drinking fluids to help thin and mobilize secretions.
- Teach coughing and deep-breathing exercises.

Home Care
- Be sure the client/family/caregiver knows how often the procedure should be done. There should be a prescription from the primary care provider.
- Most clients will not have a bed that can be placed in the Trendelenburg position.
- Demonstrate how to position the client with hips elevated on pillows, higher than the chest, or, if the client is able, to assume a knee–chest position.
- Provide the client and caregiver with contact information of healthcare personnel who can be reached for advice or emergencies.

Documentation
- Document the date and time you performed percussion, vibration, and postural drainage.
- Note the positions used and the length of time the patient maintained each position.
- Note the anatomical locations in which you performed percussion and vibration.
- Document the patient's tolerance of the procedure as well as any complications and the nursing interventions you used to treat the complication.
- Document the amount, color, odor, and consistency of sputum obtained during the procedure and whether you sent a sputum specimen to the laboratory.

Sample Documentation
00/00/0000   Percussion and vibration done over right lower lobe. Expectorated 10 mL thick, yellow, odorless mucus. Specimen to laboratory. BP 142/78, HR 98 beats/min, respirations 24 breaths/min. Few crackles auscultated over right lung base, SaO$_2$ 98% on 2 L/min nasal cannula. ——— Jeffrey Fine, RN

Practice Resources
Lippincott's Nursing Procedures (2022); Swaminathan et al. (2019).

Procedure 33-4 ■ Administering Oxygen

▶ For steps to follow in *all* procedures, refer to the Universal Steps for All Procedures on the inside back cover.

Equipment
- Oxygen source
- Flow meter
- Oxygen tubing
- Nasal cannula, oxygen mask, or face tent
- Prefilled humidification device

Delegation
The RN is responsible for assessing respiratory function and initiating oxygen therapy. However, you may delegate reapplication and maintenance of oxygen therapy (e.g., adjusting the face mask) to appropriately trained assistive personnel when necessary.

Preprocedure Assessment
- Assess the patient's understanding of oxygen therapy.
- Assessment of the patient's respiratory status; includes respiratory rate, depth, and rhythm; breath sounds; color; capillary refill and pulse oximetry results.
  Determines the need for further treatment and effectiveness of oxygen therapy.
- Assess nares for patency (if a nasal cannula is being used) and behind the ears for signs of skin breakdown.

▶ When performing the procedure, always identify your patient according to agency policy, using two identifiers, and be attentive to standard precautions, hand hygiene, patient safety and privacy, body mechanics, and documentation.

▶ *Note:* Oxygen requires a medical prescription. In an emergency, administer oxygen to the patient to prevent respiratory distress, then notify the primary care provider for a prescription.

Procedure Steps

✚ Also use Clinical Insight 33-3: Oxygen Therapy Safety Precautions.

1. **Attach the flow meter** to the wall oxygen source (in the photo the green meter on the wall). ▼

If Using a Portable Oxygen Tank
Attach the flow meter to the tank if it is not already connected. Once tubing is attached to the portable tank, check the amount of oxygen in the tank by looking at the meter.
The flow meter regulates the amount of oxygen delivered per minute. ▼

2. **Assemble the oxygen** equipment. (See the table at the end of this procedure for various oxygen delivery devices.)

3. **Attach the humidifier** to the flow meter. The humidifier is simply a small plastic container containing normal saline. If you are not using a humidifier, attach the adapter directly to the flow meter.
   The humidifier adds moisture in with the oxygen (oxygen can dry the nasal or oral cavity).

4. **Turn on the oxygen** at the flow meter, and adjust the prescribed flow rate.

Then proceed to Step 5, 7, or 10.

Procedure Variation for Nasal Cannula

Follow Steps 1 through 4.

5. **Attach the nasal cannula tubing** to the humidifier or the adapter.

6. **Place the nasal prongs** in the patient's nares—prongs curved downward—and then place the tubing around each ear.
   Properly positions the device for optimal oxygen delivery.

7. **Use the slide adjustment device** to tighten the cannula in place under the patient's chin. It must fit securely but not too tightly. **Then proceed to Step 12.**
The nasal cannula must fit securely to maximize the amount of oxygen inhaled by the patient. A good fit minimizes the amount of oxygen lost around the prongs. ▼

Procedure Variation for Face Mask

Follow Steps 1 through 4.

8. **Gently place the mask** on the patient's face, applying it from the bridge of the nose to under the chin.

9. **Secure the elastic band** around the back of the patient's head. Make sure the mask fits snugly but comfortably. **Then proceed to Step 12.**
The mask must fit snugly so that oxygen cannot escape around the edges of the mask. If the mask is too tight, it may cause skin breakdown. ▼

Procedure Variation for Face Tent

Follow Steps 1 through 4.

10. **Gently place the face tent** in front of the patient's face, making sure that it fits under the chin.

11. **Secure the elastic band** around the back of the patient's head.
To keep the face tent in place. ▼

12. **Double-check that the oxygen** equipment is set up correctly and functioning properly.
Ensures that the oxygen is delivered at the prescribed rate. Oxygen delivered at an incorrect rate can cause patient injury.

13. **Assess the patient's respiratory** status before leaving the bedside.
To be certain it is safe to leave the patient.

Evaluation

- Assess respiratory rate, depth, and effort.
- Auscultate breath sounds before leaving the bedside, then monitor every 2 to 4 hours, and as indicated.
- Monitor pulse oximetry until respiratory status improves.
- Monitor ABG results if prescribed.
- Evaluate for skin breakdown, especially behind the ears, cheekbones, and under the chin—areas that are in contact with the oxygen delivery system.
- Notify the primary provider of respiratory status, oxygen, and response and any additional prescriptions needed.

Patient Teaching

- Demonstrate oxygen administration to the patient and caregiver if the patient will be continuing oxygen therapy at home. Allow for time to answer questions, and return demonstration of attaching and placing oxygen on.
- Explain the importance of immediately reporting shortness of breath or any difficulty breathing to the nursing staff before discharge. If the patient is at home, they will need to report the difficulty to the home health and/or primary care provider and, if needed, to call 911.

Home Care

- Explain to the client and caregivers where to obtain oxygen equipment and what services are available. Make sure they choose a supplier who has 24-hour emergency services.
- Instruct the client and caregiver about oxygen therapy and its use as well as safety measures that they must institute. Safety measures include keeping oxygen away from items that may cause ignition such as lighters, cigarettes, fireplaces, and heaters.
- To demonstrate the oxygen is on, client can hold nasal prongs on the side of the cheek to feel air flow or over a glass of water to see air moving water.
- Teach the client and caregiver to clean the nasal cannula or face mask with soap and warm water when it becomes soiled, and allow the mask to air-dry.

(continued on next page)

Procedure 33-4 ■ Administering Oxygen (continued)

- Provide contact information for healthcare personnel who can be reached for advice or emergencies.
- Explain the importance of immediately reporting shortness of breath or any difficulty breathing to the home health and/or primary care provider and, if needed, to call 911.
- In the home, liquid oxygen and oxygen concentrators are more commonly used than portable oxygen tanks. Liquid oxygen may be kept in small, portable containers; an oxygen concentrator removes nitrogen from room air and concentrates O_2. It requires a battery pack or electrical outlet for power. Oxygen concentrators can deliver flow up to 4 liters per minute (L/min) to create an FIO_2 of approximately 33%. Concentrations are higher at lower flow rates (e.g., an FIO_2 of 95% at 1 L/min).

Documentation

- Document the date, time, and reason oxygen therapy was initiated.
- Note the type of oxygen delivery system used, the amount of oxygen administered, and the patient's response to oxygen therapy.
- Document vital signs, pulse oximetry values, breath sounds, skin color, and respiratory effort.

Sample Documentation

00/00/0000. Patient developed acute shortness of breath. RR 33/min & labored, P = 126 beats/min, and BP 212/110 mm Hg. Pulse ox 80% on room air. Crackles and expiratory wheezes auscultated throughout both lungs. Dr. Smith notified of patient's condition. Oxygen with partial rebreather mask @ 10 L/min and Lasix 40 mg IV prescribed and administered. Pulse ox using partial rebreather = 90%. ——————— S. Peters, RN

Practice Resources

Lippincott's Nursing Procedures (2022).

Oxygen Delivery Systems

DELIVERY METHOD	FIO₂	DISCUSSION	NURSING RESPONSIBILITIES
Nasal cannula	1 L/min = 24% 2 L/min = 28% 3 L/min = 32% 4 L/min = 33% 5 L/min = 40% 6 L/min = 44%	■ Relatively comfortable. ■ Patients can eat, talk, and cough with a nasal cannula in place. ■ Works best if the patient breathes through the nose.	■ Check frequently that the prongs are in the patient's nose. ■ Assess for dryness of the nasal mucosa. ■ Humidify flow at rates above 3 L/min (flow rates >3 L/min are drying). ■ Encourage the patient to take slow, deep breaths so they will inhale more oxygen and less room air.
Simple face mask: A clear, flexible mask that covers the nose and mouth and delivers oxygen flow into the mask.	5–10 L/min = 40%–60% FIO₂	■ Requires flow rates greater than 5 L/min to prevent accumulation and rebreathing of exhaled CO₂ from within the mask. ■ Masks are not easily tolerated because they fit tightly and keep heat from radiating from the face, making patients feel hot. ■ Talking is muffled by the mask, and it must be removed for the patient to eat or drink.	■ Place face mask securely over the mouth and nose. ■ Elastic straps fit around the head to hold the mask in place. Place the straps well above the ears to prevent skin irritation and breakdown. ■ Place gauze or other soft material beneath the straps to prevent irritation. ■ Check the skin around the mask frequently. ■ Check the skin over the ears where the mask strap rubs. ■ Encourage the patient to take slow, deep breaths so they will inhale more oxygen and less room air.

Oxygen Delivery Systems—cont'd

DELIVERY METHOD	FIO₂	DISCUSSION	NURSING RESPONSIBILITIES
Partial rebreather mask: Uses the reservoir bag to capture some exhaled gas for rebreathing.	6–15 L/min = 50%–90% FIO₂	■ Allows higher FIO₂ levels to be delivered because O₂ is collected in the reservoir bag for inhalation. ■ Exhalation ports allow most exhaled air to escape. ■ Several types are available. ■ Can deliver an FIO₂ above 50% at flow rates of 6–15 L/min. ■ Patient rebreathes some exhaled air along with O₂.	■ Maintain the flow at a high enough rate to prevent the reservoir bag from collapsing during inhalation. ■ Encourage the patient to take slow, deep breaths so they will inhale more oxygen and less room air.
Nonrebreather mask: A type of reservoir bag mask; a valve keeps exhaled air from entering the reservoir bag.	6–15 L/min = 70%–100% FIO₂	■ Contains only O₂, which allows higher FIO₂ delivery. An FIO₂ of 70%–100% can be delivered at flow rates of 6–15 L/min. ■ This mask is the only external device capable of delivering an FIO₂ of 100% (in practice, it is rare to achieve a concentration above 75% because the mask does not seal perfectly with the face).	■ Maintain the flow at a rate high enough to keep the reservoir at least one-third to one-half full during inhalation. ■ Be sure the mask fits snugly so the patient will breathe in less room air.
Venturi mask: A cone-shaped adapter that serves as a mixing valve to control the amount of O₂ and room air that flow through the mask.	24%–50% FIO₂	■ The cone-shaped adapter at the base of the mask allows a precise FIO₂ to be delivered. This is very useful for patients with chronic lung disease. ■ Exhalation ports keep CO₂ buildup to a minimum.	■ The adapter indicates the required oxygen flow rate needed to deliver the desired FIO₂. Ensure that flow is set at the rate specified to deliver the FIO₂ desired.

(continued on next page)

Procedure 33-4 ■ Administering Oxygen (continued)

Oxygen Delivery Systems—cont'd

DELIVERY METHOD	FIO_2	DISCUSSION	NURSING RESPONSIBILITIES
Face tent: A large plastic mask that fits under the chin. It is open at the top and held in place with an elastic band around the head.	8–12 L/min = 30%–55% FIO_2	■ Less reliable than a face mask for delivering precise FIO_2 levels. ■ Allows moderate- to high-density aerosol delivery for humidification. ■ Patients who feel claustrophobic in a face mask often tolerate a face tent.	■ Check the skin over the ears where the mask strap rubs.
Tracheostomy collar: A small, cup-shaped device that fits over the tracheostomy opening and is held in place with elastic straps around the neck.	4–10 L/min = 24%–100% FIO_2	■ It is possible to deliver both high FIO_2 and high humidity with a tracheostomy collar. ■ Large-bore tubing is used to deliver humidification to the trachea; however, water frequently condenses inside the tubing and can be accidentally drained into the tracheostomy. Usually, a water trap is placed in the tubing to prevent this problem.	■ Watch for water accumulation in the tubing.
T-piece: A T-shaped plastic piece; the bottom of the T fits directly and tightly onto the tracheostomy tube.	4–10 L/min = 24%–100% FIO_2	■ Oxygen and humidity are delivered into one side of the T and exhaled through the other side.	■ Take care that the oxygen delivery tubing does not pull on the T-piece, which can dislodge the tracheostomy tube and create an airway emergency.

Thinking About the Procedure

To practice applying clinical reasoning to this procedure,

➤ The video **Administering Oxygen,** along with questions and suggested responses, is available on the **Davis's *Nursing Skills Videos*** Web site at www.fadavis.com.

Procedure 33-5 ■ Performing Tracheostomy Care Using Modified Sterile Technique

▶ For steps to follow in *all* procedures, refer to the Universal Steps for All Procedures on the inside back cover.
▶ Also refer to Clinical Insight 33-4.
▶ Recall that the basic differences in sterile and modified sterile technique are that modified sterile technique uses a sterile catheter and supplies but nonsterile procedure gloves.
▶ Using tap water for procedures exposes patients to waterborne pathogens; use distilled, filtered, or sterile solution if available. This differs among institutions, so follow agency requirements.
▶ Inner cannulas (IC) can be cleaned with solutions of half- or full-strength hydrogen peroxide diluted with sterile water. Some recommendations include the use of normal saline only, especially if the IC is made of silicone as it tends to absorb cleaning products. It is important to review the manufacturer's instructions for cleaning of the IC.

Equipment

- Tracheostomy suction equipment (see Procedure 33-6)
- Tracheostomy care kit or the following sterile supplies: several cotton-tip applicators, two basins, a brush, sterile 4 in. × 4 in. gauze pads, sterile precut tracheostomy dressing
- Two pairs of procedure gloves (for sterile technique, use two pairs of sterile gloves)
- Disposable inner cannula that is the same size as the tracheostomy, if available (most tracheostomy tubes have disposable inner cannulas)
- Distilled or filtered water if agency policy allows (for sterile technique, you use sterile normal saline solution)
- Hydrogen peroxide for cleaning of reusable inner cannula only (based on manufacturer's instructions or agency policy)
- Roll of twill tape or hook-and-loop fastener (Velcro) tracheostomy holder
- Bandage scissors
- Towel or linen-saver pad
- Overbed table
- Face shield and protective gown
- Disposable prepackaged wipes, or washcloth and distilled water and soap

✚ Use only the sterile precut dressing, or open and refold a 4 in. × 4 in. gauze pad into a V-shape. Do not cut 4 in. × 4 in. gauze, and do not use cotton-filled gauze squares. The patient may aspirate the cotton or gauze fibers.

A, Nondisposable tracheostomy equipment
Outer tube with flange   Inner cannula   Obturator

B, Disposable tracheostomy equipment
Outer tube with cuff and inflating tube
Cuff
Cannula
Obturator

C, Fenestrated tracheostomy equipment
Tracheostomy tube
Inner cannula
Fenestration

Delegation

In acute care settings and with new tracheostomies, you should not delegate this procedure to the UAP. For long-standing and well-healed tracheostomies, you can safely delegate care to the UAP or LPN who is adequately trained to perform the skill. This varies by state. In some states, only RNs can perform tracheostomy care. If you are not familiar with your state's nurse practice act, contact your state board of nursing.

(continued on next page)

Procedure 33-5 ■ Performing Tracheostomy Care Using Modified Sterile Technique (continued)

Preprocedure Assessment

- Assess respiratory rate, depth, and rhythm; breath sounds; color; and pulse oximetry results.
  Helps determine whether the patient can tolerate tracheostomy care.
- Assess the tracheostomy site for drainage, redness, or swelling.
  Drainage, redness, or swelling may indicate infection.
- Determine when the patient last ate.
  It is best to schedule this procedure at least 3 hours after a meal to decrease the risk of the patient vomiting and aspirating stomach contents.

> When performing the procedure, always identify your patient according to agency policy, using two identifiers, and be attentive to standard precautions, hand hygiene, patient safety and privacy, body mechanics, and documentation.

Procedure Steps

1. **Position the patient** in semi-Fowler's position, and place a towel or linen-saver pad over the patient's chest.
   A semi-Fowler's position promotes lung expansion and prevents back strain for the nurse. A towel or linen-saver pad prevents soiling of the patient's gown.

2. **Don clean procedure gloves, gown, and face shield or mask.**

3. **Hyperoxygenate the patient as needed,** and suction the tracheostomy (see Procedure 33-6 or 33-7).
   Suctioning clears the tracheostomy of secretions that could occlude the outer cannula after the inner cannula is removed for care.

   For a Passy Muir Valve
   Remove the Passy Muir valve (PMV) before suctioning the patient to prepare for tracheostomy care. (A PMV is a device that is used to enable the patient with a tracheostomy to speak. It is attached to the end of the inner cannula at the tracheostomy site.)

4. **Remove and discard** the soiled tracheostomy dressing in the appropriate receptacle, and then remove and discard your gloves. Perform hand hygiene.

5. **Place the tracheostomy care** equipment on the overbed table, and prepare the equipment, keeping all supplies and equipment sterile.
   Ensures efficiency and helps maintain sterility during tracheostomy care.

   a. *Disposable inner cannula*—Pour filtered tap water or normal saline solution into the two sterile containers (per agency policy).

   b. *Reusable inner cannula*—Pour hydrogen peroxide (half or full strength; follow manufacturer's recommendation) into one of the sterile solution containers, and pour filtered tap water or normal saline solution into the other one. If the inner cannula is not disposable, use hydrogen peroxide solution to clean only the inner cannula. Use the filtered tap water to rinse the inner cannula and clean the faceplate and tracheostomy site.

   Steps c through g apply to both types of cannulas.

   c. Obtain and open a package of disposable prepackaged wipes for cleaning the skin around the tracheostomy site.

   d. Open one cotton-tip applicator package. Wet the applicators with normal saline solution. Wet the applicators with filtered tap water or normal saline solution.
   Prepares the applicators for cleaning the exposed surface of the outer cannula and the stoma site located under the faceplate of the tracheostomy tube, respectively.

   e. Open the package containing a new disposable inner cannula.
   Allows for quick replacement of the inner cannula.

   f. Open the package of Velcro tracheostomy ties, or cut a length of twill tape long enough to go around the patient's neck two times. Make sure to cut the end of the tape on an angle.
   Allows for quick stabilization of the tracheostomy tube, preventing dislodgement. Cutting the twill tape on an angle allows for easy insertion through the faceplate eyelets.

   g. Position a biohazard receptacle within reach.
   Allows you to dispose of contaminated supplies safely as you use them without leaving the patient or interrupting the procedure.

6. **Don clean procedure gloves.** Consider your dominant hand sterile and handle the sterile supplies with that hand only.

7. **For patients receiving oxygen:** With your nondominant hand, remove the oxygen or humidification source. Attach the oxygen source to the outer cannula, if possible. If not possible, have the respiratory therapist set up oxygen blow-by to use while you are cleaning the reusable inner cannula.
   Prevents oxygen desaturation in the patient during the procedure.

8. **Unlock and remove the inner** cannula with your nondominant (nonsterile) hand and care for it accordingly.

   For a Disposable Inner Cannula
   a. **Dispose of the inner cannula** in the biohazard receptacle according to agency policy. You should never clean and reuse a disposable inner cannula.
   Prevents contamination by bacteria contained in the inner cannula.

   b. **With your dominant hand,** insert the new inner cannula into the patient's tracheostomy in the direction of the curvature.

Following the manufacturer's instructions, lock the inner cannula in place securely to prevent it from dislodging. Remember to keep your dominant hand sterile.

For a Reusable Inner Cannula

c. Following the manufacturer's instructions, rinse the inner cannula in the basin filled with hydrogen peroxide or sterile normal saline solution.
Hydrogen peroxide helps loosen tenacious (sticky) secretions. Soaking inner cannulas is not recommended as it increases the risk of exposure to pathogens.

d. Pick up the reusable inner cannula from the basin with your nonsterile hand, and scrub it with the sterile nylon brush, using your dominant hand. ▼

e. Immerse the inner cannula in the container of filtered tap water and agitate it until it is rinsed thoroughly.
Immersing the inner cannula in filtered tap water and agitating it removes the hydrogen peroxide and debris from the inner cannula, minimizing tissue irritation.

f. Shake the cannula to remove water.
Removes excess fluid so the patient does not aspirate it when you reinsert the cannula.

g. With your dominant (clean) hand, reinsert the inner cannula into the patient's tracheostomy in the direction of the curvature. Following the manufacturer's instructions, lock the inner cannula in place securely to prevent it from dislodging. Remember to keep your dominant hand clean.

For a Passy Muir Valve

h. Swish the PMV in warm filtered tap water with mild soap.
i. Rinse the PMV thoroughly in warm filtered tap water.
j. **Key Pont:** *DO NOT use hot water, peroxide, bleach, vinegar, alcohol, brushes, or cotton-tip applicators to clean PMV, as this could damage the valve.*
k. Shake the PMV to remove excess fluid. If you are going to store the valve, be sure to air-dry the valve before placing it in a storage container.
Removes moisture, which can promote bacterial growth.
l. Set the PMV aside on clean surface to be replaced when the inner cannula is replaced.

For Patients Receiving Oxygen

m. Remove the humidification or oxygen source from the outer cannula, if indicated, using your nondominant hand.
n. Reinsert the inner cannula into the patient's tracheostomy in the direction of the curvature.
o. Following the manufacturer's instructions, lock the inner cannula in place securely. Remember to keep dominant hand clean.
Lock the inner cannula in place securely to prevent it from dislodging.

p. Reattach the humidification or oxygen source, if indicated.
Provides the patient with needed humidity or oxygen and prevents oxygen desaturation.

9. **Clean the stoma** under the faceplate with cotton-tip applicators saturated with filtered tap water or normal saline solution, using a circular motion from the stoma site outward. Use each applicator only once, and then discard it.
Prevents contamination of the cleaned area. ▼

10. **Clean the top surface** of the faceplate and the skin around it with the gauze pads saturated with filtered tap water or normal saline solution. Use each gauze pad only once, and then discard it.
Removes secretions that provide a prime medium for microbial growth; prevents contamination of cleaned areas.

11. **Dry the skin and outer** cannula surfaces by patting them lightly with the remaining dry gauze pad.
Clean, dry skin is needed to avoid skin breakdown and removes moisture, which can promote bacterial growth around the stoma site.

To finish the procedure, skip to steps 12 through 17 of Procedure 33-5A.

Procedure 33-5A ■ Performing Tracheostomy Care Using Sterile Technique

Procedure Steps

1. **Position the patient** in semi-Fowler's position and place a towel or linen-saver pad over the patient's chest.
A semi-Fowler's position promotes lung expansion and prevents back strain for the nurse. A towel or linen-saver pad prevents soiling of the patient's gown.

2. **Don clean procedure gloves.**

3. **Hyperoxygenate the patient,** as needed, and suction the tracheostomy (see Procedure 33-6 or 33-7).
Suctioning clears the tracheostomy of secretions that could occlude the outer cannula after the inner cannula is removed for care.

For a Passy Muir Valve

Remove the Passy Muir valve (PMV) before suctioning the patient to prepare for tracheostomy care. (A PMV is a device that is used to enable the patient with a tracheostomy to speak. It is attached to the end of the inner cannula at the tracheostomy site.)

(continued on next page)

Procedure 33-5 ■ Performing Tracheostomy Care Using Modified Sterile Technique (continued)

4. **Remove and discard** the soiled tracheostomy dressing in the appropriate receptacle, and then remove and discard your gloves. Perform hand hygiene.

5. **Place the tracheostomy care equipment** on the overbed table and prepare the equipment, keeping all supplies and equipment sterile.
   Ensures efficiency and helps prevent contamination during tracheostomy care.
   a. *Disposable inner cannula*—Pour sterile normal saline solution into the two sterile containers (per agency policy).
   b. *Reusable inner cannula*—Pour hydrogen peroxide (half or full strength; follow manufacturer's instructions) into one of the sterile solution containers, and pour sterile normal saline solution into the other one. If the inner cannula is not disposable, use hydrogen peroxide solution to clean only the inner cannula. Use sterile normal saline to rinse the inner cannula and clean the faceplate and tracheostomy site.

Steps c through g apply to both types of cannulas.

   c. Obtain and open two 4 in. × 4 in. sterile gauze packages. Wet the gauze in one package with sterile normal saline solution, and keep the second package dry.
   You will use the second package of gauze to dry the skin around the tracheostomy site after cleaning.
   d. Open one cotton-tip applicator package. Wet the applicators with sterile normal saline solution.
   Prepares the applicators for cleaning the exposed surface of the outer cannula and the stoma site located under the faceplate of the tracheostomy tube, respectively.
   e. Open the package containing a new disposable inner cannula.
   Allows for quick replacement of the inner cannula.
   f. Open the package of Velcro tracheostomy ties, or cut a length of twill tape long enough to go around the patient's neck two times. Make sure to cut the end of the tape on an angle.
   Allows for quick stabilization of the tracheostomy tube, preventing dislodgement. Cutting the twill tape on an angle allows for easy insertion through the faceplate eyelets.
   g. Position a biohazard bag within reach.
   Allows you to dispose of contaminated supplies safely as you use them without leaving the patient or interrupting the procedure.

6. **Don sterile gloves. Consider your dominant hand sterile and your nondominant hand clean (nonsterile).** Handle the sterile supplies with the dominant hand only.

7. **For patients receiving oxygen:** With your nondominant (nonsterile) hand, remove the oxygen or humidification source. Attach the oxygen source to the outer cannula, if possible. If not possible, have the respiratory therapist set up oxygen blow-by to use while you are cleaning the reusable inner cannula. (If not receiving oxygen, skip this step.)
   Prevents oxygen desaturation in the patient during the procedure.

8. **Unlock and remove the inner cannula** with your nondominant (nonsterile) hand and care for it accordingly.

For a Disposable Inner Cannula
   a. Dispose of the inner cannula in the biohazard receptacle according to agency policy. You should never clean and reuse a disposable inner cannula.
   Prevents contamination by bacteria contained in the inner cannula.
   b. With your dominant hand (sterile), insert the new inner cannula into the patient's tracheostomy in the direction of the curvature. Following the manufacturer's instructions, lock the inner cannula in place securely to prevent it from dislodging. Remember to keep your dominant hand sterile.

For a Reusable Inner Cannula
   c. If a reusable inner cannula was used, following manufacturer's instructions, rinse the inner cannula in the basin filled with hydrogen peroxide or normal saline solution.
   Helps loosen tenacious (sticky) secretions. Soaking inner cannulas is not recommended as it increases the risk of exposure to pathogens.
   d. Pick up the reusable inner cannula from the basin with your nondominant hand and scrub it with the sterile nylon brush, using your dominant (sterile) hand.
   e. Immerse the inner cannula in the container of sterile normal saline solution and agitate it until it is rinsed thoroughly.
   Immersing the inner cannula in sterile saline solution and agitating it removes the hydrogen peroxide and debris from the inner cannula, minimizing tissue irritation.
   f. Tap the inner cannula against the side of the container to remove water.
   Removes excess fluid so the patient does not aspirate it when you reinsert the cannula.
   g. With your dominant (sterile) hand, reinsert the inner cannula into the patient's tracheostomy in the direction of the curvature. Following the manufacturer's instructions, lock the inner cannula in place securely to prevent it from dislodging. Remember to keep your dominant hand clean.

For a Passy Muir Valve
   h. Swish the PMV in warm tap water with mild soap.
   i. Rinse the PMV thoroughly in warm filtered tap water.
   j. **Key Point:** *DO NOT use hot water, peroxide, bleach, vinegar, alcohol, brushes, or cotton-tip applicators to clean PMV, as this could damage the valve.*

k. Shake the PMV to remove excess fluid. If you are going to store the valve, be sure to air-dry the valve before placing it in a storage container.
Removes moisture, which can promote bacterial growth.

l. Set the PMV aside on clean surface to be replaced when the inner cannula is replaced.

For Patients Receiving Oxygen

m. Remove the humidification or oxygen source from the outer cannula, if indicated, using your nondominant hand.

n. Using your dominant (sterile) hand, reinsert the inner cannula into the patient's tracheostomy in the direction of the curvature.

o. Following the manufacturer's instructions, lock the inner cannula in place securely. Remember to keep dominant hand clean.
Lock the inner cannula in place securely to prevent it from dislodging.

p. Reattach the humidification or oxygen source, if indicated.
Provides the patient with needed humidity or oxygen and prevents oxygen desaturation.

9. **Clean the stoma under the faceplate** with cotton-tip applicators saturated with sterile normal saline solution, using a circular motion from the stoma site outward. Use each applicator only once and then discard it.
Prevents contamination of the cleaned area.

10. **Clean the top surface of the faceplate** and the skin around it with the gauze pads saturated in sterile normal saline solution. Use each wipe or gauze pad only once, and then discard it.
Removes secretions that provide a medium for microbial growth; prevents contamination of cleaned areas.

11. **Dry the skin and outer cannula** surfaces by patting them lightly with the remaining dry gauze pad.
Clean, dry skin is needed to avoid skin breakdown and removes moisture, which can promote bacterial growth around the stoma site.

The following steps apply to both modified sterile and sterile technique:

12. **Seek assistance from another** staff member to help with changing the tracheostomy stabilizers.
Prevents accidental dislodging should the patient begin coughing during the procedure.

13. **Remove soiled tracheostomy stabilizers.**

Removing a Soiled Velcro Tracheostomy Holder

a. With an assistant stabilizing the tracheostomy tube, disengage the Velcro on both sides of the soiled holder and remove it gently from the eyes of the faceplate. Discard the Velcro holder in the nearest biohazard receptacle.
Removing the soiled holder promotes hygiene and prevents the spread of infection.

Removing Soiled Twill Tape Tracheostomy Ties

b. With an assistant stabilizing the tracheostomy tube, cut the soiled tracheostomy ties using bandage scissors. *Do not* cut the tube of the tracheostomy balloon (if you do, the tracheostomy tube must be replaced). Remove the ties gently from the eyes of the faceplate and discard them in the nearest biohazard receptacle.
The tracheostomy balloon helps stabilize the tracheostomy in the trachea and prevents an air leak. Cutting the tube to the balloon prevents the balloon from holding air. Removing the soiled holder promotes hygiene and prevents the spread of infection.

14. **Ask the patient to flex the neck,** or, if unable, ask the assistant to hold the patient's head forward, and apply new tracheostomy ties.
Flexing the neck provides the same neck circumference as when the patient coughs and thus ensures you do not place and secure the tracheostomy stabilizers too tightly.

Using a Velcro Tracheostomy Holder

a. Unfasten the Velcro. Thread one end of the tracheostomy holder through the eyelet of the faceplate and fasten it.

b. Bring the holder around the back of the patient's neck.
The holder must be placed around the patient's neck to adequately secure the tracheostomy.

c. Thread the remaining end of the tracheostomy holder through the empty eyelet of the faceplate and fasten the Velcro, making sure that the holder fits securely. ▼

d. Place one finger under the holder to make sure that the holder is securing the tracheostomy effectively but isn't too tight.
Securing the tracheostomy too tightly might place pressure on the jugular veins, interfere with coughing, or cause necrosis at the tracheostomy insertion site.

Using Twill Tape

e. Thread one end of the twill tape into one of the eyelets on the tracheostomy faceplate.

f. Continue to thread the twill tape through the eyelet, bringing both ends of the tape together.

g. Bring both ends of the twill tape around the back of the patient's neck.
To adequately secure the tracheostomy.

(continued on next page)

Procedure 33-5 ■ Performing Tracheostomy Care Using Modified Sterile Technique (continued)

h. Thread the end of the twill tape that is closest to the patient's neck through the back of the eyelet on the faceplate.

i. Have your assistant place one finger under the twill tape while you tie the two ends together in a square knot.

Ensures you do not secure the tracheostomy too tightly.

j. Place one finger under the holder to make sure that the holder is securing the tracheostomy effectively but isn't too tight.

See step 14d.

15. **Don a new pair of sterile gloves** (after removing gloves and performing hand hygiene).

16. **Insert a precut, sterile tracheostomy dressing** under the faceplate and new tracheostomy stabilizers or fold a 4 in. × 4 in. gauze pad into a V shape (below). ▼

A

B

C

D

The new dressing absorbs secretions and prevents skin breakdown under the faceplate. Never cut the gauze to make a dressing because lint and fibers from the cut edge could enter the trachea and cause respiratory distress. ▼

17. **Dispose of the used equipment** in the appropriate biohazard receptacle according to agency policy.

Helps prevent cross-contamination.

? What if...

■ **My patient begins coughing?**

a. If the tracheostomy is still secured with ties or Velcro holder, wait to continue tracheostomy care until coughing has ended.

b. If tracheostomy is unsecured, stabilize the tube so that it does not become dislodged, being careful not to press too hard on the site. Continue with tracheostomy care when the patient finishes coughing.

Pressing too hard at the tracheostomy site will stimulate the coughing reflex.

c. If coughing continues, suspend tracheostomy care and suction the patient to remove any retained secretions.

Retained secretions may cause increased airway irritation and coughing. Removing secretions will reduce this irritation.

■ **I do not have an assistant to hold the cannula in place while replacing the soiled tracheostomy ties?**

Never cut the soiled tape before applying the clean tape. Always place the new tape/holders, be certain the tracheostomy is secured, and then cut off the soiled tape or holder.

■ **The tracheostomy tube becomes dislodged?**

a. To prevent this, plan ahead and always have another staff member with you to secure the tracheostomy tube while you change the tracheostomy ties or Velcro holder.

b. If the tracheostomy tube slips out slightly but is still in the trachea site, gently push it back into the stoma and secure it.

The pilot balloon will help to keep the tracheostomy tube from completely dislodging.

c. If the tracheostomy tube becomes completely dislodged, stay with the patient and ask your assistant to call for the respiratory therapist or trained person in your facility to insert a new tracheostomy tube.

■ **At step 9, there are crusts around the stoma when I am cleaning the stoma?**

Remove the crusts with a cotton-tip swab soaked in hydrogen peroxide, then rinse with a swab soaked in filtered tap water or normal saline. Have the patient hold their breath while you remove crusts so debris is not inhaled.

Evaluation

- Assess the area around the stoma site for signs of skin breakdown.
- Evaluate the patient's tolerance of the procedure. Note whether there were any signs of respiratory distress.

Patient Teaching

- Explain to the patient and family that bloody secretions are normal for 2 to 3 days after tracheostomy tube insertion or for 24 hours after a tracheostomy tube change.
- Tell the patient and/or family to inform the nurse immediately if the tracheostomy tube becomes dislodged.
- Teach tracheostomy care to the patient and caregiver if the tracheostomy is expected to remain long term.

Home Care

- Clean, rather than sterile, technique can be used for tracheostomy care if the tracheostomy is more than 1 month old.
- Instruct the client and caregiver about home oxygen therapy and suctioning, if necessary.
- Demonstrate tracheostomy care to the caregiver and ask for a return demonstration.
- Provide the client and caregiver with information about where to obtain tracheostomy care supplies.
- Supply the client and caregiver with contact information of healthcare personnel who can be reached for advice or emergencies.
- Recommend ways of adding moisture to the air, with a goal of maintaining a relative humidity of 50% (e.g., a large humidifier, house plants, wearing damp gauze over the stoma, closing the bathroom door and turning on the hot water to fill the room with steam).
- Instruct the patient and caregiver that the stoma should be cleaned using clean technique at least twice daily (or more often, depending on the amount of secretions).
- Stress good hand washing before and after doing any part of tracheostomy care.
- Remind client and caregiver not to use cotton or gauze. *These can leave fibers that may get into the airway and increase the incidence of infection.*

Documentation

- Document the date and time you performed tracheostomy care.
- Record the color, amount, consistency, and odor of secretions.
- Record the condition of the stoma and skin around the stoma site; note the presence of drainage, redness, or swelling.
- Document respiratory status, including respiratory rate, depth, and pattern; skin color; and breath sounds.
- Document the patient's tolerance of the procedure.
- If problems arose, document any interventions that were necessary.

Sample Documentation

NOTE: *Because this is only a partial computer screen, it may not show all the information you would need to record about the patient.* ▼

(continued on next page)

Procedure 33-5 ■ Performing Tracheostomy Care Using Modified Sterile Technique (continued)

Practice Resources
Alsunaid et al. (2021); Billington et al. (2019); John Hopkins Medicine (2020); Johnston et al. (n.d., updated 2016); Morris et al. (2013); Patton (2019); Rubin et al. (2019); Russell et al. (2019); Siegel et al. (2007).

Thinking About the Procedure
To practice applying clinical reasoning to this procedure,

The video **Performing Tracheostomy Care Using Sterile Technique,** along with questions and suggested responses, is available on the **Davis's *Nursing Skills Videos*** Web site at www.fadavis.com.

Procedure 33-6 ■ Performing Tracheostomy or Endotracheal Suctioning (Open System)

➤ For steps to follow in *all* procedures, refer to the Universal Steps for All Procedures on the inside back cover.

Equipment
- Portable or wall suction device with tubing and a collection canister
- Linen-saver pad or towel
- Resuscitation bag connected to oxygen source
- Sterile suction catheter kit: adults 12 to 18 Fr; children 8 to 10 Fr; infants 5 to 8 Fr
- If a kit isn't available, collect the following: sterile gloves, sterile suction catheter of the appropriate size, and a sterile container
- Pour bottle of sterile normal saline solution
- Sterile basin or container for fluids
- Prefilled 10-mL containers of normal saline solution
- PPE (face shield or goggles, protective gown, sterile gloves or procedure gloves; follow agency policy)

Delegation
As a rule you should not delegate tracheostomy suctioning to an LPN or UAP, because the procedure requires professional-level theoretical knowledge, assessment skills, and problem-solving ability. However, if the patient has a permanent tracheostomy tube in place and the patient will require long-term care, care can be delegated to trained personnel. Refer to individual state board of nursing for rules on delegating this procedure.

Preprocedure Assessment
- Assess the respiratory rate, depth, and rhythm; breath sounds; color; and pulse oximetry results.
- Assess for signs that indicate the need for suctioning: restlessness, cyanosis, labored respirations, decreased oxygen saturation, increased heart and respiratory rates, visible secretions in the airway, increased peak airway pressures on the ventilator, decreasing SaO_2 or PaO_2, and adventitious breath sounds during auscultation.

Suctioning should be performed only when necessary to prevent unnecessary oxygen desaturation and tissue trauma.

➤ When performing the procedure, always identify your patient according to agency policy, using two identifiers, and be attentive to standard precautions, hand hygiene, patient safety and privacy, body mechanics, and documentation.

Procedure Steps

1. **Position the patient** in semi-Fowler's position, unless contraindicated.
   Promotes lung expansion and oxygenation.

2. **Place the linen-saver pad** or towel on the patient's chest.
   Prevents soiling of the patient's gown during suctioning.

3. **Don face shield or goggles.**

4. **Turn on the wall suction** or portable suction machine, and adjust the pressure regulator according to agency policy, using the lowest possible suction pressure. Typically, this is:
   Adults: 100 to 150 mm Hg
   Children: 100 to 120 mm Hg
   Infants: 50 to 95 mm Hg
   Using the appropriate pressure prevents tissue trauma and ensures successful suctioning. Higher pressures are associated with hypoxemia, tissue trauma, and atelectasis, yet do not improve removal of secretions.

5. **Don a nonsterile glove.** Test the suction equipment by occluding the connection tubing.
   Ensures proper functioning before you insert suction catheter.

6. **Remove and discard glove.** Perform hand hygiene.

7. **Open the suction catheter kit** or (if a kit isn't available) the gathered equipment. Maintain sterility of the inside of the suction kit or the gathered equipment.

This prevents contaminating the upper airway when you introduce the suction catheter.

8. **Pour sterile saline** into the sterile container.
   Sterile saline is used to clear the suction catheter of secretions after suctioning.

9. **Premeasure the catheter insertion distance** for 0.5 to 1 cm (¼ to ½ in.) past the distal end of the endotracheal tube (ETT); the ETT normally sits 3 to 7 cm (1 to 2¾ in.) above the carina.

10. **Don sterile gloves.** Follow agency policy, as some guidelines allow for clean nonsterile rather than sterile procedure gloves. Consider your dominant hand sterile and your nondominant hand unsterile.

11. **Pick up the suction catheter** with your dominant hand, and attach it to the connection tubing. Do not touch the connection tubing with your sterile (or clean) glove.
    Prepares the suction catheter for use.

12. **Put the tip of the suction** catheter into the sterile container of normal saline solution, and suction a small amount through the suction catheter. Apply suction by placing a finger over the suction control port of the suction catheter.
    Lubricates the catheter and helps ensure that the suction equipment is functioning properly. Sterile saline is necessary to clear the suction catheter of secretions after suctioning. The outside of the saline container is not sterile; it would contaminate your dominant hand.

13. **If the patient is receiving supplemental oxygen,** hyperoxygenate the patient according to agency policy. If the patient does not require oxygen, you do not need to hyperoxygenate.
    Helps prevent hypoxia and related complications (cardiac arrhythmias, seizures, arrest) during suctioning. Suctioning clears secretions, but it also removes oxygen from airways.

If the Patient Requires Mechanical Ventilation

a. Press the 100% O_2 button on the ventilator. Some agencies require the nurse to manually hyperoxygenate the patient; follow agency policy.
   Ventilators typically have a button that allows you to hyperoxygenate the patient for a total of 2 minutes. Once this time period elapses, the ventilator automatically resumes its previous settings.

If the Patient Does Not Require Mechanical Ventilation

b. Obtain the assistance of a second provider.
c. Have your partner attach the resuscitation bag to the tracheostomy tube or endotracheal tube, and hyperoxygenate the patient by compressing the resuscitation bag three to five times as the patient inhales. Remove the resuscitation bag, and place it next to the patient when finished.
   You must perform hyperoxygenation manually if the patient does not require mechanical ventilation. ▼

14. **Perform suctioning.**
    a. Lubricate the suction catheter tip with the normal saline solution.
       Lubrication eases passage of the suction catheter through the endotracheal or tracheostomy tube.
    b. Using your dominant hand, gently but quickly insert the suction catheter into the endotracheal or tracheostomy tube. ▶

    c. ✚ Advance the suction catheter, with suction off, gently aiming downward and being careful not to force the catheter. Insert to the premeasured length: no farther than the **carina tracheae** (the ridge at the lower end of the trachea that separates the openings of the two mainstem bronchi); do not insert more than 6 inches (15 cm), and do not force against any resistance.
       Forcing the catheter during insertion may cause tissue trauma.
    d. Apply suction while you withdraw the catheter; rotate the catheter (roll it between your thumb and forefinger) as you remove it. Make sure to apply suction for no longer than 15 seconds.
       Applying suction for longer than 15 seconds causes hypoxia and may cause tissue trauma.

15. **Repeat suctioning as needed.**
    Several passes with the suction catheter may be needed to clear the airway of secretions.
    a. Allow at least 30-second intervals between suctioning.
    b. Hyperoxygenate the patient between each pass.
    c. Limit total suctioning time to 5 minutes.

16. **Coil the suction catheter** in your dominant hand (alternatively, wrap it around your dominant hand). Pull the sterile (or clean) glove off over the coiled catheter. Discard the glove containing the catheter in a fluid-resistant receptacle designated by your agency.

(continued on next page)

Procedure 33-6 ■ Performing Tracheostomy or Endotracheal Suctioning (Open System) (continued)

Prevents contaminating the environment with secretions.

17. **Replace the oxygen source** if it was removed during suctioning.
    To prevent hypoxia.

18. **Using your nondominant hand,** clear the connecting tubing of secretions by placing the tip into the container of sterile saline.
    Prepares the tubing for later reuse.

19. **Turn off** the suction units (and the oxygen, if appropriate).

20. **Remove gloves from nondominant hand,** perform hand hygiene, and don clean procedure gloves.

21. **Provide mouth care.**

22. **Reposition the patient.**
    Promotes comfort and prevents skin breakdown.

? What if . . .

- **The patient has a cuffed tracheostomy tube?**
  Check to see that it is properly inflated before suctioning. Usually this is 20 to 25 mm Hg or less, but follow the manufacturer's instructions and use a cuff manometer. See Clinical Insight 33-4 to learn how to check cuff inflation.

Evaluation

- Assess the color, amount, and consistency of secretions.
- Evaluate the patient's tolerance of the procedure (e.g., were there signs of respiratory distress during suctioning?).
- Evaluate the effectiveness of the procedure by comparing breath sounds, vital signs, and pulse oximetry before and after suctioning.

Patient Teaching

- Teach the patient and caregiver how to perform suctioning if the patient will be discharged with an artificial airway. Make sure they can successfully provide a return demonstration.
- Teach the caregiver strategies for managing the patient's airway at home.

Home Care

- Provide the family and caregiver information about where to obtain suction equipment, contact information for healthcare personnel who can be reached for advice or emergencies, and information about home oxygen therapy.
- Guidelines recommend clean technique for home care and for repeated catheter use as long as the catheter is still clear.
- Teach the family and caregiver how to clean catheters for reuse (soak in hot, soapy water; rinse inside and out with clean water; air-dry; store in a dry container).

Documentation

Document the following:
- Date, time, and reason you performed suctioning
- The size of the suction catheter you used
- Amount, color, consistency, and odor of secretions
- Patient's respiratory status before and after the procedure
- Patient's tolerance of the procedure
- Any complications that occurred as a result of the procedure and interventions you made in response

Sample Documentation

00/00/0000   0900   Pulse ox 93%, VS elevated, upper airway rhonchi auscultated. Hyperoxygenated with 100% O_2; suctioned moderate amount thick, yellow mucus with #12 Fr suction catheter. After procedure lungs clear, pulse ox 98%, VS WNL. ——————— Jackie Estes, RN

Practice Resources

Blakeman et al. (2022); Johnston et al. (n.d., updated 2016); Lavigne (2016); Lesmana (2019); Sole et al. (2015).

Thinking About the Procedure

To practice applying clinical reasoning to this procedure,

The video **Performing Endotracheal Suctioning (Open System),** along with questions and suggested responses, is available on the **Davis's *Nursing Skills Videos*** Web site at www.fadavis.com.

Procedure 33-7 ■ Performing Tracheostomy or Endotracheal Suctioning (Inline Closed System)

➤ For steps to follow in *all* procedures, refer to the Universal Steps for All Procedures on the inside back cover.

Equipment

For the once-a-day steps: Procedure gloves and inline suction catheter

When suctioning: Sterile normal saline

Inline suction catheter. (© Unomedical a/s, used with permission.)

Delegation

As a rule, you should not delegate tracheostomy or endotracheal suctioning to an LPN or UAP, because both procedures require professional-level theoretical knowledge, assessment skills, and problem-solving ability. Refer to the individual state board of nursing for rules on delegating this procedure.

Preprocedure Assessment

- Assess respiratory status, including respiratory rate, depth, and rhythm; breath sounds; color; and pulse oximetry results.
- Assess for restlessness, cyanosis, labored respirations, decreased oxygen saturation, increased heart and respiratory rates, visible secretions in the airway, and the presence of adventitious breath sounds during auscultation.
  These assessments help determine whether the patient requires suctioning. Suctioning should be performed only when necessary to prevent unnecessary oxygen desaturation and tissue trauma.

➤ When performing the procedure, always identify your patient according to agency policy, using two identifiers, and be attentive to standard precautions, hand hygiene, patient safety and privacy, body mechanics, and documentation.

➤ *Note:* This procedure uses modified sterile technique.

Daily Procedure Steps

1. An inline suction unit is available only for patients on a mechanical ventilator. Most agencies require the respiratory therapy department to set up the inline suction equipment. If this is not the agency's policy, you may need to perform these steps once per day. Open the inline suction catheter package, using sterile technique.

2. Remove the adapter on the ventilator tubing.

3. Attach the inline suction catheter equipment to the ventilator tubing.

4. Reconnect the adapter on the ventilator tubing.

5. Attach the other end of the inline suction catheter to the connection tubing placed to suction.

Suctioning Procedure Steps

1. **Place the patient in semi-Fowler's position,** unless contraindicated.
   The suction catheter is contained within a sterile unit.

2. **Don clean procedure gloves.**
   You do not need to wear sterile gloves.

3. **Place a linen-saver pad** or towel on the patient's chest.

4. **If a lock is present** on the suction control port, unlock it.

5. **Turn on the wall suction** or portable suction machine, and adjust the pressure regulator according to agency policy or provider's prescription.
   Using the appropriate pressure prevents tissue trauma and ensures successful suctioning.

6. **Pick up the catheter** with your dominant hand and use your nondominant hand for the suction port.
   Using the dominant hand improves dexterity.

7. **Unlock the inline catheter** and gently insert the suction catheter into the airway by maneuvering the catheter within the sterile sleeve. ▼

(continued on next page)

Procedure 33-7 ■ Performing Tracheostomy or Endotracheal Suctioning (Inline Closed System) (continued)

8. **Advance the suction catheter** into the airway, being careful not to force the catheter. Ask the patient to take slow, deep breaths if they can cooperate. Advance the catheter to the predetermined and premarked distance. Do not apply suction while advancing.
   Forcing the catheter during insertion may cause airway trauma.

9. **Apply suction** by depressing the button over the suction control port as you withdraw the catheter. Apply suction for no longer than 15 seconds.
   Applying suction for longer than 15 seconds causes hypoxia and may cause tissue trauma.

10. **Withdraw the inline suction** catheter completely into the sleeve. The indicator line on the catheter should appear through the sleeve.
    The indicator line is a safety mechanism designed to ensure the suction catheter is withdrawn completely to prevent airway obstruction.

11. **Attach the prefilled 10-mL** container of normal saline solution to the saline port located on the inline equipment.
    Provides a flush solution to clear the suction catheter of secretions.

12. **Squeeze the 10-mL container** while applying suction.
    Clears the catheter of secretions, preparing the catheter for repeat use. If allowed to remain in the catheter or suction line, secretions may dry and harden, reducing line suction efficiency.

13. **Lock the suction regulator port.**
    Prevents you from inadvertently applying suction.

? What if...

■ **The patient has a dysrhythmia?**
Stop suctioning and hyperoxygenate the patient. If a further attempt at suctioning promotes a dysrhythmia, notify the medical care provider.

For Evaluation, Patient Teaching, and Documentation, see Procedure 33-6. Typically, you would not be doing inline suctioning in the home.

Thinking About the Procedure

To practice applying clinical reasoning to this procedure,

The video **Performing Tracheostomy Suctioning (Inline Closed System)**, along with questions and suggested responses, is available on the **Davis's Nursing Skills Videos** Web site at www.fadavis.com.

Practice Resources
Lavigne (2016); Letchford et al. (2018).

Procedure 33-8 ■ Performing Orotracheal and Nasotracheal Suctioning (Open System)

▶ For steps to follow in *all* procedures, refer to the Universal Steps for All Procedures on the inside back cover.

▶ *Note:* This procedure uses modified sterile technique. Although the oropharynx and nasopharynx are not sterile, you should keep the suction catheter free from other contaminants as much as possible. Some facilities do use sterile gloves for this procedure.

Equipment

- Portable or wall suction device with connection tubing and a collection canister
- Linen-saver pad or towel
- Sterile, flexible, multiple-eyed suction catheter kit (12 to 18 Fr for adults, 8 to 10 Fr for children, and 5 to 8 Fr for infants); if a kit isn't available, collect the following: sterile gloves, sterile suction catheter of the appropriate size, and a sterile container for fluids
- Pour bottle of sterile water or sterile normal saline solution
- PPE (face shield or goggles and gown)
- Water-soluble lubricant for NT suctioning
- Sputum trap, if a specimen is needed
- Nasopharyngeal airway when frequent NT suctioning is required
- Resuscitation bag with mask

Delegation

You should not delegate orotracheal and nasotracheal suctioning to an LPN or UAP, because these procedures require theoretical knowledge, assessment skills, and problem-solving ability.

Preprocedure Assessment

- Assess respiratory rate, depth, and rhythm; breath sounds; skin color; and pulse oximetry results.
- Assess for signs that indicate the need for suctioning: gurgling sounds during respiration, restlessness, labored respirations, decreased oxygen saturation, increased heart and respiratory rates, and the presence of adventitious breath sounds during auscultation.

Suctioning removes oxygen from airways and can cause tissue trauma. It should be done only when essential (i.e., only when less invasive techniques have proved unsuccessful and when the secretions are causing physiological deterioration and/or distress).

- Assess the effectiveness of the cough.

▶ When performing the procedure, always identify your patient according to agency policy, using two identifiers, and be attentive to standard precautions, hand hygiene, patient safety and privacy, body mechanics, and documentation.

Procedure Steps

1. **Position the patient.**

   Variation for Orotracheal Suctioning
   a. Position the patient in semi-Fowler's position, with the head turned to face you.

   Variation for Nasotracheal Suctioning
   b. Position the patient in semi-Fowler's position, with the neck hyperextended, unless contraindicated.
   Hyperextending the neck makes it easier to insert the suction catheter. Upright position helps to prevent back strain.

2. **Place the linen-saver pad** or towel on the patient's chest.
   Prevents soiling of the patient's gown during suctioning.

3. **Don PPE (face shield or goggles and gown).**
   Protects you from contamination with secretions that may splash during suctioning.

4. **Turn on the wall suction** or portable suction machine, and adjust the pressure regulator according to agency policy. Guidelines from American Association for Respiratory Care (AARC) specify:

   Adults: 100 to 150 mm Hg
   Children: 100 to 120 mm Hg
   Infants: 80 to 100 mm Hg
   Neonates: 60 to 80 mm Hg
   The suction regulator must be set appropriately to prevent tissue trauma and hypoxia and yet remove secretions effectively.

5. **Don a procedure glove** and test the suction equipment by occluding the connection tubing. Discard the glove and perform hand hygiene.
   Testing the equipment ensures proper functioning before you insert the catheter in the patient's airway.

6. **Open the suction catheter kit** or, if a kit isn't available, the gathered equipment.

   Nasal approach: If you are using the nasal approach, open the water-soluble lubricant and a nasopharyngeal airway.

7. **Don clean nonsterile gloves.** Consider your dominant hand clean and your nondominant hand contaminated.
   Keeping the dominant hand sterile prevents contaminating the upper airways with a nonsterile suction catheter. This is a modified sterile suction technique because the catheter enters the trachea via the nose or the mouth, which are not sterile. However, take care to keep the catheter free from other contamination.

   If Using Sterile Technique
   Don sterile gloves. Consider your dominant hand sterile and your nondominant hand unsterile. Alternatively, put a sterile glove on your dominant hand and a clean procedure glove on your nondominant hand.

   Note: If you consider both hands sterile (i.e., for sterile technique), you must remove the cap from the sterile water before donning gloves.

8. **Pour sterile saline** into the sterile container, using your nondominant hand.

   Sterile saline will be used to clear the suction catheter of secretions after suctioning.

9. **Pick up the suction catheter** with your dominant hand, and attach it to the connection tubing, maintaining sterility of your hand and the catheter.
   Prepares the suction catheter for use.

10. **Put the tip of the suction** catheter into the sterile container of normal saline solution, and suction a small amount of normal saline solution through the suction catheter. Apply suction by placing a finger over the suction control port of the suction catheter.
    Lubricates the catheter and helps ensure that the suction equipment is functioning properly.

11. **Ask the patient to take several slow, deep breaths.** If patient's oxygen saturation is <94%, or if the patient is in any distress, you may need to give supplemental oxygen before, during, and after suctioning. See Procedure 33-4.
    Promotes relaxation and helps hyperoxygenate the patient before suctioning.

12. **Using your nondominant hand,** remove the oxygen delivery device, if present (for nasal suctioning only).

    For Oral Approach, Patient Receiving Nasal Oxygen
    a. If the patient is receiving nasal oxygen and you are doing orotracheal suctioning, you do not need to remove the oxygen source.

(continued on next page)

Procedure 33-8 ■ Performing Orotracheal and Nasotracheal Suctioning (Open System) (continued)

For Nasal Approach, Patient Receiving Nasal Oxygen

b. Remove the nasal oxygen and place the nasal cannula in the patient's mouth. See Procedure 33-4.

Placing the cannula in the patient's mouth makes it easier to access the nares for suctioning while still delivering oxygen to the patient (orally).

13. **Premeasure to approximate** the depth you should insert the suction catheter. For adults, insert the catheter about 15 cm (6 in.) for an oral approach, and 20 cm (8 in.) for a nasal approach. Be careful not to contaminate the catheter while you measure.

Prevents trauma at the carina and ensures suctioning of the full length of the trachea.

For Oral Approach

a. Measure the distance between the edge of the patient's mouth to the tip of the earlobe and down to the bottom of the neck. ▼

For Nasal Approach

b. Measure the distance from the tip of the nose to the tip of the earlobe and down to the bottom of the neck.

c. Insert nasopharyngeal airway gently into the nostril, with the bevel toward the septum (center of the nose), advance the airway straight in, following the floor of the nose. See Procedure 33-13.

Do not force nasopharyngeal airway into the nostril as this may cause unnecessary edema and trauma.

14. **Lubricate and insert** the suction catheter.

Lubrication makes it easier to pass a suction catheter through the nares.

For Orotracheal Suctioning

a. Lubricate the suction catheter tip with normal saline solution.

b. Using your dominant hand, gently but quickly insert the suction catheter along the side of the patient's mouth or through the endotracheal tube into the oropharynx.

Quick insertion along the side of the mouth prevents gagging.

c. When the patient inhales, advance the suction catheter to the predetermined distance, being careful not to force the catheter.

Advancing the suction catheter during inhalation ensures that the catheter enters the trachea rather than the esophagus. Forcing the catheter during insertion may cause tissue trauma.

For Nasotracheal Suctioning

d. Lubricate the catheter tip with the water-soluble lubricant.

Water-soluble lubricant is preferred because it will dissolve if it accidentally enters the lungs, whereas an oil-based lubricant (e.g., petroleum jelly) won't dissolve in the respiratory tract and causes complications if it enters the lungs.

e. Using your dominant hand, gently but quickly insert the suction catheter into the naris and down to the pharynx. When the patient inhales, advance the suction catheter, gently aiming downward to the predetermined distance, being careful not to force the catheter.

Ensures that the catheter enters the trachea. Forcing the catheter during insertion may cause tissue trauma.

15. **Place a finger or thumb** over the suction control port of the catheter. Apply suction while you withdraw the catheter, using a continuous rotating motion. Apply suction for no longer than 15 seconds.

Using a continuous rotating motion and suctioning while withdrawing the catheter prevents trauma to any one area of the airway. Limiting suctioning to less than 15 seconds prevents hypoxia. ▼

16. **After you withdraw** the catheter, clear it by placing the tip of the catheter into the container of sterile saline and applying suction. ▼

17. **Lubricate the catheter,** and repeat suctioning as needed, allowing intervals of at least 30 seconds between suctioning. Reapply oxygen between suctioning efforts, if required.
    Several passes with the suction catheter may be needed to clear the airway of secretions. Total suctioning time should be limited to 5 minutes, however, to prevent trauma and hypoxia.

18. **Replace the oxygen source.**
    Prevents hypoxia.

19. **Coil the suction catheter** in your dominant hand (alternatively, wrap it around your dominant hand). Hold the catheter while you pull the sterile glove off over it. Discard the glove containing the catheter in a biohazard receptacle (e.g., bag) designated by your agency.
    These actions prevent contaminating the environment with secretions.

20. **Using your nondominant hand,** clear the connecting tubing of secretions by placing the tip into the container of sterile saline.

21. **Dispose of equipment,** and make sure new suction supplies are readily available for future suctioning.
    The patient may require suctioning at any time, so equipment must be readily available.

22. **Remove glove from nondominant** hand and perform hand hygiene.

23. **Don clean procedure gloves** and provide mouth care.
    Promotes patient comfort and clears the mouth of any secretions the patient may have expectorated.

24. **Assist the patient** to a comfortable position, and allow them to rest.
    Comfort and rest help the patient recover from the stress of suctioning.

? What if...

- **The patient's oxygen saturation is less than 94%, or the patient is in any distress?**

    Administer supplemental oxygen before, during, and after suctioning. Notify the patient's primary provider if the patient does not respond to additional oxygen.

Evaluation

- Assess the color, consistency, and amount of secretions.
- Evaluate the patient's tolerance of the procedure. Note whether there were signs of respiratory distress during suctioning.
- Evaluate the effectiveness of the procedure by comparing breath sounds, vital signs, and pulse oximetry or blood gas data before and after the procedure.

Patient Teaching

- Explain the importance of administering supplemental oxygen or of taking several deep breaths before suctioning.
- Inform the patient that coughing typically increases with suctioning.
- Demonstrate orotracheal or nasotracheal suctioning to the caregiver, and ask for a return demonstration if suctioning will be required at home.

Home Care

- Instruct the family and caregiver about where to obtain suction equipment.
- Provide contact information of healthcare personnel who can be reached for advice or emergencies.
- Explain that the procedure can be performed using clean technique instead of sterile technique in the home.
- Instruct the caregiver that suction catheters can be cleaned for reuse by washing them with soapy water and then boiling them for 10 minutes. After they are cleaned, rinse the catheters with normal saline solution or tap water.
- Instruct to change the secretion collection container every 24 hours, or clean it according to home care agency guidelines every 24 hours.

Documentation

- Document the date, time, and reason you performed suctioning.
- Note the suction technique you used and the catheter size.
- Note the color, consistency, and odor of secretions.
- Document the patient's respiratory status before and after the procedure.
- Document the patient's tolerance of the procedure and any complications that occurred as a result of the procedure.
- Document any interventions you performed to address complications that occurred.

Sample Documentation

00/00/0000   0930 O_2 sat 89% on room air, bilateral rhonchi to bases auscultated, unproductive cough, heart rate 90, RR-18. Assistant nurse recruited for manual ventilation. Client placed in semi-Fowler's position, hyperventilated for 1 minute to 100% O_2 sat, oropharyngeal suctioning performed using sterile technique, resulting in moderate amounts of white, tenacious, yellow-tinged secretions. Improved breath sound with diminished rhonchi auscultated, O_2 sat at 97% on room air, heart rate 78, RR-14. Client smiles when asked how he feels. Bed in low position, call device and fluids in reach.——————— Kelton Jones, RN

Practice Resources

American Association for Respiratory Care (2010); Levigne (2016); Lesmana (2019).

Procedure 33-9 ■ Performing Upper Airway Suctioning

➤ For steps to follow in *all* procedures, refer to the Universal Steps for All Procedures on the inside back cover.

➤ *Note:* Upper airway suctioning may be done via the oropharyngeal or nasopharyngeal route. However, nasal suction is usually required only to improve oxygenation in infants because most adult airway obstruction occurs in the mouth and oropharynx.

✚ Vigorous nasal suction can induce epistaxis (nosebleed) and further complicate an already difficult airway.

Equipment
- Portable or wall suction device with connection tubing and a collection canister
- Linen-saver pad or towel
- Sterile suction catheter kit (12 to 18 Fr for adults, 8 to 10 Fr for children, and 5 to 8 Fr for infants); if a kit isn't available, collect the following: sterile suction catheter of the appropriate size, and a sterile container; if you plan to suction both the oropharynx and the nasopharynx, you need a separate sterile catheter for each
- Yankauer device can be used for oropharyngeal suction
- Pour bottle of sterile normal saline solution
- Sterile basin or other container for fluids
- PPE (face shield or goggles and gown)
- Procedure gloves
- Water-soluble lubricant for nasopharyngeal suctioning
- Sputum trap, if a specimen is needed
- Biohazard bag

Delegation
Do not delegate oropharyngeal and nasopharyngeal suctioning to an LPN or UAP, because these procedures require theoretical knowledge, assessment skills, and problem-solving ability. However, the UAP (and the client or family) can use a Yankauer tube to suction the oral cavity because there is less risk for trauma to mucosa than with oro- or nasopharyngeal suctioning.

Preprocedure Assessment
- Assess respiratory rate, depth, and rhythm; breath sounds; color; and pulse oximetry results. Note signs that indicate the need for suctioning: restlessness, cyanosis, labored respirations, decreased oxygen saturation, increased heart and respiratory rates, visible secretions in the airway, and the presence of adventitious breath sounds during auscultation. *You must be certain the patient requires suctioning. Suctioning should be performed only when necessary to prevent unnecessary oxygen desaturation and tissue trauma.*

➤ When performing the procedure, always identify your patient according to agency policy, using two identifiers, and be attentive to standard precautions, hand hygiene, patient safety and privacy, body mechanics, and documentation.

➤ *Note:* This procedure describes modified sterile technique: sterile supplies with clean procedure gloves. Although the oropharynx and nasopharynx are not sterile, you should keep the suction catheter free from other contaminants as much as possible. Some facilities use sterile gloves for this procedure.

Procedure Steps

1. **Position the patient.** Explain that suctioning may stimulate coughing or gagging, but that coughing helps mobilize secretions.

   Oropharyngeal Suctioning
   Position the patient in a semi-Fowler's or high-Fowler's position, with the head turned toward you.
   Facilitates insertion of the suction catheter and prevents straining your back. It also promotes lung expansion and effective coughing.

   For Nasopharyngeal Suctioning
   Position the patient in semi-Fowler's or high-Fowler's position with the neck hyperextended, unless contraindicated.

2. **Place the linen-saver pad** or towel on the patient's chest.
   Prevents soiling of the patient's gown during suctioning.

3. **Put on a face shield or goggles and gown.**
   Protects you from contamination with secretions that may splash during suctioning. Not all guidelines specify wearing a gown for this procedure.

4. **Turn on the wall suction** or portable suction machine, and adjust the pressure regulator according to agency policy, typically:
   Adults: 100 to 150 mm Hg
   Children: 100 to 120 mm Hg
   Infants: 50 to 95 mm Hg
   The suction regulator must be set appropriately to prevent tissue trauma and hypoxia and to function effectively to remove secretions. Higher pressures are associated with hypoxemia, tissue trauma, and atelectasis, yet do not improve removal of secretions.

5. **Test the suction equipment** by occluding the connection tubing.
   Ensures proper functioning before use.

6. **Open the suction catheter kit** or the gathered equipment. If you are using the nasal approach, open the water-soluble lubricant.

7. **Don procedure gloves;** consider (and keep) your dominant hand clean; consider your nondominant hand to be contaminated.
   This is not a sterile suction procedure, but care should be taken to keep the suction catheter free from other contaminants. Keeping the dominant hand clean prevents contaminating the upper airways with an unclean suction catheter.

8. **Pour sterile saline** into the sterile container, using your nondominant hand.
   Sterile saline is necessary to clear the suction catheter of secretions after suctioning. The outside of the saline container is not sterile; it would contaminate your dominant hand.

9. **Pick up the suction catheter** with your dominant hand, and use your other hand to hold the connection tubing (to suction) while you attach it.

10. **Put the tip of the suction catheter** into the sterile container of normal saline solution, and suction a small amount of normal saline solution through the suction catheter. Apply suction by placing a finger over the suction control port. When using a Yankauer-type device, the suction is continuous and there is no port to occlude.
    Ensures that the suction equipment is functioning properly. If you need to see a Yankauer device,

    ▶ Go to **Figure 33-13C** in Volume 1.

11. **Approximate the depth** to which you will insert the suction catheter.

    For Oropharyngeal Suctioning
    Measure the distance between the edge of the patient's mouth and the tip of the patient's earlobe.
    Determines the proper distance you should insert the suction catheter for oropharyngeal suctioning.

    For Nasopharyngeal Suctioning
    Measure the distance between the tip of the patient's nose and the tip of the patient's earlobe.
    Helps determine the correct distance you should insert the suction catheter for nasopharyngeal suctioning.

12. **Using your nondominant hand,** remove the oxygen delivery device, if present (for nasopharyngeal suctioning only). Have the patient take several slow, deep breaths.
    Deep breathing helps to hyperoxygenate the patient and helps prevent hypoxia during suctioning.

13. **Lubricate and insert the suction catheter.**

    For Oropharyngeal Suctioning
    a. Lubricate the catheter tip with the normal saline solution.
    b. Using your dominant hand, gently but quickly insert the suction catheter along the side of the patient's mouth into the oropharynx.
    Inserting the suction catheter along the side of the mouth prevents gagging. ▼

    c. Advance the suction catheter quickly to the premeasured distance—usually 7.5 to 10 cm (3 to 4 in.) in the adult—being careful not to force the catheter.
    Ensures that the suction catheter will reach the pharynx. Forcing the catheter during insertion may cause tissue trauma.

    For Nasopharyngeal Suctioning
    d. Lubricate the catheter tip with the water-soluble lubricant.
    Eases passage of the suction catheter through the naris. Water-soluble lubricant is preferred because it will dissolve if it accidentally enters the lungs, whereas an oil-based lubricant (e.g., petroleum jelly or lotion) will not dissolve in the respiratory tract and causes complications if it enters the lungs.

    e. Using your dominant hand, gently but quickly insert the suction catheter into the naris.
    Prevents trauma to the naris. ▼

    f. Advance the suction catheter, aiming downward to the premeasured distance—usually 13 to 15 cm (5 to 6 in.) in an adult—and being careful not to force the catheter. If you meet resistance, you may need to try the other naris.
    Advancing the suction catheter the premeasured distance ensures that the suction catheter will reach the pharynx. Forcing the catheter during insertion may cause tissue trauma.

14. **Place a finger or thumb over** the suction control port of the suction catheter, and start suctioning the patient. Apply suction as you withdraw the catheter, using a continuous rotating motion.

    ✚ Limit suctioning to 10 to 15 seconds.
    Using a continuous rotating motion while withdrawing the catheter prevents trauma to any one area of the airway. Limiting suctioning to 10 to 15 seconds prevents hypoxia.

15. **After you withdraw** the catheter, clear it by placing the tip of the catheter into the container of sterile saline and applying suction.
    Ensures patency of the catheter for repeat suctioning.

16. **Lubricate the catheter,** and repeat suctioning as needed, allowing at least 20-second intervals between suctioning. Limit total suctioning time to 5 minutes.

(continued on next page)

Procedure 33-9 ■ Performing Upper Airway Suctioning (continued)

Several passes with the suction catheter may be needed to clear the airway of secretions. The total suctioning time should be limited to 5 minutes, however, to prevent hypoxia and trauma to the mucosal membranes.

For Nasopharyngeal Suctioning

Each time you repeat suction, alternate nares.
Prevents trauma that would occur if you used only one naris.

17. **Coil the suction catheter** in your dominant hand. Pull the sterile glove off over the coiled catheter. (Alternatively, wrap the catheter around your dominant, gloved hand, and hold the catheter as you remove the glove over it.) Discard the glove containing the catheter in a biohazard receptacle designated by your agency.
Coiling the catheter inside the glove prevents contamination with secretions.

18. **Using your nondominant hand,** clear the connecting tubing of secretions by placing the tip of the tube into the container of sterile saline.
Ensures patency and prepares the equipment for future use.

19. **Dispose of equipment** in biohazard waste container/bag, and make sure new suction supplies are readily available for future suctioning needs.
The patient may require suctioning at any time, so equipment must be readily available.

20. **Provide mouth care.**
Promotes patient comfort and clears the mouth of any secretions the patient may have expectorated.

21. **Discard your other glove** and remaining supplies.

22. **Position the patient** in a comfortable position, and allow him to rest.
Promoting comfort and allowing for a period of rest help the patient recover from suctioning, which may be very tiring.

? What if . . .

- The patient's oxygen saturation is less than 94%, or the patient is in any distress?

You may need to administer supplemental oxygen before, during, and after suctioning. See Procedure 33-4.

Evaluation

- Assess the color, consistency, and amount of secretions.
- Evaluate the patient's tolerance of the procedure. Note whether there were signs of respiratory distress during the procedure.
- Evaluate the effectiveness of the procedure by comparing breath sounds, vital signs, and pulse oximetry before and after the procedure.

Patient Teaching

- Explain the importance of administering supplemental oxygen to the patient before suctioning.
- Inform the patient that coughing typically increases with suctioning.
- Demonstrate oropharyngeal or nasopharyngeal suctioning to the caregiver, and ask for a return demonstration if suctioning will be required at home.

Home Care

- Instruct the family and caregiver where to obtain suction equipment.
- Provide contact information for healthcare personnel who can be reached for advice or emergencies.
- Explain that the procedure can be performed using clean technique instead of sterile technique in the home setting.
- Instruct the caregiver that suction catheters can be cleaned for reuse by washing them with soapy water and then boiling them for 10 minutes. After they are cleaned, rinse the catheters with normal saline solution or tap water.
- Teach to change the secretion collection container every 24 hours, or clean it according to home care agency guidelines every 24 hours.

Documentation

- Document the date, time, and reason you performed suctioning.
- Note the suction technique you used and the catheter size.
- Note color, consistency, and odor of secretions.
- Document the patient's respiratory status before and after the procedure.
- Document the patient's tolerance of the procedure and any complications that occurred as a result of the procedure, with resulting interventions.

Sample Documentation

00/00/0000   2200   Resp. labored, rate 28 breaths/min. Pulse oximetry on room air 92%. Breath sounds with rhonchi scattered throughout. Gurgling audible in upper airways. Patient unable to mobilize secretions with coughing. Suctioned by nasopharyngeal route using a 14-Fr. catheter. Approximately 30 mL thin, tan, odorless secretions obtained. After suctioning, resp. nonlabored, rate 20 breaths/min, and lungs clear on auscultation, with no gurgling audible. Pulse oximetry 96%. Patient tolerated procedure with no difficulty. ———— C.F. Hiam, RN

Practice Resources

Blakeman et al. (2022); Siegel et al. (2007); Schults et al. (2021); Sole et al. (2015).

Thinking About the Procedure

To practice applying clinical reasoning to this procedure,

The video **Performing Upper Airway Suctioning: Oropharyngeal,** along with questions and suggested responses, is available on the **Davis's Nursing Skills Videos** Web site at www.fadavis.com.

Procedure 33-10 ■ Caring for Patients Requiring Mechanical Ventilation

➤ For steps to follow in *all* procedures, refer to the Universal Steps for All Procedures on the inside back cover.

TERM	EXPLANATION
FiO_2	Fraction of inspired oxygen.
Modes of ventilation	Describes the setting on the ventilator that assists the patient to breathe. Can be controlled (CMV), intermittent mandatory (IMV), or synchronized intermittent mandatory (SIMV).
Tidal volume	Amount of air delivered from the ventilator with each breath.
Assist-control mode—also known as continuous mechanical ventilation (CMV)	The preset number of breaths per minute delivered by the machine. If the patient is able to initiate breaths, the machine will deliver a breath when the patient begins to inspire. If the patient is unable to breathe on his own, the machine will deliver the preset number of breaths in a rhythmic fashion.
Intermittent mandatory ventilation	A ventilator setting that delivers a minimum number of breaths per minute if the patient does not ventilate independently.
Synchronized intermittent mandatory ventilation (SIMV)	A ventilator setting that delivers a minimum number of ventilations per minute if the patient does not ventilate independently. The ventilator breaths are synchronized with the patient's breaths. This mode is used for weaning patients from the ventilator.
Pressure support	Provides positive pressure on inspiration to decrease the workload of breathing.
Continuous positive airway pressure (CPAP)	Provides positive pressure during inspiration and expiration to keep alveoli open in a spontaneously breathing patient.
Positive end expiratory pressure (PEEP)	Provides positive pressure on expiration to keep airways open for patients on CMV or SIMV mode ventilation.

Equipment
- Two oxygen sources
- Air source that provides 50 pounds per square inch (psi)
- Mechanical ventilator
- Humidification device
- Ventilator tubing, connectors, and adaptors
- Condensation collection device
- Inline thermometer
- Resuscitation bag with oxygen connection tubing
- Pulse oximetry device
- PPE (procedure gloves, protective gown, and eye covering)
- Sterile gloves, if you will perform suctioning
- Suction equipment (possibly)
- Sterile water for the humidifier (some guidelines also recommend sterile water for rinsing the mouth)

Delegation
Care of a mechanically ventilated patient requires advanced knowledge of pulmonary anatomy and physiology and, therefore, should not be delegated to assistive personnel. In critical care settings, specially trained LPNs may provide care, but the RN is responsible for ensuring that procedures are implemented safely and effectively. RNs also provide ongoing assessment of the patient's ventilatory and oxygenation status. Patients requiring long-term ventilation are often cared for at home or in specialized long-term care units, where LPNs and family members may provide care.

Preprocedure Assessment
- Review the health record to make sure that mechanical ventilation is included in the options outlined in the patient's advance directive.
  The patient may not wish to pursue mechanical ventilation as a care option. If a patient who does not wish to be ventilated mechanically is currently on a ventilator, consult your hospital ethics committee.
- If the patient's condition allows, assess their understanding of mechanical ventilation therapy.
  Understanding helps allay anxiety and promotes cooperation.
- Assess respiratory rate, depth, and rhythm; breath sounds; color; and pulse oximetry results.
  Confirms the need for mechanical ventilation.
- Assess the oral cavity for bleeding, inflammation, odor, and presence of yeast or plaque.
  May indicate the need for more frequent oral care or for referral.
- Blood will probably be drawn for an ABG analysis.
  To establish a baseline and, after that, to monitor response to therapy.

(continued on next page)

Procedure 33-10 ■ Caring for Patients Requiring Mechanical Ventilation (continued)

➤ When performing the procedure, always identify your patient according to agency policy, using two identifiers, and be attentive to standard precautions, hand hygiene, patient safety and privacy, body mechanics, and documentation.

Procedure Steps

Initial Ventilator Setup

1. **Prepare the resuscitation bag.**
   The resuscitation bag should be readily available to provide ventilation in the event of an emergency. ▼

   a. Attach a flow meter to one of the oxygen sources.
   The flow meter helps regulate oxygen delivery.

   b. Attach an adapter to the flow meter, and connect the oxygen tubing to the adapter.

   c. Turn on the oxygen, and adjust the flow rate.

2. **Respiratory therapists** are responsible for setting up mechanical ventilation in most agencies. If you must assume the responsibility, refer to the manufacturer's instructions.

3. **Plug the ventilator into** a grounded electrical outlet and turn it on.

4. **Verify ventilator settings** and adjust as medically prescribed.
   Ventilator settings must be individualized according to the patient's need for respiratory support. Incorrect settings may cause harm (e.g., hypoxia or barotrauma) to the patient. ➤

5. **Make sure that ventilator alarm** limits are set appropriately.
   Inappropriately set alarm limits can result in harm to the patient.

6. **Make sure the humidifier** is filled with sterile distilled water.

7. **Don PPE (gloves, gown, and eye protection)** if you have not already done so.

8. **Attach the ventilator tubing** to the endotracheal tube or tracheostomy tube.

9. **Place the ventilator tubing** in the securing device.
   Prevents dislodging the endotracheal tube or tracheostomy when the patient moves.

10. **Attach a capnographic device,** if available.
    To measure levels of carbon dioxide. These data are used to confirm placement of the endotracheal tube and disconnection from or malfunction of the ventilator. Oxygen levels alone are not sufficient for the ventilated patient.

11. **Prepare the inline (closed) suction equipment** (see Procedure 33-7).
    Suctioning equipment should be readily available when the patient requires suctioning. Closed catheters are recommended to prevent ventilator-associated pneumonia.

After Initial Ventilator Setup

12. **Check respiratory status** and ABGs again about 30 minutes after setup. Also check whenever there are changes in the ventilator settings and as the patient's condition indicates.
    To be certain the patient is being adequately ventilated and not experiencing oxygen toxicity.

13. **Check the ventilator tubing** frequently for condensation. Drain the fluid into a collection device, or briefly disconnect the patient from the ventilator and empty the tubing into a waste receptacle, according to agency policy.

    ✚ Never drain the fluid into the humidifier.
    Condensation in the ventilator tubing can cause resistance to airflow. Moreover, the patient can aspirate it. The fluid should not be drained into the humidifier because the patient's secretions may have contaminated it. ▼

14. ✚ **Maintain the patient** in a semirecumbent position (head of bed elevated 30° to 45°). This is extremely important.
    To promote lung expansion, reduce gastric reflux, and prevent ventilator-associated pneumonia.

15. **Check ventilator** and humidifier settings regularly.

16. **Check the inline thermometer.**
    To ensure that the air being delivered to the patient is close to the body temperature to prevent scalding of the mucosal tissue or, instead, cooling the patient (core temperature).

17. **Provide the patient with** an alternative form of communication, such as a letter board or white board.
    A patient being mechanically ventilated is unable to speak, which can produce extreme anxiety. The patient must have a way to express needs and concerns.

18. **Reposition the patient** regularly (every 1 to 2 hours), being careful not to pull on the ventilator tubing.
    Repositioning protects skin integrity. However, pulling on the tubing creates pain. Patient comfort promotes relaxation, improving the effectiveness of the ventilator.

19. **Keep the patient's lips** moistened with a cool, damp cloth and water-based lubricant; and provide regular antiseptic oral care. A recommended regimen includes the following (American Association of Critical Care Nurses, 2017):
    - Brush the teeth twice a day for 3 or 4 minutes.
    - Use a soft toothbrush.
    - Rinse the mouth with sterile water, according to agency policy.
    - Moisturize oral mucosa and lips every 2 to 4 hours.
    - Use a chlorhexidine gluconate (0.12%) rinse twice a day for intubated patients to reduce risk of VAP (adult patients).
    - Use mouthwash twice a day for adult patients.

    Mouth care provides comfort and preserves integrity of the mucous membranes. Patients being mechanically ventilated, even for a short period, are at high risk for developing ventilator-associated pneumonia (VAP). VAP is not uncommon, and it is associated with high mortality rates. This regimen is thought to help prevent VAP.

20. **Make sure the call device** is always within reach, and answer call device and ventilator alarms promptly.
    Provides the patient with immediate access to help if a breathing problem occurs; reassures the patient and thus relieves anxiety.

21. **Monitor the tracheostomy** tube for proper cuff inflation (usually 20 to 25 mm Hg); see Clinical Insight 33-4.

22. **Check for gastric distention** and take measures to prevent aspiration.
    Aspiration creates high risk for pneumonia.

23. **Clean, disinfect, or change** ventilator tubing and equipment according to agency policy.
    There is no good evidence to indicate how often this should be done. Research so far indicates that tubing and equipment should not be routinely changed for infection control purposes (Isac et al., 2021).

24. **Give sedatives or antianxiety** drugs as prescribed.

Evaluation

- After mechanical ventilation is instituted, assess for chest expansion and auscultate for bilateral breath sounds.
- Evaluate the patient's tolerance of mechanical ventilation. Verify that the patient is being adequately ventilated and that they are breathing in synchrony with the ventilator.
- Auscultate breath sounds every 2 to 4 hours, according to agency policy.
- When monitoring vital signs, count spontaneous breaths as well as those delivered by the ventilator.
- Monitor continuous pulse oximetry, capnography, and ABGs.

Patient Teaching

- Explain mechanical ventilation to the patient and family. Include information about the alarms they will hear.
- Demonstrate an alternative form of communication to the patient and family.
- When appropriate, explain the weaning process to the patient and family.
- If the patient requires mechanical ventilation after discharge, make arrangements for a home ventilator, and teach the patient and caregiver how to use it.

Home Care

- Consult with your facility discharge planning program and/or case management for discharge plans.
- Explain to the family and caregiver where to obtain a home ventilator, resuscitation bag, and oxygen equipment and what services are available. Make sure they choose a supplier who has 24-hour emergency services available.
- Help the client and caregiver devise a backup plan for ventilating the client in the event of a power failure.
- Tell the caregiver to notify the utility company and area emergency personnel that the client is being maintained on a ventilator at home.

(continued on next page)

Procedure 33-10 ■ Caring for Patients Requiring Mechanical Ventilation (continued)

- Instruct the client and caregiver about oxygen therapy and its use as well as safety measures that they must institute.
- Teach the client and caregiver to clean the ventilator tubing with soap and warm water when it becomes soiled.
- Provide the client and caregiver with contact information of healthcare personnel who can be reached for advice or emergencies.

Documentation

- Document the date and time mechanical ventilation was initiated.
- Note the type of ventilator used and the prescribed settings used.
- Document the client's response to mechanical ventilation, including vital signs, breath sounds, ease of breathing, pulse oximetry, intake and output, skin color, and ABG and chest x-ray results.

Sample Documentation

02/26/xx   0800   Patient found difficult to rouse. Dr. Henry made aware. ABG obtained; results included pH 7.28; PCO_2 78 mm Hg; PO_2 48 mm Hg. Dr. Henry in to evaluate patient. Anesthesia called to intubate patient. Medicated with Versed 5 mg IV and intubated orally with a 7.5-Fr. ET tube. Placed on mechanical ventilator: TV 700 mL; FIO_2 80%, respiratory rate 14 breaths/min. Portable chest x-ray confirms ideal placement of ET tube as well as white-out of both lung fields. ABGs to be obtained in 30 min. Pulse oximetry 90% since being placed on ventilator. ———————— L. Houck, RN

Practice Resources

American Association of Critical-Care Nurses (2017); Atay et al. (2017); Boltey et al. (2017); Isac et al. (2021); Liu et al. (2017); Najafi Ghezeljeh et al. (2018).

Procedure 33-11 ■ Setting Up Disposable Chest Drainage Systems

▶ For steps to follow in *all* procedures, refer to the Universal Steps for All Procedures on the inside back cover.

Equipment

- Two disposable closed drainage systems
- Chest tube insertion kit (common tube size for adults is 36 Fr). Should contain povidone-iodine, local anesthetic, syringe, needles, drapes, scalpel, suture, sterile drapes, chest tube, connecting tubing, and necessary instruments.
- 5-in-1 or Y-connector for two chest tubes, if not contained in insertion kit
- Sterile water (for water-seal system)
- Two rubber-tip hemostats
- PPE (sterile gloves, masks, and sterile gowns)
- Dressings: sterile 4 in. × 4 in. gauze dressings, precut drain dressings, petroleum (or other recommended) gauze dressings, and large drainage dressings
- Tape: 2-in. silk tape, 1-in. silk tape (or nylon banding system)

For Disposable Dry-Seal Systems

- 50-mL syringe and 45 mL of sterile water or saline; some dry-seal chest drainage units (CDUs) include these

Delegation

Some agencies permit only registered nurses in the critical care units to perform dressing changes. The physician must perform dressing changes on other units. You should not delegate this procedure, because it requires advanced knowledge of pulmonary anatomy and physiology. As needed, teach the LPN and UAP how to safely provide care for the patient with chest tubes. Instruct them to notify an RN immediately if the chest drainage system becomes disconnected, the chest tube becomes dislodged, sudden bleeding occurs, or the patient develops respiratory distress.

Preprocedure Assessment

- Ensure that the patient has venous access.
- Assess vital signs.
- Assess the level of consciousness, orientation, responsiveness, anxiety, and restlessness.
  These can indicate hypoxemia.
- Assess the patient's knowledge of chest tube therapy.
  Understanding helps allay fears and anxiety.
- Assess cardiac status; respiratory rate, depth, and rhythm; breath sounds; skin color; pulse oximetry; and ABG results.
  Provides a baseline for comparison after chest tube insertion. Evaluates chest tube functioning afterward.

▶ When performing the procedure, always identify your patient according to agency policy, using two identifiers, and be attentive to standard precautions, hand hygiene, patient safety and privacy, body mechanics, and documentation.

Procedure Steps

Steps for Preparing the CDU

1. **Obtain and prepare** the prescribed chest drainage unit (CDU). ▼

Disposable water-seal system.

Disposable dry-seal system.

Procedure Variation for a Disposable Water-Seal CDU Without Suction

2. **Remove the cover** on the water-seal chamber, and, using the funnel provided, fill the second (water-seal) chamber with sterile water or normal saline. Fill the chamber to the 2-cm mark, or as indicated. (Note that some systems come prefilled.)
   The water-seal chamber allows air to exit from the pleural space during exhalation and prevents air from entering the pleural space during inspiration.

3. **Place the chest drainage unit** (CDU) upright, usually on the floor, and at least 30 cm (1 ft) below the patient's chest level.

4. **Replace the cover** on the water-seal chamber.
   Protects the chamber from contamination.

   ➤ **Go to Step 13.**

Procedure Variation for a Disposable Water-Seal CDU With Suction

5. **Remove the cover** on the water-seal chamber. If it is not a prefilled system, use a syringe or the funnel provided to fill the water-seal chamber (second chamber) with sterile water or normal saline to the 2-cm mark.
   The water-seal chamber allows air to exit from the pleural space during exhalation and prevents air from entering the pleural space during inspiration.

6. **Add sterile water or normal** saline solution to the suction control chamber. Add the amount prescribed by the clinician, typically 20 cm (7 in.). Place the CDU upright, usually on the floor, and at least 30 cm (1 ft) below the patient's chest level.
   Suction is regulated by the height of fluid in the suction control chamber.

7. **Attach the tubing** from the suction control chamber to the suction source tubing. Turn on the wall (or other) suction source. A wall suction of –80 cm H_2O is common.

   ➤ **Go to Step 13.**

Procedure Variation for a Disposable Dry-Seal CDU With Suction

8. **Remove the nonsterile** outer protective bag and the sterile inner wrapper following agency policy.

9. **Place the CDU upright,** usually on the floor, and at least 30 cm (1 ft) below the patient's chest level. Some CDUs have hangers for hanging at the bedside.

10. **If suction will be required,** attach the tubing from the suction control chamber to the connecting tubing attached to the suction source.

11. **Fill a syringe** with 45 mL of sterile water or saline (follow agency policy and the manufacturer's recommendation for type of fluid), or use the small bottle of sterile fluid in the CDU package. Fill the air leak monitor on the CDU by injecting the fluid via the needleless injection port on the back until it reaches the fill line.
    Once filled, the water may become colored for improved visibility of air leaks. Bubbles in this section of the CDU indicate an air leak.

    ➤ **Go to Step 13.**

Procedure Variation for a Heimlich Valve

12. **When a patient has little or no** drainage and does not require suction, the chest tube may be connected to a Heimlich valve instead of a CDU. These valves are attached to the end of the chest tube and allow one-way flow of air out of the chest tube. They contain "flutter" leaflets that allow air to exit but not reenter the pleural space. These valves can also be used for emergency transport until a chest drainage system is available.

    ➤ **Go to Step 13.**

(continued on next page)

Procedure 33-11 ■ Setting Up Disposable Chest Drainage Systems (continued)

Steps for Inserting and Connecting the Chest Tube

NOTE: The remaining steps apply to all variations.

13. **Position the patient** according to the indicated insertion site.
    - For removing air: second intercostal space at the midclavicular line
    - For fluid drainage: on the midaxillary line in the fifth or sixth intercostal space

14. **Open the chest tube insertion tray** and set up the sterile field. Using sterile technique, drop any necessary supplies on the field (e.g., 4 in. × 4 in. split gauze dressings, petroleum or other recommended gauze, syringes).

15. **Don a mask, gown, and sterile gloves** and organize the supplies you will need for dressing the chest tube insertion site.
    Protective clothing prevents contamination of the surgical site and protects you from splashing.

16. **Provide support to the patient** while the physician or nurse practitioner prepares the sterile field, anesthetizes the patient, and inserts and sutures the chest tube.

17. **As soon as the chest tube** is inserted, attach it to the CDU tubing, using a connector.
    Usually the nurse holds the nonsterile tubing that leads to the collection chamber and the physician attaches the sterile chest tube to it. Immediately attaching the chest tube to the drainage system prevents air from entering the pleural cavity.

18. **If suction is prescribed,** adjust the CDU suction to the level the clinician specifies, usually −20 cm H_2O. Also adjust the wall (or other) suction source, usually to −80 cm H_2O.

For a Water-Seal Drainage Unit
Adjust the suction source (e.g., wall suction) until gentle bubbling occurs in the suction control chamber. When the tube is functioning properly, the height of the fluid level in the drainage tube fluctuates with the respiratory cycle.

NOTE: Increasing suction at the suction source increases airflow through the system and creates more bubbling, but it does not increase the amount of suction placed on the chest cavity.

For a Dry-Seal Drainage Unit
Adjust the CDU suction (e.g., to −20 cm H_2O) by turning the suction control dial on the CDU. Adjust the wall (or portable) suction pressure to −80 mm Hg or greater until the display on the suction control chamber confirms adequate suction.

If Suction Is Not Prescribed
Leave the suction tubing on the drainage system open to maintain negative pressure. Follow the manufacturer's directions on the CDU, as models will differ.

Steps for Dressing the Chest Tube

19. **When the chest tube** is functioning properly, the physician or nurse practitioner will suture it in place. Then don a new pair of sterile gloves. Using sterile technique, wrap petroleum-soaked, saline-soaked, or other recommended gauze around the chest tube at the insertion site.

    (Note: Sometimes the physician dresses the site.)

    Theoretically, the moistened gauze creates a seal that prevents air from leaking around the site. However, continued use of petroleum gauze or ointments can macerate the skin, so use them with caution. Recent research suggests that saline-soaked, or even dry, gauze may be preferable to petroleum gauze; follow your agency's policy.

20. **Place a precut, sterile split-drain** dressing over the gauze around the chest tube.
    Absorbs drainage from the insertion site, thereby reducing skin irritation and possible breakdown. ➤

21. **Place a second sterile, precut** drain dressing over the first drain dressing with the opening facing in the opposite direction from the first.
    The second drain dressing helps secure the first drain dressing and provides reinforcement against drainage.

22. **Place a large drainage dressing (e.g., ABD) over the two precut drain dressings.**
    NOTE: Some guidelines recommend that instead of large amounts of tape and padding, a transparent dressing be used. This minimizes moisture collection around the site, allows nurses to inspect for leakage or infection, and does not restrict chest wall movement. Follow your agency's policy.

    The large drainage dressing covers the insertion site, protecting it from outside sources of infection.

23. **Secure the dressing in place** with wide tape, making sure to cover the dressing completely.
    Creates an occlusive dressing that protects the chest tube from becoming dislodged and provides a seal over the insertion site, protecting it from outside sources of infection.

24. **Date, time, and initial the dressing.**

    Informs other staff members when the dressing change was completed and by whom.

25. **Using the spiral taping** technique, wrap 1-in. cloth tape around the chest tube, starting above the connector and continuing below the connector. Reverse your wrapping by taping back up the tubing (using the spiral technique) until the wrapping is above the connector. The CDU may come with locking connections or bands; if so, use those.

    Ensures a tight connection between the two tubings, thereby preventing an air leak at the connection site. ▼

26. **Cut an 8-in.-long piece of 2-in. tape.** Loop one end around the top portion of the drainage tube, and secure the remaining end of the tape to the chest tube dressing.

    Prevents pulling at the chest tube site when the patient moves.

27. **Make sure the drainage tubing** lies with no kinks from the chest tube to the drainage chamber.

    Facilitates drainage and prevents fluid from accumulating in the pleural cavity. ▼

28. **Prepare the patient** for a portable chest x-ray examination.

    A chest x-ray examination should be performed after the chest tube is inserted to ensure proper placement.

29. **Institute safety measures:**
    a. Place two rubber-tip clamps at the patient's bedside for special situations.

    Rubber-tip clamps are used to clamp the chest tube to check for an air leak, to change the drainage system, and to assess whether the chest tube can be safely removed.

    b. Place a petroleum gauze dressing at the bedside.

    In case the chest tube leaks or becomes dislodged, placing a petroleum gauze dressing over the insertion site helps keep air from entering the pleural cavity.

    c. Keep a spare disposable drainage system at the patient's bedside.

    To use in case the drainage system in use is accidentally upended or the drainage collection chamber becomes filled.

30. **Position the patient for comfort,** as indicated, but with the head of the bed elevated to at least 30°.
    - If the patient received a chest tube to relieve a pneumothorax, the preferred position is semi-Fowler's position.
    - If the chest tube was inserted to promote fluid drainage, high-Fowler's position is recommended.

Evaluation

- **Evaluate the patient's** tolerance to the chest tube insertion. Determine whether the patient's respiratory status has changed.
- Auscultate breath sounds every 2 hours.
- Check chest drainage every 15 minutes for the first 2 hours, and then check as prescribed. Observe type, color, and amount.
- Monitor the chest tube insertion site for drainage and subcutaneous emphysema at least every 4 hours.

  Crepitus is a sign that air is leaking into the subcutaneous tissues. Drainage is a sign that fluid is leaking around the insertion site. Both may indicate a compromise in tube patency.
- Confirm chest tube patency and determine whether bleeding is present.
- Monitor intake and output (I&O) every 8 hours.
- Check laboratory values to evaluate blood loss and oxygenation.
- Check the disposable chest drainage system for the presence of an air leak.

  An air leak indicates that air is leaking from the chest and a tight seal has not yet formed over the site of injury.

Patient Teaching

- Teach the patient and family about chest tube insertion.
- Explain the importance of immediately reporting chest pain, shortness of breath, or tube dislodgement.

(continued on next page)

Procedure 33-11 ■ Setting Up Disposable Chest Drainage Systems (continued)

Home Care
- Explain to the client and caregiver how to care for the chest tube at home.
- Provide the client and caregiver with contact information should problems with the chest tube arise.

Documentation
- Assessment findings before, during, and after chest tube insertion (e.g., vital signs, breath sounds, cardiac status, pulse oximetry)
- Date and time of the chest tube insertion
- Name of the clinician who performed the procedure
- The location of the insertion site, the size of the chest tube, the type of drainage system, and the amount of suction applied, if any
- Any medications the patient received during the procedure
- Color and amount of drainage
- Chest tube output on the intake and output portion of the documentation record (often a flow sheet)
- Patient's tolerance of the procedure
- Presence of subcutaneous emphysema or air leak, if any
- Complications and any interventions preformed as a result of the complications
- Chest x-ray findings

Sample Documentation
00/00/0000   0230   Patient presented with acute shortness of breath, pulse ox 84%, respirations 40 breaths/min and shallow, heart rate 132 beats/min. BP 188/100 mm Hg. Breath sounds absent on right side. Patient received morphine sulfate 4 mg IVP. #36 Fr chest tube placed by Dr. Phan under sterile conditions in right anterior chest, midclavicular line, above the 2nd ICS. Chest tube attached to 20 cm of water pressure. Small air leak present, no crepitus. Portable chest x-ray obtained after procedure revealed chest tube in good placement and right lung reexpanded. Vital signs postinsertion: pulse ox 94%, BP 153/90 mm Hg, heart rate 100 beats/min, and respiratory rate 24 breaths/min. Breath sounds audible bilaterally. ——————— Pennie Bowen, RNC

Practice Resources
Graham et al. (2019); Jeffries (2017); Queiroz et al. (2022); Siegel et al. (2007).

Thinking About the Procedure
To practice applying clinical reasoning to this procedure,

➤ The video **Disposable Chest Drainage Systems: Setting Up** and **Connecting & Dressing,** along with questions and suggested responses, is available on **Davis's Nursing Skills Videos** Web site at www.fadavis.com.

Procedure 33-12 ■ Inserting an Oropharyngeal Airway

➤ For steps to follow in *all* procedures, refer to the Universal Steps for All Procedures on the inside back cover.

⊕ The American Heart Association guidelines (2019) direct that you should insert an oropharyngeal airway only if you are trained in its use.

Equipment
- Oral airways in a variety of sizes
- Tongue blade
- PPE (protective gown, face shield, goggles)
- Procedure gloves
- Suction equipment
- Resuscitation bag and oxygen source (depending on the patient's status)
- Padded tongue blade

Delegation
You should not delegate this procedure because it requires specialized knowledge, training, and assessment skills.

Preprocedure Assessments
- Determine the appropriate airway size by placing the airway on the outside of the patient's cheek. The length of the airway should extend from the front teeth to the end of the jawline.
- Assess respiratory status (breath sounds, respiratory rate and effort, skin color, and pulse oximetry findings).
  Findings confirm the need for the airway and provide a baseline for evaluating the effectiveness of the intervention.
- Assess for contraindications (e.g., patient is conscious or semiconscious; patient has loose teeth or recent oral surgery).
  An oropharyngeal airway may stimulate the gag reflex, causing vomiting or laryngospasm in a conscious patient.

➤ When performing the procedure, always identify your patient according to agency policy, using two identifiers, and be attentive to standard precautions, hand hygiene, patient safety and privacy, body mechanics, and documentation.

Procedure Steps

1. **Perform hand hygiene, don PPE** as needed, and clean procedure gloves.
   Helps prevent transfer of microorganisms and exposure to infectious material from the patient.

2. **Explain the procedure** to the patient, even if they appear to be unresponsive.
   Recall that hearing is the last sense lost, so the patient may be able to hear you. Information may help relieve the patient's anxiety, if present.

3. **Clear the mouth of any debris** or secretions. You may need to suction the mouth.

4. **Place the patient in supine** or semi-Fowler's position. Hyperextend the neck, unless contraindicated.
   Mild hyperextension allows the airway to slide naturally toward the pharynx.

5. **Gently open the mouth.** Remove dentures, if present.
   Dentures may cause further airway obstruction.

If Using Tongue Blade Technique
Open the patient's mouth and use the blade to depress the tongue.

If Using Crossed Fingers Technique
Place your thumb on the lower teeth. Cross your index finger over your thumb and place the finger on the upper teeth. Push the teeth apart.

6. **You may need to hold** the tongue down with a tongue blade as you insert the airway.

7. **Insert the airway** along the top of the tongue, in the upside-down position (the "C" faces upward toward the nose).
   Prevents pushing the tongue toward the pharynx. ▼

8. **As the airway approaches** the posterior wall of the pharynx, rotate the airway 180° so that the ends of the "C" turn downward over the back of the tongue. Continue to insert the airway until the front flange is flush with the lips. ▼

9. **Keep the patient's head tilted** slightly back and the chin elevated.
   This position helps the oropharyngeal airway to function optimally.

10. **Do not tape the airway in place.**
    You may need to remove the airway quickly for suctioning. Untaping would delay airway removal, increasing the risk of aspiration.

11. **Position the patient on their side.**
    To minimize the risk of aspiration.

12. **Provide oral hygiene** every 2 to 4 hours. Remove and cleanse the airway at that time; use hydrogen peroxide and then rinse with water.

? What if . . .

- **After inserting the airway, respirations are absent or inadequate?**

  Use a mouth-to-mask technique, a handheld resuscitation bag, or an oxygen-powered breathing device to ventilate the patient. Have someone call for help.

Evaluation

- After inserting the airway, verify patency by auscultating for bilateral breath sounds.
- Check for bleeding or tooth damage in the mouth.
  May be caused by airway insertion, especially if it must be done rapidly.
- Check to be certain the patient's lips and tongue are not caught between the teeth and the airway.
  Prevents trauma to the soft tissues.
- Monitor the airway position frequently.
  Ensures correct placement.
- Continually reassess the need for the airway. Remove it when the patient begins to cough or gag.
- Frequently assess oral mucous membranes when you remove the airway for care.
  Prolonged airway use can cause tissue irritation or ulceration.
- Keep suction available at the bedside. Suction the oropharynx as needed by inserting the suction catheter alongside the airway.

Documentation

Document the following:
- Date and time of airway insertion
- Type and size of airway (oropharyngeal or nasopharyngeal)
- Assessments before and after the procedure, including breath sounds and focused respiratory assessment
- Any suctioning performed
- Patient's tolerance of the procedure
- Adverse reactions and interventions taken

Practice Resources
American Association of Critical-Care Nurses (2016); American Heart Association (2019); Brown et al. (2022); Wyckoff et al. (2022).

Procedure 33-13 ■ Inserting a Nasopharyngeal Airway

▶ For steps to follow in *all* procedures, refer to the Universal Steps for All Procedures on the inside back cover.

✚ The American Heart Association guidelines (2015) direct that you should insert a nasopharyngeal airway only if you are trained in its use.

Equipment
- Nasopharyngeal airway of the correct size
- Tongue blade
- PPE (protective gown, face shield, goggles)
- Procedure gloves
- Water-soluble lubricant
- Penlight
- Suction equipment
- Resuscitation bag and oxygen source (depending on the patient's status)

Delegation
You should not delegate this procedure because it requires specialized knowledge, training, and assessment skills. Commonly, this procedure is performed by a respiratory therapist.

Preprocedure Assessments
- Determine the appropriate airway size: (1) Measure the diameter of the patient's nostril and use an airway that is slightly smaller than that; and (2) measure the distance from the tip of the patient's nose to the earlobe, and use an airway about 2.5 cm (1 in.) longer than that measurement. Airways are sized by their internal diameter. Generally, the larger the internal diameter, the longer the tube. Airways are available in a variety of pediatric and adult sizes.

  Small adult: 6 to 7 mm

  Medium adult: 7 to 8 mm

  Large adult: 8 to 9 mm

- Assess respiratory status (e.g., breath sounds, respiratory rate and effort, skin color, pulse oximetry findings).
  Findings confirm the need for the airway and provide a baseline for evaluating the effectiveness of the intervention.

- Assess for contraindications (e.g., anticoagulant therapy, hemorrhagic disorder, nasopharyngeal deformity, sepsis).
  Up to 30% of patients have airway bleeding after insertion of a nasopharyngeal airway.

▶ When performing the procedure, always identify your patient according to agency policy, using two identifiers, and be attentive to standard precautions, hand hygiene, patient safety and privacy, body mechanics, and documentation.

Procedure Steps

1. **Perform hand hygiene, don PPE as needed,** and don procedure gloves.
   Helps prevent transfer of microorganisms and exposure to infectious material from the patient.

2. **Position the patient supine** or in semi-Fowler's position. Explain the procedure.
   A semi-Fowler's position facilitates airway insertions. Explaining may alleviate anxiety, enabling the patient to cooperate more with the procedure.

3. **Validate that the airway size** is correct. Hold the airway next to the patient's face. The length of the airway should measure from tip of nose to jawline below the ear.

4. **Lubricate the airway** with water-soluble lubricant.
   Prevents trauma to mucosa during insertion.

5. **Tilt the patient's head backward** to hyperextend the neck. Then push up the tip of the nose and gently insert the tip of the airway into the nose.

6. **Advance the airway** along the floor of the nostril into the posterior pharynx behind the tongue—until the outer flange rests on the nostril. If you meet resistance, rotate the tube slightly to enhance passage. Do not force against resistance.
   Forcing the tube can cause tissue trauma and airway kinking.

7. **Have the patient open the mouth.** Depress the tongue with a tongue blade and inspect the pharynx for proper placement of the tube tip. Use a penlight, if necessary, for better visualization.
   When the tube is fully inserted, the outer flange of the tube should rest on the nostril, and only the tip of the tube should be visible at the top of the posterior pharynx. ▼

8. **Check for correct placement** and function: Close the patient's mouth, and place your finger close to the tube's opening to feel for air exchange.

9. **Auscultate the lungs** for the presence of bilateral breath sounds.

10. **Remove the airway** at least every 8 hours to check nasal mucous membranes for ulceration or irritation. Clean the airway at this time: Place in a basin, rinse with hydrogen peroxide, then rinse with water. Use a pipe cleaner to remove secretions, if necessary. Reinsert the airway in the other nostril.

To avoid skin and mucous membrane irritation and breakdown and to prevent infection

? What if...

- **After I insert the airway, the patient coughs, gags, vomits, or has laryngospasm?**

The tube may be too long. If the tip extends beyond the top of the posterior pharynx, remove it and insert a shorter one.

Evaluation

- Assess respiratory rate and effort.
- Assess breath sounds.
- Observe for bleeding of nasal mucosa; suction as necessary.
- If the patient is receiving artificial ventilation, monitor for gastric distention and hypoventilation.
- Provide frequent oral and nares care; assess the skin around the nostril.

Documentation

Document the following:
- Date and time of airway insertion
- Type and size of airway (nasopharyngeal)
- Assessments before and after the procedure, including breath sounds, focused respiratory assessment, and condition of the mucous membranes
- Any suctioning performed
- Patient's tolerance of the procedure
- Adverse reactions and interventions taken
- Removal of the airway, cleaning, and replacement in the other nostril

Practice Resources

American Association of Critical Care Nurses (2016); American Heart Association (n.d.; 2019); Brown et al. (2022); Wyckoff et al. (2022).

CLINICAL INSIGHTS

Clinical Insight 33-1 ▸ Tips for Obtaining Accurate Pulse Oximetry Readings

Patient Movement. A nailbed is the most common site to place the probe. However, a tremor, twitch, shivering, or movement in bed can make pulse oximetry readings inaccurate. If the patient is unable to cooperate or control movement, try using an ear probe or nasal sensor.

Acrylic Fingernails and Nail Polish. If the patient has acrylic nails, place the probe on a toe or earlobe. Many facilities stock individually packaged nail polish remover pads to remove nail polish before placing the probe. *Nail polish or acrylic nails may interfere with signal transmission, causing inaccurate SaO_2 measurement. However, a recent study found that nail polish did not cause a clinically significant change in readings in healthy people (Balaraman et al., 2020).*

Dirt and Skin Oils. Dirt and oils on the site can interfere with passage of light waves.

Poor Perfusion. A low reading may result from poor perfusion of the area where the probe is placed.
- A bent elbow, for example, may cause a slight decrease in circulation to the nailbed. If SaO_2 results are crucial to the patient's plan of care, use the earlobe to minimize the effect of movement on the reading.
- Keep the extremities warm to obtain a more accurate reading. *Vasoconstriction due to cool extremities may also limit circulation.*

- If poor perfusion is related to a disease process, use the earlobe or nose as the monitoring site.

Lighting. Bright fluorescent lighting may influence the accuracy of the reading. Dim the lights or cover the probe with bed covers or a towel to reduce error.

Anemia, Carbon Monoxide, Intravascular Dyes, and Dark Skin Color. These must be considered when interpreting oximetry readings. Because these factors cannot be controlled, watch for trend changes in the readings.

Equipment Function. Look for a displayed waveform; a reading is meaningless without the waveform. If there is a weak signal or no signal, check the patient's vital signs. If vital signs are satisfactory, check the circulation to the site. If that is satisfactory, check equipment connections.

Accuracy of the Reading. If there is an instantaneous change in saturation (e.g., from 99% to 82%), suspect an error. This is not physiologically possible. For any suspected inaccuracy, check the reading using the equipment on a healthy person. If it seems accurate, check the patient's medications and history of circulatory disorders; also check items listed previously. When in doubt, rely on your clinical judgment more than the reading from the machine.

Clinical Insight 33-2 ▸ Guidelines for Preventing Aspiration

To prevent aspiration, use the following guidelines.

For At-Risk Patients
- Position the unconscious patient on their side to protect the airway.
- Request medications in elixir or liquid form.
- Break or crush pills, when appropriate.
- Keep a suction setup available for routine and emergency use.
- If the patient is intubated, keep the endotracheal or tracheostomy cuff inflated, and suction above the cuff before deflating the cuff.
- Do not offer food or fluids if the patient is heavily sedated or in the initial recovery phase of anesthesia.

Enteral Feedings
- Check the placement of the nasogastric tube before you administer enteral feedings.

- Check gastric residual volume before administering the next enteral feeding. Hold the feeding if the residual volume is high. (Note: The amount of acceptable residual volume depends on the amount and frequency of feedings.)
- If the patient is receiving continuous tube feedings, the head of the bed must remain elevated.
- Also see Procedure 24-3 for step-by-step instructions for administering feedings through gastric and enteric tubes.

Oral Feedings
- Position the patient upright or with the head of the bed elevated for feedings or meal.
- Be sure the head of bed remains elevated for at least 30 minutes after each feeding or meal.
- Offer small, frequent meals.
- Avoid thin liquids, or use thickening agents.
- Offer foods or liquids that can be formed into a bolus before they are swallowed.
- Cut food into small pieces.

Clinical Insight 33-3 ► Oxygen Therapy Safety Precautions

- ✚ Post signs indicating that oxygen is in use.
- Do not permit smoking near oxygen delivery systems.
- Ensure that three-pronged plugs are used for electrical devices (to prevent sparks).
- Allow no open flames (e.g., candles) near oxygen.
- Do not use electrical equipment with frayed wires or loose connections.
- Do not use petroleum products, aerosol products, and products containing acetone where oxygen is in use. (These are flammable substances that are easily ignited.)
- Secure oxygen tanks to rigid stands.
- Secure portable oxygen cylinders in holders or carriers provided.

Clinical Insight 33-4 ► Caring for Patients With Endotracheal Airways

Assisting With Endotracheal Airway Insertion

- **Gather equipment.** You will need an oxygen source and a bag (e.g., Ambu or nonrebreather bag) to inflate the lungs, a laryngoscope, endotracheal tubes of various sizes, water-soluble lubricant, a syringe to inflate the cuff, and tape to secure the tube in place.
- **Keep suction at the bedside** to clear the mouth and airway if secretions are obstructing your view of the cords.
- **You will need a surgical tray** if a tracheostomy is performed to create the direct opening into the trachea.
- **Remain calm, and explain** to the patient that the airway will enable them to breathe effectively.
- **Once the airway is in place, listen to breath sounds** to establish that both lungs are ventilated.
- **Reassess breath sounds periodically.** After the airway is inserted, record the type and size, as well as the patient's response to the procedure.
- **Expect that a portable chest x-ray will be prescribed** to confirm correct placement.

Managing and Monitoring Endotracheal Airways

The following are activities associated with the care of all types of endotracheal airways.

- ✚ **Have emergency equipment,** including a duplicate tracheostomy kit, extra cannula, and suction setup, immediately available for reintubation if the tube should become dislodged.
- **Keep an extra cannula at the bedside,** as patients may accidentally decannulate.
- **Secure the endotracheal tube** with ties, Velcro tapes, or a commercial holder to prevent accidental displacement.
- **Provide tracheostomy care every 4 to 8 hours** (Alsunaid et al., 2021; Billington et al., 2019; Johnston et al. [n.d., updated 2016]).
- **Secure the orotracheal tube** to the opposite side of the mouth with each change of tape or ties to prevent skin erosion and breakdown.
- **Inspect skin around the tube** or tracheal stoma for redness, swelling, drainage, or irritation at least every 8 hours.
- **Provide skin care** around the tube and tape or holder at least daily.
- **Perform regular oral care.**
- **Inflate the cuff of the tube with a minimal occlusive volume and monitor cuff pressures** to prevent pressure necrosis inside the trachea. (This is a joint responsibility with the respiratory therapist.) Maximum acceptable tube cuff pressure is 25 mm Hg. The following is a method for checking for minimal occluding volume:
  1. Place stethoscope on patient's neck over the carotid pulse.
  2. Attach a 10-mL syringe to the pilot balloon of the inflated cuff.
  3. Remove air from the cuff (1 mL at a time) until you hear a slight leak at the peak of inspiration.
  4. When you hear the leak, inject 1 mL of air back into the cuff.
- **Monitor and document cuff pressure** once per shift and when the tube is changed or repositioned.
- **Note the centimeter reference marking** on the endotracheal tube to monitor for possible displacement.
- **Minimize pulling and traction** on the artificial airway by supporting all tubing connected to the airway and using flexible catheter mounts and swivels.
- **Remind the conscious patient not to pull on the airway.**
- **Use a bite block between the teeth** to prevent the patient from occluding an orotracheal tube.
- **Provide 100% humidification** of inspired air. Check the oxygen setup regularly.
- **Routine saline instillation** to thin secretions is no longer recommended.
- **Ensure adequate hydration** with oral or IV fluids to keep the mucosa moist and thin secretions.
- **Suction the airway** when secretions collect. Remember that the patient probably can't cough effectively to clear secretions.

Clinical Insight 33-5 ▶ Managing Chest Tubes

Monitor Breathing, Gas Exchange, and Drainage

- **Frequently assess breathing patterns, breathing effort, and breath sounds.**
- **Assess mental status, heart rate and rhythm, and pulse oximetry readings.**
  These reflect adequacy of oxygenation.
- **Monitor character, color, and amount of chest drainage.** Immediately report sudden or large increases in drainage or new onset of bright red blood, along with an assessment of the patient's condition at that time.
  Drainage is usually greatest when the chest tube is initially inserted and decreases as the lung reexpands. You must replace the chest drainage unit (CDU) when the drainage compartment is almost full.

Prevent Complications or Intervene If They Occur

- **Observe the dressing at least every 4 hours.** Make sure that the dressing around the tube insertion site is occlusive (not wet or loose). Usually, petroleum gauze is wrapped around the insertion site to ensure occlusion.
- **Inspect for excessive, abnormal, or foul-smelling drainage.**
  This may indicate hemorrhage or infection.
- **Palpate around the dressing for subcutaneous emphysema** (air in the subcutaneous tissues).
  This may be caused by an incomplete seal at the chest tube insertion site.
- **Assess for pain;** medicate as needed.
- **Reposition the patient every 2 hours** and use pillows to keep the patient's weight off the chest tube.
  To prevent occlusion of the tube, promote drainage, and preserve skin integrity.
- **Encourage the patient to use the arm on the affected side.** Assist with range-of-motion exercises, if necessary.
  To maintain joint mobility.
- ✚ **Recollapse of the lung** can occur because of loss of negative pressure within the system. This is commonly caused by air leaks, disconnections, or breaks or cracks of the bottles or chambers. If any of these occur, immediately place the disconnected end nearest the patient into a bottle of sterile water or saline.
- **Do not clamp the chest tube.** Doing so can lead to a **tension pneumothorax.** Clamp chest tubes only for changing the drainage system. Limit the clamp time and monitor respiratory status constantly until the clamp is removed.
- **If the tube is accidentally pulled out,** immediately cover the wound with a dry, sterile dressing. Listen for air leaking out of the site. If you can hear air, tape the dressing loosely so that you do not occlude the site.
  If air cannot escape from the chest, a tension pneumothorax will occur, eventually compromising cardiovascular function.

Promote Lung Reexpansion

- Encourage the patient to be as active as their condition permits.
  Chest drainage systems are bulky, but with disposable systems, patients can still get out of bed and ambulate but will need assistance to protect and monitor the system and the patient.
- **Instruct the patient to perform deep breathing and coughing every 2 hours,** unless contraindicated. Assist the patient to sit upright and splint the chest with a pillow or the hands, and provide analgesia as needed.
  These interventions help to minimize discomfort.

Key Points for Managing a One-Bottle System

- **Keep the intake tube below the fluid level in the drainage bottle.**
  To prevent drawing air into the pleural space with inhalation.
- **Maintain the tubing about 2 cm below the water level.** As tubing length below the water increases, more effort is required to exhale.
- **Take precautions to see that the bottle is not accidentally tipped over,** uncovering the long vent tube and allowing air to enter the pleural space.

Maintain the Drainage System

For All Types of CDUs:

- **Make sure the drainage system is located below the insertion site.**
  If the drainage system is higher than the insertion site, fluid may flow back into the pleural cavity, compromising the patient's respiratory status.
- **Regularly inspect tubing** to ensure that connections are airtight and tubing is not kinked or occluded.
  Kinks in the drainage tubing increase pressure in the pleural cavity and prevent fluid drainage.
- **Monitor drainage.**
  Blood or purulent matter can occlude the tubing.
- **Inspect the air vent in the drainage system** to make sure it is patent.
  If air builds up in the pleural cavity, pneumothorax may occur.
- **Monitor to ensure the system is maintaining consistent negative pressure levels.**
- ✚ Do not "milk" or strip the tubing.
  Doing so can create excess negative pressure and damage lung tissue. Always be sure to verify operation through the users' manual or with the product's vendor. Most systems will have some type of check system to ensure that the system is operating correctly.
- **To transport or ambulate a patient:** (1) Keep the CDU upright below chest level; (2) disconnect the CDU from suction source and make sure the air vent is open.

Clinical Insight 33-5 ➤ Managing Chest Tubes—cont'd

Water-Seal Drainage Systems
- **Take precautions that the CDU is not tipped over** (e.g., tape it to the floor).
- **Observe for tidaling** (fluctuations in the water-seal chamber's fluid level that correspond with respiration). The level will increase on inspiration and decrease on exhalation. This will be opposite for a patient on a mechanical ventilator.
- **Bubbling in the bottom of the water-seal chamber indicates an air leak.** When this occurs, check for poor tubing connections. A small amount of bubbling right after insertion or with exhalation or cough is normal.
- **Check the water in the suction control chamber;** replace as needed.
  The water can evaporate.
- ✚ **If the chest tube disconnects from the drainage unit,** establish a temporary water seal by immersing the open end of the chest tube in a bottle of sterile water to a depth of 2 cm until a new system can be connected. Cleanse the end of the patient connector on the drain system with alcohol and reconnect it if it has not been contaminated. If the patient connector on the drain system is contaminated, you must initiate a new CDU.

Dry-Seal Drainage Systems
- **Inspect the air vent in the drainage system** to make sure it is patent.
  The air vent must remain patent to allow air to escape. If air builds up in the pleural cavity, pneumothorax may occur.
- **Check the indicators on the CDU to be certain that suction is operating properly.**
  A dry chest drainage system doesn't use water in the suction chamber. A valve inside the regulator continuously balances the forces of suction and the atmosphere. The valve automatically responds and adjusts to changes in patient air leaks and fluctuations in suction source vacuum to deliver accurate suction to the patient. Pressure can be set from -10 cm H_2O to -40 cm H_2O by adjusting the rotary dry suction dial.
- **Observe for bubbling.**
  If the water in a dry-seal CDU is bubbling, it means there is an air leak.

ASSESSMENT GUIDELINES AND TOOLS

Focused Assessment

Oxygenation

Part I. Questions to Assess Risk for Impaired Oxygenation

Demographic Data
- What is your age?
- Where do you live?
- What is your occupation?

Health History
- What healthcare problems are you currently being treated for?
- Have you ever been hospitalized or had surgery? If so, when and for what reason?
- Do you have a history of allergies or asthma?
- What medications do you currently take?
- What over-the-counter medications or alternative treatments do you use? What do you use them for?

Respiratory History
- Have you ever been diagnosed with a respiratory problem? If so, what was the diagnosis? When was the diagnosis made?
- Have you noticed any changes in your breathing?
- How often do you cough?
- When you do cough, is it productive?
- What do the secretions you cough up look like and smell like?
- How much sputum do you produce?
- How do you treat your cough? What effect does it have?
- Do you ever wheeze or feel short of breath?
- What causes you to wheeze or feel short of breath?
- Do body positions affect your breathing pattern?
- What position do you lie in when you sleep? Do you use more than one pillow?
- Do you ever wake up short of breath?

Environmental History
- Are there pets in the house?
- What response, if any, do you have to pets, dust, pollen, or plants?
- Are you exposed to smoke or fumes in the home and workplace?

(Continued)

Focused Assessment

Oxygenation—cont'd

- Are you exposed to respiratory irritants such as asbestos, chemicals, coal dust, fungus, molds, or soot in the home or workplace?
- What type of heating, air-conditioning, or air-filtering system do you have in the home or workplace?

Lifestyle
- What is your current stress level? What are your major sources of stress?
- What is your usual diet? Is your current diet typical, or have you recently changed your eating habits?
- What is your usual activity level?
- What level of activity makes you feel short of breath?
- Do you smoke now, or have you ever smoked?
- If you smoke, how many packs per day and for how many years have you smoked?
- Do you smoke marijuana or use other substances?

Part II. Focused Physical Examination

Pulmonary System
- *Inspect* to observe respiratory patterns, signs of respiratory distress, chest structures and movement, skin and mucous membrane color, presence or absence of edema, sputum characteristics, and overall general appearance.
- *Palpate* skin temperature and areas of tenderness.
- *Percuss* over the lung fields (for consolidation or excess air pockets).
- *Auscultate* breath sounds and vascular sounds.
- *Assess breathing patterns:* eupnea, tachypnea, bradypnea, apnea, Kussmaul breathing, Biot's breathing, and Cheyne-Stokes respirations.
- *Assess cough and related symptoms:*
  - Nasal congestion, sneezing, watery eyes, and nasal discharge suggest allergies.
  - Fever, chest congestion, noisy breath sounds, sputum production suggest a URI.
  - Dyspnea, chest tightness, and wheezing suggest airway obstruction (e.g., asthma).
- *Assess/recognize cues for sputum:* appearance, color, odor, amount, and timing.
- *Obtain sputum samples* as needed.
- *Assess/recognize cues for respiratory effort:* Breathing should be effortless. Observe for shortness of breath, dyspnea, nasal flaring, head bobbing, retractions, use of accessory muscles during inspiration, grunting, needing to sit upright to breathe, paroxysmal nocturnal dyspnea, conversational dyspnea, stridor, and wheezing.

DIAGNOSTIC TESTING

Lung Volumes and Capacities

The norms presented in this table are based on averages for a young adult male patient. The following are measured by spirometry.

Title	Definition	Significance
Tidal volume (V_T)	The amount of air moved into and out of the lungs with each normal breath. Normally around 500 mL.	In a healthy state, V_T increases when oxygen demand increases. Diseases that restrict lung inflation, create muscular weakness, or paralyze the diaphragm limit the ability of the body to increase tidal volume. When such disorders become severe, V_T will fall too low to support even resting oxygen demands.
Inspiratory reserve volume (IRV)	The maximum amount of air that can be inhaled above and beyond the normal tidal volume. Ranges from 2,000 to 3,000 mL.	IRV determines how much the tidal volume can increase when oxygen demands increase.
Expiratory reserve volume (ERV)	The maximum extra amount of air that can be forcefully exhaled after the end of a normal tidal expiration. Ranges from 1,000 to 1,500 mL.	Some diseases (e.g., emphysema) cause collapse of alveoli and airways, which traps extra air in the lungs. This "trapped" air cannot be exhaled and lowers ERV.

Lung Volumes and Capacities—cont'd

Title	Definition	Significance
Residual volume (RV)	The amount of air remaining in the lungs after the most forceful exhalation. Ranges from 1,000 to 1,500 mL.	Diseases that reduce ERV lead to an increase in RV. As more air is trapped in the lungs and cannot be exhaled even with forceful attempts (ERV), it becomes part of the residual volume that is never completely exhaled.
Inspiratory capacity (IC)	The combination of the tidal volume and inspiratory reserve volume (V_T + IRV). Ranges from 2,500 to 3,500 mL.	This is the amount of air that can be inhaled with maximum effort. It reflects the capacity one has to inhale deeply.
Functional residual capacity (FRC)	The combination of expiratory reserve volume and residual volume (ERV + RV). Ranges from 2,000 to 3,000 mL. Exhalation of additional air requires effort to force more air out.	This is the amount of air that stays in the lungs at the end of a normal, passive quiet exhalation. Disorders that cause air trapping increase the FRC.
Vital capacity (VC)	The combination of inspiratory reserve volume and expiratory reserve volume (IRV + ERV). Ranges from 3,000 to 4,500 mL.	This is the maximum amount of air that can be forcefully exhaled after filling the lungs to their maximum level with the deepest possible inspiratory effort.

Tests Related to Oxygenation

Test	Purpose
Angiogram	A contrast dye is injected into a vein, and serial films are taken to assess patency of the vessels.
Arterial blood gases (ABGs)	An analysis of arterial blood that evaluates the effectiveness of gas exchange.
Bronchoscopy	Insertion of a flexible endoscope to examine the larynx, trachea, and bronchial tree.
Cardiac catheterization	A catheter is passed into the heart to assess pressures, blood flow, and the size and patency of chambers.
Chest x-ray study (CXR)	Provides an anterior–posterior or lateral view of the heart and lungs, shows tissue density (e.g., to evaluate size, masses, fluid).
Hemoglobin (Hgb)	A serum measurement that affects the oxygen-carrying capacity of the blood. May be measured separately or as part of a complete blood count.
Pulmonary function studies	A series of tests to detect lung volume and capacity.
Sputum culture	A microscopic evaluation of the sputum.
Thoracentesis	Insertion of a large-bore needle through the chest wall into the pleural space to obtain fluid specimens, to instill medication, or to drain accumulations of fluid.
Throat culture	A swab of the pharynx or tonsils is performed to assess pathogens present in the pharynx.
Ventilation–perfusion scan	Used to assess for pulmonary embolus, this scan entails injection of a radioactive substance that allows blood flow to the lungs to be evaluated. A second substance is inhaled that maps out oxygen distribution in the lungs.
White blood cell (WBC) count	A serum measure to assess for the presence of infection.

Diagnostic Testing

Reading a Tuberculin Skin Test Result

Size of Induration	Considered Positive For
>5 mm	People who have had recent close contact with someone with active TB
	People who have HIV or risk factors for HIV
	People with history of TB
	People who use IV drug and are known to be HIV-negative
>10 mm	People with medical conditions that increase the risk of progressing from latent TB to active TB (e.g., diabetes mellitus, use of steroids, chronic renal failure, some malignancies)
	Residents and employees of high-risk congregate settings: prisons, skilled nursing facilities (SNFs) and other long-term facilities, healthcare facilities, and homeless shelters
	Foreign-born persons recently arrived (i.e., within the past 5 yr) from countries having a high incidence of TB
	People in low-income groups
	Children younger than 4 years of age or exposed to adults in high-risk categories
>15 mm	People who do not meet any of the previously mentioned criteria

CLINICAL REASONING
Applying the Full-Spectrum Nursing Model

PATIENT SITUATION

Haley, a 15-year-old female high school student, was admitted to the hospital with shortness of breath and right-side chest pain when breathing. She states that she has had "the flu" for 3 days. She has a history of asthma since age 6 and smokes half a pack of cigarettes a day. Both her parents are heavy smokers. An IV was initiated, and she is receiving 800 mg of vancomycin (an antibiotic) intravenously every 12 hours. She is not on oxygen therapy but receives 10 incentive spirometer treatments per hour while awake. Her heart rate is 80 beats/min, respiratory rate 24 breaths/min, and blood pressure 110/70 mm Hg. Her skin is pale but warm, and capillary refill time is 2 seconds. She has no clubbing of the fingers. She is urinating approximately 400 mL of clear yellow urine every 8 hours and maintaining a normal bowel elimination pattern. Laboratory results are:

Red blood cell count (RBCs): 3.56×10^6 (3.56 million/mm^3)
White blood cell count (WBCs): 11,800/mm^3
Hemoglobin: 11.2 g/dL
Hematocrit: 32.7%
Haley says, "I feel really tired, and too weak to even pick up a glass of water." Her cough produces white, thick sputum. Sputum culture on admission confirms a diagnosis of streptococcal pneumonia.

THINKING

1. *Theoretical Knowledge:*

   a. According to the Centers for Disease Control and Prevention, should Haley have received a pneumonia immunization? Why or why not?

   b. What is clubbing of the fingers? You may wish to refer to Chapter 19 for review, or to a medical-surgical nursing text.

2. *Critical Thinking (Analyzing Cues):*

   a. Why is it a positive finding for Haley that she does not have clubbed fingers?

DOING

3. *Practical Knowledge:*
   Twenty-four hours after the antibiotics were started, Haley's respiratory status becomes worse. She says, "It's so hard to breathe." It is decided to begin administering oxygen. Another sputum culture is prescribed. You are to collect a sputum specimen from the patient.

   a. What position should Haley assume for this procedure?

   b. What kind of protective clothing do you need for this procedure?

   c. You remove the lid from the specimen container. When you hand it to Haley, she touches the inside of the container with her fingers. What should you do?

   d. What would you tell Haley to do in order to expectorate the sputum specimen?

4. *Nursing Process (Assessment/Recognizing Cues):*

   a. In the admission data, what important information is missing regarding her respiratory status?

CARING

5. *Self-Knowledge:*

   a. Describe one or two patient care experiences you might draw on to help you in caring for Haley. In what ways were those patients similar to Haley, and how might that help you?

6. *Ethical Knowledge:*

   a. After you finish collecting the sputum specimen, what do you think Haley's biggest concern is right now?

Critical Thinking and Clinical Judgment

1. Recall the three patients discussed in the Meet Your Patients scenario in your textbook in Volume 1:

   - Mary is a 4-year-old patient with a history of asthma. Her mother, Ms. Green, has brought her in because of an "asthma attack." Mary is sitting on her mother's lap and breathing rapidly through an open mouth. Her cough sounds congested and wheezy. The nurse practitioner has ordered a nebulized treatment containing albuterol (Proventil) and ipratropium bromide (Atrovent).

   - Mr. Chu is a 78-year-old patient complaining of cough, sore throat, fatigue, and weakness. His temperature is 100.4°F (38°C), pulse is 90 beats/min, respirations are 26/min, and blood pressure (BP) is 166/82 mm Hg.

   - William is a 19-year-old male patient who has had a sudden onset of right-side chest pain and shortness of breath. His chest x-ray revealed a right pneumothorax, and he is currently receiving 35% oxygen by face mask while waiting for an ambulance to transport him to the hospital for further evaluation.

   a. Which patients are having problems with ventilation? Explain your answer.

   b. Which patient appears to be having problems with hypoxia? Does the problem appear to be related to oxygenation or perfusion? Explain your answers.

   c. Mr. Chu has smoked two packs of cigarettes per day for 50 years. ABGs reveal a low Po_2 and a high Pco_2 consistent with chronic lung disease. He is diagnosed with an acute exacerbation of chronic bronchitis. He is placed on oral antibiotics and long-acting bronchodilators by metered-dose inhaler (MDI). What teaching could you offer to help Mr. Chu mobilize and expectorate secretions?

d. Mary receives her nebulizer treatment and markedly improves. The physician has prescribed a variety of take-home medications that you must teach Mary's mother about. The treatment plan includes a protocol based on peak expiratory flow monitoring. Discuss how you might involve Mary in her own care.

e. William's chest x-ray film reveals a spontaneous pneumothorax. There is no apparent fluid in the pleural space. What chest tube systems can be used to treat his pneumothorax? Explain your thinking.

2. You are caring for a 68-year-old woman during the night shift. Earlier today she had an abdominal hysterectomy under general anesthesia. You note that her respiratory rate has steadily risen from 16 to 26 and that she has developed a mild, nonproductive cough. When you listen to her chest, you hear crackles throughout. She has a 40-pack-per-year cigarette smoking history. Identify an appropriate nursing diagnosis for this patient. Explain the reasons for your choice.

3. For each of the following concepts, use critical thinking to describe how or why it is important to nursing, patient care, or oxygenation. Note that these are not to be merely definitions.

Ventilation

Gas exchange

Artificial airways

Suctioning

Negative pressure in the chest

Hypoventilation

Hyperventilation

Supplemental oxygen

Pulse oximetry

What Are the Main Points in This Chapter?

- The structures of the airways, lungs, chest cavity, heart, and blood vessels function together to supply oxygen to the tissues; thus, abnormalities in any of these structures can interfere with tissue oxygenation.
- Developmental stage, environment, individual characteristics, lifestyle, medications, and pathological factors can interfere with ventilation, circulation, or gas exchange, leading to problems with tissue oxygenation.
- A health assessment related to oxygenation includes assessment of ventilation (breathing), circulation (blood flow), and gas exchange (exchange of oxygen and carbon dioxide). The length and focus of the assessment vary with the purpose and urgency of the clinical situation.
- A physical examination related to adequacy of oxygenation includes observations of adequacy of breathing, circulation, and gas exchange.
- Pulse oximetry and arterial blood gases are used to monitor oxygen saturation.
- Small changes in oxygen saturation are associated with large shifts in the amount of oxygen available to the tissues and organs.
- Interventions to promote optimal respiratory function include deep regular breathing, flu and pneumonia immunizations for at-risk individuals, frequent position changes, incentive spirometry, and preventing aspiration.

- Deep breathing, coughing exercises, and hydration promote deep inhalation and forceful expulsion of secretions.
- Supplemental oxygen is used to prevent hypoxemia. It may be delivered by a variety of methods.
- Artificial airways provide an open airway for patients who cannot maintain their own airway. The most common artificial airways are oropharyngeal, nasopharyngeal, and endotracheal.
- Airways can be suctioned to remove secretions and maintain patency. Signs that indicate the need for suctioning include gurgling sounds during respiration, restlessness, labored respirations, decreased oxygen saturation, increased heart and respiratory rates, and the presence of adventitious breath sounds during auscultation.
- Mechanical ventilation with a positive pressure ventilator requires the patient to have an artificial airway.
- Chest tubes remove air or fluid from the pleural space so that the lungs can fully expand. Chest tubes should be clamped only for changing the drainage system; clamping can lead to tension pneumothorax.
- Respiratory medications promote ventilation and oxygenation by their effects on the respiratory system. The major types of respiratory medicines include bronchodilators, corticosteroids, cough preparations, decongestants, antihistamines, and mucolytics.

Knowledge Map

Oxygenation

PULMONARY/LUNG COMPONENT

- **AIRWAYS**
  - Upper
  - Lower
    - Trachea
    - Bronchi
    - Bronchioles
- **LUNGS**
  - Alveoli
  - Surfactant
  - Pleura
- **VENTILATION**
  - Inhalation
  - Exhalation
- **RESPIRATION**
  - External
  - Internal

FACTORS AFFECTING
- Developmental stage
- Environment
- Stress
- Lifestyle: occupation, pregnancy nutrition, obesity; exercise; smoking, substance abuse
- Medications

ALTERATIONS IN OXYGENATION
- Hypoxemia
- Hypoxia
- Hypercarbia/capnia
- Hypocarbia/capnia

Caused by:
- Structural abnormalities
- Airway inflammation/obstruction
- Infection
- Alveolar-capillary membrane disorders
- Atelectasis
- Pulmonary embolus
- Pulmonary hypertension

NURSING

Promoting optimal respiratory function

IMMUNIZATION/SCREENING
Influenza, pneumonia, tuberculosis
- Prevent URIs
- Position for maximum ventilation
- Teach/assist with incentive spirometry
- Implement aspiration precautions

MOBILIZE SECRETIONS
- Cough/deep-breathe; hydration; chest PT
- Supplemental oxygen
- CPR
- Pharmacotherapy

ASSESSMENTS
- Breathing pattern
- Cough
- Respiratory effort: retractions, orthopnea, dyspnea, stridor
- Adventitious breath sounds
- Pulse oximetry

ARTIFICIAL AIRWAY MANAGEMENT
- Oropharyngeal; nasopharyngeal; endotracheal; tracheostomy
- Care includes maintaining placement; suctioning

MECHANICAL VENTILATION
- Intubation; maintaining proper settings; troubleshooting problems
- Can be used long term in home settings

CHEST TUBES
- Monitor breathing/gas exchange and drainage
- Keep drainage system intact and functioning properly
- Promote lung expansion
- Prevent tension pneumothorax; recollapse of lung

CHAPTER 34

Circulation & Perfusion

STUDENT RESOURCES

The questions and exercises in this book allow you to practice the kind of thinking you will use as a full-spectrum nurse. Critical-thinking questions usually have more than one right answer, so we do not provide "correct" answers for these features. Try to answer these questions yourself. It is more important to develop your nursing judgment than to just cover content. You will learn more by discussing the questions with your peers. If you are still unsure, see the Davis Advantage chapter resources for suggested responses.

To explore learning resources for this chapter,

Go to www.DavisAdvantage.com and find:

Answers and Suggested Responses for all questions in this chapter
Concept Map
Knowledge Map
References and Bibliography

Key Concepts

Circulation
Perfusion

Related Concepts

See the Concept Map on Davis Advantage.

Example Client Condition

Decreased Cardiac Output

Caring for the Williams Family

Charlene Williams, Stanley's mother, has been complaining she feels tired all the time; she just can't do what she normally does. She describes having a hard time catching her breath as she walks up stairs and goes about her day. Stanley has noticed that his mother's ankles are more swollen than he has ever seen them. He schedules an appointment for his mother at the family clinic where you are the nurse. Mrs. Williams appears pale and not her usual energetic self. Stanley tells you that his mom is "not right" and seems to be confused about things at home, which is not like her. She has a history of chronic congestive heart failure.

A. What additional health history data would be useful to gather at this time?

B. During her visit at the clinic, you observe that Mrs. Williams has a cough. She spits a small amount of pink, frothy mucus into a tissue. Mrs. Williams' vital signs are as follows: BP, 142/90 mm Hg; pulse, 96 beats/min and with some irregular beats; respirations, 38 breaths/min and shallow; temperature, 97.8°F (36.5°C) oral.

- Which of these symptoms and vital signs is/are not within normal limits?
- For each abnormal finding, explain why you think it is occurring.

Caring for the Williams Family (continued)

C. You decide to include a nursing diagnosis of acute confusion in Mrs. Williams' plan of care.
- What symptoms does she have that support this nursing diagnosis?
- What physiological changes are causing these symptoms?

D. In addition to angiotensin-converting enzyme (ACE) inhibitor, beta blocker, diuretic, and digoxin, what therapies do you anticipate the physician will prescribe?

E. Mrs. Williams asks you, "What can I do to make sure I never get this sick again?" How would you answer this question?

Practical Knowledge
clinical application

PROCEDURES

In this section you will find the procedures necessary for supporting circulation and perfusion. As you perform the procedures, apply the theoretical knowledge and concepts you obtained in Volume 1. The registered nurse is responsible for assessing patients' circulation and perfusion and their responses to procedures.

Procedure 34-1 ■ Performing Cardiac Monitoring

➤ For steps to follow in *all* procedures, refer to the Universal Steps for All Procedures on the inside back cover.

Equipment
- Alcohol pads
- Gauze dressing
- Washcloth
- Shaving supplies or scissors, if necessary
- Disposable electrodes

For Hardwire Monitoring, Add:
- Cardiac monitor
- Cable with lead wires
- Safety pin
- 1-in. tape

For Telemetry, Add:
- Transmitter with lead wires (with a new battery inserted before each use)
- Pouch to carry transmitter

Delegation
You should not delegate this procedure to the licensed practical nurse or unlicensed assistive personnel because it requires knowledge of anatomy, physiology, and advanced assessment techniques.

Preprocedure Assessment
- Assess cardiovascular status, including heart sounds, pulse rate, and blood pressure, and check for the presence of pain.
- Assess skin integrity of the chest before applying electrodes. *Skin lesions contraindicate the application of leads to the affected area.*
- Assess for history of dysrhythmias. *Early recognition of dysrhythmias allows for prompt treatment, which improves patient outcomes.*

➤ When performing the procedure, always identify your patient according to agency policy, using two identifiers, and be attentive to standard precautions, hand hygiene, patient safety and privacy, body mechanics, and documentation.

Procedure Steps

1. **Prepare the monitoring equipment.**

    For Hardwire Monitoring
    a. Plug the cardiac monitor into an electrical outlet and turn it on.
    Allows the monitor to warm up while you prepare the patient for monitoring.
    b. Connect the cable with lead wires into the monitor.
    The cable and lead wires must be properly connected to the monitor to obtain an accurate electrocardiogram (ECG) tracing. Most are color coded.

    For Telemetry Monitoring
    c. Insert a new battery into the transmitter.
    A new battery should be inserted with each use to ensure transmitter function.
    d. Turn on the transmitter.
    Tests the unit to make sure that the battery is functional.

(continued on next page)

Procedure 34-1 ■ Performing Cardiac Monitoring (continued)

e. Connect the lead wires to the transmitter, if they are not permanently attached. Be sure to attach each one to its correct outlet.
   The lead wires must be properly connected to the transmitter to obtain an accurate ECG tracing.

2. **Expose the patient's chest** and identify electrode sites based on the monitoring system being used and the patient's anatomy. Gently rub the placement sites with a washcloth or gauze pad until the skin reddens slightly.
   The monitoring system will dictate lead placement. Sites over soft tissues or close to bone provide accurate waveforms; sites over bony prominences, thick muscles, and skinfolds can produce artifact. ▼

3. **If the patient's chest has dense hair,** shave or clip the hair with scissors at each electrode site.
   Hair may interfere with electrical contact, preventing accurate ECG waveform transmission.

4. **With an alcohol pad** clean the areas chosen for electrode placement, and allow them to dry.
   Alcohol removes oil on the skin that may prevent the electrodes from adhering.

5. **Remove the electrode backing** and make sure the gel is moist. Discard the electrode if the gel is dry. The number of electrodes needed will depend on the monitoring system being used. It will be three to five electrodes.
   A dry electrode will not conduct electrical activity.

6. **Attach the lead wires** to the electrodes by snapping or clipping them in place.

7. **Apply the electrode** to the site by pressing it firmly. Repeat with the remaining electrodes.
   Pressing the electrode firmly creates a tight seal, which ensures electrical contact.

8. **Secure the monitoring equipment.**

   For Hardwire Monitoring
   a. Wrap a piece of 1-in. tape around the cable, and secure it to the patient's gown with a safety pin.
      Secures the cable so leads are not disconnected with patient movement.

   For Telemetry Monitoring
   b. Place the transmitter in the pouch, and tie it around the patient's neck. Place the transmitter into the patient's robe or gown pocket if a pouch is not available.
      Allows the patient independence with ambulation.

9. **Check the patient's ECG** tracing on the monitor. If necessary, adjust the gain to increase the waveform size.
   The ECG tracing should be large enough to accurately assess all of the waveform components.

   For Telemetry Monitoring
   You may need to call a monitoring room to verify ECG tracing and rhythm.

10. **Set the upper and lower** heart rate alarm limits according to agency policy or patient condition, and turn them on.

11. **Obtain a rhythm strip** by pressing the "record" button.
    You must obtain a rhythm strip to document the patient's cardiac rhythm.

    For Hardwire Monitoring
    a. Press the "record" button on the bedside monitor.
       The "record" button, located on the monitor at the bedside, allows you to print a rhythm strip immediately when cardiac symptoms occur.

    For Telemetry Monitoring
    b. Press the "record" button on the transmitter of the telemetry unit, or call the monitoring room to have the ECG trip printed.
       The "record" button on the telemetry transmitter allows you or the patient to print a rhythm strip immediately when cardiac symptoms occur.

12. **Interpret the rhythm strip,** and then mount it appropriately (e.g., with transparent tape) in the patient's record.
    Provides a permanent record of the patient's heart activity; identifies rhythm abnormalities in the patient's rhythm.

? What if...

■ **The patient is diaphoretic?**

   Remove electrodes, clean the area with alcohol, allow the area to dry, and then reapply electrodes.
   To obtain an accurate ECG tracing.

■ **The patient is receiving a cardiac medication?**

   Print a strip before giving medication and after giving medication. You may also need to call the telemetry station to have the ECG monitored.
   To assess and monitor effects of medication.

■ **I am not getting a good reading on the monitor?**

   Recheck the leads; replace leads or move leads if necessary.

Evaluation

- Evaluate changes in the patient's cardiac rhythm.
- Check skin integrity, and replace the electrodes at least every 24 hours.
  Avoids skin irritation at the electrode sites. In addition, the gel begins to dry, so replacement ensures an adequate waveform.

Patient Teaching

- Explain the rationale for cardiac monitoring.
- Teach the patient that if they have symptoms (e.g., shortness of breath, chest pain, dizziness, palpitations) the patient should notify the nurse immediately so a rhythm strip can be recorded.
- Tell the patient being monitored by telemetry to remove the transmitter before showering. Ask the patient to inform you before removing it.
- Discuss home telemetry monitoring with the patient and caregiver if the patient requires telemetry monitoring after discharge.

Home Care

- Evaluate the client's and caregiver's ability to continue telemetry monitoring at home with help from an outside agency.
- Help the client and caregiver contact the monitoring agency and arrange for home telemetry monitoring.
- Explain to the caregiver and patient that the emergency medical service will be notified by the monitoring agency if a dysrhythmia develops.
- Instruct the caregiver and patient about proper lead placement and the need to rotate electrode sites to prevent skin breakdown.

Documentation

- Document the date and time that monitoring was instituted.
- Note the monitoring lead selected.
- Document a rhythm strip every 8 hours and with changes in the patient's condition according to agency policy. Label the rhythm strip (if the monitor does not label it for you) with the date, time, patient's name, and room number. Indicate on the strip when symptoms and treatment interventions occurred.
- Document the patient's response to treatment.

Practice Resources

Ajmal et al. (2021); Hancock et al. (2009); Ladha et al. (2018).

ASSESSMENT GUIDELINES & TOOLS

Assessing Circulation

Part I. Questions to Assess Risk for Impaired Circulation

Demographic Data
- What is your age?
- Where do you live?
- What is your occupation?

Health History
- Do you have current health problems? Describe.
- Do you have past health problems? Describe.
- Have you ever been hospitalized or had surgery. If so, when and for what reason?
- Do you take medication for your heart, blood pressure, cholesterol, erectile dysfunction, diabetes, breathing difficulty, or other conditions?
- Do you have chronic fatigue, heartburn, anxiety, swelling of the ankles, difficulty breathing, chest discomfort, palpitations, dizziness or fainting spells, dental problems, pain in the calf when walking that stops with rest, chronic cough or wheezing, shortness of breath, or unexplained weight loss?
- Do you take over-the-counter products, such as vitamins, supplements, or aspirin?
- What else do you want to tell me about your physical or mental health history?

Family History
- Did your father or a brother develop coronary artery disease or have a heart attack before the age of 55?
- Did your mother or sister develop coronary artery disease or have a heart attack before the age of 65?

Cardiovascular History
- Have you ever had or been diagnosed with a heart attack, angina, coronary artery disease, peripheral artery disease, stroke, or aortic aneurysm?
- Do you have high or low blood pressure? Do you feel dizzy if you stand up quickly?
- Have you ever had chest pain? If so, describe the circumstances. What was done to relieve the symptoms? What measures do you take to prevent the pain?
- Do you become easily fatigued or feel your heart rate is rapid? Do you ever feel heart palpitations?

(Continued)

Focused Assessment

Assessing Circulation—cont'd

- Do you have pain in your legs when you are walking uphill or walking for a long time?
- Do you ever have cold hands and feet? If so, how often?
- Do you have pain or tingling in your feet or toes with exercise? Do they feel numb when you are at rest? Does the pain worsen when your leg is elevated and/or improve when you dangle your legs over the side of the bed?
- Do you have pain in your leg, foot, or toes that is so severe that shoes or the weight of a sheet at night is painful?
- If you are male, do you have impotence?
- Do you have ulcers that do not heal?

Female-Specific Assessment

- Do you have a systemic autoimmune inflammatory disease (SLE, RA)?
- Do you have a history of gestational diabetes mellitus (GDM)?
- Do you have a history of pregnancy-induced hypertension, preeclampsia, and/or eclampsia?
- Did you deliver a preterm or small for gestational-age baby?
- Do you have a history of stillbirth or miscarriage? If so, how many?
- At what age was the onset of menopause?
- Do you have a history of depression or anxiety?

Nutrition History

- In a typical day, how many servings of whole grains, fruits, vegetables, dairy products, eggs, nuts, and red meat or fish do you eat or drink per day?
- How many meals per week do you eat fast food or other high-fat food?
- How many sugar-sweetened soft drinks and sodas do you drink per day?
- How many meals per week do you eat out? Where?
- How many times per day do you add salt or eat salty foods?
- How many times per week do you skip a meal?
- Do you have diabetes or prediabetes? Are you a normal weight?

Lifestyle and Health Promotion Activities

- What is your current stress level? What are your major sources of stress? How do you relieve stress?
- What is your usual diet? Is your current diet typical, or have you recently changed your eating habits?
- What is your usual activity level? Do you exercise regularly? If so, how many minutes per week of moderate to vigorous physical activity do you get?
- Do you check your lipid profile (cholesterol and triglycerides) and blood sugar (fasting blood sugar and hemoglobin A_{1C}) on a regular basis?
- Do you smoke now, or have you ever smoked? If you smoke, how much (packs per day or e-cigarettes) and for how many years have you smoked?
- Do you use crack cocaine or other illicit substances?

Social Determinants of Health

Specialized screening tools allow healthcare providers to assess and monitor social needs and risk factors of all persons seeking healthcare. For an example of screening tools:

- Go to the Health-Related Social Needs (HRSN) Screening Tool at https://innovation.cms.gov/files/worksheets/ahcm-screeningtool.pdf
- Go to PRAPARE Implementation and Action Toolkit at https://aapcho.org/prapare-implementation-and-action-toolkit/
- Go to the HealthBegins screening tool at https://www.aamc.org/system/files/c/2/442878-chahandout1.pdf

Part II. Focused Physical Examination

Cardiovascular System

- Review **Procedure 19-13: Assessing the Heart and Vascular System.**
- *Inspect the neck* for carotid and jugular pulsations. Palpate each carotid separately. Auscultate the carotid arteries and jugular veins for bruits and hums.
- *Inspect the precordium* for pulsations. Palpate for pulsations, lifts, heaves, and thrills. Auscultate for heart sounds.
- *Assess peripheral circulation:* Palpate peripheral pulses, assess skin color and temperature, and note hair distribution on extremities. Inspect for skin ulcers and edema of the feet and ankles.
- *Inspect* for venous valve competence.
- *Perform the capillary refill test* anywhere you note signs of diminished blood flow.

DIAGNOSTIC TESTING

Tests Related to Circulation

Test	Purpose
Angiogram	A contrast dye is injected into a vein, and serial films are taken to assess patency of the vessels.
Arterial blood gases (ABG)	An analysis of arterial blood evaluates the effectiveness of gas exchange and perfusion.
Cardiac catheterization	A catheter is threaded through the blood vessels into the heart to assess pressures, blood flow, and the size and patency of chambers.
Chest x-ray study (CXR)	Provides an anterior–posterior or lateral view of the heart and lungs, shows tissue density (e.g., to evaluate size, masses, fluid).
Cholesterol, lipid profile	Indicates risk for cardiovascular disease long term.
Creatine kinase-MB (CK-MB)	The MB isoenzyme is present only in the heart muscle. A serum measurement of the MB band is used to detect a myocardial infarction (MI). Levels rise with an acute MI.
Echocardiogram	An ultrasound evaluation of the heart that examines heart function and blood flow
Electrocardiogram (ECG)	Electrodes placed on the extremities and chest wall conduct electrical activity from the heart. ECG illustrates heart rate, rhythm, and size and helps evaluate heart damage.
Hemoglobin (Hgb)	A serum measurement that affects the oxygen-carrying capacity of the blood. May be measured separately or as part of a complete blood count.
Holter monitor	A continuous ECG tracing used to correlate symptoms and cardiac activity. Typically the tracing lasts 48 hours to 7 days.
Magnetic resonance angiography (MRA)	Powerful magnetic field and radio frequency waves are used to evaluate blood vessels and help identify abnormalities. This examination is noninvasive and does not use radiation.
Technetium scan	Technetium-99m sestamibi is injected intravenously. Approximately 90 to 120 minutes later, the heart is scanned. Areas of myocardial damage appear as "hot spots" on the scan.
Treadmill test	Evaluates the effect of exercise on the heart and circulation via continuous ECG and vital sign monitoring during exercise.
Troponin	A serum evaluation of a complex of proteins is used to detect MI. Levels of these contractile proteins remain elevated for up to 7 days after MI.
Ultrasound (Doppler)	A transducer, which directs high-frequency sound waves to the artery of vein, is used to examine blood flow. A normal result shows no areas of narrowing or closure in the blood vessel.
Venography	Using dye and x-ray technology, a narrow tube (catheter) is inserted into a large vein to identify any blood clots or unusual narrowing or blockage of venous blood flow.
VQ scan	Used to detect a blood clot in the lungs.

CLINICAL REASONING
Applying the Full-Spectrum Nursing Model

PATIENT SITUATION

Margarita, a 62-year-old director of management technology for a large company, was admitted to the hospital with shortness of breath, sudden and intense fatigue, and intense chest pressure that she describes as feeling like a steel band tightening around her rib cage. She reports the pain moved up to her jaw. The pain began suddenly but lasted approximately 5 to 7 minutes. During the episode, her husband tells you that Margarita acted as though she had a feeling of doom.

Margarita also has a history of sudden-onset neck pain that seems to be triggered by heightened stress at work. Margarita is pale and clammy. She states she feels nauseated and has burning in her epigastric area. Her heart rate is 80 beats/min, respiratory rate 12 breaths/min, and blood pressure 168/92 mm Hg. Skin is pale but warm, and capillary refill time is 4 seconds. Height is 5 ft 4 in. Weight is 156 lb. Body mass index (BMI) is 29.2. Waist circumference is 36 in.

The health history includes type 2 diabetes mellitus, high blood pressure, and tobacco use (half a pack of cigarettes a day). Margarita's mother had a heart attack in her 50s.

Laboratory work before admission:

Fasting lipids: total cholesterol, 288 mg/dL; LDL, 148 mg/dL; HDL, 44 mg/dL; triglycerides, 222 mg/dL
Serum glucose: 244 mg/dL
Hs-CRP: 3.1 mg/dL

THINKING

1. *Theoretical Knowledge:*

   a. What predisposing factors increase Margarita's risk for myocardial infarction?

   b. What does it mean to have infarcted myocardial tissue?

2. *Critical Thinking (Analyzing Assumptions):*
   Based on your knowledge of vascular causes of myocardial infarction, what are the most likely causes in this patient?

DOING

3. *Practical Knowledge:*
   After your patient's vital signs are stable and her pain is controlled, the emergency physician prescribes further diagnostic testing to determine the extent of damage to her heart.

   a. What tests would you expect your patient to have?

   b. You attempt to adhere electrodes for cardiac monitoring to Margarita's chest. The ECG tracing shows a great deal of artifact rather than a clear ECG tracing. What should you do to obtain an accurate tracing?

   c. You notice your patient has multiple "runs" of aberrant heartbeats. What should you do in response to the abnormal ECG tracing?

4. *Nursing Process (Assessment/Recognizing Cues):*
   In the admission data, what important information is missing regarding her cardiac status?

CARING

5. *Self-Knowledge:*
   Describe a personal experience involving someone in your own family or a friend who had a life-threatening event. How did you feel when your loved one was faced with a potentially life-altering heart condition? How might you draw on this experience to help you in caring for Margarita?

6. *Ethical Knowledge:*

   a. After Margarita is finished with the last diagnostic test, what do you think her biggest concern is likely to be?

   b. Margarita tells you that she does not want anyone to know she has a heart problem. Yet her husband wants to tell other family members. How do you best respond to her concerns for privacy?

Critical Thinking and Clinical Judgment

1. Recall the patient discussed in the Meet Your Patient scenario in Volume 1 of your textbook:
   Ms. Saunders is a 55-year-old accountant. Ms. Saunders complains of being extremely tired, easily becomes short of breath, and is unable to complete chores without frequent rest breaks. Ms. Saunders is pale and seems tired. Vital signs are as follows: temperature, 98.4°F (36.7°C); pulse, 86 beats/min; respirations, 24 breaths/min and unlabored; BP, 136/78 mm Hg; and pulse oximetry, 98% on room air. Ms. Saunders is now waiting for her laboratory results, which include a complete blood count (CBC).
   Which of the following nursing diagnoses can you make, based on the patient data given here? Use a nursing diagnosis handbook as needed.

   Decreased cardiac output

   Risk for impaired cardiac tissue perfusion

   Impaired peripheral tissue perfusion

   Activity Iintolerance

2. Ms. Saunders is diagnosed with severe anemia and is hospitalized with a hemoglobin value of 8.9 g/dL. How will this affect Ms. Saunders' oxygenation? What interventions/nursing actions would improve the fatigue?

3. For the following concepts, use critical thinking to describe how or why they are important to nursing, patient care, or oxygenation. Note that these are *not* to be merely definitions.

   Circulation

   Perfusion

What Are the Main Points in This Chapter?

- The structures of the airways, lungs, chest cavity, heart, and blood vessels function together to supply oxygen to the tissues; thus, abnormalities in any of these structures can interfere with tissue oxygenation.
- Developmental stage, environment, individual characteristics, lifestyle, medications, and pathological factors can interfere with circulation and perfusion, leading to problems with tissue oxygenation.
- A health assessment related to circulation includes assessment of ventilation (breathing), circulation (blood flow), perfusion, and gas exchange (exchange of oxygen and carbon dioxide). The length and focus of the assessment vary with the purpose and urgency of the clinical situation.
- A physical examination to assess adequacy of circulation includes collecting objective data using the techniques of inspection, palpation, percussion, and auscultation as appropriate.
- Cardiovascular function is influenced by developmental stage; environment; lifestyle; substance abuse; medications; and pathophysiological conditions such as heart failure, coronary artery disease, and peripheral vascular disorders.
- The purposes of cardiac monitoring are to identify the patient's baseline rhythm and rate, recognize significant changes in the baseline rhythm and rate, and recognize life-threatening dysrhythmias that require immediate intervention.
- Promoting circulation ensures that oxygenated blood reaches tissues and organs and venous blood returns to the heart. Activities that promote venous return and peripheral arterial circulation and prevent clot formation assist with circulation.
- Cardiovascular drugs are used to enhance cardiac output, thus providing increased blood flow and oxygenation to organs and tissues. They include vasodilators, beta-adrenergic blocking agents, diuretics, and positive inotropes.

Knowledge Map

OXYGENATION CARDIOVASCULAR

CIRCULATION:
- Oxygenated blood to tissues
- Deoxygenated blood to heart/lungs

HEART:
- 4 Chambers
- Electrical Conduction

PULMONARY:
- Circulation
- Peripheral Vessels
- Arteries
- Veins

FACTORS AFFECTING:
- Developmental stage
- Environment
- Stress
- Lifestyle
- Medications

ALTERATIONS IN OXYGENATION
- Hypoxemia
- Hypoxia
- Hypercarbia/capnia
- Hypocarbia/capnia

Caused by

HEART FAILURE
- Cardiomyopathy
- Cardiac Ischemia: MI, angina
- Dysrhythmias
- Valve Abnormalities
- Anemia
- CO poisoning
- Peripheral Vascular Disease

NURSING

Promoting Optimum Circulation

ASSESSMENT
- Carotid & Jugular Pulsations
- Inspect Precordium
- Palpate Peripheral pulses
- Skin color/temperature
- Hair distribution
- Capillary refill test

PREVENTION/DIAGNOSTICS
IMMUNIZATION/SCREENINGS:
- Influenza, Pneumonia, Tuberculosis

DIAGNOSTIC TESTS:
- Angiogram
- Cardiac catheterization
- Creatine kinase MB/Troponin
- Echocardiogram

PROMOTE VENOUS RETURN
- Ambulation
- Positioning
- ROM
- Compression devices

PREVENT CLOT FORMATION
CPR
PHARMACOTHERAPY

CHAPTER 35

Hydration & Homeostasis

STUDENT RESOURCES

The questions and exercises in Volume 2 allow you to practice the kind of thinking you will use as a full-spectrum nurse. Critical-thinking questions usually have more than one right answer, so we do not provide "correct" answers for these features. Try to answer these questions yourself. It is more important to develop your nursing judgment than to just cover content. You will learn by discussing the questions with your peers. If you are still unsure, see the Davis Advantage chapter resources for suggested responses.

To explore learning resources for this chapter,

Go to www.DavisAdvantage.com and find:

Answers and Suggested Responses for all questions in this chapter
Concept Map
Knowledge Map
References and Bibliography

Key Concepts

Acid–base balance
Electrolyte balance
Fluid balance

Related Concepts

See the Concept Map on Davis Advantage.

Example Client Conditions

Fluid, electrolyte, and acid–base imbalances

767

Caring for the Williams Family

Stanley Williams has been prescribed the following medicines:

lisinopril 20 mg PO daily
hydrochlorothiazide 25 mg PO daily in the a.m.
metformin 500 mg PO before breakfast and lunch

Today he had blood drawn for analysis. Following are the electrolyte panel results.

Sodium	136 mEq/L
Potassium	3.0 mEq/L
Chloride	96 mEq/L
Bicarbonate	24 mEq/L
Blood urea nitrogen (BUN)	18 mg/dL
Creatinine	0.8 mg/dL

A. Review the laboratory results. Compare Stanley's laboratory work with the established norms for these values. Based on the laboratory results, what kind of assessment questions would be appropriate to ask Stanley?

B. Use your pharmacology text to review Stanley's medications. Which, if any, of these medicines might be contributing to Stanley's laboratory results?

C. What teaching would be appropriate for Stanley?

Practical Knowledge clinical application

To prevent, identify, and treat fluid, electrolyte, and acid–base problems, you will need to be skilled at initiating and managing intravenous infusions of fluids and blood, performing focused history and physical assessments, and interpreting arterial blood gas (ABG) values. When performing the procedures, apply the concepts and other theoretical knowledge you have learned.

PROCEDURES

Procedure 35-1 ■ Initiating a Peripheral Intravenous Infusion

▶ For steps to follow in *all* procedures, refer to the Universal Steps for All Procedures on the inside back cover.

Equipment
- IV solution
- Administration set or IV lock and injection caps (for a glass solution container, use vented tubing; for a plastic container you may use either vented or nonvented tubing)
- Extension tubing with or without saline lock
- Appropriately sized intravenous (IV) catheter
- Prefilled syringe to prime extension tubing
- Clean, unsterile gloves
- Scissors
- Antiseptic swabs that contain solutions such as chlorhexidine (preferred INS, 2021) or 70% alcohol wipes
- Tourniquet (nonlatex, if available)
- Sterile manufactured catheter stabilization device or ½-in. tape
- Transparent semipermeable occlusive dressing (preferred) and/or 2-in. × 2-in. sterile gauze
- 1-in. nonallergenic tape, preferably clear
- Labels, time tape
- Linen-saver pad
- Arm board, if necessary

Delegation
In some states and agencies, you can delegate peripheral IV catheter insertion to a licensed practical nurse (LPN) who is adequately trained in the procedure.

Preprocedure Assessment
- Assess the patient's need for IV therapy by checking vital signs, laboratory values, urine output, skin turgor, breath sounds, and the condition of mucous membranes.
- Check for any situations that may contraindicate administering the prescribed fluids to the patient.
- Assess for allergy to tape.
- Assess the veins on the arms and hands for a potential insertion site.
  The upper extremities are preferred because of better blood flow, easier access, and less potential for complications than in other locations.
- Check the medical record for factors such as anticoagulant therapy, bleeding disorders, or low platelet count.
  These factors place the patient at risk of bleeding during IV catheter insertion.

▶ When performing the procedure, always identify your patient according to agency policy, using two identifiers, and be attentive to standard precautions, hand hygiene, patient safety and privacy, body mechanics, and documentation.

(continued on next page)

Procedure 35-1 ■ Initiating a Peripheral Intravenous Infusion (continued)

Procedure Steps

✚ *Note:* Maintain scrupulous aseptic technique throughout this procedure. *Any microorganisms introduced can cause infection at the site, which could quickly migrate into the bloodstream and cause sepsis.*

1. **Place the patient in** a comfortable position, the bed at a comfortable working height, and supplies within reach. Explain the procedure to the patient.
   Makes the procedure safer and easier and decreases the risk for the nurse to develop back problems from improper body mechanics.

2. **Prepare the IV solution** and administration set or IV lock.
   a. Following the rights of medication administration, check the IV solution to make sure that you have the proper solution with the prescribed additives.
   IV solution is considered medication, and you should check it carefully to avoid administration and compatibility errors.
   b. Check the expiration date on the IV solution. Do not use IV solution after the expiration date.
   c. Check the IV solution for discoloration or particulate matter.
   Indicates contamination and should not be used.
   d. Label the IV solution container with the patient's name, date, and your initials. Place a time tape on the solution container with the prescribed infusion rate, time the infusion begins, and time it is to be completed.
   Policies govern when solution containers, administration sets, dressings, and IV catheters need to be changed to avoid complications such as infection. Although not all agencies require a time tape, labeling infusion rates on the solution containers in this manner will alert others and makes it easy to see at a glance whether the solution is infusing on time. ▶
   e. Take the administration set from the package and close the roller clamp by rolling it downward. Label the tubing with the date and time.
   Ensures that fluid does not flow through inadvertently after the bag is spiked.
   f. Remove the protective cover from the solution container port.
   g. Remove the protective cover from the spike on the IV administration set, keeping the spike sterile. Insert the spike into the port of the solution container. ▼

When Using a Glass Bottle
Clean the rubber stopper on the top of the bottle with an alcohol pad. Then insert the spike of the administration set through the stopper.
   h. Be certain the tubing is clamped. Hang the IV solution container on an IV pole.
   Clamping prevents leakage of fluid.
   i. Lightly compress the drip chamber, and allow it to fill up halfway.
   Overfilling the drip chamber will impair your ability to see the drips and adequately regulate the IV flow rate. ▼

When Not Using Extension Tubing
Prime the tubing by opening the roller clamp and allowing the fluid to slowly fill the tubing. When tubing is filled, close the clamp.

When Using Extension Tubing
Either attach it to the end of the administration set now and prime it with the rest of the IV line, or prime it separately, as follows:
   j. Scrub the injection port of the extension tubing with an antiseptic pad and let it dry.
   k. Attach a flush syringe filled with normal saline to the injection port or to the nonluer-lock end and slowly push the fluid through the tubing until completely primed. (Consult packaging instructions for the amount of saline needed to flush the tubing.)
   l. Leave flush syringe attached to the extension tubing.
   IV extension tubing makes it easier to convert an IV to a saline lock without disturbing the IV dressing and catheter. Manipulation of the IV catheter increases the risk of complications such as phlebitis, inflammation, infection, and infiltration.
   m. Inspect the tubing for air. If air bubbles remain in the tubing, flick the tubing with a fingertip to mobilize them into the drip chamber. Recap the end of the tubing firmly.
   Air in the tubing creates the potential for air embolism.

Performing the Venipuncture

3. **Place a linen-saver pad** under the patient's arm.
   Protects the bed from soiling during venipuncture.

4. **Place the patient's arm** in a dependent position.
   Gravity helps fill and dilate the vein, making venipuncture easier.

5. **Apply a tourniquet** 10 to 20 cm (4 to 8 in.) above the selected site. Palpate the radial pulse. If no pulse is present, loosen the tourniquet, and reapply it with less tension.
   Occluding the arterial flow diminishes venous filling, making venipuncture difficult.

6. **Locate a vein for inserting the IV** catheter. Select the best vein. For adults, use the veins located on the dorsal and ventral surfaces of the upper arm, including the metacarpal, cephalic, basilic, and medial veins (INS, 2021). Hand veins should be used only for therapy less than 24 hours. Check with the medical provider before using an arm or hand that contains a dialysis graft or fistula, or the affected arm of a patient who has undergone a mastectomy. See Clinical Insight 35-3 for more guidelines.
   Choose the most distal veins on the hand or arm so that you can perform subsequent venipunctures proximal to the previous site. This preserves veins for long-term therapy and prevents extravasation of fluid and medicines.

7. **Palpate the vein and press it** downward, making sure that it rebounds quickly. If the vein is not adequately dilated, ask the patient to open and close the fist; apply heat (e.g., a warm towel, a warming mitt); lightly tap the vein site; or stroke the extremity from distal to proximal, beginning below the selected venipuncture site. If available in your agency, use an infrared or other visualization device to assist in locating a vein.
   These actions bring blood to the local area to dilate the vein, making it easier to locate and making venipuncture easier.

8. **Loosen the tourniquet.** If excessive hair is present at the venipuncture site, clip it with scissors.
   Loosening the tourniquet restores blood flow and allows for patient comfort while preparing for venipuncture. Clipping the hair helps the dressings to adhere after catheter insertion. Shaving is not recommended because it may abrade the skin, providing a portal of entry for pathogens.

9. **Don clean nonsterile gloves.**
   Provides protection from inadvertent exposure to blood. Note that some nurses don gloves routinely, even when preparing supplies and equipment. However, there is no risk for coming in contact with body fluids before this step, so strictly speaking, CDC standard precautions require gloves only from this step forward.

10. **Select an IV catheter** appropriate for the size of the vein, the solution to be infused, and the expected duration of therapy. Using aseptic technique, open the package by touching only the outside of it.
    Reduces the risk of extravasation and phlebitis. Always use the smallest diameter and shortest catheter that will deliver the desired solution flow. For most adults this will be a 20- to 24-gauge to minimize venous irritation and promote blood flow around the catheter. Aseptic handling reduces the risk of infection.

11. **Gently reapply the tourniquet** and scrub the site, using an antiseptic swab that contains alcohol-based chlorhexidine solution (INS, 2021); if this is not available, or if contraindicated, use 70% alcohol wipes. Cleansing by using a back-and-forth motion for 30 seconds is recommended. If povidone iodine must be used, apply with an applicator and allow to remain on the skin for 1.5 to 2 minutes until completely dry. Remove with sterile normal saline or sterile water for patients with compromised skin integrity.
    Removes microorganisms from the skin so that they do not enter the venous system during venipuncture. ▶

12. **Allow the antiseptic to air-dry.** Do not fan.
    The antiseptic promotes adherence of the dressing. Fanning can cause contamination of the skin.

13. **Pick up the catheter and inspect the tip.**
    There should be no burrs (rough spots, ridges) on the needle or peeling of the catheter material.

14. **Inform the patient** that you are about to insert the catheter and that it may be uncomfortable.
    Keeping the patient informed promotes cooperation and lessens anxiety.

Variation: If Using a Wing-Tipped Catheter (Butterfly)

15. **Grasp the catheter by the wings,** using the thumb and forefinger of your dominant hand, making sure that the bevel is up. Remove the protective cap from the needle.
    Stabilizes the catheter for insertion. Inserting the needle bevel up makes it less likely that you will pierce both vein walls (go "through" the vein) and will make piercing the skin less painful for the patient. ▼

(continued on next page)

Procedure 35-1 ■ Initiating a Peripheral Intravenous Infusion (continued)

Variation: If Using an Over-the-Needle Catheter

16. **Grasp the catheter by the hub,** using the thumb and forefinger of your dominant hand, making sure that the bevel is up.
    See Wing-Tipped Catheter rationale, preceding. ▼

17. **Using your nondominant hand,** stabilize the vein by continuously pulling the skin taut below the puncture area (pull downward toward the hand or fingers). Do not press too hard, and make sure not to contaminate the insertion site.
    Stabilizing the vein eases insertion, prevents damage to the underside of the vein, and prevents the vein from rolling. Pressing too hard compresses blood flow in the vein and causes it to collapse. ▼

18. **Holding the catheter at** a 30° to 45° angle, pierce the skin directly over the vein. Penetrate all layers of the vein with one quick, smooth motion.
    A 30° to 45° angle allows you to pierce the skin without inadvertently passing through the vein and allows backflow of blood into the catheter.

19. **Look for a flashback of blood** into the chamber of the catheter or the tubing of the winged catheter.
    The flashback of blood indicates that the vein has been entered, but only by the needle when using an over-the-needle catheter.

20. **Lower the angle of the catheter** and needle to skin level and advance them into the vein.

    For a Wing-Tip Catheter
    Fully advance the catheter.

    For an Over-the-Needle Catheter
    Still maintaining traction on the skin with your nondominant hand, hold the catheter hub with your thumb and middle finger, and use your index finger to advance the catheter to at least half of its length before you begin withdrawing the needle. When a steady backflow of blood occurs, partially withdraw the needle while advancing the catheter fully into the vein.
    Withdrawing the needle too early will result in the catheter not fully entering the vein, only the needle. There will be no bleeding from the catheter and infiltration will occur when starting the IV solution. The patient will also have pain. ▼

21. **While holding the catheter** in place with one hand, release the tourniquet and remove or retract the needle.

    For an Over-the-Needle Catheter
    Hold the catheter in place by placing light pressure on the catheter, away from the hub and venipuncture site.

    ✚ Never attempt to reinsert the needle after it is withdrawn. This can damage the catheter and even cause bits of it to break off within the vein.

    For a Winged Needle
    Place a finger lightly on the same area plus a finger farther along the vein away from the needle so the needle does not go through the vein.
    Releasing the tourniquet restores full circulation to the patient's extremity and prevents injury. Placing light pressure on the catheter or vein minimizes bleeding from the catheter or needle while you complete the procedure.

22. **Quickly connect** the administration set to the IV catheter, using aseptic technique.
    To minimize bleeding and prevent infection. ▼

    If Using a Peripheral IV Lock
    Once the lock is connected, flush with normal saline and then disconnect the flush. A common amount is 1 to 2 mL, but tubing varies, so check package instructions for the exact amount needed.
    Flushing the catheter both clears it and keeps it sterile.

23. **While still stabilizing the catheter** in place, slowly open the roller clamp. Observe that flow is achieved. Adjust the drip to the prescribed flow rate.

24. **Secure the connection** between the tubing and the catheter. Many sets have luer-lock connections, so no further securing is needed. If not using luer-lock tubing, clasping devices and threaded devices can be used. Do not use tape.
    Secure the connection to prevent separation of tubing from the hub.

    ✚ Taping is not recommended because the junction is not visible under tape; therefore, the tubing could separate from the catheter without being discovered, possibly leading to air embolism, bleeding, or infection.

25. **Stabilize the catheter** to directly hold it in place on the skin. Use an agency-approved device. Catheter stabilization devices include manufactured devices (such as StatLok) or tape.

When Stabilizing With Tape
Place a narrow (¼-in.) strip of tape under the catheter hub and crisscross the ends over the hub to form a chevron. Apply tape only to the catheter hub, not to the catheter itself, and do not apply tape directly to the site where the catheter enters the skin.

Luer locks are designed to prevent accidental disengagement of tubing and catheter; they do not stabilize the catheter. Catheter stabilization (or primary securement) is important to minimize catheter movement and help prevent complications such as phlebitis, inflammation, infiltration, and infection.

26. **Dress the site,** following agency policy. If needed, clean the site with an antiseptic swab and allow it to dry before applying the dressing.

If Using a Transparent Dressing (Preferred)
a. Open the package containing the dressing. Remove the protective backing from the dressing, making sure not to touch the sterile surface.
b. Cover the insertion site and the hub or winged portion of the catheter with the dressing. Do not cover the junction with the administration tubing. ▼

c. Gently pinch the transparent dressing around the catheter hub to secure the hub further (primary securement). Smooth the remainder of the dressing so that it adheres to the skin. ▶

— Secondary securement
— Primary securement

The INS (2021) recommends that the butterfly catheter be used for venipunctures or an intermittent infusion. It should not be used for regular infusions.

If You Must Use a Gauze Dressing
d. Fold a 2-in. × 2-in. sterile gauze dressing in half, cover it with 1-in. tape (about 3 in. long).
e. Place under the tubing–hub junction and press down on the tape. *Raises hub off the skin and prevents pressure on the skin.*
f. Place a sterile gauze pad over the insertion site and catheter hub—but not over the catheter–hub junction.
g. Secure all edges with tape.

27. **Label the dressing** with the date and time of insertion, catheter size, and your initials.
A label lets nurses see at a glance how long the dressing has been in place.

28. **Secure the IV administration** tubing by looping and taping the tubing to the skin (secondary securement). See Step 26c, preceding.
Helps prevent the IV catheter from becoming dislodged and decreases movement of the catheter, thereby decreasing the risk of phlebitis, inflammation, and infiltration.

29. **Place an arm board** under the joint and secure it with tape if the insertion site is located near a joint. *An arm board stabilizes the joint and helps prevent the catheter from becoming dislodged. However, avoid inserting an IV near a joint when possible, as there is increased potential for movement of the IV catheter, leading to an increased risk of complications. IVs placed in the antecubital fossa are difficult to assess for infiltration. Arm boards are not widely used because of the high acuity of inpatients, many of whom have central lines instead of peripheral IVs.*

30. **Dispose of all supplies,** including sharps, into appropriate receptacles; raise the side rail; lower the bed; and be sure the patient call system is within reach. Wash your hands.
Prevents infection and ensures patient and staff safety.

❓ What if . . .

■ **The patient is an older adult?**

Do not scrub skin too vigorously. *This can damage fragile surface tissue, creating a portal for pathogens.*

Use a softer tourniquet and do not apply tightly; for well-dilated veins, do not use 1 at all. *This decreases the risk of rupture of fragile veins.*

Use the smallest catheter possible to meet the infusion needs.

Insert the needle at an almost flat angle (10° to 20°). *In most older adults, veins are close to the skin surface.*

Before penetrating the skin, apply traction to the vein below the insertion site. *Stabilizes the vein and makes it easier and less painful for the needle to enter the skin.*

Insert the catheter on top of the vein; do not use the side access technique. If bleeding occurs, hold gentle pressure longer than for younger patients. *A clot may take longer to form.*

(continued on next page)

Procedure 35-1 ■ Initiating a Peripheral Intravenous Infusion (continued)

- **The patient is an infant younger than 2 months old?**
  Allow the antiseptic to air-dry on the skin. Do not fan.
  Increases the antiseptic's effectiveness; promotes patient comfort on puncture of the skin; promotes adherence of dressing. Fanning increases exposure to airborne microbes.

- ✚ **The patient is allergic to iodine or shellfish?**
  Use 70% alcohol or chlorhexidine for 30 seconds to cleanse the site (not povidl-iodine or iodine).

- **I am not successful with the first venipuncture attempt?**
  Use a new cannula and make a second attempt on the other arm; if unsuccessful, place it higher up on the same arm. Do not make more than two attempts without seeking assistance.

- ✚ **When I insert the needle and catheter and connect the tubing, I see bright red blood quickly appear and start to advance up the tubing?**
  You may have inadvertently entered an artery. If this occurs, remove the catheter and apply direct pressure for at least 5 minutes. Notify the primary care provider. Monitor the extremity distal to the insertion site for pulses, color, and temperature.

Evaluation

- Monitor the IV site and flow rate regularly (many agency standards require hourly) while IV fluid is infusing. Check for signs of infiltration, inflammation, and phlebitis.
- Monitor the patient's tolerance of IV therapy by auscultating breath sounds and monitoring vital signs, urine output, laboratory values, and neck vein distention. Report to the primary provider any signs of fluid overload, such as crackles, edema, shortness of breath, diminished urine output, increased blood pressure, increased heart rate with bounding pulse, and distended neck veins. Fluid overload can lead to pulmonary edema and heart failure.

Patient Teaching

- Instruct the patient about IV therapy.
- ✚ Teach the patient the importance of notifying staff immediately if the catheter or administration set becomes dislodged; the insertion site becomes tender, red, or swollen; or the patient notices moisture or fluid leakage.
- Explain the desired and adverse effects of IV therapy, and tell the patient to notify staff if they develop discomfort or breathing difficulty.
- Teach the patient measures to avoid dislodging the catheter.

Home Care

- Explain home IV therapy to the client and caregiver, and teach them how to identify complications.
- Provide the client with the name and phone numbers of people to contact in case problems arise with the catheter site or if there is a change in level of comfort (e.g., increased pain, swelling).

Documentation

- Date and time of insertion, gauge and type of catheter, number of attempts, and location of the insertion site
- Tourniquet use (or nonuse)
- Blood return in catheter, whether the IV flushes, and type and amount of flush solution used
- Dressing and tape type used
- Method of securing or stabilizing the IV line
- Type and rate of the IV fluid infusing
- Patient's tolerance of the procedure, any adverse reactions to the insertion or IV therapy, and the interventions required
- Patient teaching
- Often, IV care is documented on a flowsheet; fluids infused are documented on the intake and output (I&O) record as well

Sample Documentation

00/00/0000-0200. 20-gauge, winged catheter inserted in cephalic vein, with tourniquet, without difficulty on first attempt. Obtained blood return. Catheter flushed easily. Dressed site with a transparent, semipermeable dressing and clear tape. Catheter stabilized with fixation device. 1 L of D_5/NS hung at 125 mL/hr. Patient tolerated venipuncture with no difficulty. Instructed to notify nursing staff immediately if pain or swelling occurs at the site. Also taught precautions to take to avoid dislodging IV catheter and importance of notifying staff immediately should it become dislodged. ————————————S. Jiminez, RN

Practice Resources
Czajka et al. (2018); INS (2021); Shlamovitz (2021).

Thinking About the Procedure

The video **Initiating a Peripheral Intravenous Infusion**, along with questions and suggested responses, is available on the **Davis's *Nursing Skills Videos*** Web site at www.fadavis.com.

Procedure 35-2 ■ Regulating the IV Flow Rate

➤ For steps to follow in *all* procedures, refer to the Universal Steps for All Procedures on the inside back cover.

Equipment
- IV solution hanging on an IV pole and attached to an administration set
- Watch with a second hand or digital seconds
- Time tape

Delegation
Refer to your state nurse practice act and agency policy regarding delegation of this task to an LPN.

Preprocedure Assessment
- Assess the IV catheter for patency and date of insertion before starting the infusion and then regularly (many agencies specify hourly) while the IV fluid infuses.
  Decreases risk of complications related to incorrect infusion rate, expired infusion solution, tubing, or catheter dwell time.

- Assess the IV site for signs of phlebitis, infiltration, infection, or inflammation.
  You must change the IV catheter before regulating the flow rate if any of these complications occur.

- Confirm the patient's need for IV therapy by verifying the prescription and checking laboratory values, urine output, vital signs, and breath sounds.
  Ensures that the patient still needs IV fluids and that the solution is correct. Laboratory values and assessment findings verify the need for the IV treatment plan. IV therapy creates a risk for fluid overload.

➤ When performing the procedure, always identify your patient according to agency policy, using two identifiers, and be attentive to standard precautions, hand hygiene, patient safety and privacy, body mechanics, and documentation.

Procedure Steps

1. **Follow all the checks and rights** of medication administration, including verifying the prescription. Check the solution to make sure that you have the proper IV fluid hanging with the prescribed additives and that there is no discoloration of or particles or crystallization in the fluid. Also verify the infusion rate.
   IV solution is considered medication, and you should check it carefully to avoid administration and compatibility errors. Do not simply pull a bag of fluid from a shelf assuming that the shelf is labeled properly, as bags are often misplaced, and this is a potential source of error.

2. **Calculate the hourly rate** if it is not specified in the prescription. Divide the volume to be infused by the number of hours it is to be infused. For example, if the provider prescribes 1,000 mL to run over the course of 4 hours, the infusion rate is 250 mL/hr.
   You must carefully calculate the infusion rate to ensure that the patient receives the correct volume of fluid.

   Note: If you are using a volume-control pump, you can omit Steps 3 and 4.

3. **Calculate the drip rate** by multiplying the number of milliliters to be infused in 60 minutes by the drop factor in drops [gtts]/per milliliter; then divide by 60 minutes:

   $$\frac{\text{Hourly rate in mL} \times (\text{gtts/mL})}{60 \text{ minutes}} = \text{drip rate}$$

   For example, an hourly rate of 100 mL multiplied by 15 gtts/mL and divided by 60 minutes equals 25. Therefore, the drip rate equals 25 gtts/min. Each administration set has a drip factor that is determined by the manufacturer. The drip factor is the number of drops necessary to deliver 1 mL of solution. Microdrip tubing has a drip factor of 60 gtts/mL; blood administration tubing typically has a drip factor of 10 gtts/mL; macrodrip tubing has a drip factor of 15 gtts/mL.

4. **Verify your calculations.**
   To prevent dosage errors, either have a second person verify your calculations or check them a second time yourself.

5. **Apply a time tape** when hanging a new bag to the IV solution container next to the volume markings. Mark the time tape with the time that the infusion was started. Continue to mark 1-hour intervals on the time tape until you reach the bottom of the container.
   The time tape allows all nurses to accurately monitor the rate of administration.

6. **Open the roller clamp** so that IV fluid begins to flow (when hanging a new bag).
   The roller clamp must be opened to allow the flow of fluid.

7. **Set the rate.**

   For Gravity Drip
   Using a watch placed next to the drip chamber, count the number of drops entering the drip chamber in 1 minute. Adjust the roller clamp by increasing or decreasing the flow until you achieve the prescribed drip rate.
   Timing the drip rate for 1 minute helps to accurately achieve the correct drip rate, and having the watch next to what you are

   (continued on next page)

Procedure 35-2 ■ Regulating the IV Flow Rate (continued)

counting will ensure that you do not miss seeing any drops. ▼

For a Volume-Control Pump
Program the prescribed rate into the pump.
IV solution is considered a medication and must infuse at the prescribed rate.

8. **Monitor manually regulated** infusion rates closely for the first 15 minutes after you begin an infusion; then monitor at least hourly by counting drops per minute or reading the numbers on the pumps.
Changes in the patient's position may speed up or slow down the infusion rate; frequent monitoring of the infusion rate ensures that the correct volume of fluid infuses over the correct length of time.

? What if...

- **The prescription for the IV flow rate changes?**
Recalculate the new flow rate and adjust the drops per minute to obtain the desired new flow rate. Also, remove the old time tape and place a new time tape with the new rate of infusion.

- **When I check the rate, I discover that the IV has been running too slowly for the past hour?**
Adjust to the correct rate, but do not attempt to catch up by adjusting the flow to a rate higher than prescribed. *Too-rapid IV infusion can lead to fluid overload for patients with congestive heart failure or other cardiopulmonary problems.*

- **When I check the rate, I discover that the IV has been running too fast for the past hour?**
Slow the rate and assess the patient for signs of fluid volume excess.

Evaluation
- Evaluate the patient's response to IV therapy by checking for signs of excessive or deficient fluid volume.
- Evaluate the IV site for signs of infiltration, inflammation, infection, and phlebitis.
- Check laboratory studies to help evaluate the effectiveness of IV therapy.
- Monitor for correct IV rate at least hourly.
- Evaluate the tubing for kinks or patient lying on the tubing. *Kinked tubing will interfere with the flow rate.*

Patient Teaching
- Explain the desired and adverse effects of IV therapy.
- Discuss the importance of notifying staff immediately if the catheter or administration set becomes dislodged; if the insertion site becomes tender, red, or swollen; if the patient notices moisture or fluid leakage; or if they have difficulty breathing.
- Teach safety measures if the patient is permitted to ambulate while the IV is infusing.

Home Care
- Explain home IV therapy to the client and caregiver. Teach them how to identify complications.
- Provide the client and caregiver with the name and phone numbers of people to contact in case problems arise with the catheter, insertion site, or level of comfort.

Documentation
Often IV care is documented on a flowsheet and includes the following:
- Date and time the infusion was started
- Type of IV fluid, rate of infusion, and IV catheter site
- Whether rate is manual or pump controlled
- Patient's tolerance of IV therapy, any complications, and the interventions taken
- Document the volume infused on the intake and output (I&O) record.

Practice Resources
INS (2021); Shlamovitz (2021).

Thinking About the Procedure

The video **Regulating the IV Flow Rate,** along with questions and suggested responses, is available on the **Davis's Nursing Skills Videos** Web site at www.fadavis.com.

Procedure 35-3 ■ Setting Up and Using Volume-Control Pumps

➤ For steps to follow in *all* procedures, refer to the Universal Steps for All Procedures on the inside back cover.

Equipment
- Nonsterile gloves
- Alcohol wipes or chlorhexidine/alcohol antiseptic product
- Volume-control pump and IV pole
- Administration set appropriate for the pump
- IV fluid or medicated solution
- Tape for IV fluid solution time tape

Delegation
You can delegate the task of setting up a volume-control pump to an LPN who is specially trained in IV therapy, if covered by the agency's policy. Do not delegate this task to unlicensed assistive personnel (UAP). Do, however, instruct the UAP to notify you of any pump alarms that sound.

Preprocedure Assessment
- Confirm the patient's need for IV therapy by checking vital signs, laboratory values, urine output, skin turgor, breath sounds, and the moisture of mucous membranes.
  IV therapy creates a risk for fluid overload and electrolyte imbalance, which may be revealed by assessment data.
- Assess the existing IV catheter for patency.
  Occlusion of the IV catheter prevents the infusion of IV fluid. If it is not patent, you will need to change the IV.
- Assess the IV site hourly for signs of phlebitis, infiltration, infection, and inflammation.
  Complications of IV therapy interfere with the therapeutic benefit of the fluids and increase medical concerns and treatment cost for the patient. You must change the IV catheter and site if any of these complications occur.

➤ When performing the procedure, always identify your patient according to agency policy, using two identifiers, and be attentive to standard precautions, hand hygiene, patient safety and privacy, body mechanics, and documentation.

Procedure Steps

1. **Calculate the infusion rate** by dividing the volume to be infused by the number of hours it is to be infused. For example, if the prescription states 1,000 mL to run over 8 hours, divide 1,000 mL by 8 hours to determine the infusion rate of 125 mL/hr.
   This ensures that the patient receives the correct dose. Pumps are usually programmed in milliliters per hour instead of drops per minute.

2. **Verify your calculations.**
   To prevent dosage errors, either ask a second person to verify your calculations or check them a second time yourself.

3. **Attach the pump to the IV pole,** and plug it into the nearest electrical outlet.
   ✛ Check to be sure that the infusion pump has a safety sticker on it and that the cord and plug are intact.
   Volume-control pumps need regular maintenance checks. Using an electrical outlet saves battery power if needed for transport or electrical outage. As with gravity flow, the IV solution container needs to remain above the pump to prevent occlusion and for proper drainage of the container. ➤

4. **Take the administration set** from the package and close the clamp on it.
   To prevent inadvertent loss of fluid.

5. **Attach a filter to the end** of the administration set, if required.
   Filters are sometimes used to filter minute particles from the solution.

6. **Remove the protective covers,** and spike the port of the solution container with the administration set, maintaining sterility. Label the IV tubing and solution container with the date and time, and place a time tape on the solution container. Hang the container on the IV pole.
   Labeling the administration set with the date and time informs the nursing staff when the administration set should be changed. The time tape allows you and other nurses to see at a glance whether the correct volume is infusing.

7. **Compress the drip chamber** of the administration set and allow it to fill halfway. Consult the manufacturer's instructions for setup, as pumps differ. (On older gravity pumps, place the electronic eye on the drip chamber between the fluid level and the origin of the drop.)
   Prepares the administration set for priming and prevents air from entering the tubing with the solution. Infusion pumps compress the tubing to move fluid; they measure the amount internally. On older gravity-type pumps, an electronic eye counts the number of drops to ensure the proper rate.

8. **Prime the administration set** with fluid by opening the roller clamp and allowing the fluid to flow slowly through the tubing. Close the clamp.
   Priming removes air from the tubing to prevent air embolus.

(continued on next page)

Procedure 35-3 ■ Setting Up and Using Volume-Control Pumps (continued)

9. **Inspect the tubing** for air. If air bubbles remain in the tubing, flick the tubing with a fingertip to mobilize the bubbles into the drip chamber.
   Air bubbles in the administration tubing interrupt flow and can cause air emboli, which can be dangerous to the patient if they accumulate in the circulation.

10. **Turn on the pump,** and load the administration tubing into the pump according to the manufacturer's instructions.
    Note: This process differs among manufacturers; thus, consult their instructions. ▼

11. **Program the pump** with the prescribed information: total hours, infusion rate (hourly rate) and the volume to be infused (usually the total amount in the IV bag). NOTE: Some pumps have only total hours and volume to infuse and do not have a feature that allows you to program in the infusion rate. ➤

12. **Don clean nonsterile gloves,** check the IV site for patency, and scrub all surfaces of the primary line injection port or needleless connector, including the threads, with an antiseptic pad for at least 15 seconds. Allow it to dry.
    Clean nonsterile gloves protect from exposure to body fluids when you connect the tubing to the IV catheter or port. Scrubbing the port helps prevent infection.

13. **Connect the administration set adapter** to the injection port, keeping the connecting ends sterile.
    Aseptic technique decreases the risk for contamination.

14. **Unclamp the administration set tubing** (open the roller clamp all the way), and press the start button on the pump.
    Allows the IV fluid to flow through the administration set.

15. **Make sure the alarms** are turned on and audible.
    The alarms must be functioning so that the pump can alert you of problems, such as kinks, air in the tubing, or catheter occlusion.

    Key Point: Do not depend completely on the pump alarms to indicate IV patency. Pumps can infuse fluid, even if the line is clogged or infiltrated into the surrounding tissue.

16. **Check the pump regularly** to make sure the correct volume is infusing. Checks are commonly done hourly.
    Infusion pumps sometimes malfunction, so frequent monitoring is essential.

17. **At the end of your shift** (or at the time specified by your healthcare facility), clear the pump of the volume infused and record the volume on the patient's I&O form.
    This helps the oncoming shift accurately monitor the fluid infused during their shift.

? What if...

■ **I later find the IV free flowing and not running via the pump setting?**

Immediately slow the IV fluid down. At the same time, begin assessing the patient: vital signs, mental awareness, lung sounds, pulse oximetry. Depending on the type of fluid running, you may need to make other assessments. Calculate the amount of IV fluid actually infused compared with the prescribed amount. Notify the provider and write out an occurrence report. If the pump is malfunctioning, set it aside, label it as "not working," and notify biomedical engineering so they can repair it.
Labeling the pump will prevent others from using it until it can be repaired.

Evaluation

- Monitor the correct functioning of the pump regularly, perhaps hourly.
- Assess the IV site hourly for signs of phlebitis, infiltration, infection, and inflammation.

Complications of IV therapy interfere with the therapeutic benefit of the fluids and increase medical concerns and treatment costs for the patient. You must change the IV catheter and document if any of these complications occur.

Patient Teaching

- Explain use of the IV infusion pump to the patient.
- Teach the patient the importance of notifying staff immediately if the infusion pump alarm sounds; the catheter or administration set becomes dislodged; the insertion site becomes tender, red, or swollen; or the dressing becomes wet.
- Teach the patient safety measures if they are able to ambulate while the infusion pump is in use.

Home Care

- Explain home IV infusion pump use to the client and caregiver, and teach them how to identify complications. Most home infusion pumps are smaller than institutional pumps.
- Provide the client with the names and phone numbers of people to contact in case problems arise with the catheter, insertion site, IV infusion pump, or other equipment.

Documentation

- Type and volume of IV fluid infusing, along with the infusion rate
- Use of the infusion pump and patient's tolerance of IV therapy
- Any complications of IV therapy and the interventions taken
- Volume infused on the patient's I&O record and/or an IV flowsheet

Sample Documentation

00/00/0000- 0600   Patient admitted from the ED with dehydration. NSS infusing at 250 mL/hr via infusion pump through an 18-gauge catheter. No signs of infiltration. No tenderness, redness, or swelling at the insertion site. Temp 102.6°F orally. HR 118 beats/min, RR 24 breaths/min, and BP 90/46. ————————————————————R. Brill, RN

Practice Resources
Franklin (2017); Giuliano et al. (2021); INS (2021); Phillips & Gorski (2018).

Thinking About the Procedure

The video **Setting Up and Using Volume-Control Pumps,** along with questions and suggested responses, is available on the **Davis's *Nursing Skills Videos*** Web site at www.fadavis.com.

Procedure 35-4 ■ Changing IV Solutions and Tubing

▶ For steps to follow in *all* procedures, refer to the Universal Steps for All Procedures on the inside back cover.

Equipment

- Nonsterile gloves
- Administration set
- IV solution
- IV pole
- Antiseptic swabs that contain solutions such as 70% alcohol or alcohol-based chlorhexidine solution (you may use iodine-based products if alcohol or chlorhexidine is contraindicated and the patient is not allergic to iodine; check manufacturer's guidelines or agency policy neonates and infants)
- 1-in. nonallergenic tape
- Time tape
- Watch with a second hand or digital seconds

Delegation

You can delegate the tasks of changing IV solutions and tubing to an LPN who is specially trained in IV therapy. The task should not be delegated to a UAP. However, do instruct the UAP to notify you of any problems that occur with IV therapy, such as the disconnecting of the administration set; catheter dislodging; or complaints of pain, swelling, or redness at the insertion site.

Preprocedure Assessments

- Assess the IV catheter for patency before changing the solution container or administration set.
- Assess the IV site for signs of phlebitis, infiltration, infection, or inflammation.
If any of these complications occur, discontinue the IV and start a new IV at a different site.
- Check IV catheter insertion date.
IV catheters are replaced per agency guidelines, which are based on the INS and CDC recommendations of changing a peripheral IV site when clinically indicated (e.g., signs of phlebitis, infiltration, irritation).

(continued on next page)

Procedure 35-4 ■ Changing IV Solutions and Tubing (continued)

Procedure 35-4A ■ Changing the IV Solution

▶ When performing the procedure, always identify your patient according to agency policy, using two identifiers, and be attentive to standard precautions, hand hygiene, patient safety and privacy, body mechanics, and documentation.

Procedure Steps

1. **Following the rights** of medication administration, prepare and label your next container of IV solution at least 1 hour before the present infusion is scheduled to finish.
   Preparing the next IV solution container reduces the risk of the present container running dry, thereby causing clots to form that would occlude the catheter.

2. **Close the roller clamp** on the infusing administration set.
   Prevents air from entering the tubing while changing the IV solution container.

3. **Wearing clean nonsterile gloves,** remove the old IV solution container from the IV pole. Remove the spike from the bag, keeping the spike sterile.
   The spike must remain sterile to prevent contamination of the new IV fluid. Clean nonsterile gloves protect you from exposure to body fluids.

4. **Remove the protective cover** from the new IV solution container port.

5. **Place the spike into the port** of the new solution container.

For a Glass Bottle
First scrub the rubber stopper on the top of the bottle with an antiseptic pad, then insert the spike of the administration set through the rubber stopper.
Cleansing the stopper removes particulate matter and microbes.

6. **Hang the IV solution** container on the IV pole.
   Allows the fluid to infuse by gravity.

7. **Inspect the tubing** to be sure that it is free of air bubbles and the drip chamber remains half-filled. Flick the tubing with a finger to mobilize the bubbles into the drip chamber.
   Prevents air from entering the system as the new solution is hung. If the drip chamber becomes too full, it will be difficult to impossible to count the drip rate properly and regulate the IV.

8. **Open the roller clamp** and adjust the drip rate, as prescribed.
   IV solution is considered a medication and must infuse at the prescribed rate for therapeutic effect and to prevent fluid overload.

9. **Affix the time tape** to the new IV solution container, if practiced within your agency. Mark the tape with the time the infusion was started, and mark 1-hour intervals on the tape until you reach the bottom of the container.
   The time tape allows you and other nurses to monitor the rate of administration easily.

10. **Dispose of used supplies** into appropriate receptacles according to agency policy in line with INS and CDC guidelines.

Thinking About the Procedure

▶ The video **Changing the IV Solution,** along with questions and suggested responses, is available on the **Davis's** *Nursing Skills Videos* Web site at www.fadavis.com.

Procedure 35-4B ■ Changing the IV Administration Tubing and Solution

▶ When performing the procedure, always identify your patient according to agency policy, using two identifiers, and be attentive to standard precautions, hand hygiene, patient safety and privacy, body mechanics, and documentation.

Procedure Steps

1. **Prepare the IV solution** and tubing as you would when initiating a new IV. (See Procedure 35-1, Step 2.)

2. **Hang the new administration** set on the IV pole.

3. **Close the roller clamp** on the old administration set.
   Stops the flow of fluid from the old container.

4. **Disconnect the old tubing.**
   a. Wearing clean nonsterile gloves, place a sterile swab under the catheter hub.
      The swab absorbs any leakage from the catheter hub when you disconnect the tubing.
   b. Apply pressure to the vein about 3 inches above the insertion site, using the fourth or fifth finger of your nondominant hand. Hold the catheter hub firmly with the thumb and index finger of that hand, but do not apply downward pressure.
      Prevents blood from leaking out of the catheter during the tubing change. Holding the hub firmly keeps the catheter from moving about and traumatizing the vein.
   c. Then carefully remove the device securing the connection between the catheter and tubing. This may be as simple as unscrewing a luer lock. The connection should not be covered by tape, but if it is, remove it so you can access the connection.

5. **Remove the protective cover** from the distal end of the new administration set.
   Cover keeps the distal end sterile until you are ready to connect it to the IV catheter.

6. **Continue to stabilize the IV** catheter with your nondominant hand while applying pressure over the vein. ▶

7. **Gently disengage the used tubing** from the IV catheter and place it in a basin or other receptacle. Quickly insert the new tubing into the catheter hub.
   The INS recommends IV tubing be changed no less than 96-hour intervals, but at least every 7 days, depending on agency policy and solution. Certain solutions (e.g., blood, blood products, fat emulsions) require more tubing changes within 24 hours of initiating the infusion (INS, 2021). Change it quickly to prevent microorganisms from entering the IV catheter.

8. **Open the roller clamp** on the new administration set, and allow the IV solution to infuse.
   This clears the IV catheter of blood, preventing catheter occlusion.

9. **Program and turn on** the volume-control pump. Or, for a gravity drip, use the roller clamp to adjust the flow to the prescribed rate.
   IV solution is considered a medication and must infuse at the prescribed rate.

10. **Cleanse the IV site** and secure the IV catheter and tubing connection.
    Removes microorganisms and media for growth; helps preserve the integrity of the intact line; and prevents air and microorganisms from entering the line.

11. **Loop and tape tubing** to patient's skin.
    Helps minimize catheter movement, which contributes to phlebitis.

12. **Label tubing and solution** with date, initials, rate, and time tape.
    Alerts staff to when tubing and solution were changed and to when they will need to be changed again to decrease the incidence of infection.

13. **Dispose of used supplies** into appropriate receptacles according to agency policy in line with CDC guidelines.

? What if...

- **The drip chamber becomes too full (over half) so that drops cannot be adequately counted?**
  Close the roller clamp, invert the bag or bottle, and squeeze the excess fluid back into the bag/bottle.

- **The tubing will not separate from the catheter connection when I attempt to disconnect it?**
  If the lock does not twist off, gently try using a hemostat ("mosquito" clamp) to twist the lock. Do not lock the hemostat; merely use it lightly as a grip. After the lock is off, if the tubing will not separate, use the hemostat to gently twist the tubing back and forth. If the catheter needs to be stabilized, wear a sterile glove or use a sterile hemostat.

Evaluation

- Assess the IV insertion site for signs of infiltration, inflammation, infection, and phlebitis.
- Evaluate the effectiveness of IV therapy by assessing the patient's hydration status or expected effect of the intravenous medication/solution.
- Monitor the IV rate regularly (usually hourly).

Patient Teaching

- Discuss the importance of notifying staff immediately if the catheter or administration set becomes dislodged; if the insertion site becomes tender, red, or swollen; or if the IV dressing becomes wet.

Home Care

- Explain home IV therapy to the client and caregiver and teach them how to identify complications.
- Obtain a return demonstration to ensure the caregiver can perform fluid and tubing changes, when necessary.

Documentation

- Fluid and tubing changes are usually documented on a flowsheet.
- Document the date and time the IV fluid and tubing were changed, type of IV fluid and rate of infusion, and the location and condition of the IV catheter insertion site.
- Any complications of IV therapy and the interventions taken.

(continued on next page)

Procedure 35-4 ■ Changing IV Solutions and Tubing (continued)

Sample Documentation

[Screenshot of IV Assessment documentation screen showing: Right Ventral Cephalic (Forearm); Type of IV Access: Peripheral checked; Site Assessment: Insertion site clean and dry, No redness or swelling noted checked; Dressing Type: Dressing change per hospital protocol, Transparent dressing placed over IV site and dated, IV tubing change per hospital protocol; dated checked; IV Used For / Flush: Patent, flushes easily checked; Infusion Pump In Use checked; IV Notes: 2300 - 1 Liter 0.9% normal saline hung at 100 mL/hr through a 20-gauge angiocath.]

Practice Resources
INS (2021); Philips & Gorski (2018).

Thinking About the Procedure

The video **Setting Up and Using Volume-Control Pumps,** along with questions and suggested responses, is available on the **Davis's *Nursing Skills Videos*** Web site at www.fadavis.com.

Procedure 35-5 ■ Changing IV Dressings

➤ For steps to follow in *all* procedures, refer to the Universal Steps for All Procedures on the inside back cover. For this procedure, also refer to Clinical Insights 20-1 through 20-4 and Procedures 20-7 and 20-8 if you need to review information about medical and surgical asepsis.

Equipment

Peripheral IV Dressings
- Clean nonsterile gloves
- Sterile transparent semipermeable dressing or dressing specified by institution
- Antiseptic swabs: alcohol or alcohol-based chlorhexidine solution

  NOTE: Use iodine-based products only if the preferred antiseptics cannot be used. Check manufacturer and agency policy for neonates and infants.

- 1-inch nonallergenic tape or manufactured stabilization device

Central Line Dressings
- Clean nonsterile gloves
- Central line dressing kit (it should include sterile gloves, a mask, a sterile transparent semipermeable dressing, sterile tape, an antimicrobial agent, and a sterile catheter stabilization device; if it does not, obtain them)

  NOTE: It is acceptable to use povidone-iodine followed by alcohol as the antimicrobial if the preferred chlorhexidine solution is contraindicated.

- A sponge containing the antimicrobial agent chlorhexidine may be used as a part of the dressing, as well.
  To reduce the risk for catheter-related infection

- Mask for patient (possibly)

  NOTE: Some institutions do not include this in their procedure, and a few patients cannot tolerate wearing a mask.

Delegation

You can delegate the tasks of changing dressings to an LPN who is specially trained in IV therapy. The task should not be delegated to a UAP. Do, however, instruct the UAP to notify you of any problems that occur with dressing such as soiling, blood, leakage, or loosening.

Preprocedure Assessments

- Assess the IV catheter for patency before changing the dressing.
  Ensure that the IV is still working properly.

- Assess the IV site for signs of phlebitis, infiltration, infection, or inflammation.
  If any of these complications exist, the current IV will need to be discontinued and a new IV started.

- Assess for allergy to tape.
- Assess IV catheter start date.
  Vascular access devices or changes when clinically indicated (INS, 2021) or per agency policy. There is no known optimal dwell time.

Procedure 35-5A ■ Peripheral IV Dressings

➤ When performing the procedure, always identify your patient according to agency policy, using two identifiers, and be attentive to standard precautions, hand hygiene, patient safety and privacy, body mechanics, and documentation.

➤ NOTE: This procedure is usually performed at the same time the IV tubing is changed because the old dressing may need to be removed to do that. The INS recommends that dressing be changed when damp, loosened, or visibly soiled. You should follow your agency's policy.

Procedure Steps

1. **Wearing clean nonsterile gloves,** stabilize the catheter with your nondominant hand, avoiding direct pressure on the catheter–hub junction, and carefully remove and discard the dressing and the catheter stabilization device.
   Remove the dressing gently to avoid dislodging the catheter.

2. **Inspect the insertion site.** Look for erythema and drainage, and note any tenderness. Remove procedure gloves and perform hand hygiene.
   If signs of infection, phlebitis, or infiltration are present, you must remove the IV catheter.

3. **Don a clean pair of nonsterile gloves.**

4. **Cleanse the insertion site,** and then allow the antiseptic to dry on the skin. Do not fan.

   If Using Chlorhexidine
   Apply using a back-and-forth motion and friction for at least 30 seconds.

   If Using Alcohol or 2% Tincture of Iodine
   Using a circular motion, start at the insertion site and work outward 2 to 3 inches. Do not go back over any cleansed area.
   Removes microorganisms from the skin to minimize the risk of their entering the venipuncture site. Allowing the antiseptic to dry increases its effectiveness.

(continued on next page)

Procedure 35-5 ■ Changing IV Dressings (continued)

5. **Perform hand hygiene** and change procedure gloves. Apply a new sterile catheter stabilization device and dressing. For illustrations, see Procedure 35-1.

If Using a Transparent Dressing
   a. Open the package containing the sterile, semipermeable, transparent dressing. Remove the protective backing from the dressing, making sure not to touch the sterile surface.
   b. Cover the insertion site and the hub with the dressing. Do not cover the junction with the tubing of the administration set.
   c. Gently pinch the transparent dressing around the catheter hub to secure the hub. Smooth the remainder of the dressing so that it adheres to the skin.
   Pinching the dressing around the hub prevents pressure of the hub on the underlying skin.

If Using a Gauze Dressing
   d. Fold a 2-in. × 2-in. sterile gauze dressing in half, and cover it with 1-inch tape (about 3 in. long).
   e. Place under the tubing–hub junction and press down on the tape.
   Raises the hub to prevent pressure on the skin.
   f. Place a sterile gauze pad over the insertion site and catheter hub—but not over the catheter–hub junction.
   g. Secure all edges with tape.

6. **Secure the connection between** the catheter and the tubing, but do not cover the catheter–tubing junction with tape.
   Securing the connection helps maintain a closed system and prevents entry of microorganisms. You should not cover the junction with tape because removing the tape may interfere with your ability to disconnect the tubing from the hub quickly, should you need to do so. Removing tape requires much manipulation; the more the catheter is manipulated, the higher the risk for infection and dislodging.

7. **Secure the IV administration** tubing by looping and taping the tubing to the skin (referred to as *secondary securement*). See Procedure 35-1, Step 26C.
   Looping the tubing provides slack to prevent the IV catheter from becoming dislodged.

8. **Label the dressing with the date** and time of insertion, catheter size, date the dressing was changed, and your initials.
   Peripheral IV catheters should be replaced as clinically indicated (e.g., phlebitis, infiltration, irritation) to prevent complications. Labeling the dressing with the date and time of insertion helps communicate to other nurses the date of the IV insertion and dressing change.

9. **Discard all supplies** in the appropriate containers according to agency policy in line with CDC guidelines.

? What if . . .

- **The patient is immunocompromised? Or the peripheral midline catheter must be in the same site for an extended time?**

  Use sterile gloves and a mask when changing the dressing and giving site care.

Thinking About the Procedure

The video **Peripheral IV Dressings**, along with questions and suggested responses, is available on the **Davis's Nursing Skills Videos** Web site at www.fadavis.com.

Procedure 35-5B ■ Central Line Dressings

➤ When performing the procedure, always identify your patient according to agency policy, using two identifiers, and be attentive to standard precautions, hand hygiene, patient safety and privacy, body mechanics, and documentation.

➤ **NOTE:** This procedure focuses on dressing change. Refer to Clinical Insight 35-4 for assessments and maintenance of CVCs.

Procedure Steps

1. **Obtain a sterile central line** dressing kit (or equivalent supplies if there is no kit) and mask for the patient, if one is needed.
   Because central lines have direct access to the central circulation, the risk of systemic infection is greater. Therefore, the procedure uses aseptic technique. All supplies must be sterile. A kit standardizes the procedure and promotes efficiency (INS, 2021).

2. **Place the patient** in a semi-Fowler's position, if tolerated. Lower the side rail and adjust the bed to working height.
   Semi-Fowler's position and bed adjustments facilitate site cleansing and dressing application and reduce strain on the nurse's back.

3. **Explain the procedure** and ask the patient to turn their head to the opposite side from the insertion site. If they cannot cooperate, place a mask on the patient.
   Explanation may reduce anxiety and enhance cooperation; turning helps prevent contamination of the insertion site.

4. **Put on your mask** and clean non-sterile gloves. Carefully remove the old dressing and catheter stabilization device, if present.

5. **Inspect the site** for signs and symptoms of infection and other complications.
   If a complication is suspected, notify the person who placed the central line.

6. **Measure the external CVAD length** to access for malposition.
   Comparing the CVAD length to that at insertion helps to detect dislodgement or malposition (INS, 2021).

7. **Remove and discard your gloves,** along with the soiled dressing. Perform hand hygiene.

8. **Set up a sterile field** and open the dressing kit.
   To prevent contamination of the insertion site and the sterile supplies.

9. **Don the sterile gloves** contained in the kit and arrange sterile supplies as needed.

10. **Scrub the insertion site** and surrounding skin with an antiseptic swab.

    ### If Using Chlorhexidine
    Use a back-and-forth motion with friction and scrub for at least 30 seconds.

    ### If Using Povidone-Iodine and Alcohol
    The kit should contain three swabs of each. Beginning with a povidone-iodine swab, start at the insertion site and work outward several inches from site (clean) outward. Repeat with the other two povidone-iodine swabs. Then, using the same method, clean with the three alcohol swabs. With each swab, do not "go back over" an area you have just cleaned with that swab.
    To rid the site of any potential infectious microorganisms, work "from clean to contaminated."

11. **Scrub the sutures (if any),** and the catheter from insertion site to the hub or bifurcation, for at least 15 seconds with an alcohol swab or chlorhexidine-alcohol antiseptic product.

12. **Allow the site to dry**—do not fan.
    Allows the antiseptic time to work completely and allows the dressing to stick properly. Povidone-iodine requires 1 minute to air-dry completely; chlorhexidine requires 30 seconds.

13. **Apply the transparent dressing** that comes in the kit.

    ### If You Place Gauze Under the Catheter Hub
    You may first place a small piece of folded sterile gauze under the catheter hub.
    To reduce pressure on the skin under the hub.

    A chlorhexidine-impregnated dressing is recommended for adults 18 years and older with short-term nontunneled CVADs (INS, 2021).
    Apply the dressing directly over the catheter insertion site, ensuring that it is in full contact with the skin. Then apply the transparent dressing over the sponge.
    Reduces the risk for catheter-related infection, especially in units with high infection rates or in high-risk patients (INS, 2021).

14. **Apply a new catheter** stabilization device, if one is used.

15. **Remove the drape,** if you used one.

16. **Loop the catheter gently** and secure it with tape to the skin. Avoid securing it to the dressing. Or, depending on type of CVC, place a piece of clear tape across the ends of the catheter lumens, near but not on the hubs.
    Ensures that accidental tugging on the catheter does not dislodge the catheter. Do not cover the hubs, as you may need to access them.

17. **Label the dressing** with the date changed, time, and your initials.
    Alerts staff to when the next dressing change will be due.

18. **Dispose of supplies** into the appropriate receptacles according to agency policy in line with CDC guidelines.

19. **Place the patient in** a comfortable position, raise the side rail, and be sure the call device is accessible.

20. **Remove your mask and gloves** and the patient's mask.

Thinking About the Procedure

The video **Central Line Dressings,** along with questions and suggested responses, is available on the **Davis's Nursing Skills Videos** Web site at www.fadavis.com.

(continued on next page)

Procedure 35-5 ■ Changing IV Dressings (continued)

Procedure 35-5C ■ PICC Line Dressings

> When performing the procedure, always identify your patient according to agency policy, using two identifiers, and be attentive to standard precautions, hand hygiene, patient safety and privacy, body mechanics, and documentation.

Procedure Steps

1. **Obtain a sterile PICC** (central) line dressing kit (or equivalent supplies if there is no kit) and mask for the patient, if one is needed.
   Because central lines have direct access to the central circulation, the risk of systemic infection is greater. Therefore, this procedure uses aseptic technique, even though the insertion site is peripheral. All supplies must be sterile.

2. **Place the patient in a semi-Fowler's position,** if tolerated. Lower the side rail and adjust the bed to working height.
   Semi-Fowler's position and bed adjustments facilitate site cleansing and dressing application and reduce strain on the nurse's back.

3. **Explain the procedure** and ask the patient to turn their head to the opposite side from the insertion site. If the patient cannot cooperate, place a mask on them, if consistent with agency policy.
   Explanation may reduce anxiety and enhance cooperation; turning helps prevent contamination of the insertion site from nasal and oral airborne secretions.

4. **Inspect the site** for signs and symptoms of infection and catheter migration.

5. **Put on your mask and** clean nonsterile gloves and carefully remove the old dressing by pulling toward the insertion site and catheter stabilization device, if present. Discard your gloves with the dressing.
   The mask helps prevent contamination of the insertion site from the nurse's nasal and oral airborne secretions. Pulling toward the insertion site minimizes the possibility of dislodging the catheter.

6. **Perform hand hygiene,** open the kit, and remove and don the sterile gloves.

7. **Unfold drape and establish your sterile field.** Transfer items from kit to your sterile field.
   Ensures that strict sterile technique is maintained.

8. **Use a sterile tape measure** to compare the external length of the PICC with the baseline insertion length.
   Detects catheter migration, which may indicate that the PICC line is not in the correct location. The Infusion Nurse Society recommends measuring the CVAD and comparing it with the original insertion length to detect malposition (INS, 2021).

9. **Scrub the insertion site** and surrounding skin with an antiseptic solution. Ensure that blood or encrustations are removed from the site and catheter. (Refer to Procedure 38-5B: Central Line Dressings, Steps 9 and 10.)

10. **If you are using a chlorhexidine-impregnated dressing** as part of the dressing, apply it directly over the catheter insertion site, ensuring that it is in direct contact with the skin.
    Minimizes the proliferation of microorganisms.

11. **Allow the site to air-dry.**

12. **Apply a commercial stabilization** device, if applicable.

13. **Apply a transparent dressing** over catheter site. ➤

14. **Label the dressing** with the date, time, and your initials.
    Used to identify the next scheduled dressing change.

15. **Loop and anchor the catheter tubing, as needed;** secure it with tape.
    Reduces the risk of accidental dislodgement.

16. **Place the patient** in a comfortable position, raise the side rails, and place the call light so it is accessible to patient.

17. **Dispose of used supplies** into the appropriate receptacles according to agency policy and consistent with CDC guidelines.

Evaluation

- Evaluate the IV insertion site and surrounding tissue for signs of infiltration, inflammation, infection, and phlebitis.
- Monitor the dressing for dampness, blood, soiling, or loosening.
  If these occur, the dressing must be changed.

Patient Teaching

- Explain the importance of notifying staff if the IV dressing becomes soiled, dampened, or loosened.
- Remind the patient to notify staff immediately for bleeding, pain, or swelling around the catheter or dressing area or discomfort in the hand, arm, or shoulder on the same side as the catheter.

Home Care

- Explain home IV therapy to the client and caregiver and teach them how to identify complications.
- Obtain a return demonstration by the client or caregiver to ensure competent performance of fluid, tubing, and dressing changes when necessary.

Documentation

- Document the date and time the dressing was changed. Document the location and condition of the IV catheter insertion site.
- Document any complications of IV therapy and the interventions taken.
- Document the dressing change on your IV record. Often, IV care is documented on a flowsheet.

Sample Documentation

00/00/0000—2300   New transparent semipermeable dressing applied over PICC insertion site in left forearm. No redness, tenderness, swelling, or exudate at the site.————————————Mary Teu, RN

Practice Resources
Gonzalez & Cassaro (2021); INS (2021).

Thinking About the Procedure

The video **PICC Line Dressings,** along with questions and suggested responses, is available on the **Davis's *Nursing Skills Videos*** Web site at www.fadavis.com.

Procedure 35-6 ■ Converting a Primary Line to a Peripheral IV Lock

➤ For steps to follow in *all* procedures, refer to the Universal Steps for All Procedures on the inside back cover.

Equipment

- Clean nonsterile gloves
- Peripheral intermittent IV lock adapter
- For short and long PIVCs and midline catheters, the Infusion Nurse Society recommends single-dose systems (e.g., prefilled labeled syringe; single-dose vial) of preservative-free 0.9% sodium chloride for adults (INS, 2021) (either preservative-free 0.9% sodium chloride or heparine 10 units/mL are recommended to lock CVADs; follow agency policy).
- Linen-saver pad
- Transparent semipermeable dressing
- Alcohol or chlorhexidine/alcohol or other antiseptic swab

Delegation

You can delegate the task of converting a primary IV line to an intermittent lock device to an LPN who is specially trained in IV therapy. The task should not be delegated to unlicensed assistive personnel (UAP). However, you should instruct the UAP to notify you of any problems with the intermittent lock device, such as dislodging of the catheter or client complaints of pain, swelling, or redness at the insertion site.

Preprocedure Assessment

- Assess the patient's readiness to have the IV fluid discontinued (e.g., tolerating oral fluids, adequate urine output, and laboratory values within normal limits).
  If the patient's condition indicates that they still require IV fluids, notify the primary care provider and do not discontinue the IV line.
- Assess for allergy to tape.
- Assess the IV site for signs of phlebitis, infiltration, extravasation, or infection.
  If complications are present, remove the IV catheter instead of converting it to an intermittent lock.

➤ When performing the procedure, always identify your patient according to agency policy, using two identifiers, and be attentive to standard precautions, hand hygiene, patient safety and privacy, body mechanics, and documentation.

➤ Maintain sterility of supplies and equipment (e.g., do not touch catheter opening or ends of the IV lock; keep flush syringe connector sterile).

(continued on next page)

Procedure 35-6 ■ Converting a Primary Line to a Peripheral IV Lock (continued)

Procedure Steps

1. **Help the client assume** a comfortable position that provides access to the IV site.
   Promotes cooperation and facilitates your ability to perform the procedure.

2. **Lower side rails, raise the bed** to working height, and place linen-saver pad under extremity with the IV.
   Protects linens from blood and fluid that might leak from the vessel during catheter removal and ensures good body mechanics.

3. **Don clean nonsterile gloves.** Remove the IV lock from the package and flush the adapter with the first syringe of saline or dilute heparin, according to agency policy. Place the lock back loosely inside the sterile package, keeping it sterile. **Continue with Step 4.**
   Removes air from the lock. ▼

Variation for Primary Tubing Setup With Extension Tubing With a Lock

Discontinue the IV solution and disconnect the primary tubing from the extension tubing with lock. Then, flush extension tubing per agency policy and **skip to Step 13.**

4. **Carefully remove the IV dressing** and the tape that is securing the tubing.
   Provides access to the IV catheter.

5. **Close the roller clamp** on the administration set.
   Prevents loss of IV fluid during the procedure.

6. **With the side of your nondominant hand,** apply pressure over the vein just above the insertion site but not directly on the catheter–hub junction. At the same time, stabilize the catheter hub with your thumb and forefinger.
   Applying pressure over the vein stops blood from flowing from the catheter as you change the administration tubing.

7. **Gently disengage the used tubing** from the IV catheter. If the tubing does not separate from the catheter, see the What If... section at the end of Step 12.

8. **Quickly insert the lock adapter** into the IV catheter and turn it to lock it in place.
   Insert the adapter quickly to prevent bleeding from the IV catheter. ▼

9. **With the attached syringe of saline or dilute heparin,** flush the catheter using the method recommended according to agency policy (e.g., push-stop-push or a slow, steady push). Scrub the injection port of the adapter with an antiseptic pad.
   The Infusion Nurse Society recommends a pulsatile flushing technique (short boluses of 1 mL) to flush the VAD (INS, 2021). Follow agency policy regarding the flushing technique. ▶

10. **Using aseptic technique,** cover the insertion site and catheter hub with a sterile transparent semipermeable dressing. Do not cover the junction of the catheter hub and the IV lock. See Procedure 35-5A for review of dressings.
    Secures the IV catheter and prevents contamination of the site.

11. **Label the dressing** with the date changed and your initials.

12. **Discard used supplies** into appropriate receptacles according to agency policy in line with CDC guidelines.
Discarding used equipment properly keeps the healthcare environment safe.

? What if...

- **At Step 7, the tubing will not separate from the catheter?**

First, if it is a luer-lock connection, be sure you have twisted the luer-lock "open." If so, place a hemostat ("mosquito" clamp) on the IV tubing and gently twist back and forth to loosen the connection. Then if the IV tubing still does not come loose, use the hemostat to gently twist the lock back and forth to loosen the connection. Do not lock the hemostat; merely use it lightly as a grip.
Use of hemostat may help loosen tubing from the catheter, but placement is critical so that the IV catheter and connector are not damaged.

- **At Step 7, the IV catheter becomes dislodged while trying to disconnect the tubing?**

If you can see as much as three-fourths of the catheter emerging from the site, you must remove it and start a new IV at a different site.
Trying to readvance the catheter might cause it to pierce through the vein as well as increase the risk of infection from reinserting a catheter that is no longer sterile. It also causes tissue trauma and increases the risk of phlebitis from catheter manipulation.

Evaluation

- Assess the patency of the catheter before each use according to institutional policy. Patency check and flushing are usually done every 8 to 24 hours. The Infusion Nurse Society recommends every 24 hours for peripheral intravenous catheters (PIVCs) and midline catheters not being used (INS, 2021).
- Evaluate the patient's tolerance to intermittent IV therapy.
- Inspect the insertion site for signs of complications.

Patient Teaching

Explain the importance of notifying staff if the IV site becomes red, painful, or swollen or if the dressing becomes soiled, damp, or loosened (indicating that the catheter has become dislodged or the connection is loose). Include the family in the teaching, as the patient may not be able to assess their own IV therapy.

Home Care

- Explain home use of the intermittent lock to the patient and caregiver. Teach them how to flush the catheter before and after administering prescribed medications.
- Provide the patient and caregiver with the name and phone numbers of people to contact in case problems arise with the catheter or insertion site.

Documentation

- Document the date and time the IV line was converted to an intermittent lock device.
- Note the size and location of the catheter as well as the type and amount of flush solution used.
- Record on the I&O the amount of IV fluid infused.
- Document the condition of the IV site and any complications noted.
- Often, IV care is documented on a flowsheet or the electronic patient record.

Practice Resources
Cullinane (2019); INS (2021).

Thinking About the Procedure

The video **Converting a Primary Line to a Peripheral IV Lock,** along with questions and suggested responses, is available on the **Davis's *Nursing Skills Videos*** Web site at www.fadavis.com.

Procedure 35-7 ■ Discontinuing a Peripheral IV

➤ For steps to follow in *all* procedures, refer to the Universal Steps for All Procedures on the inside back cover.

Equipment
- Clean nonsterile gloves
- Sterile 2-in. × 2-in. gauze dressings
- 1-in. tape or transparent semipermeable dressing
- Linen-saver pad

Delegation
You can delegate the task of discontinuing an IV to an LPN who is specially trained in IV therapy. The task should not be delegated to unlicensed assistive personnel (UAP). However, you should instruct the UAP to notify you of any bleeding from the insertion site.

Preprocedure Assessment
- Assess the patient's readiness to have the IV fluid discontinued and verify the prescription. For example, determine whether they are tolerating oral fluids and have adequate urine output and whether laboratory values are within normal limits.

  If the patient's condition indicates that they still require IV fluids, notify the provider and do not discontinue the IV line.

➤ When performing the procedure, always identify your patient according to agency policy, using two identifiers, and be attentive to standard precautions, hand hygiene, patient safety and privacy, body mechanics, and documentation.

Procedure Steps

1. **Assist the client to a** comfortable position and raise the bed to working height.
   Helps ensure patient cooperation with the procedure; supports good body mechanics for the nurse.

2. **Place a linen-saver pad** under the extremity with the IV.
   Protects linens from blood and fluid that might leak from the vein during catheter removal

3. **Don clean nonsterile gloves** and close the roller clamp on the administration set.
   Closing the roller prevents IV fluid from spilling onto the bed or client during catheter removal. Procedure gloves protect you from body fluid exposure.

4. **Carefully remove the IV dressing,** catheter stabilization device, and the tape that is securing the tubing.
   Removing tape and dressings can be painful especially if over hair or sensitive or thin skin.

If the IV Is Running Through an Extension Tubing or a Saline Lock
Disconnect the administration set tubing and close the slide clamp on the extension tubing.

5. **Scrub the catheter–skin junction** with an alcohol prep pad or chlorhexidine-alcohol antiseptic product for at least 15 seconds.
   Removes microorganisms from the skin entry site.

6. **Apply a sterile 2-in. × 2-in. gauze** pad above the IV insertion site and gently remove the catheter, directing it straight along the vein. Do not press down on the gauze pad while removing the catheter.
   Directing the catheter along the vein prevents vein injury while you are removing the catheter. ▼

7. **Immediately apply firm pressure** with the gauze pad over the insertion site. Hold pressure for 1 to 3 minutes; hold longer if bleeding persists.
   This typically stops bleeding by hastening clot formation.

8. **Remove the soiled 2-in. × 2-in.** gauze pad, and replace it with a sterile 2-in. × 2-in. gauze pad folded over to form a pressure dressing. Secure it with 1-inch tape or a transparent semipermeable dressing.
   Protects the site from contamination.

9. **Return the bed to a low position.** Discard all supplies in the appropriate receptacles according to agency policy in line with CDC guidelines.

Evaluation

- Assess the integrity of the removed catheter; compare the length with the original insertion length to ensure the entire catheter is removed. If a catheter defect is noted, report to the manufacturer and regulatory agencies and complete an incident report according to agency policy.
- Evaluate the patient's response to oral fluids after IV therapy is discontinued.
- Monitor for changes in the patient's condition to assess whether IV therapy should be reestablished.

Patient Teaching

- Instruct the client and family to notify staff if bleeding or discomfort occurs at the insertion site.
- Teach the importance of drinking adequate amounts of fluid, within the prescribed treatment plan, to prevent dehydration. (Some patients have fluid restrictions.)

Documentation

- Document the date and time that IV therapy was discontinued.
- Note the condition of the site, including the presence of any complications. If complications are present, document your interventions, including provider notification.
- Often you will document this procedure on a flow sheet or in the electronic patient record.

Sample Documentation

00/00/0000-2100   Discontinued RA#2, 22-gauge catheter. Site without redness, swelling, tenderness, or exudates. Pressure applied to site for 3 minutes. Bleeding stopped and sterile 2 in. × 2 in. gauze dressing applied. Informed patient to notify staff if bleeding or discomfort occurs. —————————————————S. Horowitz, RN

Practice Resources
INS (2021).

Thinking About the Procedure

The video **Discontinuing a Peripheral IV,** along with questions and suggested responses, is available on the **Davis's** *Nursing Skills Videos* Web site at www.fadavis.com.

Procedure 35-8 ■ Administering a Blood Transfusion

▶ For steps to follow in *all* procedures, refer to the Universal Steps for All Procedures on the inside back cover.

Equipment

- Clean nonsterile gloves
- Blood product
- Normal saline IV solution, 250 mL

    Key Point: *Normal saline solution is the only solution that is compatible with blood products; other IV solutions cause hemolysis of blood cells.*

- Blood administration set (with a 200-micrometer filter and luer-lock connection). If there is no filter on the tubing, you must attach one.
- IV pole
- Watch with a second hand or digital seconds
- Thermometer
- Blood pressure cuff with sphygmomanometer
- Stethoscope

Delegation

Do not delegate this procedure to the LPN or UAP, because blood product administration requires advanced assessment and critical-thinking skills. The LPN and UAP can assist by monitoring vital signs. Instruct both about the complications associated with blood product administration and instruct them to inform you if any occur.

Preprocedure Assessment

- Confirm the patient's need for blood products by assessing vital signs, urine output, and laboratory studies.
    Blood products may cause life-threatening complications; therefore, they should be administered only when needed. Vital signs should be obtained within 30 minutes before the infusion (INS, 2021).
- Check the patient's history for previous blood transfusions and reactions and verify their blood type.
    If the patient has a history of a reaction to blood transfusion, precautions must be taken before they receive additional transfusions. For example, they may need premedication with acetaminophen, a corticosteroid, and diphenhydramine; specially treated blood products; and the use of a specialized administration set with greater filtering capabilities.
- Assess patency of the existing IV catheter, and make sure that it is the proper size for blood product administration.
    Nurses often use a 20-gauge catheter for blood administration. However, for routine transfusion, a 22-gauge or even a 24-gauge catheter can be used. You would need an 18- or 20-gauge catheter when large amounts of blood must be transfused rapidly. The primary consideration should be the size of the patient's veins and not an arbitrary catheter size.
- Assess for allergy to tape.

(continued on next page)

Procedure 35-8 ■ Administering a Blood Transfusion (continued)

Procedure 35-8A ■ Administering Blood and Blood Products

➤ When performing the procedure, always identify your patient according to agency policy, using two identifiers, and be attentive to standard precautions, hand hygiene, patient safety and privacy, body mechanics, and documentation.

Procedure Steps

1. **Verify that informed consent** has been obtained.
   Informed consent is required for blood product administration, as for any invasive or risk-bearing procedure.

2. **Verify the medical prescription,** noting the indication, rate of infusion, and any medications. If there are any pretransfusion medications, administer them as prescribed.
   Helps prevent administration errors.

3. **Ensure patient has a patent IV line or lock** and obtain a blood administration set and 250 mL of IV normal saline solution or as prescribed. Some agencies may require a flush with normal saline between infusions.

4. **Obtain infusion pump,** if possible, and blood warmer, if necessary.
   Having all supplies and equipment on hand minimizes delays in starting the transfusion.

5. **Obtain the blood product** from the blood bank, according to your institution's policy. Wear clean nonsterile gloves whenever handling blood products.
   Some blood banks require a pickup slip that verifies the presence of a functioning IV catheter, signed informed consent, and a prescription, because blood must be discarded after it has been out of refrigeration for 30 minutes.

6. **Verify that the blood product** matches the prescription. Inspect the blood. If you note any of the following abnormalities, return the blood to the blood bank and obtain a new bag:
   a. Pink plasma indicates hemolysis.
   b. The red blood cells should be red, not purple or black.
   c. There should be no large clots visible.
   d. There should be no leakage.

7. Verify **the patient and blood product identification** with another qualified staff member (as deemed by your institution).
   The Infusion Nurse Society recommends an independent double check by two adults trained in blood components and patient identification in the presence of the patient (INS, 2021).
   The Joint Commission (2021) requires the second verifier to be competent in conducting the identification verification process for blood and blood product, according to the organization.

   a. Use two patient coidentifiers (e.g., ask the patient to tell you their full name and date of birth) and compare it with the name and date of birth located on the blood bank form and patient ID band.
   Allowing the patient to confirm their identity and comparing the information against the blood bank form are safety measures to ensure that the correct patient is receiving the correct blood product.

   b. Compare the patient name and hospital identification number on the patient's identification bracelet with the patient name and hospital identification number on the blood bank form attached to the blood product.
   Verifies that the correct patient is receiving the correct blood product.

   c. Compare the unit identification number located on the blood bank form with the identification number printed on the blood product container.
   Verifies that the blood bank has dispensed the correct blood product. ➤

   d. Compare the patient's blood type listed on the blood bank form with the blood type listed on the blood product container.
   Verifies that the blood type of the product matches the patient's blood type.

   e. If all verifications agree, both staff members should sign the blood bank form attached to the blood product container.

   ✚ Contact the blood bank immediately if any discrepancies occur during the identification process. If there are any discrepancies, do not administer the blood product.
   Signing the blood bank form confirms that the blood product was identified and verified by two qualified staff members.

   f. Document on the blood bank form the date and time that the transfusion was started.
   Blood cannot be infused past the expiration time; documenting the start time alerts the nurse of the expiration time.

   g. Make sure that the blood bank form remains attached to the blood product container until administration is complete.
   Ensures product identity should a transfusion reaction occur.

8. **Remove the blood** administration set from the package and label the tubing with the date and time. Then, close all clamps on the administration set.
Labeling the administration set with the date and time informs the nursing staff when the administration set should be changed.

9. **Remove the protective covers** from the normal saline solution container port and from one of the spikes located on the "Y" of the blood product administration set. Place the spike into the port of the solution container.

10. **Hang the normal saline solution** container on the IV pole. Refer to the photo in Step 16.

11. **Compress the drip chamber** of the saline administration set and allow it to fill halfway.
Prevents air from entering the tubing with the solution.

12. **Open the roller clamp** and prime the administration set tubing with normal saline.
Removes air from the tubing.

13. **Close the roller clamp.** Inspect the tubing for air. If air bubbles are in the tubing, flick the tubing with a fingertip to mobilize the bubbles up into the drip chamber.
Air bubbles in the administration tubing can cause an air embolus.

14. **Gently invert the blood** product container several times, but do not shake the bag.
Mixes the blood product with the preservatives that are added to the container without causing trauma (lysis) to the cells.

15. **Hang the blood product bag** on the IV pole and thread the line through the infusion pump.
Enables the blood to flow by gravity.

16. **Remove the protective covers** from the blood spike on the blood tubing and the blood product port. Carefully spike the blood product container through the port.
Prevents inadvertent puncturing of the container. ▶

17. **Obtain and document** the patient's vital signs, including temperature, pulse, and blood pressure, before beginning the transfusion.
Establishes a baseline to help monitor for transfusion reactions.

18. **Using aseptic technique,** attach the distal end of the administration set to the IV catheter.
Prevents contamination of the IV catheter and administration set.

19. **Slowly open the roller clamp** closest to the blood product.
Allows the blood product to slowly fill that side of the "Y" of the administration set tubing.

20. **Set the infusion rate.** Start the infusion rate slowly for the first 15 minutes (INS, 2021). If no reaction occurs after 50 mL has infused, set it to the prescribed rate.
Major reactions usually occur before 50 mL has been infused. A unit of blood cannot hang for more than 4 hours; otherwise, bacterial growth may occur.

For a Volume-Control Infusion Pump
Program the rate. Push "Start." Start the rate slowly until 50 mL has infused. If no reaction occurs, set it to the prescribed rate.

For Gravity Flow
Using the roller clamp, adjust the drip rate. Keep in mind that blood administration sets have a drip factor of 10 gtts/mL.

NOTE: *When using a 24-gauge needle, you will usually (but not always) use gravity infusion instead of a pump.*

Forcing red blood cells through a smaller catheter could result in some cell damage. Allowing the blood to flow by gravity allows time for the cells to change shape as they naturally do when flowing through small capillaries. However, only pumps that have been approved for blood transfusions should be used, because they prevent hemolysis.

21. **Remain with or near the patient** until 50 mL has infused and assess vital signs. Assess the patient every 30 minutes throughout the transfusion for any adverse reactions.
The literature indicates that most severe blood transfusion reactions occur during the transfusion of the initial 50 mL of blood.

22. **Ensure that the patient's** call device is readily available and have them alert you immediately of any signs or symptoms of a transfusion reaction, such as back pain, chills, itching, or shortness of breath.
If the patient alerts you immediately, you should be able to stop the transfusion in time to prevent serious complications.

23. **Obtain vital signs** again in 15 minutes (follow agency procedures), then again in 30 minutes, and then hourly while the transfusion infuses. Vital signs should be monitored every 15 to 30 minutes initially to detect adverse reactions (Suddock & Crookston, 2022). The Infusion Nurse Society (2021) recommends that the patient's vital signs be checked 15 minutes after starting the transfusion, upon completion of the infusion, and again at 1 hour after completion.
Blood and blood product infusions must be completed within 4 hours (AABB, 2018; INS, 2021).
Frequent monitoring alerts you to detect early signs of transfusion reaction or fluid overload. Research shows that the average time to react is over 1.5 hours into the blood infusion (Cortez-Gann et al., 2017).

(continued on next page)

Procedure 35-8 ■ Administering a Blood Transfusion (continued)

24. **After the unit has infused,** close the roller clamp to the blood product container and open the roller clamp to the normal saline solution to flush the administration set with normal saline solution.
Flushing the tubing with normal saline solution clears the tubing of any blood and avoids wasting any of the blood product.

25. **Close the roller clamp** to the normal saline and then disconnect the blood administration set from the IV catheter, if an additional unit of blood has not been prescribed.

26. **If another unit of blood** is required, change the transfusion administration set and filter after the completion of each unit.
This practice promotes safety.

27. **Discard the empty blood** container and administration set in a biohazard receptacle, according to your institution's policy.
Promotes a safer healthcare environment.

? What if...

- Two individuals are not available to verify that the blood and the patient are a match, and the blood must be hung now?

In this instance, if it is available, an automated identification technology (e.g., bar coding) may be used.

Thinking About the Procedure

The video **Administering Blood and Blood Products,** along with questions and suggested responses, is available on the **Davis's** *Nursing Skills Videos* Web site at www.fadavis.com.

Procedure 35-8B ■ Managing a Transfusion Reaction

▶ When performing the procedure, always identify your patient according to agency policy, using two identifiers, and be attentive to standard precautions, hand hygiene, patient safety and privacy, body mechanics, and documentation.

Procedure Steps

1. **If signs or symptoms of a transfusion reaction occur, stop the transfusion immediately. Do not flush the tubing.**
Flushing the tubing causes the patient to receive the blood that remains in the tubing.

2. **Disconnect the administration** set from the IV catheter. Call for help. Obtain vital signs and auscultate heart and breath sounds.
Severe transfusion reactions may cause respiratory distress and shock; early recognition and treatment improve patient outcomes.

3. **Maintain patency of the IV** catheter by hanging a new infusion of normal saline solution, using new tubing.
Maintaining a patent IV catheter with normal saline solution provides IV access in which emergency medication can be administered if necessary.

4. **Notify the primary provider** as soon as you have stopped the blood, assessed the patient, and hung the new normal saline solution.

5. **Place the administration set** and blood product container, with the blood bank form attached, inside a biohazard bag. Send the bag to the blood bank immediately.
The remainder of the blood must be sent to the blood bank, where it can be analyzed to help determine the cause of the reaction.

6. **Obtain blood** (from the extremity opposite the transfusion site) and urine specimens according to your institution's policy.
Blood banks typically require (a) a specimen for a type and crossmatch to compare with the pretransfusion type and crossmatch, (b) a specimen for free hemoglobin, and (c) a specimen for serum bilirubin level. A urine sample should also be sent to check for hemoglobinuria, a sign of acute hemolytic reactions.

7. **Continue to monitor vital signs** frequently, at least every 15 minutes for the first hour. Continue to monitor the patient for 4 to 6 hours after the reaction.
To quickly detect worsening of the patient's condition.

8. **Administer medications,** as prescribed.
Medications will vary depending on the type of transfusion reaction.

? What if...

- At Step 3, I do not have a new bag of normal saline to hang?

Clamp the normal saline line until you can obtain a new bag of normal saline, then disconnect the old normal saline. Do this as quickly as possible.
Preserves the patency of the IV catheter.

Evaluation

- Evaluate the patient's response to the blood transfusion by checking for changes in blood pressure and oxygenation, improvement in color, or signs of fluid overload.
- Monitor for signs and symptoms of transfusion reaction.
- Assess the IV insertion site for signs of infiltration, phlebitis, infection, or inflammation.
- Monitor laboratory studies, such as complete blood count, to help evaluate the effectiveness of therapy and/or transfusion reaction.

Patient Teaching

- Explain the signs and symptoms of transfusion reactions and tell the client and family to notify staff immediately should they occur.
- Warn the client or family to notify staff immediately if tenderness, redness, or swelling occurs at the IV catheter insertion site.
- Explain the importance of notifying staff immediately if the administration set becomes disconnected from the IV catheter or the IV catheter becomes dislodged.

Documentation

- Document the date, time, and reason the transfusion was started.
- Document transfusion vital signs according to institution policy (many institutions have a special form for transfusion vital signs).
- Record the amount of blood transfused on the I&O record.
- Document any complications and the interventions taken.

Sample Documentation

00/00/0000   0600,   1 unit (250 mL) PRBCs hung at 0300 and infused through 20-gauge catheter in LA, for Hgb of 8.3 mg/dL. Pretransfusion vital signs: T 98.9°F, BP 100/68 mm Hg, HR 114 beats/min, and RR, 22 breaths/min. See frequent vital sign sheet for other transfusion vital signs. Breath sounds remained clear throughout the transfusion. No evidence of reaction. Post-transfusion laboratory due at 1200. ————————————————L. Gilmore, RN

Practice Resources
Cortez-Gann et al. (2017); INS (2021); Suddock & Crookston (2022).

Thinking About the Procedure

The video **Manage a Transfusion Reaction,** along with questions and suggested responses, is available on the **Davis's** *Nursing Skills Videos* Web site at www.fadavis.com.

Procedure 35-9 ■ Assisting With Percutaneous Central Venous Catheter Placement

➤ For steps to follow in *all* procedures, refer to the Universal Steps for All Procedures on the inside back cover.

Equipment

- Sterile gloves (two or three pairs)
- Masks, hats, barrier gowns
- 10-mL vials of normal saline (three or four)
- Syringes with 1-in. needle (two or three)
- 25-gauge ⅝-in. and 18-gauge 1½-in. needles (two or three of each)
- Central venous catheter (CVC) kit containing: an introducer, antiseptic solution/swabs, sterile drapes, 10-mL syringe, 1% or 2% Xylocaine without epinephrine, suture, sterile scissors and needle holder, CVC kit (single- or multilumen)
- Injection caps
- Alcohol wipes

Delegation

Do not delegate this procedure because complex assessment and support skills are needed. The nurse must be alert to changes in the patient's condition and signs of developing complications. CVC placement at the bedside is associated with pneumothorax, hemothorax, cardiac tamponade, and air emboli.

Preprocedure Assessments

- Obtain baseline vital signs.
- Verify that informed consent has been given.
- Assess for allergy to tape.

➤ When performing the procedure, always identify your patient according to agency policy, using two identifiers, and be attentive to standard precautions, hand hygiene, patient safety and privacy, body mechanics, and documentation.

(continued on next page)

Procedure 35-9 ■ Assisting With Percutaneous Central Venous Catheter Placement (continued)

Procedure Steps

1. **Explain the procedure** to the patient.
   To relieve anxiety and increase the patient's ability to cooperate with the procedure.

2. **Verify informed consent** and obtain vital signs.

3. **Gather supplies and perform** meticulous hand hygiene.
   Promotes efficiency; removes contaminants to help prevent infection.

4. **Set up the sterile field** and add supplies. Position the table so it is easily accessible by the provider during the procedure.
   Promotes efficiency and makes the procedure faster and therefore less burdensome for the patient.

5. **Position the patient** to facilitate the procedure, usually in the Trendelenburg position with a rolled towel between the shoulders.
   To prevent air embolism and dilate neck veins.

6. **Offer mask, gown, and sterile gloves** (and possibly hat, depending on agency policy) to the provider after they perform hand hygiene.
   Maximum barrier precautions are required for central line placement.

7. **Don mask and then sterile gloves.**
   To prevent contamination of sterile areas and of the insertion site as you cleanse it. Don mask first to keep gloves sterile.

8. **Prep the marked site** with alcohol-based chlorhexidine preparation (INS, 2021), using a friction scrub.
   a. Use a back-and-forth motion to scrub an area 20 to 25 cm (8 to 10 in.) in diameter. Do not go back over an area with the same applicator.
   b. Repeat with three applicators. Total scrub should take at least 30 seconds (2 minutes for a moist site such as the femoral vein).
   c. Allow site to air-dry completely (about 2 minutes). Never wipe or blot dry.
   Insertion kits and agency policies may vary. Follow agency policy. If it does not conform to evidence-based guidelines, work for policy change.

9. **Drape the insertion site** with a large sterile drape, exposing only the prepared skin area. Use other large drapes to cover the patient from head to toe. If your agency does not have a policy that the patient wears a mask, have the patient turn their head in the opposite direction of insertion site.
   Creates a sterile field and decreases the chance of contamination by the patient's exhalations. Turning the head to the opposite side also helps to make it easier to advance the catheter when it passes through the subclavian site.

10. **Observe while the provider** performs the following steps:
    a. Anesthetizes the area with lidocaine.
    b. Primes the central venous catheter with saline.
    c. Performs venipuncture with the insertion needle (in the internal jugular or subclavian site). The femoral site may be used in emergencies, but it is associated with a higher rate of complications than other sites.
    d. Attaches a syringe to the needle and aspirates for blood.
    To ensure the needle is in the vein.
    e. After obtaining blood return, removes syringe from the needle and inserts a guidewire through the needle.
    The guidewire guides the flexible catheter into the vein.
    f. Aspirates all air out of the catheter lumens and then flushes them with normal saline.
    To reduce the risk of air embolism.
    g. Places injection caps on each lumen.
    To prevent blood loss and maintain sterility of the lumens
    h. Sutures the catheter in place.
    To minimize movement and prevent catheter migration (in or out).

11. **Apply sterile transparent dressing** over the site after the provider is finished.
    Minimizes contamination of the site. The most common route of infection is via migration of skin organisms at the insertion site into the cutaneous catheter tract with colonization of the catheter tip. Transparent dressing allows for observation of the site without removing the dressing and manipulating the catheter.

12. **If there are clamps** on the lumens, close them.

13. **Place tape over the lumens** near the ends, but not on the injection caps.
    To minimize movement of the catheter that increases the risk of dislodgement.

14. **Remove sterile drape** and assist the patient to a comfortable position. Monitor for complications, especially respiratory distress.

15. **Dispose of used supplies** and equipment in the appropriate receptacles according to agency policy in line with CDC guidelines.

16. **Remove and dispose of mask and gloves.** Perform hand hygiene.
    Observes standard precaution guidelines.

17. **Follow provider's prescriptions** (e.g., obtain chest x-ray).

Guidelines

- The patient and all staff in the room should wear a mask.
- A health professional who has received appropriate education (e.g., a nurse) should observe the CVC insertion to ensure that aseptic technique is maintained.
- This person should stop the procedure if aseptic technique errors are made.
- A central line checklist should be used during the procedure. You may be responsible for auditing the procedure and completing the checklist.

? What if...

- **In Step 9, a large sterile drape is not available?**

   Use two small drapes to cover the patient from head to toe.
   Evidence-based guidelines advise maximal barrier precautions for insertion of CVCs.

Evaluation

- Obtain vital signs.
- Auscultate the lungs and assess for respiratory distress, sharp chest pain, and coughing. Monitor for 24 hours for these signs.
   To detect pneumothorax or cardiac tamponade.
- Obtain a chest x-ray.
   To verify correct location of catheter tip in the distal third of the superior vena cava as well as absence of thorax and cardiac puncture.
- Assess the patient daily to determine continuing need for the CVC.
   Risk of infection is closely related to the length of time the CVC is in place.
- For further evaluation and follow-up, refer to Clinical Insight 35-4: Caring for Patients With a Central Venous Access Device (CVAD): CVC and PICC; and Procedure 35-5B: Central Line Dressings.

Documentation

- Date and time of catheter insertion
- Catheter type and size
- Site location
- Assessments and interventions performed at insertion and immediately after
- Patient's tolerance of procedure (subjective and objective data)
- x-ray verification of catheter placement

Practice Resources

INS (2021); Suddock & Crookston (2022).

Thinking About the Procedure

The video **Assisting With Percutaneous Central Venous Catheter Placement,** along with questions and suggested responses, is on the **Davis's *Nursing Skills Videos*** Web site at www.fadavis.com.

CLINICAL INSIGHTS

Clinical Insight 35-1 ▸ Assessing for Trousseau's and Chvostek's Signs

Positive Trousseau's and Chvostek's signs are signs of hypocalcemia. To check for these signs, follow these instructions.

Trousseau's Sign
Inflate a blood pressure cuff above systolic pressure. Flexion of the wrist and hand constitutes a positive sign.

Chvostek's Sign
Tap the face in front of the ear and below the zygomatic bone (cheek bone). Facial twitching constitutes a positive sign.

Clinical Insight 35-2 ▸ Guidelines for Measuring Intake and Output (I&O)

General Guidelines
Assessing
- Identify factors that can affect the patient's fluid intake or output (e.g., surgery, medical condition, or medications such as diuretics).
- Measure all fluids the patient consumes or excretes.
- Enlist the patient's help in keeping track of I&O if they are able.
- If you delegate the task of recording intake and output:
  - Be sure the assistive person understands its importance and knows how to perform the procedure correctly.
  - Be certain to evaluate the totals and the fluid sources. A patient or UAP can collect the data, but an RN must make the assessments.
- For accuracy, use a graduated container and hold it at eye level when measuring fluids.

Recording
- You will usually record measurements on a bedside I&O form and transfer the 8-hr total to a graphic sheet or the 24-hr I&O on the patient's record. You may sometimes need hourly measurements. See Chapter 17, "Intake and Output Records," and Figure 17-2.
- Document your findings in milliliters (mL). Describe any fluid restrictions and the patient's compliance with them.

Measuring Intake
It is most accurate to premeasure fluids before they are consumed. However, if that is not possible, you can use the following estimates:

Equivalents
1 oz = 30 mL
1 teaspoon = 5 mL
1 tablespoon = 15 mL
1 home measuring cup of fluid = 8 oz (240 mL)
1 pint of fluid = 16 oz (480 mL)
1 quart of fluid = 32 oz (960 mL)

Various Containers
Record ice chips as fluid at half their volume (1 cup ice = ½ cup fluid)

Clinical Insight 35-2 ▶ Guidelines for Measuring Intake and Output (I&O)—cont'd

Bowl (soup) = 180 mL
Creamer (small) = 30 mL
Custard cup = 100 mL
Drinking cup = 180 mL
Coffee mug = 240 mL
Gelatin cup = 100 mL
Ice cream serving = 120 mL
Juice glass = 120 mL
Paper cup, large = 200 mL
Paper cup, small = 120 mL
Water glass = 200 mL
Water pitcher = 1,000 mL

Examples of Fast-Food Drinks

Child-size drink = 12 oz
Small drink = 16 oz
Medium drink = 21 oz
Large drink = 32 oz

Assessing

- Fluid intake includes the following:
  Oral fluids, including the liquid in prepared foods
  Soups
  Everything that melts into liquid at room temperature (e.g., gelatin, custard, ice cream, and ice)
  Liquid medications and fluids used to take tablets or capsules
  IV fluids
  Enteral or parenteral nutrition fluids
  Instillations into the gastrointestinal tract
  Bladder irrigations
- Measure oral fluids according to agency policy.
- For increased accuracy, use a graduated cup to measure and record fluid amounts before the patient consumes them. Subtract from the total any fluid that the patient throws away or saves for future consumption.
- Wash the measuring cup after each use, except after measuring water.
- Measure and teach the patient to measure and record the amount of fluid they drink with each meal, with medicine, and between meals.
- In the home, cups come in many sizes, so do the following:
  Explain to use a measuring cup to measure how much the drinking cups and glasses hold.
  Specify to always use the same drinking cup or glass.
  Explain that the labels on cans and bottles will help to determine precise fluid amounts.

Recording

- At least every 8 hours, record the type and amount of all fluids the patient has received and indicate the route (oral, parenteral, rectal, or enteric tube).
- Record all forms of intake except blood and blood products.

Measuring Output

Assessing

Fluid output includes everything that leaves the body in fluid form: urine, watery stool, vomitus, wound drainage, surgical drains, NG tubes, chest tubes, and any fluid aspirated from a body cavity.

- Use a calibrated container to measure fluids. Observe it at eye level and take the reading at the bottom of the fluid meniscus.
- Use a different graduated container for each patient; clean after use.
- Teach the patient to keep toilet paper out of the urine for accurate measurement.
- If irrigating an NG tube or the bladder, measure the amount instilled and subtract it from total output.
- You will need to empty wound drains or other devices to measure this volume.
- If a wound is draining, but the fluid is not collected in a drainage device, you may measure the amount of fluid lost by weighing dressings before and after they are applied. If measuring the exact volume is not crucial, you may evaluate the degree of saturation of the dressing.

Recording

- Record the type, route, and amount of all fluids the patient loses.
- Insensible fluid losses can't be easily quantified. However, unusual losses (e.g., saturated dressing, excessive perspiration, rapid breathing patterns, and large burn areas) should be objectively described in narrative documentation.

Tips for Analyzing I&O

- Measure and record all intake and output.
- Determine whether output is more or less than intake.
- Evaluate trends over a period of 24 to 48 hours.
- To identify problems, when evaluating total urine output, ask how many times the patient voided. For example, was a total of 300 mL obtained from 2 voids or from 10 voids of 30 mL each?
- Evaluate patterns and values outside the normal range (e.g., frequent voiding, infrequent voiding), keeping in mind the normal range for 24-hour intake and output.
- The amount of output is important, but consider color, color changes, and odor.
- Analyze intake and output holistically. Take into account the patient's usual pattern and amounts, age, medical problem, and type of surgical procedure.
- You must correlate I&O with daily weights to accurately determine overall fluid status (Antonio et al., 2021; Davies et al., 2018; Shells & Morrell-Scott, 2018).

Clinical Insight 35-3 ▶ Guidelines for Selecting a Peripheral Venipuncture Site

- As a general rule, select the most distal vein on an upper extremity.
- If available, use visualization technologies such as portable ultrasound or imaging devices.
  This minimizes the number of needlesticks the patient must undergo.
- For adults, use the veins located on the dorsal and ventral surfaces of the upper arm, including the metacarpal, cephalic, basilic, and medial (INS, 2021). Hand veins should be used only for therapy less than 24 hours. For infants, veins in the scalp or dorsum of the foot can also be used.
- If possible, select a vein on the patient's nondominant hand or arm.
  Helps to preserve functional ability.

A Superficial veins of the hand
(Cephalic vein, Basilic vein, Dorsal venous arch, Metacarpal veins, Digital veins)

B Superficial veins of the forearm
(Cephalic vein, Basilic vein, Median cubital vein, Accessory cephalic vein, Medial antebrachial vein)

- Look for a vein that has a firm, round appearance with a relatively straight pathway. Do not use a red, hot, or hard vein.
- Avoid veins that are highly visible; they tend to roll.
- The cephalic vein of the arm is one of the best veins to use because it is relatively large, and the forearm provides a natural splint.
- The dorsal veins of the hand are easy to access and are splinted by the metacarpals, but these veins are often quite small and fragile.
- Avoid the antecubital veins if possible. If the patient flexes their arm, the IV catheter may become displaced, so you would probably need to splint the elbow to prevent that. Furthermore, if a PICC line is needed later, you will still have the antecubital veins available for it.
- For the following situations, you need to use the largest vein available, keeping other selection criteria in mind:
  - Hypertonic solutions, viscous solutions, or irritating medications
  - Rapid rates (also require a larger IV catheter)
- If the infusion is to be ongoing, begin the infusion with the best lowest vein and move proximal to the previous site (toward the heart) for subsequent insertions. Peripheral IV catheters are changed as clinically indicated (INS, 2021). If you start the next IV below an already used site (i.e., to change the site or after a failed attempt at insertion), fluid may leak from the old site.
- Avoid areas at which the vein crosses over joints. If you must use such an area, splint the joint to limit movement.
  Splinting the joint helps preserve the vein for use, but it limits functional ability.
- Avoid areas with scarring or with impaired circulation or neurological status (e.g., the affected arm after a mastectomy; an area with signs of infection, previous infiltration, or thrombosis; an arm with an arteriovenous fistula [shunt for dialysis]; or the affected side after cerebrovascular accident [stroke, brain attack]).
  Key Point: *If you must use such an area, first obtain a medical prescription.*
- Do not use veins in the legs and feet unless there is no other option.
  Peripheral circulation may not be adequate in the lower limbs, so there is increased danger of thrombus formation. In adults, this location also interferes with mobility. Foot veins may be used for infants if the IV is taped securely.

Clinical Insight 35-4 ▶ Caring for Patients With a Central Venous Access Device (CVAD): CVC and PICC

✚ Asepsis

- **Use good hand hygiene and follow agency protocols** for site care.
  To protect yourself and the patient.
- **Use strict aseptic technique** when manipulating injection ports, catheter hub and extension legs, needleless connectors, insertion site, and dressing. This includes sterile gloves and supplies, mask, and in some agencies a mask for the patient.
  To minimize line contamination and infection.
- **Scrub injection ports, extension legs, and catheter hubs** vigorously for at least 15 seconds, preferably with 70% alcohol, alcohol-based chlorhexidine solution, or iodophors (i.e., povidl-iodine) preparation, before accessing them (INS, 2021).
- **Appropriate antiseptics** include alcohol and chlorhexidine gluconate (CHG). Do not use povidl-iodine and tincture of iodine to scrub ports unless there is some reason alcohol or CHG-alcohol combination products can't be used.
- **Do not apply organic solvents,** such as acetl or acetl-based products, to the skin before insertion of a catheter or during dressing changes.

✚ Assessments

- **Check the patient record for radiographic confirmation** of correct tip location before beginning prescribed therapies.
- **Inspect catheter–skin junction sites** through the transparent dressing and palpate for tenderness daily.
- **Do not remove transparent dressing except** when dressing change is required. If site is dressed with gauze, remove it to inspect the site.
  A high-risk route of infection is via migration of skin organisms at the insertion site into the cutaneous catheter tract, with colonization of the catheter tip.
- **Observe for excessive bleeding** at the insertion site.
  You may need to obtain a prescription for a topical hemostatic agent and use with a pressure dressing.
- **If symptoms of infection occur** (e.g., fever without obvious cause, redness, edema, induration, exudates, or tenderness at the site), remove the dressing and inspect the site directly. Anticipate that blood cultures will be needed from both the peripheral site and the central catheter.
- **Be aware that risk of infection is higher** with femoral catheters and with multilumen catheters.
  Multilumen catheters require more manipulation, which encourages more colonization and bacterial growth within the catheter lumen.
- **Assess for compromised catheter integrity** (wet dressing; kinked, cracked, or leaking external catheter).
- **Inspect catheter connections** and pump function, including flow rate.
- **Observe for symptoms of catheter migration** to the right atrium or ventricle (i.e., mid- to lower sternal pain, dysrhythmias).
- **If there are signs of complications,** notify the medical provider.
- **Assess the patient daily** for indications that the CVC or PICC line is still needed.
  CVCs or PICC line should be removed as soon as possible because the infection rate is closely related to the length of time the catheter is in place.

Maintenance Interventions

- **The site should be covered** with a semipermeable transparent dressing, the catheter secured with a sterile commercially manufactured stabilizer (instead of tape), and the lumens anchored near the ports with clear tape.
- **Keep dressings dry, intact, and air occlusive.** Protocols generally require a dressing change every 7 days for transparent dressings, unless it is damp, loosened, or soiled, or if the site must be examined (e.g., because of pain or odor). A dressing change every 2 days is required for a gauze and tape dressing.
- **Perform site care with each dressing change.** Cleanse the catheter–skin junction with an appropriate antiseptic solution, apply a sterile stabilizer, and apply a new sterile dressing.
- **Manipulate the catheter hub as little as possible.**
  To minimize catheter movement, phlebitis, and contamination of the line. Less catheter manipulation is associated with fewer bloodstream infections.
- **Flush catheters before and after any infusions** or per agency protocol. The Infusion Nurse Society recommends 24 hours when not in use.
  - **Flush volume** should be twice the volume of the catheter and add-on devices (consult package label).
  - **Use a syringe size recommended** by the catheter manufacturer (10 mL is the smallest size recommended because of the pressure generated).
  - **Type of flush solution depends on agency policy** (saline versus heparin). The Infusion Nurse Society (2021) recommends preservative-free 0.9% sodium chloride for short and long PIVC and midline catheters.
  - **Use single-use, labeled syringes of flush solution** to prevent cross-contamination.
  - **If you have trouble flushing,** the catheter may be kinked or malpositioned, the inline filter may be clogged, or a clamp may need to be released. You can correct these problems.
  - ✚ **Never flush against resistance.**
    The catheter might be clogged and you would risk dislodging a small clot. This could also rupture the catheter.

(Continued)

Clinical Insight 35-4 ➤ Caring for Patients With a Central Venous Access Device (CVAD): CVC and PICC—cont'd

- ✚ **If the patient has a PICC line,** take blood pressures on the alternate arm.

  Using the arm with the PICC can cause bleeding at the site, thrombus formation, retrograde blood flow, and increased risk of catheter occlusion.

- **If the patient is receiving parenteral nutrition,** reserve and label one lumen just for that purpose.

Documentation

- **Document routine assessments and the condition of the catheter–skin junction site.** When site care is given, also document the patient's response and any actions taken to correct or prevent adverse reactions.

Related Information

- **For information about dressing changes,** refer to Procedure 35-5B: Central Line Dressings.
- **For information about administering medications** through a CVAD, see Procedure 23-18: Administering Medication Through a Central Venous Access Device.

Practice Resources

Hicks & Lopez (2022); INS (2021).

Clinical Insight 35-5 ➤ Managing Infiltration and Extravasation

- ✚ At the first sign or symptom of infiltration or extravasation, stop the IV. Symptoms include slowed or stopped flow, swelling, tenderness, pallor, hardness, and coolness at the site. The patient may complain of pain or a burning sensation in the area.

For a Central Venous Access Device: CVC or PICC

- Clamp and cap the catheter hub.
- Do not remove the catheter.
- Follow agency policy when you suspect infiltration or extravasation.
- If the patient has an implanted port, aspirate, remove the port access needle, and apply a dressing.
- Notify the provider who inserted the catheter, who may prescribe an x-ray to help determine the cause of the problem.

For a Short Peripheral Catheter

- Assess capillary refill, sensation, and motion distal to the infiltrated site.
- Disconnect the tubing from the catheter hub; attach a 3- to 5-mL syringe and try to aspirate fluid from the catheter lumen. Use aseptic technique.
- Photograph the site to create a record of its condition, if agency policy allows.
- Wearing gloves, remove the catheter and hold a dry gauze pad over the site to stop the bleeding. Apply a dry dressing.
- ✚ Do not apply excessive pressure to the site.
- Use a skin marker to outline the areas of infiltration/extravasation to monitor changes.
- If you need to start a new IV, use the other arm, if possible. If it is not possible, start it in a more proximal location on the same arm.
- Measure the circumference of the arm and compare it with the opposite arm.

- ✚ Apply cold or warm compresses depending on which fluid has escaped into the tissues.
  - Avoid wet compresses that can lead to maceration.
  - For DNA binding agents, use dry, cold compresses for vasoconstriction to reduce inflammation and localize the infiltrate.
  - For non-DNA binding agents, use dry, warm compresses for vasodilation to increase blood flow to the area.
  - For isotonic or hypotonic fluids or medications, choose either heat or cold, or alternate them, based on patient comfort.
- Apply compresses for 15 to 30 minutes every 4 to 6 hours, or as prescribed by the provider.
- Estimate the volume of fluid that escaped into the tissues; notify the prescriber.
- Some medications leaked into the surrounding tissue can cause damage and even necrosis. For instance, when dopamine extravasates, you might need to give a prescribed amount of antidote (e.g., regitine injected subcutaneously) as well as hydrocortisone and an anti-inflammatory to minimize tissue damage. Be sure to check the protocol at your facility.
- Elevate the extremity and advise the patient to rest.
- Document all fluids and medications involved, equipment being used (e.g., pump), size and type of the catheter, description of the site (including location, size, and color), methods used to assess the site before administering the fluids (e.g., aspiration), patient's signs and symptoms, interventions, notifications, and patient teaching.
- Complete an occurrence (or incident) report, as required by your facility.

Practice Resources

Gahart & Nazareno (2019); INS (2021).

ASSESSMENT GUIDELINES AND TOOLS

Assessing Fluids, Electrolytes, and Acid–Base Balance

Nursing History

Demographic Data
Age, sex, height, weight, body mass index

Medical History
- Have you ever been hospitalized or had surgery? If so, when and for what reason?
- For what healthcare problems are you currently being treated?
- Have you ever been diagnosed with kidney disease, high blood pressure, diabetes, or thyroid or parathyroid problems?

Current Health Concerns
- What symptoms do you currently have?
- Have you recently had any of the following symptoms?

Excessive thirst	Difficulty breathing
Fever	Swelling of hands, feet, or ankles
Excessive perspiration	Dizziness or feeling faint
Nausea, vomiting, or diarrhea	Muscle weakness
Dry skin or mucous membranes	Excessive fatigue
Dark, concentrated urine	Numbness, tingling, or cramping sensations
Limited amounts of urine	

- Is your weight stable? Have you had any recent changes in your weight?
- Do you believe you have any problems with fluid loss?

Food and Fluid Intake
- How much fluid do you usually drink in a 24-hour period?
- Do you believe you drink adequate amounts of fluid?
- Describe your usual diet.
- Have you recently changed your diet or fluid intake?
- Are you following a special diet?
- Have you ever been placed on a restricted diet?
- Have you had any recent changes in your appetite or thirst?
- Do you salt your food?
- Do you ever use a salt substitute?

Fluid Elimination
- How often do you urinate in a 24-hour period? Has that changed recently?
- How often do you get up during the night to urinate?
- Have you noticed any recent changes in the amount or appearance of your urine?
- How often do you have vomiting, diarrhea, or constipation? Describe your experience.

- Do you have any wounds? If so, where are they and how did they happen? What is the color of drainage and how much drainage do you have?
- Do you have any breaks in your skin? If so, describe the problem and show me the area.

Medications
- What prescribed medications do you currently take?
- What over-the-counter medications or alternative treatments do you use? Why do you use them?
- How often do you take laxatives or antacids?
- What vitamins, herbals, or supplements do you take?

Lifestyle
- What is your usual activity level?
- What type of exercise do you engage in? How often?
- How much fluid do you consume before, during, and after exercise?
- Do you drink alcohol? If so, how much do you consume in a day? In a week?
- Do you smoke? If so, how much? For how long have you smoked?
- Do you use any illegal medications or drugs?

Physical Assessments

Skin
Assess the skin for the following:
- Color and temperature may be cues to the presence of fever and circulation status.
- Moisture content offers some indication of fluid status. A diaphoretic client is losing fluid at a faster rate than a client with dry skin. Dry, scaling skin may indicate a fluid deficit. Any breaks in the skin are potential areas for fluid loss.
- Turgor varies with age, weight, and skin condition but does offer information on fluid status. Pinch the skin over the sternum. Normally skin immediately returns to its usual position. In fluid volume deficit or malnutrition the skin may remain "tented" before returning to its original position. You must, however, correlate skin turgor with context and other clinical signs. For example, the skin loses elasticity with aging, so clients older than age 65 often have decreased turgor, which is normal for them.
- Edema in dependent areas is a cue for fluid volume excess. In an ambulatory client, assess the lower extremities and hands. In a bedridden client, edema will shift as the client is turned.
- To grade edema (on a scale +1 to +4, +1 represents minimal edema and +4 represents the most severe edema).

(Continued)

Assessing Fluids, Electrolytes, and Acid–Base Balance—cont'd

Mucous Membranes
- Inspect the tongue and buccal mucosa. Mouth breathing alone usually does not change these areas.
- Assess tongue turgor in all age groups because it is not affected by age.
- Assess the color, moisture, and continuity of the mucous membranes
- Dry, cracked, or dull mucous membranes are signs of fluid volume deficit.

Cardiovascular System
- Assess vital signs (see later section).
- Pulse and blood pressure are affected by fluid and electrolyte status.
- If you suspect fluid volume deficit, assess for orthostatic hypotension:
  - Assess blood pressure while client is lying or sitting.
  - Have the client rise to a seated or standing position, and reassess the blood pressure (BP).
  - A drop in systolic BP of >15 mm Hg is a sign of orthostatic hypotension.
- Check capillary refill. Delayed capillary refill is a sign of fluid volume deficit; rapid capillary refill indicates adequate circulation and volume. If capillary refill is delayed, evaluate feet and hands bilaterally. Delays in just one area indicate impaired circulation to the extremity rather than volume changes.
- Assess venous filling by observing the jugular and hand veins. Flat jugular or hand veins indicate low fluid volume. Distended vessels are a sign of overload.
- Assess peripheral edema (discussed previously).

Respiratory System
- Assess respiratory rate, depth, and pattern. The respiratory system rapidly responds to changes in pH. Similarly, alterations in gas exchange at the alveolar–capillary membrane may trigger pH changes.
- Assess breath sounds. Crackles or moist rales may indicate fluid overload. Areas of consolidation indicate impaired gas exchange.

Neurological System
- Assess level of consciousness and orientation.
- Assess neuromuscular irritability.
- Assess energy level and fatigue.
- Assess reflexes.

For specific neurological cues to alterations in fluid, electrolyte, or acid–base balance,

➡ Go to **Chapter 35, Table 35-5: Electrolyte Imbalances** and **Table 35-7: Acid-Base Imbalances,** in Volume 1.

Vital Signs
- Temperature. An elevated body temperature increases the loss of body fluids.
  - In hypernatremia, body temperature elevates because less fluid is available for sweating.
  - In uncomplicated fluid volume deficit, body temperature decreases.
- Pulse
  - Tachycardia is an early sign of fluid volume deficit.
  - Pulse rate is affected by fluid status and some electrolytes (primarily sodium, potassium, calcium, and magnesium).
  - Dysrhythmias are seen with potassium and magnesium imbalances.
  - The pulse volume is directly affected by fluid status. As fluid volume increases, the pulse volume also increases. Similarly, a drop in fluid volume leads to a drop in pulse volume.
- Respiratory rate. Alterations in respiratory rate may cause acid–base imbalances or be associated with compensation for a metabolic disorder.
- Blood pressure
  - Assess for orthostatic hypotension (a drop in the systolic BP from lying or sitting to standing positions greater than or equal to 20 mm Hg).
  - Blood pressure rises and falls with fluid volume.
  - Blood pressure is elevated by hypernatremia and fluid volume excess.
  - Respiratory acidosis causes increased heart rate, resulting in BP elevation.
  - High potassium intake may lower blood pressure.

Daily Weights
Daily weights are an accurate method of assessing fluid status.
- Use the same balanced scale each day to monitor fluid status accurately.
- Weigh the client at the same time of day, making sure that the client is wearing the same amount of clothing.
- Each kilogram (2.2 lb) of weight is equivalent to 1 liter (1,000 mL) of fluid.
- For clients undergoing hemodialysis (blood cleansing through an artificial kidney), weigh the client before and after dialysis treatments. Many lose 3 to 4 kg (6.6 to 8.8 lb) after several hours of dialysis.
- You may institute weight monitoring as an independent nursing prescription, which can be delegated to a UAP.
- This is important when it is impractical or impossible to measure I&O accurately (breastfeeding intake, incontinence, draining wounds).

Fluid Intake and Output
See Clinical Insight 35-2.

DIAGNOSTIC TESTING

Assessing Fluid, Electrolyte, and Acid–Base Balances

Venous Blood Sample	Normal Ranges
Sodium	135–145 mEq/L
Potassium	3.5–5 mEq/L
Chloride	97–107 mEq/L
Bicarbonate	22–26 mEq/L
BUN	10–31 mg/dL
Creatinine	0.5–1.2 mg/dL
Serum osmolality	275–295 mOsm/kg
Urine osmolality	250–900 mOsm/kg
Hematocrit	43%–49% in men
	38%–44% in menstruating women
Freshly Voided Urine Sample	
pH	5.0–9.0
Specific gravity	1.001–1.029
Arterial Blood Sample	
pH	7.35–7.45
P_{CO_2}	35–45 mm Hg
HCO_3^-	22–26 mEq/L

CLINICAL REASONING
Applying the Full-Spectrum Nursing Model

PATIENT SITUATION

Darlene Malone, age 42, has been admitted to the emergency department with complaints of fatigue, extreme weakness, and heart palpitations. She says she has not seen a healthcare provider in nearly 10 years. Suddenly, she slumps and falls over. She is not breathing, has no pulse, and does not respond to verbal stimuli. She is resuscitated with cardiopulmonary resuscitation (CPR) and IV epinephrine, and an endotracheal tube is placed. STAT laboratory results show a potassium level of 7.7 mEq/L, BUN of 102 mg/dL, and creatinine of 5 mg/dL. A provider diagnoses acute renal failure. Among other interventions, an IV is started to administer 10% calcium chloride solution, 1000 mg, by slow IV push to counteract the toxic effects of hyperkalemia on the cell membranes. The nurse used a 20-gauge over-the-needle catheter in Ms. Malone's right median antebrachial vein.

THINKING

1. *Theoretical Knowledge:*

   a. Which laboratory results are abnormal? Are they high or low?

   b. Which laboratory results directly reflect her renal failure?

   c. What term correctly describes serum potassium of 7.7 mEq/L?

2. *Critical Thinking (Considering Alternatives):*

   a. What do you think is causing Ms. Malone to have hyperkalemia? You should be able to think this through and make a reasonable guess even if you have not studied pathophysiology.

   b. Ms. Malone is to be given 50 mEq of sodium bicarbonate by slow IV push for an acid–base imbalance that is often associated with hyperkalemia. Which imbalance do you think would be treated with sodium bicarbonate: metabolic acidosis or metabolic alkalosis?

DOING

3. *Practical Knowledge:*

   a. When you prepare to administer the sodium bicarbonate (in question 2b), you notice that the IV infusion is barely flowing and that the insertion site is swollen and pale. What is the first thing you should do?

   b. You aspirate the catheter and do not obtain a blood return. Ms. Malone absolutely must have this medication. Describe what you would do in the order you would do it.

4. *Nursing Process (Planning Goals):* The outcome best suited to evaluate Ms. Malone's hyperkalemia is electrolyte and acid–base imbalance. Based on the function of this electrolyte, what is the primary indicator that you could use to evaluate her goal achievement for this problem?

CARING

5. *Self-Knowledge:* Ms. Malone will need dialysis to replace her inadequate renal function and control her serum potassium level. It is likely that her renal failure was brought on by years of illegal drug abuse. She has never held a full-time job and has not worked at all for the past 7 years. Her dialysis treatments will need to be paid for by the government-funded program Medicaid. How do you feel about this—specifically, how do you feel about the issues of (a) a person's responsibility for their own health and (b) compassion for people who cannot afford to pay for healthcare? Focus on your own feelings, not on issues of what "should" be done.

Critical Thinking and Clinical Judgment

1. Recall the Meet Your Patients scenario in Volume 1. When you review Jackson LaGuardia's medical records to prepare for the clinical day, you find that he is in the emergency department (ED) with four other members of the LaGuardia family. All of them have come to the ED complaining of nausea, vomiting, and diarrhea related to severe gastroenteritis, a viral intestinal disorder. The family members include the following:

   8-month-old Jason, grandson of Jackson

   26-year-old Susanna, Jackson's daughter and Jason's mother

   60-year-old Jackson

   58-year-old Gemma, Jackson's wife

   82-year-old Martha, Jackson's mother

   Jason, Jackson, and Martha are being admitted to the hospital. However, Susanna and Gemma have been asked to follow up tomorrow in the urgent care clinic. The following questions pertain to this scenario.

   a. Martha LaGuardia's prescriptions call for lactated Ringer's solution with 20 mEq KCl per liter to infuse at 150 mL/hr. After 4 hours of infusion, Martha begins to complain of shortness of breath and develops a cough. What do you suspect may be happening? What actions should you take?

   b. What theoretical knowledge will you use in caring for Ms. LaGuardia's immediate problem?

c. Jason LaGuardia has been prescribed 250 mL of 0.9% saline solution over 8 hours. What type of equipment should you consider using?

d. Calculate the drip rate for Jason's infusion if a gravity flow device is used. What further information do you need to perform this calculation?

e. As you may recall, Jackson LaGuardia has end-stage renal disease. His laboratory work reveals a hemoglobin of 7.6 mg/dL and a hematocrit of 21%. He has been prescribed two units of packed red blood cells over 8 hours. Given his condition, for what fluid balance problem is he at risk? What additional parameters should you assess while he is receiving the transfusion?

2. You are asked to administer an antibiotic intravenously via piggyback. You are not familiar with the equipment that this facility uses. As a student, what approach should you take to solve this problem?

3. Identify techniques that you have observed that may contribute to contamination of an IV site.

4. Interpret the following ABG results. Explain your thinking.

   a. pH 7.47 Pco_2 45 mm Hg HCO_3^- 32 mEq/L

   b. pH 7.32 Pco_2 50 mm Hg HCO_3^- 25 mEq/L

   c. pH 7.30 Pco_2 41 mm Hg HCO_3^- 18 mEq/L

   d. pH 7.45 Pco_2 30 mm Hg HCO_3^- 22 mEq/L

5. For each of the following concepts, use critical thinking to describe how or why it is important to nursing; patient care; or fluids, electrolytes, and acid–base balance. Note that these are *not* to be merely definitions.

   Homeostasis

   Selectively permeable membranes

   Fluid imbalance

   Electrolyte imbalances

   Acid–base imbalances

   Parenteral fluid and electrolyte replacement

What Are the Main Points in This Chapter?

- Water is the largest single constituent of the body. Total body water content varies with age, sex, and the number of fat cells.
- Intracellular fluid (ICF) is contained within the cells. It is essential for cell function and metabolism and accounts for approximately 40% of body weight.
- Extracellular fluid (ECF) consists of three types of fluid: interstitial, intravascular, and transcellular fluid. ECF carries water, electrolytes, nutrients, and oxygen to the cells and removes the waste products of cell metabolism. ECF accounts for 20% of body weight.
- Electrolytes that carry a positive charge are called cations. These include sodium (Na^+), potassium (K^+), calcium (Ca^{2+}), and magnesium (Mg^{2+}). Electrolytes that carry a negative charge are called anions.

- Potassium and magnesium are the major cations in the ICF. Phosphate and sulfate are the major anions.
- The major electrolytes of ECF are sodium, chloride, and bicarbonate. Albumin is also present in the ECF.
- The functions of the major electrolytes include the following:
  - Sodium is essential to regulate fluid volume.
  - Chloride works with sodium to regulate osmotic pressure and with the bicarbonate buffer system to regulate acid–base balance.
  - Potassium is essential for cellular metabolism.
  - Calcium is responsible for bone health and neuromuscular and cardiac function and is an essential factor in blood clotting.
  - Magnesium is a mineral used in more than 300 biochemical reactions in the body.
  - Phosphorus is important in the formation of bones and teeth and has an inverse relationship with calcium.
- Osmosis, diffusion, filtration, and active transport are mechanisms used to maintain a balance between fluids and solutes in the body.
- General recommendations for total fluid intake are 2700 mL per day for females and 3700 mL per day for males.
- When the body is in a healthy state, fluid losses through urine, skin, insensible losses, and feces are equivalent to fluid intake.
- Fluid volume deficit occurs when there is a proportional loss of water and electrolytes from the ECF.
- Fluid volume excess involves excessive retention of sodium and water in the ECF.
- Bicarbonate is important in acid–base regulation and is regulated by the kidneys to maintain pH.
- The amount of acid or base present in a solution is measured as pH. The pH is reported on a scale of 1 to 14, with 1 to 6.9 being acidic, 7 neutral, and 7.1 to 14 basic, or alkaline. Normal blood pH is slightly alkalotic, between 7.35 and 7.45.
- A buffer system consists of a weak acid and a weak base. These molecules react with strong acids or bases to keep them from altering the pH by either absorbing free hydrogen ions or releasing free hydrogen ions. The principal buffer system in the ECF is the carbonic acid (H_2CO_3) and sodium bicarbonate ($NaHCO_3^-$) system.
- When the serum pH falls below 7.35, the patient is acidotic. When the serum pH increases above 7.45, the patient is alkalotic. ABGs are used to monitor acid–base balance.
- When the serum pH is too acidic (pH is low), the lungs remove carbon dioxide through rapid, deep breathing. If the serum pH is too alkaline (pH is high), the lungs try to conserve carbon dioxide through shallow respirations.
- The kidneys affect pH by regulating the amount of bicarbonate (base) that is kept in the body.
- Assessment of a client's fluid, electrolyte, and acid–base balance includes history; laboratory data; physical examination of the skin, mucous membranes, and neurological status; and assessment of cardiovascular and respiratory systems.
- I&O are monitored to assess fluid status. To monitor, measure all fluids consumed and excreted in a 24-hour period.
- Tests used to monitor fluid, electrolyte, and acid–base balance include serum electrolytes and osmolality, complete blood count, urinalysis, and measurement of arterial blood gases.
- Nursing actions for patients with alterations in fluid, electrolyte, or acid–base balance include preventing imbalances by modifying oral intake, providing parenteral replacement, and transfusing blood products.
- Intravenous fluids are classified as isotonic, hypotonic, and hypertonic solutions, based on their comparison to the osmolality of blood serum.
- Vascular access devices may provide access to peripheral or central veins.
- Intravenous equipment consists of the IV catheter, an administration set, extension tubing, and the IV solution.
- Nurses are responsible for using established formulas to calculate and maintain the correct rate of flow and for monitoring the client's response to the infusion.
- Assess for local IV site complications (e.g., infiltration, extravasation, infection, thrombus, and thrombophlebitis) and systemic complications (e.g., fluid volume excess, sepsis, and embolus).
- Meticulous aseptic technique is required for initiation and care of intravenous infusions to prevent bloodstream infection.
- Blood products are infused when the client has had significant blood loss, diminished oxygen-carrying capacity, or a deficiency in one of the blood components.
- Nurses must administer the correct blood type to patients to prevent a hemolytic reaction.

Knowledge Map

CHAPTER 35 Hydration & Homeostasis

HOMEOSTASIS: BALANCE

BODY FLUIDS

Imbalances:
- **FLUID VOLUME DEFICIT:**
  - Hypovolemia
  - Dehydration
- **FLUID VOLUME EXCESS:**
  - Hypervolemia
  - Fluid overload

Locations:
- Interstitial
- Intravascular
- Transcellular

Functions:
- Maintain blood volume
- Regulate temperature
- Cellular transport/metabolism
- Digestion/excretion

Movement:
- Active transport
- Passive transport; osmosis, diffusion, and filtration

Regulation:
- OUTPUT
- INTAKE
- HORMONAL REGULATION

ELECTROLYTES

Imbalances: Excesses or deficits in the ICF or ECF

- **ICF:** K^+, Mg, phosphate, sulfate
- **ECF:** Na^+, chloride, bicarb, albumin

Functions:
- Fluid volume
- Impulse conduction
- Muscle contraction
- Acid–base balance
- Cellular activity/metabolism

NURSING CARE

Assessment:
- Skin, mucous membranes, CV, neuro, respiratory
- Vital signs
- Weight/I&O
- Labs/ABGs

Prevention:
- Dietary changes
- Oral electrolyte supplements
- Facilitate fluid restriction or intake

PARENTERAL

ACID–BASE

Regulation:
- **ACID:** H^+ donor
- **BASE:** H^+ acceptor
- **BUFFERS:**
  - Carbonic acid/bicarb
  - Phosphate system
  - Protein system
- **RESPIRATORY:**
  - Carbon dioxide
  - Retention/elimination
- **RENAL:**
  - Conserve/excrete bicarb
  - Ammonium formation

Imbalances:
- **ACIDOSIS:**
  - Respiratory
  - Metabolic
- **ALKALOSIS:**
  - Respiratory
  - Metabolic

CHAPTER 36

Caring for the Surgical Patient

STUDENT RESOURCES

The questions and exercises in this book allow you to practice the kind of thinking you will use as a full-spectrum nurse. Critical-thinking questions usually have more than one right answer, so we do not provide "correct" answers for these features. Try to answer these questions yourself. It is more important to develop your nursing judgment than to just cover content. You will learn more by discussing the questions with your peers. If you are still unsure, see the Davis Advantage chapter resources for suggested responses.

To explore learning resources for this chapter,

Go to www.DavisAdvantage.com and find:

Answers and Suggested Responses for all questions in this chapter
Concept Map
Knowledge Map
References and Bibliography

Key Concepts

Intraoperative care
Perioperative nursing
Preoperative care
Postoperative care

Related Concepts

See the Concept Map on Davis Advantage.

Caring for the Williams Family

Charlene Williams, the mother of Stanley Williams, has been having blurred vision and decreased visual acuity. A local ophthalmologist diagnosed bilateral cataracts. The ophthalmologist has recommended cataract removal in the left eye, with insertion of an intraocular lens. The ophthalmologist told Mrs. Williams to schedule the surgery "at your convenience" and explained that the surgery would be performed on an outpatient basis. The ophthalmologist gave Mrs. Williams the following list of activities to prepare for the surgery:

- Schedule a date for your surgery. My receptionist will set up a time for your surgery. All surgeries are performed at Western Medical Center Same-Day Surgery Department.
- Please arrange to be seen by your primary care provider 1 to 2 weeks before the surgery to receive clearance for surgery.
- Make an appointment with the Preoperative Center at Western Medical Center Same-Day Surgery Department 1 to 2 days before surgery.
- Arrange to have a ride to and from the surgery.

Caring for the Williams Family (continued)

A. What preoperative testing is Mrs. Williams likely to undergo? Explain your rationale.

B. The preoperative list states that the patient must be seen by the primary care provider to receive clearance for surgery. Why is this an essential part of the preoperative period?

C. What theoretical knowledge do you need to perform preoperative teaching for Mrs. Williams? How could you obtain that information? Be specific about your sources.

D. What content would you include in Mrs. Williams' preoperative teaching?

E. The ophthalmologist has planned anesthesia via conscious sedation. What factors, if any, might keep Mrs. Williams from receiving this form of anesthesia? What additional information do you need to answer this question?

Practical Knowledge clinical application

Caring for the surgical patient includes procedures and techniques designed for prevention and early detection of complications. Recall that full-spectrum nursing involves thinking, doing, and caring—all are equally important in perioperative as well as other settings.

PROCEDURES

The procedures in this section will help you to prevent postoperative complications. Preoperative teaching of coughing, deep breathing, moving in bed, and leg exercises helps to prevent thrombophlebitis, atelectasis, and pneumonia. Antiembolism stockings and sequential compression devices are designed to promote peripheral circulation and prevent thrombus formation. Gastrointestinal suction is used to relieve or prevent abdominal distention.

Procedure 36-1 ■ Teaching a Patient to Deep-Breathe, Cough, Move in Bed, and Perform Leg Exercises

➤ For steps to follow in *all* procedures, refer to the Universal Steps for All Procedures on the inside back cover.

Equipment

For Teaching Deep Breathing and Coughing
- Folded blanket or a pillow (if teaching will include splinting of a surgical incision site)
- Tissues

For Moving in Bed
- Small pillow or folded blanket
- Pillows

Delegation

You or another RN should perform the initial teaching. You may delegate reinforcement of the teaching to a licensed vocational/practical nurse (LVN/LPN), or unlicensed assistive personnel (UAP).

Preprocedure Assessments

- Assess the patient's cognitive level and level of consciousness.
  Helps assess the patient's ability to understand and follow directions and select the appropriate teaching method.
- Assess the patient's pain level.
  Even preoperatively, pain must be well controlled to ensure full patient participation.
- Determine whether the surgical procedure and/or a physical disability will limit the patient's participation.
  For example, a fractured arm that has not yet been repaired will impair the patient's ability to hold a pillow for splinting.
- Determine whether the surgical procedure will entail special exercises or equipment. In addition, assess for any special equipment, such as braces, slings, or abductor wedges, that may be needed when turning a patient in bed.

(continued on next page)

Procedure 36-1 ■ Teaching a Patient to Deep-Breathe, Cough, Move in Bed, and Perform Leg Exercises (continued)

> Knee and hip surgeries often involve special exercises or equipment postoperatively. Consult the surgeon before teaching the patient any leg exercises. Spinal and neurological surgeries often limit movement in the postoperative period. For example, some spinal surgeries require the patient to logroll (move from head to toe as one unit). Some neurological procedures require limiting the time the patient's head of bed is above 30°. Identify these restrictions preoperatively, and inform the patient and family about them during your teaching session.

- Assess the patient's belief about the ability of the surgical incision to remain intact.
  If the patient believes that the incision will not stay together with coughing or moving, the patient is less likely to comply.

Procedure 36-1A ■ Teaching a Patient to Deep-Breathe and Cough

> When performing the procedure, always identify your patient according to agency policy, using two identifiers, and be attentive to standard precautions, hand hygiene, patient safety and privacy, body mechanics, and documentation.

Deep breathing and coughing expand the lungs, improve ventilation, promote gas exchange, and help prevent atelectasis and pneumonia. Coughing after deep breathing mobilizes secretions, which keeps airways and alveoli open and provides greater surface area for gas exchange.

Procedure Steps

1. **Assist the patient to a Fowler's or semi-Fowler's position**, with the shoulders relaxed.
   Allows for best chest and lung expansion.

2. **Assist the patient who will have a chest or abdominal incision** to practice splinting the site with a folded blanket or pillow.
   Counterpressure supports the incision and decreases pain. ▼

3. **Teach the patient diaphragmatic/deep breathing.** Tell the patient to:
   a. Place hands anteriorly, along the lower end of the rib cage. The tips of the third fingers should touch at the midline.
   b. Slowly take a deep breath in through the nose. Tell the patient that they should feel their chest expanding as the diaphragm moves down.
   c. Hold the breath for 2 to 5 seconds.
      Stimulates surfactant production and helps prevent alveolar collapse.
   d. Slowly and completely exhale the breath through the mouth.

4. **Teach the patient to cough** in conjunction with diaphragmatic breathing. Instruct the patient to:
   a. Complete two or three cycles of diaphragmatic breathing.
   b. On the next breath in, have the patient lean forward and cough rapidly, through an open mouth, using the muscles of the abdomen, thighs, and buttocks. Cough several times on that breath.
      This information helps the patient to distinguish coughing from merely clearing the throat.

   For a Patient With Weakness

   If the patient is too weak to perform this maneuver, have the patient inhale deeply, bend forward slightly, and perform three or four "huffs" against an open glottis to move secretions forward.

Procedure 36-1B ■ Teaching a Patient to Move in Bed

> When performing the procedure, always identify your patient according to agency policy, using two identifiers, and be attentive to standard precautions, hand hygiene, patient safety and privacy, body mechanics, and documentation.

Moving in bed promotes blood circulation, stimulates respiratory function, and helps mobilize gas in the intestines.

Procedure Steps

1. **Start with the patient in** supine position, bed rails up. Then instruct the patient as follows.

2. **To turn to the left side:** Bend the right leg, sliding the foot flat along the bed and flexing the knee.
   Enables the patient to push their body over to the opposite side.

3. **Reach the right arm across the chest,** and grasp the opposite bed rail.
   Helps the patient to turn, reduces the need to use the abdominal muscles for turning, and minimizes incision pain.

4. **Breathe deeply, and practice splinting** any potential abdominal or chest incisions. Assist the patient to practice as needed.
   Facilitates comfort during movement.

5. **Pull on the bed rail** while pushing off with the right foot.
   Assists patient to turn to the left. ▼

6. **If the patient cannot maintain** this position independently, place a folded pillow or blanket along the back for support.

7. **Teach the patient to change** positions every 2 hours, repeating the turning process with the opposite arm and leg. For patients who need pillows placed for support, you will need to assist with turning.

Procedure 36-1C ■ Teaching Leg Exercises

➤ When performing the procedure, always identify your patient according to agency policy, using two identifiers, and be attentive to standard precautions, hand hygiene, patient safety and privacy, body mechanics, and documentation.

Leg exercises flex and extend the leg muscles to increase peripheral circulation and help prevent thrombus formation. Thrombus formation is a common postoperative complication.

Procedure Steps

1. **Instruct the patient to lie supine** in the bed.

   Note: *Although these exercises can be done when the patient is up in a chair, the effect will be diminished by gravity.*

2. **Perform ankle circles.** Instruct the patient to:
   a. Start with one foot in the dorsi-flexed position.
   b. Slowly rotate the ankle clockwise.
   c. After three rotations, repeat the procedure in a counterclockwise direction.
   d. Repeat this exercise at least three times in each direction, then switch and exercise the other ankle. ➤

3. **Perform ankle pumps.** Instruct the patient to:
   a. Start with one foot, leg extended.
   b. Point the toe until foot is plantar flexed.
   c. Pull the toes back toward the head until the foot is dorsiflexed; at the same time, press the back of the knee into the bed.
   d. Make sure the patient feels a pull, or a stretch, in the calf.
   e. Repeat the alternation between plantar flexion and dorsiflexion several times.
   f. Repeat the cycle with the other foot.

4. **Perform leg exercises.** Instruct the patient to:
   a. Lie supine in the bed.
   b. Slowly begin bending one knee, sliding the sole of the foot along the bed until the knee is in a flexed position. ▼

   c. Reverse the motion, extending the knee until the leg is once again flat on the bed. ▼

(continued on next page)

814 UNIT 4 Supporting Physiological Functioning

Procedure 36-1 ■ Teaching a Patient to Deep-Breathe, Cough, Move in Bed, and Perform Leg Exercises (continued)

d. Repeat several times.
e. Repeat using the opposite leg.

? What if . . .

■ **The patient has had knee, hip, or back surgery?**

Leg exercises may be contraindicated in patients having knee, hip, or back surgery. Check the surgeon's prescriptions and/or collaborate with the physical therapist.

■ **The patient has had nasal, ophthalmic, or neurological surgery?**

Coughing and deep-breathing exercises are contraindicated.
To avoid increasing intracranial pressure.

Evaluation

Make sure that the patient performs correctly a return demonstration of the procedures taught.

Documentation

In many healthcare facilities, checklists and charts have special areas in which to document patient teaching. Documentation should identify the person who completed the teaching, the person to whom the procedures were taught, what procedures were taught, and whether the patient understood the teaching. Also include the name and type of any printed materials given.

Sample Electronic Documentation

Note that because this is just one screen of a documentation system, not all of the information is visible. For example, you cannot see the date or the name of the nurse.

Practice Resources

Mekdad (2022); Saraceni et al. (2022); Vancouver Coastal Health (2014); Xin et al. (2022).

Thinking About the Procedure

The video **Teaching a Patient to Deep-Breathe and Cough, Teaching a Patient to Move in Bed,** and **Teaching Leg Exercises,** along with questions and suggested responses, is available on the **Davis's Nursing Skills Videos** Web site at www.fadavis.com.

CHAPTER 36 Caring for the Surgical Patient   815

Procedure 36-2 ■ Applying Antiembolism Stockings

▶ For steps to follow in *all* procedures, refer to the Universal Steps for All Procedures on the inside back cover.

Equipment
- Measuring tape
- Antiembolism stockings
- Disposable wipes or washcloth and towel (if needed to cleanse legs)
- Talcum powder (optional; check manufacturer's recommendations)

Delegation
You can delegate application of antiembolism stockings to unlicensed assistive personnel who have been trained in the task. Instruct the UAP as follows:
- Report the presence of any abnormalities on the lower extremities, such as lesions, sores, or redness, before applying the stockings.
- Instruct the patient to maintain a recumbent position for at least 15 minutes before applying the stockings.
- Do not massage the legs.
- Make sure there are no wrinkles in the stockings once they have been applied.

Preprocedure Assessment
- Assess the level of consciousness and cognitive ability.
  If the patient is unconscious or confused, you will need to call for assistance to hold and stabilize the lower extremities as you apply the stockings.
- Assess for signs and symptoms of severe peripheral arterial disease, such as weak or absent pulses, discoloration or cyanosis, or gangrene.
  Antiembolism stockings should not be used in patients with any of these findings because stockings compress the vessels and, therefore, further impede the already compromised arterial flow.
- Assess skin condition. Note lesions, dermatitis, or major edema, as evidenced by shiny, taut skin.
  If skin is overstretched by edema, antiembolism stockings may irritate or worsen skin conditions and cause skin breakdown.
- Note the patient's position and length of time they have been in that position.
  Place the patient supine for at least 15 minutes before stocking application. This prevents trapping of pooled venous blood.

▶ When performing the procedure, always identify your patient according to agency policy, using two identifiers, and be attentive to standard precautions, hand hygiene, patient safety and privacy, body mechanics, and documentation.

▶ If possible, apply stockings in the morning, before the patient gets out of bed. This prevents venous distention and edema that occur when the patient is sitting or standing.

Procedure Steps

1. **Measure the patient's lower extremities** to obtain the correct size stockings. This is critical to their effectiveness.
   Stockings must be sized correctly in order to apply the correct amounts of pressure at the ankle, midcalf, and upper thigh. If they are not tight enough, they will not improve venous return effectively. If they are too tight, they may compress the veins and impair circulation to the skin. ▼

For Thigh-High Stockings

✚ *Note:* Thigh-high elastic stockings have not proved to be more effective in preventing thromboembolism than knee-high ones, and should probably be avoided because of the tendency to roll and have a tourniquet effect (Gerhard-Herman et al., 2017).

   a. Measure the circumference of the upper thigh at the gluteal fold.
   The manufacturer of TED stockings recommends that thigh-high stockings not be applied if the thigh circumference exceeds 82 cm (32 in.). Use knee-high stockings instead.
   b. Measure the calf circumference at the widest section.
   c. Measure the distance from the gluteal fold to the base of the heel.

For Knee-High Stockings
   d. Measure the circumference of the calf at the widest section.
   e. Measure the distance from the base of the heel to the middle of the knee joint.
   Evidence is not conclusive, but increasingly supports the use of knee-high instead of thigh-high hose.

2. **Assist the patient to a supine** position, and instruct them to maintain that position for at least 15 minutes before you apply the stockings.
   Prevents trapping of pooled venous blood by the antiembolism stockings.

3. **Cleanse the patient's legs and** feet if necessary. Dry well.
   Removing surface dirt and bacteria will decrease the likelihood of infection and odor.

(continued on next page)

Procedure 36-2 ■ Applying Antiembolism Stockings (continued)

4. **Lightly dust the legs and feet** with talcum powder to ease the application of the stockings, if recommended by the manufacturer. **Key Point:** *Do not use powder if the patient is or is likely to become diaphoretic. Powder eases the application of the stockings, but perspiration will cause the powder to clump.*

5. **Holding one stocking at the top** cuff in your dominant hand, slide your nondominant arm down and into the stocking until your hand reaches the heel of the stocking.

6. **Grasp the center of the heel** with your hand inside the stocking, and then slowly turn the stocking inside out to the level of the heel with your other hand.
   The elastic in the stockings is very strong; this method is the easiest way to fit it over the foot and calf. ▼

7. **Ask the patient to point their toes** as you grasp the turned foot of the stocking and ease it onto their foot and heel (like putting on a sock). Center the patient's heel in the heel of the stocking.
   Ensures that the pressure of the stocking is over the correct anatomical areas.

8. **Gradually pull the remainder** of the stocking up and over the leg, turning it right side out as you proceed. Be certain the stocking is straight. ▼

For Knee-High Stockings
   a. Pull up to 2.5 to 5 cm (1 to 2 in.) below the knee.

For Thigh-High Stockings
   b. Pull up to the gluteal fold of the thigh, rotating inward so the gusset (triangular insert at the seam) is centered over the femoral artery, slightly toward the inside of the leg.
   Stockings apply varying amounts of compression between ankle, calf, and thigh areas. Keeping the stocking straight ensures that the pressure occurs over the correct areas.

9. **Smooth out any excess** material; keep stockings free of wrinkles and bunching.
   Decreases the risk of skin breakdown and areas of inappropriate and potentially dangerous constriction.

10. **When using stockings with closed toes,** tug gently on the stocking toe to create a small space between the end of the toes and the stocking.
    Prevents compression of small vessels in the toes, which may impede circulation.

11. **Repeat the procedure** on the other leg.

12. **Remove the stockings** and bathe and dry the legs daily.

13. **Launder the stockings** at least every 3 days; dry them on a flat surface.
    Soiled stockings can irritate the skin; dry flat to prevent stretching.

? What if...

- **Both legs do not measure the same?**
  Order two different sizes of stockings and use one from each package to make two pairs.

Evaluation

- Evaluate patient comfort.
  Severe, continuous discomfort may indicate that the stockings are the wrong size.
- Check the stockings for wrinkles and/or rolling down at the top, especially when sitting.
  Wrinkles and rolling down can cause skin breakdown and areas of constriction.
- Evaluate and monitor skin condition.
  Elastic stockings should be removed for 20 to 30 minutes every 8 to 12 hours to allow you to inspect the patient's skin and evaluate the adequacy of circulation.
- Evaluate the patient's ability to ambulate.
  It is important to reduce the time the patient is immobile due to pain, sedation, mechanical ventilation, and so on.
- Remeasure the legs regularly.
  To prevent complications related to swelling and weight gain.

Home Care

- Teach the client and/or caregiver to apply the stockings.
- Encourage the client to have two pairs of stockings on hand so that one pair can be used while the other is being laundered.
- Instruct the client to follow the manufacturer's directions for washing the stockings.
- Teach the client not to roll down the tops of the stockings.

Documentation

- To provide a baseline, document leg measurements and size of the stockings used.
- Document the time and date applied.
- Note the condition of the skin, including any abnormalities.

Sample Electronic Documentation

Note that because this is just one screen of a documentation system, not all of the information is visible. For example, you cannot see the date or the name of the nurse.

Practice Resources
Akyüz et al. (2021); American Association of Critical-Care Nurses (2016); Gee (2019).

Thinking About the Procedure

The video **Applying Antiembolism Stockings,** along with questions and suggested responses, is available on the **Davis's Nursing Skills Videos** Web site at www.fadavis.com.

Procedure 36-3 ■ Applying Sequential Compression Devices

> For steps to follow in *all* procedures, refer to the Universal Steps for All Procedures on the inside back cover.

Equipment

Note: Sequential compression devices may be referred to by several brand names, including SCDS (sequential compression decompression stockings), Flowtrons, and PAS (pneumatic air stockings).

- Compression pump, motor, or machine
- Connecting tubing, if applicable (in some devices, the tubing is preconnected to the sleeves)
- Compression sleeve (knee-high or thigh-high, depending on the order and the type of device)
- Elastic stockings (if also prescribed)
- Disposable wipes or washcloth and towel as needed to cleanse the lower extremities
- Measuring tape

Delegation

You may delegate the application of the sequential compression device to a UAP who has had training in that task. Instruct the UAP to report any redness, irritation, or open areas on the lower extremities. SCDs should not be removed for long periods because they are needed to support the patient's peripheral circulation. Instruct the UAP to ensure that all cords and connecting tubing are in a place that will not create a fall risk for the patient or visitors.

Preprocedure Assessment

- Assess cognitive level and level of consciousness.
  Patients with altered cognition may be at higher risk for falls related to the presence of the connecting tubing and attachment to the

(continued on next page)

Procedure 36-3 ■ Applying Sequential Compression Devices (continued)

compression pump. Patients who are unconscious will not be able to report a device that is creating too much pressure.

- Assess signs and symptoms of severe peripheral arterial disease, such as weak or absent pulses, discoloration or cyanosis, or gangrene.
  Increased compression of vessels by the sequential device may further impede arterial flow.

- Assess skin condition. Note lesions, dermatitis, or major edema, as evidenced by shiny, taut skin.
  If skin is overstretched by edema, the sequential compression sleeve may irritate or worsen skin conditions and cause skin breakdown.

> When performing the procedure, always identify your patient according to agency policy, using two identifiers, and be attentive to standard precautions, hand hygiene, patient safety and privacy, body mechanics, and documentation.

Procedure Steps

1. **Position the patient supine.**
   Prevents venous pooling. Allows for easier application of the compression sleeve.

2. **For thigh-high SCD sleeves,** measure the circumference and length of both thighs to ensure that the sleeves are of the proper size. Follow the manufacturer's instructions.

3. **Cleanse the lower extremities,** if necessary.
   Removes surface dirt and bacteria to decrease the likelihood of infection and odor.

4. **Apply elastic stockings** if they have been ordered in conjunction with the sequential compression device, following the steps in Procedure 36-2.

5. ✚ **Place the compression device pump** in a location near an electrical outlet so that the cord will not pose a fall risk. Plug in the pump.

   Note: Many compression pumps come equipped with hangers so you can hang the device at the bottom of the patient's bed.

6. **Apply the compression sleeve.** ▼

   For Knee-High length
   a. Open the Velcro fasteners on the sleeve.
   b. Place the sleeve under the lower leg below the knee, with the "air bladder" side down on the bed.
   c. Bring the ends of the sleeve up, and wrap them around the lower leg, leaving one to two fingerbreadths of space between the leg and the sleeve.
   Prevents excess pressure and overcompression.

   For Thigh-High Length
   d. Open the Velcro fasteners on the sleeve.
   e. Place the sleeve under the leg, ensuring that the knee opening is at the level of the knee joint and that the fastener will close on the anterior surface.
   Ensures that compression occurs over the correct structures. Prevents restricted range of motion (ROM) of the knee joint.
   f. Bring the ends of the sleeve up, and wrap them around the leg, leaving one to two fingerbreadths of space between the leg and the sleeve.
   Prevents excess pressure and overcompression.

7. **Connect the sleeve** to the compression pump.

8. **Turn the pump on** and, if applicable, set the compression pressure on the pump device to the manufacturer's recommended setting.

   Note: In some facilities, the compression pressure amount is preset and can be changed only by the central supply/equipment department.

Evaluation

After applying the device, make the following ongoing assessments:
- Inflation and deflation of the sleeve
  Ensures that the device is actually working.
- Kinking or pinching of the connecting tubing
  Interferes with inflation of sleeves and may cause overheating or malfunction of the unit.
- Circulation, sensation, and motion of the foot, including skin color, pulses, temperature, capillary refill, motion, and sensation

- Patient comfort
  Increasing discomfort may indicate excess or incorrect pressure.
- Skin condition. Remove the compression sleeves at intervals so that you can inspect skin and evaluate the adequacy of circulation.

  Note: If elastic stockings are being used in conjunction with the sequential compression device, follow the recommendations in Procedure 36-2.

- Signs and symptoms of deep vein thrombosis
  Even with sequential compression device therapy, a patient can still develop thrombi.

Patient Teaching

✚ Teach the patient to call for assistance when disconnecting the tubing from the compression pump to ambulate. *Prevents patient falls. The SCD tubing is a tripping hazard, and injuries from falls involving SCDs are likely to be more severe than injuries associated with general patient falls* (Edwards, et al., 2017).

Documentation

- Document the date and time you applied the device.
- Note the type and size (if applicable) of the compression sleeve used.
- Document the skin condition, including any abnormalities.

Sample Documentation

00/00/0000   1100.   Knee-high SCD applied per order. Skin warm, dry, and intact at time of application. Peripheral pulses palpable. Pt's wife instructed on use of SCD. Pt unresponsive. No evidence of discomfort, no grimace or movement with application. ——————— S. Bee, RN

Practice Resources

Edwards, et al. (2017); Sadaghianloo et al. (2016).

Thinking About the Procedure

➤ The video **Applying Sequential Compression Devices**, along with questions and suggested responses, is available on the **Davis's *Nursing Skills Videos*** Web site at www.fadavis.com.

Procedure 36-4 ■ Managing Gastric Suction

➤ For steps to follow in *all* procedures, refer to the Universal Steps for All Procedures on the inside back cover.

Equipment

Procedure 36-4A Initial Equipment Setup

- Nonsterile procedure gloves
- Suction source (either a portable machine or piped-in wall source)
- Suction container and tubing
- Stopcock (to connect the NG tube to suction tubing)

Procedure 36-4B Emptying the Suction Container

- PPE (gown, mask, face shield, clean nonsterile procedure gloves)
- Graduated container
  To measure gastric output when emptying the suction container. Not needed if suction canister is marked for measuring.
- Alcohol wipes or chlorhexidine-alcohol antiseptic product

Procedure 36-4C Irrigating the Nasogastric Tubing

- PPE (gown, mask, face shield, clean nonsterile procedure gloves)
- Irrigating set (basin and bulb syringe or catheter-tipped syringe)
- Normal saline irrigant (unless another irrigant is prescribed)
- Linen-saver pads

Procedure 36-4D Providing Comfort Measures

- Nonsterile procedure gloves
- Emesis basin, cup, and water for mouth care
- Water-soluble lubricant
- Cotton-tip applicators
- Tissues or damp washcloth

Note: This procedure assumes an NG or other enteric tube is already in place and that its correct placement has already been verified. If you need to insert an NG tube or check placement, refer to Chapter 24. Tubes for gastric decompression are typically large-lumen tubes such as a Salem sump or Levin tube. See the table at the end of this procedure for more information about tubes. ▼

(continued on next page)

Procedure 36-4 ■ Managing Gastric Suction (continued)

Delegation
A registered nurse should do the initial setup and any subsequent irrigation. You may delegate the UAP to empty and measure drainage and perform comfort measures. You must monitor equipment functioning and the patient's responses to the decompression. Instruct the UAP about observations that should be reported to you.

Preprocedure Assessments
- Determine that the NG tube has been inserted and placement has been verified.
- Verify the prescriber's order for type of tube and whether it is to be placed to suction or a drainage bag; also verify the type of suction to be used (low, high, continuous, intermittent).
- Auscultate for bowel sounds.
- Assess the patient's ability to cooperate with the procedure and understand explanations.
- Refer to the Evaluation section of this procedure. This procedure assumes an NG tube is already in place, so assessments are ongoing.

Procedure 36-4A ■ Initial Equipment Setup

➤ When performing the procedure, always identify your patient according to agency policy, using two identifiers, and be attentive to standard precautions, hand hygiene, patient safety and privacy, body mechanics, and documentation.

Procedure Steps

1. **Place the collection container** in the holder (either on the portable suction machine or on the wall). Plug the power cord into a grounded outlet if using a portable suction machine.

2. **Connect the short tubing** between the container and the suction source. In some systems, the port will be marked "vacuum."

3. **Connect the long suction tubing** to the container (it may be marked "patient"); if one is available, connect a stopcock to the open end nearest the patient.

4. **Don PPE as needed or per agency policy.**
   Helps prevent contaminations with body secretions and transfer of microorganisms.

5. **After the NG tube has been inserted** and placement verified, attach the end of the NG tube to the suction tubing.
   See Chapter 24 to review importance of tube placement. You must be certain the NG tube is in the stomach, not in the esophagus or airways.

6. **If the patient has a double-lumen** tube (e.g., Salem sump), instill 10 to 20 mL of air into the vent lumen to make sure it is patent. This should create a soft hissing sound.

7. **Check that the NG tube is secured** to the patient's nose and gown, or secure if needed (see Chapter 24 to review).
   Minimizes movement of the tube, helping to prevent irritation of the nares or other insertion site, as well as helping to keep the tube from migrating up out of the stomach.

8. **Turn on the suction source** to the prescribed amount. In an emergency when there is no order, always use low suction. Open the stopcock; note the direction of the arrows.

9. **Observe that drainage appears** in the collection container.
   It may take up to 5 minutes for air to be removed from the canister before the stomach contents will drain. ➤

Procedure 36-4B ■ Emptying the Suction Container

➤ When performing the procedure, always identify your patient according to agency policy, using two identifiers, and be attentive to standard precautions, hand hygiene, patient safety and privacy, body mechanics, and documentation.

1. **Don PPE as needed or according to agency policy.**
   Limits contamination with body secretions and the transfer of microorganisms.

2. **Turn off the suction source** and close the stopcock on the tubing (or clamp the tubing, if there is no stopcock).
   Prevents suction flow during emptying of the container.

3. **Empty the suction canister.**

   For a Suction Container Marked With Measurements
   Note the amount, color, and odor of the contents. Empty and rinse the container.

   For a Suction Container Not Marked Incrementally
   Remove the cap from the lid of the suction container and pour the drainage into a graduated measuring container. Note color, odor, and amount. Empty and rinse the container.
   A container with graduated markings enables you to monitor intake and output (I&O) accurately. Rinsing removes organic material that could be a reservoir for microorganisms.

4. **Wipe the port of the suction** container with an alcohol wipe. Place the suction container back in its holder and close the stopper on the lid.

5. **Turn on the suction source** to the prescribed amount. Note the direction of the arrows and turn the stopcock to the "on" position. If there is no stopcock, unclamp the tubing.

6. **Observe for proper functioning** of the suction and patency of the tubing.
   Prevents complications that would result from malfunction.

7. **Remove and discard your PPE.** Perform hand hygiene.

Procedure 36-4C ■ Irrigating the Nasogastric Tubing

➤ When performing the procedure, always identify your patient according to agency policy, using two identifiers, and be attentive to standard precautions, hand hygiene, patient safety and privacy, body mechanics, and documentation.

1. **Place a linen-saver pad** on the bed under the NG tube.

2. **Open the irrigation set** and pour saline into the basin.
   Water is not used because it may cause electrolyte imbalances.

3. **Place patient at a 30° to 45° elevation** (unless contraindicated or not tolerated).
   This position helps avoid gastric reflux of irrigant.

4. **Don PPE as needed or according to agency policy.**
   Limits contamination by body secretions and the transfer of microorganisms.

5. **Check for correct placement** of the NG tube using at least two bedside methods (see Chapter 24 as needed).
   Prevents accidental instillation of irrigant into the airways.

6. **Fill the syringe with 10 to 30 mL** of saline and place it on the linen-saver pad.

7. **Clamp the NG tube** or turn off the stopcock connected to the suction tubing. Then disconnect the NG tube from the suction tubing.
   Prevents backflow of drainage and soiling of linens and clothing.

8. **Hold the drainage tubing up** until suction clears it. Then place it on the linen-saver pad or hook it over the suction machine.
   Keeps secretions from soiling the bed linens or clothing.

9. **Turn off the suction machine.**

10. **Unclamp the NG tube** or turn on the stopcock.

11. **Unpin the NG tube** (or remove tape) from the patient's clothing.

12. **Attach the syringe and instill** the irrigant slowly into the NG tube. Do not force the solution. Be careful not to instill fluid into the air vent.
    Clears the NG tube of gastric contents to keep it patent and helps keep the tube from adhering to the gastric mucosa. Partially digested food, clotted blood, or tissue debris may clog the tube and prevent effective drainage.

13. **Lower the end of the NG tube** and then release the syringe bulb (or, depending on the type of syringe, pull back the plunger) to withdraw fluid. Instill and withdraw until fluid flows in and out freely.
    Uses the force of gravity with negative pressure to withdraw instilled fluid and gastric contents.

    For a Double-Lumen NG Tube
    Draw 30 mL of air into the syringe and inject it into the "pigtail" (the smaller-bore tube). Follow agency policy for this.
    This clears the air-vent tube of any secretions. It must be patent in order to equalize pressure and prevent gastric tissue trauma at the drainage ports. The air also keeps the tube from draining fluid out of the stomach by capillary action.

(continued on next page)

UNIT 4 Supporting Physiological Functioning

Procedure 36-4 ■ Managing Gastric Suction (continued)

14. **Reclamp the NG tube** or turn off the stopcock.
    Prevents backflow of drainage.

15. **Reconnect the NG tube** to the suction tube. Then release the clamp or turn on the stopcock.

16. **Reattach the NG tube** to the patient's clothing (with a pin or tape—see Chapter 24 as needed).
    Prevents pulling on and irritating the patient's nostril.

17. **Provide comfort measures** (e.g., mouth care).

18. **Remove and discard PPE.** Perform hand hygiene.

Procedure 36-4D ■ Providing Comfort Measures

➤ When performing the procedure, always identify your patient according to agency policy, using two identifiers, and be attentive to standard precautions, hand hygiene, patient safety and privacy, body mechanics, and documentation.

1. **Don PPE as needed or according to agency policy.**

2. **Provide mouth care** (see Procedures 22-6, 22-7, and 22-8 if you need to review). Use mouthwash as desired. Avoid using lemon-glycerine swabs. Apply water-soluble lubricant to the lips if they become dry and crusty.
   The patient most likely has a dry mouth from not receiving oral intake and from mouth breathing. Lemon-glycerine swabs cause even more drying of tissues.

3. **Remove nasal secretions** with a tissue or a damp washcloth. Moisten a cotton-tip applicator and wipe the inside of each nostril. If secretions are encrusted, moisten the applicator with hydrogen peroxide, then follow with an applicator moistened with water.
   To soften, dissolve, and remove secretions and prevent tissue irritation.

4. **Apply a small amount of** water-soluble lubricant to the inside of each nostril.
   Soothes and softens dried skin. Avoid petroleum-based lubricants, as complications may occur if they are inhaled.

5. **Check that the tape or tube** fixation device is secure. If it is not, replace it (see Procedure 24-2 as needed).
   Prevents irritation of the nasal skin and mucosa. Helps prevent migration of the NG tube from the stomach.

? What if...

■ **I get resistance when irrigating the NG tube?**

Check the tubing for kinks or evidence of obstruction. Have the patient turn to the left side.
Turning to one side changes the position of the distal tip of the NG tube.

■ **The patient complains that the NG tube is pulling against the nostril?**

The tube may not be properly anchored to their clothing. Reattach the safety pin (or tape) closer to the nose so that there is more slack in the tube.

■ **The NG tube causes excoriation of the nares?**

Remove the tape or fixation device from the nose. Remove the residual adhesive from the skin. Apply skin sealant and anchor the tube so that the adhesive touches in a different place on the skin. Keep the excoriated areas clean and dry.

■ **The NG tube does not drain?**

Check tubing for kinks or blockage. Check the suction apparatus. If the collection container is higher than the patient's abdomen, lower it. If these aspects are working properly, irrigate the tube (see Procedure 36-4C, preceding). If the tube still is not draining and the patient is uncomfortable, document and notify the primary care provider. Encourage the patient to relax and breathe slowly through the nose. If the patient has abdominal distention, pain, or vomiting, notify the provider immediately.

✚ *If the container is too high, the negative pressure of low suction may not be enough to overcome the force of gravity. Abdominal distention, pain, or vomiting may mean the system is not working. Continued distention creates undue strain on the suture line. You should notify the care provider of these symptoms even when the mechanical aspects of the suction seem in working order.*

Gastric Decompression Tubes

TYPE	LUMEN(S)	USE	MANAGEMENT	DISCUSSION
Levin	1, unvented	Decompression, feedings, or irrigation	Use low intermittent suction; may require irrigation.	If the tube opening(s) rest(s) against the gastric mucosa, the suction may irritate or injure the tissue.
Salem Sump	2	Decompression, suction, gastric lavage	Vented. May use high continuous suction.	The air vent helps keep the tube away from the gastric mucosa during suction.
Sengsten–Blakemore	3	Decompression; treatment of active bleeding from esophageal or gastric varices	Use low intermittent suction.	Gastric or esophageal balloons hold the tube in place.
Cantor	1, unvented	Decompression	Use intermittent suction.	Distal end is weighted with a balloon. Used in bowel obstruction. Rarely used because of the hazard posed by the mercury in the weighted balloon.
Miller–Abbott	2	Decompression	Use intermittent suction.	Distal end weighted with a balloon. Used in bowel obstruction. Rarely used because it contains mercury in the weighted balloon.
Ewald or other very large-bore tube		May be passed orally for emergency evacuation of stomach contents to prevent absorption of ingested medications, poisons, or products. A piston-tip syringe is placed on the end of the tube for manual suction. Typically the stomach is washed repeatedly with saline and all contents are withdrawn. Because of its large diameter, this type of tube is not tolerated by patients who are alert, and is not left in place after lavage is completed.		
Weighted small-bore tubes (e.g., Keofeed)		For feedings only. Suction collapses the tube.		

Evaluation and Maintenance

- Periodically assess placement of the tube by a combination of methods (i.e., by checking pH of aspirate, by listening over the stomach with a stethoscope while injecting air into the tube, and by reviewing radiographic reports). See Chapter 24 for review, as needed.
- Monitor patency of the tube and the effectiveness of the suction. Check tube connections.
- Monitor patient comfort (e.g., sore throat).
  The continuing presence of a tube in the nose and throat is bothersome to patients. The major nuisance is the pressure of the tube against the internal mucous membranes, irritating the nostril, pharynx, and esophagus.
- Auscultate for bowel sounds; turn off suction while auscultating.
  Bowel sounds indicate the return of peristalsis and the success of gastric decompression. You may hear the sound of the suction apparatus and misinterpret it as bowel sounds.
- Monitor for gastric distention, vomiting, and abdominal pain.
  These symptoms probably indicate the suction is not working effectively. See the What If... section, preceding.
- Examine skin and mucous membranes around the insertion site (e.g., nares, abdomen).
- Follow agency policy or the primary care provider's prescription for irrigation of the gastric tube. It is common to irrigate with 10 to 30 mL of normal saline every 3 to 4 hours.
- Monitor the color of the drainage (should be green to gold). If there is blood in the drainage, notify the primary care provider.
- For patients undergoing prolonged GI suction, observe for signs and symptoms of hyponatremia and hypokalemia (i.e., fatigue, lethargy, confusion, seizures, muscle weakness, paresthesia, and cardiac dysrhythmias). Review laboratory results and report any symptoms to the primary care provider.

(continued on next page)

Procedure 36-4 ■ Managing Gastric Suction (continued)

- Assess the patient's ability to move about in bed while attached to the suction source.

Patient Teaching
- Instruct the patient to notify you of any discomfort and to not tug on or try to reposition the NG tube if it becomes uncomfortable.
- Instruct the patient to notify you if feeling nauseated. *This could mean the tube is blocked and not draining effectively.*

Home Care
Usually, gastric suction is performed in a hospital. If the client is to go home with gastric suction (e.g., a terminally ill person who has a bowel obstruction and wants to be in his or her own home), teach the family how to use the device before discharge. Also arrange for home healthcare.

Documentation
- Record all drainage as output on the I&O record.
- Record the time, type, and volume of irrigations and the drainage returned.
- Be sure to include irrigation fluids as input on the I&O record.
- Note color, odor, and consistency of drainage.
- Document patient's emotional and physical responses to NG intubation.
- Document any evidence of tube or equipment malfunction.
- Document epigastric pain, discomfort, distention, or vomiting.

Practice Resources
Best practices: Evidence-based nursing procedures (2nd ed.) (2007); Hayes & Hayes (2018); Liu et al. (2021); Thompson (2019).

Thinking About the Procedure

The video **Managing Gastric Suction: Initial Equipment Setup, Emptying the Suction Container, and Irrigating the Nasogastric Tubing,** along with questions and suggested responses, is available on the **Davis's *Nursing Skills Videos*** Web site at www.fadavis.com.

CLINICAL INSIGHTS

Clinical Insight 36-1 ➤ Preoperative Teaching

Explain What to Expect Before Surgery

- Explain the planned preoperative testing—laboratory tests, x-ray studies, ECG, and so on.
- Discuss skin preparation, including preoperative wash with an antibacterial product, if this is included in the treatment plan.
- Discuss prescribed preoperative medications.
- Outline activities that will occur before surgery, such as insertion of an IV, placement of a urinary catheter, or cardiac monitoring.
- Review the preoperative restriction of fluid and food.
- Tell the patient that a member of the anesthesia team will speak to them about the proposed anesthesia before surgery.
- If the patient is having surgery on the gastrointestinal (GI) tract, an additional bowel prep may be ordered (e.g., a low-residue diet beginning 1 week before surgery, and a liquid diet for the 48 hours preceding surgery). Patients having GI surgery also may have enemas before surgery.
- Explain the need to remove jewelry, makeup, hearing aids, glasses, contact lenses, and any removable dental prostheses before being transported to the operating suite. It is best to have a family member take valuable belongings home for safekeeping.
- Give the patient and family a tentative schedule for the operative day, including the time to arrive at the hospital or surgery center.

Explain What to Expect in the Operative Suite

- Inform the patient and family where they can go to wait during surgery.
- Describe the operating room and the activities that the patient may anticipate before the surgery.
- Describe the types of people who may be present in the operative suite. This is particularly important if the patient is not receiving a general anesthetic.
- Explain that the anesthesiologist or nurse anesthetist will monitor the patient and is responsible for keeping the patient comfortable with medications throughout the entire procedure.
- Describe the activities that may occur in the preoperative holding area.

Explain What to Expect After Surgery

- Explain that the patient will initially be cared for in the postanesthesia care unit. After a period of observation, the patient will be transferred to the surgical unit. Note that some patients may be transferred directly to a critical care unit after surgery. If this is expected, tell the patient and family about this preoperatively.
- Family may visit after the patient has been admitted and assessed on the surgical unit.
- Tell the patient what to expect in terms of dressings, equipment, and monitoring devices.
- Describe the types of assessments that will be performed.
- Explain that pain medication will be given to keep the patient comfortable. If the patient has pain, tell the nursing staff.
- Discuss the usual progression of recovery, including activity level, deep breathing, coughing, leg exercises, and dietary intake.
- Discuss the usual progression of recovery, including activity level, deep breathing and coughing, leg exercises, and dietary intake.
- Discuss the anticipated length of stay.
- Teach the patient how to move into and out of bed after surgery.
- Teach the importance of deep breathing and coughing, especially after general anesthesia. Demonstrate how to splint the incision to facilitate deep breathing and coughing. Refer to Procedure 36-1.
- Teach and emphasize the importance of leg exercises to minimize the risk of thrombus formation. Refer to Procedure 36-1.
- If decreased activity or prolonged bedrest is anticipated, explain the use of antiembolism stockings or sequential compression devices. Refer to Procedure 36-2.

Note: If the patient is to be discharged the day of surgery, inform the patient in advance about what to wear to the facility, and explain that they must arrange for a responsible adult to drive home.

Clinical Insight 36-2 ▶ Preparing a Room for a Patient's Return From Surgery

In many institutions, the patient is transported to surgery using the bed that is in his hospital room, so these steps may vary.
- Put clean linens on the bed, including pads to protect the linen from drainage.
- Fold the linens back to the end of the bed.
- Raise the bed to stretcher height, and lock the wheels.
- Move furniture and equipment so that the stretcher can be placed directly against the bed.
- If needed, set up suction, oxygen, or other special equipment.
- Place the following equipment in the room:
  - Stethoscope, manometer, thermometer (to measure vital signs)
  - IV pole
  - Emesis basin
  - Tissues
  - A clean gown, washcloth, and towel
  - Extra pillows for positioning the patient

Clinical Insight 36-3 ▶ Creating an Operative Field

- A nonsterile team member (usually the circulating nurse) performs a surgical prep, using a scrub agent and "paint," to cleanse the operative site. Antiseptic agents must be approved by the U.S. Food and Drug Administration and by the agency's infection control professional. Chlorhexidine and povidone-iodine solutions are most commonly used.
- The **operative field** encompasses the patient and the immediate surrounding area.
- Creation of the sterile field proceeds as follows:
  - Don head covering and shoe covers before entering the surgical suite.
  - Perform a surgical scrub.
- Don sterile gown, gloves, and other surgical attire (e.g., mask).
- Cover the area surrounding the operative site with sterile drapes so that only the patient's operative area is exposed.
- Place sterile draping over the remainder of the patient's body.
- In most cases, suspend a vertical drape at neck level so the patient's head and airway are accessible to the anesthesiologist or nurse anesthetist (who is not sterile). For neurosurgery, even the head is draped, and the anesthesiologist or nurse anesthetist sits to the side of the head.

ASSESSMENT GUIDELINES AND TOOLS

Example of a Preoperative Checklist (AORN)

Focused Assessment

AORN SAMPLE Preoperative Assessment Form *(Facility Name and Address)* NOTE: This record is a sample only. Clinical records should be customized to incorporate data fields that represent the setting, facility, procedure, and patient. Reproductions and variations are encouraged, provided credit is given to AORN.	Addressograph (Patient Information: name, age, gender, medical record number, date)

Date:_____

Structural Data:

Admitted via: ☐ Ambulatory ☐ Wheelchair ☐ Stretcher ☐ Other assistive devices:_____ Admitted from: ☐ Home ☐ Transferring hospital ☐ Acute rehab facility ☐ Extended/skilled care facility	Identity confirmed (I26): ☐ Yes ☐ No Advance directive signed: ☐ Yes ☐ No Location:_____

Date of preoperative assessment:_____
 	
Planned procedure:_____
 	
Language(s) spoken: ☐ English ☐ Spanish ☐ Other:____
	Operative procedure, surgical site, and laterality verified (I143): ☐ Yes ☐ No
	Consent for planned procedures verified (I124):
	  ☐ Yes ☐ No
	NPO status verified (I138): ☐ Yes ☐ No
	  Since: (date/time)_____

☐ Patient's records, belongings, valuables secured (I115) Belonging inventory: ☐ Watch ☐ Jewelry ☐ Contacts/glasses ☐ Dentures/partial(s) ☐ Hearing aid	Preadmission testing ☐ CBC_____ ☐ Urinalysis_____ ☐ Potassium level___ ☐ EKG_____ ☐ CXR_____ ☐ Pregnancy test:_____ ☐ Type and cross # of units:_____

Nursing Data Elements:

General health status: (check when present)
☐ Diabetes ☐ Cancer ☐ Obesity ☐ Pregnancy
☐ Hematologic disorders (anemia, sickle cell disease or conditions)
 	
☐ Vital signs:
  Temperature:_____ Pulse:_____ BP:_____
  Respirations:_____ Height:_____ Weight:_____
 	
☐ Allergies verified (note type of reaction) (I123)
  Latex allergy: ☐ Yes ☐ No
  Medications: ☐ Yes:_____ ☐ No
  _____
  _____
  Food: ☐ Yes:_____ ☐ No
  _____
 	
☐ Daily medications (prescription, OTC, vitamins, alternative medication, herbal remedies, chemotherapy):
_____
_____
_____
Medications taken day of surgery:_____
 	
☐ Alcohol/Drug social use:_____
 	
☐ **Neurologic assessment:** ☐ Alert and oriented
  ☐ Speech intact ☐ Follows simple commands
  ☐ Risk of falls ☐ History of seizures
  LOC: ☐ Alert/oriented ☐ Drowsy ☐ Sedated
    ☐ Asleep ☐ Unresponsive ☐ Disoriented
    ☐ Other:_____
 	
☐ **Sensory assessment:**
  ☐ No limitations ☐ Hearing impairment ☐ Visual impairment
	☐ **Cardiovascular assessment:**
	  ☐ Pacemaker ☐ Implanted defibrillator
	  ☐ Chest pain
	  ☐ Peripheral edema: Location:_____
	  ☐ DVT/PE risk:
	    ☐ None ☐ Low ☐ Med ☐ High
	  _____
	  _____
	
	☐ **Respiratory assessment:**
	  ☐ Tracheotomy
	  ☐ Intubated
	  ☐ Chest tube
	  Respirations: ☐ Regular ☐ Labored
	  Smoking history ☐ Yes ☐ No
	    Packs/day:____ Years smoked:_____
	    Quit date:_____
	  ☐ Cough ☐ Cold symptoms
	  ☐ Current or recent respiratory infection
	  ☐ Preexisting respiratory problems (specify):
	    _____
	    _____
	
	☐ **Musculoskeletal assessment:**
	  ☐ No limitations
	  ☐ Paralysis
	  ☐ Traction
	  ☐ Limited ROM
	  ☐ Amputation:_____
	  ☐ Prosthesis:_____

(Continued)

Example of a Preoperative Checklist (AORN)—cont'd

Nursing Data Elements (continued):

☐ **Skin assessment:**
  ☐ Cool ☐ Warm ☐ Intact
  ☐ Dry ☐ Moist
  ☐ Body jewelry removed
  ☐ Makeup removed
  ☐ Tattoos: _____
  ☐ Rash: _____
  ☐ Bruises: _____
  ☐ Wounds: _____
  ☐ Ostomy: _____
  ☐ Catheter/Drain: _____
  ☐ Venous access device: _____

☐ **Gastrointestinal assessment:**
  Last bowel movement (date/time): _____
  Usual diet: _____
  _____

  Recent unexplained weight loss
  ☐ Yes: Amount: _____ Time frame: _____
  ☐ No
  Problems chewing or swallowing
  ☐ Yes ☐ No
  Special needs:
  ☐ Chewing ☐ Swallowing
  ☐ Appetite ☐ Diet preferences

☐ **Genitourinary/Gynecology assessment:**
  ☐ Voided on call to OR
    Time: _____ Amount: _____
  ☐ Urinary catheter: Amount in bag: _____
  ☐ Urinary incontinence

☐ **Psychosocial assessment:**
  ☐ Calm/relaxed ☐ Anxious ☐ Talkative
  ☐ Crying ☐ Restless ☐ Withdrawn
  ☐ Other: _____
  ☐ Concerns regarding surgery or hospitalization:
  _____
  ☐ Religious/cultural concerns/requests:
  _____
  ☐ Receives help from:
    ☐ Children ☐ Support person
    ☐ Other (specify):
  _____
  ☐ Patient cares for:
    ☐ Children: Ages: _____
    ☐ Self ☐ Spouse
    ☐ Other (specify):
  _____

☐ Determine level of knowledge (I135):
  ☐ Barriers to learning: _____
  ☐ Motivation to learn
    ☐ excellent ☐ average ☐ limited

☐ Abuse screening
  Have you ever felt threatened verbally, emotionally, or physically in any of your relationships?
  ☐ Yes ☐ No
  Have you been hit, slapped, kicked, or otherwise physically hurt by an intimate partner?
  ☐ Yes ☐ No
  Are you afraid of your partner or anyone you live with?
  ☐ Yes ☐ No
  If yes, describe and make appropriate referral

☐ **Pain assessment**
  ☐ Instructed on use of pain scale
  ☐ Pain assessment (0-10): _____
    Location: _____

☐ **Discharge planning**
  Will require assistance after discharge
  ☐ Yes ☐ No
  Discharge plan:
  ☐ Home
  ☐ Home nursing service
  ☐ Short-term care facility
  ☐ Extended care facility
  ☐ Other: _____

Individual who will escort patient home:
Name: _____
Phone number: _____
Relationship: _____

Comments:
_____
_____
_____
_____

Preoperative nursing diagnoses
☐ Anxiety/fear (X4)
☐ Therapeutic regimen management ineffective (X33)
☐ Deficient knowledge (X30)
☐ Risk for injury (X29)
☐ Pain (X38)
☐ Other: _____

Comments:

RN Signature:
X

Source: Reprinted with permission from AORN Perioperative Patient-Focused Model. Copyright 2011 AORN, Inc, 2170 Paker Rd., Suite 300, Denver, CO 80231. All rights reserved.

Focused Assessment

Intraoperative Care Questionnaire

Common nursing interview questions include the following:
- What is your name?
- What type of surgery are you going to have today?
- Is someone here with you?
- Are you allergic to any medications, latex, or tape?
- When is the last time that you had anything to eat or drink?
- Do you have false teeth, contact lenses, or any other prostheses that need to be removed?
- Have you taken any medications today?
- Do you have any implants, such as metal plates or a pacemaker?
- Do you have any scratches, bruises, or other wounds on your body at this time?
- Are there any parts of your body that are painful, such as a stiff shoulder or leg?

Also see the WHO Surgical Safety Checklist, following.

Focused Assessment

Example of a Surgical Safety Checklist

Surgical Safety Checklist — World Health Organization | Patient Safety — A World Alliance for Safer Health Care

Before induction of anaesthesia → **Before skin incision** → **Before patient leaves operating room**

(with at least nurse and anaesthetist) | (with nurse, anaesthetist and surgeon) | (with nurse, anaesthetist and surgeon)

Before induction of anaesthesia

Has the patient confirmed his/her identity, site, procedure, and consent?
☐ Yes

Is the site marked?
☐ Yes
☐ Not applicable

Is the anaesthesia machine and medication check complete?
☐ Yes

Is the pulse oximeter on the patient and functioning?
☐ Yes

Does the patient have a:

Known allergy?
☐ No
☐ Yes

Difficult airway or aspiration risk?
☐ No
☐ Yes, and equipment/assistance available

Risk of >500ml blood loss (7ml/kg in children)?
☐ No
☐ Yes, and two IVs/central access and fluids planned

Before skin incision

☐ Confirm all team members have introduced themselves by name and role.

☐ Confirm the patient's name, procedure, and where the incision will be made.

Has antibiotic prophylaxis been given within the last 60 minutes?
☐ Yes
☐ Not applicable

Anticipated Critical Events

To Surgeon:
☐ What are the critical or non-routine steps?
☐ How long will the case take?
☐ What is the anticipated blood loss?

To Anaesthetist:
☐ Are there any patient-specific concerns?

To Nursing Team:
☐ Has sterility (including indicator results) been confirmed?
☐ Are there equipment issues or any concerns?

Is essential imaging displayed?
☐ Yes
☐ Not applicable

Before patient leaves operating room

Nurse Verbally Confirms:
☐ The name of the procedure
☐ Completion of instrument, sponge and needle counts
☐ Specimen labelling (read specimen labels aloud, including patient name)
☐ Whether there are any equipment problems to be addressed

To Surgeon, Anaesthetist and Nurse:
☐ What are the key concerns for recovery and management of this patient?

This checklist is not intended to be comprehensive. Additions and modifications to fit local practice are encouraged.

Revised 1 / 2009 © WHO, 2009

Source: Reprinted with permission from the World Health Organization. Retrieved from http://apps.who.int/iris/bitstream/10665/44186/2/9789241598590_eng_Checklist.pdf

Focused Assessment

Postanesthesia Assessment: Essential Elements

The Association of periOperative Registered Nurses (AORN) (2020) has identified the essential elements of assessment in the PACU.

- **Vital signs**
  - Blood pressure, cuff or arterial
  - Respiratory rate, respiratory competence, and breath sounds
  - Respiratory adequacy, including skin color and condition
  - Temperature (record type of measurement used, for example, skin, tympanic, oral)
  - Pulse (apical and peripheral)
  - Oxygen saturation (e.g., pulse oximeter reading)
- **Peripheral circulation** (postoperative tissue perfusion), for example, peripheral pulses and sensation at extremities
- **Neurological status,** including pupil response and intracranial pressure (if indicated)
- **Mental status,** including level of consciousness, alertness, lucidity, orientation
- **Intravenous therapy,** including patency, location of sites, rates of solution(s), and/or blood products infusing
- **Allergies and sensitivities**
- **Pain**
- **Motor abilities,** including return of sensory and motor control in areas affected by local or regional anesthetics
- **Skin integrity**
- **Temperature regulation**
- **Positioning**
- **Surgical incision site,** including condition of suture line(s) if visible
- **Nausea and vomiting**
- **Fluid and electrolyte balance**
- **Safety needs** (e.g., side rails raised)
- **Central venous pressure (CVP), pulmonary wedge pressure**
- **Airway:** patency, presence of artificial airway, mechanical ventilator settings
- **Condition of dressing(s)**
- **Drainage,** including type; patency; and amount and type of drainage from dressings, tubes, and catheters

DIAGNOSTIC TESTING

Common Preoperative Screening Tests

Test	Uses
Urinalysis	To detect urinary tract infections (UTIs) and the presence of glucose or protein in the urine, which may indicate poorly controlled diabetes or renal disease
Complete blood count (CBC)	To detect irregularities in hemoglobin (Hgb) and hematocrit (Hct)
	A low Hgb level is an indication of anemia, which may place the client at risk if significant blood loss occurs
	Measures white blood cell (WBC) count as an indicator of immune function
	Measures platelet count, which affects clotting ability
ECG	To detect cardiac dysrhythmias (electrocardiogram) and other cardiac pathology
Chest x-ray	To detect for or evaluate underlying pulmonary disease; also to reveal heart size as an indicator of heart function
Blood type and crossmatch	To identify blood type in the event that blood transfusion becomes necessary
Serum electrolytes	To detect sodium, potassium, chloride, magnesium, calcium, and pH imbalances, which affect cardiac and other organ function and fluid balance
Fasting blood sugar	To detect diabetes or poorly controlled diabetes
Comprehensive metabolic panel	Includes electrolytes, blood glucose, liver function tests (ALT, AST), serum albumin and protein, and renal function tests (BUN and creatinine); used to detect underlying health problems that may affect surgical risk or outcome

CLINICAL REASONING
Applying the Full-Spectrum Nursing Model

PATIENT SITUATION

Recall Nishad Singh (Meet Your Patient, in Volume 1). He is a 68-year-old patient who came to the emergency department (ED) with sudden-onset of rectal bleeding. He had been "tired and dragging for several months." The ED nurse identified nursing diagnoses of mild anxiety, pain, and risk for bleeding. Preoperatively, his vital signs were as follows:

BP: 138/88 mm Hg
Pulse: 104 beats/min and regular; 120 beats/min; 134 beats/min
Respiratory rate: 20 breaths/min
Temperature: 36.7°C (98.0°F)
Oxygen saturation: 98%

Mr. Singh was admitted to the hospital where he received an IV of 1,000 mL of lactated Ringer's solution and a unit of packed red blood cells. He was to undergo emergency colon resection surgery; however, a left hemicolectomy including the sigmoid colon and the anus was required. He spent 4 hours in the PACU, until his vital signs stabilized. Mr. Singh now has a colostomy high in his descending colon, with a stoma on his left abdomen slightly superior to the level of his umbilicus. He also has an abdominal incision that was made for exploration. On the next day after the surgery, the surgeon informed Mr. Singh that he has widespread adenocarcinoma (cancer) of the colon with metastasis to the liver. The nurse has identified these four nursing diagnoses (among others):

Knowledge deficit (colostomy care) r/t lack of prior experience and no preparation before surgery
Fear r/t diagnosis of colon cancer, liver metastasis, and possible terminal illness
Pain secondary to surgical incision and manipulation of abdominal organs during the surgical procedure
Risk for impaired skin integrity r/t irritation from fecal drainage and ostomy pouch

THINKING

1. *Theoretical Knowledge:*

   a. What is a left hemicolectomy? If you do not know the answer, consult an appropriate reference.

   b. What does metastasis to the liver mean? If you do not know the answer, consult an appropriate reference.

2. *Critical Thinking (Inquiry):*

   a. Why might Mr. Singh have needed a colostomy instead of having his transverse colon reconnected to the remaining lower colon or rectum? State the reference you used to answer this question.

   b. Why do you think Mr. Singh has a colostomy above the level of the umbilicus and not lower down in his abdomen? State the reference you used to answer this question.

DOING

3. *Practical Knowledge:* Mr. Singh returned from surgery with knee-high antiembolism stockings.

   a. You notice that the stockings have slid down and become wrinkled between his knees and ankles. After you straighten them and pull them up, the tops reach to about 7.6 cm (3 in.) below Mr. Singh's knees. What does this probably mean, and what should you do?

   b. Which of the following instructions should you give when delegating care of Mr. Singh's antiembolism stockings to the nursing assistant? (Mr. Singh's stockings have closed toes.)

   - Remove the stockings and bathe and dry the legs every 8 to 12 hours.

   - Massage the legs after removing Mr. Singh's stockings.

   - Before reapplying stockings, report the presence of any lesions, sores, or redness of the lower extremities.

- Instruct the patient to remain supine for at least 15 minutes after removing the stockings.

- Make sure there are no wrinkles in the stockings once they have been applied.

- Tug gently on the end of the stocking to create a small space between the end of the toes and the stocking.

4. *Nursing Process (Nursing Diagnosis/Analyzing Cues):* List Mr. Singh's four nursing diagnoses in order of priority. List the highest priority first. Explain how you decided the priorities.

CARING

5. *Self-Knowledge:*

    a. If you were assigned to care for Mr. Singh today, what aspect of care would you feel best prepared to give? Explain your thinking.

    b. What aspect of Mr. Singh's care would you be most uncomfortable providing? Explain your thinking.

6. *Ethical Knowledge:* You want to provide culturally competent care. What is the first thing you will need to do to address Mr. Singh's cultural needs? Review Chapter 12 if you need to.

Critical Thinking and Clinical Judgment

1. You are speaking with several classmates about an upcoming surgical rotation. During the rotation, you will have an opportunity to work with a circulating nurse and a scrub nurse. One of your classmates says that they are very nervous. "I don't know whether I will be able to handle this rotation. I'm afraid I might not be able to watch the surgery. I've never really seen anything gross like that before." Another classmate confides that they are worried that they will contaminate everything and put the patient at risk. What advice can you give your classmates, and what actions can you take to prepare yourself for your experience in the OR?

2. You are working on a busy surgical unit on the evening shift. There is one UAP on the unit this evening. You are caring for the following patients:

    - Mr. Singh (Meet Your Patient, in Volume 1), underwent a colon resection and colostomy for colon cancer. He is now in postoperative day 2. Mr. Singh is complaining of chest pain and shortness of breath.

    - Ms. Yasmin is a 52-year-old patient admitted to the unit from PACU 1 hour ago after total abdominal hysterectomy and bilateral salpingo-oophrectomy (TAH-BSO—removal of the uterus, ovaries, and fallopian tubes).

    - Steven Stellanski, a 16-year-old patient with trisomy 21, underwent an emergency appendectomy early this morning.

    The PACU calls to inform you that they are ready to transport Mrs. Bauer back to the unit. She is an 87-year-old patient from the local skilled nursing facility who underwent an extensive debridement of a stage IV pressure injury on the coccyx. The PACU nurse tells you Mrs. Bauer is confused and agitated and will need close monitoring.

    a. What problem(s) does admission of this new patient present for you? To answer this question, identify the priority nursing activity for each of the three patients you already have, as well as for Mrs. Bauer.

    b. How will you handle this situation? Identify three options, and explain their advantages and disadvantages.

3. You will be caring for a 23-year-old patient who underwent emergency surgery after an automobile accident. He has had no preoperative teaching. What concerns does this raise for you? How will you address these concerns?

4. For each of the following concepts, use critical thinking to describe how or why it is important to nursing, patient care, or perioperative nursing. Note that these are *not* to be merely definitions.

Preoperative teaching

Preoperative physical preparation

Intraoperative safety measures

Anesthesia

Postoperative complications

What Are the Main Points in This Chapter?

- Perioperative nursing includes care of patients during the preoperative, intraoperative, and postoperative phases.
- Caring for the surgical patient requires the systematic integration and synthesis of the nursing process with established standards of practice.
- The Association of periOperative Registered Nurses (AORN) is the organization that developed the standards of care that inform perioperative nursing and the standardized language, the Perioperative Nursing Data Set (PNDS).
- "Never events" are serious and costly errors resulting in severe consequences for the patient and are mostly preventable. Medicare will not reimburse institutions for care related to complications caused by never events.
- Surgical risk is associated with the type of surgery and the condition of the patient (e.g., age, general health, personal habits).
- During the preoperative period, it is essential to determine whether the patient is physiologically, cognitively, and psychologically prepared for the intraoperative and postoperative phases of surgery.
- Preoperative care includes assessment, preoperative teaching, confirming that surgical consent has been obtained; preventing wrong patient, wrong site, wrong surgery; communicating with the surgical team; preparing the patient physically for surgery; transferring the patient to the operative suite; and preparing the postoperative room on the surgical unit.
- The surgical consent form is a witnessed legal document that ensures that the surgical patient has given informed consent for the surgical procedure. The physician is legally responsible for obtaining informed consent; however, the nurse sometimes obtains the patient's signature on the form after verifying that the patient has been informed.
- A great deal of perioperative nursing care is standardized, aimed at preventing potential complications, and applicable to all patients having surgery.
- General anesthesia produces rapid unconsciousness and loss of sensation. Regional anesthesia produces loss of pain sensation without loss of consciousness.
- Intraoperative care includes skin preparation, positioning the patient for surgery, and protective measures to ensure patient safety during surgery.
- The PACU RN integrates knowledge of common complications of surgery, well-established nursing diagnoses for the postoperative patient, and data from an individualized comprehensive postoperative assessment to plan and implement appropriate outcomes and interventions for the patient during the postoperative stage.
- Assessments during postoperative recovery are the same as those performed in the PACU, but they can be performed less frequently.
- Antiembolism stockings and sequential compression devices may be used to help prevent thrombophlebitis.
- Incentive spirometry may be used to help prevent atelectasis and pneumonia.
- Gastrointestinal suction may be used for gastric decompression after certain surgeries to prevent gastric distention, which can increase respiratory complications, place a strain on suture lines, and interfere with wound closure.

Knowledge Map

THE PERIOPERATIVE EXPERIENCE

PREOPERATIVE PHASE: Preparing the client for surgery

NURSING ASSESSMENTS:
- Health history: allergies, medications, alcohol/drug use
- Surgical risk factors
- Culture/spiritual factors
- Access to resources
- Coping strategies
- Understanding of surgery and anesthesia

PHYSICAL PREP:
- NPO
- Skin prep
- Bowel and bladder
- Pre-op medication
  - Routine meds
- Prosthesis management
- Antiembolism stockings

SAFETY:
- Signed/informed surgical consent

TEACHING:
- Based on the type of surgery
- Explanation of care pre-, during and postsurgery
- At patient's level; using appropriate language
- Written instructions; discussion

FACTORS AFFECTING SURGICAL RISK:
- Age
- Wounds present
- Preexisting conditions
- Mental status
- Medications: (e.g., anticoagulants; steroids)
- Personal/lifestyle habits
- Allergies

SURGERIES: CLASSIFIED BY:
- Body system involved
- Purpose (e.g., diagnostic, cosmetic)
- Urgency:
  - Emergency, urgent, elective
- Risk involved:
  - Major; minor

INTRAOPERATIVE PHASE

STERILE TEAM:
- Surgeon
- Surgical assistant
- Scrub person

CLEAN TEAM:
- Anesthesiologist
- Circulating nurse
- Technicians

ADMINISTRATION OF ANESTHESIA:
- General
- Conscious sedation
- Regional

SAFETY:
- Positioning
- Maintaining sterile fields
- Monitoring I&O
- Handling specimens
- Sponge/instrument count
- Documentation

POSTOPERATIVE PHASE

POST ANESTHESIA CARE UNIT: PACU
- Focused physical assessments
- Frequent monitoring:
  - Vital signs
  - Airway
  - LOC
  - Positioning
  - Wound/sutures
  - Dressings/drainage devices
  - IV therapy
  - Comfort

THE SURGICAL UNIT
- Continued frequent monitoring
- Patient/family teaching
- Prevention early detection of potential complications

Patient/family teaching:
- Ambulation
- Incentive spirometer
- SCDs
- Diet
- Activity
- Signs/symptoms to report
- Follow-up appointment

Potential complications:
- Aspiration pneumonia/pneumonia
- Atelectasis
- DVT/PE
- Hemorrhage
- Hypovolemia
- Nausea/vomiting; distention
- Constipation/ileus
- Urinary retention/infection
- Renal failure
- Dehydration
- Evisceration
- Infection

UNIT 5

Nursing Functions

37 **Community & Home Health Nursing**

38 **Informatics**

39 **Legal Accountability**

40 **Leading & Managing**

CHAPTER 37

Community & Home Health Nursing

STUDENT RESOURCES

The questions and exercises in this book allow you to practice the kind of thinking you will use as a full-spectrum nurse. Critical-thinking questions usually have more than one right answer, so we do not provide "correct" answers for these features. Try to answer these questions yourself. It is more important to develop your nursing judgment than to just cover content. You will learn more by discussing the questions with your peers. If you are still unsure, see the Davis Advantage chapter resources for suggested responses.

To explore learning resources for this chapter,

Go to www.DavisAdvantage.com and find:

Answers and Suggested Responses for all questions in this chapter
Concept Map
Knowledge Map
References and Bibliography

Key Concepts

Community nursing
Home healthcare
Population

Related Concepts

See the Concept Map on Davis Advantage.

Caring for the Williams Family

Nadine Williams works as a preschool teacher in her community. Luna is a 4-year-old girl in her class. Over the past few months, she has noticed that Luna has many bruises in various stages of healing. The child seems withdrawn and does not interact much with the other children. Nadine is concerned that Luna might be a victim of child abuse, but Nadine is reluctant to make that accusation, especially because the classroom assistant doesn't seem to have noticed anything amiss.

Nadine talks to her husband, Stanley, about her concerns: "I'm worried about a child at school, but I'm afraid to say anything. What if I'm wrong? I'd probably lose my job. But if I'm right and I don't say anything, I could still lose my job, and this girl could be hurt even worse." Stanley suggests that she contact the clinic nurse at the Family Medicine Center for confidential advice on how to proceed.

(Continued)

837

Caring for the Williams Family (continued)

A. Imagine that you are the clinic nurse. Use the full-spectrum nursing model to identify at least 10 questions that you would need to answer to investigate Nadine's concerns further.

B. *Self-knowledge:* What personal values do you have that would affect the way you handle this situation? Explain.

C. *Ethical knowledge:* What is the most important ethical issue in this situation? That is, what is the most important goal? Note that there may be several moral and legal issues, but you are being asked to identify the *most* important one. Note also that you are not being asked what the nurse *can* do but rather what the nurse ideally *must* do.

D. You share the questions you have with Nadine. She believes that there is a need to investigate child abuse. You advise her to call the local child protective services (CPS) agency. Based on your knowledge of community and public health nursing, what aspects of the community health role will the nurse from CPS use as she investigates this situation?

Practical Knowledge
clinical application

Practical knowledge in community and home-care nursing requires you to apply the nursing process to individuals, families, and groups.

CLINICAL INSIGHTS

Clinical Insight 37-1 ▸ Safety Considerations in Home Care

Before the Visit

- **Plan ahead.** Know where you are headed. Use a map or global positioning system (GPS). Contact the client or caregiver for directions if it is unclear where you are headed. File a visit plan with your office each day.
- **Dress in appropriate clothing** as dictated by your agency. Wear a nametag clearly identifying you and the agency. Wear shoes that will allow you to run if necessary.
- **Carry a cell phone.** Check to be sure it is fully charged. Program 911 into it in case of emergency.
- **Do not carry a purse into the home.** Leave it out of sight in a locked vehicle. Carry enough money or a credit card for emergency transportation, telephone numbers for clients and home health agency, and emergency contact information.
- **Keep your vehicle in good repair** and always have enough fuel in the tank or with sufficient charge if driving an electric vehicle. Be prepared for inclement weather, and always carry emergency safety equipment.
- **Do not get out of your vehicle for any reason if driving in an area that might not be safe.** Carjacking involves minor car impact as a strategy to get a person to exit the vehicle, leaving you vulnerable for attack, assault, or theft.
- **Observe your surroundings** as you drive to the visit. Notice the location of emergency services, local gas stations, and public places if help is required.
- **Carry mace or other items to aid in self-defense** in situations in which you feel threatened.
- **Park as close to your destination as possible.** If possible, park your car facing the direction you wish to go when you leave. Never enter dead-end streets or alleys.
- **Check your surroundings before you leave your car.** If you feel unsafe, leave the area immediately and call your office.
- **Prepare your bag while you are still in the car.**
- **Carry your equipment bag on one arm. In the opposite hand, carry your keys.** Always have them ready. You may need them if you decide to exit quickly. Also, you can use keys to defend yourself by placing the pointed ends of the keys between your fingers.
- **Walk directly to the client's house.** Walk in the middle of the sidewalk. Use common walkways. Avoid isolated and poorly lit areas. Do not take shortcuts.
- **Knock or ring the doorbell before entering.** Never enter without being invited. If there is no answer at the door, use your cell phone to call the patient.
- **If for any reason you feel that the neighborhood is unsafe, do not get out of the vehicle.** Instead, leave the neighborhood immediately and call your agency.

During the Visit

- **Introduce yourself** and clearly identify your agency. Show your name badge.
- **Perform patient care where you have access to an exit.** When you enter the home, note all exits.
- **Pay attention to who is present in the home. Request introductions.** This information is useful for planning care as well as for ensuring safety.
- **Leave immediately if you suspect substance use,** drug dealing, or intoxicated behavior.
- **Leave immediately if there is aggressive behavior in the home.** Do not attempt to intervene. When you return to your vehicle, use your cell phone to dial 911. You may need to drive to a safe location to place the call.
- **Request pets be kept in another room** while you make your visit.
- **If weapons are visible, require that they be put away immediately.** Leave the home if this request is not met.
- **If household members interfere with the visit,** discuss the problem with the client. You may need to request they refrain from interruptions or leave the room. You might have to reschedule the visit when they are not present.

After the Visit

- **Continue to observe the safety precautions** you used when arriving for the visit. Do not let down your guard as you return to your car.
- **If you are in an unsafe neighborhood or poorly lit area, leave immediately and do not consult the map** for directions to your next visit. Drive to a secure public location, and then consult the map.
- **Inform your agency** if you believe the home or neighborhood is potentially hazardous.
- **Request a security escort service** if future visits are required.
- **Document your assessments** and the care delivered.
- **Report abuse** if you suspect it in the home.

Other

You also need to protect yourself from infection and accidental injury, as you would in a hospital (see Clinical Insight 37-2).

- Use safe lifting techniques, especially because you might have to improvise more than in the hospital. There will probably be no one to assist with patient transfer, ambulation, or lifting. Mechanical lifts are likely not available.
- Do not dispose of loose sharps in household trash containers, toilets, or recycling bins. Place them immediately in a sharp disposal container. If this is not available, use a puncture- and leak-resistant plastic household container.

Clinical Insight 37-2 ➤ Infection Control in the Home

The following suggestions can help you maintain infection control during a home visit.

Hand Hygiene
- Keep antibacterial cleanser and personal protective equipment in your nursing bag.
- Perform hand hygiene using soap and warm water or an antibacterial handrub at the beginning and end of each visit and before and after any treatment and before handling your equipment bag.

Supplies
- Leave your nursing bag in the car; bring only the supplies you need for the visit.
- If necessary, use antiseptic spray or wipes to disinfect surfaces or equipment in the home.
- When placing clean supplies on a soft surface that cannot be disinfected, open a clean, disposable towel to cover the surface. Avoid using paper towels, newspaper, or other products that may wick moisture from the environmental surface.

Equipment Bag Hygiene
- Do not bring the bag into the home in any of the following circumstances. The home is:
  - Known to be colonized with a multidrug-resistant organism (e.g., MRSA, *C. difficile, S. aureus*)
  - Infested with bedbugs, pests, vermin
  - Soiled with human or pet urine or feces (McGoldrick, 2017)
- **Nonwheeled bag**—Place on an impermeable surface barrier with antimicrobial additives to protect the bag from contact with microorganisms. In the car, you should place it on a visibly clean, dry surface.
- **Wheeled bag**—If the bag is brought into the home, keep it on the floor and do not allow the front flap to have contact with the surface of the floor.
- If you use items from your equipment bag during the visit, always clean them with an approved antibacterial wipe or solution before placing them back into your bag.
- Clean the interior and exterior surfaces of the bag monthly when a surface barrier is used.

Biohazard and Sharps Disposal
- Flush wound irrigation or potentially contaminated liquids down the toilet while wearing gloves and any other appropriate protective equipment.
- Double-bag dressings, equipment, or disposable supplies that have been contaminated with body secretions to prevent leakage. The bags should be labeled *Biohazard*.
- Carry small biohazard sharps containers. Place syringes and sharp items in the container without recapping them. If clients or family must use syringes or sharps, you may wish to leave a safety disposal container in the home. An alternative solution is to have them use a metal coffee can with lid, for example.

Client Teaching
- Provide instruction on home cleanliness, hygiene, hand hygiene, and food preparation and instructions to avoid contact with persons who are ill, as needed.
- If the client is immunocompromised, teach the signs and symptoms of infection. Advise the client to immediately notify the primary care provider of any changes.

Special Situations
- If the patient has a multidrug-resistant infection or pulmonary tuberculosis, use appropriate barrier precautions, including an N95 respirator. Leave reusable equipment in the home; and if possible, schedule these clients as the last appointment of the day.

CLINICAL REASONING
Applying the Full-Spectrum Nursing Model

PATIENT SITUATION

Lorenzo and Elvia are healthy adults. They learn they have been exposed to SARS-CoV-2 (coronavirus; COVID-19). They are concerned about the possibility of contracting the virus and becoming ill.

THINKING

1. *Theoretical Knowledge:*

   a. How is COVID-19 spread?

2. *Critical Thinking (Contextual Awareness):*

   a. Why is it important to detect and treat COVID-19 infection?

   b. Who is at the greatest risk for COVID-19 infection?

DOING

3. *Nursing Process (Assessment):*

   How might you assess the extent of the COVID-19 infections within the area where they live?

4. *Practical Knowledge:*

   a. As the community health nurse, you design a *primary* intervention program to prevent COVID-19 virus infection in the local community. What might you do for this program?

   b. What *secondary* interventions would you include in your patient education?

CARING

5. *Self-Knowledge:*

   a. When showing compassion for your clients, what information about COVID-19 might you offer?

   b. How would you feel if you were exposed to COVID-19?

Critical Thinking and Clinical Judgment

1. You are nearing completion of your fundamentals course. One night while you are preparing for your next clinical, your neighbor Stephanie calls you on your mobile phone. Her 20-month-old daughter, Tiffany, attends day care. Tiffany came home with a letter from the school nurse stating that another child in the class was ill with respiratory syncytial virus (RSV) and other children in the day care room had been exposed to this contagious virus.

   Stephanie is concerned about the risks to Tiffany and the rest of the family. There is currently no vaccine available to protect against RSV. Stephanie is 8 months pregnant. She states that because you are a nursing student, she thought you might know what she should do or where she might go for assistance.

   What are the key pieces of information (both theoretical knowledge and patient data) you need to solve your neighbor's situation?

2. You are a nurse in a public health clinic providing routine childhood immunizations. A 16-year-old client comes into the clinic requesting "shots" for her newborn baby as well as a birth control "shot." She indicates that she has no money to pay for the shots because her 20-year-old boyfriend gave her only enough to get to the clinic.

   Which of the following is your nursing priority for this situation?

   What will you do next?

   Explain *how* you have chosen your priority diagnosis.

   On what did you base your choice?

   - Give the newborn the immunizations, and arrange for the client to meet with the social worker regarding securing healthcare coverage.

   - Educate the mother about birth control.

   - Take the client and child to a private room and discuss the general health of the newborn and the plans for a healthcare provider to see the child. Also ask about the health needs of the mother.

   - Ask the client whether she is being abused and report the incident if so.

3. Your assignment is to conduct a community assessment of your own neighborhood.

   How will your membership in the community affect your assessment? What activities could you delete from the assessment?

4. You are driving home from nursing school clinical day and happen upon a car overturned along a deserted country road. You recall what you learned about the Good Samaritan laws.

   Under these circumstances, are you liable for the care you provide? What is your best course of intervention?

5. As a beginning home health nurse, you have been assigned to visit the following clients today:

   - Roland Escobar (Meet Your Patients, Volume 1), a 78-year-old man recovering from a cerebrovascular accident (stroke)

   - Sally Littlemoon, a 48-year-old woman with diabetes mellitus, blindness, and lower extremity cellulitis (a skin infection)

   - Beatrice Wayne, a 67-year-old woman who has undergone elective coronary artery bypass graft surgery (open-heart surgery)

   - Kent Churchill, an 80-year-old man with a recent hip fracture and surgical repair

   - Chana Padir, a 50-year-old woman with severe pain secondary to breast cancer with extensive metastases. She is receiving hospice care.

   a. Explore some alternatives for your schedule. How would you prepare to make these five visits in 1 day? How would you determine how to arrange your schedule?

   b. The report you receive from the home health supervisor includes the following information:

      - Ms. Littlemoon and Mr. Churchill require dressing changes.

      - Mr. Escobar and Ms. Wayne require teaching about their medications.

      - Mr. Escobar, Ms. Littlemoon, and Mr. Churchill require venipuncture for laboratory work.

- Ms. Padir is having increasing pain.

    Based on this information, what else do you need to know and/or do before you begin your visits?

    What practical knowledge will you need to provide care for these clients?

c. How might the care you deliver to Ms. Wayne differ from the care you give to Ms. Padir? To answer the question, consider the context for each woman. How are their situations different?

d. When visiting Ms. Padir, you realize that her husband and children are very fearful of her impending death. They seem overwhelmed by the care she requires.

   What values and beliefs do you have about death and dying that might influence your care of the Padir family? (Review Chapters 12, 13, and 14 in Volume 1, if necessary.)

   What must you consider when planning your interventions? How might you intervene?

e. When you arrive at the home of Ms. Wayne, she is dressed and out of bed. She tells you she can walk around her house independently with very little pain. She can identify the medications she is receiving, their purpose, and their schedule for administration. Her chest wound is healing nicely, and her breath sounds are clear. She informs you that she is planning on going to her cabin in the mountains this upcoming weekend with her husband and children.

   What actions must you take to continue her home visits? Why?

   What rules/guidelines will influence your choice of action?

6. For each of the following concepts, use critical thinking and summarize how or why it is important to nursing, patient care, or community nursing. Note that these are *not* to be merely definitions.

Community	Primary intervention
Aggregates	Secondary intervention
Census tracts	Tertiary intervention
Vulnerable populations	Disaster preparedness
Healthy People 2030	Omaha System
Windshield survey	

7. For each of the following concepts, use critical thinking to describe how or why it is important to nurses, patient care, or nursing in the home. Note that these are *not* to be merely definitions.

Delivering healthcare in the home setting	Developing rapport at the home visit
Skilled services	Assessment of the home environment
Caregiver role strain	Documentation of home healthcare services
Preparing for the home visit	Clinical Care Classification System

What Are the Main Points in This Chapter?

- A community can be defined as a place with defined boundaries and a group of people with a common language, rituals, or customs.
- Each community determines the meaning of health and nursing activities to promote health.
- A vulnerable population is defined as an aggregate that is at increased risk of adverse health outcomes. Members of vulnerable groups have a higher probability of developing illness.
- The community nurse assesses three general dimensions of a community: structure, status, and process.
- Common practice areas for community-based nurses include schools, churches, prison systems, disaster relief services, occupational and public health clinics, and international relief organizations.
- Community health nursing focuses on the health of individuals, families, and groups and how their individual health affects the community as a whole.
- Public health nursing focuses on the community at large and the eventual effect of the community's health status on the health of individuals, families, and groups.
- Community-oriented nursing combines components of community and public health. Nurses practicing community-oriented nursing are fluid in their approach. Their focus is a comprehensive look at the individual, family, group, and community at large. Community-based nurses serve as advocates, educators, collaborators, counselors, and effective communicators.
- Community-based nurses may provide care at three levels: primary (preventive), secondary (early detection and early treatment), and tertiary (halt disease progression). The focus is on primary prevention.
- The Omaha System is a commonly used documentation system for generating a care plan for a community or an individual within the community setting.
- A community health nurse might practice as a school nurse, public health nurse, parish or prison nurse, international health nurse, or disaster service nurse.
- Home healthcare is delivered in the community setting.
- Home health nursing fosters client and family independence and promotes self-care.
- In the home setting, many factors, such as cleanliness and noise level, are not within the nurse's control. In addition, the home health nurse works without immediate on-site access to other healthcare professionals.
- Home health agencies may be public, voluntary, proprietary, or hospital-based agencies. They may provide direct or indirect care and may specialize in certain types of clients.
- As a full-spectrum nurse working in home healthcare, you will function in the following roles: communicator, direct care provider, client/family educator, client advocate, and care coordinator (case manager).
- Hospice nurses work in hospitals, special hospice facilities, or the homes of patients who are dying. The goal of their care is to provide comfort and manage symptoms.
- Home healthcare is reimbursed by Medicare, by Medicaid, and by private insurance, or paid for through direct payment from the client. Medicare and Medicaid are the largest payers.
- To be eligible for continuing care under most government healthcare programs and private insurers, a client must be homebound and require skilled nursing care.
- Preparation for a home visit includes obtaining information from the referral, identifying the purpose of the visit, gathering required supplies, contacting the client to arrange the visit, and providing for your own safety.
- During a home visit, you will establish a rapport with the client and family, assess the needs of the client and caregivers, develop and discuss the plan of care and needed services with the client and caregivers, provide skilled care, and evaluate the need for continued services.
- Medicare requires specific client assessments using a form called the Outcome and Assessment Information Set (OASIS). It must be completed at the start of care, with each recertification (every 60 days), and at the termination of care.
- The Clinical Care Classification (CCC) system is a system of care and documentation used by most home-care agencies.
- Interventions to reduce caregiver strain include providing emotional support and arranging additional home and community services to support the client and caregiver.
- As a nurse delivering home care, you will need to follow standard precautions but recognize how infection control techniques may be modified to the home environment.
- In addition to infection control, nursing interventions usually include assisting with medication management, assessing and supporting home safety, and providing caregiver support.
- After a home visit you must document care, coordinate services for the client, and prepare for future visits.

Knowledge Map

CHAPTER 37 Community & Home Health Nursing

COMMUNITY AND HOME NURSING

Vulnerable population

Who:
- Low income and/or impoverished individuals/families
- Migrants
- The disabled
- Individuals with unwanted pregnancy
- Substance abusers
- Victims
- Untreated mentally ill
- Chemically ill
- The very old and very young
- Certain geographic communities

Why:
- Low income and/or impoverished individuals/families
- Age
- Chronic disease
- History of abuse or trauma

Assess to determine: Structure, Status, Process

- General characteristics
- Biological, Emotional, Social components
- Overall effectiveness level

Aspects: Structure, Status, Process

COMMUNITY-BASED CARE

FOUNDERS
- Florence Nightingale
- Lillian Wald
- Clara Barton
- Margaret Sanger

- Community health nursing: focus on individuals
- Public health nursing: focus on community at large
- Community-oriented nursing: flexible focus

COMMUNITY NURSES
- HOSPICE NURSES
- HOME NURSES

ROLES
- Client advocate
- Educator
- Collaborator
- Counselor
- Case manager

OPPORTUNITIES
- School nursing
- Parish nursing
- Occupational health nursing
- Corrections facilities nursing
- Disaster services
- International nursing
- Forensics (sexual assault/violence)

Interventions

FUNCTIONS
- Medication management
- Pain control
- Infection control
- Safety

- Primary (Preventative)
- Secondary (detection or early treatment)
- Tertiary (halt progression)

CHAPTER 38

Informatics

STUDENT RESOURCES

The questions and exercises in this book allow you to practice the kind of thinking you will use as a full-spectrum nurse. Critical-thinking questions usually have more than one right answer, so we do not provide "correct" answers for these features. Try to answer these questions yourself. It is more important to develop your nursing judgment than to just cover content. You will learn more by discussing the questions with your peers. If you are still unsure, see the Davis Advantage chapter resources for suggested responses.

To explore learning resources for this chapter,

Go to www.DavisAdvantage.com and find:

Answers and Suggested Responses for all questions in this chapter
Concept Map
Knowledge Map
References and Bibliography

Key Concepts

Electronic communication
Informatics
Healthcare technology

Caring for the Williams Family

Stanley Williams, a patient you have been caring for at the Family Medicine Center, has been devastated by his recent diagnoses of type 2 diabetes mellitus and hypertension. "Oh, my, this is bad. Diabetes can kill you. I don't understand what I did to cause this," he says with a sigh. He is having difficulty following his medication regimen and says he doesn't understand what he is supposed to do. You have supplied him with information at each of his clinic visits as well as handouts, medication information, and a reminder sheet for his medicines. Stanley asks you whether there is any information available on the Internet.

A. What advice would you give Stanley about looking up medical information on the Internet?

B. What sources would you recommend to Stanley?

CLINICAL REASONING
Applying the Full-Spectrum Nursing Model

PATIENT SITUATION

Sarita, a nurse working in the surgical intensive care unit (ICU), is ordering patient laboratory testing and documenting patient information in the electronic health record (EHR). While she is at the computer terminal, a surgeon walks over to her and requests an update on a patient's condition after surgery. Before she logs out, they go to the bedside to assess the patient's color and perfusion. Another nurse, Janelle, needs to order a STAT x-ray using the central computer in the unit. When Sarita goes back to the computer screen to order laboratory work and finish her documentation, Janelle has stepped in and is now accessing another patient's record.

THINKING

1. *Theoretical Knowledge:*
   a. Name five benefits of using an EHR for storing and retrieving patient data in a busy critical care unit.
   b. List five potential areas of difficulty in using this same EHR terminal as others use.

2. *Critical Thinking (Considering Alternatives):*
   a. Brainstorm about possible solutions for dealing with bottlenecks among staff using a centralized computer.

DOING

3. *Practical Knowledge:*
   a. Where would you look to find out who has accessed the patient record?

CARING

4. *Ethical Knowledge:*
   a. What violation has Sarita committed in this situation? What should she have done instead?
   b. What is the nurse's responsibility in protecting patient information in the EHR? What kinds of things should the nurse do?

5. *Self-Knowledge:*
   a. Have you ever been so busy that you felt as though you just needed to take a "necessary" shortcut to save time? Describe your experience.

Critical Thinking and Clinical Judgment

1. Refer to the following table. For each of the uses listed, what kind of information do you think the database should provide? That is, what kind of data would you need? For example, look at the first item under In Nursing Practice. For "Literature access and retrieval," you would use a database that contains information about journals, books, reports, and their content, perhaps CINAHL. What kind of database would you use? What kind of information would you need? The first one is done for you.

Work with your classmates. Share your knowledge and experience to answer these questions. Consult your instructor as needed.

USE IN NURSING PRACTICE	TYPE OF INFORMATION NEEDED
Literature access and retrieval	*Suggested response:* CINAHL; Google Scholar, MEDLINE, Cochrane Library, National Guideline Clearinghouse, US National Library of Medicine, Standard, PsycINFO, Scopus, Sage Research Methods, PubMed, National Institute for Health & Care Excellence (NICE) Guidelines, Essential Evidence Plus, Joanna Briggs Institute, Virginia Henderson Global Nursing e-Repository, Up-to-Date Clinical Decision Support Tool, PLOS Medicine.
Care planning	*Clues:* What information would you need for care planning? Where would you find it? *Suggested response:*
Patient health records	
Telehealth	
Case management	
USE IN NURSING EDUCATION	**TYPE OF INFORMATION NEEDED**
Literature access and retrieval	
Instructional technology	
Virtual learning	
Testing and evaluation	
Student records	
USE IN NURSING ADMINISTRATION	**TYPE OF INFORMATION NEEDED**
Quality improvement (QI) programs	*Clues:* What information would you need to monitor, analyze, and improve the quality of care in your institution? What are the best practices for conducting a QI program?
Employee records (e.g., licensure and certifications, immunizations)	
Staffing patterns, hiring	
Facilities management	
Budgetary planning	
Accreditation reviews	
USE IN NURSING RESEARCH	**TYPE OF INFORMATION NEEDED**
Literature review	
Data collection	
Data analysis	
Research dissemination	
Grant application	

2. Search for online nursing journals on the Internet. Make a list of nursing journals that provide full-text articles that are available on the Internet at no charge.

3. For each of the following concepts, use critical thinking to describe how or why it is important to nursing, patients, or nursing informatics. Note these are *not* to be merely definitions.

Nursing informatics	Connectivity
Data	Group messaging by text or application
Knowledge	Telehealth
Wisdom	Electronic health records
Evidence-based practice	Standardized nursing language
Computers	Literature databases
Hardware	Evaluating Internet sites
Storage media	

What Are the Main Points in This Chapter?

- Whatever their roles—staff nurse, administrator, educator, researcher, primary care provider—nurses use data, information, and knowledge in their daily work.
- Informatics is the processing and management of data, information, and knowledge necessary for making practice decisions.
- Nursing informatics specialists use nursing science, computer science, and information science to manage and communicate data, information, knowledge, and wisdom in nursing practice.
- A computer has four main functions: input, processing, output, and storage. Together they are known as information processing (or data processing).
- *Connectivity* is a term referring to the ways in which computers and other hardware communicate and share information.
- Some forms of electronic communication include electronic mail and text and application-based messaging, web conferencing and webinars, online forums, social networking, and telehealth applications.
- Electronic health records (EHRs) are a platform for communication among the interdisciplinary healthcare team regarding patient healthcare needs, patient data, and plan for care.
- EHRs allow clinicians to create, store, edit, and retrieve patient charts via the Internet or local intranet software.
- Benefits of EHRs include reduced errors resulting from illegible handwriting, efficiency of medication ordering, convenience of patient communication, and service of patient scheduling and reminders.
- EHRs equip providers with clinical support tools to conveniently access information to assist with clinical decision-making.
- Computer- and application-based tools for providing and managing care, including tracking patients and equipment and managing workflow, reduce errors with automation and aid patients in self-care.
- Standardized languages within the EHR facilitate research to improve healthcare. They also aid in billing, record-keeping, and scheduling follow-up care.
- It is important to use and protect passwords to guard the privacy of patient records.
- Computer illiteracy and discomfort with technology are common reasons for resisting use of an EHR. Many claim documentation in the system is time consuming, especially when less familiar with the system.
- Evidence-based practice requires the ability to organize and manage information to identify a clinical problem, search the literature, evaluate the evidence, and plan an intervention.
- An information-literate person seeks authoritative, current, and reliable sources of information from trusted Internet sources.
- CINAHL, MEDLINE, and Google Scholar are commonly used databases for searching the health literature.

Knowledge Map

CONNECTIVITY
- Wired
- Wireless
- Modem
- Cable
- DSL
- Internet

enables

ELECTRONIC COMMUNICATION
- POTS
- Videoconference
- Fax
- E-mail
- Telehealth

COMPUTER SYSTEM
- Microchips
- Process
- Storage

Input → Output

ONLINE NURSING RESEARCH
- Textbooks
- Journal articles
- Scholarly journals
- Periodicals
- WWW

LITERATURE DATABASES
- MEDLINE
- CINAHL

INFORMATICS

APPLICATIONS
- Practice
- Education
- Research

Wisdom uses → Data, Information, Knowledge — needed for → **EVIDENCE-BASED NURSING PRACTICE**

to → Manage or solve human problems

involves:
- Identifying the problem
- Performing literature search
- Evaluating the evidence
- Choosing interventions

NURSING INFORMATICS

ELECTRONIC HEALTH RECORD

needs

STANDARDIZED NURSING LANGUAGE

ETHICAL FACTORS
- Passwords
- Audit trails
- HIPAA

CHAPTER 39

Legal Accountability

STUDENT RESOURCES

The questions and exercises in this book allow you to practice the kind of thinking you will use as a full-spectrum nurse. Critical-thinking questions usually have more than one right answer, so we do not provide "correct" answers for these features. Try to answer these questions yourself. It is more important to develop your nursing judgment than to just cover content. You will learn more by discussing the questions with your peers. If you are still unsure, see the Davis Advantage chapter resources for suggested responses.

To explore learning resources for this chapter,

Go to www.DavisAdvantage.com and find:

Answers and Suggested Responses for all questions in this chapter
Concept Map
Knowledge Map
References and Bibliography

Key Concepts

Law
Liability
Malpractice

Related Concepts

See the Concept Map on Davis Advantage

Caring for the Williams Family

Stanley and Nadine Williams have requested an appointment with you, the nurse at the Family Medicine Clinic, to discuss advance directives. Their experience with Stanley's mother, Charlene, has created concerns about end-of-life care.

A. Stanley asks you, "Do you think it's appropriate to create an advance directive at my age?" How would you respond?

B. Stanley tells you that he believes in "natural death." He states, "I don't want extraordinary measures, and I never want to be resuscitated." Nadine responds that she is extremely uncomfortable with blanket statements about treatment. "If he got hit by a car or had some accident, I would want you to do everything in your power to treat him. I couldn't carry out his wishes," she states. What actions should you take to help Stanley and Nadine resolve this discrepancy?

Practical Knowledge clinical application

CLINICAL INSIGHTS

Clinical Insight 39-1 ▸ Tips for Avoiding Malpractice

Patient Relationships

- **Develop open, honest, respectful, and caring relationships** with patients and families. Patients are less likely to sue if they feel that you were caring and professional.
- **Maintain patient privacy and confidentiality.**
- **Recognize "problem" patients.** Try to identify the basic problem or complaint and intervene to resolve it. Angry patients who feel mistreated are more likely to bring a malpractice lawsuit.

Professional Interactions

- **Don't blame or criticize other healthcare providers** in the presence of patients (e.g., "Sorry you didn't get your pain medication. The night shift was a little short-staffed last night").
- **Don't make statements that may appear to be an admission of guilt** (e.g., "Oh, my gosh, I forgot to shut off that IV!"). Errors should not be included on the patient's health record but instead recorded in an incident report.

Patient Assessments

- **Perform timely assessments and recognize significant assessment cues;** notify primary care providers of changes in the patient's condition or patient complaints.
- **Use the proper chain of command** to ensure appropriate and timely care when the primary healthcare provider is not available.
- **Perform fall risk assessments,** document, and take measures to ensure client safety. Falls are a common cause of patient injury.

Documentation

- **Careful, thorough documentation** is the best defense if a lawsuit does occur:
  - Use and document all steps of the nursing process.
- Be especially thorough when documenting care for patients who will not comply with treatments or who complain a lot.
- Courts assume that if care is not documented, it was not given.
- **Document the time and content of telephone conversations with other healthcare providers.**
- **Send copies only,** never originals, of records and reports requested by other professionals.

Competent Practice

- **Know and follow applicable laws:** (1) federal and state laws, (2) your state's NPA (perform only the activities within your scope of practice and competence).
- **Know and follow agency policies and procedures.**
- **Know and follow standards of care** set forth in the state NPA, by professional organizations, in professional literature, by agency policy, and so on.
- **Stay competent in your area of practice.** For example, attend continuing education, webinars, and in-service programs to improve your knowledge and skills.
- **Don't accept a clinical assignment that you think you are not competent to perform.** Evaluate your assignment with your supervisor if there is a question.

Medication Administration

- **Follow the "rights" of medication administration** (see Chapter 23).
- **Follow medical prescriptions,** but clarify them as needed. Do not implement a questionable prescription or one you do not understand.

Practice Resources

Brown (2016); Fall Documentation and Injury Prevention (2018); Ghaith et al. (2022); Gleason et al. (2021); Oyeleye (2019); Pierce (2019).

Clinical Insight 39-2 ▶ Using Equipment Safely

The following will help you to ensure proper and safe use of equipment:
- Obtain appropriate training on equipment use.
- Follow the healthcare agency's protocols, policies, and procedures on the use of the equipment.
- Follow the manufacturer's operating instructions.
- Be sure medical equipment has been properly inspected.
- Perform safety checks regularly and before each use.
- Position and use equipment properly during treatment.
- Know how the equipment functions. Be alert to signs that it is not working properly.
- Make sure rooms are not cluttered with equipment.
- Follow agency policies regarding equipment brought from the patient's home (e.g., hair dryers, electric shavers, radios); usually these should be inspected for proper grounding and safe cords.
- Remove and label equipment that is malfunctioning to prevent others from using it until it can be repaired or replaced.
- Advocate for replacement of essential equipment (e.g., bed alarms).

Practice Resources
Brous (2019a, 2019b); Mattox (2012); Watson (2014).

Clinical Insight 39-3 ▶ Guidelines for Documenting Care

To be accurate and complete, your reporting and documentation of client care must address the following:
- Patient status (e.g., symptoms and responses to treatments)
- The nursing care given
- Providers' prescriptions
- Medications and treatments
- Patient responses
- Consultations with other members of the healthcare team regarding patient status

You might find the 5 Cs mnemonic helpful for documenting care. Documentation should be:
- **C**omplete
- **C**lear
- **C**orrect
- **C**omprehensive
- **C**hronological

Practice Resources
Brown (2016); Ghaith et al. (2022); Malpractice outcome could hinge on what ED nurses documented (2017); Reiner (n.d.).

CLINICAL REASONING
Applying the Full-Spectrum Nursing Model

PATIENT SITUATION

A nurse employed by a temporary agency is assigned to a neurology unit for a 12-hour shift. On arrival, they discover that the registered nurse (RN) assigned for the shift called in sick, leaving the nurse with two unlicensed assistive personnel (UAPs) to provide client care and administer medication, including controlled substances. The nursing supervisor informs the nurse that they will be responsible for the unit with 22 clients, 12 of whom are acutely ill and require close observation and frequent care. The nursing supervisor is not available to work on the unit and has no additional RNs to provide client care. The nurse decides not to accept the assignment, to report the decision and reasons to the agency supervisor, and to leave the neurology unit immediately before starting the shift.

THINKING

1. *Theoretical Knowledge:*

    a. In addition to protecting their nursing license, what other factors should the nurse have considered in deciding whether to stay on or leave the unit?

    b. Because the nurse decided not to accept the assignment, would this have been considered abandonment?

    c. What standards, guidelines, and laws would apply to determine whether the nurse's behavior was in accordance with standards of practice?

2. *Critical Thinking (Contextual Awareness):*

   a. Which statements in the American Nurses Association (ANA) Nurses' Bill of Rights should the nurse have considered before deciding whether to accept the assignment?

   b. What factors in this situation could create legal problems for the nurse?

DOING

3. *Nursing Process (Planning/Generating Solutions; Implementation/Taking Actions):* The nurse's action (leaving the unit) might be viewed under some laws in some situations as abandonment of clients. What are some alternative actions the nurse might have taken to avoid that risk?

CARING

4. *Self-Knowledge:* Have you ever been in a situation in which you felt a moral obligation to help, yet you knew you would be in over your head? Describe your experience.

5. *Ethical Knowledge:* In your opinion, did the nurse do the right thing when they decided not to accept the assignment and to leave the nursing unit immediately? Explain your thinking.

Critical Thinking and Clinical Judgment

1. Think about the Meet Your Nurse Role Model scenario you read at the beginning of the chapter in Volume 1. A nurse with 3 years of experience on a medical-surgical unit arrives to work and discovers that two of her colleagues called in sick, including the charge nurse. The nursing supervisor informs the nurse that she will need to assume the charge nurse role in addition to assuming care for three clients. Feeling frustrated, the nurse ponders whether she should just quit and find another job, but then decides to accept the assignment. Two hours into the shift, one of her clients begins to have complications, requiring blood glucose checks every 2 hours and frequent monitoring. In addition, one of the nurses becomes ill and is replaced by a float nurse from the labor and delivery unit, who spends her time continuously texting on her cell phone. The nurse contacts the nursing supervisor and requests additional assistance but is told no other nurse is available and that the supervisor is involved with an emergency situation on another unit. The nurse begins to analyze this situation from a legal perspective to determine the best course of action.

   Use the critical-thinking model to identify questions to ask yourself in reflecting and deciding what to do.

   Go to Chapter 2, **Box 2-2: Critical-Thinking Model,** in Volume 1.

   a. What questions do you need to ask about context?

   b. What knowledge do you need to make an informed and credible decision?

   c. What questions do you need to ask when considering alternatives?

   d. What questions do you need to ask about analyzing your assumptions?

   e. What questions do you need to ask about reflecting and deciding?

2. Analyze this passage:
   Nursys is the national database for verification of nurse licensure and contains information on disciplinary information for RNs and LVN/LPNs [licensed vocational nurses/licensed practical nurses]. The e-Notify feature of Nursys provides free real-time information to employers about their nurse employees (https://www.nursys.com/).

   - Do you think there is a need for Nursys?

   - What rights does it help protect?

3. Imagine that you are working in a large medical center in an area where there have been several robberies and assaults in the past 6 months, mostly late at night. Although the parking lot is nearly a block from the employees' exit and is not well lit, there is only one security guard on duty outside the hospital after 10 p.m. Despite repeated requests from employees all the way up the chain of command, no efforts are being made to improve lighting or to hire more security guards. What standards and laws might be helpful to the employees?

4. George Agnew, 75 years old, is admitted to the emergency department after being involved in a serious car accident. His wife is with him, and she is very upset—to the point of being hysterical. It is likely that Mr. Agnew will die, but providers are considering whether he will need a ventilator in the next hour or so. You need to know Mr. Agnew's wishes on this issue, but he is not conscious. The charge nurse tells you not to ask Mrs. Agnew because it will just upset her more.

   a. What is happening in the situation that may influence the outcome?

   b. What factors may influence your behavior and the behavior of others in this situation?

   c. What values or biases do you have that influence your behavior in this situation?

   d. Where might you get the information you need instead of asking Mrs. Agnew?

   e. What would you do? What legal support, if any, do you have?

5. Compare the following definitions of practical nursing and professional nursing taken from the nurse practice act in Missouri and then discuss the differences in the scope of practice for the LPN/LVN and the RN. Identify two tasks/responsibilities that only the RN can perform.
   DEFINITION 1. Practical nursing is the performance for compensation of selected acts for the promotion of health and in the care of persons who are ill, injured, or experiencing alterations in normal health processes. Such performance requires substantial specialized skill, judgment, and knowledge. All such nursing care shall be given under the direction of a person licensed by a state regulatory board to prescribe medications and treatments or under the direction of a registered professional nurse. For the purposes of this chapter, the term "direction" shall mean guidance or supervision provided by a person licensed by a state regulatory board to prescribe medications and treatments or a registered professional nurse, including, but not limited to, oral, written, or otherwise communicated orders or directives for patient care. When practical nursing care is delivered pursuant to the direction of a person licensed by a state regulatory board to prescribe medications and treatments or under the direction of a registered professional nurse, such care may be delivered by a licensed practical nurse without direct physical oversight.
   DEFINITION 2. Professional nursing is the performance for compensation of any act which requires substantial specialized education, judgment, and skill based on knowledge and application of principles derived from the biological, physical, social, and nursing sciences, including, but not limited to:

   a. Responsibility for the teaching of health care and the prevention of illness to the patient and his or her family

   b. Assessment, nursing diagnosis, nursing care, and counsel of persons who are ill, injured, or experiencing alterations in normal health processes

   c. The administration of medications and treatments as prescribed by a person licensed by a state regulatory board to prescribe medications and treatments

   d. The coordination and assistance in the delivery of a plan of health care with all members of a health team

   e. The teaching and supervision of other persons in the performance of any of the foregoing (Missouri Revised Statutes, 2013)

6. The patient was an older adult with various medical conditions and receiving multiple medications. The nurse determined the patient was a high fall risk, 8 on a scale of 0 to 10. The nurse decided to initiate the hospital's fall prevention plan, which meant raising the side rails and placing restraints on the patient without a prescription from the provider. Hospital policy, however, did require a nurse who initiated restraints on a patient for fall prevention to notify a provider within 1 hour after doing so.

   The next day, another nurse, seeing that no prescriptions for restraints had been received, removed the restraints. The patient was getting up out of bed on his own. His nursing neurological assessment showed signs of dementia and confusion. His oxygen saturation was low, and his heartbeat was irregular. The provider was notified by phone but declined to prescribe restraints. Later that evening the patient was found on the floor with a closed-head injury. He was transferred to a university hospital, where he died a few weeks later. The case was dismissed against the hospital (*Sturgill v. Ashe Memorial Hosp.*, 2008).

   a. In this case, the nurse was caring for a patient at high risk for fall but did not have a prescription to use restraints. Why do you think the court dismissed the case against the hospital?

   b. What other action might the nurse have taken to prevent this patient's fall?

7. For each of the following concepts, use critical thinking to describe how or why it is important to nurses, patients, or legal issues. Note that these are *not* to be merely definitions.

   Civil law

   The U.S. Constitution Bill of Rights and the Patient Care Partnership

   The ANA Code of Ethics; the ANA Standards of Practice; and the ANA Nurses' Bill of Rights

   Patient advocacy

   Battery

   Vicarious liability

What Are the Main Points in This Chapter?

- The law is a binding practice, rule, or code of conduct that guides a community or society and is enforced by a controlling authority.
- Laws are primarily derived from four sources: (1) the Constitution, (2) statutes, (3) administrative bodies, and (4) the courts.
- The right of privacy comes from the Bill of Rights.
- A living will gives directions to others about a person's wishes regarding life-prolonging treatments if the person becomes unable to make those decisions; it must be prepared when the person is alert and oriented (competent).
- A durable power of attorney for healthcare identifies a person who will make healthcare decisions in the event the client is unable to do so.
- State laws affecting nursing practice include mandatory reporting laws, Good Samaritan laws, safe harbor laws, and nurse practice acts.
- The ANA Code of Ethics describes the standards of professional responsibility for nurses and provides insight into ethical and acceptable behavior.
- The ANA Nurses' Bill of Rights identifies the rights nurses should expect from their workplace and work environment that are necessary for sound professional practice.
- A primary function of the medical malpractice system is to encourage healthcare providers to adhere to standards of practice and perform their responsibilities in a competent manner.
- Standards of practice look to what a reasonable and prudent nurse would do in the same or similar situation.
- Nurse practice acts are established by state boards of nursing to govern the practice of nursing.
- In most states, nurses are obligated legally to report suspected or actual client abuse, impaired health professionals, and communicable diseases.
- State boards of nursing are empowered under the nurse practice act to approve prelicensure nursing education programs, determine the criteria for licensure, define the practice of nursing, and establish grounds for disciplinary actions against nurses.

- Criminal law deals with wrongs or offenses against society. Civil law deals with wrongs to individuals.
- Intentional torts include assault, battery, false imprisonment, fraud, and invasion of privacy.
- Quasiintentional torts involve those actions that injure a person's reputation.
- Unintentional torts that involve healthcare professionals are negligence and malpractice.
- Negligence is a wrong committed against an individual by one who has failed to use ordinary care.
- Malpractice is negligence committed against an individual by a licensed professional involving a duty, breach of that duty, an injury, and damages.
- Litigation is the formal process whereby the legal issues, rights, and duties between the parties are heard and decided. The stages include (1) pleading and pretrial motions, (2) discovery, (3) alternative dispute resolution, (4) trial, and (5) appeal.
- Malpractice claims, in general, result from failure to maintain the standard of practice, including failure to assess, diagnose, plan, implement, and evaluate client responses to care.
- Nurses can help reduce their legal risks by developing open, honest, respectful, caring relationships with clients and families; observing standards of care; and accurate documentation.
- You may witness a client's signature on a consent form, but you are not legally responsible for explaining the treatments and options, nor are you responsible for evaluating whether the provider has adequately explained them.

Knowledge Map

LAWS AND REGULATIONS

STATE LAWS
- Mandatory reporting
- Good Samaritan
- Nurse Practice Acts
  - Credentialing
  - Licensing
  - Discipline

STANDARDS OF PRACTICE
- What a reasonable and prudent nurse would do
- Mandatory = Nurse Practice Act
- Voluntary = ANA

FEDERAL LAWS
- Bill of Rights
- EMTALA
- ADA
- Patient Self-Determination Act
- HIPAA

OTHER GUIDELINES
- Agency policies and procedures
- Nursing Code of Ethics
- Patient Care Partnership
- ANA Bill of Rights for Nurses

CRIMINAL LAW
- Misdemeanor
- Felony

CIVIL LAW
- Contract law
- Tort law
  - Negligence
  - Malpractice

COMMON NURSING MALPRACTICE CLAIMS
Failure to:
- Assess and diagnose
- Plan
- Implement plan
- Evaluate

How to avoid
- Observe standards of care
- Avoid medication/treatment errors
- Report/document
- Obtain informed consent
- Attend to safety
- Maintain confidentiality
- Provide education
- Delegate correctly
- Observe boundaries

TYPES OF TORTS
Quasi-intentional:
- Defamation
- Slander
- Libel

Intentional:
- Assault and battery
- False imprisonment
- Fraud
- Invasion of privacy

CHAPTER 40

Leading & Managing

STUDENT RESOURCES

The questions and exercises in this book allow you to practice the kind of thinking you will use as a full-spectrum nurse. Critical-thinking questions usually have more than one right answer, so we do not provide "correct" answers for these features. Try to answer these questions yourself. It is more important to develop your nursing judgment than to just cover content. You will learn more by discussing the questions with your peers. If you are still unsure, see the Davis Advantage chapter resources for suggested responses.

To explore learning resources for this chapter,

Go to www.DavisAdvantage.com and find:

Answers and Suggested Responses for all questions in this chapter

Concept Map

Knowledge Map

References and Bibliography

Key Concepts

Change
Followership
Leadership
Management

Related Concepts

See the Concept Map on Davis Advantage.

Caring for the Williams Family

Naomi Jackson, Stanley's sister, is scheduled for outpatient cataract surgery later this week at the local hospital. Stanley reports to the clinic wishing to discuss the plan for his sister's surgery "with whoever is the boss." Stanley is concerned that his sister will not be staying at the hospital. "She's having surgery. I don't understand this! She's 65 years old. She's going to need help. This doesn't make sense. You have to change things. It won't be safe to do this as planned."

Stanley tells you he has discussed his concerns with the ophthalmologist. He tells you that the ophthalmologist told him he was "overreacting. We always do it this way. You just don't understand." Stanley is visibly upset. He believes that his sister is receiving inadequate care. He appeals to you to help him take care of his sister. "This is where my sister gets her care. You know her. You have to change this."

Naomi Jackson has been seen at the family clinic several times over the past few years. She takes a medication for osteoporosis and has been counseled about the need for exercise and weight loss. She has also begun to have problems with "accidents" (i.e., urine leakage). She has never had surgery in the past, and her only hospitalizations have been for childbirth. Ms. Jackson's husband recently passed away, and she has been living alone since then.

A. Devise a plan to resolve this conflict with Stanley.

CLINICAL REASONING
Applying the Full-Spectrum Nursing Model

ORGANIZATIONAL SITUATION

A small, not-for-profit hospice center in a small community has received a generous memorial gift from the family of a client who recently died. The family asked only that the money be "put to the best possible use." Everyone in the facility has an opinion about the best use for the money.

The administrator wants to renovate their old, run-down headquarters. The financial officer wants to put the money in the bank "for a rainy day." The chaplain wants to add a small chapel to the building. The nurses want to create a food bank to help the poorest of their clients. The social workers want to buy a van to transport clients to healthcare providers. The staff has agreed that all the ideas have merit, and all the needs are important. Unfortunately, there is enough money to fund only one of them.

The more the staff members discuss how to use this gift, the more insistent each group becomes about defending its own idea. At the last meeting, some members became angry and frustrated. A shouting match even occurred between the administrator and the financial officer.

THINKING

1. *Theoretical Knowledge:*

   Which is appropriate at this point, a problem-solving approach or informal negotiation? Explain your answer.

DOING

2. *Practical Knowledge:*

   If you were to conduct the informal negotiation, list the steps of the plan you would follow.

CARING

3. *Self-Knowledge:*

   Which idea do you think has the most merit? Why did you select the one you did?

4. *Ethical Knowledge:*

   Which groups or individuals seem to demonstrate the value of caring for clients? Explain your thinking.

Critical Thinking and Clinical Judgment

1. Identify a personal or professional change that you would like to see take place, and outline the steps needed to implement the change.

2. Eleanor, an LPN returning to school to obtain her associate's degree in nursing, is faced with a multitude of responsibilities. A wife, mother of two toddlers, and full-time staff member at a local hospital, Eleanor suddenly finds herself in a situation in which there are not enough hours in a day. She is convinced that becoming a registered nurse is an impossible goal. You are Eleanor's mentor. When you ask where she wants to be in 5 years, she answers, "At this moment, I think, in Tahiti!"

   a. Help Eleanor develop a personal time inventory. To help her determine specifically what to include, make your own personal time inventory to share with her as an example.

   b. Once Eleanor has finished her time plan, how would you advise her to use it to make better use of her time? Make specific suggestions.

3. What strategies could you use to better manage your time?

4. Why is it important to learn good time management habits while you are a student?

5. This is your first semester in the nursing program. Although you have attended college to complete the prerequisite courses, this seems to be so different. Now you have to attend clinical rotations in addition to classes. And you must prepare ahead of time for the clinical experience, even going to the hospital the night before to obtain information related to your patients. You feel like you are drowning! What can you do?

    Refer to Table 40-5, Components of Time Management, in Volume 1. Work through the table, asking yourself questions such as the following. Be very specific in your answers; give examples.

    a. *Prioritizing:*
        - What tasks do you have to complete on a daily basis? Weekly? During the semester?
        - List the tasks in order of importance.
        - Which of the tasks do you have control over (e.g., scheduling a haircut or setting aside time to read the next assignment versus taking a test that is scheduled)?

    b. *Assigning priorities:* Assign priorities to the tasks you have identified.

    c. *Questioning effectiveness, efficiency:* Ask yourself, "How can I accomplish these tasks in the shortest time but to the best of my ability?"

    d. *Rechecking:* Review your plan. Mentally and physically recheck the plan. Revise the plan as needed.

    e. *Self-reliance:* Carry out your plan. Use critical-thinking skills, and adapt the plan as needed so that you "go with the flow."

    f. *Treating:* Be good to yourself but commit yourself to time management and excellence. How can you do that? What treats will you give yourself?

6. For each of the following concepts, use critical thinking to describe how or why it is important to nursing, patient care, or managing or leading. Note that these are *not* to be merely definitions.

    Leadership skills   Time management

    Management skills   Resolving conflicts

    Becoming a mentor   Delegating appropriately

    Being a mentee   Understanding the change process

What Are the Main Points in This Chapter?

- Leadership is the ability to influence other people.
- Transformational leaders communicate their vision in a way that reduces negativity and inspires commitment in people.
- Three common behavioral leadership styles are authoritarian, democratic, and laissez-faire.
- A manager is an employee of an organization who has power, authority, and responsibility for planning and directing the work of others.
- Effective managers have a combination of qualities: leadership skills, clinical expertise, and business sense.
- A manager's activities are generally organizational, interpersonal, and informational.
- Not all leaders should be managers, but all managers should be leaders.
- It is never too early in your career to develop a SWOT or SOAR analysis. Throughout your nursing program, revisit the analysis, and update it as you gain new knowledge and skills.
- A mentor is a role model who develops the novice nurse to be a professional by coaching, encouraging, supporting, and guiding them.
- Learn from nurses who demonstrate strong mentor qualities. Do not be afraid to ask for their support and guidance. Develop mentor qualities of your own so you can also mentor a new graduate nurse.
- At times throughout your nursing career, you will assume the role of follower.
- Followers need to be self-directing, actively participating experts who work on behalf of the organization.
- Sources of power include authority, reward, expertise, and coercion.
- Nurses have expertise, power, and authority over other healthcare workers. It is important that you understand your sources of power and use them wisely.
- Empowerment is the feeling of self-determination, competence, and recognition that your expertise and power within the healthcare system can have a positive impact.
- Evaluative feedback is a leadership responsibility that reinforces constructive behavior, provides recognition, and develops employee skills.
- Delegation of patient care tasks to other healthcare workers is an important responsibility of the registered nurse.
- Nurses must understand change and act as change agents within today's healthcare setting.
- Managing change involves recognizing and decreasing resistance.
- Conflict is inevitable, but it does not need to be destructive.
- One of a manager's responsibilities is to facilitate conflict resolution and, if necessary, function as an informal negotiator.
- Effective time management is essential to planning safe, effective patient care and demonstrating management skills.
- Time management includes goal setting and organizing and streamlining your work.
- Do not forget to get rest and take time off when managing time.

CHAPTER 40 Leading & Managing

Knowledge Map

TRAITS
- Interpersonal skills
- Self-esteem
- Creativity

BEHAVIORAL
- Autocratic
- Democratic
- Laissez-faire

SITUATIONAL
- Flexible
- Dependent on needs of the group

THEORIES

TASK/RELATIONSHIP
- Get it done versus getting along

SCIENTIFIC
- Motivate with properly designed tasks and sufficient incentive

THEORIES

HUMAN RELATIONS
- Motivate by keeping morale high

ACTIVITIES
- Interpersonal
- Decision
- Informational

QUALITIES
- Leadership
- Clinical
- Expertise
- Business sense

LEADER ⇠ ⇢ **MANAGER**

MENTORS; PRECEPTORS

CHALLENGES
- Economic climate
- Nursing labor market

SOURCES OF POWER
- Authority • Reward
- Expertise • Coercion

EMPOWERMENT

SOURCES OF POWER
- Enhance expertise
- Share expertise

SKILLS FOR EFFECTIVE GROUP FUNCTIONING
- Communicate clearly
- Delegate appropriately
- Manage change
- Deal with conflict
- Manage time effectively

Credits

Note: Unless cited here, text credits appear within the text.

CHAPTER 3

Unnumbered figure 3-1: Courtesy of Shawnee Mission Health System, Shawnee Mission, KS.

Unnumbered figure 3-2: With permission from the National Council of State Boards of Nursing (NCSBN), Chicago, IL (1997).

Evaluation checklist: From Wilkinson, J. (2001). *Nursing Process and Critical Thinking* (5th ed.). Upper Saddle River, NJ: Prentice Hall.

CHAPTER 8

Discharge Assessment/Instructions, Patient Education Form: Fisherman's Hospital, Marathon, FL. Used with permission.

CHAPTER 17

Adult Admission History Electronic Screening: Courtesy of Cerner Corporation.

Nursing Assessment Flowsheet: Courtesy of Teton Hospital, Driggs, ID.

CHAPTER 19

Procedure 19-3, Step 1b, Pediculosis; 19-6, Step 6b, Hordeolum; 19-6, Step 6e, Pterygium; 19-6, Step 6e, Subconjunctival hemorrhage: Courtesy of Wills Eye Hospital, Philadelphia, PA.

Procedure 19-7, Step 3d, Normal TM, left ear: Courtesy of Ann Marie Ramsey, RN, MSN, CPNP.

Procedure 19-7, Step 3e, Otitis Media and Perforated TM: Courtesy of Welch Allyn, Skaneateles Falls, NY.

Procedure 19-9, Step 3: Courtesy Robert A. Levine, DDS, and Sheryl Radin, DDS.

Procedure 19-9, Step 4, Geographic Tongue, Leukoplakia, and Cancer of the Tongue: Courtesy of Tina S. Liang, DMD.

Procedure 19-9 Step 4, Black Hairy Tongue; 19-15, Step 7a, Heberden's Nodes; 19-15, Step 7b, Rheumatoid Arthritis; 19-17, Step3d, Syphilitic Chancre; 19-17, Step 3d, Genital Warts: Courtesy MCP-Hahnemann University Department of Dermatology, Philadelphia, PA.

Procedure 19-17, Stages 1-5 and 19-18; MSF Stages 1-5: Adapted from Tanner, JM (1962), *Growth and Adolescence* (2nd ed.). Oxford: Blackwell Scientific Publications

CHAPTER 20

Procedure 20-1b, Step 3: © iStockphoto.

CHAPTER 21

Procedure 24-1, Step 1: Infrared-Beam Detector, Cord-Activated Sensor: Courtesy of Smart Caregiver Corporation.

Safety Assessment Scale: With Permission from Dr. Louise Poulin de Courval, CLSC Cote-des-Nieges.

CHAPTER 22

Procedure 22-7 Equipment: Courtesy of Sage Products, Inc., Cary, IL.

CHAPTER 23

Procedure 23-6 Equipment: With Permission from Hospi Macy Catheter, https://www.macycatheter.com/.

Procedure 23-10 Equipment 1: Courtesy of Edward Lin, MD, Ingenious Technologies Corporation. Training video link: http://ingenious.com/NS/ns.htm.

Procedure 23-17A, Step 7: Dr. Brian Oxhorn, Roseman University, Henderson, NV. Used with permission.

CHAPTER 24

Procedure 24-3, Step 5h: Nestle Healthcare Nutrition Inc.

Procedure 24-5 Equipment: Permission for use granted by Cook Medical Incorporated, Bloomington, IN.

CHAPTER 26

Procedure 26-8 Equipment and Procedure 26-8B, Steps 8 and 11: Courtesy of Hollister Incorporated, Libertyville, IL.

CHAPTER 32

Procedure 32-11 Documentation: Renee Fransen, RN, BSN; David McIntosh, Graphics Designer; and Daniel Tucker, RN, BS; at NurseSquared (a division of Elsevier, Inc); Bergeron, J.D., Bizjak, G., Le Badour, G., et al. (2009); Rolstad, B. S., & Ovington, L. G. (2011).

Braden Scale for Predicting Pressure Ulcer Score Risk: Copyright © Barbara Braden and Nancy Bergstrom, 1988. Reprinted with permission.

Norton Scale for Assessing Risk of Pressure Ulcers: Copyright © D. Norton, R. McLaren, & A. N. Exton-Smith. 1975. Reprinted with permission.

The PUSH Tool for Evaluation of Pressure Ulcers: Copyright © D. National Pressure Ulcer Advisory Panel (NPUAP). 1998. Reprinted with permission.

CHAPTER 33

Procedure 33-2, Step 6: iStockphoto.

Procedure 33-7 Equipment: With permission from Unomedical a/s.

CHAPTER 36

Procedure 36-4 Equipment 1: Courtesy of Allied Healthcare Products, St. Louis, MO.

Perioperative Checklist: Reprinted with permission from AORN Perioperative Patient-Focused Model. Copyright AORN, Inc, 2170 Parker Rd., Suite 300, Denver, CO 80231. All rights reserved.

Surgical Safety Checklist: Reprinted with permission from the World Health Organization. Retrieved from http://apps.who.int/iris/bitstream/10665/44186/2/9789241598590_eng_Checklist.pdf.

INDEX

References are to volume and page number(s). Page numbers followed by *f* refer to figures; page numbers followed by *t* refer to tables; page numbers followed by *b* refer to boxes; page numbers followed by *p* refer to procedures

A

AACN. *See* American Association of Colleges of Nursing (AACN)
AB blood group, (V1) 1068, (V1) 1068*t*
Abbreviations
　commonly used in healthcare, (V2) 163–165, (V2) 426
　medication-related, (V2) 459
Abdomen
　assessment of, (V2) 257–263*p*
　auscultation of, (V1) 503
　four quadrants of, (V1) 502, (V1) 503*f*
　inspection of, (V1) 503
　palpation of, (V1) 503
　percussion of, (V1) 503
　physical examination of, (V1) 502–503, (V1) 503*f*, (V1) 510, (V1) 512*p*
　variations in shape of, (V1) 503*f*
Abdominal binders, (V1) 972
Abdominal circumference, (V1) 696
Abdominal distention, as postoperative complication, (V1) 1100*t*
Abdominal flat plate, (V2) 587
ABG. *See* Arterial blood gases (ABG)
Ablative surgery, (V1) 1078
A blood group, (V1) 1068, (V1) 1068*t*
Abnormal sensitivity to drugs, (V1) 621
ABO blood type, (V1) 1068
Abrasion, (V1) 582, (V1) 945*t*
Abscess, (V1) 945*t*
Absent or weak pulse, (V1) 461
Absorbent sutures, (V1) 948
Absorption, drug, (V1) 611
Abstinence, (V1) 896, (V2) 642
Abuse and neglect
　assessing for, (V1) 161*p*, (V2) 43–47*p*
　　after the examination, (V2) 45*p*
　　focused health history in, (V2) 43*p*
　　focused physical assessment in, (V2) 44–45*p*
　　for psychological abuse, (V2) 44*p*
　　for sexual abuse, (V2) 43*p*
　of children (*See* Child abuse and neglect)
　communicable diseases and, (V1) 1178
　flow chart of possible, (V2) 42
　of older adults, (V1) 198, (V1) 199–200
　vulnerable populations and, (V1) 1113
Accelerated BSN programs, (V1) 11
Acceptable macronutrient distribution range (AMDR), (V1) 667
Accessory muscles and inspiration, (V1) 994
Access to care, (V1) 310, (V1) 479
Accidents. *See* Safety
Accommodation, (V1) 147, (V1) 327
Accountability, (V1) 553
　legal (*See* Law and legal liability)
Accreditation, (V1) 1165
Acculturation, (V1) 313
Accumulation of drugs in tissues, (V1) 621
Acetaminophen, (V1) 828, (V1) 834
Achondroplasia, (V1) 857

Acid-base balance, (V1) 671, (V1) 1045, (V1) 1049
　acidosis and alkalosis and, (V1) 1047, (V1) 1050*t*
　assessment of, (V1) 1052–1053, (V2) 803–804
　critical thinking and clinical judgment on, (V2) 806–807
　diagnostic testing of, (V2) 805
　full-spectrum nursing model applied to, (V2) 805–806
　knowledge map on, (V2) 809
　management of, (V1) 1054
Acidosis, (V1) 1047, (V1) 1050*t*, (V1) 1052
Acne, (V1) 582
　newborn, (V1) 941
Acromegaly, (V1) 491
Actigraph, (V1) 932
Active B cells, (V1) 524
Active euthanasia, (V1) 361
Active involvement in patient learning, (V1) 400
Active listening, (V1) 343, (V1) 387–388, (V1) 388*f*, (V1) 1191
Active prewarming, (V1) 1086
Active range of motion (AROM), (V1) 845
　exercises for, (V1) 875–876
Active release therapy (ART), (V1) 824
Active resistance, (V1) 1193
Active T cells, (V1) 524
Active transport, (V1) 1039–1040, (V1) 1040*f*
Activities of daily living (ADLs), (V1) 198, (V1) 576, (V1) 578
　ambulation exercises and, (V1) 876, (V1) 877*f*
　assessment of, (V1) 200
　　Katz Index of ADL scale, (V2) 17, (V2) 384–385
　　special needs, (V2) 18
　pain and, (V1) 821
Activity theory, (V1) 191
Activity tolerance, (V1) 865, (V1) 866
Actual loss, (V1) 348
Acupressure, (V1) 824
Acupuncture, (V1) 261, (V1) 824
　for acute postoperative pain, (V1) 1102
　for neuropathic pain, (V1) 917
Acute bronchitis, (V1) 985
Acute care, (V1) 16
Acute illness, (V1) 219
Acute infections, (V1) 519
Acute pain, (V1) 812, (V1) 817, (V1) 821
Acute wounds, (V1) 944
Adaptation, (V1) 147
　See also Stress
　assessment of, (V1) 254
　　guidelines and tools for, (V2) 82–84
　burnout and, (V1) 253–254, (V1) 254*b*
　to change as hardiness, (V1) 220
　crisis and, (V1) 252–253, (V1) 253*f*
　crisis intervention, (V1) 263, (V2) 81
　critical thinking and clinical judgment on, (V2) 85–86

defined, (V1) 239
full-spectrum nursing model applied to, (V2) 84–85
general adaptation syndrome (GAS), (V1) 242–245, (V1) 243–244*f*
health promotion activities for, (V1) 258–259
knowledge map on, (V2) 88
local adaptation syndrome, (V1) 245–246, (V1) 245*b*
as outcome of stress, (V1) 241, (V1) 241*f*
personal factors influencing, (V1) 241–242
planning for, (V1) 257–258
problems related to failure of, (V1) 251–254, (V1) 252*t*, (V1) 253*f*, (V1) 254*b*
relation to stress, (V1) 240–242, (V1) 241*f*
sleep and, (V1) 917
somatoform disorders and, (V1) 251
to stimuli, (V1) 784, (V1) 786
stress-induced chronic responses and, (V1) 251
stress-induced psychological responses and, (V1) 251–253
Adapted physical activity (APA), (V1) 191
Adaptive coping, (V1) 240
A-delta fibers, (V1) 813, (V1) 814–815, (V1) 815*f*
Adenosine, (V1) 923
Adenosine trisphosphate (ATP), (V1) 1040
Adequate intake (AI), (V1) 667
Adhesive strips, (V1) 948
Adhesive tape, (V1) 971
Adjuvant analgesics, (V1) 828
Administration set, IV infusion, (V1) 1061–1062, (V1) 1062*f*
　changing, (V1) 1067
Administrative law, (V1) 1156, (V1) 1157*t*
Admission, (V1) 236*p*
　critical thinking and clinical judgment on, (V2) 76–77
　data form, (V1) 430–431, (V2) 166
　full-spectrum nursing model applied to, (V2) 75–76
　of patient to nursing unit, (V1) 236*p*, (V2) 60–62*p*
　preparing room for, (V2) 69
Adolescents
　assessment of, (V1) 176–179
　blood pressure in, (V1) 469
　breast self-examination in, (V1) 178
　cardiovascular function in, (V1) 1020
　common health problems of, (V1) 172–176
　communication by, (V1) 380
　depression in, (V1) 172
　development of
　　cognitive, (V1) 171
　　physical, (V1) 171, (V1) 171*b*
　　psychosocial, (V1) 171–172, (V1) 172*f*
　　sexuality, (V1) 887–888
　drowning of, (V1) 549
　eating disorders in, (V1) 172, (V1) 174
　emerging sexual orientation in, (V1) 172
　energy needs of, (V1) 683

866

gender and sexual identity in, (V1) 888
grief in, (V1) 353
group acceptance among, (V1) 171–172
health risks in families with, (V1) 297, (V1) 298f
hearing in, (V1) 787
hygiene and, (V1) 576
immunization in, (V1) 178
implementation for, (V1) 177–179
loss in, (V1) 348
nutrition in, (V1) 686
onset of puberty in, (V1) 171
overweight and obesity in, (V1) 174–175, (V1) 177–178
physical activity guidelines for, (V1) 852b
physical examination of, (V1) 485
poisoning in, (V1) 548
pregnancy in, (V1) 151, (V1) 176, (V1) 178, (V1) 299
psychomotor skills in, (V1) 787
pulmonary function in, (V1) 980
risk sexual behaviors in, (V1) 175
safety of, (V1) 547
sexually transmitted infections (STIs) in, (V1) 175–176
skin of, (V1) 583, (V1) 941
sleep requirements and characteristics in, (V1) 918t, (V1) 923
social skills in, (V1) 787
stressors in, (V1) 240b
substance abuse by, (V1) 172, (V1) 173–174
suicide by, (V1) 172
surgical risk in, (V1) 1078
tattoos and piercings in, (V1) 172
testicular self-examination in, (V1) 178
vision in, (V1) 787
Adrenaline, (V1) 243
Adrenocorticotropic hormone (ACTH), (V1) 242
Adults
blood pressure in, (V1) 469
bowel elimination in, (V1) 758
cohabitating, (V1) 293
grief in, (V1) 353
home safety interventions for, (V1) 563
hygiene and, (V1) 576
middle age (*See* Middle adulthood)
normal pulse in, (V1) 460
older (*See* Older adults)
physical activity guidelines for, (V1) 852b
poisoning in, (V1) 548
respiration in, (V1) 463
safety of, (V1) 547
self-concept formation in, (V1) 267
sensory function in, (V1) 787
sexuality in, (V1) 888–889, (V1) 889f
single, (V1) 292
skin of, (V1) 941
young (*See* Young adults)
Advance directives, (V1) 139, (V1) 358–359, (V1) 421, (V1) 1159–1160
Advanced practice registered nurses (APRNs), (V1) 12, (V1) 26
Adverse reactions
to blood infusions, (V1) 1069–1070, (V1) 1070t
to drugs, (V1) 621
Advice, offering, as barrier to therapeutic communication, (V1) 390

Advocacy
client, (V1) 138–139, (V1) 1115, (V1) 1124–1125
ethical, (V2) 33
by managers, (V1) 1185
Aerobic conditioning, (V1) 852
Aerobic exercise, (V1) 852
Aerosol sprayers, (V1) 641
Aerosol sprays or foams, (V1) 613t, (V1) 614t
Aesthetic needs, (V1) 102f
Affective learning, (V1) 398t, (V1) 399
Affordable Care Act (ACA), (V1) 21
African diets, (V1) 667–668
Against medical advice (AMA), (V1) 1167
Age
body temperature and, (V1) 448
pharmacokinetics and, (V1) 619
physical examination modifications by, (V1) 485–486
pulse and, (V1) 457
safety and accidents and, (V1) 546–547
skin and, (V1) 193t, (V1) 488, (V1) 941
sleep and, (V1) 923
surgical risk and, (V1) 1078–1079
total body fluid and, (V1) 1037, (V1) 1037t
vulnerable populations and, (V1) 1113
Age-friendly communities, (V1) 188–189
Age-friendly residences, (V1) 188
Ageism, (V1) 198
Agency for Healthcare Research and Quality (AHRQ), (V1) 516
Agglutination, (V1) 524
Aggregate groups, (V1) 1111
Aggressive communication style, (V1) 382–383
Aging
changes in sexual response with, (V1) 894t
distinguishing changes of dementia from typical, (V1) 197t
life expectancy and, (V1) 186–187
life-span perspective of, (V1) 187
migration and distribution of age groups and, (V1) 187
normal changes in, (V1) 193–194t
percentage of total population of different groups and, (V1) 187
perspectives on, (V1) 186–187
in place and alternatives, (V1) 187–190
sensory function changes with, (V1) 787t
theories of, (V1) 190
Agonist-antagonist opioids, (V1) 828
AHA. *See* American Heart Association (AHA)
AI. *See* Adequate intake (AI)
Air embolus, as complication of intravenous therapy, (V1) 1066t
Air pollution, (V1) 551, (V1) 570
pulmonary function and, (V1) 981
Airway, (V1) 976–977, (V1) 976f
artificial, (V1) 1005, (V1) 1005–1006, (V1) 1005f
endotracheal, (V1) 1005, (V1) 1005f
caring for patients with, (V2) 749
suctioning of, (V1) 1007, (V2) 726–730p
nasopharyngeal, (V1) 1005, (V1) 1015p
insertion of, (V2) 746–747p
oropharyngeal, (V1) 1005, (V1) 1014p
insertion of, (V2) 744–745p
suctioning of, (V1) 1006–1007, (V1) 1007f, (V1) 1012–1013p, (V2) 726–736p

Airway resistance, (V1) 978
Alarm fatigue, (V1) 554, (V1) 574
Alarm safety, (V1) 554
Alarm stage in stress, (V1) 242–244, (V1) 243–244f
Albumin, (V1) 698
Alcohol use
cardiovascular function and, (V1) 1022
host susceptibility to infection and, (V1) 525, (V1) 528
influence on health and wellness, (V1) 213
nutrition and, (V1) 690, (V1) 693
osteoporosis and, (V1) 867
PICOT questions, (V1) 296
during pregnancy, (V1) 150
sleep and, (V1) 924
urinary elimination and, (V1) 723
Aldosterone, (V1) 242, (V1) 1041
Algor mortis, (V1) 367
Alignment, body, (V1) 844, (V1) 844f
Alkalosis, (V1) 1047, (V1) 1050t
Allergies and allergic reactions
to blood infusions, (V1) 1070t
cardiovascular function and, (V1) 1021
cough and, (V1) 995
to drugs, (V1) 621, (V1) 622, (V1) 622t, (V1) 623f
food, (V1) 761
pulmonary function and, (V1) 981
in school-age children, (V1) 169
surgical risk and, (V1) 1080
testing for, (V1) 996
Allodynia, (V1) 814
Allopathic medicine, (V1) 317
Alopecia, (V1) 490, (V1) 598, (V1) 943
Alpha waves, (V1) 920, (V1) 920f, (V1) 920t
Alternative care providers, (V1) 19
Alternative dispute resolution, (V1) 1170
Alternative healing systems, (V1) 319–320
Alternatives
in choosing interventions, (V1) 79b
in critical thinking, (V1) 40b, (V1) 41, (V1) 41f
Altitude
cardiovascular function and, (V1) 1021
pulmonary function and, (V1) 981–982
Alveolar-capillary membrane disorders, (V1) 989
Alveoli, (V1) 977, (V1) 977f
Ambulation
assisting with, (V1) 876–878, (V1) 876–878f, (V2) 625–628p
walking aids for, (V1) 877–878, (V1) 877–878f
physical conditioning exercises to prepare for, (V2) 629
Ambulatory care centers, (V1) 17, (V1) 17f
AMDR. *See* Acceptable macronutrient distribution range (AMDR)
American Association of Colleges of Nursing (AACN), (V1) 6
on collaborative professional communication, (V2) 143
core competencies for professional nursing, (V1) 8
American Heart Association (AHA), (V1) 672t, (V1) 691

American Hospital Association (AHA), (V1) 132
  Patient Care Partnership, (V1) 132, (V1) 132b, (V1) 138, (V1) 397
American Nurses Association (ANA), (V1) 14
  Code of Ethics for Nurses, (V1) 13, (V1) 86, (V1) 118, (V1) 119, (V1) 132, (V1) 396, (V1) 1161–1162
  on collaborative professional communication, (V2) 142
  on cultural competency, (V1) 320
  definition of nursing, (V1) 8–9
  on documentation, (V1) 420
  on do-not-resuscitate (DNR) prescription, (V1) 360, (V1) 360b
  on infection prevention, (V1) 516
  Nurses' Bill of Rights, (V1) 1162
  on nursing research, (V1) 105
  Nursing: Scope and Standards of Practice, (V1) 52, (V1) 132, (V1) 396, (V1) 420, (V1) 516
  on patient safety, (V1) 545
  Principles for Health System Transformation, (V1) 22
  Standards for Community Health Nursing, (V1) 1119
  Standards of Practice, (V1) 1162
  on teaching responsibilities, (V1) 396–397
American Nurses Credentialing Center (ANCC), (V1) 1183
American Psychiatric Association (APA), (V1) 62
American Red Cross, (V1) 6
Americans with Disabilities Act (ADA), (V1) 300, (V1) 1160
Amino acids, (V1) 669–670
Amphetamines, (V1) 924
Amphiarthroses, (V1) 842
Ampules, (V1) 645, (V1) 646f, (V1) 659p
ANA. *See* American Nurses Association (ANA)
Anabolism, (V1) 669, (V1) 942
Anaerobic exercise, (V1) 852
Analgesics
  adjuvant, (V1) 828
  dosage and administration, (V1) 826–827
  epidural catheter for, (V2) 609
  nonopioid, (V1) 827–828, (V1) 834
  opioid, (V1) 828–831, (V1) 829b, (V1) 831f, (V1) 834
  patient-controlled analgesia (PCA), (V1) 831–832, (V1) 831f, (V2) 606–608p
  urinary elimination and, (V1) 723
  use in older adults, (V1) 823
Anal intercourse, (V1) 896
Anal sphincter surgery, (V1) 760
Anal stage, in psychoanalytic theory, (V1) 147t, (V1) 163
Anal stimulation, (V1) 895–896
Analytic reading, (V1) 111, (V1) 112–113
Anastomose tissue, (V1) 948
Andropause, (V1) 181
Anemia, (V1) 1025
  nutrition and, (V1) 678
  respiration and, (V1) 464
Anesthesia
  bowel elimination and, (V1) 759–760
  conscious sedation, (V1) 1091
  epidural, (V1) 1092, (V1) 1092f
  general, (V1) 1091

local, (V1) 832, (V1) 1092
recovery from, (V1) 1095–1096, (V1) 1096b
regional, (V1) 1091–1092, (V1) 1092f
spinal, (V1) 1092, (V1) 1092f
topical, (V1) 832
urinary elimination and, (V1) 723–724
Anesthesiologist, (V1) 1090
Anger
  dealing with patients experiencing, (V2) 80
  management of, (V1) 260
  in response to stress, (V1) 250
Angina, (V1) 1024
Angiocaths, (V1) 1057, (V1) 1057f
Angiogram, (V2) 753, (V2) 763
Anilingus, (V1) 895
Animal-assisted therapy, (V1) 826
Animals, pathogens from, (V1) 550
Anions, (V1) 1037
Anisocoria, (V1) 493
Ankylosing spondylitis, (V1) 858
Anorexia nervosa, (V1) 172, (V1) 174
Antacids, (V1) 759
Antagonistic drug relationship, (V1) 623
Antalgic gait, (V1) 865
Anterior chest, (V1) 496
Anthropometric measurements, (V1) 696–697, (V1) 697b
Antibiotics
  bowel elimination and, (V1) 759
  preoperative, (V1) 1087, (V1) 1087t
  skin effects of, (V1) 943
Antibodies, (V1) 524
Anticholesterol medications, (V1) 1033
Anticholinergics
  preoperative, (V1) 1087t
  urinary elimination and, (V1) 723
Anticipated life changes, as health disruption, (V1) 217
Anticipatory grief, (V1) 354
Anticipatory stressors, (V1) 239
Anticoagulants, (V1) 1033
  skin effects of, (V1) 943
  subcutaneous administration of, (V2) 458
Anticonvulsants, (V1) 926
Antidepressants
  sleep and, (V1) 924, (V1) 935
  urinary elimination and, (V1) 723
Antidiuretic hormone (ADH), (V1) 242, (V1) 718, (V1) 1041
Antiembolism stockings, (V1) 1032, (V1) 1088f, (V1) 1104p, (V2) 815–817p
  postoperative, (V1) 1103–1104
  preoperative, (V1) 1088
Antigen-avoidance diets, (V1) 695
Antigen-presenting cell (APC), (V1) 524
Antigens, (V1) 524
Antihistamines, (V1) 936, (V1) 984t
  preoperative, (V1) 1087t
Antimicrobial-coated catheters, (V1) 735
Antimotility drugs and bowel elimination, (V1) 759
Antiseptic solutions, (V1) 960
Antispasmodics and urinary elimination, (V1) 723
Anus, (V1) 756, (V1) 756f
  assessment of, (V2) 294–295p
  physical examination of, (V1) 509, (V1) 513p
  as primary defense against infection, (V1) 521

Anxiety
  assessment of, (V2) 93
  cardiovascular system and, (V1) 1025–1026, (V1) 1032
  coping with, (V1) 277–279
  defense mechanisms for, (V1) 278–279
  levels of, (V1) 277, (V1) 278t
  mild to moderate, (V1) 248, (V1) 278t
  nursing care for, (V1) 279–281
  pain and, (V1) 816
  panic, (V1) 248, (V1) 249–250, (V1) 278t
  in patients with confusion, (V1) 289, (V1) 805
  relieving, (V1) 259–260
  in response to stress, (V1) 246
  severe, (V1) 248, (V1) 278t
  sleep and, (V1) 917, (V1) 924
  urinary elimination and, (V1) 722
Anxiolytics, preoperative, (V1) 1087t
AORN SAMPLE preoperative assessment form, (V2) 827–828
Apex, heart, (V1) 1017, (V1) 1017f
Apgar scoring, (V1) 155, (V2) 50
Apical pulse, (V1) 452p, (V1) 459, (V1) 460, (V1) 460f
  assessment of, (V2) 184–185p
Apical-radial pulse
  deficit, (V1) 452p, (V1) 460, (V2) 186–187p
  when to take, (V1) 460
Apnea, (V1) 465t, (V1) 994
Apothecary system, (V1) 624
Appeal, legal, (V1) 1170
Appearance
  body image and, (V1) 268
  facial, (V1) 491
  in general survey, (V1) 487
Appendix, (V1) 755
Appetite loss, (V1) 702
Appetite suppression, (V1) 693
Approval or disapproval, expressions of, (V1) 390
APRNs. *See* Advanced practice registered nurses (APRNs)
Aqueous solutions, (V1) 614–615t, (V1) 614t
Arbitration, (V1) 1170
Archetypes, cultural, (V1) 315
Arm exercises, (V1) 876
Aromatherapy, (V1) 786
Arousal in level of consciousness (LOC), (V1) 505
Arousal mechanism, (V1) 784–785
Art activities, (V1) 262
Arterial blood carbon dioxide, (V1) 998
Arterial blood gases (ABG), (V1) 1050t, (V1) 1051, (V1) 1053, (V2) 753, (V2) 763
  interpretation of, (V1) 1049
  sampling of, (V1) 466, (V1) 997
Arterial compliance and blood pressure, (V1) 469
Arterial oxygen saturation, (V1) 466
Arterial size and blood pressure, (V1) 468
Arterial ulcers, (V1) 946t
Arteries, (V1) 502, (V1) 1018
  abnormalities of, (V1) 1025
  auscultation of major, (V1) 503
  coronary, (V1) 1018–1019, (V1) 1019f
Arteriosclerosis, (V1) 469
Articular cartilage, (V1) 842
Articulation, joint, (V1) 841
Artificial active immunity, (V1) 523b

Artificial airways, (V1) 1005, (V1) 1005–1006
Artificial eyes, (V1) 600, (V1) 603p, (V2) 374–375p, (V2) 603p
Artificial intelligence (AI), (V1) 1145
Artificial passive immunity, (V1) 523b
Ascending colon, (V1) 755
Ascorbic acid. *See* Vitamin C
Asepsis
  critical thinking and clinical judgment on, (V2) 328
  full-spectrum nursing model applied to, (V2) 327–328
  hand hygiene for, (V1) 1076, (V1) 1076b, (V2) 303–304p
    infection prevention and, (V1) 531, (V1) 533, (V1) 539p
    preschoolers and, (V1) 166
    surgical, (V1) 539p
    types of, (V1) 537t
  knowledge map on, (V2) 330
  medical, (V1) 533–536, (V1) 535t, (V1) 536f
  surgical, (V1) 536–539, (V1) 537t, (V1) 540b
  wound care and, (V1) 972
Asian diet, (V1) 667–668, (V1) 691–692
Asphyxia, birth, (V1) 155
Asphyxiation, (V1) 549
Aspiration, (V1) 703, (V1) 706
  precautions for, (V1) 1002
  prevention of, (V2) 748
Aspiration pneumonia, (V1) 1098t
Aspirin, (V1) 759, (V1) 827–828
  cardiovascular function and, (V1) 1022
  sensory function and, (V1) 788
Assault, (V1) 1166
  sexual, (V1) 897, (V1) 900, (V2) 639
Assault and battery, (V1) 1167
Assertive communication style, (V1) 383, (V1) 388
Assessment, (V1) 47–50
  abuse, (V1) 161p, (V2) 43–47p
  activity and exercise, (V2) 632–633
  adolescent, (V1) 176–179
  age-related changes, (V1) 193–194t
  anus and rectum, (V2) 294–295p
  anxiety, (V2) 93
  Apgar scoring, (V1) 155, (V2) 50
  blood pressure, (V1) 470–471f, (V1) 470–474, (V1) 473f, (V1) 473t
  body composition, (V1) 683, (V1) 696–697, (V1) 697b
  body temperature, (V1) 450–454, (V1) 452–454t, (V1) 452p, (V2) 173–179p
  bowel elimination, (V1) 763–764t, (V1) 763–766, (V2) 585
  brief bedside, (V1) 513p, (V2) 295–296p
  cardiovascular system, (V1) 1025–1028, (V1) 1028f
  caregiver role strain, (V1) 302b, (V1) 304–307
  chest and lungs, (V2) 244–250p
  circulation, (V2) 761–762
  client's environment, (V1) 601
  communication, (V1) 387, (V2) 144–145
  community nursing, (V1) 1119–1120
  cultural, (V1) 322–324
  death and dying, (V1) 362, (V2) 132–133
  depression, (V1) 200, (V1) 282, (V1) 287f, (V2) 92, (V1) 94–95
  discharge, (V2) 70–71
  ears, (V2) 227–231p
  eyes, (V1) 599, (V2) 220–227p
  for falls, (V1) 557–561, (V1) 562f
  family health, (V1) 302–304, (V1) 303b, (V1) 303f, (V2) 102–103
    beliefs, (V1) 302–303
    communication patterns, (V1) 304
    coping processes, (V1) 304
    genetics, (V1) 302, (V1) 303b, (V1) 303f
    guidelines and tools for, (V1) 103–104
  female genitourinary system, (V2) 290–293p
  fetal development, (V2) 48–49
  fluid, electrolytes, and acid-base balance, (V1) 1052–1053, (V2) 803–804
  foot, (V1) 589
  full-spectrum nursing model applied to, (V2) 50
  functional ability, (V1) 50, (V1) 200, (V2) 17
  genetic history, (V1) 302
  guidelines and tools, (V2) 13–14
  hair, (V1) 597, (V2) 215–216p
  head and face, (V2) 218–219p
  health (*See* Health assessment)
  health beliefs, (V1) 227–228
  health promotion, (V1) 226
  health screening, (V1) 228–229
  hearing, (V1) 493–494, (V1) 511p, (V2) 227–231p
  heart, (V1) 1025–1026, (V2) 250–257p
  history and physical examination, (V1) 226
  home healthcare, (V1) 1129
  home safety, (V1) 561
  hygiene, (V1) 577, (V2) 384–385
  infant, (V1) 160
  infections, (V1) 529–530
  learning, (V2) 150–151
  life stress review, (V1) 227
  lifestyle and risk, (V1) 227, (V2) 73–75
  male genitourinary system, (V2) 285–289p
  for medication administration, (V1) 630–631
  middle adulthood, (V1) 182–183
  mobility and exercise, (V1) 863–865, (V1) 864b
  multicultural populations, (V2) 111–112
  musculoskeletal system, (V2) 263–272p
  nails, (V1) 590, (V2) 216–218p
  neonatal, (V1) 155–156
  nose and sinuses, (V1) 511p, (V2) 232–234p
  nursing skills in, (V1) 48–49, (V1) 48b
  nutritional, (V1) 50, (V1) 228, (V1) 695–699, (V1) 697b, (V1) 698b, (V2) 505–509
  older adults, (V1) 198–201, (V1) 201f, (V2) 54–55
  oral cavity, (V1) 594
  oxygenation, (V1) 993–998, (V1) 995b, (V1) 996–998f, (V2) 751–752
  pain, (V1) 50, (V1) 818–821, (V1) 820t, (V2) 610–612
  patient education, (V1) 408, (V2) 150–151
  perception, (V2) 599–601
  physical, (V1) 48 (*See also* Physical examination)
    cultural competence and, (V1) 323–324
    genitourinary system, (V1) 507–509
  physical fitness, (V1) 226–227, (V2) 72
  postanesthesia, (V2) 830
  postoperative, (V1) 1097
  preoperative phase, (V1) 1081–1082, (V1) 1093, (V2) 827–828
  preschooler, (V1) 166
  psychosocial health, (V1) 270–271
  pulse, (V1) 452p, (V1) 458–461, (V1) 459–460f
  respiration, (V1) 452p, (V1) 464–467, (V1) 465t, (V2) 187–189p
  risk for violence, (V1) 561
  safety, (V1) 557–561, (V1) 562f
  school-age children, (V1) 169
  self-care, (V1) 577
  self-concept disturbance and low self-esteem, (V1) 272–273, (V2) 90–91
  sensory system, (V1) 802–803, (V2) 599–601
  sexual health, (V1) 902, (V2) 644–645
  skin, (V1) 323–324, (V1) 510p, (V1) 584, (V2) 206–214p, (V2) 694–699
  sleep, (V1) 931–932
  sleep and rest, (V2) 652–653
  special needs, (V1) 49–50, (V2) 18
  spirituality, (V1) 340–341, (V2) 121–122
  stress and adaptation, (V1) 254, (V1) 257b, (V2) 82–84
  theory applied to, (V1) 103
  toddler, (V1) 164
  types and sources of data in, (V1) 47–48, (V1) 48t
  types of, (V1) 49–50
  urinary elimination, (V1) 724, (V1) 727–730, (V1) 728f, (V1) 729b, (V1) 730f, (V2) 545–546
  wellness, (V1) 50, (V1) 223, (V1) 226–229
  wound, (V1) 952–953, (V1) 954–957t, (V1) 956–959, (V2) 694–699
  young adults, (V1) 180
Assimilation, (V1) 147, (V1) 313
Assist bath, (V1) 585
Assisted-living facilities (ALFs), (V1) 17, (V1) 189
Assisted suicide, (V1) 361
Associate degree nursing programs, (V1) 11
  nursing research and, (V1) 106
Association of Perioperative Registered Nurses (AORN), (V1) 1076, (V1) 1077
Assumptions
  in choosing interventions, (V1) 79b
  in critical thinking, (V1) 40b, (V1) 41, (V1) 41f
  defined, (V1) 94
Asthma, (V1) 981
  childhood, (V1) 168
    teaching about, (V1) 170
  sleep and, (V1) 931
Asymmetry of head, (V1) 491
Ataxic gait, (V1) 865
Atelectasis, (V1) 989, (V1) 1098t
Atheism, (V1) 337
Athletic performance and nutrition, (V1) 690–691
Atomizers, (V1) 641
Atria, (V1) 1017, (V1) 1017f
Atrial natriuretic peptide (ANP), (V1) 1041
Atrioventricular (AV) node, (V1) 1018
Atrophy, (V1) 864b
Attitudes
  critical thinking, (V1) 37–38
  leaders and, (V1) 1191
  values, beliefs, and, (V1) 124–126
Audio-recorded reports, (V1) 437
Audio recordings, (V1) 389
Audit trails, (V1) 1150

Auscultation, (V2) 298
  abdomen, (V1) 503
  blood pressure, (V1) 472–473, (V1) 473f
    with palpation, (V1) 473–474
  heart, (V1) 501, (V1) 501f, (V1) 501t
  in physical examination, (V1) 484
  respiratory function, (V1) 993
Authoritarian leadership, (V1) 1182
Authority and tradition, (V1) 107
Autoimmune reaction, (V1) 190
Autologous donation of blood, (V1) 1069
Autolytic débridement, (V1) 967
Automated dispensing cabinets (ADCs), (V1) 610, (V1) 629
Automated dispensing systems, (V1) 610
Automaticity, heart, (V1) 1018
Automatic stop dates, prescription, (V1) 625
Automation for error-prevention, (V1) 1142–1143
Automobiles
  accidents in, (V1) 157, (V1) 550
    adolescents and, (V1) 172, (V1) 177, (V1) 179
  car seats, (V1) 161, (V1) 167, (V1) 567–568t
  safety and, (V1) 567, (V1) 567–568t
Autonomic nervous system, (V1) 457, (V1) 843–844, (V1) 1019–1020
Autonomy
  as ethical concept, (V1) 128–129
  intellectual, in critical thinking, (V1) 37
  versus shame and doubt, in psychosocial development theory, (V1) 148, (V1) 162–163
Autonomy model, (V1) 138
Autopsy, (V1) 361
Avoidance
  as defense mechanism, (V1) 247t
  of maladaptive behaviors, (V1) 259
Axillae, (V1) 495, (V1) 511p
  assessment of, (V1) 511p, (V2) 240–243p
Axillary body temperature measurement, (V1) 456t, (V2) 174p
Axillary crutches, (V1) 878, (V1) 878f
Ayurveda, (V1) 320

B

Babinski reflex, (V1) 154
Baccalaureate degree nursing (BSN) programs, (V1) 11
  nursing research and, (V1) 106
Bacillus, (V1) 517
Back injury
  in healthcare workers, (V1) 556
  teaching patients how to prevent, (V1) 856
Back massage, (V1) 585
Bacteremia, (V1) 519
Bacteria, wound drainage, (V1) 949
Bacterial growth with enteral nutrition, (V1) 706
Bacterial infections with blood infusions, (V1) 1070t
Bag bath, (V1) 585
Balance
  body mechanics of, (V1) 844, (V1) 845f
  family, (V1) 295
  problems with, (V1) 504

Balanitis, (V1) 901
Bandages, (V1) 972–973, (V2) 684–687p
Barbiturates, (V1) 935
  preoperative, (V1) 1087t
Barcode medication administration, (V1) 628
Bariatric surgery, (V1) 693
Barium enema (BE), (V2) 587
Baroreceptors, (V1) 1020
Barton, Clara, (V1) 6, (V1) 1114
Basal ganglia, (V1) 845
Basal metabolic rate (BMR), (V1) 447
  defined, (V1) 682
  direct measurement of, (V1) 682
  factors affecting, (V1) 682–683
  indirect calculation of, (V1) 682, (V1) 683b
Base, heart, (V1) 1017, (V1) 1017f
Baseline activity, (V1) 851
Baseline data, (V1) 479
Base of support, (V1) 844, (V1) 845f
Basic needs, (V1) 98–99, (V1) 99b
Basin and water bath, (V1) 585–586
Bathing
  bed baths and modified bed baths, (V1) 585–586
  guidelines for, (V1) 586b
  NIC interventions, (V1) 79b
  of older adults, (V1) 588–589
  patients who have dementia, (V1) 587
  patients who have morbid obesity, (V1) 588
  perineal care, (V1) 587, (V1) 602p, (V2) 352–355
  providing a complete bed bath using prepacked bathing product, (V2) 346–351p
  purposes of, (V1) 585
  showers, (V1) 586, (V2) 383
  therapeutic bath, (V1) 586–587
  tub, (V1) 586, (V2) 383
  using a basin and water, (V2) 351–352p
Bathwater, (V1) 586
Battery, (V1) 1166–1167
B blood group, (V1) 1068, (V1) 1068t
Beard and mustache care, (V1) 598, (V1) 602p, (V2) 369–370p
Bed and chair monitoring devices, (V1) 573p, (V2) 332–334p
Bed baths, (V1) 585–586
Bed making, (V1) 604–605
  occupied, (V1) 603p, (V2) 380–382p
  unoccupied, (V1) 603p, (V2) 377–380p
Bedpans, placing and removing, (V2) 562–565p
Bedrest
  assisting with ambulation after, (V1) 876–878, (V1) 877–878f
  physical activity by persons on, (V1) 860
Beds, (V1) 604–605
  adjustable, (V1) 868–869
  moving patients in, (V1) 873, (V1) 873f, (V2) 617–621p
  pillows on, (V1) 869, (V1) 869f
  positioning in, (V1) 871–872t
  siderails on, (V1) 555, (V1) 604, (V1) 604f, (V1) 869
  smart, (V1) 1145
  specialized, (V1) 869
  transferring patients out of, (V1) 874–875, (V1) 874–875f, (V2) 622–625p
  trapeze bars on, (V1) 869

Bedside assessment, (V1) 513p, (V2) 295–296p
Bedside equipment, (V1) 603–604
Bedside reports, (V1) 437
Behavioral learning theory, (V1) 397
Behavioral theories, (V1) 1182
Behaviors
  assessment of, (V2) 273p
  dealing with inappropriate sexual, (V1) 907–908
  unintentional injury and, (V1) 547, (V1) 547t
Behavior(s)
  avoidance of maladaptive, (V1) 259
  control of temperature by, (V1) 447
  in general survey, (V1) 487
  health promotion and, (V1) 222
  sick role, (V1) 218
  stages of illness, (V1) 218–219
  violent (*See* Violence)
Beliefs, (V1) 124
  defined, (V1) 314
  health, (V1) 227–228, (V1) 318
    assessment of family, (V1) 302–303
  religious (*See* Religion(s))
  spiritual (*See* Spirituality)
Bell stethoscopes, (V1) 458, (V1) 459f
Beneficence, (V1) 129–130, (V1) 130f
Benner, Patricia, (V1) 99
  model of development of expertise of, (V1) 12–13, (V1) 94, (V1) 94f, (V1) 99
  primacy of caring model of, (V1) 99
Benzodiazepines, (V1) 926, (V1) 935
Bereavement, (V1) 348
Beta-adrenergic blockers, (V1) 1023t, (V1) 1033
Beta blockers, (V1) 924
Beta waves, (V1) 920, (V1) 920f, (V1) 920t
Biases, (V1) 61, (V1) 321, (V1) 338
Bibliotherapy, (V1) 364
Bicarbonate, (V1) 1019
  electrolytes, (V1) 1043t, (V1) 1044
Bicultural persons, (V1) 312–313
Bier (intravenous) block, (V1) 1091
Bilateral equality of, (V1) 461
Bill of Rights, (V1) 1157
Binders, (V1) 972, (V2) 682–684p
Bioavailability, (V1) 611
Bioethics, (V1) 117
Biofeedback, (V1) 261
Biofilm, (V1) 964
Biological data, (V1) 1111
Biological half-life of drugs, (V1) 619
Biological hazards in healthcare facilities
  back injury, (V1) 556
  to healthcare workers, (V1) 556
  needlestick injury, (V1) 556
  radiation injury, (V1) 556–557
  violence, (V1) 557
Biological variations and culture, (V1) 316
Biopsy, tissue, (V1) 958, (V2) 700
Biorhythms, (V1) 919
Biosensors, (V1) 1144
Bioterrorism, (V1) 541
Biotherapy (Maggot) débridement therapy, (V1) 967
Biot respirations, (V1) 465t, (V1) 994
Birth asphyxia, (V1) 155
Birth defects, screening for, (V1) 151
Birth injuries, (V1) 155
Birthmarks, (V1) 490
Black clients, hair care for, (V1) 598
Bladder irrigation, (V1) 739, (V2) 540–543p

Blended families, (V1) 293
Blood, testing stool for occult, (V2) 560–562p
Bloodborne pathogens exposure, (V1) 540, (V1) 540b
Blood cholesterol, (V1) 672t
Blood clots, as complication of parenteral nutrition, (V1) 715
Blood flow
 drug distribution and, (V1) 616–617
 medication administration and, (V1) 616
Blood glucose screening, (V1) 182, (V1) 698, (V2) 480–483p
Blood infection, central-line associated, (V1) 1058–1059
Blood infusions, (V2) 791–795p
 autologous donation of blood for, (V1) 1069
 blood groups and, (V1) 1068, (V1) 1068t
 blood products for, (V1) 1069
 blood typing and crossmatching for, (V1) 1068–1069
 changing administration sets for, (V1) 1067
 donating blood for, (V1) 1068
 initiation of, (V1) 1069
 procedure for, (V1) 1073p
 reactions to, (V1) 1069–1070, (V1) 1070t
Blood pressure
 assessment of, (V1) 470–471f, (V1) 470–474, (V1) 473f, (V1) 473t
 auscultating, (V1) 472–473, (V1) 473f
 blood volume and, (V1) 469
 body regulation of, (V1) 467–469
 cardiac function and, (V1) 467–468
 classification of, (V1) 467, (V1) 468t
 cuff size for measuring, (V1) 471–472, (V1) 473t, (V2) 193
 defined, (V1) 467
 equipment for measuring, (V1) 470–471, (V1) 470–472f
 factors influencing, (V1) 469
 full-spectrum nursing model applied to, (V2) 194
 hypertension, (V1) 469, (V1) 474–475
  alternative therapies for, (V1) 475
 hypotension, (V1) 474
 implementation for, (V1) 475–476
 measurement of, (V1) 452p, (V2) 189–193p
  accuracy of, (V2) 193
 nursing diagnosis and, (V1) 474–475
 palpating, (V1) 473–474
 peripheral resistance and, (V1) 468–469
 planning for, (V1) 475
 skin effects of medications for, (V1) 943
 which site to use for measuring, (V1) 472
Blood studies, urinary elimination, (V1) 727, (V2) 548–550
Blood sugar, fasting, (V2) 830
Blood transfusions, (V2) 791–795p
Blood types and crossmatching, (V1) 1068–1069, (V2) 830
Blood urea nitrogen (BUN), (V1) 727, (V2) 548
Blood vessels, (V1) 1018
Blood viscosity, (V1) 468
Blood volume, (V1) 469
Bloom's domains of learning, (V1) 398–399, (V1) 398t, (V1) 399f
BMI. *See* Body mass index (BMI)
BMR. *See* Basal metabolic rate (BMR)
Body alignment, (V1) 844, (V1) 844f
Body composition analysis, (V1) 683, (V1) 696–697, (V1) 697b, (V2) 500–501

Body fluids and solutes
 acid-base balance regulation, (V1) 671, (V1) 1045
 balance of, (V1) 1040–1041
 compartments of, (V1) 1037
 electrolytes, (V1) 1037–1038
  major, (V1) 1041–1045, (V1) 1042–1044t
 fluid intake and, (V1) 1040
 fluid output and, (V1) 1040–1041
 movement in the body, (V1) 1038–1040, (V1) 1038–1040f, (V1) 1040t
 total, in relation to sex and age, (V1) 1037, (V1) 1037t
 types of, (V1) 1037
Body image, (V1) 268
 promoting positive, (V1) 276–277
Body language, (V1) 388–389
Body mass index (BMI), (V1) 487–488, (V1) 588, (V1) 696–697, (V1) 697b, (V2) 508–509
 oxygenation and, (V1) 982
 in school-age children, (V1) 169
Body mechanics, (V2) 628
 balance, (V1) 844, (V1) 845f
 body alignment, (V1) 844, (V1) 844f
 coordination, (V1) 845
 guidelines for, (V1) 845
 range of motion, (V1) 845, (V1) 846–851t
Body shape and symmetry, (V1) 504
Body structure and form, water in, (V1) 681
Body systems approach in physical examination, (V1) 480
Body temperature
 assessment of, (V1) 450–454, (V1) 452–454t, (V1) 452p, (V2) 173–179p
 axillary, (V1) 456t, (V2) 174p
 behavioral control of, (V1) 447
 chemical strip thermometer for, (V2) 178p
 decreases in, (V1) 447
 defined, (V1) 445–446
 disadvantages and contraindications of various sites for measuring, (V1) 455–456t
 equipment for measuring, (V1) 451, (V1) 452–453t, (V1) 454
 evidence-based practice and, (V1) 458
 exercise rand, (V1) 854
 factors influencing, (V1) 448–449
 fever and, (V1) 449–450
 heat exchange between the body and environment and, (V1) 448, (V1) 448f
 heat production in the body and, (V1) 447
 hyperthermia/heatstroke, (V1) 450–451
 hypothermia and, (V1) 450
 increases in, (V1) 447
 infections and, (V1) 530
 measurement scales for, (V1) 450–451, (V1) 451f
 normal, (V1) 446–447, (V1) 446t, (V1) 447f
 normothermia maintenance, (V1) 1086
 oral, (V1) 455t, (V2) 175p
 rectal, (V1) 455t, (V2) 175–176p
 response to variations in, (V1) 447–448, (V1) 448f
 sites to use for measuring, (V1) 454
 skin function in regulating, (V1) 582
 temporal artery, (V1) 455t, (V2) 176–177p
 thermoregulation and, (V1) 446
 tympanic membrane, (V1) 456t, (V2) 177–178p

 variations in, (V1) 446–447, (V1) 447f, (V1) 454
 water and, (V1) 681
Bolus method, (V1) 713
Bones, (V1) 841, (V1) 842f
 diseases related to formation and metabolism of, (V1) 857
 interventions for, (V1) 866
 problems affecting integrity of, (V1) 858
 trauma to, (V1) 858–859, (V1) 860f
 tumors of, (V1) 858, (V1) 866
Borg Rate of Perceived Exertion Scale, (V1) 853b
Borrowed servant doctrine, (V1) 1169
Boswellia, (V1) 823
Botulinum toxin and urinary elimination, (V1) 723
Boundaries, professional, (V1) 1176, (V1) 1176b
Bowel diversion, (V1) 761–762, (V1) 762f
 caring for patients with, (V1) 775–782, (V1) 778f, (V1) 780–781b
Bowel elimination
 anatomy of gastrointestinal tract and, (V1) 754–756, (V1) 754–756f
 assessment of, (V1) 763–764t, (V1) 763–766
  guidelines and tools for, (V2) 585
 bowel diversion and, (V1) 761–762, (V1) 762f
 caring for patient with indwelling fecal drainage device, (V2) 583
 critical thinking and clinical judgment on, (V2) 592
 defecation in, (V1) 757
 diagnostic testing of, (V2) 586–588
 factors affecting
  developmental stage, (V1) 757–758
  medications, (V1) 759, (V1) 759b
  nutrition, hydration, and activity level, (V1) 758
  pathological conditions, (V1) 760–761
  personal and sociocultural, (V1) 758
  pregnancy, (V1) 760
  probiotics, (V1) 759
  surgery and procedures, (V1) 759–760
 feces and, (V1) 756–757
 full-spectrum nursing model applied to, (V2) 591
 key concepts on, (V1) 754
 knowledge map on, (V2) 594
 neonatal, (V1) 153
 nursing care plan for, (V2) 589–590
 nursing diagnosis, (V1) 766
 ostomy care guidelines, (V2) 584
 preoperative, (V1) 1087
 prior to death, (V1) 357
 procedures
  administering an enema, (V2) 565–569p
  colostomy irrigation, (V2) 577–579p
  ostomy appliance changing, (V2) 573–576p
  placing and removing bedpans, (V2) 562–565p
  placing fecal drainage devices, (V2) 579–582p
  rectal tube insertion, (V2) 571–572p
  removing stool digitally, (V2) 569–571p
  testing stool for occult blood, (V2) 560–562p
 promoting normal or regular, (V1) 767–768

Bowel incontinence, (V1) 766, (V1) 776–778
  bowel training for, (V1) 775
  caring for patients with diversions for, (V1) 775–782
  fecal collection and drainage devices, (V1) 775
Bowel sounds, (V1) 503
Bowel training, (V1) 775
Bowlby, John, (V1) 350t
Bowman's capsule, (V1) 717, (V1) 718
Braces, (V1) 878
Brachial artery
  blood pressure measurement and, (V1) 472
  pulse measurement and, (V1) 459, (V2) 180p
Braden Scale for Predicting Pressure Sore Risk, (V2) 696
Bradycardia, (V1) 460
Bradypnea, (V1) 465t, (V1) 994
Brain, the
  and brain waves during sleep, (V1) 919, (V1) 920t
  death and, (V1) 354, (V1) 356
  locus of control and, (V1) 228, (V1) 268
  pain transmission to, (V1) 814
  protecting health of, (V1) 804
  responding to sensations, (V1) 785–786, (V1) 785f
  reticular activating system (RAS) in, (V1) 784–785, (V1) 920, (V1) 920f
  seizures and, (V1) 794, (V1) 797, (V1) 805–809
  sensory function and injury to, (V1) 788
  and skull in school-age children, (V1) 167
Brain natriuretic peptide (BNP), (V1) 1041
Brainstem centers, (V1) 1020
Breach of duty, (V1) 1168
Breast cancer, (V1) 182
  prevention of, (V1) 180
  screening for, (V1) 180, (V1) 182, (V1) 228–229, (V1) 495–496
Breastfeeding, (V1) 156
Breasts, (V1) 882–883
  assessment of, (V2) 240–243p
  clinical breast examination of, (V1) 495, (V1) 906
  mammography of, (V1) 180, (V1) 182, (V1) 495–496
  physical examination of, (V1) 495, (V1) 495f, (V1) 510, (V1) 511p
  vasocongestion and, (V1) 893
Breast self-examination, (V1) 229, (V1) 495
  adolescents and, (V1) 178
  young adults and, (V1) 180
Breathing
  control of, (V1) 979
  deep, (V1) 1002
  diaphragmatic, (V1) 826
  mechanics of, (V1) 463, (V1) 463f
  respiratory function and patterns of, (V1) 994
Breath sounds, (V1) 465–466, (V1) 496, (V1) 499–500f
Brevity in communication, (V1) 378
Brewster, Mary, (V1) 6
Brief bedside assessment, (V1) 513p, (V2) 295–296p
Brisk walking, (V1) 853
Bronchi, (V1) 977
Bronchioles, (V1) 977

Bronchodilators, (V1) 984t
Bronchoscopy, (V2) 753
Bronchospasm, (V1) 977
Brushing and flossing, (V1) 595, (V1) 595f, (V1) 602p, (V2) 358–361p
Bruxism, (V1) 930
Buccal medications, (V1) 636
Buccal mucosa, (V1) 494, (V1) 494f
Buddhism, (V1) 332, (V1) 337, (V1) 337f
Buffers, (V1) 1045
Bulimia, (V1) 174
Bullying, (V1) 168, (V1) 382
Bunions, (V1) 589
Burnout, (V1) 220, (V1) 253–254, (V1) 254b
Burns and scalds, (V1) 548–549, (V1) 582
Bursae, (V1) 504, (V1) 504f
Business sense of managers, (V1) 1184
Butterfly needle, (V1) 1057, (V1) 1057f

C

Cadence in communication, (V1) 377
Café-au-lait spots, (V1) 488, (V1) 941
Caffeine
  nutrition and, (V1) 690
  for pain management, (V1) 823
  sleep and, (V1) 924
  urinary elimination and, (V1) 723
Calcium, (V1) 678, (V1) 679t
  bone formation and, (V1) 857
  bowel elimination and, (V1) 758
  electrolytes, (V1) 1042t, (V1) 1043–1044
  osteoporosis and, (V1) 866–867
  recommended daily allowance for, (V1) 1044t, (V1) 1055
  supplementation of, (V1) 700
Calcium-channel blockers, (V1) 1023t
Calluses, (V1) 589
Calorie-protein push, (V1) 695
Calorie-restricted diets, (V1) 694
Calories, (V1) 682
  skin and, (V1) 942
Canaliculi, (V1) 841
Cancer
  breast, (V1) 182, (V1) 228–229
    prevention of, (V1) 180
    self-examination and, (V1) 178, (V1) 180, (V1) 229
  cervical, (V1) 229
  colorectal, (V1) 182
  fistula from, (V1) 951
  leukemia, (V1) 529
  lung, (V1) 181
  in middle adulthood, (V1) 181–182
  oral, (V1) 594
  prostate, (V1) 182, (V1) 229
  renal, (V1) 724
  sexuality and, (V1) 891
  skin, (V1) 229
  testicular, (V1) 229, (V1) 906
    self-examination and, (V1) 178, (V1) 180
Candida albicans, (V1) 517
Canes, (V1) 877, (V1) 877f
Cannabidiol (CBD), (V1) 823, (V1) 937
Capillaries, (V1) 497, (V1) 1018
Capillary hemangiomas, (V1) 488
Capnography, (V1) 996–997f, (V1) 996–998
Capsicum/capsaicin, (V1) 823
Capsules, (V1) 612t
Captain of the ship principle, (V1) 1169

Caput succedaneum, (V1) 155
Carbohydrates, (V1) 669, (V1) 670t
  sleep and, (V1) 923
Carbon dioxide, (V1) 979
  cardiovascular system transport of, (V1) 1019
Carbonic acid-sodium bicarbonate system, (V1) 1045
Carbon monoxide exposure, (V1) 548, (V1) 1025
  preventing, (V1) 564
Cardiac arrest, (V1) 1033–1034
Cardiac catheterization, (V2) 753, (V2) 763
Cardiac cycle, (V1) 499, (V1) 1017, (V1) 1018f, (V1) 1028
Cardiac injury from exercise, (V1) 854
Cardiac ischemia, (V1) 1024
Cardiac monitoring, (V1) 1028, (V1) 1028f, (V2) 759–761p
Cardiac output, (V1) 457
  alteration in, (V1) 461
  blood pressure and, (V1) 467–468
Cardiac sphincter, (V1) 754
Cardioinhibitory center, (V1) 1020
Cardiomyopathy, (V1) 1024
Cardiopulmonary resuscitation (CPR), (V1) 360, (V1) 1033–1034
Cardiorespiratory fitness assessment, (V1) 226–227
Cardiovascular disease (CVD), (V1) 182
  evidence-based practice on, (V1) 1023
  sexuality and, (V1) 891
  urinary elimination and, (V1) 724
Cardiovascular system, (V1) 496–499
  abnormalities of, (V1) 1024–1025
  age-related changes in, (V1) 193t
  assessment of, (V1) 1025–1028, (V1) 1028f
  autonomic nervous system and, (V1) 1019–1020
  brainstem centers and, (V1) 1020
  cardiopulmonary resuscitation (CPR) and, (V1) 360, (V1) 1033–1034
  coronary arteries, (V1) 1018–1019, (V1) 1019f
  diagnostic testing of, (V1) 1027–1028, (V1) 1028f
  function of, (V1) 1019–1020
    factors influencing, (V1) 1020–1025, (V1) 1023–1024t
  heart, (V1) 499
    auscultation of, (V1) 501, (V1) 501f, (V1) 501t
    cardiac cycle and, (V1) 499
    inspection and palpation of, (V1) 499, (V1) 501
    sounds of, (V1) 501
    structures of, (V1) 1017–1018, (V1) 1017–1018f
  interventions for, (V1) 1031–1035
  in neonates, (V1) 153
  nursing diagnosis and, (V1) 1029
  oxygen and carbon dioxide transport, (V1) 1019
  physical examination of, (V1) 509, (V1) 511–512p
  responses related to failure of adaptation, (V1) 252t
  response to stress, (V1) 244
  structures of, (V1) 1017–1019, (V1) 1017–1019f

systemic and pulmonary blood vessels, (V1) 1018
unrelieved pain and, (V1) 817
vascular system, (V1) 502
Caregiver role strain, (V1) 302b, (V1) 304–307, (V1) 1129
Caregiver support, (V1) 205, (V1) 1135
Care maps
  pain management, (V1) 838
  urinary catheterization, (V1) 751
Care plans, (V1) 67–71, (V1) 68f, (V1) 70f, (V1) 422
  bowel elimination, (V2) 589–590
  computer-generated, (V1) 69, (V1) 74, (V1) 78
  critical pathways in, (V1) 69, (V1) 70f
  evaluating and revising, (V1) 89–90
  individualized, (V1) 69, (V1) 71
  integrated plans of care (IPOCs) in, (V1) 69–71
  pain, (V1) 837–838
  policies and procedures in, (V1) 67
  protocols in, (V1) 67
  special discharge or teaching, (V1) 69
  standardized, (V1) 67–71, (V1) 68f, (V1) 70f
  standardized (model) nursing care plans, (V1) 67, (V1) 68f
  student, (V1) 69
    mind-mapping, (V1) 71
  unit standards of care in, (V1) 67
  urinary catheterization, (V1) 748–751
  urinary elimination, (V2) 551–554
  wound, (V1) 959–974
Caring, (V1) 42, (V1) 43t
  for the family, (V1) 104
  for oneself, (V1) 149
  for others, (V1) 149
  as respecting personhood and dignity, (V1) 204
  for self and others, (V1) 149
Carminative enemas, (V1) 771
Carotid arteries, (V1) 502
  pulse measurement using, (V1) 459, (V2) 181p
Car seats, (V1) 161, (V1) 167, (V1) 567–568t
Cartilage, (V1) 504, (V1) 504f, (V1) 843
Case management, (V1) 22
  community nursing, (V1) 1115
Case manager, role and function of, (V1) 7t
Case method of care, (V1) 16
Casts, care of, (V1) 859
Catabolism, (V1) 669, (V1) 942
Catalyst, water as, (V1) 681
Cataplexy, (V1) 926
Cataracts, congenital, (V1) 492–493
Catheter embolus, as complication of intravenous therapy, (V1) 1067t
Catheterization, cardiac, (V2) 753, (V2) 763
Catheter lumens, (V1) 657, (V1) 657f
Catheters
  butterfly needle, (V1) 1057, (V1) 1057f
  central venous access, (V1) 656–657, (V1) 657f, (V1) 661p, (V1) 1058–1060, (V1) 1059–1060f, (V2) 801–802
    catheter lumens, (V1) 657, (V1) 657f
    internal or implantable ports, (V1) 657, (V1) 657f
    placement of, (V2) 795–797p
  epidural, (V2) 609

indwelling urinary, (V1) 728, (V1) 735, (V1) 736f, (V1) 1087
  caring for patient with, (V1) 737–739, (V1) 738f
inside-the-needle, (V1) 1057, (V1) 1057f
irrigation of, (V2) 540–543p
midline peripheral, (V1) 1058
over-the-needle, (V1) 1057, (V1) 1057f
peripheral intravenous lock, (V1) 1058, (V1) 1058f
selection of, (V1) 1061
Cations, (V1) 1037
Causation, (V1) 1168
CCC. See Clinical Care Classification (CCC)
Cecum, (V1) 755
Celecoxib, (V1) 827–828
Celibacy, (V1) 896
Cellular immunity, (V1) 524, (V1) 524f
Cellular malfunction, (V1) 190
Cellular response to stress, (V1) 245
Centenarians, (V1) 191
Center of gravity, (V1) 844, (V1) 845f
Centers for Disease Control and Prevention (CDC), (V1) 515–516
  on accidents, (V1) 545
  guidelines for preventing transmission of pathogens, (V1) 534–536, (V1) 535t, (V1) 536f
  on standard precautions, (V2) 323–324
Centigrade scale, (V1) 450–451, (V1) 451f
Central chemoreceptors, (V1) 463
Central nervous system (CNS)
  abnormalities of, (V1) 992
  depressants of, (V1) 788
  disorders of, (V1) 859–860
Central venous access devices (CVAD), (V1) 656–657, (V1) 657f, (V1) 661p, (V1) 1058–1060, (V1) 1059–1060f
  caring for patients with, (V2) 801–802
  catheter lumens, (V1) 657, (V1) 657f
  internal or implantable ports, (V1) 657, (V1) 657f
  medication administration through, (V2) 450–453p
  placement of, (V2) 795–797p
Central vessels, (V1) 502
Cephalocaudal development, (V1) 144
Cephalocaudal growth, (V1) 144
Cerebellum, (V1) 845
Cerebral cortex, (V1) 845
Cerebral function, (V1) 505–506
Cerebrovascular accident, (V1) 859
  oxygenation and, (V1) 992
Certification, (V1) 1165
Certified nurse midwife (CNM), (V1) 26
Certified registered nurse anesthetist (CRNA), (V1) 26, (V1) 1090
Cerumen, (V1) 493, (V1) 600–601
Cervical cancer screening, (V1) 229
Cervical lymph nodes, (V1) 495
C fibers, (V1) 814, (V1) 815f
Chain of infection, (V1) 516–519, (V1) 517f
Chamomile, (V1) 937
Change
  comfort zone and, (V1) 1192–1193, (V1) 1192–1193f
  commanding, (V1) 1193
  implementation of, (V1) 1194
  integration of, (V1) 1194

providing psychological safety during, (V1) 1194, (V1) 1194b
refuting currently held beliefs and, (V1) 1193–1194
resistance to, (V1) 1193–1194
role and function of agents in, (V1) 7t
sharing information about, (V1) 1193
Changing the subject, (V1) 390
Channel, communication, (V1) 376
Charitable organizations, as payors of healthcare, (V1) 21
Charting by exception (CBE), (V1) 422–423
Checklists, (V1) 384, (V1) 432, (V1) 433f
  evaluation, (V2) 15–17
Cheilosis, (V1) 594
Chemical burns, (V1) 549
Chemical pain relief measures, (V1) 832
Chemical reagent testing of urine, (V1) 729
Chemical respiration, (V1) 462
Chemical strip thermometers, (V2) 178p
Chemoreceptors, (V1) 784, (V1) 979, (V1) 1020
  respiration and, (V1) 463
Chemotherapeutic effects, (V1) 620
  skin and, (V1) 943
Chemotherapy, (V1) 693
Chest
  and abdomen movement with breathing, (V1) 466
  assessment of, (V2) 244–250p
  landmarks of, (V1) 496, (V1) 497–498f
  physical examination of, (V1) 496, (V1) 497–499f, (V1) 511p
  shape and size of, (V1) 496
Chest drainage systems, (V2) 740–744p
Chest physiotherapy, (V1) 1003
Chest radiology, (V1) 1082
Chest tubes, (V1) 1009–1010, (V1) 1009–1010f, (V1) 1014p, (V2) 750–751p
Chest x-ray study, (V2) 753, (V2) 763, (V2) 830
Chewing and swallowing, (V1) 693
Cheyne-Stokes respirations, (V1) 357, (V1) 465t, (V1) 994
Child abuse and neglect, (V1) 301
  assessing for, (V1) 161p
  flow chart of possible, (V2) 42
  of infants, (V1) 158–160
    detecting and preventing, (V1) 161
  of preschoolers, (V1) 166
Childcare, (V1) 296
Childproofing, parent teaching about, (V1) 164
Children
  blood pressure in, (V1) 469
  bowel elimination in, (V1) 757
  cholesterol screening for, (V1) 1027–1028
  dealing with loss, (V1) 367, (V1) 368
  energy needs of, (V1) 683
  grief in, (V1) 353
  health risk factors in families with young, (V1) 296–297, (V1) 297f
  hearing in, (V1) 787
  home safety interventions for, (V1) 563
  hygiene and, (V1) 576
  married adults without, (V1) 292
  neurological system examination in, (V1) 505
  oral hygiene for, (V1) 595
  oral medications for, (V1) 637, (V1) 638
  pain response in, (V1) 816, (V1) 819
  pharmacokinetics in, (V1) 620f

physical activity guidelines for, (V1) 852b
poisoning in, (V1) 548, (V1) 548b
preoperative teaching for, (V1) 1086
preschool-age (*See* Preschooler(s))
psychomotor skills in, (V1) 787
school-age (*See* School-age children)
self-concept in, (V1) 21
sex education for, (V1) 891
skin of, (V1) 583, (V1) 941
social skills in, (V1) 787
stressors in, (V1) 240b
suffocation/asphyxiation of, (V1) 549
teaching, (V1) 403, (V1) 405
   about sexual predators, (V1) 908
toddler-age (*See* Toddler(s))
vision in, (V1) 787
Chiropractic adjustment, (V1) 261
Chlamydia trachomatis, (V1) 896, (V1) 898t
Chloride electrolytes, (V1) 1043t, (V1) 1044
Choking, (V1) 549
  rescue for, (V1) 565, (V1) 566f, (V2) 338
Cholesterol
  dietary, (V1) 672t
  screening for, (V1) 182, (V1) 1027–1028, (V2) 763
  skin and, (V1) 942
Chondroitin, (V1) 823
Chorionic gonadotropin, (V1) 883
Christianity, (V1) 332, (V1) 335
Christian Science, (V1) 336t
Chronic grief, (V1) 354
Chronic illness, (V1) 219
  as challenge to family health, (V1) 300
  in families with young children, (V1) 297
  host susceptibility to infection and, (V1) 529
  nutrition and, (V1) 692–693
  in older adults, (V1) 195
  physical activity and, (V1) 856
  physical activity guidelines for patients with, (V1) 852b
  in school-age children, (V1) 168
  and self-management through telehealth, (V1) 216
  stress-induced, (V1) 251
  vulnerable populations and, (V1) 1113
Chronic infections, (V1) 519
Chronic obstructive pulmonary disease (COPD), (V1) 496, (V1) 499f
  sleep and, (V1) 931
Chronic pain, (V1) 812
Chronic wounds, (V1) 945, (V1) 945f, (V1) 946t
Chvostek's sign, (V2) 798
Cigarette smoking. *See* Smoking
Cilia, (V1) 977
Circadian rhythms
  body temperature and, (V1) 449
  disorders of, (V1) 925
  sleep and, (V1) 919
Circulating nurse, (V1) 1090
Circulation
  cardiac monitoring, (V1) 1028, (V1) 1028f, (V2) 759–761p
  critical thinking and clinical judgment on, (V2) 765
  defined, (V1) 1017
  diagnostic testing of, (V2) 763
  full-spectrum nursing model applied to, (V2) 764

impaired, (V1) 490
  physical activity and, (V1) 860
  skin and, (V1) 583, (V1) 943
  interventions to promote, (V1) 1032
  knowledge map on, (V2) 766
  pathophysiological conditions and, (V1) 1024–1025
  peripheral arterial, (V1) 1032
Circulatory overload due to blood infusions, (V1) 1070t
Circumcision, (V1) 508
  female, (V1) 889–890
Circumferences, body, (V1) 696
Cisgender, (V1) 886
Civil law
  litigation and, (V1) 1169–1170
  quasi-intentional torts, (V1) 1166
Claims-made liability insurance, (V1) 1178
Clarity in communication, (V1) 378, (V1) 388
Clark's Rule, (V2) 469
Clary sage, (V1) 786
Classifications, drug, (V1) 608
Classification systems, (V1) 62
Clavicle fracture, (V1) 155
Clean, nongranulating wounds, (V1) 957t
Clean-catch specimen, (V1) 728
Clean-contaminated wounds, (V1) 945
Cleaning, (V1) 534
Cleansing, wound, (V1) 960
Clean team, (V1) 1090
Clean technique, (V1) 537
  for artificial airway, (V1) 1006
  home healthcare, (V1) 1132
Clean wounds, (V1) 945
Client advocate, role and function of, (V1) 7t
Client/family educator, role and function of, (V1) 7t
Clients
  advocacy for, (V1) 138–139
  asking how to address, (V1) 387
  consequences of unhealthy homes for, (V1) 1133
  education for (*See* Patient education)
  goals/outcomes planning for, (V1) 71–74, (V1) 73t
  maintaining trust of, (V1) 235–236
  power of, (V1) 1190
  prayer with, (V2) 120
  preparing for implementation, (V1) 82
  preparing for physical examination, (V1) 480–481
  promoting participation and adherence by, (V1) 82–83, (V1) 83b
  restraints on, (V1) 554–555, (V1) 571–572, (V1) 573p, (V2) 334–337p, (V2) 339
  self-monitoring of blood pressure by, (V1) 471
  with speech impairments, (V1) 392–393
  uniqueness of, (V1) 38–39
  verifying problems with, (V1) 59
Clinical breast examination, (V1) 495, (V1) 906
Clinical Care Classification (CCC), (V1) 62, (V1) 79, (V1) 324
  community nursing and, (V1) 1120
  home healthcare and, (V1) 1130
Clinical expertise of managers, (V1) 1184
Clinical judgment, (V1) 7–11
  applying the full-spectrum nursing model, (V2) 8–10

on asepsis and infection prevention, (V2) 328
on bowel elimination, (V2) 592
caring and, (V1) 42, (V1) 43t
on circulation, (V2) 765
on communication, (V2) 146–147
on death and dying, (V2) 134–136
definitions of, (V1) 29–30
different kinds of nursing knowledge and, (V1) 30–36
on documentation, (V2) 168–169
documentation and, (V1) 425–426
ethics and values, (V2) 33–36
evidence-based practice (EBP) and, (V1) 36, (V2) 26–28
evolution of nursing thought and action, (V2) 4
on family health, (V2) 105–106
on fluids, electrolytes, and acid-base balance, (V2) 806–807
on growth and development, (V2) 50–51
on home healthcare, (V2) 841–843
on hospital admission and discharge, (V2) 76–77
on hygiene, (V2) 386–388
key concepts in, (V1) 29
on leading and managing, (V2) 860–861
on legal accountability, (V2) 854–856
on medication administration, (V2) 470–473
minimizing malpractice risks, (V1) 1172
models of, (V1) 30–34, (V1) 31t, (V1) 32f, (V1) 33–35t
on multicultural populations, (V2) 114–115
on nursing informatics, (V2) 847–849
nursing process and, (V1) 42, (V1) 42t, (V2) 20–22
on nutrition, (V2) 511–513
on older adults, (V2) 56
on oxygenation, (V2) 755–756
on pain, (V2) 613–614
on patient education, (V2) 152–153
on physical activity and exercise, (V2) 635
on psychosocial health, (V2) 96–99
on safety, (V2) 342–343
on sensation and perception, (V2) 602–603
on sexual health, (V2) 646–648
on skin and wound healing, (V2) 701–702
on sleep and rest, (V2) 654–655
on spirituality, (V2) 123–124
on stress and adaptation, (V2) 85–86
on surgical patient care, (V2) 832–833
on urinary elimination, (V2) 556
on vital signs, (V2) 195–196
Clinical nurse specialist (CNS), (V1) 26
Clinical practice guidelines, (V1) 76
Clinical practice theories, (V1) 98
Clinical support tools (CSTs), (V1) 1147
Clitoris, (V1) 882, (V1) 893, (V1) 894
Clonus, (V1) 864b
Closed feeding systems, (V1) 713
Closed gloving, (V1) 538, (V1) 539p
Closed head injury, (V1) 788
Closed-loop communication, (V1) 384
Closed questions, (V1) 50
Closed systems, (V1) 103
Closed-wound drainage system, (V2) 691–692p
Closed wounds, (V1) 944
Clostridium difficile, (V1) 515, (V1) 517
Clostridium tetani, (V1) 517

Closures, wound, (V1) 948–949, (V1) 949f, (V2) 680–681p
Cloth bandages, (V1) 973
Cloudy pupils, (V1) 493
Clubbing, nail, (V1) 491
CNS. *See* Central nervous system (CNS)
Coaching, employee, (V1) 1185
Coagulation studies, (V2) 700
Cocaine, (V1) 150
Codes of ethics, (V1) 13, (V1) 86, (V1) 118, (V1) 119, (V1) 131–132, (V1) 396, (V1) 1161–1162
Cognition and cognitive development
   adolescent, (V1) 171
   age-related changes in, (V1) 194t
   and assessing cognitive status in older adults, (V1) 198, (V1) 200
   communicating with clients who have impaired, (V1) 393, (V1) 393–394b
   hygiene and, (V1) 576
   infant, (V1) 156–157
   middle adulthood, (V1) 181
   neonate, (V1) 154–155
   nutrition and, (V1) 693
   older adults, (V1) 191
     promotion of, (V1) 203
   pain and, (V1) 816–817, (V1) 820
   patient education and, (V1) 402–408, (V1) 403–405t, (V1) 406b
   preschooler, (V1) 165
   prior to death, (V1) 357
   school-age children, (V1) 167–168
   self-care ability and, (V1) 577
   skin and diminished, (V1) 942–943
   surgical risk and, (V1) 1080
   toddler, (V1) 162
   urinary elimination and, (V1) 724
   young adult, (V1) 179
Cognitive-behavioral therapy (CBT) for pain, (V1) 825
Cognitive development theory, (V1) 147, (V1) 148t, (V1) 402–403
Cognitive learning, (V1) 398, (V1) 398t
Cognitive needs, (V1) 102f
Cognitive restructuring, (V1) 262
Cognitive theory, (V1) 397
Cohabitating adults, (V1) 293
Coinsurance, (V1) 19
Coitus, (V1) 895
Cold and cardiovascular function, (V1) 1021
Cold laser therapy, (V1) 824
Colds
   holistic healing for, (V1) 1000
   medicines for, (V1) 1000
Cold therapy
   for pain, (V1) 824–825
   for wound care, (V1) 973–974, (V1) 973–974f, (V1) 974, (V2) 694
Colic, (V1) 157, (V1) 160
Collaboration, (V1) 327
   communication and, (V1) 382–384, (V2) 142–143
   community nursing, (V1) 1115
   in teaching clients, (V1) 401
   in wound care, (V1) 957
Collaborative problems
   evaluating, (V1) 88–89
   interventions for, (V1) 75, (V1) 83
Collaborative wound treatments, (V1) 949
Collecting tubule, (V1) 718

Colloids, (V1) 1039
Colon, (V1) 755–756
Colon cancer screening, (V1) 228
Colonoscopy, fiberoptic, (V2) 586–587
Colorectal cancer, (V1) 182
Color vision, (V1) 492
Colostomy, (V1) 761–762, (V1) 762f
   evidence-based practice on, (V1) 782
   irrigation of, (V2) 577–579p
   sexuality and, (V1) 891
Colostomy irrigation, (V1) 781
Coma, (V1) 356, (V1) 506
Comeback diseases, (V1) 300
Comfort, (V1) 104
   parenteral medications and, (V1) 648
COMFORT Scale, (V1) 820
Comfrey extract, (V1) 823
Commercial irrigation systems, (V1) 964
Commodity Supplemental Food Program (CSFP), (V1) 701
Common health problems
   in adolescents, (V1) 172–176
   in infants, (V1) 157–158
   in middle adulthood, (V1) 181–182
   in neonates, (V1) 155–156
   in older adults, (V1) 195, (V1) 195b, (V1) 198
   in preschoolers, (V1) 166
   in school-age children, (V1) 168–169
   in toddlers, (V1) 163–164
Common (judicial) law, (V1) 1156–1157, (V1) 1157t
Common sense, (V1) 107
Communicable diseases
   abuse and, (V1) 1178
   in preschoolers, (V1) 166
Communication
   assessment of, (V1) 387, (V2) 275–276p
   family patterns in, (V1) 304
   guidelines and tools for, (V2) 144–145
   with clients from other cultures, (V1) 391–392, (V2) 144
   with clients who are hearing impaired, (V2) 598–599
   with clients who are visually impaired, (V2) 598
   with clients who have impaired cognition or reduced level of consciousness, (V1) 393, (V1) 393–394b
   with clients who have impaired speech, (V1) 392–393
   with clients who speak a different language, (V1) 325–326, (V1) 327b, (V2) 110
   with clients with confusion, (V1) 805
   collaborative professional, (V1) 382–384, (V2) 142–143
   critical thinking and clinical judgment on, (V2) 146–147
   culture and, (V1) 315
   in culture of safety, (V1) 553
   defined, (V1) 375
   diagnosis of problems in, (V1) 387
   documentation in, (V1) 420
   electronic, in nursing informatics, (V1) 1140
   as etiology of other nursing diagnoses, (V1) 387
   factors affecting
     environment, (V1) 380
     life span variations, (V1) 380
   of feelings of grief, (V1) 363–364, (V1) 364f

   full-spectrum nursing model applied to, (V2) 145–146
   gender and, (V1) 380–381
   in group helping relationships, (V1) 385–386, (V1) 386b
   impaired, (V1) 387
     urinary elimination and, (V1) 724
   implementation for, (V1) 387
   importance of good, (V1) 374, (V1) 374b
   involving content, (V1) 375
   key concepts in, (V1) 375
   knowledge map on, (V2) 148
   by leaders, (V1) 1191
   levels of, (V1) 375
   nonverbal, (V1) 378–380, (V1) 379f, (V1) 380b, (V1) 383
   with older adults, (V1) 204
   pain and, (V1) 816–817, (V2) 610
   for patient learning, (V1) 402
   patient rounds approach to, (V1) 384
   with people who are grieving, (V2) 127
   personal space and, (V1) 381, (V1) 381f
   with persons with cognitive defects, (V1) 204–205
   planning for, (V1) 387
   as process, (V1) 375–377, (V1) 376f
   roles and relationships and, (V1) 382
   SBARQ model, (V1) 384, (V2) 143
   sexuality and, (V1) 892
   sociocultural factors in, (V1) 382
   standardized tools for, (V1) 384
   styles of, (V1) 382–384
   surgical team, (V1) 1081, (V1) 1088–1089
   territoriality and, (V1) 381
   therapeutic, (V1) 363, (V1) 364b
     barriers to, (V1) 389–391
     enhancing, (V1) 387–389, (V1) 388f
     in groups, (V1) 385–386, (V1) 386b
     key characteristics of, (V1) 385
   verbal, (V1) 377–378, (V2) 159
Communication styles
   aggressive, (V1) 382–383
   assertive, (V1) 383
   passive, (V1) 382
   passive aggressive, (V1) 382
Communicator, role and function of, (V1) 7t
Community-based nursing
   See also Home healthcare
   applying the nursing process in, (V1) 1121–1122
   career opportunities in, (V1) 1116–1118, (V1) 1118b, (V1) 1118f
   care settings for, (V1) 1113
   community health nursing, (V1) 1113
   community-oriented nursing, (V1) 1114, (V1) 1114f
   pioneers of, (V1) 1114
Community care, standardized languages for, (V1) 79
Community health nursing, (V1) 1113
Community(ies)
   assessment of, (V1) 50
   components of, (V1) 1111
   health of, (V1) 1111–1112, (V1) 1112f
   population and, (V1) 1110–1111, (V1) 1111f
   social and community context of, (V1) 1112
   vulnerable populations in, (V1) 314, (V1) 1112–1113
   working within, (V1) 1114–1118, (V1) 1116f, (V1) 1118b, (V1) 1118f

Community nursing, (V1) 1110
  applying the nursing process in, (V1) 1121–1122
  assessment in, (V1) 1119–1120
  in correctional facilities, (V1) 1117
  disaster services nursing, (V1) 1117–1118, (V1) 1118b
  faith, (V1) 1117
  international nursing, (V1) 1118, (V1) 1118f
  interventions in, (V1) 1121
  levels of care in, (V1) 1115–1116, (V1) 1116f
  nursing diagnosis in, (V1) 1120–1121
  occupational health, (V1) 1117
  primary interventions in, (V1) 1116
  in public health clinics, (V1) 1117
  roles in, (V1) 1115
  school, (V1) 1116–1117
  secondary interventions, (V1) 1116, (V1) 1116f
  tertiary interventions, (V1) 1116
Community-oriented nursing, (V1) 1114, (V1) 1114f
Community/public health centers, (V1) 18
Compensation
  as defense mechanism, (V1) 247t
  pH, (V1) 1045, (V1) 1051
Compensatory justice, (V1) 131
Competing demands, as health disruption, (V1) 217
Complementary and alternative medicine (CAM), (V1) 24–25, (V1) 320
  aromatherapy, (V1) 786
  for depression, (V1) 288
  for pain relief, (V1) 823–824
  stress-management techniques, (V1) 260, (V1) 261
Complement cascade, (V1) 521, (V1) 524
Complete bath, (V1) 585
Complete blood count (CBC), (V1) 1082, (V2) 830
Complete proteins, (V1) 670
Complex carbohydrates, (V1) 669
Complicated grief, (V1) 354, (V1) 355–356
  interventions for, (V1) 368, (V1) 369
Comprehensive assessments, (V1) 49
Comprehensive Drug Abuse Prevention and Control Act, (V1) 609
Comprehensive metabolic panel, (V2) 830
Comprehensive nursing care plan, (V1) 67–71, (V1) 68f, (V1) 70f
Comprehensive physical examination, (V1) 479
Compression devices, (V1) 1032
Compromise, (V1) 383
Computed tomography (CT), (V2) 587–588
Computer-assisted diagnosis, (V1) 60
Computerized care plans, (V1) 69, (V1) 74, (V1) 78
  using NIC in, (V1) 79
Computerized prescriber order entry (CPOE), (V1) 628
Computers
  See also Internet, the
  interoperability, (V1) 1147
  in nursing informatics, (V1) 1140
  password management for, (V1) 1150b
  for providing and managing care, (V1) 1142–1146, (V1) 1143f, (V1) 1146f, (V1) 1146t

  simulations using, (V1) 1145–1146
  supporting evidence-based practice, (V1) 1149–1153, (V1) 1153–1154b
  use in different nursing areas, (V1) 1146t
Concentric exercise, (V1) 851
Concepts, (V1) 94–95
Conceptual framework, (V1) 95
Conceptual models, (V1) 95
Concreteness, (V1) 385
Concrete operations stage, in cognitive development theory, (V1) 148t, (V1) 402
Concussion, (V1) 169
Condoms
  adolescents and, (V1) 175
  male and female, (V2) 642
  teaching patients about, (V2) 641
Conduction, (V1) 448
Confidence in reasoning, (V1) 38
Conflict, (V1) 1184
  informal negotiation on, (V1) 1196
  occurring at all levels, (V1) 1195
  steps in resolving, (V1) 1195–1196
  "win-win" resolutions to, (V1) 1195
Confrontation, (V1) 385
Confusion
  anxiety in patients with, (V1) 289
  caring for patients with, (V1) 804–805
  pain and, (V1) 815–816
Congenital anomalies, (V1) 155
  maternal age effects on, (V1) 151
  mobility interventions and, (V1) 866
  musculoskeletal system, (V1) 857
Congenital cataracts, (V1) 492–493
Congenital dermal melanocytosis, (V1) 153, (V1) 488
Congenital nevi, (V1) 941
Conjunctiva, (V1) 492
Connotative meaning, (V1) 377
Consciousness, (V1) 805
Conscious sedation, (V1) 1091
Consequentialism, (V1) 126–127
Constipation, (V1) 703, (V1) 766, (V1) 768–769, (V1) 773–774
  as postoperative complication, (V1) 1100t
Constitutional law, (V1) 1156, (V1) 1157t
Constructive affirmation, (V1) 375
Consumers, healthcare, (V1) 24
Contact burns, (V1) 548–549
Contact lenses, (V1) 600, (V1) 603p, (V2) 372–373p, (V2) 603p
Contaminated wounds, (V1) 945
Contamination, wound, (V1) 943–944, (V1) 945
Content, teaching, (V1) 410
Content of communication, (V1) 375
Contextual awareness, (V2) 9
  in choosing interventions, (V1) 79b
  in critical thinking, (V1) 39, (V1) 40b, (V1) 41f
Continent ileostomy, (V1) 761
Continent urinary reservoir, (V1) 740
Continuing care retirement communities (CCRCs), (V1) 189
Continuing education (CE), (V1) 12
  minimizing malpractice risks, (V1) 1176
Continuity of care
  for clients with confusion, (V1) 805
  documentation in, (V1) 420

Continuous infusions, (V1) 711, (V1) 1067
Continuous irrigations, (V1) 964
Continuous passive motion (CPM), (V1) 876
Continuous quality improvement (CQI) programs, (V1) 23
Continuous tube feedings, (V1) 637
Contraception, (V1) 689, (V1) 907, (V2) 641, (V2) 642
  methods of, (V2) 642–643
Contraceptive sponge, (V2) 642
Contracting, (V1) 232
Contract law, (V1) 1166
Contralateral stimulation, (V1) 825
Controlled substances regulation, (V1) 609–610, (V1) 610f
Contusion, (V1) 945t
Convalescence, infection, (V1) 520
Convection, (V1) 448
Conventional healthcare system, (V1) 317
Conventional stage, in moral development theory, (V1) 148
Conventional urostomy, (V1) 740
Conversational dyspnea, (V1) 994
Conversion, as defense mechanism, (V1) 247t
Coordination, body, (V1) 845
Coordination of care, (V1) 83
  home healthcare, (V1) 1125
Coordination problems, (V1) 504
Copayments, (V1) 19
Coping, (V1) 212, (V1) 239, (V1) 262
  adaptive, (V1) 240
  with anxiety, (V1) 277–279
  assessment of family processes for, (V1) 304
  common approaches to, (V1) 241
  impairments in, (V1) 271
  maladaptive, (V1) 240–241
  relation to stress, (V1) 240–242, (V1) 241f
  strategies for, (V1) 240
Copper, (V1) 680t
  skin and, (V1) 942
Cordotomy, (V1) 832
Core temperature, (V1) 446, (V1) 454, (V1) 1086
Corn, epidermis, (V1) 589
Cornea, (V1) 492
Coronary arteries, (V1) 1018–1019, (V1) 1019f
Coronary artery disease, (V1) 931, (V1) 1024
Coronary circulation, (V1) 497
Correctional facilities, nursing in, (V1) 1117
Corticotropin-releasing hormone (CRH), (V1) 242
Cortisol, (V1) 242, (V1) 243f
Cosmetic surgery, (V1) 1078
Cost containment, (V1) 122
Cough, (V1) 466
  assessment of, (V1) 994–995, (V1) 995b
  incentive spirometry for, (V1) 1103, (V1) 1103f
  medicines for, (V1) 1000
  mobilizing secretions and, (V1) 1002–1003, (V1) 1003f
  surgical patients and, (V2) 811–814p
Cough preparations, (V1) 984t
Counseling
  community nursing, (V1) 1115
  individual, (V1) 232
  minimizing malpractice risks, (V1) 1175
  for sexual problems, (V1) 907
  using technology for, (V1) 232–233

Counselor, role and function of, (V1) 7t
Countershock phase in stress, (V1) 242
Courage, intellectual, (V1) 37
COVID-19 pandemic, (V1) 321–322, (V1) 520
  children's fears related to, (V1) 368
  physical activity and, (V1) 856
  remote patient care during, (V1) 1141
Crack cocaine, (V1) 150
Crackles, (V1) 466
Cradle boards, (V1) 869
Cranial nerves, (V1) 492, (V1) 492f, (V1) 506t
  assessing function of, (V1) 506, (V2) 276–278p
  origin of, (V1) 507f
Crawling reflex, (V1) 153–154, (V1) 154f
C-reactive protein, (V1) 1027
Creams, (V1) 613t, (V1) 614t, (V1) 637
Create Your Plate, (V1) 668
Creatine kinase-MB, (V2) 763
Creatinine, (V1) 699, (V1) 727, (V2) 548
Credentialing, (V1) 1165
Credibility in communication, (V1) 378
Credible sources
  in choosing interventions, (V1) 79b
  in critical thinking, (V1) 39, (V1) 41f
  ethical decision making and, (V1) 140
Crepitus, (V1) 858, (V1) 953
Crimean War, (V1) 3
Criminal law, (V1) 1165–1166
Crisis, (V1) 252–253, (V1) 253f
Crisis intervention, (V1) 263, (V2) 81
Critical Care Pain Observation Tool (CPOT), (V1) 820
Critical colonization, (V1) 944
Critical (CUS) language, (V1) 383–384
Critically ill patients, oral care for, (V1) 596
Critical pathways, (V1) 22, (V1) 69, (V1) 70f
  evidence-based practice and, (V1) 75
Critical thinking, (V1) 8
  on asepsis and infection prevention, (V2) 328
  attitudes in, (V1) 37–38
  on bowel elimination, (V2) 592
  caring and, (V1) 42
  on circulation, (V2) 765
  on communication, (V2) 146–147
  on death and dying, (V2) 134–136
  defined, (V1) 37
  on documentation, (V2) 168–169
  on ethics and values, (V2) 34–36
  evidence-based practice (EBP) and, (V1) 37, (V2) 26–28
  evolution of nursing thought and action, (V2) 4
  on family health, (V2) 105–106
  on fluids, electrolytes, and acid-base balance, (V2) 806–807
  full-spectrum nursing model and, (V2) 9–10
  on growth and development, (V2) 50–51
  on home healthcare, (V2) 841–843
  on hospital admission and discharge, (V2) 76–77
  on hygiene, (V2) 386–388
  importance of, (V1) 38–39
  knowledge map for, (V2) 11
  on leading and managing, (V2) 860–861
  on legal accountability, (V2) 854–856
  on medication administration, (V2) 470–473
  medication error avoidance and, (V1) 628
  model for, (V1) 39–41, (V1) 40b, (V1) 41f

  on multicultural populations, (V2) 114–115
  on nursing informatics, (V2) 847–849
  nursing process and, (V1) 41–42, (V2) 20–22
  on nutrition, (V2) 511–513
  on older adults, (V2) 56
  on oxygenation, (V2) 755–756
  on pain, (V2) 613–614
  on patient education, (V2) 152–153
  on physical activity and exercise, (V2) 635
  on psychosocial health, (V2) 96–99
  on safety, (V2) 342–343
  on sensation and perception, (V2) 602–603
  on sexual health, (V1) 908–909, (V2) 646–648
  skills in, (V1) 37
  on skin and wound healing, (V2) 701–702
  on sleep and rest, (V2) 654–655
  on spirituality, (V2) 123–124
  on stress and adaptation, (V2) 85–86
  on surgical patient care, (V2) 832–833
  on urinary elimination, (V2) 556
  on vital signs, (V2) 195–196
Criticism, (V1) 383
Crossmatching, blood, (V1) 1069
Crushing tables, (V1) 637
Crushing wounds, (V1) 945t
Crust, (V2) 214p
Crutches, (V1) 878, (V1) 878f
Crying and colic, (V1) 157, (V1) 160
  due to pain, (V1) 816
Crystalloids, (V1) 1039
C-type natriuretic peptide (CNP), (V1) 1041
Cultural archetypes, (V1) 315
Cultural assessment, (V1) 50, (V2) 111–112
  health history in, (V1) 323
  models and tools for, (V1) 324
  physical, (V1) 323–324
Cultural awareness, (V1) 320
Cultural brokerage, (V1) 325
Cultural competence, (V1) 320, (V1) 321
  developing one's, (V1) 327–328
  with dying patients, (V1) 366, (V1) 366f
  evidence-based practice in, (V1) 323
  implementation and, (V1) 325
  Leininger and, (V1) 99–100
  nursing diagnosis and, (V1) 324
  planning and, (V1) 324–325
  theory applied to, (V1) 104
Cultural humility, (V1) 322
Culturally and linguistically appropriate services (CLAS) standards, (V1) 326
Culturally competent care, (V1) 310–311
  American Nurses Association on, (V1) 320
  assessment for, (V1) 322–324
  barriers to, (V1) 321–322
  defined, (V1) 320
  nursing strategies for providing, (V1) 325–327, (V1) 326t, (V1) 327b
  pain assessment, (V1) 819
  patient teaching, (V1) 406b
  safe, effective nursing care (SENC) and, (V1) 320–321
Culturally congruent care, (V1) 321
Culturally sensitive care, (V1) 80
Cultural sensitivity, (V1) 320
Cultural stereotypes, (V1) 315, (V1) 321
Culture
  See also Multicultural populations
  affecting health, (V1) 314–317
  biological variations and, (V1) 316
  characteristics of, (V1) 311, (V1) 311f

  communication and, (V1) 315, (V1) 382, (V1) 391–392, (V2) 110
  concepts related to, (V1) 312–314, (V1) 313f
  defined, (V1) 311
  dominant, (V1) 313
  environmental control and, (V1) 316, (V1) 327b
  ethnicity, race, and religion and, (V1) 312
  healthcare, (V1) 317–320, (V1) 317t, (V1) 552
  hygiene and, (V1) 576
  influence on health and illness, (V1) 214
  of nursing, (V1) 318–319
  patient education and, (V1) 316, (V1) 405, (V1) 406b
  rituals in, (V1) 315, (V1) 315f
  sensory function and, (V1) 788
  sexuality and, (V1) 889–890
  socialization, acculturation, and assimilation and, (V1) 313
  social organization and, (V1) 316, (V1) 327b
  space and, (V1) 315, (V1) 327b
  subcultures, (V1) 313–314
  time orientation and, (V1) 315–316, (V1) 327b
  underrepresented (minority) groups and, (V1) 314
  why learn about, (V1) 309–311, (V1) 309f, (V1) 310b
Culture commonalities, (V1) 314
Culture diversities, (V1) 315
Culture specifics, (V1) 315
Culture universals, (V1) 314
Cumulative effects of drugs, (V1) 623
Cunnilingus, (V1) 895
Cures, (V1) 333
Curiosity, intellectual, (V1) 37
Current Opioid Misuse Measure (COMM), (V1) 835
Current Procedural Terminology (CPT), (V1) 62
Custodial care, (V1) 17
Cutaneous pain, (V1) 811
Cutaneous stimulation, (V1) 824
Cutaneous ureterostomy, (V1) 740
CVAD. See Central venous access devices (CVAD)
Cyanocobalamin, (V1) 677–678t
Cyanosis, (V1) 461, (V1) 466, (V1) 489t, (V1) 584
Cyclic feedings, (V1) 713
Cyst, (V2) 212p
Cytomegalovirus (CMV), (V1) 151
Cytotoxic (killer) T cells, (V1) 524

D

Daily stresses, (V1) 227
Damages, (V1) 1168
Dampness, skin, (V1) 582–583
Dance and stress, (V1) 262
Dandruff, (V1) 597–598
Dangling, (V1) 876
Data
  about healthcare services, (V1) 1111
  admission, (V1) 421, (V2) 166
  analyzing and interpreting, (V1) 56, (V1) 58
  baseline, (V1) 479
  biological, (V1) 1111
  in community nursing, (V1) 1121–1122
  demographic, (V1) 1111

diagnostic reasoning and, (V1) 56–60, (V1) 58b, (V1) 58f
documentation of, (V1) 52, (V1) 53f
electronic health records (EHRs) (*See* Electronic health records (EHRs))
emotional, (V1) 1111
gaps in, (V1) 58
graphic, (V1) 421, (V1) 431–432
home healthcare, (V1) 1128
inconsistencies in, (V1) 58
laboratory, (V1) 478
in nursing informatics, (V1) 1139
organization of, (V1) 52
pulse, (V1) 460–461
reassessment, (V1) 87–88
respiration, (V1) 464–466, (V1) 465t
on skin condition, (V1) 584
social, (V1) 1111
sources of spiritual, (V1) 340
types and source of, (V1) 47–48, (V1) 48t
validation of, (V1) 51–52
Databases, (V1) 110, (V1) 112t, (V1) 422
Date rape, (V1) 900
Death and dying
See also Grief
analysis/diagnosis, (V1) 362
assessment of, (V1) 362
guidelines and tools for, (V2) 132–133
cardiovascular disease and, (V1) 1025
caring for the patient facing, (V1) 365–367, (V1) 366f, (V2) 128–130
causes of adolescent, (V1) 172
of a child, as health disruption, (V1) 217
coma and persistent vegetative state and, (V1) 356
critical thinking and clinical judgment on, (V2) 134–136
definitions of, (V1) 354, (V1) 356
end-of-life care and, (V1) 18, (V1) 358–362, (V1) 360b
evidence-based practice on, (V1) 366
from firearms injuries, (V1) 549
from fires, (V1) 549
full-spectrum nursing model applied to, (V2) 134
helping families of patients facing, (V1) 365, (V2) 127–128
higher-brain, (V1) 354
impending, (V1) 216–217
interventions/implementation for, (V1) 363
complicated grief, (V1) 368, (V1) 369
knowledge map on, (V2) 138
leading causes of, in older adults, (V1) 195b
organ donation after, (V1) 361
planning outcomes/evaluation in, (V1) 362–363
poisoning, (V1) 548
postmortem care after, (V1) 367, (V2) 130–131
autopsy in, (V1) 361
stages of
physiological, (V1) 356–357
psychological, (V1) 357
sudden infant death syndrome (SIDS), (V1) 150, (V1) 157–158, (V1) 160
from suffocation, (V1) 549
Débridement, wound, (V1) 966–967
Debriefs, end of shift, (V1) 384

Decisional conflict, (V1) 133, (V1) 341
Decision making, (V1) 123–132
ethical, (V1) 134–140
Decision-making activities by managers, (V1) 1185
Decline, infection, (V1) 520
Decreased cardiac output, (V1) 1029–1031
Deductive reasoning, (V1) 96–97, (V1) 96f
Deep breathing, (V1) 1002, (V2) 811–814p
Deep sensations, testing, (V2) 279p
Deep sleep, (V1) 920
Deep somatic pain, (V1) 811
Deep tendon reflexes (DTRs), (V1) 506–507
testing, (V2) 281–282p
Deep vein thrombosis (DVT), (V1) 1026, (V1) 1088
Defecation, (V1) 757
promoting normal or regular, (V1) 767–768
Defense mechanisms, (V1) 147, (V1) 247–248t
for anxiety, (V1) 278–279
Defervescence, (V1) 450
Deficient knowledge, (V1) 408–409
Definitions, (V1) 95
Dehiscence, (V1) 950, (V1) 950f
as postoperative complication, (V1) 1101t
Dehydration
from exercise, (V1) 854
oral problems with, (V1) 594
skin and, (V1) 583
Delayed grief, (V1) 354
Delayed primary closure, (V1) 947, (V1) 947f
Delegation, (V1) 82–84, (V1) 85b
documentation, (V1) 442
ear cleaning and hearing aid care, (V1) 601
focused nutritional assessment, (V1) 699
hygiene care, (V1) 578–579, (V1) 579f
incentive spirometry, (V1) 1002
by leaders and managers, (V1) 1191–1192, (V1) 1192b
minimizing malpractice risks, (V1) 1175
pain management, (V1) 823, (V1) 823b
safety interventions, (V1) 557
vital signs, (V1) 476
wound assessment, (V1) 958–959
Delirium, (V1) 282, (V1) 804
Delta waves, (V1) 920, (V1) 920–921t, (V1) 920f
Deltoid injection site, (V1) 652, (V1) 652f
Dementia, (V1) 195, (V1) 196–197, (V1) 282, (V1) 804
bathing patients who have, (V1) 587
differentiated from depression, (V2) 95
distinguishing changes of typical aging from, (V1) 197t
oral care for patients who have, (V1) 596–597
Pain Assessment in Advanced Dementia (PAINAD) Scale and, (V1) 820, (V1) 820t
PICOT questions, (V1) 901
Democratic leadership, (V1) 1182
Demographic changes, (V1) 309–310
influence on contemporary nursing, (V1) 24
Demographic data, (V1) 1111
Demonstration and return demonstration, for patient teaching, (V1) 411
Denial, (V1) 279
as defense mechanism, (V1) 247t
Denotative meaning, (V1) 377
Dental caries, (V1) 593, (V1) 595
Dental health screening, (V1) 228

Dental hygiene
in adolescents, (V1) 179
in infants, (V1) 157
in preschoolers, (V1) 166
in school-age children, (V1) 169
Denture care, (V1) 595–596, (V1) 596f, (V1) 602p, (V2) 361–363p
Denver Developmental Screening Test, (V1) 160
Deontology, (V1) 127
Deoxygenated blood, (V1) 1017
Dependence
drug, (V1) 624
on others during illness, (V1) 218
Dependent interventions, (V1) 75
Depilatory products, (V1) 599
Depo-Provera injections, (V2) 643
Depositions, (V1) 1170
Depression
in adolescents, (V1) 172
assessment for, (V1) 200, (V1) 282, (V1) 287f, (V2) 92, (V2) 94–95
complementary and alternative medicine (CAM) for, (V1) 288
differentiated from dementia, (V2) 95
evidence-base practice on, (V1) 289
flat affect in, (V1) 282, (V1) 282f
grief versus, (V1) 362
nursing care for, (V1) 282–287, (V1) 287b, (V1) 287t
in older adults, (V1) 198
pain and, (V1) 816
prevalence of, (V1) 281
in response to stress, (V1) 251
sexuality and, (V1) 892
sleep and, (V1) 924, (V1) 931
suicide risk and, (V1) 287b
truths and myths about, (V1) 281t
Dermatitis, (V1) 943
Dermatoses, (V1) 943
Dermis, (V1) 579, (V1) 941
neonatal, (V1) 153
Descending colon, (V1) 755
Designated workstation computers, (V1) 1150
Desire in sexual response cycle, (V1) 893, (V1) 894t
Desquamates, (V1) 579
Development
adolescent, (V1) 171–179, (V1) 171b, (V1) 172f
assessment of family, (V2) 103–104
critical thinking and clinical judgment on, (V2) 50–51
gestational period, (V1) 149–152, (V1) 151f
in health and wellness, (V1) 212
infant, (V1) 156–162, (V1) 157b
knowledge map on, (V2) 52
middle adulthood, (V1) 181–183, (V1) 181f
nature versus nurture in, (V1) 144
neonate, (V1) 152–154f, (V1) 152–156
older adults, (V1) 191–198
pain and delayed, (V1) 820
preschool stage, (V1) 164–167, (V1) 165b, (V1) 165f
principles of growth and, (V1) 144
school-age child, (V1) 167–171, (V1) 167b, (V1) 168f
sexuality, (V1) 886–889, (V1) 887f, (V1) 889f
spirituality, (V1) 341

theories of, (V1) 103, (V1) 145–148t, (V1) 145–149
toddler, (V1) 162–164, (V1) 162f, (V1) 163b
young adulthood, (V1) 179–181
Developmental dysplasia of the hip (DDH), (V1) 857
Developmental stage
  blood pressure and, (V1) 469
  body temperature and, (V1) 448
  bowel elimination and, (V1) 757–758
  cardiovascular function and, (V1) 1020–1021
  exercise and, (V1) 856
  host susceptibility to infection and, (V1) 525
  hygiene and, (V1) 576
  nutrition and, (V1) 684–689
  pain and, (V1) 816
  patient education and, (V1) 402
  pulmonary function and, (V1) 980–981
  pulse rate and, (V1) 457
  respiration and, (V1) 463
  safety and, (V1) 546–547, (V1) 547t
  self-concept and, (V1) 267
  skin and, (V1) 583
  urinary elimination and, (V1) 721–722
Developmental stressors, (V1) 239
Developmental task theory, (V1) 145, (V1) 145–146t
Developmental theories of families, (V1) 295–296
Diabetes
  Diabetes Food Plate, (V1) 668
  diets for, (V1) 694
  foot care with, (V1) 590
  foot ulcer with, (V1) 945f, (V1) 959
  sexuality and, (V1) 891
  sleep and, (V1) 931
  teaching about, (V1) 170
  when to assess for, (V1) 698, (V1) 698b
Diabetes Food Plate, (V1) 668
Diabetic foot ulcers, (V1) 945f, (V1) 946t, (V1) 959
Diabetic retinopathy, (V1) 788
Diagnostic and Statistical Manual of Mental Disorders, Fifth Edition (DSM-5), (V1) 62, (V1) 924
Diagnostic reasoning, (V1) 56–60, (V1) 58b, (V1) 58f
  reflecting critically on, (V1) 60–61, (V1) 61b
Diagnostic-related groups (DRGs), (V1) 21–22
Diagnostic statements, (V1) 62–65
  basic three-part statement, (V1) 64
  basic two-part statement, (V1) 64
  collaborative problems, (V1) 65
  connecting phrase in, (V1) 64
  etiology in, (V1) 62, (V1) 64, (V1) 65
  formats for, (V1) 64–65
  one-part statement, (V1) 64
  other format variations, (V1) 64–65
  problem in, (V1) 62, (V1) 65
Diagnostic studies, (V1) 421
Diagnostic (exploratory) surgery, (V1) 1078
Diagnostic testing
  bowel elimination, (V2) 586–588
  cardiovascular system, (V1) 1027–1028, (V1) 1028f
  circulation, (V2) 763
  for evaluating presence or risk of infections, (V2) 327
  fluids, electrolytes, and acid-base balance, (V2) 805

  lung volume and capacities, (V2) 752–754
  nutrition status, (V2) 510
  oxygenation, (V1) 995–998, (V1) 996–998f, (V2) 753
  preoperative care, (V1) 1082, (V2) 830
  respiratory function, (V1) 995–998, (V1) 996–998f
  tuberculin skin testing, (V1) 996, (V2) 754
  urinary elimination, (V2) 547–550
  wounds, (V2) 700
Diaphragm, (V1) 978
Diaphragm (contraception), (V2) 643
Diaphragmatic breathing, (V1) 826
Diaphragm stethoscopes, (V1) 458, (V1) 459f
Diarrhea, (V1) 766, (V1) 768, (V1) 770–771
Diarthroses, (V1) 842
Diastole, (V1) 457, (V1) 499
Diastolic pressure, (V1) 467, (V1) 473
Dietary Approaches to Stop Hypertension (DASH), (V1) 691
Dietary fiber, (V1) 669
Dietary intake, interventions for impaired, (V1) 701–702
Dietary reference intakes (DRI), (V1) 666–667, (V1) 673, (V1) 674–678t
Diet(s)
  See also Nutrition
  Asian, Latin American, Mediterranean, and African heritage, (V1) 667–668, (V1) 691–692
  bowel elimination and, (V1) 758, (V1) 767–768
  Buddhism and, (V1) 337
  calorie-restricted, (V1) 691, (V1) 694
  cardiovascular function and, (V1) 1022
  Christians and, (V1) 335
  Dietary Guidelines for Americans, (V1) 230–231
  drug interactions and, (V1) 623
  energy balance and, (V1) 682–683, (V1) 683b
  ethnic, cultural, and religious practices related to, (V1) 691–692
  evidence-based practice on, (V1) 692
  fluid and electrolyte balance and, (V1) 1055
  fluid restriction and, (V1) 1055–1056
  Hinduism and, (V1) 336
  Islam and, (V1) 335
  Judaism and, (V1) 335
  modified by consistency, (V1) 694, (V1) 694t
  modified for disease, (V1) 694–695
  NPO, (V1) 694, (V1) 702
  oral problems and, (V1) 593
  with ostomies, (V1) 780–781b
  for preventing and treating osteoporosis, (V1) 866–867
  pulse rate and, (V1) 457
  regular, (V1) 694
  restless legs syndrome (RLS) and, (V1) 925
  skin and, (V1) 944
  sleep and, (V1) 923
  special, (V1) 694–695, (V1) 694t
  urinary elimination and, (V1) 723
  vegetarian/vegan, (V1) 667–668, (V1) 690
Differentiated practice, (V1) 16
Diffusion, (V1) 1039, (V1) 1039f
Digestive function, impaired, (V1) 703
Digital rectal examination, (V1) 182
Digital sources of information, for patient teaching, (V1) 411

Digital stethoscopes, (V1) 459
Dignity, (V1) 129, (V1) 204
  urinary elimination and loss of, (V1) 723
Diploma nursing programs, (V1) 11
  nursing research and, (V1) 106
Direct auscultation, (V1) 484
Direct-care
  interventions planning in, (V1) 74
  recipients of, (V1) 14
Direct care agencies, (V1) 1124
Direct care providers, role and function of, (V1) 7t
Direct-entry doctorate programs, (V1) 11–12
Direct-entry master's degree programs, (V1) 11
Direct hernias, (V1) 508
Directive interview, (V1) 51t
Direct method for measuring blood pressure, (V1) 470
Direct payment of services, (V1) 19
Direct-to-consumer marketing, (V1) 24
Disability
  Americans with Disabilities Act (ADA) and, (V1) 300, (V1) 1160
  as challenge to family health, (V1) 300
  in families with young children, (V1) 297
  physical examination modifications for persons with, (V1) 486
  sexuality and, (V1) 892
Disaccharides, (V1) 669
Disaster services nursing, (V1) 1117–1118, (V1) 1118b
Discharge
  critical thinking and clinical judgment on, (V2) 76–77
  forms for, (V2) 70–71
  full-spectrum nursing model applied to, (V2) 75–76
  from healthcare facility, (V1) 237p, (V2) 66–68p
  maintaining trust of client during, (V1) 236
Discharge planning, (V1) 66–67, (V1) 421, (V1) 431, (V1) 431f
Discharge summary, (V1) 431, (V1) 431f
Disciplinary actions, (V1) 1164–1165
Discovery phase, (V1) 1169–1170
Discrimination, (V1) 321
Discriminatory sensations, testing, (V2) 280p
Disease. *See* Illness and disease
Disease-specific studies, (V1) 226
Disenfranchised grief, (V1) 354
Disengagement theory, (V1) 191
Disinfection, (V1) 534
Displacement, (V1) 279
  as defense mechanism, (V1) 247t
Disposable chemical thermometers, (V1) 453t, (V1) 454
Disruptions to health, (V1) 209
Dissociation, as defense mechanism, (V1) 247t
Distal and collecting tubules, (V1) 718
Distance vision, (V1) 491
Distention, (V1) 503
Distilled water, (V1) 963
Distraction for pain, (V1) 825–826
Distress/eustress, (V1) 239
Distribution, drug, (V1) 616–617
Distributive justice, (V1) 131
Diuretics, (V1) 1033
  promoting circulation, (V1) 1024t
  urinary elimination and, (V1) 723

Index

Diurnal variations and blood pressure, (V1) 469
Diversity. *See* Multicultural populations
Diverticulosis, (V1) 761
Dix, Dorothea, (V1) 6
Dock, Lavinia, (V1) 6
Doctoral programs, (V1) 11–12
   nursing research and, (V1) 106
Doctor of nursing practice (DNP), (V1) 12
Doctor of philosophy (PhD), (V1) 12
Documentation
   cerebral function, (V1) 506
   clinical judgment and, (V1) 425–426
   critical thinking and clinical judgment on, (V2) 168–169
   data, (V1) 52, (V1) 53*f*, (V2) 166–167
   defined, (V1) 420
   delegation of, (V1) 442
   evidence-based practice on, (V1) 441
   as final step of implementation, (V1) 84
   forms for, (V2) 166–167
      additional information about medications, (V1) 432, (V1) 434–435
      checklist, (V1) 432, (V1) 433*f*
      discharge summary, (V1) 431, (V1) 431*f*
      flowsheets and graphic records, (V1) 431–432
      intake and output records, (V1) 432
      integrated plans of care (IPOCs), (V1) 69–71, (V1) 435–436
      medication administration records (MARs), (V1) 432, (V1) 434*f*, (V1) 434*t*
      nursing admission data, (V1) 430–431
      occurrence reports, (V1) 436, (V1) 436*b*
      patient care summary, (V1) 435, (V1) 435*f*
   full-spectrum nursing model applied to, (V2) 168
   guidelines for, (V1) 440–442, (V1) 440*b*, (V2) 159–162
   guidelines for documentation of, (V2) 853
   health records systems
      charting by exception (CBE), (V1) 422–423
      defined, (V1) 421
      electronic health records (EHRs), (V1) 420, (V1) 421, (V1) 423–425, (V1) 424*f*
      paper records, (V1) 425, (V1) 425*b*, (V2) 163
      problem-oriented record (POR) systems, (V1) 422, (V1) 422*f*
      source-oriented, (V1) 421–422
   in home healthcare, (V1) 436–437
   how healthcare providers use, (V1) 420–421
   incident reports, (V1) 1173–1174
   key concepts in, (V1) 420
   knowledge map on, (V2) 171
   minimizing malpractice risks, (V1) 1172–1174
   pain management, (V1) 836
   of patient education, (V1) 418
   physical examination findings, (V1) 509–513
   progress notes, (V1) 421, (V1) 422
      "do no use" list for, (V1) 426*t*
      electronic entry, (V1) 429–430, (V1) 430*f*
      FACT system, (V1) 429
      Focus Charting, (V1) 428
      narrative format, (V1) 426–427
      problem-intervention-evaluation (PIE) system, (V1) 427
      SOAP format, (V1) 427–428
      use of abbreviations in, (V1) 426

standardized nursing languages and (*See* Standardized nursing languages)
   of verbal and telephone prescriptions, (V1) 438–439, (V2) 159
   vital signs (VS), (V1) 445
Domestic violence. *See* Intimate partner violence (IPV)
Dominant culture, (V1) 313
Donation, blood, (V1) 1068
Do-not-resuscitate (DNR) prescription, (V1) 360, (V1) 360*b*
"Do not use" list, (V1) 426*t*
Dopaminergic agents, (V1) 925
Doppler ultrasound, (V2) 763
Dorsalis pedis pulse, (V1) 460, (V2) 181*p*
Dorsal recumbent position, (V1) 872–873
Dorsogluteal injection site, (V1) 652
Dosage, medication
   calculating and measuring, (V1) 624, (V2) 466–469
   Institute for Safe Medication Practices (ISMP) List of Error-Prone Abbreviations, Symbols, and Dose Designations, (V2) 460–465
   measured when changing needles, (V2) 456–457
   medication measurement systems for, (V1) 624, (V2) 466–467
Dose-related adverse reactions, (V1) 621
Double-lumen stethoscopes, (V1) 458
Douches, (V1) 640
Douching, (V1) 905
Down syndrome, (V1) 151
Drainage
   chest tubes, (V1) 1009–1010, (V1) 1009–1010*f*, (V1) 1014*p*
   postural, (V1) 1003, (V1) 1003*f*, (V1) 1011*p*
   wound, (V1) 949, (V1) 956–957, (V1) 965, (V1) 965*f*
Dress, grooming, and hygiene in general survey, (V1) 487
Dressings
   hydrating, (V2) 678–680*p*
   intravenous, (V1) 1064, (V1) 1067, (V1) 1072*p*, (V2) 783–787*p*
   removing and applying dry, (V2) 666–668*p*
   removing and applying wet-to-damp, (V2) 668–670*p*
   taping, (V2) 665–666*p*
   transparent film, (V2) 676–678*p*
   wound, (V1) 972
      for controlling infections, (V1) 971–972, (V1) 972*f*
      primary, (V1) 971, (V1) 971*f*
      securing, (V1) 971, (V1) 971*f*
      types of, (V1) 967, (V1) 968–970*t*
DRIs. *See* Dietary reference intakes (DRI)
Drowning, (V1) 565
Drug Enforcement Agency (DEA), (V1) 609
Drugs. *See* Medications
Dry dressings, (V2) 666–668*p*
Dry heat, (V1) 973–974, (V1) 974*f*
Dry mouth, (V1) 594, (V1) 703
Dry powder inhalers, (V1) 641–642, (V1) 641*f*
Dry skin, (V1) 582
Dual-earner families, (V1) 292
Dunn's health grid, (V1) 210, (V1) 210*f*
Duodenum, (V1) 755
Durable medical equipment (DME), (V1) 1124

Durable power of attorney (DPOA), (V1) 359, (V1) 1159–1160
Durham-Humphrey Amendment, (V1) 609
Duty, (V1) 1168
Dynamic self, (V1) 267
Dysfunctional grief, (V1) 354
Dysmenorrhea, (V1) 897
Dyspareunia, (V1) 901
Dysphagia, (V1) 703
Dyspnea, (V1) 465
   assessment of, (V1) 994
   cardiovascular disease and, (V1) 1026
Dysrhythmias, (V1) 461, (V1) 462, (V1) 1024, (V1) 1028

E

EAR. *See* Estimated average requirement (EAR)
Early childhood. *See* Preschooler(s)
Early term fetus, (V1) 150
Ears
   assessment of, (V1) 511*p*, (V2) 227–231*p*
   care of, (V1) 600–601, (V1) 601*f*
   hearing aids for, (V1) 601, (V2) 375–377*p*, (V2) 603*p*
   hearing assessment and, (V1) 493–494
   irrigation of, (V2) 596–598*p*
   otic medications for, (V1) 640
      procedure for administering, (V1) 658*p*
   physical examination of external and middle, (V1) 493, (V1) 493*f*, (V1) 509, (V1) 511*p*
Eating disorders, (V1) 172, (V1) 174
EBP. *See* Evidence-based practice (EBP)
Eccentric exercise, (V1) 851
Ecchymosis, (V1) 489*t*
Echocardiogram, (V2) 763
E-cigarettes, (V1) 983
Economic climate of healthcare, (V1) 1188–1189
Ectropion, (V1) 492
Edentulism, (V1) 191
Education
   nursing (*See* Nursing education)
   patient (*See* Patient education)
Ego, (V1) 146–147
   integrity versus despair, in psychosocial development theory, (V1) 148, (V1) 194
Ejaculation, (V1) 883, (V1) 894
   premature, (V1) 902
   retrograde, (V1) 902
Elastic bandages, (V1) 973
Elder abuse, (V1) 198, (V1) 199–200
Elective surgery, (V1) 1078
Electrical conduction, heart, (V1) 1018, (V1) 1018*f*
Electrical hazards, (V1) 571
Electrocardiogram (ECG), (V1) 461, (V1) 1028, (V1) 1028*f*, (V2) 763, (V2) 830
   preoperative care, (V1) 1082
Electroencephalogram (EEG), (V1) 920, (V1) 920*f*
Electrolytes, (V1) 1037–1038
   assessment of, (V1) 1052–1053, (V2) 803–804
   critical thinking and clinical judgment on, (V2) 806–807
   diagnostic testing of, (V2) 805

full-spectrum nursing model applied to, (V2) 805–806
  imbalance in, (V1) 1047, (V1) 1047–1049t
    prevention of, (V1) 1054–1056
    self-care on, (V1) 1054
  knowledge map on, (V2) 809
  management of, (V1) 1054
  movement of, (V1) 1038–1040, (V1) 1038–1040f, (V1) 1040t
Electronic blood pressure monitors, (V1) 470–471
Electronic communication, (V1) 1140
Electronic entry, progress notes, (V1) 429–430, (V1) 430f
Electronic health records (EHRs), (V1) 420, (V1) 421, (V1) 423–425, (V1) 424f, (V1) 1146, (V2) 189p
  See also Nursing informatics
  barriers to adoption of, (V1) 1149
  benefits of, (V1) 1147, (V1) 1149
  ethical use of, (V1) 1149–1150, (V1) 1149f
  evidence-based practice on, (V1) 441
  guidelines for, (V1) 440–441, (V1) 440b
  in home care, (V1) 1142
  interoperability and standardized nursing languages and, (V1) 1147
  professional standards for, (V1) 1150, (V1) 1151b
Electronic infrared thermometers, (V1) 453t, (V1) 454
Electronic thermometers, (V1) 451, (V1) 453t
Elimination
  bowel (*See* Bowel elimination)
  by neonate, (V1) 153
  urinary (*See* Urinary elimination)
Elixirs, (V1) 612t
Embolus
  air, as complication of intravenous therapy, (V1) 1066t
  catheter, as complication of intravenous therapy, (V1) 1067t
  as postoperative complication, (V1) 1099t
  pulmonary, (V1) 992
    as postoperative complication, (V1) 1098t
Embryonic phase, (V1) 149
Emergency care triage, (V1) 1141
Emergency Medical Treatment and Active Labor Act (EMTALA), (V1) 1158
Emergency surgery, (V1) 1078
Emerging pathogens and diseases, (V1) 520
Emojis, (V1) 377
Emoticons, (V1) 377
Emotional data, (V1) 1111
Emotional distress, as vital sign, (V1) 444
Emotional intelligence theory, (V1) 1182
Emotions
  See also Stress
  body temperature and, (V1) 449
  communication of grieving, (V1) 363–364, (V1) 364f
  pain and, (V1) 815–816, (V1) 821
  vital signs and, (V1) 444
Empathy, (V1) 1182
  intellectual, (V1) 37
  in therapeutic relationship, (V1) 385
Employee development, (V1) 1185
Employment-based private insurance, (V1) 19
Empowerment, (V1) 1190
Empty nest, (V1) 298
Emulsions, lipid, (V1) 714

Encoding, (V1) 375, (V1) 376f
Encopresis, (V1) 166
Encryption, (V1) 1150
Endemic, (V1) 520
Endocrine system
  age-related changes in, (V1) 194t
  responses related to failure of adaptation, (V1) 252t
  responses to stressors, (V1) 242–243, (V1) 244f
  unrelieved pain and, (V1) 817
End-of-life care, (V1) 18
  See also Death and dying
  assisted suicide in, (V1) 361
  competencies in, (V1) 357–358
  defined, (V1) 357
  euthanasia in, (V1) 361
  hospice care in, (V1) 358
  legal and ethical considerations in, (V1) 358–361, (V1) 360b
  palliative care in, (V1) 358
  palliative sedation in, (V1) 361
  therapeutic communication in, (V1) 363, (V1) 364b
Endogenous analgesia system, (V1) 814
Endogenous infections, (V1) 519
Endogenous opioids, (V1) 814
Endorphins, (V1) 242
Endotracheal airways, (V1) 1005, (V1) 1005f
  caring for patients with, (V2) 749
  suctioning of, (V1) 1007, (V2) 726–730p
Enemas, (V1) 769, (V1) 771, (V1) 1087
  administration of, (V2) 565–569p
  barium, (V2) 587
  solutions for, (V1) 771, (V1) 772t
Energy, health as expression of, (V1) 208, (V1) 210, (V1) 211f
Energy balance, (V1) 682–683, (V1) 683b
Energy nutrients
  carbohydrates, (V1) 669, (V1) 670t
  defined, (V1) 669
  energy balance and, (V1) 682–683, (V1) 683b
  lipids, (V1) 670t, (V1) 671–673, (V1) 672t
  proteins, (V1) 669–671, (V1) 670t
Energy requirements, daily, (V1) 683
Engel, George, (V1) 350t
Enteral medications, (V1) 637
Enteral nutrition
  contamination of, (V1) 713–714
  enteric tubes for, (V1) 706
  feeding schedules, (V1) 710, (V1) 713
  monitoring patients receiving, (V1) 713, (V2) 503
  open and closed feeding systems, (V1) 713
  removing feeding tubes for, (V1) 714
  risks associated with, (V1) 706
  selecting feeding tube for, (V1) 706
  types of feeding solutions, (V1) 710
Enteral tube suction, (V1) 637
Enteric-coated drugs, (V1) 616
Enteric tubes, (V1) 706
Entropion, (V1) 492
Enuresis, (V1) 166, (V1) 721
  nocturnal, (V1) 721–722
Environment
  adaptation to hospital, (V1) 803
  cardiovascular function and, (V1) 1021
  client's
    noise in, (V1) 603

preventing and eliminating odors in, (V1) 601, (V1) 603
providing clean, (V2) 322
room temperature in, (V1) 603
standard bedside equipment in, (V1) 603–604
communication and, (V1) 380
culture and, (V1) 316, (V1) 327b
heat exchange between body and, (V1) 448, (V1) 448f
host susceptibility to infection and, (V1) 528
influence on body temperature, (V1) 448
maintaining clean, (V1) 533–534
pharmacokinetics and, (V1) 619
physical activity and, (V1) 856
pulmonary function and, (V1) 981–982
sensory deficits and assessment of, (V1) 803
sleep and, (V1) 924
supportive to microbes, (V1) 517–518
Environmental loss, (V1) 348
Environmental pollutants
  health promotion and, (V1) 222
  influence on health, (V1) 214–215
Environmental tobacco smoke (ETS), (V1) 983
Enzymatic débridement, (V1) 967
Enzyme secretion, (V1) 693
EOMs, (V1) 492
Epibole, wound, (V1) 953
Epidemics, (V1) 520, (V1) 541
Epidermis, (V1) 579, (V1) 941
  neonatal, (V1) 153
Epidural anesthesia, (V1) 1092, (V1) 1092f
Epidural catheter, (V2) 609
Epidural injections, (V1) 615t
  opioid, (V1) 831, (V1) 831f
  pain, (V1) 831–832
Epiglottis, (V1) 754, (V1) 977
Epilepsy and sleep, (V1) 931
Epinephrine, (V1) 244f
Epithelial healing, (V1) 946
Epithelialization, (V1) 948, (V1) 948f
Epithelial tissue in wounds, (V1) 957t
Equianalgesia, (V1) 830
Equipment and supplies, (V1) 21
  accidents related to, (V1) 553–554
  antiembolism stockings, (V1) 1032, (V1) 1088, (V1) 1088f, (V1) 1103–1104, (V1) 1104p, (V2) 815–817p
  catheters
    butterfly needle, (V1) 1057, (V1) 1057f
    epidural, (V2) 609
    indwelling urinary, (V1) 728, (V1) 735, (V1) 736f, (V1) 1087
      caring for patient with, (V1) 737–739, (V1) 738f
    inside-the-needle, (V1) 1057, (V1) 1057f
    midline peripheral, (V1) 1058
    over-the-needle, (V1) 1057, (V1) 1057f
    peripheral intravenous lock, (V1) 1058, (V1) 1058f
    selection of, (V1) 1061
  control of potentially contaminated, (V1) 536
  disposal of used, (V1) 536
  dressings, (V1) 972
  gastric and enteric tubes, (V2) 488–492p
  gastric suction, (V2) 819–824p
  intravenous infusion, (V1) 1061–1062, (V1) 1062f

legal accountability and safe use of, (V2) 853
for measuring blood pressure, (V1) 470–471, (V1) 470–472f
for measuring respiratory rate, (V1) 464
medication, (V1) 633
for moving patients in bed, (V1) 873, (V1) 873f
nasogastric and nasoenteric tubes, (V2) 483–487p
negative pressure wound therapy (NPWT), (V2) 671–676p
parenteral medications, (V1) 642–645, (V1) 643–645f, (V1) 643t
patient-controlled analgesia (PCA), (V1) 831–832, (V1) 831f, (V2) 606–608p
sequential compression devices (SCDs), (V1) 1032, (V1) 1103–1104, (V1) 1104p, (V2) 817–819p
speculum, (V2) 298–299
standard bedside, (V1) 603–604
sterile technique for, (V1) 538
stethoscopes, (V1) 458–459, (V1) 459f, (V1) 465–466
thermometers, (V1) 451, (V1) 452–453t
tracheostomy care, (V2) 719–726p
tracheostomy or endotracheal suctioning, (V2) 726–730p
tracking patients and, (V1) 1142
for transferring patients out of bed, (V1) 874–875, (V1) 874–875f
walking aids, (V1) 877–878, (V1) 877–878f
Erectile dysfunction (ED), (V1) 889, (V1) 892, (V1) 892t, (V1) 901
Erection, (V1) 893
Erickson, Erik, (V1) 266
Erosion, skin, (V2) 213p
Erotic dreams, (V1) 895
Erythema, (V1) 489t, (V1) 584, (V1) 953
Erythema toxicum, (V1) 941
Erythrocyte sedimentation rate (ESR), (V2) 700
Eschar, (V1) 953, (V1) 957t
Eschatology, (V1) 331
Esophagogastroduodenoscopy (EGD), (V2) 586
Esophagus, (V1) 754, (V1) 754f
Essential fatty acids, (V1) 673
Essential oils, (V1) 786
Essentials: Core Competencies for Professional Nursing Education, The, (V1) 6
Estimated average requirement (EAR), (V1) 666
Estrogen and urinary elimination, (V1) 723
Ethical concepts and principles, (V1) 128–131
autonomy, (V1) 128–129
beneficence, (V1) 129–130, (V1) 130f
fidelity, (V1) 130
guidelines for advocacy, (V2) 33
justice, (V1) 131
nonmaleficence, (V1) 129
in use of electronic health records (EHRs), (V1) 1149–1150, (V1) 1149f
veracity, (V1) 130–131
Ethical decision making, (V1) 134–140
improving one's, (V1) 139–140
MORAL model, (V1) 135–138, (V2) 32
nurses' obligations in, (V1) 138–140
problem or dilemma in, (V1) 135

Ethical frameworks, (V1) 126–128
Ethics, (V1) 30
See also Values
codes of, (V1) 13, (V1) 86, (V1) 118, (V1) 119, (V1) 131–132, (V1) 396, (V1) 1161–1162
end-of-life care, (V1) 358–362, (V1) 360b
ethical agency and, (V1) 118
ethical frameworks and, (V1) 126–128
external and internal factors and, (V1) 118
factors affecting moral decisions and, (V1) 123–132
full-spectrum nursing model applied to, (V2) 33–34
impaired nursing practice and, (V1) 119
institutional ethics committees and, (V1) 138
issues in healthcare, (V1) 132–133
key concepts in, (V1) 116
knowledge map for, (V2) 38
the law and, (V1) 116
moral distress and, (V1) 118–119, (V1) 119f, (V1) 120
morals and, (V1) 116
nature of nursing work and, (V1) 122–123
nursing, (V1) 117
professional guidelines on, (V1) 131–132, (V1) 132b
reasons to study, (V1) 117–118
related to values, (V1) 125
and sources of ethical problems for nurses, (V1) 119, (V1) 121–123
whistleblowing and, (V1) 119, (V1) 121, (V1) 122
Ethics-of-care, (V1) 128
Ethnicity. *See* Race and ethnicity
Ethnocentrism, (V1) 321
Etiologies, (V1) 59, (V1) 65
Eucalyptus, (V1) 786
Eupnea, (V1) 465t, (V1) 994
Euthanasia, (V1) 361
Evaluation, (V1) 47, (V1) 84–91
abuse, (V2) 46p
body composition analysis, (V1) 683, (V1) 696–697, (V1) 697b, (V2) 500–501
checklist for, (V2) 15–17
documentation of, (V1) 420
as essential to full-spectrum nursing, (V1) 85–86
ethical decision making and, (V1) 140
evaluative statement and, (V1) 88
pain, (V1) 836
of patient learning, (V1) 417–418
patient progress, (V1) 87–89, (V1) 89f
quality of care, (V1) 91
reflecting critically about, (V1) 90
relation to other steps of nursing process, (V1) 84–85
and revision of care plans, (V1) 89–90
standards and criteria used in, (V1) 86
types of, (V1) 86–87
vital signs, (V1) 476
Evaporation, (V1) 448
Evidence-based practice (EBP)
body temperature, (V1) 458
cardiovascular disease, (V1) 1023
choosing interventions based on, (V1) 75–76
clinical judgment and, (V1) 36, (V2) 26–28
colostomy, (V1) 782
critical thinking and, (V1) 37, (V2) 26–28

cultural competence, (V1) 323
death and dying care, (V1) 366
depression treatment, (V1) 289
diet, (V1) 692
electronic health records (EHRs), (V1) 441
ethics and, (V1) 122
fall prevention, (V1) 15, (V1) 76
family nursing, (V1) 294
full-spectrum nursing model applied to, (V1) 93, (V2) 26
health promotion activities to reduce anxiety and, (V1) 260
home-delivered meals and risk of falls, (V1) 205
home healthcare, (V1) 1133–1134
infection prevention, (V1) 542–543
key concepts in, (V1) 93
knowledge map for, (V2) 30
malpractice, (V1) 1168
meaningful work and physical activity, (V1) 260
medication errors, (V1) 630
missed nursing care, (V1) 1195
music and surgery, (V1) 1090
nursing informatics to support, (V1) 1150–1153, (V1) 1153–1154b
nursing research and, (V1) 105, (V1) 109–114, (V1) 112b, (V1) 112t
oral care, (V1) 597
pain management, (V1) 827
parenteral therapy, (V1) 1061
patient education, (V1) 407
pneumonia, (V1) 1008
SBAR tool, (V1) 553
sensory function, (V1) 806
sexuality and, (V1) 890
sleep disorders, (V1) 927
social determinants of health and postoperative complications of vertical sleeve gastrectomy, (V1) 230
spirituality and, (V1) 334
standardization supporting, (V1) 1147, (V1) 1148b
therapeutic communication, (V1) 392
urinary catheter insertion, (V1) 737
wearable devices, (V1) 1143–1145
weight-related health behaviors in adolescents, (V1) 176
wound care, (V1) 966
Evisceration, wound, (V1) 950–951, (V1) 951f
as postoperative complication, (V1) 1101t
Evolution of nursing, (V2) 3–5
knowledge map for, (V2) 6
Excitement in sexual response cycle, (V1) 893–894, (V1) 894t
Excoriation, (V1) 582, (V1) 943, (V1) 945t, (V2) 213p
Excretion, drug, (V1) 617–618
Exercise, (V1) 841
See also Physical activity
aerobic, (V1) 852
anaerobic, (V1) 852
assessment of, (V1) 863–865, (V1) 864b
guidelines and tools for, (V2) 632–633
benefits of regular, (V1) 853, (V1) 855b
cardiovascular function and, (V1) 1021, (V1) 1022
critical thinking and clinical judgment on, (V2) 635

full-spectrum nursing model applied to, (V2) 634
isokinetic, (V1) 852
isometric, (V1) 851
isotonic, (V1) 851
knowledge map on, (V2) 637
osteoporosis and, (V1) 867
overcoming objections to, (V1) 868b
oxygenation and, (V1) 982
pain with, (V1) 1032
physiology of movement and, (V1) 841–844, (V1) 842–843f, (V1) 843t
planning and evaluating fitness program for, (V1) 852–853, (V1) 852b, (V1) 853b
to prepare for ambulation, (V2) 629
promotion of, (V1) 867, (V1) 868b
range-of-motion, (V1) 875–876, (V2) 629
risks associated with, (V1) 853–855
types of, (V1) 851–852
Exercises, for assisting with ambulation, (V1) 876–878, (V1) 877–878f
Exhalation, (V1) 978
Exhaustion stage of stress, (V1) 244
Exocrine glands and drug excretion, (V1) 618
Exogenous infections, (V1) 519
Exophthalmos, (V1) 492
Expertise and empowerment, (V1) 1190
Expiration, (V1) 463, (V1) 463f
Expiratory reserve volume, (V2) 752
Exploring meaning, as spiritual intervention, (V1) 343
Expressive writing for pain, (V1) 826
Extended care facilities, (V1) 17
Extended families, (V1) 293
Extension tubing, IV, (V1) 1062
External central venous access devices, (V1) 657
External ear, (V1) 493
External gas exchange, heart, (V1) 1017
External loss, (V1) 348
External respiration, (V1) 462, (V1) 979, (V1) 979f
External sphincter, (V1) 756, (V1) 756f
External stressors, (V1) 239
External (condom) urinary catheter, (V2) 535–537p
Extinguishers, fire, (V1) 571
Extracellular fluid (ECF), (V1) 681, (V1) 1037, (V1) 1038
Extracts, (V1) 612t
Extravasation, as complication of intravenous therapy, (V1) 1065t
management of, (V2) 802
Exudate, (V1) 949
change in, (V1) 957t
Exudate formation, (V1) 245
Eyeglasses, (V1) 600
Eyelashes, (V1) 492, (V1) 492f
Eyelids, (V1) 492, (V1) 492f
Eyes
altered level of consciousness and, (V1) 805
artificial, (V1) 600, (V1) 603p, (V2) 374–375p, (V2) 603p
assessment of, (V2) 220–227p
care of, (V1) 599–600
contact lenses and, (V1) 600, (V2) 372–373p, (V2) 603p
external structures of, (V1) 492–493, (V1) 492f

internal structures of, (V1) 493
ophthalmic medications for, (V1) 639–640
procedure for administering, (V1) 658p
physical examination of, (V1) 491–493, (V1) 492f, (V1) 509, (V1) 511p
as primary defense against infection, (V1) 521
visual acuity and, (V1) 491–492
Eye shields, (V1) 536f

F
Face
assessment of, (V2) 218–219p
physical examination of, (V1) 491, (V1) 510p
Face masks, (V1) 536f
Face-to-face oral reports, (V1) 437
Facial appearance, (V1) 491
Facial expression, (V1) 379, (V1) 379f
FACT system, (V1) 429
Fahrenheit scale, (V1) 450–451, (V1) 451f
Failing to probe, (V1) 390
Failure to assess/recognize cues and diagnose/formulate hypotheses, (V1) 1170–1171
Failure to evaluate, (V1) 1171
Failure to implement a plan of care/take action, (V1) 1171, (V1) 1171b
Failure to plan/generate solutions, (V1) 1171
Failure to thrive, (V1) 157
Fair-mindedness, (V1) 38
Faith, (V1) 332
Faith community nursing, (V1) 1117
Fallopian tubes, (V1) 882
Falls
assessment for, (V1) 557–561, (V1) 562f, (V1) 877
in infants, (V1) 157
in older adults, (V1) 201, (V1) 549, (V1) 877
prevention of, (V1) 15, (V1) 76
in healthcare facilities, (V1) 571
home-delivered meals and, (V1) 205
False imprisonment, (V1) 1167
False reassurance, (V1) 390–391
Families
assessment of, (V1) 302–304, (V1) 303b, (V1) 303f
blended and step-, (V1) 293
caregiver role strain in, (V1) 302b, (V1) 304–307, (V1) 307b
caring for, (V1) 104, (V1) 293f
families as context for care in, (V1) 294
families as unit of care in, (V1) 294
family as system in, (V1) 294
theories in, (V1) 295–296
changes in structures of, (V1) 292–293
characteristics of healthy, (V1) 306b
cohabitating adults and, (V1) 293
coping impairment in, (V1) 271
dual-earner, (V1) 292
of dying patients, (V1) 365
evidence-based practice for, (V1) 294
extended, (V1) 293
family nursing approaches for, (V1) 293–294, (V1) 293f
forms of, (V1) 292
foster, (V1) 293
grandparent, (V1) 292
health challenges in, (V1) 299–307
chronic illness and disability, (V1) 300

homelessness, (V1) 300–301, (V1) 301f
infectious diseases, (V1) 300
poverty and unemployment, (V1) 299
violence and neglect, (V1) 301–302
health risk factors in, (V1) 296–299, (V1) 297–298f
with adolescents, (V1) 297, (V1) 298f
with middle-aged adults, (V1) 298
with older adults, (V1) 298–299, (V1) 298f
with young adults, (V1) 297–298, (V1) 298f
with young children, (V1) 296–297, (V1) 297f
key concepts on, (V1) 292
LGBTQ+, (V1) 293
low-income, (V1) 299
married adults without children, (V1) 292
middle-income, (V1) 299
military, (V1) 292
multigenerational/intergenerational, (V1) 293
pain education for, (V1) 835–836
relationships in
assessment of, (V1) 50
self-concept and, (V1) 267–268
sandwich, (V1) 293, (V1) 297
single adults and, (V1) 292
single parent, (V1) 292, (V1) 299
traditional, (V1) 292
Family health
assessment of, (V1) 302–304, (V1) 303b, (V1) 303f, (V2) 102–103
beliefs, (V1) 302–303
communication patterns, (V1) 304
coping processes, (V1) 304
genetics, (V1) 302, (V1) 303b, (V1) 303f
guidelines and tools for, (V2) 103–104
full-spectrum nursing model applied to, (V2) 104–105
knowledge map on, (V2) 107
Family interactional theory, (V1) 295
Family nursing, (V1) 293–294, (V1) 293f
Fantasies, sexual, (V1) 895
Fasting blood sugar, (V2) 830
Fatigue
cardiovascular disease and, (V1) 1026
physical activity and, (V1) 860, (V1) 877
and sleep deprivation among healthcare workers, (V1) 919
Fat-restricted diets, (V1) 694
Fats, dietary, (V1) 670t, (V1) 671–673, (V1) 672t
sleep and, (V1) 923
Fat-soluble vitamins, (V1) 673, (V1) 674–675t
Fatty acids, (V1) 671
Fear
pain and, (V1) 815
in response to stress, (V1) 248, (V1) 250
sleep and, (V1) 924
Febrile episode, (V1) 449
after blood infusions, (V1) 1070t
Fecal drainage devices
caring for patient with, (V2) 583
procedure for placing, (V2) 579–582p
Fecal impaction, (V1) 766, (V1) 768–769, (V1) 773–774
Fecal occult blood testing, (V1) 765
Feces, (V1) 756–757, (V1) 763, (V1) 763–764t
fluid loss via, (V1) 1041

Federal law, Bill of Rights, (V1) 1157
Feedback
  in communication, (V1) 377
  leaders providing evaluative, (V1) 1191
  in patient learning, (V1) 400
  in systems theory, (V1) 103
Feeding
  assisting patients with meals and, (V2) 502
  infant, (V1) 156
  through gastric and enteric tubes, (V2) 488–492p
Feet
  care of, (V1) 602p, (V2) 355–358p
    teaching client about, (V1) 591
  deformities of, (V1) 857
  odor of, (V1) 589
  problems in, (V1) 589–590
    common, (V1) 589
    in older adults, (V1) 589
  ulcers, diabetic, (V1) 945f, (V1) 946t
Fellatio, (V1) 895
Felony, (V1) 1165
Female circumcision, (V1) 889–890
Female genital mutilation, (V1) 889–890
Female genitourinary system, (V1) 508, (V1) 512–513p
  assessment of, (V2) 290–293p
  speculum examination, (V2) 298–299
Female reproductive organs, (V1) 882–883, (V1) 883f
  menstrual cycle and, (V1) 883, (V1) 884f
Female sterilization, (V2) 643
Feminist ethics, (V1) 127–128
Femoral artery pulse, (V1) 460, (V2) 182p
Fencing reflex, (V1) 153
Fertility awareness, (V2) 642
Fertilization, (V1) 149
Festinating gait, (V1) 865
Fetal alcohol spectrum disorders (FASDs), (V1) 150
Fetal alcohol syndrome (FAS), (V1) 150
Fetal development, (V1) 149–150, (V2) 48–49
Fever, (V1) 449–450
  after blood infusions, (V1) 1070t
  causes of, (V1) 449
  constant (sustained), (V1) 450
  intermittent, (V1) 450
  pulse rate and, (V1) 457
  relapsing (recurrent), (V1) 450
  remittent, (V1) 450
  respiration and, (V1) 464
  as secondary defense against infection, (V1) 521
  skin and, (V1) 943
  sweating due to, (V1) 943
  three phases of, (V1) 449–450
Fiber, dietary, (V1) 669, (V1) 758, (V1) 767
Fiberoptic colonoscopy, (V2) 586–587
Fibroblasts, (V1) 948, (V1) 948f
Fidelity, (V1) 130
Fight or flight response, (V1) 242–244, (V1) 243–244f
Filters, IV infusion, (V1) 1062
Filtration, (V1) 1039, (V1) 1039f
Filtration pressure, (V1) 1039
Finances, influence on health and illness, (V1) 215
Fine motor skills, toddler, (V1) 162
Fingernails, hygiene for, (V2) 321

Firearm injuries, (V1) 549
  prevention of, (V1) 564
Fire-hosing information, (V1) 389
Fires
  and electrical hazards in healthcare facilities, (V1) 554, (V1) 571
  in the home, (V1) 549, (V1) 564–565
First heart sound, (V1) 501
First impressions, (V1) 379
First-pass effect, (V1) 617
First trimester
  fetal development during, (V1) 149
  maternal changes during, (V1) 150
Fissure, (V2) 213p
Fistulas, (V1) 951, (V1) 951f
Fitness, (V1) 841
Fitness programs, (V1) 852–853, (V1) 852b, (V1) 853b
  teaching clients how to set up, (V1) 854
Flaccidity, (V1) 864b
Flattening, skull, (V1) 491
Flatus, (V1) 757, (V1) 768
Flexibility assessment, (V1) 227
Flexibility training, (V1) 852
Flow rates, IV infusion, (V1) 1063–1064, (V1) 1064b, (V2) 775–776p
Flowsheets, (V1) 431–432, (V2) 167
Flu. See Influenza
Fluid(s)
  See also Hydration
  active transport of, (V1) 1039–1040, (V1) 1040f
  assessment of, (V1) 1052–1053, (V2) 803–804
  balance of, (V1) 1040–1041
    PICOT questions, (V1) 682
    proteins and, (V1) 671
    water and, (V1) 681–682
  critical thinking and clinical judgment on, (V2) 806–807
  diagnostic testing of, (V2) 805
  diffusion of, (V1) 1039, (V1) 1039f
  extracellular, (V1) 681, (V1) 1037, (V1) 1038
  extracts, (V1) 612t
  filtration of, (V1) 1039, (V1) 1039f
  full-spectrum nursing model applied to, (V2) 805–806
  hypertonic, (V1) 1039
  hypotonic, (V1) 1039
  imbalances of
    acid-base, (V1) 1047, (V1) 1050t, (V1) 1051
    arterial blood gas (ABG) and, (V1) 1049, (V1) 1050t
    electrolyte, (V1) 1047, (V1) 1047–1049t
    nursing diagnosis of, (V1) 1053
    prevention of, (V1) 1054–1056
    self-care on, (V1) 1054
  intake of
    bowel elimination and, (V1) 758, (V1) 767–768
    facilitating, (V1) 1055
    pharmacokinetics and, (V1) 619
    urinary elimination and, (V1) 732
  interstitial, (V1) 1037
  intracellular, (V1) 681, (V1) 1037, (V1) 1038
  intravenous (See Intravenous fluids)
  isotonic, (V1) 1039
  knowledge map on, (V2) 809
  management of, (V1) 1054
  osmosis, (V1) 1038–1039, (V1) 1038f
  overload, as complication of intravenous therapy, (V1) 1066t

  restriction of, (V1) 1055–1056
  volume of
    deficit, (V1) 461, (V1) 1053
    excess, (V1) 461, (V1) 1053
Fluoride, (V1) 680t
Flushing, (V1) 489t
Foam skin cleansers, (V1) 964
Foam tape, (V1) 971
Focus Charting, (V1) 428
Focused assessments, (V1) 49
  intraoperative care, (V2) 829
  nutrition, (V2) 506–509
Folate, (V1) 677t
Folic acid
  deficiency in, (V1) 151
  supplementation of, (V1) 700
Folk medicine, (V1) 319
Follicle-stimulating hormone (FSH), (V1) 883
Follicular phase, (V1) 883
Followership, (V1) 1188
Fontanels, (V1) 152, (V1) 153f
Food and Drug Administration (FDA), (V1) 609, (V1) 621
  Nutrition Facts labels and, (V1) 668–669, (V1) 668f
Food-borne pathogens, (V1) 550
Food deserts, (V1) 211
Food frequency questionnaire, (V1) 696
Food guides, (V1) 666
Food insecurity, (V1) 211
Food intake and pulse rate, (V1) 457
Food record, (V1) 696
Food(s)
  allergies to, bowel elimination and, (V1) 761
  diabetes food plate, (V1) 668
  intolerances of, bowel elimination and, (V1) 761
  limited budgets for nutritious, (V1) 702
Food safety, (V1) 568, (V1) 569
Footboards, (V1) 869
Foot cradles, (V1) 869
Forearm support crutches, (V1) 878, (V1) 878f
Forgiveness facilitation, (V1) 343–344
Formal education, (V1) 10–12
Formal operations stage, in cognitive development theory, (V1) 148t, (V1) 402
Formula feeding, (V1) 156
Formularies, (V1) 608
Formulas, enteral feeding, (V1) 710
Foster families, (V1) 293
Fourth heart sound, (V1) 501
Fowler, James, (V1) 149
Fowler's position, (V1) 870, (V1) 871t, (V1) 871f
Fraction of inspired oxygen, (V1) 997
Fractures, (V1) 858–859
  casts for, (V1) 859
  clavicle, (V1) 155
  types of, (V1) 860f
Frail elderly adults, (V1) 191, (V1) 192–193, (V1) 687
Framingham studies, (V1) 93
Frankl, Victor, (V1) 213
Fraud, (V1) 1167
Freckles, (V1) 490
Freud, Sigmund, (V1) 145–147, (V1) 147t, (V1) 163, (V1) 165–166
Friction-reducing devices, (V1) 873
Friendships. See Peer relationships/friendships

Frontal cortex, (V1) 814
Full compensation, (V1) 1051
Full Outline of UnResponsiveness (FOUR), (V1) 506, (V2) 285
Full-spectrum nursing model, (V1) 6–8, (V1) 42–45, (V1) 43t, (V1) 44f, (V2) 19–20
   activity and exercise and, (V2) 634
   asepsis and infection prevention and, (V2) 327–328
   blood pressure and, (V2) 194
   bowel elimination and, (V2) 591
   circulation, (V2) 764
   clinical judgment in applying, (V2) 9–10
   communication and, (V2) 145–146
   death and dying and, (V2) 134
   defined, (V1) 42
   documentation and, (V2) 168
   ethics and values and, (V2) 33–34
   evaluation as essential to, (V1) 85–86
   evidence-based practice (EBP) and, (V1) 93, (V2) 26
   family health and, (V2) 104–105
   fluids, electrolytes, and acid-base balance and, (V2) 805–806
   growth and development and, (V2) 50
   home healthcare and, (V2) 841
   hospital admission and discharge and, (V2) 75–76
   hygiene and, (V2) 386
   as jigsaw puzzle, (V1) 93, (V1) 93f
   leading and managing and, (V2) 860
   legal accountability and, (V2) 853–854
   medication administration and, (V2) 469–470
   multicultural populations and, (V2) 113
   nursing informatics and, (V2) 847
   nutrition, (V2) 510–511
   older adults and, (V2) 55–56
   oxygenation, (V2) 754–755
   pain and, (V2) 613
   patient education and, (V2) 151
   psychosocial health and, (V2) 95–96
   restraints and, (V2) 341–342
   sensation and perception and, (V2) 601–602
   sexual health and, (V2) 645–646
   skin and wound healing and, (V2) 701
   sleep and rest and, (V2) 653–654
   spirituality and, (V2) 123
   stress and adaptation and, (V2) 84–85
   surgical patient care, (V2) 831–832
   urinary elimination, (V2) 555
Full term newborn, (V1) 150, (V1) 156
Full-thickness wounds, (V1) 946
Functional ability
   assessment of, (V1) 50, (V2) 17
   in older adults, (V1) 200
   limitations of oldest-old adults, (V1) 191
   losses in older adults, (V1) 299
   promotion in older adults, (V1) 202–203
Functional nursing, (V1) 16
Functional residual capacity, (V2) 753
Furosemide, (V1) 788

G

Gabapentin, (V1) 834
Gait, (V1) 379, (V1) 504, (V1) 865
Gallbladder, (V1) 693
   disease of, as complication of parenteral nutrition, (V1) 715

Gases, (V1) 614t
Gas transport, (V1) 462
Gastric lipase, (V1) 754
Gastric secretions, decreased, (V1) 703
Gastric suction, (V2) 819–824p
Gastric ulcers, (V1) 931
Gastroesophageal reflux, (V1) 703
Gastroesophageal sphincter, (V1) 754
Gastrointestinal motility alteration, (V1) 766
Gastrointestinal suction, postoperative, (V1) 1104, (V1) 1105p
Gastrointestinal system
   age-related changes in, (V1) 193t
   bowel incontinence, (V1) 775–782
   constipation, (V1) 703, (V1) 766, (V1) 768–769, (V1) 773–774
   constipation and impaction, (V1) 768–769
   diarrhea, (V1) 766, (V1) 768, (V1) 770–771
   drug excretion and, (V1) 617
   in neonates, (V1) 153
   as primary defense against infection, (V1) 521
   responses related to failure of adaptation, (V1) 252t
   response to stress, (V1) 244
   in school-age children, (V1) 167
   unrelieved pain and, (V1) 818
Gastrointestinal tract, (V1) 754f
   large intestine, (V1) 755–756, (V1) 756f
   rectum and anus, (V1) 756, (V1) 756f
   small intestine, (V1) 755, (V1) 755f
   upper, (V1) 754
   visualization studies of
     direct, (V2) 586–587
     indirect, (V2) 588–589
Gastrostomy button (G-button), (V1) 708, (V1) 710f
Gastrostomy tube (G-tube), (V1) 637, (V1) 708
Gate-control theory, (V1) 814–815, (V1) 815f, (V1) 824
Gauze, (V1) 973
Gels, (V1) 613t
Gender
   blood pressure and, (V1) 469
   body temperature and, (V1) 448–449
   cardiovascular disease and, (V1) 1025
   communication and, (V1) 380–381
   diversity, in nursing, (V1) 24
   energy needs and, (V1) 683
   homelessness and, (V1) 301
   illness and, (V1) 212
   life expectancy and, (V1) 186
   pharmacokinetics and, (V1) 619
   pulse rate and, (V1) 457
   self-concept and, (V1) 267
   sexual identity and, (V1) 888
   as subculture, (V1) 314
   total body fluid and, (V1) 1037, (V1) 1037t
Gender binary, (V1) 886
Gender identity, (V1) 885–886
Gender nonbinary, (V1) 886
Gender roles, (V1) 885
Gender transition, (V1) 886
General adaptation syndrome (GAS), (V1) 242–245, (V1) 243–244f

General anesthesia, (V1) 1091
General survey, (V1) 486–488, (V1) 487f, (V1) 509, (V1) 510p, (V2) 200–205p
General systems theory, (V1) 295
Generativity versus stagnation, in psychosocial development theory, (V1) 148, (V1) 181
Genetic-behavior-environment interaction, (V1) 187
Genetic makeup
   assessment of family history and, (V1) 302, (V1) 303b, (V1) 303f
   biological variations in, (V1) 109
   blood pressure and, (V1) 469
   illness and, (V1) 212
   pharmacokinetics and, (V1) 619
Genetic theories, (V1) 190
Genital herpes, (V1) 151, (V1) 898t
Genital stage, in psychoanalytic theory, (V1) 147t
Genitourinary system
   age-related changes in, (V1) 193t
   female, (V1) 508
   male, (V1) 507–508
   physical examination of, (V1) 507–508, (V1) 510, (V1) 512–513p
   as primary defense against infection, (V1) 521
   unrelieved pain and, (V1) 817–818
Genograms, (V1) 302
Genomics, (V1) 302
Genuineness, (V1) 385
Geopolitical boundaries, (V1) 1111
Geranium, (V1) 786
Gestation
   See also Pregnancy
   common health problems during, (V1) 150–152, (V1) 151f
   fetal development during, (V1) 149–150
   maternal changes during, (V1) 150
Gestational diabetes, screening for, (V1) 151
Gestures, (V1) 379
Get Up and Go test, (V1) 557
Gilligan, Carol, (V1) 149
Gingivitis, (V1) 593
Gingiva, (V1) 494, (V1) 494f
Ginkgo biloba, (V1) 288
Ginseng, (V1) 288, (V1) 823
Glasgow Coma Scale (GCS), (V1) 506, (V2) 284
Glass thermometers, (V1) 451, (V1) 452t
Global positioning systems (GPS), (V1) 1142
Globulin, (V1) 699
Glomerular filtration, (V1) 717, (V1) 720f
Glomerular filtration rate (GFR), (V1) 718
Glomerulus, (V1) 717
Glossitis, (V1) 594
Gloving, (V1) 538, (V1) 539p
   closed method, (V2) 314–3153p
   open method, (V2) 316–317p
Glucosamine, (V1) 823
Glucose intolerance, (V1) 703
Glucose testing, (V1) 1027
Gluteal drills, (V1) 876
Gluten-free diet, (V1) 695
Glycerides, (V1) 671
Glycerol, (V1) 671
Glycogen, (V1) 669

Index

Goals
    patient, (V1) 71–74, (V1) 73t
        judging achievement of, (V1) 87–88
    time management and, (V1) 1197
Gonorrhea, (V1) 151, (V1) 896, (V1) 898t
Good Samaritan laws, (V1) 1160–1161
Gout, (V1) 858, (V1) 858f
Government (public) financing of healthcare, (V1) 19–20
Government/military personnel, licensure of, (V1) 1163
Government subsidized home healthcare, (V1) 1125–1126
Graduate nursing education, (V1) 12
Grandparent families, (V1) 292
Grand theory, (V1) 98
Granulation tissue, (V1) 947, (V1) 947f, (V1) 948, (V1) 948f, (V1) 956, (V1) 957t
Graphic flow sheet, (V1) 53f
Graphic records form, (V1) 431–432
Grasp reflex, (V1) 153, (V1) 154f
Gravity feedings, (V1) 713
Gravity flow, (V1) 1063
Green tea and cardiovascular function, (V1) 1022
Grief, (V1) 298
    See also Death and dying; Loss
    anticipatory, (V1) 354
    assessment of, (V2) 132–133
    communicating with people experiencing, (V2) 127
    complicated, (V1) 354, (V1) 355–356, (V1) 368, (V1) 369
    defined, (V1) 348–349
    depression versus, (V1) 362
    developmental stages and, (V1) 353
    diagnoses related to, (V1) 362
    disenfranchised, (V1) 354
    as etiology, (V1) 362
    facilitating work on, (V1) 363–365, (V1) 364b, (V1) 364f
    factors affecting, (V1) 349–353, (V1) 350–352t
    host susceptibility to infection and, (V1) 529
    patient education on, (V1) 367
    theoretical foundations of, (V1) 349
    types of, (V1) 354
    uncomplicated, (V1) 354
Gross motor skills, toddler, (V1) 162, (V1) 162f
Group acceptance, adolescent, (V1) 171–172
Group B streptococcus, screening for, (V1) 152
Group communication, (V1) 375, (V1) 385–386, (V1) 386b
Group insurance, (V1) 19
Group meetings, for patient teaching, (V1) 411
Group rape, (V1) 900
Groupthink, (V1) 385–386
Growth
    of adolescents, (V1) 171
    critical thinking and clinical judgement on, (V2) 50–51
    defined, (V1) 144
    effect of sleep on, (V1) 916
    fetal, (V1) 149–150
    of infants, (V1) 156
    knowledge map on, (V2) 52
    of neonates, (V1) 152, (V1) 152f
    of preschoolers, (V1) 164–165
    of school-age children, (V1) 167
    of toddlers, (V1) 162
    of young adults, (V1) 179

Grunting, (V1) 994
Gua sha, (V1) 488
Guided imagery, (V1) 826, (V1) 934

H

H1N1 influenza, (V1) 520
H_2 receptor antagonists, preoperative, (V1) 1087t
Hacking cough, (V1) 466
Hair, (V1) 490, (V1) 510p
    assessment of, (V2) 215–216p
    care of, (V1) 597–599, (V1) 602p, (V2) 366–369p
Hair cells, (V1) 784
Half-and-half nails, (V1) 491
Halitosis, (V1) 594
Hand and wrist splints, (V1) 869, (V1) 870f
Hand hygiene, (V1) 1076, (V1) 1076b, (V2) 303–304p
    guidelines for, (V2) 321
    infection prevention and, (V1) 531, (V1) 533, (V1) 539p
    preschoolers and, (V1) 166
    surgical hand washing, (V1) 539p
        brushless system, (V2) 311–313p
        traditional method, (V2) 309–311p
    types of, (V1) 537t
Handoff reports, (V1) 384, (V1) 437–438
Handoffs, (V1) 235
Hand rolls, (V1) 869
Hardiness, (V1) 208, (V1) 219–220, (V1) 220f, (V1) 227
    adaptation and, (V1) 242
Harris flush, (V1) 771
Harrison Narcotics Act, (V1) 609
Haustral churning, (V1) 756
Havighurst, Robert, (V1) 145, (V1) 145–146t
Hay fever, (V1) 981
Hazardous waste, (V1) 570
Head
    assessment of, (V2) 218–219p
    concussion to, (V1) 169
    injury to, (V1) 859
    neonatal, (V1) 152, (V1) 153f
    physical examination of, (V1) 491–493, (V1) 492f, (V1) 509, (V1) 510p
Head-to-toe approach in physical examination, (V1) 480
Healing
    cellular and tissue, (V1) 245
    spiritual, (V1) 333
Healing presence, (V1) 208, (V1) 235–236
Health, (V1) 208
    See also Illness; Wellness
    as the ability of the soul to cope, (V1) 209
    biological factors in, (V1) 212
    cultural values and beliefs and, (V1) 314–317, (V1) 318
    defined, (V1) 208–209
    disruptions to, (V1) 209
    Dunn's health grid and, (V1) 210, (V1) 210f
    as expression of living energy, (V1) 208, (V1) 210, (V1) 211f
    factors that disrupt, (V1) 215–218
    hardiness and, (V1) 219–220, (V1) 220f
    how people experience, (V1) 212–215, (V1) 214t
    how to honor each client's unique experience with, (V1) 233–235

    as individual experience, (V1) 209
    influence of body image on, (V1) 268
    influence of culture on, (V1) 214
    influence of environmental factors on, (V1) 214–215
    influence of finances on, (V1) 215
    influence of lifestyle on, (V1) 213
    influence of nutrition on, (V1) 212–213
    influence of personal relationships on, (V1) 213–214, (V1) 214t
    influence of religion and spirituality on, (V1) 214
    influence of spiritual beliefs on, (V1) 333
    key concepts of, (V1) 208–209
    knowledge map on, (V2) 78
    meaningful work and, (V1) 213
    psychosocial (See Psychosocial health)
    screening for, (V1) 224–226t
    sexual (See Sexual health)
    sexuality and, (V1) 891–892, (V1) 892t
    social determinants of, (V1) 210–212, (V1) 211f
    three elements of, (V1) 208
    using conceptual models to understand, (V1) 209–210, (V1) 210f
Health assessment, (V2) 199
    abdomen, (V2) 257–263p
    anus and rectum, (V2) 294–295p
    breasts and axillae, (V2) 240–243p
    brief bedside, (V1) 513p, (V2) 295–296p
    chest and lungs, (V2) 244–250p
    ears and hearing, (V1) 511p, (V2) 227–231p
    eyes, (V2) 220–227p
    female genitourinary system, (V2) 290–293p
    general survey, (V2) 200–205p
    hair, (V2) 215–216p
    head and face, (V2) 218–219p
    heart and vascular system, (V2) 250–257p
    key concepts in, (V1) 479
    laboratory data in, (V1) 478
    male genitourinary system, (V2) 285–289p
    mouth and oropharynx, (V1) 511p, (V2) 234–238p
    musculoskeletal system, (V2) 263–272p
    nails, (V2) 216–218p
    neck, (V2) 238–240p
    nose and sinuses, (V1) 511p, (V2) 232–234p
    physical examination in (See Physical examination)
    sensory-neurological system, (V2) 272–285p
    skin, (V2) 206–214p
Health beliefs, (V1) 227–228
    assessment of, (V1) 302–303
    cultural values and, (V1) 314–317
Healthcare, (V1) 16–23
    abbreviations commonly used in, (V1) 426, (V2) 163–165
    alternative healing systems of, (V1) 319–320
    care settings in, (V1) 16–18, (V1) 17f
    classification systems used in, (V1) 62
    conventional system, (V1) 317
    cost containment in, (V1) 122
    culture of, (V1) 317–320, (V1) 317t
    economic climate of, (V1) 1188–1189
    ethical issues in, (V1) 132–133
    financing of, (V1) 19–21, (V1) 19f
    holistic, (V1) 319
    Indigenous, (V1) 317–318
    influence of finances on, (V1) 215
    jargon of, (V1) 322

members of interprofessional healthcare team in, (V1) 18–19, (V1) 18f
organization of, (V1) 18–19
providers and facilities ensuring quality care in, (V1) 23
reforms of, (V1) 21–23
regulation of, (V1) 21
as right or privilege, (V1) 22–23
supplies and equipment in, (V1) 21
trends in nursing and, (V1) 24–27
types of care in, (V1) 16
Healthcare-associated infections (HAIs), (V1) 515, (V1) 516
Healthcare-associated pneumonia (HCaP), (V1) 1000
Healthcare facilities
accidents and deaths in, (V1) 551–552
alarm safety in, (V1) 554, (V1) 574
biological hazards in, (V1) 556–557
culture of safety in, (V1) 553
equipment-related accidents in, (V1) 553–554
fires and electrical hazards in, (V1) 554, (V1) 571
healthcare culture in, (V1) 552
mercury exposure in, (V1) 555, (V1) 555t, (V1) 572, (V1) 573b
never events in, (V1) 552
quality nursing care in, (V1) 552
restraints in, (V1) 554–555, (V1) 571–572
safety promotion in, (V1) 571–574, (V1) 573b
understanding errors in, (V1) 552
violence in, (V1) 557, (V1) 574
Healthcare financing, (V1) 19–21, (V1) 19f, (V1) 122, (V1) 316
Healthcare reform
effects on care, (V1) 21–22
issues related to, (V1) 22–23
Healthcare teams, (V1) 18–19, (V1) 18f
Healthcare workers
computers and mobile devices for supporting, (V1) 1145–1146, (V1) 1146f
fatigue and sleep deprivation among, (V1) 919
operative personnel, (V1) 1089–1090
violence against, (V1) 557, (V1) 574
Health disparities, (V1) 211, (V1) 310
Health disruptions, (V1) 215–218
Health education, (V1) 233
Health equity, (V1) 211
Health history, (V1) 50–52, (V1) 51t, (V1) 226, (V1) 421
adolescent, (V1) 176–177
bowel elimination, (V2) 585
cardiovascular function and, (V1) 1021
cultural competence and, (V1) 323
fluids, electrolytes, and acid-base balance, (V2) 803
infections assessment and, (V1) 529–530
medication administration and, (V1) 631
nutrition, (V2) 506–507
oxygenation, (V2) 751–752
pain, (V2) 610
sexual, (V1) 902, (V2) 640
skin and wound, (V2) 694
sleep, (V2) 652–653
urinary elimination, (V2) 545

Health illiteracy, (V1) 405
Health-illness continuum, (V1) 209–210, (V1) 210f
Health Information Technology for Economic and Clinical Health (HITECH) Act, (V1) 1158
Health insurance, (V1) 299
home healthcare, (V1) 1126
Health Insurance Portability and Accountability Act (HIPAA), (V1) 439, (V1) 1140–1141, (V1) 1157–1158
electronic health records (EHRs) and, (V1) 1150
Health literacy, (V1) 405–406
Health maintenance organizations (HMOs), (V1) 22
Health policy, (V1) 27
Health practices, (V1) 318
Health promotion, (V1) 18, (V1) 208
assessment of, (V1) 226
attaining healthy life and, (V1) 236–237
critical thinking and clinical judgment on, (V2) 76–77
defined, (V1) 208–209
exercise, (V1) 867, (V1) 868b
full-spectrum nursing model applied to, (V2) 75–76
health literacy, (V1) 406
versus health protection, (V1) 220
implementation for, (V1) 230–231
information dissemination for, (V1) 222
interventions for adolescents, (V1) 177–179
interventions for toddlers, (V1) 164
knowledge map on, (V2) 78
models of, (V1) 221–222f, (V1) 221–223
nursing diagnosis and, (V1) 229
nursing process used in, (V1) 223–237
physical fitness assessment, (V1) 226–227, (V2) 72
PICOT questions for, (V1) 232
planning/prioritizing hypothesis/generating solutions for, (V1) 229–230
programs of, (V1) 222
providing counseling on, (V1) 232–233
role modeling and, (V1) 231–232
self-concept and self-esteem, (V1) 276–277
settings for, (V1) 223
for stress, (V1) 258–259
to support host defense against infections, (V1) 531–533
throughout the life span, (V1) 223, (V1) 224–226t
Health protection, (V1) 208, (V1) 220
levels of prevention in, (V1) 220
Health records systems
charting by exception (CBE), (V1) 422–423
defined, (V1) 421
electronic health records (EHRs), (V1) 420, (V1) 421, (V1) 423–425, (V1) 424f
paper records, (V1) 425, (V1) 425b, (V2) 163
problem-oriented record (POR) systems, (V1) 422, (V1) 422f
source-oriented, (V1) 421–422
Health restoration, (V1) 18
Health risks, (V1) 234
appraisal of, (V1) 223, (V1) 227
family, (V1) 296–299, (V1) 297–298f
with adolescents, (V1) 297, (V1) 298f
with middle-aged adults, (V1) 298

with older adults, (V1) 298–299, (V1) 298f
with young adults, (V1) 297–298, (V1) 298f
with young children, (V1) 296–297, (V1) 297f
loneliness, (V1) 271
spiritual distress, (V1) 341, (V1) 342b
Health status
disparities and, (V1) 310
drawing conclusions about, (V1) 58–59
hygiene and, (V1) 576–577
influencing adaptation, (V1) 241
physical examination for monitoring, (V1) 479
skin problems and, (V1) 582–583
Health System domain, (V1) 1081
Healthy People 2030 goals, (V1) 229–230, (V1) 231b
Hearing
assessment of, (V1) 493–494, (V1) 511p, (V2) 227–231p
communicating with client with impaired, (V2) 598–599
in infants, (V1) 787
in neonates, (V1) 154–155, (V1) 786
in oldest-old adults, (V1) 191
screening older adults', (V2) 599
in toddlers, (V1) 162
Hearing aids, (V1) 601, (V1) 603p, (V2) 375–377p, (V2) 603p
Hearing Handicap Inventory for the Elderly Screening Version (HHIE-S), (V2) 599
Heart, (V1) 499, (V1) 511–512p, (V1) 1017, (V1) 1017f
assessment of, (V1) 1025–1026, (V2) 250–257p
auscultation of, (V1) 501, (V1) 501f, (V1) 501t
autonomic nervous system and, (V1) 1019
cardiac arrest and, (V1) 1033–1034
cardiac cycle and, (V1) 499, (V1) 1017, (V1) 1018f
cardiac monitoring of, (V1) 1028, (V1) 1028f
decreased cardiac output, (V1) 1029–1031
dysrhythmias, (V1) 1028
electrical conduction of, (V1) 1018, (V1) 1018f
inspection and palpation of, (V1) 499, (V1) 501
sounds of, (V1) 501
Heart failure, (V1) 1024
Heart valve abnormalities, (V1) 1024–1025
Heat
cardiovascular function and, (V1) 1021
exchange between the body and environment, (V1) 448, (V1) 448f
production in the body, (V1) 447
for wound care, (V1) 973–974, (V1) 973–974f, (V2) 693
Heat exhaustion, (V1) 854
Heating equipment fires, (V1) 549
Heat packs for pain, (V1) 824–825
Heatstroke, (V1) 450–451
HEENT, (V1) 491
Height and weight measurements in general survey, (V1) 487, (V1) 487f
Height and weight tables, (V1) 683
Helper cells, (V1) 524
Helper T cells, (V1) 524
Helplessness and pain, (V1) 815–816

Index

Hemangiomas, (V1) 941
Hematocrit, (V1) 468
Hematoma, (V1) 950
    as complication of intravenous therapy, (V1) 1065t
Hemiplegia, (V1) 864b
Hemoglobin, (V1) 699, (V1) 997, (V2) 753, (V2) 763
    carbon dioxide and, (V1) 1019
    production of, (V1) 982
    respiration and, (V1) 464
Hemolytic reactions to blood infusions, (V1) 1070t
Hemorrhage
    as postoperative complication, (V1) 1099t
    pulse rate and, (V1) 457
    wound, (V1) 949–950
Hemorrhoids, (V1) 509, (V1) 756
Hemostasis, (V1) 949
Hemothorax, (V1) 1009
Hemovac drains, (V1) 965, (V1) 965f
Henderson, Virginia, (V1) 98–99, (V1) 99b
Heparin, (V1) 624
    administration of, (V1) 650–651
Hepatitis B, (V1) 899t
Herbal supplements, (V1) 261
    for relaxation and sleep, (V1) 937
Hernias, (V1) 508
Heroin, (V1) 150
Hierarchy of needs, (V1) 100, (V1) 102, (V1) 102f, (V1) 266–267
Higher-brain death, (V1) 354, (V1) 356
High-fidelity mannequins, (V1) 1146, (V1) 1146f
High-Fowler's position, (V1) 870
Hinduism, (V1) 332, (V1) 336–337
Hip abduction pillows, (V1) 869–870
Hirsutism, (V1) 490
Hispanic diet, (V1) 692
Historical context of nursing, (V1) 4–8, (V1) 106, (V1) 1114
    spirituality in, (V1) 330
HIV. See Human immunodeficiency virus (HIV)
Hoarseness, (V1) 487
Holistic belief system, (V1) 318
Holistic healing, (V1) 39, (V1) 104, (V1) 319
    acupuncture for acute postoperative pain, (V1) 1102
    alternative therapies for lowering blood pressure, (V1) 475
    common cold, (V1) 1000
    end-of-life care, (V1) 359
    essential oils, (V1) 786
    hospice and, (V1) 358
    intercessory prayer in, (V1) 345
    natural sleep aids, (V1) 937
    pain management, (V1) 823, (V1) 824–826
    standardized language and, (V1) 80
Holmes-Rahe Social Readjustment Scale, (V2) 82
Holter monitor, (V2) 763
Home fires, (V1) 549, (V1) 564–565
Home health agencies, (V1) 1123–1124
Home healthcare, (V1) 1110
    See also Community-based nursing agencies for, (V1) 17–18
    apical-radial pulse deficit, (V2) 187p
    assessment in, (V1) 1129

    for patient with mobility concerns, (V1) 865
    assisting with medication management, (V1) 1131–1132, (V1) 1132f
    blood pressure, (V2) 192p
    body temperature, (V2) 178–179p
    caregiver support in, (V1) 205, (V1) 1135
    caring for urinary diversion, (V1) 745
    for casts, (V1) 859
    controlling infections in, (V1) 1132, (V1) 1134–1135, (V1) 1134f
    critical thinking and clinical judgment on, (V1) 841–843
    defined, (V1) 1122
    distinctive features of, (V1) 1122–1123, (V1) 1123b, (V1) 1123f
    documentation in, (V1) 436–437
    encouraging toddlers to eat, (V1) 685
    evidence-based practice on, (V1) 1133–1134
    full-spectrum nursing model applied to, (V2) 841
    future of, (V1) 1126
    goals of, (V1) 1122
    home health nurses in, (V1) 1124–1125
    home nutritional support, (V1) 708
    home visits in, (V1) 1127–1128, (V1) 1127–1128f
    hospice care, (V1) 1125, (V1) 1125t
    infections and, (V1) 532, (V1) 1132, (V1) 1134–1135, (V1) 1134f, (V2) 840
    interventions in, (V1) 1131–1135, (V1) 1132f, (V1) 1134f
    knowledge map on, (V2) 845
    managing nocturnal enuresis in children, (V1) 722
    nursing diagnosis in, (V1) 1129–1130
    nursing process in, (V1) 1129
    patient self-monitoring of blood pressure, (V1) 471
    payment for, (V1) 1125–1126
    peak flow meter use, (V1) 999
    peripheral pulse, (V2) 183p
    personal protective equipment (PPE), (V2) 307p
    potential abuse and, (V2) 46p
    preoperative assessment for surgical client who will be discharged to home, (V1) 1082
    preventing infection, (V1) 532
    preventing poisoning, (V1) 564
    promoting safety in the home, (V1) 1134–1135
    providers of, (V1) 1123–1125, (V1) 1125t
    referral of clients to, (V1) 1126
    respiration assessment, (V2) 188p
    safety considerations in, (V1) 1127, (V2) 839
    standardized languages for, (V1) 79
    standardized nursing interventions in, (V1) 1131
    surgical hand washing, (V2) 313p
    unhealthy home may mean poor health and, (V1) 1133
    use of informatics in, (V1) 1142
Home health monitoring, (V1) 1141
Homelessness, (V1) 300–301, (V1) 301f
Homeostasis, (V1) 239
    See also Acid-base balance; Electrolytes; Fluid(s); Hydration
    knowledge map on, (V2) 809

Home oxygen administration equipment fires, (V1) 549
Home safety
    hazards in, (V1) 547–549, (V1) 548b, (V1) 561
    interventions for, (V1) 563–567, (V1) 566f
Home visits, (V1) 1127–1128, (V1) 1127–1128f
Honesty, (V1) 378, (V1) 383
Honoring personhood, (V1) 104
Hope, (V1) 332–333
    inspiration of, (V1) 344
HOPE approach to spiritual assessment, (V1) 340–341, (V2) 121
Hops, (V1) 937
Hormonal implant (contraception), (V2) 643
Hormonal regulation of fluid and electrolyte balance, (V1) 1041
Hormone replacement therapy (HRT), (V1) 183, (V1) 906
Hospice and Palliative Nurses Association (HPNA), (V1) 361
Hospice care, (V1) 358
    home healthcare, (V1) 1125, (V1) 1125t
Hospital Accreditation Standards, (V1) 52
Hospital-based agencies, (V1) 1124
Hospitalization
    admitting patient to nursing unit, (V1) 236p, (V2) 60–62p
    critical thinking and clinical judgment on, (V2) 76–77
    discharge
        forms, (V2) 70–71
        from healthcare facility, (V1) 237p, (V2) 66–68p
        maintaining trust of client during, (V1) 236
        planning, (V1) 66–67, (V1) 421, (V1) 431, (V1) 431f
        summary, (V1) 431
    full-spectrum nursing model applied to, (V2) 75–76
    interventions to help families cope with, (V1) 307, (V1) 307b
    preparing room for admission, (V2) 69
    reducing stress of, (V1) 263
    restraints used in, (V1) 554–555, (V1) 571–572, (V1) 573p, (V2) 334–337p, (V2) 339
    of school-age children, (V1) 170–171
    self-concept and, (V1) 268
    transfer of patient to another unit, (V1) 236p, (V2) 63–64p
    transfer of patient to long-term care facility, (V1) 237p, (V2) 64–65p
Hospitals, (V1) 16–17, (V1) 17f
    adaptation to environment in, (V1) 803
    beds in, (V1) 604–605, (V1) 604f, (V1) 868–869
    recovery rooms, (V1) 1089, (V1) 1095, (V1) 1095f
    surgical holding areas in, (V1) 1089, (V1) 1089f
Hostility, (V1) 250
Host susceptibility to infections, (V1) 525, (V1) 528–529
Household system for medication measurement, (V1) 624
Housing and aging, (V1) 187–190
HPV. See Human papillomavirus (HPV)
HRT. See Hormone replacement therapy (HRT)

Human immunodeficiency virus (HIV), (V1) 300, (V1) 899t
   host susceptibility to infection and, (V1) 529
Humanism, (V1) 397–398
Human papillomavirus (HPV), (V1) 896–897, (V1) 898t
Human relations-based management, (V1) 1184
Humidifiers, (V1) 1002
Humidity, (V1) 448
   pulmonary function and, (V1) 982
Humility
   cultural, (V1) 322
   intellectual, (V1) 37
Humor, (V1) 261–262, (V1) 262f, (V1) 378, (V1) 826
Humoral immunity, (V1) 524, (V1) 525f
Hydrating dressing, (V2) 678–680p
Hydration
   See also Fluid(s); Water
   body fluids and solutes
     acid-base balance regulation, (V1) 671, (V1) 1045
     balance of, (V1) 1040–1041
     compartments of, (V1) 1037
     electrolytes, (V1) 1037–1038
       major, (V1) 1041–1045, (V1) 1042–1044t
     fluid intake and, (V1) 1040
     fluid output and, (V1) 1040–1041
     movement in the body, (V1) 1038–1040, (V1) 1038–1040f, (V1) 1040t
     total, in relation to sex and age, (V1) 1037, (V1) 1037t
     types of, (V1) 1037
   bowel elimination and, (V1) 758, (V1) 767–768
   intake and output (I&O)
     guidelines for measuring, (V2) 798–799
     records of, (V1) 432
   key concepts in, (V1) 1037
   mobilizing secretions, (V1) 1002–1003
   in older adults, (V1) 299
   procedures
     assisting with percutaneous central venous catheter placement, (V2) 795–797p
     changing IV dressings, (V2) 783–787p
     changing IV solutions and tubing, (V2) 779–782p
     discontinuing peripheral IV, (V2) 790–791p
     initiating a peripheral intravenous infusion, (V2) 769–774p
     regulating IV flow rate, (V2) 775–776p
     setting up and using volume-control pumps, (V2) 777–779p
   skin and, (V1) 942
   urinary elimination and, (V1) 732
Hydrocephalus, (V1) 491
Hydrocolloid dressing, (V2) 678–680p
Hydrodensitometry, (V1) 697
Hydrogel-coated catheters, (V1) 735
Hydrogel dressing, (V2) 678–680p
Hydrogenated vegetable oils, (V1) 672
Hydrophilic medications, (V1) 637
Hydrostatic pressure, (V1) 1039
Hydrotherapy, (V1) 967
Hygiene
   See also Self-care
   assessment of, (V1) 577
     guidelines and tools for, (V2) 384–385

bathing
   providing a complete bed bath using prepackaged bathing product, (V2) 346–351p
   using a basin and water, (V2) 351–352p
   beard and mustache care, (V1) 598, (V1) 602p, (V2) 369–370p
   in clients with morbid obesity, (V1) 588
   critical thinking and clinical judgment on, (V2) 386–388
   delegating responsibility for patient, (V1) 578–579, (V1) 579f
   denture care, (V1) 602p, (V2) 361–363p
   factors influencing, (V1) 576
   foot care, (V1) 591, (V1) 602p, (V2) 355–358p
   full-spectrum nursing model applied to, (V2) 386
   hand, (V1) 1076, (V1) 1076b
     infection prevention and, (V1) 531, (V1) 533, (V1) 539p
     preschoolers and, (V1) 166
     surgical, (V1) 539p
     types of, (V1) 537t
   implementation for, (V1) 578–579, (V1) 579f
   key concepts on, (V1) 576
   knowledge map on, (V2) 390
   nursing diagnosis and, (V1) 577–578
   oral care for unconscious patients, (V1) 602p, (V2) 363–366p
   perineal care, (V1) 602p, (V2) 352–355p
   planning for, (V1) 578
   shampooing the hair, (V1) 598, (V1) 602p, (V2) 366–369p
   shaving a patient, (V1) 599, (V2) 370–372p, (V2) 602–603p
   showers or tub baths, (V1) 586, (V2) 383
   skin, (V1) 944
   teeth care, (V1) 595–596, (V1) 595f, (V1) 602p, (V2) 358–361p
   types of scheduled, (V1) 578
   urinary elimination and, (V1) 732
Hyperalgesia, (V1) 814
Hyperbaric oxygen therapy (HBOT), (V1) 949
Hypercalcemia, (V1) 1048t
Hypercarbia, (V1) 985b, (V1) 998
Hyperglycemia, (V1) 698
Hyperkalemia, (V1) 1048t
Hypermagnesemia, (V1) 1049t
Hypermania, (V1) 892
Hypernatremia, (V1) 1047t
Hyperphosphatemia, (V1) 1049t
Hyperpyrexia, (V1) 449
Hypersomnia, (V1) 926
Hypertension, (V1) 469, (V1) 474–475
   alternative therapies for, (V1) 475
   patient education on, (V2) 194
   pulmonary, (V1) 992
   sensory function and, (V1) 788
Hyperthermia, (V1) 450–451, (V1) 854
Hyperthyroidism, (V1) 447, 488
   sleep and, (V1) 931
Hypertonic fluids, (V1) 1057
Hypertonic solutions, (V1) 1039
Hypertrophy
   muscle, (V1) 864b
   prostate gland, (V1) 724
Hyperventilation, (V1) 467, (V1) 978
Hypnosis, (V1) 826
Hypnotics, preoperative, (V1) 1087t
Hypocalcemia, (V1) 1048t, (V2) 798

Hypocarbia, (V1) 985b, (V1) 998
Hypochondriasis, (V1) 251
Hypoglycemia, (V1) 698
Hypokalemia, (V1) 1048t
Hypomagnesemia, (V1) 1049t
Hyponatremia, (V1) 1047t
Hypophosphatemia, (V1) 1049t
Hypotension, (V1) 474
   orthostatic, (V1) 876
Hypothalamus, (V1) 242
   fever and, (V1) 449
Hypothermia, (V1) 450, (V1) 451, (V1) 855
Hypothetical thinking, (V1) 149
Hypothyroidism, (V1) 447
   sleep and, (V1) 931
Hypotonic fluids, (V1) 1039
Hypotonic solutions, (V1) 1039, (V1) 1056–1057
Hypoventilation, (V1) 467, (V1) 978
Hypovolemia, as postoperative complication, (V1) 1099t
Hypoxemia, (V1) 979, (V1) 985b
Hypoxia, (V1) 466, (V1) 467, (V1) 978, (V1) 985b
Hysterectomy, (V1) 891

I

Ibuprofen, (V1) 827–828
ICN. See International Council of Nurses (ICN)
Id, the, (V1) 146
Ideal weight, (V1) 683
Identification, as defense mechanism, (V1) 247t
Identity
   personal, (V1) 269
   versus role inferiority, in psychosocial development theory, (V1) 148
Idiosyncratic reactions to drugs, (V1) 623
Ileocecal valve, (V1) 755
Ileostomy, (V1) 761
Ileum, (V1) 755
Ileus, as postoperative complication, (V1) 1100t
Illicit drugs, (V1) 624
   See also Substance abuse
   cardiovascular function and, (V1) 1022
   oxygenation and, (V1) 982
Illness and disease
   See also Health
   acute, (V1) 219
   beliefs about, (V1) 318
   biological factors in, (V1) 212
   blood pressure and, (V1) 469
   bowel elimination and, (V1) 760–761
   chronic (See Chronic illness)
   congenital (See Congenital anomalies)
   effects on physical activity, (V1) 857–860, (V1) 858f, (V1) 860f
   emerging, (V1) 520
   environmental pollutants and, (V1) 214–215
   hardiness and, (V1) 219–220, (V1) 220f
   as health disruption, (V1) 216, (V1) 217
   host susceptibility to infection and, (V1) 525
   how people experience, (V1) 212–215, (V1) 214t, (V1) 218–223
   how to honor each client's unique experience with, (V1) 233–235

as individual experience, (V1) 209
intensity, duration, and multiplicity of disruption due to, (V1) 220
knowledge map on, (V2) 78
nature of, (V1) 219, (V1) 219b
as outcome of stress, (V1) 241, (V1) 241f
pharmacokinetics and, (V1) 619
prevention of, (V1) 18, (V1) 208
　for older adults, (V1) 203–204
psychosocial (See Psychosocial illness)
pulse rate and, (V1) 457
respiration and, (V1) 464
self-concept and, (V1) 268
sensory function and, (V1) 788
sexuality and, (V1) 891–892, (V1) 892t
skin diseases, (V1) 583
sleep and, (V1) 917, (V1) 917f, (V1) 924
somatoform, (V1) 251
stages of behavior in, (V1) 218–219
stress-induced chronic, (V1) 251
urinary elimination and, (V1) 724
Illness practices, (V1) 318
Illness stage, infections, (V1) 520
Imagery, (V1) 260–261
Imbalance, as health disruption, (V1) 217–218
Immature breathing patterns and oxygenation, (V1) 992
Immediate drug reactions, (V1) 622
Immobility
　See also Mobility
　altered level of consciousness and, (V1) 805
　bowel elimination and, (V1) 760
　prolonged, (V1) 860–863
　urinary elimination and, (V1) 724
Immobilization and traction for pain, (V1) 825
Immune system
　host susceptibility to infection and deficiency in, (V1) 529
　protein role in, (V1) 671
　responses related to failure of adaptation, (V1) 252t
　in school-age children, (V1) 167
Immunity
　artificial active, (V1) 523b
　artificial passive, (V1) 523b
　cellular, (V1) 524, (V1) 524f
　humoral, (V1) 524, (V1) 525f
　Immunoglobulin (Ig) classes, (V1) 524, (V1) 525b
　natural active, (V1) 522b
　natural passive, (V1) 523b
Immunizations, (V1) 297
　adolescent, (V1) 178
　infant, (V1) 161
　infection prevention and, (V1) 533
　influenza and pneumonia, (V1) 1001
　middle adulthood, (V1) 183
　needle size for, (V1) 653, (V1) 653t
　older adults, (V1) 203–204
　preschooler, (V1) 166
　school-age child, (V1) 169
　tetanus, (V1) 958
　toddler, (V1) 163
Immunoglobulin (Ig) classes, (V1) 524, (V1) 525b
Impaired nurses, (V1) 1177, (V1) 1177b
Impetigo, (V1) 583
Implantable ports, (V1) 657, (V1) 657f

Implanted ports, (V1) 1059–1060, (V1) 1060f
Implementation, (V1) 47
　change, (V1) 1194
　choosing, (V1) 77–78t
　computer-generated, (V1) 78
　defined, (V1) 81
　doing or delegating in, (V1) 82–84, (V1) 85b
　in health promotion, (V1) 230–231
　planning, (V1) 74–75
　　theory-based, (V1) 104
　planning theory-based, (V1) 104
　preparing for, (V1) 81–82
　problem status and, (V1) 76
　process for generating and selecting, (V1) 76–78, (V1) 78t
　theory applied to, (V1) 103
　using standardized language to plan, (V1) 78–80, (V1) 79b
Incentive spirometry, (V1) 1002, (V1) 1103, (V1) 1103f
Incident reports, (V1) 1173–1174
Incision, (V1) 945t
Incisors, (V1) 592
Incivility, (V1) 382
Incompatibilities, drug, (V1) 623
Incomplete proteins, (V1) 671
Incubation, infection, (V1) 519
Independent interventions, (V1) 75
Independent living facilities, (V1) 18
Indexes, (V1) 110
Indian diet, (V1) 692
Indigenous healthcare system, (V1) 317–318
Indigenous religions, (V1) 337, (V1) 338f
Indirect auscultation, (V1) 484
Indirect care, (V1) 15
　interventions planning in, (V1) 74
Indirect hernias, (V1) 508
Indirect method for measuring blood pressure, (V1) 470
Indirect service agencies, (V1) 1124
Individual coping, impaired, (V1) 271
Individual counseling, (V1) 232
Individualized nursing care plans, (V1) 69, (V1) 71
Individual private insurance, (V1) 19
Individuals, as payors of healthcare, (V1) 19
Inductive reasoning, (V1) 96–97, (V1) 96f
Industry versus inferiority, in psychosocial development theory, (V1) 148, (V1) 168
Indwelling urinary catheter, (V1) 728, (V1) 735, (V1) 736f, (V1) 1087
　caring for patient with, (V1) 737–739, (V1) 738f
　insertion of, (V2) 529–535p
　removal of, (V2) 537–539p
Infants
　See also Neonates
　abnormal shape or flattening of skull in, (V1) 491
　abuse, neglect, and violence involving, (V1) 158–160, (V1) 161, (V2) 42
　assessment of, (V1) 160
　body temperature in, (V1) 448
　bowel elimination in, (V1) 757
　cardiovascular function in, (V1) 1020
　car seats for, (V1) 161
　common health problems of, (V1) 157–158
　communication by, (V1) 380
　congenital cataracts in, (V1) 492–493

crying and colic in, (V1) 157, (V1) 160
dental caries in, (V1) 157
development of
　cognitive, (V1) 156–157
　physical, (V1) 156, (V1) 157b
　psychosocial, (V1) 157
　sexuality, (V1) 886–887, (V1) 887f
failure to thrive in, (V1) 157
hearing in, (V1) 787
hygiene and, (V1) 576
immunizations for, (V1) 161
implementation for, (V1) 160–162
loss in, (V1) 348
neurological system examination in, (V1) 505
nutrition in, (V1) 684–685
pain response in, (V1) 816, (V1) 819
physical examination of, (V1) 485
play and, (V1) 161
pulmonary function in, (V1) 980
pulse rate in, (V1) 457
safe sleep of, (V1) 935
safety of, (V1) 546
self-concept in, (V1) 267
sensory function in, (V1) 787
skin of, (V1) 583, (V1) 941
sleep requirements and characteristics in, (V1) 918t
sudden infant death syndrome (SIDS) in, (V1) 150, (V1) 157–158, (V1) 160
suffocation of, (V1) 549
surgical risk in, (V1) 1078
touch sense in, (V1) 787
unintentional injury in, (V1) 157, (V1) 161
urinary elimination in, (V1) 721–722
vision in, (V1) 787
Infection prevention nurse, (V1) 540
Infections
　See also Medical asepsis
　CDC guidelines for preventing transmission of, (V1) 534–536, (V1) 535t, (V1) 536f
　central-line associated bloodstream, (V1) 1058–1059
　as challenge to family health, (V1) 300
　characteristics of environments supportive to microbes and, (V1) 517–518
　classified by location and duration, (V1) 519
　as complication of intravenous therapy, (V1) 1066t
　as complication of parenteral nutrition, (V1) 715
　control and prevention
　　for healthcare workers, (V1) 540–543, (V1) 540b
　　in the home, (V2) 840
　critical thinking and clinical judgment on, (V2) 328
　defenses against, (V1) 520–521
　　primary, (V1) 521, (V1) 525
　　promoting wellness to support, (V1) 531–533
　　secondary, (V1) 521, (V1) 522t
　　tertiary, (V1) 521, (V1) 522–523b, (V1) 524, (V1) 524f, (V1) 525b, (V1) 525f
　developing in response to a chain of factors, (V1) 516–519, (V1) 517f
　diagnostic testing for, (V2) 327
　due to bioterrorism and epidemics, (V1) 541

due to multidrug-resistant organisms, (V1) 520, (V1) 526–528
effects on pregnancy, (V1) 151
emerging, (V1) 520
evidence-based practice on, (V1) 542–543
in families with young children, (V1) 296
full-spectrum nursing model applied to, (V2) 327–328
healthcare-associated (HAIs), (V1) 515, (V1) 516
home healthcare and, (V1) 532, (V1) 1132, (V1) 1134–1135, (V1) 1134f, (V2) 840
host susceptibility to, (V1) 525, (V1) 528–529
immunity against
  artificial active, (V1) 523b
  artificial passive, (V1) 523b
  cellular, (V1) 524, (V1) 524f
  humoral, (V1) 524, (V1) 525f
  Immunoglobulin (Ig) classes, (V1) 524, (V1) 525b
  natural active, (V1) 522b
  natural passive, (V1) 523b
implementation for, (V1) 531
infectious agents and, (V1) 516–517
key concepts on, (V1) 515
knowledge map on, (V2) 330
limiting the spread of, (V1) 516, (V1) 541–542
methicillin-resistant *Staphylococcus aureus* (MRSA), (V1) 164
mode of transmission of, (V1) 517–518
in neonates, (V1) 155
nursing diagnosis and, (V1) 530
pathogens and, (V1) 517
PICOT questions on, (V1) 517
portal of entry, (V1) 519
portal of exit, (V1) 517
predictable stages of, (V1) 519–520
in preschoolers, (V1) 166
professional standards and guidelines on, (V1) 515–516
reservoirs of, (V1) 517
respiratory, oxygenation and, (V1) 982, (V1) 985–989
sexually transmitted (*See* Sexually transmitted infections (STIs))
skin, (V1) 943–944
surgical site, (V1) 1080, (V1) 1085
susceptible host for, (V1) 519
teaching clients and caregivers about preventing, (V1) 531
in toddlers, (V1) 163
transmission-based precautions for, (V1) 535, (V1) 535t, (V1) 536, (V2) 325–326
urinary elimination and, (V1) 724
urinary tract, (V1) 725–726, (V1) 737–738, (V1) 738f
vancomycin-resistant enterococci (VRE), (V1) 164
wound, (V1) 943–944, (V1) 945, (V1) 950
  dressings for controlling, (V1) 971–972, (V1) 972f
  as postoperative complication, (V1) 1101t
Inferences, (V1) 58–59
Infibulation, (V1) 890
Infiltration, as complication of intravenous therapy, (V1) 1065t
  management of, (V2) 802

Inflammation
airway, (V1) 989
in phases of wound healing, (V1) 947–948, (V1) 948f
as secondary defense against infection, (V1) 521
urinary elimination and, (V1) 724
Inflammatory bowel disease (IBD), fistulas with, (V1) 951
Inflammatory chemicals, (V1) 524
Inflammatory disorders, (V1) 168
Inflammatory phase in wound healing, (V1) 947–948, (V1) 948f
Inflammatory response to stress, (V1) 245–246, (V1) 245b
Influenza, (V1) 300, (V1) 985–989
immunization for, (V1) 1001
Informal education, (V1) 12–13
Informatics. *See* Nursing informatics
Informational responsibilities of managers, (V1) 1185
about change, (V1) 1193
Information-literacy, (V1) 1150, (V1) 1151b
Informed consent, (V1) 109, (V1) 128
minimizing malpractice risks, (V1) 1174–1175
for surgery, (V1) 1084–1085
Infusion kit, (V1) 1061–1062
Infusion pumps, (V1) 1063, (V1) 1071p
Infusions
blood, (V2) 791–795p
  autologous donation of blood for, (V1) 1069
  blood groups and, (V1) 1068, (V1) 1068t
  blood products for, (V1) 1069
  blood typing and crossmatching for, (V1) 1068–1069
  changing administration sets for, (V1) 1067
  donating blood for, (V1) 1068
  initiation of, (V1) 1069
  procedure for, (V1) 1073p
  reactions to, (V1) 1069–1070, (V1) 1070t
intermittent, (V1) 655, (V1) 655f, (V1) 661p
intravenous
  complications of, (V1) 1064, (V1) 1065–1067t
  discontinuing, (V1) 1068
  equipment and supplies for starting, (V1) 1060–1063, (V1) 1062f
  regulating and maintaining, (V1) 1063–1067, (V1) 1064b, (V1) 1065–1067t
  solutions, tubing, and dressings for, (V1) 1064
  peripheral intravenous, (V1) 1058, (V1) 1058f, (V1) 1067–1068, (V2) 769–774p, (V2) 790–791p
subcutaneous, (V1) 1060, (V1) 1061f
volume-control, (V1) 656, (V1) 656f
Ingrown toenail, (V1) 589
Inguinal hernia, (V1) 508
Inhalation, (V1) 977–978, (V1) 978f
mobilizing secretions, (V1) 1002–1003, (V1) 1003f
In-hospital cardiac arrests, (V1) 1034
Initial assessment, (V1) 49, (V1) 49t, (V1) 480
discharge planning beginning at, (V1) 66

Initiative versus guilt, in psychosocial development theory, (V1) 148, (V1) 165
Injection port, IV infusion, (V1) 1062
Injections
intradermal, (V1) 648, (V1) 648–649f, (V2) 428–430p
intramuscular, (V1) 651–652f, (V1) 651–654, (V1) 653t, (V1) 660–661p
subcutaneous, (V1) 649–651, (V1) 649f, (V1) 660p, (V1) 830, (V2) 431–434p
Injury
automobile accidents (*See* Automobiles)
back, (V1) 556
  in healthcare workers, (V1) 556
  teaching patients how to prevent, (V1) 856
birth, (V1) 155
bone, ligament, and tendon, (V1) 858–859
brain, sensory function and, (V1) 788
carbon monoxide exposure, (V1) 548, (V1) 564
choking, (V1) 549, (V1) 565, (V1) 566f, (V2) 338
developmental stage and, (V1) 546–547
from exercise, (V1) 854
fall, (V1) 201, (V1) 549
fire, (V1) 549, (V1) 564–565
firearm, (V1) 549, (V1) 564
head and spine, (V1) 859
as health disruption, (V1) 215
in the home, (V1) 547–549, (V1) 548b
needlestick, (V1) 556, (V1) 647, (V1) 647f, (V2) 338–339
nerve, as complication of intravenous therapy, (V1) 1066t
nutrition and, (V1) 693
poisoning, (V1) 166, (V1) 548, (V1) 548b
polypharmacy, (V1) 631
pressure, (V1) 111, (V1) 582, (V1) 588, (V1) 589, (V1) 805
  care plan for, (V1) 959–974
  PICOT questions on, (V1) 942
  skin integrity and, (V1) 951–952, (V1) 951–952f
radiation, (V1) 556–557
scalds and burns, (V1) 548–549, (V1) 565, (V1) 582
skin, (V1) 582
spinal cord, (V1) 859, (V1) 891, (V1) 992
suffocation/asphyxiation, (V1) 549
unintentional
  in infants, (V1) 157, (V1) 161
  in school-age children, (V1) 168–169
  in toddlers, (V1) 163
Inner ear, (V1) 493, (V1) 493f
Inpatient care, (V1) 16
Inquiry, in critical thinking, (V1) 40b
Insects, (V1) 550, (V1) 568, (V1) 570
Insensible loss, (V1) 448
In-service education, (V1) 12
Inside-the-needle catheters, (V1) 1057, (V1) 1057f
Insomnia, (V1) 924–925
Inspection, (V1) 481
abdomen, (V1) 503
heart, (V1) 499, (V1) 501
respiratory function, (V1) 993
Inspiration, (V1) 463, (V1) 463f
Inspiratory capacity, (V2) 753

Inspiratory reserve volume, (V2) 752
Institute for Healthcare Improvement, (V1) 1077
Institute for Safe Medication Practices (ISMP), (V2) 460–465
Institute for Safe Medication Practices (ISMP) List of Error-Prone Abbreviations, Symbols, and Dose Designations, (V2) 460–465
Institute of Medicine (IOM), (V1) 5, (V1) 6, (V1) 105–106, (V1) 374
　on patient safety, (V1) 545
Institutional ethics committees, (V1) 138
Institutional policies and procedures, (V1) 1161
Institutional review boards (IRB), (V1) 109
Instructional materials, for patient teaching, (V1) 411
Instrumental activities of daily living (IADLs), (V1) 198
　assessment of, (V1) 200
　　Lawton Instrumental Activities of Daily Living (IADL) scale, (V2) 17
Insulin, (V1) 624
　categories of, (V1) 650
　injectors for, (V1) 650
　mixing two kinds of, in one syringe, (V2) 457–458
　timing of administration of, (V1) 650
Insurance deductibles, (V1) 19
Intake and output (I&O)
　guidelines for measuring, (V2) 798–799
　records of, (V1) 432
Integrated delivery networks (IDNs), (V1) 22
Integrated plans of care (IPOCs), (V1) 69–71, (V1) 435–436
Integration of change, (V1) 1194
Integrative healthcare, (V1) 320
Integument
　age-related changes in, (V1) 193t
　care for pressure injury to, (V1) 111
　in neonates, (V1) 153
Integumentary system
　anatomy and physiology of, (V1) 579
　hair, (V1) 490, (V1) 597–599
　nails, (V1) 491, (V1) 590–591
　skin, (V1) 488–490, (V1) 489t (See also Skin)
Intellectual autonomy, (V1) 37
Intellectual courage, (V1) 37
Intellectual curiosity, (V1) 37
Intellectual empathy, (V1) 37
Intellectual humility, (V1) 37
Intellectualization, as defense mechanism, (V1) 247t
Intellectual perseverance, (V1) 37
Intensity, pain, (V1) 813
Intensive care unit, sensory overload in, (V1) 793
Intensivists, (V1) 1141
Intentional torts, (V1) 1166–1167
Interaction, drug, (V1) 623–624
Interaction in families, (V1) 295
Intercostal muscles, (V1) 978
Intercostal retraction, (V1) 466
Interdisciplinary collaboration, (V1) 25–26
Interleukins, (V1) 524
Intermittent claudication, (V1) 1032
Intermittent fever, (V1) 450
Intermittent infusions, (V1) 655, (V1) 655f, (V1) 661p, (V1) 1067, (V2) 446–449p

Intermittent mechanical traction, (V1) 825
Intermittent urinary catheter, (V2) 523–529p
Internal loss, (V1) 348
Internal ports, (V1) 657, (V1) 657f
Internal respiration, (V1) 462, (V1) 979
Internal sphincter, (V1) 756, (V1) 756f
Internal stressors, (V1) 239
International Classification for Nursing Practice (ICNP), (V1) 62
International Council of Nurses (ICN), (V1) 8–10, (V1) 14
　Code of Ethics, (V1) 131–132
International normalized ratio (INR), (V2) 700
International nursing, (V1) 1118, (V1) 1118f
International Statistical Classification of Diseases and Related Health Problems (ICD-10), (V1) 62
Internet, the
　See also Computers
　electronic communications and, (V1) 1140
　online forums and, (V1) 1141
　social networking and, (V1) 1140–1141
　telehealth nursing and, (V1) 25, (V1) 216, (V1) 1141, (V1) 1141f
　use by healthcare consumers, (V1) 24
　web conferencing and webinars and, (V1) 1141
Interoperability, (V1) 1147
Interpersonal activities of managers, (V1) 1184–1185
Interpersonal communication, (V1) 375
Interpersonal role conflict, (V1) 269
Interpreters, (V1) 326, (V2) 110
Interrogatories, (V1) 1170
Interrole conflict, (V1) 269
Intersex, (V1) 886
Interstitial fluid, (V1) 1037
Interviews, nursing, (V1) 49, (V1) 50–52, (V1) 51t
　of school-age children, (V1) 169
　sensory-perceptual assessment in, (V1) 802
Intestinal surface area and nutrition, (V1) 693
Intestinal ulcers, (V1) 931
Intimate distance, (V1) 381
Intimate partner violence (IPV), (V1) 180, (V1) 301–302, (V1) 897
Intimate relationships, (V1) 895
In-toeing, (V1) 865
Intonation in communication, (V1) 377
Intra-articular pain pumps, (V1) 831, (V1) 831f
Intracellular fluid (ICF), (V1) 681, (V1) 1037, (V1) 1038
Intractable pain, (V1) 812
Intradermal injections, (V1) 648, (V1) 648–649f, (V2) 428–430p
Intramuscular injections, (V1) 651–652f, (V1) 651–654, (V1) 653t, (V1) 660–661p, (V2) 434–440p
　opioid, (V1) 830
Intramuscular stimulation, (V1) 824
Intraoperative care
　operative personnel and, (V1) 1089–1090
　questionnaire on, (V2) 829
　safety measures in, (V1) 1095
　types of anesthesia in, (V1) 1091–1093, (V1) 1092f
Intraosseous devices, (V1) 1060
Intrapersonal communication, (V1) 375
Intraspinal injections, (V1) 615t
Intrathecal injections, (V1) 615t

Intrauterine device (IUD), (V2) 643
Intravenous fat emulsions, (V1) 1067
Intravenous fluids
　added to IV bags, (V1) 654, (V1) 654f, (V1) 661p
　central venous access devices, (V1) 656–657, (V1) 657f, (V1) 661p
　changing, (V2) 779–782p
　intermittent infusion, (V1) 655, (V1) 655f, (V1) 661p
　IV push medications, (V1) 654, (V1) 654f
　needleless connections, (V1) 655–656, (V1) 656f
　opioid, (V1) 830–831
　volume-control infusion sets, (V1) 656, (V1) 656f
Intravenous infusions
　blood infusions
　　autologous donation of blood for, (V1) 1069
　　blood groups and, (V1) 1068, (V1) 1068t
　　blood products for, (V1) 1069
　　blood typing and crossmatching for, (V1) 1068–1069
　　changing administration sets for, (V1) 1067
　　donating blood for, (V1) 1068
　　initiation of, (V1) 1069
　　reactions to, (V1) 1069–1070, (V1) 1070t
　complications of, (V1) 1064, (V1) 1065–1067t
　discontinuing, (V1) 1068
　equipment and supplies for starting, (V1) 1060–1063, (V1) 1062f
　regulating and maintaining, (V1) 1063–1067, (V1) 1064b, (V1) 1065–1067t
　solutions, tubing, and dressings for, (V1) 1064, (V2) 779–789p
Intuition and inspiration, (V1) 107
Intuitive thought stage, (V1) 165
Iodine, (V1) 680t
IPASS format, (V1) 438
IPV. See Intimate partner violence (IPV)
Iron, (V1) 680t
　bowel elimination and, (V1) 759
　deficiency in, (V1) 678
　supplementation of, (V1) 700
Irrigations and instillations
　bladder or catheter, (V2) 540–543p
　colostomy, (V1) 781, (V2) 577–579p
　defined, (V1) 639
　nasal medications, (V1) 640, (V1) 658p
　ophthalmic medications, (V1) 639–640, (V1) 658p
　otic, (V2) 596–598p
　otic medications, (V1) 640, (V1) 658p
　rectal medications, (V1) 640, (V1) 659p
　vaginal medications, (V1) 640, (V1) 658–659p
　wound, (V1) 964–965, (V2) 662–664p
Irritable bowel syndrome, (V1) 758
Ishihara cards, (V1) 492
Islam, (V1) 332, (V1) 335–336
Isokinetic exercise, (V1) 852
Isolation
　as health disruption, (V1) 218
　homelessness and, (V1) 300–301
　protective, (V1) 536
　as psychosocial diagnosis, (V1) 271
　transmission-based, (V1) 536

Isometric exercise, (V1) 851
Isotonic exercise, (V1) 851
Isotonic fluids, (V1) 1056
Isotonic solutions, (V1) 1039
I statements, (V1) 383
IV flow rates, (V1) 1063–1064, (V1) 1064*b*, (V2) 775–776*p*
IV push (bolus) medications, (V1) 654, (V1) 654*f*, (V1) 661*p*, (V2) 441–446*p*

J

Jackson-Pratt drains, (V1) 965, (V1) 965*f*
JAREL spiritual well-being scale, (V1) 341
Jargon, (V1) 322
Jaundice, (V1) 155, (V1) 489*t*, (V1) 583, (V1) 584
Jehovah's Witness, (V1) 336*t*
Jejunal tubes, (V1) 637
Jejunostomy tube (J-tube, PEJ), (V1) 708
Jejunum, (V1) 755
Jellies, (V1) 613*t*, (V1) 614*t*
Jewelry, removal of, (V2) 321
Joint Commission, The, (V1) 52, (V1) 86, (V1) 132, (V1) 374, (V1) 374*b*, (V1) 1077
   on collaborative professional communication, (V2) 143
   "do not use" list, (V1) 426*t*
   on infection prevention, (V1) 516
   on nurses' teaching responsibilities, (V1) 397
   on patient safety, (V1) 545, (V1) 551*b*
Joint mobility, (V1) 504
Joints, (V1) 841–842, (V1) 843*t*
   mobility of, (V1) 845
      diseases affecting, (V1) 857–858, (V1) 858*f*
      interventions for, (V1) 866
Journals, (V1) 110
   for stress, (V1) 262
Judaism, (V1) 332, (V1) 334–335
Jugular veins, (V1) 502
Justice, (V1) 131

K

Karnofsky Performance scale, (V2) 17
Katz Index of ADL scale, (V2) 17, (V2) 384–385
Kava, (V1) 937
Kayser-Jones Brief Oral Health Status Examination (BOHSE), (V1) 594
K-complexes, (V1) 920, (V1) 920*t*
Keloid, (V2) 214*p*
Keratinocytes, (V1) 941
Ketogenic diet, (V1) 694–695
Kidneys, (V1) 718*f*
   drug excretion and, (V1) 617
   failure, as postoperative complication, (V1) 1100*t*
   function of, (V1) 717
   neonatal, (V1) 153
Kidney stones, (V1) 724
Kilocalories (kcal), (V1) 682
Kinesthetic sensations, testing, (V2) 280*p*
Klass, Dennis, (V1) 352*t*
Knowledge
   nursing, (V1) 30–36, (V1) 60–61
      method of gaining, (V1) 107
      in nursing informatics, (V1) 1139, (V1) 1139*f*
   nursing research and, (V1) 106–114
   psychosocial health, (V2) 100
   sleep and rest, (V2) 657
   skills, and attitudes (KSAs), (V1) 13
Knowledge deficit and home healthcare, (V1) 1129–1130
Knowledge maps
   asepsis and infection prevention, (V2) 330
   bowel elimination, (V2) 594
   circulation, (V2) 766
   communication, (V2) 148
   critical thinking, (V2) 11
   death and dying, (V2) 138
   documentation, (V2) 171
   ethics and values, (V2) 38
   evidence-based practice (EBP), (V2) 30
   evolution of nursing thought and action, (V2) 6
   family health, (V2) 107
   fluids, electrolytes, and acid-base balance, (V2) 809
   growth and development, (V2) 52
   home healthcare, (V2) 845
   hygiene, (V2) 390
   leading and managing, (V2) 863
   legal accountability, (V2) 858
   medication administration, (V2) 475
   multicultural populations, (V2) 117
   nursing informatics, (V2) 850
   nursing process, (V2) 24
   nutrition, (V2) 515
   older adults, (V2) 58
   oxygenation, (V2) 757
   pain, (V2) 615
   patient education, (V2) 155
   physical activity and immobility, (V2) 637
   physical examination, (V2) 301
   safety, (V2) 344
   sensation and perception, (V2) 604
   sexual health, (V2) 649
   on skin and wound healing, (V2) 704
   sleep and rest, (V2) 657
   spirituality, (V2) 125
   stress and adaptation, (V2) 88
   surgical patient care, (V2) 834
   urinary elimination, (V2) 558
   vital signs, (V2) 197
   wellness, health, and illness, (V2) 78
Knowledge map, bowel elimination, (V2) 594
Kock pouch, (V1) 761
Kohlberg, Lawrence, (V1) 123–124, (V1) 148–149
Korotkoff sounds, (V1) 473, (V1) 473*f*
Kübler-Ross, Elisabeth, (V1) 357
   on grief, (V1) 351–352*t*
Kussmaul respirations, (V1) 465*t*, (V1) 994

L

Labia majora, (V1) 882, (V1) 893
Labia minora, (V1) 882
Laboratory data, (V1) 421
   reflecting nutritional status, (V1) 697–699, (V1) 698*b*
   serum protein levels, (V1) 698–699
   wound assessment, (V1) 958
Laboratory specimens, handling of, (V1) 536
Laboratory studies, (V1) 226
   bowel elimination, (V1) 765
      occult blood, (V2) 560–562*p*
   cardiovascular system, (V1) 1027–1028
   fluid, electrolytes, and acid-base balance, (V1) 1052–1053
Labor market, nursing, (V1) 1189
Laceration, (V1) 945*t*
Lactating patients, nutrition for, (V1) 686
Laissez-faire leadership, (V1) 1182
Lamellae, (V1) 841
Langerhans cells, (V1) 941
Language, patronizing, (V1) 391
Language barriers, (V1) 322, (V1) 325–326, (V1) 327*b*, (V1) 391–392
   and communication with clients who speak a different language, (V1) 325–326, (V1) 327*b*, (V2) 110
   in general survey, (V1) 487
Large-bore NG tubes, (V1) 707–708
Large intestine, (V1) 755–756, (V1) 756*f*
Lasater clinical judgment rubric (LCJR), (V1) 31
Latency stage, in psychoanalytic theory, (V1) 147*t*
Latent infections, (V1) 519
Lateral chest, (V1) 496
Lateral position, (V1) 870, (V1) 871*t*, (V1) 871*f*
Lateral recumbent position, (V1) 870
Late term fetus, (V1) 150
Latin American diets, (V1) 667–668
Laughter, (V1) 261–262, (V1) 262*f*
Lavage, (V1) 964
Lavender, (V1) 786
Law and legal liability
   advance directives, (V1) 139, (V1) 358–359
   civil, (V1) 1166–1169
      litigation and, (V1) 1169–1170
   criminal, (V1) 1165–1166
   critical thinking and clinical judgment on, (V2) 854–856
   on definition of death, (V1) 356, (V1) 356*b*
   documentation and, (V1) 420, (V2) 853
   do-not-resuscitate (DNR) prescription, (V1) 360, (V1) 360*b*
   drug administration, (V1) 609
   ethics and, (V1) 116
      at end of life, (V1) 358–362, (V1) 360*b*
   full-spectrum nursing model applied to, (V2) 853–854
   Good Samaritan, (V1) 1160–1161
   guiding nursing practice
      federal, (V1) 1157–1160, (V1) 1159*b*
      other guidelines, (V1) 1161–1162
      state, (V1) 1160–1161
   key concepts in, (V1) 1156
   knowledge map on, (V2) 858
   malpractice, (V1) 1161, (V1) 1167–1169
      common claims in, (V1) 1170–1172, (V1) 1171*b*
      minimizing risks of, (V1) 1172–1179, (V1) 1176*b*, (V1) 1177*b*
      professional liability insurance for, (V1) 1178–1179
      tips for avoiding, (V2) 852
   mandatory reporting, (V1) 896, (V1) 1160
   medical aid in dying (MAiD), (V1) 360
   nurse practice acts, (V1) 13, (V1) 609, (V1) 1161, (V1) 1162–1165
   safe harbor, (V1) 1178
   sources and types of, (V1) 1156–1157, (V1) 1157*t*
   using equipment safely and, (V2) 853

Lawton Instrumental Activities of Daily Living (IADL) scale, (V2) 17
Laxatives and bowel elimination, (V1) 759, (V1) 759b, (V1) 769
Leadership
  See also Management
  career growth and, (V1) 1187–1188
  by effective managers, (V1) 1184
  followership and, (V1) 1188
  key concepts in, (V1) 1181
  power and empowerment in, (V1) 1189–1190
  preceptors and mentors and, (V1) 1187, (V1) 1187b
  servant, (V1) 1184
  theories of, (V1) 1181–1183, (V1) 1183t
Leading and managing
  of change, (V1) 1192–1193f, (V1) 1192–1194, (V1) 1194b
  communication in, (V1) 1191
  critical thinking and clinical judgment on, (V2) 860–861
  delegation in, (V1) 1191–1192, (V1) 1192b
  effective
    activities of, (V1) 1184–1185
    challenges to being, (V1) 1188–1189
    qualities of, (V1) 1184
  full-spectrum nursing model applied to, (V2) 860
  knowledge map on, (V2) 863
  managing conflict, (V1) 1194–1196
  power of, (V1) 1189
  preparation for, (V1) 1185–1188, (V1) 1185b, (V1) 1186t, (V1) 1187b, (V1) 1187f
  role and function in, (V1) 7t
  time management in, (V1) 1196–1200, (V1) 1198–1199t, (V1) 1200t
Learning
  See also Patient education
  assessment of, (V2) 150–151
  environment for, (V1) 400–401, (V1) 401b
  evaluation of, (V1) 417–418
  occurring in three domains, (V1) 398–399, (V1) 398t, (V1) 399f
  sleep and, (V1) 917
  theories of, (V1) 397–398
Lecture, for patient teaching, (V1) 411
Left-sided heart failure, (V1) 1024
Legal accountability. See Law and legal liability
Leg exercises for surgical patients, (V2) 811–814p
Legislation
  advance directives, (V1) 359
  Controlled Substances Act, (V1) 609
  influence on contemporary nursing, (V1) 24
  U.S. drug, (V1) 609
Legislators, in healthcare regulation, (V1) 21
Leininger, Madeleine, (V1) 99–100, (V1) 321
Leisure activities and stress, (V1) 259
Lemon, (V1) 786
Lens, eye, (V1) 492
Lesions, skin, (V1) 490, (V2) 209–214p
Leukemia, (V1) 529
Leukocytes. See White blood cells (WBCs)
Level of arousal (LOA) assessment, (V2) 273p
Level of consciousness (LOC), (V1) 505
  assessment of, (V1) 802
  caring for patients with altered, (V1) 805

clients with reduced, (V1) 393, (V1) 393–394b
Lewis, C. S., (V1) 332
LGBTQ+ persons, (V1) 293, (V1) 886, (V1) 888
Liability insurance, (V1) 1178–1179
Libel, (V1) 1166
Libido, (V1) 893
  low, (V1) 900–901
Licensed nutritionists, (V1) 18–19
Licensed practical nurses (LPNs), (V1) 10–11, (V1) 609, (V1) 1185
  on healthcare team, (V1) 18
Licensed vocational nurses (LVNs), (V1) 10–11, (V1) 1185
Licensure
  requirements for, (V1) 1163
  special cases of, (V1) 1163
Life care communities, (V1) 189
Life expectancy, (V1) 186–187
Life review, (V1) 364
Life span
  in adolescence, (V1) 171–179, (V1) 171b, (V1) 172f
  development over, (V1) 144–149, (V1) 145–148t
  gestational period in, (V1) 149–152, (V1) 151f
  health promotion throughout, (V1) 223, (V1) 224–226t
  in infancy, (V1) 156–162, (V1) 157b
  key concepts on, (V1) 144
  in middle adulthood, (V1) 181–183, (V1) 181f
  in neonatal period, (V1) 152–154f, (V1) 152–156
  in older adulthood, (V1) 185–206
  pain and, (V1) 816
  perspective on aging, (V1) 187
  pharmacokinetics and, (V1) 619, (V1) 620f
  in preschoolers, (V1) 164–167, (V1) 165b, (V1) 165f
  in school-age children, (V1) 167–171, (V1) 167b, (V1) 168f
  sensory function and, (V1) 786–787
  in toddlerhood, (V1) 162–164, (V1) 162f, (V1) 163b
  variations in communication across, (V1) 380
  in young adulthood, (V1) 179–181
Life stress review, (V1) 227
Lifestyle
  blood pressure and, (V1) 469
  cardiovascular function and, (V1) 1021–1022
  health promotion and, (V1) 222
  influence on health and illness, (V1) 213
  nutrition and, (V1) 689–690
  oxygenation and, (V1) 982–983, (V1) 983b
  physical activity and, (V1) 856
  providing and facilitating support for changes in, (V1) 233
  recommendations for health promotion, (V1) 231
  and risk assessment, (V1) 227, (V2) 73–75
  sedentary, (V1) 856
  sensory function and, (V1) 788
  sexuality and, (V1) 890–891
  skin and, (V1) 583, (V1) 944
  sleep and, (V1) 923–924
  surgical risk and, (V1) 1080
  urinary elimination and, (V1) 723

Ligaments, (V1) 504, (V1) 504f, (V1) 842
  sprains and strains of, (V1) 859
Light and sleep, (V1) 924
Limbic system, (V1) 814
Limited mobility and self-care, (V1) 577
Line of gravity, (V1) 844, (V1) 845f
Liniments, (V1) 613t
Lipid emulsions, (V1) 714
  administration of, (V2) 498–500p
Lipid panel screening, (V1) 182, (V1) 228, (V1) 1027, (V2) 763
Lipids
  functions of, (V1) 673
  types of, (V1) 671–673, (V1) 672t
Lipid-soluble drugs, (V1) 616
Lipid-soluble lozenges, (V1) 613t
Lipoproteins, (V1) 671–672
Lips, (V1) 494, (V1) 494f
Liquid skin cleansers, (V1) 964
Listening, (V1) 104
  active, (V1) 343, (V1) 387–388, (V1) 388f
Literature, nursing, (V1) 110–114, (V1) 112t
Litigation in civil claims, (V1) 1169–1170
Lived experience, (V1) 209
Liver
  drug excretion and, (V1) 617
  dysfunction, as complication of parenteral nutrition, (V1) 715
  nutrition and, (V1) 693
Living wills, (V1) 359, (V1) 1159, (V1) 1159b
Livor mortis, (V1) 367
Local adaptation syndrome, (V1) 245–246, (V1) 245b
Local anesthesia, (V1) 832, (V1) 1092
Local effects, drug, (V1) 612, (V1) 637
Local infections, (V1) 519
Localized reactions to drugs, (V1) 621
Locus of control, (V1) 228
  self-concept and, (V1) 268
Log, sleep, (V2) 653
Logical reasoning, (V1) 107
  in spiritual development theory, (V1) 149
Logrolling, (V1) 873
Loneliness, (V1) 271
Long-term care, documentation in, (V1) 437
Long-term care facility, transfer of patient to, (V1) 237p, (V2) 64–65p
Long-term support services, (V1) 16
Loop of Henle, (V1) 717
Loss
  See also Grief
  actual versus perceived, (V1) 348
  of aspects of self, (V1) 348
  assessment of, (V2) 132–133
  categories of, (V1) 348
  and communicating with people who are grieving, (V2) 127
  defined, (V1) 348
  diagnoses related to, (V1) 362
  environmental, (V1) 348
  as etiology, (V1) 362
  external versus internal, (V1) 348
  in families with older adults, (V1) 298
  as health disruption, (V1) 216
  helping children deal with, (V1) 367
  key concepts on, (V1) 348
  physical versus psychological, (V1) 348
  of significant relationships, (V1) 348

Lotions, (V1) 613t, (V1) 637
Love, (V1) 333
  and belonging needs, (V1) 102, (V1) 102f
Low-density lipoproteins (LDLs), (V1) 671
Lower airway, (V1) 977
  infections of, (V1) 980
Low-FODMAP diet, (V1) 695
Low-income families, (V1) 299
Low-level laser therapy (LLLT), (V1) 824
LPNs. See Licensed practical nurses (LPNs)
L-tryptophan, (V1) 923
Lubricant, water as, (V1) 681
Lumen, catheter, (V1) 736, (V1) 736f
Lung cancer, (V1) 181
Lung receptors, (V1) 979
Lungs, (V1) 977, (V1) 977f
  abnormal sounds of, (V2) 249–250p
  assessment of, (V2) 244–250p
  breath sounds and, (V1) 465–466, (V1) 496,
    (V1) 499–500f
  compliance of, (V1) 978
  drug excretion and, (V1) 617
  elasticity of, (V1) 978
  expansion of, (V1) 978
  fluid loss via, (V1) 1041
  normal sounds of, (V2) 249p
  physical examination of, (V1) 496, (V1)
    511p
  structure of, (V1) 977, (V1) 977f
  volumes and capacities testing, (V2)
    752–753
Luteal phase, (V1) 883
Luteinizing hormone (LH), (V1) 883
LVNs. See Licensed vocational nurses (LVNs)
Lymph nodes, (V1) 530
Lymphocytes, (V1) 524, (V1) 699
Lyon, Edward, (V1) 6

M

Maceration, (V1) 582, (V1) 953
Macrominerals, (V1) 673, (V1) 679–680t
Macronutrients, (V1) 669
Macrosomia, (V1) 151
Macule, (V2) 211p
Magical thinking, (V1) 353
Magico-religious system, (V1) 318, (V1) 319
Magnesium, (V1) 678, (V1) 679t
  bowel elimination and, (V1) 758
  electrolytes, (V1) 1042t, (V1) 1044
  for pain management, (V1) 823
  sleep and, (V1) 937
Magnetic resonance angiography (MRA), (V2)
  763
Magnetic resonance imaging (MRI), (V2)
  588
Magnolia bark, (V1) 937
Mahoney, Mary, (V1) 6
Mainstream smoke, (V1) 983
Major surgery, (V1) 1078
Maladaptive coping, (V1) 240–241, (V1) 259
Male genitourinary system, (V1) 507–508, (V1)
  512p
  assessment of, (V2) 285–289p
Male reproductive organs, (V1) 883–885, (V1)
  884f
Male sterilization, (V2) 643
Malignant hyperthermia, (V1) 1091
Malingering, (V1) 251
Malnutrition and underweight, (V1) 703–706

Malpractice, (V1) 1161, (V1) 1167–1169
  common claims in, (V1) 1170–1172, (V1)
    1171b
  minimizing risks of, (V1) 1172–1179, (V1)
    1176b, (V1) 1177b
  professional liability insurance for, (V1)
    1178–1179
  tips for avoiding, (V2) 852
Mammary glands, (V1) 882–883
Mammography, (V1) 180, (V1) 182, (V1)
  495–496
Managed care organizations (MCOs), (V1) 22
Management
  See also Leadership
  change, (V1) 1192–1193f, (V1) 1192–1194,
    (V1) 1194b
  defined, (V1) 1183
  human relations-based, (V1) 1184
  key concepts in, (V1) 1181
  scientific, (V1) 1184
  theories of, (V1) 1183–1184
Mandatory reporting laws, (V1) 1160
  minimizing malpractice risks, (V1)
    1176–1178, (V1) 1177b
  on sexually transmitted infections (STIs),
    (V1) 896
Mania, (V1) 892
Mannequins, (V1) 1146, (V1) 1146f
Man's Search for Meaning, (V1) 213
Manual traction, (V1) 825
Marital relationship health risks, (V1) 297
Marriage and family therapists, (V1) 18
Marriage rituals, (V1) 315, (V1) 315f
Married adults without children, (V1) 292
Masked grief, (V1) 354
Maslow, Abraham, (V1) 100, (V1) 102, (V1)
  102f, (V1) 266–267
Maslow's hierarchy of needs, (V1) 100, (V1)
  102, (V1) 102f, (V1) 266–267, (V1)
  1193
Massage, (V1) 261, (V1) 824
  back, (V1) 585
Mass peristalsis, (V1) 756
Mastectomy, (V1) 891
Master's degree programs, (V1) 12
  nursing research and, (V1) 106
Masturbation, (V1) 895
Maternal changes during pregnancy, (V1) 150
Maternal diabetes, (V1) 151
Mathematical and calculation skills,
  assessment of, (V2) 274p
Mattresses and linens, (V1) 604–605
Maturation phase in wound healing, (V1) 948,
  (V1) 948f
MDI. See Metered-dose inhalers (MDI)
Meaning
  denotative and connotative, (V1) 377
  end-of-life care and finding, (V1) 364
Meaningful work, (V1) 213, (V1) 260
Mechanical débridement, (V1) 967
Mechanical lifts, (V1) 874, (V1) 874–875f
Mechanical respiration, (V1) 462, (V1) 531
  pain and, (V1) 820
Mechanical ventilation, (V1) 1008–1009, (V1)
  1008f, (V1) 1014p
  caring for patients requiring, (V2) 737–740p
Mechanoreceptors, (V1) 784
Meconium, (V1) 153, (V1) 757
Mediastinum, (V1) 977
Mediation, (V1) 1170

Medicaid, (V1) 19–20
  home healthcare, (V1) 1126
Medical aid in dying (MAiD), (V1) 360
Medical asepsis
  See also Infections
  cleaning and, (V1) 534
  defined, (V1) 533
  disinfecting and, (V1) 534
  maintaining clean environments, (V1)
    533–534
  maintaining clean hands, (V1) 533
  sterilizing and, (V1) 534
Medical errors, (V1) 1142–1143
  minimizing malpractice risks and, (V1) 1172
  "never events," (V1) 545, (V1) 552, (V1) 1077
  reduction with electronic health records
    (EHRs), (V1) 1147
Medical malpractice. See Malpractice
Medical orders, electronic transmission of,
  (V1) 1140
Medicare, (V1) 19
  home healthcare, (V1) 1125–1126
  on "never events," (V1) 545
  reforms to, (V1) 21–22
Medicated enemas, (V1) 771
Medication administration
  abbreviations related to, (V2) 459
  assessment for, (V1) 630–631
  blood flow and, (V1) 616
  critical thinking and clinical judgment on,
    (V2) 470–473
  dosage
    calculating, (V1) 624, (V2) 467–469
    Institute for Safe Medication Practices
      (ISMP) List of Error-Prone
      Abbreviations, Symbols, and Dose
      Designations, (V2) 460–465
    measured when changing needles, (V2)
      456–457
  medication measurement systems for,
    (V1) 624, (V2) 466–467
  full-spectrum nursing model applied to,
    (V2) 469–470
  intermittent infusion, (V1) 661p, (V2)
    446–449p
  intradermal, (V2) 428–430p
  intramuscular, (V1) 660–661p, (V2) 434–440p
  intravenous medications
    added to IV bags, (V1) 654, (V1) 654f, (V1)
      661p, (V2) 440–441p
    central venous access devices, (V1)
      656–657, (V1) 657f, (V1) 661p
    intermittent infusion, (V1) 655, (V1) 655f,
      (V1) 661p
    IV push medications, (V1) 654, (V1) 654f
    needleless connections, (V1) 655–656,
      (V1) 656f
    volume-control infusion sets, (V1) 656,
      (V1) 656f
  irrigations and instillations
    defined, (V1) 639
    nasal medications, (V1) 640, (V1) 658p
    ophthalmic medications, (V1) 639–640,
      (V1) 658p
    otic medications, (V1) 640, (V1) 658p
    rectal medications, (V1) 640, (V1) 659p
    vaginal medications, (V1) 640, (V1)
      658–659p, (V1) 658p
  IV push (bolus) medications, (V1) 654, (V1)
    654f, (V1) 661p, (V2) 441–446p

key concepts in, (V1) 607
knowledge map on, (V2) 475
legal considerations with, (V1) 609
medication errors
　avoidance of, (V1) 627–629
　causes of, (V1) 627, (V1) 627b
　defined, (V1) 627
　evidence-based practice on, (V1) 630
　in older adults, (V1) 639b
metabolism of, (V1) 617
metered-dose inhalers (MDI), (V1) 659p, (V2) 415–417p
mixing two kinds of insulin in one syringe, (V2) 457–458
nasal, (V2) 405–407p
nonadherence to, (V1) 631
onset, peak, and duration of action of, (V1) 618, (V1) 618f
ophthalmic, (V1) 658p, (V2) 400–403p
oral
　buccal and sublingual, (V1) 636
　for children, (V1) 637, (V1) 638
　enteral, (V1) 637
　for older adults, (V1) 637–638
　pouring, (V1) 636, (V1) 636f
　procedure for administering, (V1) 658p, (V2) 396–400p
　special situations, (V1) 637
oral problems with, (V1) 593
otic, (V1) 658p, (V2) 403–405p
parenteral medications
　comfort and safety considerations with, (V1) 648
　defined, (V1) 642
　drawing up and mixing, (V1) 645–647, (V1) 646f, (V1) 659–660p
　equipment for, (V1) 642–645, (V1) 643–645f, (V1) 643t
　intradermal injections, (V1) 648, (V1) 648–649f
　intramuscular injections, (V1) 651–652f, (V1) 651–654, (V1) 653t, (V1) 660–661p
　preventing needlestick injuries with, (V1) 647, (V1) 647f
　subcutaneous injections, (V1) 649–651, (V1) 649f, (V1) 660p
　subcutaneous medications, (V1) 660p, (V2) 431–434p
pH and ionization effects on, (V1) 616
pharmacodynamics (See Pharmacodynamics)
pharmacokinetics of (See Pharmacokinetics)
PICOT questions on, (V1) 628
polypharmacy and, (V1) 195, (V1) 198, (V1) 631
preparing, drawing up, and mixing medications, (V1) 659–660p, (V2) 417–425p
prescriptions, (V1) 625, (V1) 625f
　abbreviations used in, (V1) 625
　communication of, (V1) 626, (V1) 626b
　questioning of, (V1) 439
　receiving and documenting verbal and telephone, (V1) 438–439
　types of, (V1) 625–626
　what to do about incorrect, (V1) 626–627
pulse rate and, (V1) 457
pupil size and, (V1) 493

quality and safety of, (V1) 608–611, (V1) 610f
recapping needles using one-handed technique, (V1) 660p, (V2) 426–428p
rectal, (V1) 659p, (V2) 409–412p
respiration and, (V1) 464
respiratory inhalations
　metered-dose inhalers and dry powder inhalers, (V1) 641–642, (V1) 641f, (V1) 659p
　types of nebulizers for, (V1) 641, (V1) 641f
routes of administration, (V1) 611, (V1) 612–615t, (V1) 619
safe, (V1) 633–636, (V1) 635f
skin, (V1) 659p, (V2) 412–414p
solubility of, (V1) 612, (V1) 616
steps to follow for, (V2) 392–396p
storage and distribution of, (V1) 610, (V1) 610f
subcutaneous injections, (V1) 660p, (V2) 431–434p
　anticoagulants, (V2) 458
teaching patients about, (V1) 632–633
therapeutic range of, (V1) 618–619
through central venous access device (CVAD), (V2) 450–453p
topical
　lotions, creams, and ointments, (V1) 637
　procedure for administering, (V1) 659p
　transdermal, (V1) 637, (V1) 639f
using prefilled unit-dose system, (V2) 454
vaginal, (V1) 658p, (V2) 407–409p
Medication administration records (MARs), (V1) 432, (V1) 434f, (V1) 434t, (V1) 635–636, (V1) 635f
Medication errors
　avoidance of, (V1) 627–629
　causes of, (V1) 627, (V1) 627b
　defined, (V1) 627
　evidence-based practice on, (V1) 630
　minimizing malpractice risks and, (V1) 1172
　in older adults, (V1) 639b
　taking action after, (V2) 453
Medications
　abuse or misuse of, (V1) 624
　administration of (See Medication administration)
　allergic reactions to, (V1) 621, (V1) 622, (V1) 622t, (V1) 623f
　biological half-life of, (V1) 619
　blood pressure and, (V1) 469
　bowel elimination and, (V1) 759, (V1) 759b
　cardiovascular, (V1) 1033
　cardiovascular function and, (V1) 1022, (V1) 1023–1024t
　concentration at target sites, (V1) 619
　controlled substances, (V1) 609–610, (V1) 610f
　cough and cold, (V1) 1000
　death from, (V1) 548
　distribution throughout the body, (V1) 616–617
　documenting additional information about, (V1) 432, (V1) 434–435
　drug listings and directories, (V1) 608
　drug names and classification, (V1) 607–608
　effects on gestation, (V1) 151
　effects on sexuality, (V1) 892, (V1) 892t
　excretion from the body, (V1) 617–618

home healthcare and, (V1) 1131–1132, (V1) 1132f
hormone replacement therapy (HRT), (V1) 183
host susceptibility to infection and, (V1) 529
interactions of, (V1) 623–624
nutrition and, (V1) 693
osteoporosis and, (V1) 867
oxygenation and, (V1) 982, (V1) 983–984
pain, (V1) 826–835, (V1) 829b, (V1) 831f
patient-controlled analgesia (PCA), (V1) 831–832, (V1) 831f, (V2) 606–608p
premenstrual syndrome, (V1) 906
preoperative, (V1) 1087–1088, (V1) 1087t
reconstitution of, (V1) 646, (V2) 455
respiratory, (V1) 1000
safe disposal of, (V1) 1132
sensory function and, (V1) 788, (V1) 789f
skin reactions to, (V1) 943, (V1) 943f
sleep
　natural, (V1) 937
　nonprescription, (V1) 935–936
　prescription, (V1) 935
sleep and, (V1) 924
surgical risk and, (V1) 1080, (V1) 1080b
urinary elimination and, (V1) 723, (V1) 723b
Meditation, (V1) 260
Mediterranean diet, (V1) 667–668, (V1) 691
Mees' lines, (V1) 491
Melanin, (V1) 579, (V1) 941
Melanocytes, (V1) 941
Melatonin, (V1) 935, (V1) 937
Membrane permeability, (V1) 617
Memory
　age-related changes in, (V1) 194t, (V1) 299
　assessment of, (V2) 274p
　consolidation during NREM sleep, (V1) 920
　grieving patients and recalling of, (V1) 364
Memory cells, (V1) 524
Memory T cells, (V1) 524
Menarche, (V1) 887
Menopause, (V1) 181, (V1) 888
　hormone replacement therapy (HRT) and, (V1) 906
　osteoporosis prevention in, (V1) 867
　sexuality after, (V1) 889
　sleep and, (V1) 923
Menstrual phase, (V1) 883
Menstruation
　menarche, (V1) 887
　menstrual cycle, (V1) 883, (V1) 884f, (V1) 905
　premenstrual dysphoric disorder (PMDD) and, (V1) 897
　premenstrual syndrome (PMS) and, (V1) 897, (V1) 905–906
　puberty and, (V1) 887
Mental health
　in adolescents, (V1) 172–175
　self-care ability and, (V1) 577
　sexuality and, (V1) 892
Mental illness
　as health disruption, (V1) 215
　substance abuse and, (V1) 287, (V1) 290
Mental status
　assessment of, (V1) 802
　cognitive function and, (V1) 505–506
　in general survey, (V1) 487
　screening of, (V2) 283p
　surgical risk and, (V1) 1080

Mentors, (V1) 1187, (V1) 1187b
Mercury exposure, (V1) 555, (V1) 555t, (V1) 572, (V1) 573b
Message in communication, (V1) 375–376, (V1) 376f
Metabolic acidosis, (V1) 1050t, (V1) 1052
Metabolic alkalosis, (V1) 1050t
Metabolic disorders and urinary elimination, (V1) 724
Metabolism, (V1) 666
　drug, (V1) 617
　drugs that alter, (V1) 693
　heat production and, (V1) 447
　protein, (V1) 671
　protein role in, (V1) 671
　response to stress, (V1) 244
　sleep and, (V1) 916–917
Metered-dose inhalers (MDI), (V1) 641, (V1) 641f
　administration of, (V1) 659p, (V2) 415–417p
Methadone, (V1) 150
Methamphetamines, (V1) 150
Methicillin-resistant *Staphylococcus aureus* (MRSA), (V1) 164, (V1) 300
Metric system, (V1) 624
Microcephaly, (V1) 491
Micronutrients, (V1) 669
　defined, (V1) 673
　minerals, (V1) 673, (V1) 678–681, (V1) 679–681t
　vegetarianism and, (V1) 690
　vitamins, (V1) 673, (V1) 674–678t
Microsleep, (V1) 925
Microwave use and burns, (V1) 548
Middle adulthood
　assessment in, (V1) 182–183
　cardiovascular disease (CVD) in, (V1) 182
　cardiovascular function in, (V1) 1021
　common health problems in, (V1) 181–182
　development in
　　cognitive, (V1) 181
　　physical, (V1) 181
　　psychosocial, (V1) 181, (V1) 181f
　exercise in, (V1) 183
　health risks in families during, (V1) 298
　hormone replacement therapy (HRT) in, (V1) 183
　immunizations in, (V1) 183
　implementation for, (V1) 183
　loss in, (V1) 348
　nursing diagnosis and, (V1) 183
　nutrition in, (V1) 183, (V1) 686
　obesity in, (V1) 182
　physical examination of, (V1) 485–486
　pulmonary function in, (V1) 981
　sexuality in, (V1) 888
　sleep requirements and characteristics in, (V1) 918t, (V1) 923
　stressors in, (V1) 240b
Middle childhood. *See* School-age children
Middle ear, (V1) 493
Middle-income families, (V1) 299
Middle-old adults, (V1) 191
　assessment of, (V1) 201, (V1) 201f
　implementation for, (V1) 202
Midlife crisis, (V1) 298
Midline peripheral catheter, (V1) 1058
Midrange theory, (V1) 98
Midupper arm circumference, (V1) 696
Mild anxiety, (V1) 278t

Milia, (V1) 153, (V1) 490, (V1) 941
Military families, (V1) 292
Milliequivalents (mEq), (V1) 624
Mindfulness, (V1) 260
Mind-mapping student care plans, (V1) 71
Minerals, (V1) 673, (V1) 678–681, (V1) 679–681t
　bowel elimination and, (V1) 758
　cardiovascular function and, (V1) 1022
　osteoporosis and, (V1) 867
　teaching clients about supplementation with, (V1) 700–701
Minimization, as defense mechanism, (V1) 247t
Minimum data set (MDS), (V1) 437
Mini-Nutritional Assessment (MNA), (V1) 695, (V2) 506
Minor surgery, (V1) 1078
Miosis, (V1) 493
Miracles, (V1) 333
Misdemeanor, (V1) 1165
Missed nursing care, (V1) 1195
Mobility
　See also Immobility
　assessment of, (V1) 863–865, (V1) 864b
　　in wound assessment, (V1) 953
　assisting with ambulation and, (V1) 876–878, (V1) 877–878f
　body mechanics and, (V2) 628
　bowel elimination and, (V1) 760
　defined, (V1) 841, (V1) 855
　factors affecting, (V1) 855–860, (V1) 858f, (V1) 860f
　gait and, (V1) 379, (V1) 504, (V1) 865
　interventions for (*See* Mobility interventions)
　joint, (V1) 845
　　diseases affecting, (V1) 857–858, (V1) 858f
　pain and, (V1) 821
　range-of-motion exercises for, (V1) 875–876, (V2) 629
　self-care and, (V1) 577
　skin and impaired, (V1) 942
　surgical patients and, (V2) 811–814p
　urine specimen collection and, (V1) 728
　walking aids for, (V1) 877–878, (V1) 877–878f, (V2) 630–631
Mobility interventions
　assisting with ambulation, (V2) 625–628p
　exercise promotion, (V1) 867, (V1) 868b
　moving and turning patients in bed, (V2) 617–621p
　osteoporosis prevention, (V1) 866–867
　for patients with specific disease and abnormalities, (V1) 866–867
　positioning patients for, (V1) 867–873, (V1) 869–870f, (V1) 871–872t
　transferring patients, (V2) 622–625p
Models
　Benner's, (V1) 94, (V1) 94f
　clinical judgment, (V1) 30–33, (V1) 31t, (V1) 32f, (V1) 33–35t
　conceptual, (V1) 95
　critical thinking, (V1) 39–41, (V1) 40b, (V1) 41f
　defined, (V1) 95
　ethical dilemma, (V1) 138
　health promotion, (V1) 221–222f, (V1) 221–223

stress, (V1) 240
　transtheoretical model of change, (V1) 222
Mode of transmission of infections, (V1) 517–518
Moderate-intensity walking, (V1) 853
Modified bed baths, (V1) 585–586
Modified sterile technique, (V1) 537
　for artificial airway, (V1) 1006
Modulation, pain, (V1) 814–815, (V1) 815f
Moist heat, (V1) 973, (V1) 974f
Moisture and skin infections, (V1) 588
Moisture-associated skin damage (MASD), (V1) 943
Molars, (V1) 592
Mongolian spots, (V1) 941
Monitoring by managers, (V1) 1185
Monosaccharides, (V1) 669
Monounsaturated fat, (V1) 672, (V1) 672t
Mons pubis, (V1) 882
Montgomery straps, (V1) 971, (V1) 972f
Moral agency, (V1) 118
Moral decisions, (V1) 123–132
Moral development, (V1) 123–124
Moral development theory
　Gilligan's, (V1) 149
　Kohlberg's, (V1) 148–149
Moral distress, (V1) 118–119, (V1) 119f, (V1) 120, (V1) 133, (V1) 342b
Moral frameworks, (V1) 126–128
MORAL model, (V1) 135–138, (V2) 32
Moral outrage, (V1) 119
Morals, (V1) 116
Mormonism, (V1) 336t
Moro reflex, (V1) 153
Morphine, (V1) 150
Morse Fall Scale, (V1) 557
Mosquitoes, (V1) 550, (V1) 568, (V1) 570
Motivation in patient learning, (V1) 399–400
Motor and cerebellar function, (V1) 507
Motor cortex, (V1) 979
Motor development, infant, (V1) 156
Motor nervous system, (V1) 843–844
Motor vehicles. *See* Automobiles
Mottling, (V1) 489t
Mourning, (V1) 348
Mouth, (V1) 754, (V1) 754f
　assessment of, (V1) 594, (V2) 234–238p
　common problems of, (V1) 593–595
　denture care, (V1) 602p, (V2) 361–363p
　dry, (V1) 594, (V1) 703
　implementation for, (V1) 594–595
　nursing diagnosis of, (V1) 594
　physical examination of, (V1) 494, (V1) 494f, (V1) 509, (V1) 511p
　planning for, (V1) 594
　as primary defense against infection, (V1) 521
Movement
　body mechanics and, (V1) 844–845, (V1) 844f, (V1) 845f, (V1) 846–851t
　of patients in bed, (V1) 873, (V1) 873f
　physiology of, (V1) 841–844, (V1) 842–843f, (V1) 843t
　problems with, (V1) 504
　transferring patients out of bed, (V1) 874–875, (V1) 874–875f
MRSA. *See* Methicillin-resistant *Staphylococcus aureus* (MRSA)
Mu agonist opioids, (V1) 828
Muffled blood pressure sound, (V1) 473

Multicultural populations
See also Culture
assessment of, (V2) 111–112
and communication with clients who speak a different language, (V1) 325–326, (V1) 327b, (V2) 110
critical thinking and clinical judgment on, (V2) 114–115
cultural knowledge for, (V1) 309–311, (V1) 309f, (V1) 310b
definitions of, (V1) 312–313
diversity of, (V1) 121, (V1) 309–310, (V1) 310b
ethics and, (V1) 121
full-spectrum nursing model applied to, (V2) 113
knowledge map on, (V2) 117
understanding biological variations in, (V2) 109
Multidimensional Health Locus of Control (MHLC) scale, (V1) 228
Multidrug-resistant organisms, (V1) 520, (V1) 526–528
Multigenerational/intergenerational families, (V1) 293
Multiple IV lines, management of, (V1) 1064
Multiple sclerosis, (V1) 859
Murmurs, (V1) 501
Muscarinic receptor antagonists and urinary elimination, (V1) 723
Muscles
function of, (V1) 504, (V1) 843f
respiratory, (V1) 978
sprains and strains of, (V1) 859
types of, (V1) 843
Muscular fitness assessment, (V1) 227
Musculoskeletal system
age-related changes in, (V1) 193t
assessment of, (V2) 263–272p
balance, coordination, and movement, (V1) 504
body mechanics, (V1) 844–845, (V1) 844f, (V1) 845f, (V1) 846–851t
body shape and symmetry, (V1) 504
bones, (V1) 504, (V1) 504f
congenital abnormalities of, (V1) 857
heat production and, (V1) 447
injury from exercise, (V1) 854
joint mobility and muscle function, (V1) 504
motor nervous system, (V1) 843–844
muscles
function of, (V1) 504, (V1) 843f
types of, (V1) 843
in oldest-old adults, (V1) 191
physical examination of, (V1) 504, (V1) 504f, (V1) 510, (V1) 512p
physiology of movement and, (V1) 841–844, (V1) 842–843f, (V1) 843t
prior to death, (V1) 357
responses related to failure of adaptation, (V1) 252t
response to stress, (V1) 244
in school-age children, (V1) 167
unrelieved pain and, (V1) 817
Music during and after surgery, (V1) 1090
Music therapy, (V1) 262, (V1) 934
Mutual masturbation, (V1) 895
Mutual recognition model (MRM), (V1) 1163
Myasthenia gravis, (V1) 859

Mydriasis, (V1) 493
Myofascial release therapy, (V1) 824
Myofascial trigger point dry needling, (V1) 824
Myopia, (V1) 491–492
MyPlate, (V1) 230–231, (V1) 667, (V1) 668f
for older adults, (V1) 667
in Spanish, (V1) 667
MyVeganPlate, (V1) 690, (V1) 691f

N

Nails, (V1) 491, (V1) 510p
assessment of, (V2) 216–218p
care of, (V1) 590–591
ingrown, (V1) 589
Names, drug, (V1) 607–608
NANDA-I diagnostic classification system, (V1) 62, (V1) 63t, (V1) 1120
on caregiver role strain, (V1) 304
communication problems, (V1) 387
ethical issues in, (V1) 133
health promotion and, (V1) 229
infections and, (V1) 530
self-neglect and, (V1) 577
stress and, (V1) 257
Naproxen, (V1) 827–828
Narcolepsy, (V1) 926
Narcotics, (V1) 150
Narrative format progress notes, (V1) 426–427
Nasal decongestants, (V1) 984t
Nasal flaring, (V1) 994
Nasal medications, (V1) 640
administration of, (V2) 405–407p
opioid, (V1) 830
Nasoenteric tubes, (V2) 483–487p
Nasogastric tubes, (V1) 601, (V1) 637, (V1) 709f
checking placement of, (V1) 710, (V1) 711–712b
insertion of, (V2) 483–487p
large-bore, (V1) 707–708
small-bore, (V1) 707
Nasopharyngeal airways, (V1) 1005, (V1) 1015p
insertion of, (V2) 746–747p
Nasotracheal approach to airway suctioning, (V1) 1007, (V2) 730–733p
National Academy of Medicine (NAM), (V1) 374
Core Competencies, (V1) 5, (V1) 6, (V1) 105–106
National Council Licensure Examination (NCLEX), (V1) 10, (V1) 11
National Council of State Boards of Nursing (NCSBN), (V1) 29
clinical judgment measurement (CJM) model, (V1) 31–33, (V1) 32f, (V1) 33–35t
National economy influence on contemporary nursing, (V1) 24
National Institute for Occupational Safety and Health (NIOSH), (V1) 549
National League for Nursing (NLN), (V1) 14, (V1) 375
National Pressure Injury Advisory Panel (NPIAP), (V1) 952
National Quality Partners Leadership Consortium, (V1) 1077

National School Lunch and Breakfast Programs, (V1) 701
National Student Nurses' Association (NSNA), (V1) 14
National Survey of Family Growth (NSFG), (V1) 887
Native American religions, (V1) 337, (V1) 338f
Natural active immunity, (V1) 522b
Naturally occurring retirement community (NORC), (V1) 189
Natural passive immunity, (V1) 523b
Natural sleep aids, (V1) 937
Nature versus nurture, (V1) 144
Nausea and vomiting, (V1) 701–702
as postoperative complication, (V1) 1100t
NCLEX examination, (V1) 1185
Near vision, (V1) 492
Nebulization, (V1) 641, (V1) 641f, (V1) 1003
Nebulizers, (V1) 641, (V1) 641f
Neck, (V1) 495, (V1) 509, (V1) 511p
assessment of, (V2) 238–240p
Necrotic tissue, (V1) 956
Needle aspiration, wound, (V1) 958
Needles, (V1) 642, (V1) 643–644f, (V1) 644
dead space in, (V1) 646–647
intramuscular, (V1) 653, (V1) 653t
measuring dosage when changing, (V2) 456–457
recapping of, (V1) 426–428p, (V1) 660p
transfer, (V1) 654, (V1) 654f
Needless connections, (V1) 655–656, (V1) 656f
Needlestick injury, (V1) 556, (V1) 647, (V1) 647f, (V2) 338–339
Negative nitrogen balance, (V1) 671
Negative pressure ventilators, (V1) 1008
Negative pressure wound therapy (NPWT) device, (V2) 671–676p
Negative self-talk, (V1) 375
Neglect. *See* Abuse and neglect
Negligence, (V1) 1167–1169
Negotiation, (V1) 325, (V1) 327, (V1) 1170
Neighborhood conditions and physical activity, (V1) 856
Neimeyer, Robert, (V1) 352t
Neobladder, (V1) 744
Neonates
See also Infants
Apgar scoring of, (V1) 155, (V2) 50t
assessment of, (V1) 155
birth injuries in, (V1) 155
blood pressure in, (V1) 469
cardiovascular system in, (V1) 153
common health problems of, (V1) 155–156
congenital anomalies in, (V1) 151, (V1) 155
development of
cognitive, (V1) 154–155
physical, (V1) 152–154, (V1) 152–154f
psychosocial, (V1) 155
elimination in, (V1) 153
growth of, (V1) 152, (V1) 152f
hearing and smell in, (V1) 154–155, (V1) 786
implementation for, (V1) 156
infections in, (V1) 155
jaundice in, (V1) 155
neuromuscular system, (V1) 153–154, (V1) 154f
pain response in, (V1) 816
pulse rate in, (V1) 457
respiration in, (V1) 152–153, (V1) 153f, (V1) 463

respiratory distress in, (V1) 155
sensory function in, (V1) 786–787
skin of, (V1) 941
sleep requirements and characteristics in, (V1) 918t
thermoregulation in, (V1) 153
touch sense in, (V1) 155, (V1) 786–787
transition to extrauterine life, (V1) 155
vision in, (V1) 154, (V1) 786
Nephrons, (V1) 717–718, (V1) 719f
NERDS, wound, (V1) 950
Nerve blocks, (V1) 832
Nerve injury, as complication of intravenous therapy, (V1) 1066t
Nervous system
  age-related changes in, (V1) 193t
  motor, (V1) 843–844
  urinary elimination and, (V1) 724
NE tubes, (V1) 707, (V1) 709f
  checking placement of, (V1) 710
Networking by managers, (V1) 1184
Neuman, Betty, (V1) 208, (V1) 210, (V1) 211f
Neural tube defects, (V1) 151
Neurectomy, (V1) 833
Neurogenic bladder, (V1) 724
Neuroleptics, preoperative, (V1) 1087t
Neurological system
  assessment of, (V2) 272–285p
  cerebral function in, (V1) 505–506
  cranial nerves assessment, (V1) 506, (V1) 506t, (V1) 507f
  development considerations in examination of, (V1) 505
  motor and cerebellar function, (V1) 507
  physical examination of, (V1) 510, (V1) 512p
  reflex function, (V1) 506–507
  sensory function, (V1) 507, (V1) 788
Neuromuscular system
  neonatal, (V1) 153–154, (V1) 154f
  oxygenation and abnormalities of, (V1) 992
Neuropathic pain, (V1) 812
  acupuncture for, (V1) 917
Neurotransmitters, (V1) 814
"Never events," (V1) 545, (V1) 552, (V1) 1077
Nevi (moles), (V1) 490
  congenital, (V1) 941
Newly identified diseases, (V1) 520
Niacin, (V1) 676–677t
NIC. See Nursing Interventions Classification (NIC)
Nicotine, (V1) 150
  sleep and, (V1) 923
Nightingale, Florence, (V1) 3, (V1) 4–6, (V1) 6f, (V1) 94, (V1) 98, (V1) 1114
Night terrors, (V1) 930–931
Nitrogen balance, (V1) 671
NLN. See National League for Nursing (NLN)
NOC. See Nursing outcomes classification (NOC)
Nociceptive pain, (V1) 812
Nocturnal enuresis, (V1) 721–722, (V1) 931
Nocturnal feedings, (V1) 713
Noise
  in client's environment, (V1) 603
  sleep and, (V1) 924
Noise pollution, (V1) 551, (V1) 570
Nomograms, (V2) 469
Nonabsorbent sutures, (V1) 949
Nonadherence, (V1) 341, (V1) 631
  to fitness programs, (V1) 853

Nonallergenic tape, (V1) 971
Nonbenzodiazepines, (V1) 935
Noncommunicating Children's Pain Checklist-Revised (NCCPC-R), (V1) 820
Nondirective interview, (V1) 51t
Nonelectrolytes, (V1) 1037
Nonessential amino acids, (V1) 670
Nonessential fatty acids, (V1) 673
Nonmaleficence, (V1) 129
Nonopioid analgesics, (V1) 827–828
  in older adults, (V1) 834
Nonshivering thermogenesis, (V1) 447
Nonsteroidal anti-inflammatory drugs (NSAIDs), (V1) 759, (V1) 827–828, (V1) 834
  postoperative, (V1) 1102
  skin effects of, (V1) 943
Nontunneled central venous catheters, (V1) 657, (V1) 1059, (V1) 1059f
Nonverbal communication, (V1) 378–380, (V1) 379f, (V1) 380b, (V1) 383
  of pain, (V1) 820–821, (V2) 610
Norepinephrine, (V1) 243, (V1) 244f
Normal flora, (V1) 516–517, (V1) 521
Normal/functional grief, (V1) 354
Normal life changes, as health disruption, (V1) 217
Normal saline, (V1) 960, (V1) 963
Normal temperature, (V1) 446–447, (V1) 446t, (V1) 447f
Normothermia, (V1) 1086
Norton Pressure Sore Risk Assessment Scale, (V2) 697
Nose, (V1) 494, (V1) 494f, (V1) 509, (V1) 511p
  assessment of, (V1) 511p, (V2) 232–234p
  care of, (V1) 601
  procedure for administering medication to, (V1) 658p
Notes on Hospitals, (V1) 6
Nothing by mouth (NPO), (V1) 694, (V1) 702, (V1) 1086
NREM sleep, (V1) 920–921, (V1) 921t
NSNA. See National Student Nurses' Association (NSNA)
Numerical Rating Scale (NRS), (V2) 610
Nurse administrator, (V1) 26
Nurse educator, (V1) 26
Nurse entrepreneur, (V1) 26
Nurse informaticist, (V1) 26
Nurse licensure compact, (V1) 1163
Nurse practice acts, (V1) 13, (V1) 1161, (V1) 1162–1165
  credentialing, (V1) 1165
  disciplinary actions, (V1) 1164–1165
  medications and, (V1) 609
  requirements for licensure, (V1) 1163
  safe harbor laws, (V1) 1178
  scope of practice, (V1) 1163–1164
  special cases of licensure, (V1) 1163
Nurse practitioner (NP), (V1) 18, (V1) 26
Nurse researcher, (V1) 26
Nurse(s)
  application of knowledge, skill, and caring by, (V1) 7
  dealing with complex situations, (V1) 38
  desirable job skills for, (V1) 1185b
  education of (See Nursing education)
  expanded career roles for, (V1) 26
  followership and, (V1) 1188

home health (See Home healthcare)
honoring each client's unique experience with wellness, health, and illness, (V1) 233–235
impaired, (V1) 1177, (V1) 1177b
important qualities of, (V1) 10b
infection prevention, (V1) 540
influence on health policy, (V1) 27
preceptors and mentors for, (V1) 1187, (V1) 1187b
professional boundaries for, (V1) 1176, (V1) 1176b
providing healing presence, (V1) 208, (V1) 235–236
qualifications for assignments, (V1) 1176
roles and functions of, (V1) 7t, (V1) 29
taking care of self when caring for dying persons, (V1) 367–368
teaching responsibilities of, (V1) 396–397
understanding wellness, health, and illness as individual experiences, (V1) 209
using conceptual models to understand health and illness, (V1) 209–210, (V1) 210f
Nurses' Bill of Rights, (V1) 1162
Nurses' notes, (V1) 421
Nursing
  codes of ethics for, (V1) 13, (V1) 86, (V1) 118, (V1) 119, (V1) 131–132
  community-based (See Community-based nursing)
  community-oriented, (V1) 1114, (V1) 1114f
  in correctional facilities, (V1) 1117
  definition of, (V1) 9b
    American Nursing Association (ANA), (V1) 8–9
    importance of, (V1) 9, (V1) 10b
    International Council of Nurses (ICN), (V1) 8–10
  disaster services, (V1) 1117–1118, (V1) 1118b
  end-of-life care and, (V1) 18
  ethical problems in, (V1) 122–123
  evolution of, (V2) 3–5
    knowledge map for, (V2) 6
  faith community, (V1) 1117
  family, (V1) 293–294, (V1) 293f
  full-spectrum (See Full-spectrum nursing)
  gender diversity in, (V1) 24
  and healthcare trends, (V1) 24–27
  health promotion and, (V1) 18
  health restoration and, (V1) 18
  historical context of, (V1) 4–8, (V1) 106
  illness prevention and, (V1) 18
  interdisciplinary collaboration in, (V1) 25–26
  international, (V1) 1118, (V1) 1118f
  key concepts in, (V1) 4
  labor market changes for, (V1) 1189
  occupational health, (V1) 1117
  and other professional subcultures, (V1) 318–319
  perioperative, (V1) 1076–1077, (V1) 1076b
  as profession, discipline, or occupation, (V1) 9–10, (V1) 11t
  public health, (V1) 1113–1114, (V1) 1114f, (V1) 1117
  school, (V1) 1116–1117
  student garb in, (V1) 25f
  telehealth, (V1) 25, (V1) 216, (V1) 1141, (V1) 1141f

types of knowledge in, (V1) 30–36
values and behaviors, (V1) 13b
Nursing care
  for caregiver role strain, (V1) 302b, (V1) 304–307, (V1) 307b
  caring for clients, (V1) 14–16
  continuity of, (V1) 420
  of dying persons, (V1) 365–367, (V1) 366f
  guidelines for documenting, (V1) 440–442, (V1) 440b
  holistic, (V1) 39
  models of, (V1) 16
  patient care plans for, (V1) 67–71, (V1) 68f, (V1) 70f
  to promote psychosocial health, (V1) 270–271, (V1) 272t
  for promoting family wellness, (V1) 307, (V1) 307b
  purposes of, (V1) 15
  recipients of, (V1) 14–15
  safe, effective nursing care (SENC), (V1) 5
  for self-concept disturbance and low self-esteem, (V1) 272–277
  settings for, (V1) 16–18, (V1) 17f, (V1) 25
  strategies for culturally competent, (V1) 325–327, (V1) 326t, (V1) 327b
  types of, (V1) 16
  using sterile technique in, (V1) 538
Nursing care facilities, (V1) 17, (V1) 189–190
Nursing diagnoses, (V1) 47, (V1) 183
  blood pressure, (V1) 474–475
  bowel elimination, (V1) 766
  cardiovascular system, (V1) 1029
  communication problems, (V1) 387
  community nursing, (V1) 1120–1121
  cultural competence and, (V1) 324
  death and dying, (V1) 362
  eyes, (V1) 599
  fluid, electrolytes, and acid-base balance, (V1) 1053
  foot problems, (V1) 589
  goals and, (V1) 72–74, (V1) 73t
  hair, (V1) 597–598
  health promotion and, (V1) 229
  home healthcare, (V1) 1129–1130
  hygiene and, (V1) 577–578
  infections, (V1) 530
  medication administration, (V1) 631
  mobility and exercise, (V1) 866
  nails, (V1) 590
  nutrition problems, (V1) 699
  for older adults, (V1) 201
  oral cavity, (V1) 594
  origins of, (V1) 53
  pain, (V1) 821
  patient education, (V1) 408–409
  physical examination for identifying, (V1) 479
  planning for, (V1) 183–184
  postoperative care, (V1) 1097
  preoperative care, (V1) 1082–1083, (V1) 1084t
  preoperative phase, (V1) 1093
  psychosocial health, (V1) 271, (V1) 272t
  pulmonary function, (V1) 998–999
  pulse, (V1) 461
  relation to outcomes and interventions, (V1) 65
  respiration and, (V1) 467
  safety problems, (V1) 562
  self-care, (V1) 577
  self-concept disturbance and low self-esteem, (V1) 272–277
  self-neglect, (V1) 577
  sensory system, (V1) 803
  sexual health, (V1) 903–904, (V1) 904f
  skin problems, (V1) 584
  sleep, (V1) 932–933
  spirituality and religious, (V1) 341, (V1) 342b
  stress and adaptation, (V1) 257
  theory applied to, (V1) 103
  types of, (V1) 56, (V1) 57t
  when to use, (V1) 54–56, (V1) 55f
  wounds, (V1) 959
  writing diagnostic statements in, (V1) 62–65
Nursing education, (V1) 6, (V1) 8–16
  continuing, (V1) 12
  formal, (V1) 10–12
    graduate nursing, (V1) 12
    practical and vocational, (V1) 10–11
    registered nursing entry education, (V1) 11–12
  informal, (V1) 12–13
    Benner's model, (V1) 12–13
  in-service, (V1) 12
  nursing organization guidelines on, (V1) 13
  nursing research and, (V1) 106
  use of nursing theory in, (V1) 98
Nursing ethics, defined, (V1) 117
Nursing history
  bowel elimination, (V1) 763
  mobility and exercise, (V1) 864
  preoperative care, (V1) 1081
  wound assessment, (V1) 952
Nursing homes, (V1) 17, (V1) 189–190
Nursing informatics
  See also Electronic health records (EHRs)
  aiding patients in self-care, (V1) 1143
  biosensors, (V1) 1144
  computer- and application-based tools for providing and managing care, (V1) 1142–1146, (V1) 1143f, (V1) 1146f, (V1) 1146t
  computer basics for, (V1) 1140
  critical thinking and clinical judgment on, (V2) 847–849
  data in, (V1) 1139
  defined, (V1) 1138–1140, (V1) 1139f
  electronic messaging in, (V1) 1140
  full-spectrum nursing model applied to, (V2) 847
  information in, (V1) 1139
  Internet-based software and applications, (V1) 1143–1144
  key concepts in, (V1) 1138
  knowledge in, (V1) 1139, (V1) 1139f
  knowledge map on, (V2) 850
  managing staffing and workflow, (V1) 1142
  reducing error with automation, (V1) 1142–1143
  social networking and, (V1) 1140–1141
  supporting evidence-based practice, (V1) 1150–1153, (V1) 1153–1154b
  supporting healthcare professional, (V1) 1145–1146, (V1) 1146f
  telehealth, (V1) 1141, (V1) 1141f
  tracking patients and equipment, (V1) 1142
  use in home care, (V1) 1142
  wearable devices, (V1) 1143–1144
  wisdom in, (V1) 1139
Nursing informatics specialists (NISs), (V1) 1139
Nursing interventions
  adolescent, (V1) 177–179
  blood pressure, (V1) 475–476
  bowel elimination, (V1) 767–768
  for bowel elimination problems, (V1) 768–782, (V1) 772t, (V1) 778f, (V1) 780–781b
  cardiovascular system, (V1) 1031–1035
  choosing, (V1) 75–78
  communication problems, (V1) 387
  community nursing, (V1) 1115–1116, (V1) 1116f, (V1) 1121
  complicated grief, (V1) 368, (V1) 369
  for coping with hospitalization, (V1) 307, (V1) 307b
  cultural competence and, (V1) 325
  death and dying, (V1) 363
  eyes, (V1) 599–600
  fluid, electrolytes, and acid-base balance, (V1) 1054
  foot care, (V1) 590
  hair care, (V1) 598–599
  home healthcare, (V1) 1131–1135, (V1) 1132f, (V1) 1134f
  hygiene, (V1) 578–579, (V1) 579f
  infant, (V1) 160–162
  infections, (V1) 531
  medication administration, (V1) 632
  middle adulthood, (V1) 183
  mobility (See Mobility interventions)
  nail care, (V1) 591
  neonatal period, (V1) 156
  nutrition problems, (V1) 700–701
  older adults, (V1) 201–205
  oral cavity, (V1) 594–595
  oxygenation, (V1) 999–1003, (V1) 1001b, (V1) 1003f
  pain, (V1) 822–836
  patient education, (V1) 409–417
  postoperative care, (V1) 1098–1101t, (V1) 1098–1104
  preoperative care, (V1) 1083–1089, (V1) 1087t, (V1) 1088–1089f
  preoperative phase, (V1) 1094–1095
  preschooler, (V1) 166–167
  problem status and, (V1) 77t
  pulse problems, (V1) 462
  safety, (V1) 563–574
    choking rescue, (V1) 565, (V1) 566f
    general, (V1) 563
    home care, (V1) 563–567, (V1) 566f
    preventing carbon monoxide poisoning, (V1) 564
    preventing drowning, (V1) 565
    preventing firearm injuries, (V1) 564
    preventing home fires, (V1) 549, (V1) 564–565
    preventing scalds and burns, (V1) 564
    preventing suffocation, (V1) 564–565, (V1) 566f
    preventing take-home toxins, (V1) 565
  school-age children, (V1) 169–171
  self-care, (V1) 578
  self-concept disturbance and low self-esteem, (V1) 276–277
  sensory system, (V1) 804–809
  sexual health, (V1) 904–908
  skin problems, (V1) 585–587, (V1) 586b

sleep, (V1) 933–937, (V1) 934f
spiritual, (V1) 343–345, (V1) 344f
stress and adaptation, (V1) 258
toddler, (V1) 164
urinary catheterization, (V1) 732–740, (V1) 736f, (V1) 738f
for urinary elimination problems, (V1) 731
wellness, (V1) 80
wound care, (V1) 959
young adults, (V1) 180
young-old adults, (V1) 201–202
Nursing Interventions Classification (NIC), (V1) 78–79, (V1) 79b
interventions in, (V1) 104
theory and, (V1) 104
Nursing orders, (V1) 80–81
Nursing outcomes
blood pressure, (V1) 475
bowel elimination, (V1) 766
cardiovascular system, (V1) 1029
client's environment, (V1) 601
community nursing, (V1) 1121
eyes, (V1) 599
fluid, electrolytes, and acid-base balance, (V1) 1053
foot problems, (V1) 589–590
hair, (V1) 598
home healthcare, (V1) 1130–1131
medication administration, (V1) 631–632
mobility and exercise, (V1) 866
nails, (V1) 590
nutrition problems, (V1) 699–700
oral cavity, (V1) 594
pain, (V1) 821–822
postoperative care, (V1) 1097–1098
preoperative care, (V1) 1083
preoperative phase, (V1) 1094
pulmonary function, (V1) 999
self-care deficit, (V1) 578
sensory system, (V1) 803–804
sexual health, (V1) 904
skin problems, (V1) 585
sleep, (V1) 933
urinary elimination, (V1) 731
wound care, (V1) 959
Nursing outcomes classification (NOC), (V1) 229
components of, (V1) 74
computerized care plans and, (V1) 74
goals for wellness diagnoses, (V1) 74
Nursing practice, (V1) 6
factors influencing contemporary, (V1) 23–27
impaired, (V1) 119
laws and regulations guiding, federal, (V1) 1157–1160, (V1) 1159b
nurse practice acts, (V1) 13
nursing care in, (V1) 14–16
regulation of, (V1) 21
standards of practice, (V1) 13
use of nursing theory in, (V1) 97–98
Nursing process, (V1) 47
analysis/diagnosis in, (V1) 47, (V1) 53–56, (V1) 54f, (V1) 55f
assessment in, (V1) 47–50, (V1) 48b, (V1) 48t, (V1) 49t
guidelines and tools for, (V2) 13–14
clinical judgment and, (V1) 42, (V1) 42t, (V2) 20–22
in community-based care, (V1) 1121–1122

critical thinking and, (V1) 41–42, (V2) 20–22
diagnostic reasoning in, (V1) 56–60, (V1) 58b, (V1) 58f
documenting in, (V1) 52, (V1) 53f, (V1) 84
drawing conclusions about health status in, (V1) 58–59
evaluation in, (V1) 47, (V1) 84–91
checklist for, (V2) 15–17
in home healthcare, (V1) 1129
implementation in, (V1) 47, (V1) 81–84, (V1) 83b
interventions in, (V1) 74–75
choosing, (V1) 75–78, (V1) 77–78t
interviewing in, (V1) 50–52, (V1) 51t
key concepts in, (V1) 47
knowledge map for, (V2) 24
minimizing malpractice risks, (V1) 1172
nursing orders in, (V1) 80–81
organization of data in, (V1) 52
pain management, (V1) 836–839
planning in, (V1) 47, (V1) 65–67
nursing interventions, (V1) 74–75
patient care plans, (V1) 67–71, (V1) 68f, (V1) 70f
patient goals/outcomes, (V1) 71–74, (V1) 73t
reflecting critically on diagnostic reasoning in, (V1) 60–61, (V1) 61b
sexual health and, (V1) 909
standardized nursing languages in, (V1) 61–62
steps of, (V2) 12–17
used in health promotion, (V1) 223–237
validation of data in, (V1) 51–52
writing diagnostic statements in, (V1) 62–65
Nursing: Scope and Standards of Practice, (V1) 52, (V1) 132, (V1) 396, (V1) 420, (V1) 516
Nursing theory, (V1) 93–94, (V1) 94f
See also Theory/theories
components of, (V1) 94–95, (V1) 95b
conceptual framework in, (V1) 95
conceptual models in, (V1) 95
development of, (V1) 96–97, (V1) 96f
essential concepts of, (V1) 97, (V1) 97f
family care and, (V1) 295–296
importance of, (V1) 93–94, (V1) 94f
important nurse theorists and, (V1) 98–100, (V1) 99b, (V1) 101t
models in, (V1) 95
paradigms in, (V1) 95
planning interventions/implementation based on, (V1) 104
uses of, (V1) 97–98
Nutrition
See also Diet(s)
adolescent, (V1) 177, (V1) 178–179
assessment of, (V1) 50, (V1) 228, (V1) 695–699, (V1) 697b, (V1) 698b
guidelines and tools for, (V2) 505–509
assisting patients with meals, (V2) 502
body composition analysis and, (V1) 683, (V1) 696–697, (V1) 697b, (V2) 500–501
bowel elimination and, (V1) 758
cardiovascular function and, (V1) 1021, (V1) 1022
childhood obesity and, (V1) 168
critical thinking and clinical judgment on, (V2) 511–513
diagnostic testing and, (V2) 510

dietary reference intakes (DRI), (V1) 666–667
disease processes and functional limitations and, (V1) 692–693
energy nutrients, (V1) 669–673, (V1) 670t, (V1) 672t
carbohydrates, (V1) 669, (V1) 670t
defined, (V1) 669
lipids, (V1) 670t, (V1) 671–673, (V1) 672t
proteins, (V1) 669–671, (V1) 670t
enteral
contamination of, (V1) 713–714
enteric tubes for, (V1) 706
feeding schedules, (V1) 710, (V1) 713
monitoring patients receiving, (V1) 713, (V2) 503
open and closed feeding systems, (V1) 713
removing feeding tubes for, (V1) 714
risks associated with, (V1) 706
selecting feeding tube for, (V1) 706
types of feeding solutions, (V1) 710
evidence-based practice on, (V1) 692
factors affecting
developmental stage, (V1) 684–689
lifestyle choices, (V1) 689–690
facts labels, (V1) 668–669, (V1) 668f
food deserts and, (V1) 211
food insecurity and, (V1) 211
full-spectrum nursing model applied to, (V2) 510–511
for health and athletic performance, (V1) 690–691
home-delivered meals and, (V1) 205
host susceptibility to infection and, (V1) 529, (V1) 531
infant, (V1) 160
influence on health, (V1) 212–213
interventions
for impaired dietary intake, (V1) 701–702
for patients with impaired digestive function, (V1) 703
for patients with impaired swallowing, (V1) 702–703, (V1) 703f
for patients with underweight and nutrition, (V1) 703–706
teaching clients about vitamin and mineral supplementation, (V1) 700–701
key concepts in, (V1) 666
knowledge map on, (V2) 515
maternal, (V1) 151, (V1) 151f
middle adulthood, (V1) 183
MyPlate, (V1) 667, (V1) 668f
nursing diagnosis and, (V1) 699
obesity and, (V1) 168, (V1) 177
in older adults, (V1) 299
in oldest-old adults, (V1) 191
oral problems with, (V1) 593
oxygenation and, (V1) 982
parenteral, (V1) 714–715, (V1) 714f, (V2) 494–498p
monitoring patients receiving, (V2) 504
physical activity and, (V1) 856
preoperative, (V1) 1086
in preschoolers, (V1) 166, (V1) 167
procedures
administering feedings through gastric and enteric tubes, (V2) 488–492p

administering parenteral nutrition, (V2) 494–498p
checking fingerstick blood glucose levels, (V2) 480–483p
inserting nasogastric and nasoenteric tubes, (V2) 483–487p
lipid administration, (V2) 498–500p
removing nasogastric and nasoenteric tubes, (V2) 493–494p
in school-age children, (V1) 169
skin and, (V1) 583, (V1) 942
stress and, (V1) 258
teaching about, to school-age children, (V1) 170
urinary elimination and, (V1) 732
USDA *Dietary Guidelines for Americans 2020–2025,* (V1) 667, (V1) 667Ib
wound healing and, (V1) 958
Nutritional assessment, (V1) 50, (V1) 228
assessing body composition in, (V1) 696–697, (V1) 697b
delegation of, (V1) 699
dietary history in, (V1) 695–696
focused, (V1) 695
assessing body composition in, (V1) 696–697, (V1) 697b
as cues to nutrient imbalance, (V1) 697
delegation of, (V1) 699
dietary history in, (V1) 695–696
laboratory values reflecting nutritional status in, (V1) 697–699, (V1) 698b
physical examination in, (V1) 696
laboratory values reflecting nutritional status in, (V1) 697–699, (V1) 698b
physical examination in, (V1) 696
as cues to nutrient imbalance, (V1) 697
Nutrition Screening Initiative (NSI), (V1) 695, (V2) 505
Nutritive enemas, (V1) 771

O

Obesity and overweight, (V1) 687–689
in adolescents, (V1) 174–175, (V1) 177–178
bathing patients who have, (V1) 588
blood pressure and, (V1) 469
calorie-restricted diets for, (V1) 691, (V1) 694
cardiovascular function and, (V1) 1020, (V1) 1022
childhood, (V1) 168
in middle adulthood, (V1) 182
oxygenation and, (V1) 982
physical activity and, (V1) 856
in young adults, (V1) 180
Objective data, (V1) 47–48, (V1) 48t
Oblique position, (V1) 870, (V1) 872f
O blood group, (V1) 1068, (V1) 1068t
Observations, (V1) 48
sharing of, (V1) 388–389
Obstruction, airway, (V1) 989
Occult blood testing, (V2) 560–562p
Occupational hazards and oxygenation, (V1) 982
Occupational health nursing, (V1) 1117
Occupational therapists (OTs), (V1) 18
Occupied bed making, (V1) 603p, (V2) 380–382p
Occurrence reports, (V1) 436, (V1) 436b
Occurrence-type liability insurance, (V1) 1178

Odors
foot, (V1) 589
preventing and eliminating, (V1) 601, (V1) 603
Oil-retention enemas, (V1) 771
Oils, (V1) 671
Ointments, (V1) 613t, (V1) 637
Old diseases, (V1) 300
Older adults
abuse of, (V1) 198, (V1) 199–200
aging in place, (V1) 187–190
assessment of, (V1) 198–201, (V1) 201f
guidelines and tools for, (V2) 54–55
oral cavity, (V1) 594
assisting with ambulation by, (V1) 877
automobile accidents in, (V1) 567
bathing of, (V1) 588–589
benefits of walking for, (V1) 853
blood pressure in, (V1) 469
body temperature in, (V1) 448
bowel elimination in, (V1) 758
calcium intake of, (V1) 1055
cardiovascular function in, (V1) 1021
chest shape and size in, (V1) 496
chronic diseases in, (V1) 195
common health problems in, (V1) 195, (V1) 195b, (V1) 198
communicating with, (V1) 204
communication by, (V1) 380
deep vein thrombosis in, (V1) 1088
dementia in, (V1) 195, (V1) 196–197, (V1) 804
depression in, (V1) 198, (V1) 200
developmental changes in, (V1) 191–198
cognitive, (V1) 191, (V1) 194t
physical, (V1) 191
psychosocial, (V1) 194–195t, (V1) 195f
discharge planning for, (V1) 66–67
drug misuse by, (V1) 624
ectropion in, (V1) 492
energy needs of, (V1) 683
falls in, (V1) 201, (V1) 549, (V1) 877
fever in, (V1) 449
fluid intake in, (V1) 1040
frailty in, (V1) 191, (V1) 192–193, (V1) 687
full-spectrum nursing model applied to, (V2) 55–56
functional status assessment in, (V1) 200
general anesthesia and, (V1) 1091
genitourinary system in, (V1) 508
glomerular filtration in, (V1) 718
grief in, (V1) 353
health risks in families with, (V1) 298–299, (V1) 298f
hearing screening in, (V2) 599
home healthcare for, (V1) 1122
home safety interventions for, (V1) 563
host susceptibility to infection in, (V1) 525
hygiene and, (V1) 576
illness prevention for, (V1) 203–204
immunizations in, (V1) 203–204
implementation for, (V1) 201–205
influence on contemporary nursing, (V1) 24
insomnia in, (V1) 925
key concepts on, (V1) 186
knowledge map on, (V2) 58
as least active age-group, (V1) 856
loss in, (V1) 348
medication containers for, (V1) 633, (V1) 1132

medication errors in, (V1) 639b
medication schedules for, (V1) 632
mental state in, (V1) 487
MyPlate for, (V1) 667
neurological system examination in, (V1) 505
nonadherence to medications in, (V1) 1131
nonsteroidal anti-inflammatory drugs (NSAIDs) and, (V1) 828
normal aging changes in, (V1) 193–194t
NPO for, (V1) 702
nutritional assessment of, (V1) 695
nutrition in, (V1) 686–687
nutrition interventions for, (V1) 702
opioid use in, (V1) 834
oral medications for, (V1) 637–638
osteoporosis in, (V1) 195
prevention of, (V1) 867
pain in, (V1) 816
analgesics for, (V1) 823
management of, (V1) 833–834
misconceptions about, (V1) 833
perspectives on aging and, (V1) 186–187
pharmacokinetics in, (V1) 620f
physical activity guidelines for, (V1) 852b
physical examination of, (V1) 486
polypharmacy in, (V1) 195, (V1) 198, (V1) 631
postoperative pain control in, (V1) 1102
pregnancy in, (V1) 151
preoperative nursing diagnosis for, (V1) 1083, (V1) 1084t
preoperative physical assessment of, (V1) 1082
preoperative teaching for, (V1) 1086
pressure injury in, (V1) 111
promoting cognitive function in, (V1) 203
promoting independence and maintaining functional ability in, (V1) 202–203
providing support to caregivers of, (V1) 205
pulmonary function in, (V1) 981
putting plans together for, (V1) 205–206
respiration in, (V1) 463
restless legs syndrome (RLS) in, (V1) 925
safety of, (V1) 547
self-catheterization by, (V1) 740
sensory function in, (V1) 787, (V1) 787t
sexuality in, (V1) 888–889, (V1) 889f
skin of, (V1) 583, (V1) 583t, (V1) 941
sleep medications for, (V1) 935
sleep requirements and characteristics in, (V1) 918t, (V1) 923
smoking by, (V1) 1022
stages of, (V1) 190–191
stressors in, (V1) 240b
as subculture, (V1) 314
surgical risk in, (V1) 1078–1079
surgical site infection in, (V1) 1080
taping a dressing on, (V1) 971
teaching for, (V1) 203, (V1) 402–403, (V1) 403–405t
teeth and gums in, (V1) 592
theories of aging and, (V1) 190
transfer reports for, (V1) 438
urinary elimination in, (V1) 722
Oldest-old adults, (V1) 191
assessment of, (V1) 201
implementation for, (V1) 202
Olfaction, (V1) 484
Olfactory receptors, (V1) 784

Omaha System, (V1) 62, (V1) 79, (V1) 1120–1121
Omega-3 fatty acids, (V1) 823
One-to-one instruction, for patient teaching, (V1) 411
Ongoing assessment, (V1) 49, (V1) 49t, (V1) 479
Ongoing groups, (V1) 386
Online forums, (V1) 1141
Open-ended questions, (V1) 51, (V1) 389
Open feeding systems, (V1) 713
Open gloving, (V1) 538, (V1) 539p
Open systems, (V1) 103, (V1) 295
Open wounds, (V1) 944
Operational definition, (V1) 95
Operative field, (V2) 826
Operative personnel, (V1) 1089–1090
Operative suite, (V1) 1089, (V1) 1089f
Ophthalmic medications, (V1) 639–640
  administration of, (V1) 658p, (V2) 400–403p
Opioid analgesics, (V1) 788, (V1) 814
  abuse of, (V1) 834–835
  administration routes of, (V1) 830–831, (V1) 831f
  effectiveness of, (V1) 828–829
  equianalgesia and, (V1) 830
  in older adults, (V1) 834
  postoperative, (V1) 1101–1102
  preoperative, (V1) 1087t
  side effects of, (V1) 829–830, (V1) 829b
  sleep and, (V1) 924
  types of, (V1) 828
  use in older adults, (V1) 834
Opioid Risk Tool (ORT), (V1) 834, (V2) 612
Oral body temperature measurement, (V1) 455t, (V2) 175p
Oral care
  for children, (V1) 595
  for critically ill patients, (V1) 596
  denture care, (V1) 602p, (V2) 361–363p
  evidence-based practice in, (V1) 597
  for patients who have dementia, (V1) 596–597
  self-care, (V1) 595–596, (V1) 595–596f
  teeth care, (V1) 595–596, (V1) 595f, (V1) 602p, (V2) 358–361p
  for unconscious patients, (V1) 596, (V2) 363–366p
Oral communication, impaired, (V1) 387
Oral contraceptives, (V1) 689, (V2) 642
Oral electrolyte supplements, (V1) 1055
Oral-genital stimulation, (V1) 895
Oral health
  See also Teeth
  altered level of consciousness and, (V1) 805
  assessment of, (V1) 594
  care of, (V1) 602p
  common problems of the mouth, (V1) 593–595
  hygiene for, (V1) 592
  implementation for, (V1) 594–595
  nursing diagnosis of, (V1) 594
  patient education on, (V1) 595–596, (V1) 595f
  planning for, (V1) 594
  risk factors for, (V1) 592–593
Oral medications
  buccal and sublingual, (V1) 636
  for children, (V1) 637, (V1) 638
  enteral, (V1) 637

  for older adults, (V1) 637–638
  opioid, (V1) 830
  pouring, (V1) 636, (V1) 636f
  procedure for administering, (V1) 658p, (V2) 396–400p
  special situations, (V1) 637
Oral reporting, (V2) 157–158
  handoff reports in, (V1) 384, (V1) 437–438
  key concepts in, (V1) 420
  questioning prescriptions, (V1) 439
  receiving and documenting verbal and telephone prescriptions, (V1) 438–439
  standardized formats for, (V1) 437–438
  transfer reports in, (V1) 438
Oral sex, adolescents and, (V1) 175
Oral stage, in psychoanalytic theory, (V1) 147t
Oral sucrose, (V1) 825
Orchiectomy, (V1) 891
Orders, nursing, (V1) 80–81
Organ donation, (V1) 361
Organizations, nursing, (V1) 13–14
  American Nurses Association (ANA), (V1) 14
  International Council of Nurses (ICN), (V1) 14
  National League for Nursing (NLN), (V1) 14
  National Student Nurses' Association (NSNA), (V1) 14
  Sigma Theta Tau International (STTI), (V1) 14
  specialty organizations, (V1) 14
Orgasm, (V1) 894, (V1) 894t
Orgasmic disorders, (V1) 901–902
Orientation, promoting, (V1) 805
Orientation in level of consciousness (LOC), (V1) 505, (V2) 273–274p
Orientation phase of communication, (V1) 384–385
Oropharyngeal airways, (V1) 1005, (V1) 1014p
  insertion of, (V2) 744–745p
Oropharynx, (V1) 494, (V1) 494f, (V1) 511p
  assessment of, (V1) 511p, (V2) 234–238p
Orotracheal approach to airway suctioning, (V1) 1007, (V2) 730–733p
Orthopnea, (V1) 465
Orthopneic position, (V1) 870, (V1) 872f
Orthostatic hypotension, (V1) 876
Osmolality, (V1) 1039, (V1) 1053
Osmosis, (V1) 1038–1039, (V1) 1038f
Osmotic pressure, (V1) 1039
Osteoarthritis (OA), (V1) 858
Osteoblasts, (V1) 841
Osteoclasts, (V1) 841
Osteocytes, (V1) 841
Osteogenesis imperfecta (OI), (V1) 857
Osteomyelitis, (V1) 858, (V1) 866
Osteoporosis, (V1) 195, (V1) 496, (V1) 858
  calcium and, (V1) 678
  preventing and treating, (V1) 866–867
  screening for, (V1) 183
Ostomy care, (V1) 775–782, (V1) 778f, (V1) 780–781b
  appliance changing, (V2) 573–576p
  guidelines for, (V2) 584
Otic irrigation, (V2) 596–598p
Otic medications, (V1) 640
  administration of, (V1) 658p, (V2) 403–405p
Otoscopic examination, (V1) 493
Outbreaks, (V1) 520, (V1) 541

Outcomes, patient
  evaluation of, (V1) 23, (V1) 87–89, (V1) 89f
  goals and, (V1) 71–74, (V1) 73t
  related to death and dying, (V1) 362–363
  theory applied to, (V1) 103
Out-of-pocket expenses, (V1) 19
Outpatient care, (V1) 16
Output, in systems theory, (V1) 103
Out-toeing, (V1) 865
Ova (eggs), (V1) 882
Overdosing, (V1) 621
Over-the-counter (OTC) medications and oxygenation, (V1) 982
Over-the-needle catheters, (V1) 1057, (V1) 1057f
Overweight. See Obesity and overweight
Ovulation, (V1) 883
Ovulatory phase, (V1) 883
Oxygen, (V1) 979, (V1) 1011p
  administration of, (V1) 1011p, (V2) 714–718p
  safe, (V1) 1004, (V2) 749
  cardiovascular system transport of, (V1) 1019
  measuring arterial blood, (V1) 997
  transport abnormalities, (V1) 1025
Oxygenated blood, (V1) 1017
Oxygenation, (V1) 444
  See also Respiratory system
  assessment of, (V1) 993–998, (V1) 995b, (V1) 996–998f
  guidelines and tools for, (V2) 751–752
  breathing control, (V1) 979
  critical thinking and clinical judgment on, (V2) 755–756
  developmental stage and, (V1) 980–981
  diagnostic testing of, (V1) 995–998, (V1) 996–998f, (V2) 753
  environment and, (V1) 981–982
  full-spectrum nursing model applied to, (V2) 754–755
  interventions for, (V1) 999–1003, (V1) 1001b, (V1) 1003f
  key concepts on, (V1) 976
  knowledge map on, (V2) 757
  lifestyle and, (V1) 982–983, (V1) 983b
  medications and, (V1) 983–984, (V1) 984t
  nursing diagnosis and, (V1) 999
  pathophysiological conditions altering, (V1) 984–993, (V1) 984t, (V1) 985b
  procedures
    caring for patients requiring mechanical ventilation, (V2) 737–740p
    collecting sputum specimen, (V1) 1011p, (V2) 706–709p
    inserting nasopharyngeal airway, (V2) 746–747p
    inserting oropharyngeal airway, (V2) 744–745p
    orotracheal and nasotracheal suctioning, (V2) 730–733p
    oxygen administration, (V1) 1011p, (V2) 714–718p
    percussion, vibration, and postural drainage, (V2) 712–713p
    pulse oximetry monitoring, (V2) 709–711p
    setting up disposable chest drainage system, (V2) 740–744p
    tracheostomy care using modified sterile technique, (V2) 719–726p

tracheostomy or endotracheal suctioning, (V2) 726–730p
upper airway suctioning, (V2) 734–736p
pulmonary system and
  abnormalities of, (V1) 989
  components of, (V1) 976–977, (V1) 976–977f
  factors influencing, (V1) 980–984, (V1) 983b
  functions of, (V1) 977–979, (V1) 978–979f
  respiration (See Respiration)
  tests of blood, (V1) 1027
Oxygen saturation, (V1) 444, (V1) 466
  sensory function and, (V1) 788
Oxygen therapy, (V1) 1003–1004, (V1) 1003–1004f

P

PACE format, (V1) 438
Pacing in communication, (V1) 377
Paget disease, (V1) 857
Pain
  acute, (V1) 812, (V1) 817, (V1) 821
  assessment of, (V1) 50, (V1) 818–821, (V1) 820t
    guidelines and tools for, (V2) 610–612
  blood pressure and, (V1) 469
  body reaction to, (V1) 817–818, (V1) 818b
  cardiac, (V1) 1026
  cause of, (V1) 812
  chronic, (V1) 812
  client pain relief diary, (V2) 611
  critical thinking and clinical judgment on, (V2) 613–614
  cutaneous or superficial, (V1) 811
  deep somatic, (V1) 811
  defined, (V1) 811
  duration of, (V1) 812
  epidural catheter for, (V2) 609
  evaluation of, (V1) 836
  evidence-based practice on, (V1) 827
  with exercise, (V1) 1032
  factors influencing
    communication and cognitive impairments, (V1) 816–817
    emotions, (V1) 815–816
    life stage, (V1) 816
    sociocultural, (V1) 816
  as fifth vital sign, (V1) 444, (V1) 819
  full-spectrum nursing model applied to, (V2) 613
  gate-control theory of, (V1) 814–815, (V1) 815f, (V1) 824
  as health disruption, (V1) 216
  indicators of, (V1) 817
  in infants and children, (V1) 819
  intensity scales for, (V1) 819
  during intercourse, (V1) 889
  interventions for, (V1) 822–823
    chemical, (V1) 832
    documentation of, (V1) 836
    holistic healing, (V1) 824–826
    nonpharmacological, (V1) 823–824
    in older patients, (V1) 833–834
    patient-controlled analgesia (PCA), (V1) 831–832, (V1) 831f, (V2) 606–608p
    in patients who are difficult to assess, (V1) 819–820
    perception of, (V1) 814

phantom, (V1) 811–812
pharmacological, (V1) 826–835, (V1) 829b, (V1) 831f
PICOT questions for, (V1) 917
placebos for, (V1) 835
postoperative management of, (V1) 1101–1102, (V1) 1102f
previous experience with, (V1) 816
psychogenic, (V1) 812
quality of, (V1) 812–813
radiating, (V1) 811
radiofrequency ablation, (V1) 832
referred, (V1) 811
reflex pain response, (V1) 245
respiration and, (V1) 464
respiratory function and, (V1) 994
at rest, (V1) 1032
self-care ability and, (V1) 577
self-reporting of, (V1) 818–819
sleep and, (V1) 917, (V1) 931
somatic, (V1) 812
somatoform, (V1) 251
spiritual, (V1) 342b, (V1) 342f
surgical interruption of pain conduction pathways, (V1) 832–833
threshold of, (V1) 814
tolerance of, (V1) 814
transduction of, (V1) 813
transmission of, (V1) 813–814, (V1) 813f
unrelieved, (V1) 817–818
visceral, (V1) 811, (V1) 812
what happens with, (V1) 813–815, (V1) 813f, (V1) 815f
wound and tissue, (V1) 958
intractable, (V1) 812
and joy in life, (V1) 234
key concepts on, (V1) 811
knowledge map on, (V2) 615
misconceptions about, (V1) 833, (V1) 833t
modulation of, (V1) 814–815, (V1) 815f
neuropathic, (V1) 812, (V1) 917
nociceptive, (V1) 812
nonverbal signs of, (V1) 820–821, (V2) 610
nursing process for, (V1) 836–839
origin of, (V1) 811–812, (V1) 812f
parenteral medications and, (V1) 648
patient and family teaching about, (V1) 835–836
taking history on, (V2) 610
Pain Assessment in Advanced Dementia (PAINAD) Scale, (V1) 820, (V1) 820t
Pain medications, bowel elimination and, (V1) 759
Pain pumps, (V1) 831, (V1) 831f
Pain scales, (V2) 610–611
Paleo diet, (V1) 691
Palliative care, (V1) 358, (V1) 769
  sedation in, (V1) 361
Palliative surgery, (V1) 1078
Pallor, (V1) 461, (V1) 489t, (V1) 584
Palpation, (V1) 458
  abdomen, (V1) 503, (V2) 263p
  blood pressure, (V1) 473–474
  heart, (V1) 499, (V1) 501
  in physical examination, (V1) 484
  respiratory function, (V1) 993
Pancreas, (V1) 693
Pandemics, (V1) 520, (V1) 541
Panic, (V1) 248, (V1) 249–250, (V1) 278t
Pantothenic acid, (V1) 677t

Paper records, (V1) 425, (V1) 425b, (V2) 163
Paper tape, (V1) 971
Pap smear, (V1) 508
Papule, (V2) 211p
Paradigm, (V1) 95
Paralytic ileus, (V1) 760
Paraplegia, (V1) 864b
Parasomnias, (V1) 927, (V1) 930–931
Parasympathetic fibers, (V1) 1019
Parasympathetic nervous system and pain, (V1) 817
Parental role conflict, (V1) 271
Parenteral medications
  comfort and safety considerations with, (V1) 648
  defined, (V1) 642
  drawing up and mixing, (V1) 645–647, (V1) 646f, (V1) 659–660p, (V1) 659p
  equipment for, (V1) 642–645, (V1) 643–645f, (V1) 643t
  intradermal injections, (V1) 648, (V1) 648–649f
  intramuscular injections, (V1) 651–652f, (V1) 651–654, (V1) 653t, (V1) 660–661p
  preventing needlestick injuries with, (V1) 647, (V1) 647f
  subcutaneous injections, (V1) 649–651, (V1) 649f, (V1) 660p
Parenteral therapy, (V1) 714–715, (V1) 714f
  blood infusions
    autologous donation of blood for, (V1) 1069
    blood groups and, (V1) 1068, (V1) 1068t
    blood products for, (V1) 1069
    blood typing and crossmatching for, (V1) 1068–1069
    changing administration sets for, (V1) 1067
    donating blood for, (V1) 1068
    initiation of, (V1) 1069
    reactions to, (V1) 1069–1070, (V1) 1070t
  central venous access devices, (V1) 1058–1060, (V1) 1059–1060f
  evidence-based practice on, (V1) 1061
  intraosseous devices, (V1) 1060
  intravenous infusions
    complications of, (V1) 1064, (V1) 1065–1067t
    discontinuing, (V1) 1068
    equipment and supplies for starting, (V1) 1060–1063, (V1) 1062f
    regulating and maintaining, (V1) 1063–1067, (V1) 1064b, (V1) 1065–1067t
    solutions, tubing, and dressings for, (V1) 1064
  monitoring patients receiving, (V2) 504
  peripheral vascular access devices, (V1) 1057–1058, (V1) 1057–1058f
  safe use of, (V1) 708
  subcutaneous infusion, (V1) 1060, (V1) 1061f
  types of IV solutions for, (V1) 1056–1057
Paresis, (V1) 864b
Paresthesia, (V1) 864b
Paroxysmal nocturnal dyspnea, (V1) 994
Partial bath, (V1) 585
Partial compensation, (V1) 1051
Partial pressure of oxygen, (V1) 997
Partial-thickness wounds, (V1) 946

Index

Partial thromboplastin time, activated (aPTT), (V2) 700
Passionflower, (V1) 937
Passive aggressive communication style, (V1) 382
Passive communication style, (V1) 382
Passive euthanasia, (V1) 361
Passive range of motion (PROM), (V1) 845, (V1) 876
Passive relaxation, (V1) 260
Passive resistance, (V1) 1193
Passive thermal care, (V1) 1086
Passive transport, (V1) 1038–1039, (V1) 1038–1039f
Passwords, (V1) 1149–1150, (V1) 1150b
Pastes, (V1) 613t
Paternalism, (V1) 130, (V1) 130f
Pathogens, (V1) 517
  CDC guidelines for preventing transmission of, (V1) 534–536, (V1) 535t, (V1) 536f
  cellular immunity and, (V1) 524
  exposure to bloodborne, (V1) 540, (V1) 540b
  food-borne, (V1) 550
  vector-borne, (V1) 550
Patient benefit model, (V1) 138
Patient Care Partnership (PCP), (V1) 132, (V1) 132b, (V1) 138, (V1) 397, (V1) 1162
Patient care summary, (V1) 435
Patient-controlled analgesia (PCA), (V1) 831–832, (V1) 831f, (V2) 606–608p
Patient education
  about clean, intermittent self-catheterization, (V2) 544
  about sexual health, (V1) 904–907
  assessment of, (V1) 408
    guidelines and tools for, (V2) 150–151
  barriers to, (V1) 406–408
  on blood pressure, (V2) 192p, (V2) 194
  on body temperature, (V2) 178p
  bowel elimination problems, (V1) 768
  cardiovascular system, (V1) 1032–1033
  for children, (V1) 403, (V1) 405
  on cleaning and storing contact lenses, (V1) 600
  community nursing, (V1) 1115
  condom use, (V2) 641
  creating teaching materials for, (V1) 417, (V1) 418f
  critical thinking and clinical judgment on, (V2) 152–153
  culture and, (V1) 316, (V1) 405, (V1) 406b
  documentation of, (V1) 418
  evaluation of learning in, (V1) 417–418
  evidence-based practice in, (V1) 407
  factors affecting
    active involvement, (V1) 400
    amount and complexity of content, (V1) 401–402
    communication, (V1) 402
    cultural, (V1) 405
    developmental stage, (V1) 402
    feedback, (V1) 400
    health literacy, (V1) 405–406
    learning environment, (V1) 400–401, (V1) 401b
    motivation, (V1) 399–400
    readiness, (V1) 400
    repetition, (V1) 400
    in special populations, (V1) 402
    timing, (V1) 400
  five rights of teaching and, (V1) 397b
  on food safety, (V1) 570, (V1) 571
  foot care, (V1) 590
  formats for, (V1) 415–416t
  full-spectrum nursing model applied to, (V2) 151
  general tips for effective, (V1) 410
  grief, (V1) 367
  home healthcare, (V1) 1124, (V1) 1131–1132
  on hypertension, (V2) 194
  interventions for
    selecting specific teaching strategies, (V1) 411, (V1) 417
    teaching plans, (V1) 409–414, (V1) 410t, (V1) 411f
  key concepts on, (V1) 396
  knowledge map on, (V2) 155
  learning occurring in three domains and, (V1) 398–399, (V1) 398t, (V1) 399f
  learning theories in, (V1) 397–398
  medication self-administration, (V1) 632–633
  minimizing malpractice risks, (V1) 1175
  on motor vehicle safety, (V1) 567, (V1) 567–568t
  nail care, (V1) 591
  nurses' teaching responsibilities for, (V1) 396–397
  nursing diagnoses and, (V1) 408–409
  for older adults, (V1) 203, (V1) 402–403, (V1) 403–405t
  oral hygiene, (V1) 595–596, (V1) 595f
  on pain, (V1) 835–836
  planning for, (V1) 409
  postoperative, (V1) 1102–1103
  preoperative, (V1) 1085–1086, (V2) 825
  on preventing fluid and electrolyte imbalances, (V1) 1054
  on prevention of infections, (V1) 531
  safety self-care, (V1) 567–571
  on sleep, (V1) 935–937
  on speaking up, (V1) 374, (V1) 374b
  stages of cognitive development and, (V1) 402–408, (V1) 403–405t, (V1) 406b
  on vector-borne pathogens, (V1) 568, (V1) 570
  on vitamin and mineral supplementation, (V1) 700–701
  on walking aids, (V2) 630–631
  on weather hazards, (V1) 570–571
  who are the learners in, (V1) 396
Patient Health Questionnaire (PHQ-9), (V2) 94
Patient Protection and Affordable Care Act of 2010, (V1) 405, (V1) 545
Patient rounding, (V1) 384
Patients. See Clients
Patient Self-Determination Act (PSDA), (V1) 359, (V1) 1159–1160, (V1) 1159b
Patient sensitivity drug reactions, (V1) 621
Patronizing language, (V1) 391
Peak flow monitoring, (V1) 998, (V1) 998f, (V1) 999
Pedal pulse, (V1) 460
Pediculosis, (V1) 490, (V1) 598
Peer relationships/friendships
  among adolescents, (V1) 171–172
  among school-age children, (V1) 168, (V1) 168f
  self-concept and, (V1) 267–268
Pelvic inflammatory disease (PID), (V1) 897
Pender's Health Promotion Model (HPM), (V1) 221, (V1) 221f
Penetrating injury, (V1) 788, (V1) 945t
Penicillin, (V1) 624
Penis, (V1) 883, (V1) 884f, (V1) 893
Penrose drains, (V1) 965, (V1) 965f
Peplau, Hildegard, (V1) 99
Peppermint, (V1) 786
Pepsin, (V1) 754
Perceived loss, (V1) 348
Perception
  See also Sensation
  assessment of, (V2) 599–601
  critical thinking and clinical judgment on, (V2) 602–603
  defined, (V1) 784
  developmental influences on, (V1) 212
  full-spectrum nursing model applied to, (V2) 601–602
  knowledge map on, (V2) 604
  pain, (V1) 814
  of stimuli, (V1) 784
Percussion, (V1) 484, (V2) 297, (V2) 712–713p
  abdomen, (V1) 503
  chest, (V1) 1003, (V1) 1011p
  respiratory function, (V1) 993
Percutaneous electrical stimulation (PENS), (V1) 824
Percutaneous endoscopic gastrostomy tube (PEG), (V1) 708, (V1) 709f
Perfusion, (V1) 444
  defined, (V1) 1017
  pathophysiological conditions and, (V1) 1024–1025
Perimenopausal symptoms, (V1) 181
Perineal care, (V1) 587, (V1) 602p, (V2) 352–355p
Perineal surgery, (V1) 760
Periodic feedings, (V1) 713
Periodicity, pain, (V1) 812
Periodic limb movement disorder (PLMD), (V1) 925
Periodontal disease, (V1) 592, (V1) 593, (V1) 595
Perioperative nursing, (V1) 1076–1077, (V1) 1076b
Perioperative Nursing Data Set (PNDS), (V1) 62, (V1) 1081
Perioperative Patient-Focused Model, (V1) 1081
Peripheral arterial disease, (V1) 1032
Peripheral chemoreceptors, (V1) 463
Peripheral circulation
  assessment of, (V1) 1026
  host susceptibility to infection and, (V1) 529
  prior to death, (V1) 357
Peripheral intravenous infusion
  discontinuing, (V2) 790–791p
  initiation of, (V2) 769–774p
  lock for, (V1) 1058, (V1) 1058f, (V1) 1067–1068, (V1) 1072–1073p
  site selection for, (V1) 1062
Peripherally inserted central catheters (PICCs), (V1) 657, (V1) 1059, (V1) 1059f
  caring for patient with, (V2) 801–802

Peripheral nerve block, (V1) 1091
Peripheral nerve catheter, (V1) 831
Peripheral pulses, (V1) 452p, (V1) 459
    assessment of, (V2) 179–183p
Peripheral resistance and blood pressure, (V1) 468–469
Peripheral vascular access devices, (V1) 1057–1058, (V1) 1057–1058f
    procedure for initiating, (V1) 1071p
Peripheral venipuncture site selection, (V2) 800
Peripheral vessels, (V1) 502
    abnormalities of, (V1) 1025
Peripheral vision, (V1) 492
Peristalsis, (V1) 693
Peritubular capillaries, (V1) 718
Periwound area, (V1) 953
Permanent bowel diversions, (V1) 761
Permanent drug reactions, (V1) 622
PERRLA, (V1) 492
Perseverance, intellectual, (V1) 37
Persistent vegetative state, (V1) 356
Peristalsis, (V1) 756
Personal and sociocultural factors
    bowel elimination, (V1) 758
    physical activity and, (V1) 856
    urinary elimination, (V1) 722–723
Personal appearance, (V1) 379
Personal distance, (V1) 381, (V1) 381f
Personal identity, (V1) 269
    in general survey, (V1) 487
Personality
    age-related changes in, (V1) 194t
    in preschoolers, (V1) 165
    sensory function and, (V1) 788
Personal presence, (V1) 104
Personal protective equipment (PPE), (V1) 535, (V1) 536f, (V1) 539p
    donning, (V2) 305–307p
    removing, (V2) 307–309p
Personal relationships, impact on health and wellness, (V1) 213–214, (V1) 214t
Personal space, (V1) 315, (V1) 327b
    communication and, (V1) 381, (V1) 381f
Personal values, (V1) 125, (V1) 314
Personhood, honoring, (V1) 104, (V1) 204
Petechiae, (V1) 489t
Phagocytosis, (V1) 521, (V1) 522t, (V1) 947
Phallic stage, in psychoanalytic theory, (V1) 147t, (V1) 165–166
PH and drug absorption, (V1) 616
Phantom pain, (V1) 811–812
Pharmacists, (V1) 18
Pharmacodynamics
    defined, (V1) 619
    primary effects, (V1) 619–621
    secondary effects, (V1) 621–623, (V1) 621b, (V1) 622t, (V1) 623f
Pharmacogenomics, (V1) 195
Pharmacokinetics
    defined, (V1) 611, (V1) 611f
    drug distribution throughout the body, (V1) 616–617
    drug effectiveness, (V1) 618–619, (V1) 618f
    drug excretion from the body, (V1) 617–618
    drug metabolism in the body, (V1) 617
    factors affecting, (V1) 619, (V1) 620f
    factors affecting drug absorption, (V1) 611–616, (V1) 612f–615t

Pharmacopoeia, (V1) 608
Pharyngeal airway, (V1) 1005
Pharynx, (V1) 754, (V1) 754f, (V1) 977
Phenomena, (V1) 94
Phlebitis, as complication of intravenous therapy, (V1) 1065t
PH measurement, (V1) 1045, (V1) 1049f
Phosphate electrolytes, (V1) 1043t, (V1) 1044
Phosphate system, (V1) 1045
Phospholipids, (V1) 671
Phosphorus, (V1) 679t
Photoreceptors, (V1) 784
Photosensitivity, (V1) 943
Physiatrists, (V1) 18
Physical activity
    See also Exercise
    adapted physical activity (APA) programs, (V1) 191
    in adolescents, (V1) 177–178
    assessment of, (V2) 632–633
    benefits of regular, (V1) 853, (V1) 855b
    blood pressure and, (V1) 469
    body mechanics and, (V1) 844–845, (V1) 844f, (V1) 845f, (V1) 846–851t
    body temperature and, (V1) 449
    bowel elimination and, (V1) 758, (V1) 768
    critical thinking and clinical judgment on, (V2) 635
    defined, (V1) 851
    diseases and abnormalities and, (V1) 857–860, (V1) 858f, (V1) 860f
    factors affecting, (V1) 855–860, (V1) 858f, (V1) 860f
    full-spectrum nursing model applied to, (V2) 634
    guidelines for Americans, (V1) 852b
    host susceptibility to infection and, (V1) 529, (V1) 533
    influence on health, (V1) 213
    key concepts on, (V1) 841
    knowledge map on, (V2) 637
    in middle adulthood, (V1) 183
    by middle-old adults, (V1) 191
    by older adults, (V1) 183, (V1) 202, (V1) 203, (V1) 857
    physiology of movement and, (V1) 841–844, (V1) 842–843f, (V1) 843t
    PICOT questions for, (V1) 203
    pulse rate and, (V1) 457
    recommendations for health promotion, (V1) 231, (V1) 231f
    respiration and, (V1) 463
    in school-age children, (V1) 170
    skin and, (V1) 944
    sleep and, (V1) 923
    stress and, (V1) 258–259, (V1) 260
    wound assessment and, (V1) 953
    in young adults, (V1) 180
    in young-older adults, (V1) 202
Physical development
    adolescent, (V1) 171, (V1) 171b
    infant, (V1) 156, (V1) 157b
    middle adulthood, (V1) 181
    neonate, (V1) 152–154, (V1) 152–154f
    older adults, (V1) 191
    preschooler, (V1) 164–165, (V1) 165b
    school-age children, (V1) 167, (V1) 167b
    toddler, (V1) 162, (V1) 162f, (V1) 163b
    young adult, (V1) 179

Physical disease, as health disruption, (V1) 215
Physical examination, (V1) 50–52, (V1) 51t, (V1) 226, (V1) 421
    abdomen, (V1) 502–503, (V1) 503f, (V1) 510
    adolescent, (V1) 176–177
    bowel elimination, (V1) 763, (V1) 763–764t, (V2) 585
    breasts and axillae, (V1) 495–496, (V1) 495f, (V1) 510
    cardiovascular system, (V1) 496–499, (V1) 509, (V1) 1026
    chest and lungs, (V1) 496, (V1) 497–499f, (V1) 499–500f
    documenting findings of, (V1) 509–513
    ears and hearing, (V1) 493–494, (V1) 493f, (V1) 509
    eyes, (V1) 491–493, (V1) 492f, (V1) 509
    fluids, electrolytes, and acid-base balance, (V2) 803–804
    general survey, (V1) 486–488, (V1) 487f, (V1) 509, (V1) 510p, (V2) 200–205p
    genitourinary system, (V1) 507–508, (V1) 510
    head, (V1) 491–493, (V1) 492f, (V1) 509
    heart, (V1) 499–501, (V1) 501f, (V1) 501t
    for infections, (V1) 530
    integumentary system, (V1) 488–491, (V1) 489t
    knowledge map on, (V2) 301
    for medication administration, (V1) 631
    mobility and exercise, (V1) 864–865
    modifications in
        for clients with disabilities, (V1) 486
        for different-age groups, (V1) 485–486
    mouth and oropharynx, (V1) 494, (V1) 494f, (V1) 509
    musculoskeletal system, (V1) 504, (V1) 504f, (V1) 510
    neck, (V1) 495, (V1) 509
    neurological system, (V1) 505–507, (V1) 506t, (V1) 507f, (V1) 510
    nose, (V1) 494, (V1) 494f, (V1) 509
    nutritional assessment, (V1) 696, (V2) 507
    oxygenation, (V2) 752
    positioning the client for, (V1) 481, (V1) 482–484t
    preparing to perform, (V1) 480–481
    purposes of, (V1) 479
    respiratory function, (V1) 993–995, (V1) 995b
    sensory system, (V1) 802–803
    sexual health assessment, (V1) 902
    techniques in
        auscultation, (V1) 484
        inspection, (V1) 481
        olfaction, (V1) 484
        palpation, (V1) 484
        percussion, (V1) 484
    throat, (V1) 509
    types of, (V1) 479
    urinary elimination, (V2) 546
    wound assessment, (V1) 952–953, (V1) 954–956t, (V1) 956–958, (V1) 957t, (V2) 695
Physical fitness assessment, (V1) 226–227, (V2) 72
Physical loss, (V1) 348
Physical therapists (PTs), (V1) 18
Physician assistants (PAs), (V1) 18

Physicians, (V1) 18
    shortage of, (V1) 1141
Physician's Desk Reference (PDR), (V1) 608
Physiological needs, (V1) 100, (V1) 102f
    during active dying, (V1) 365
Physiological stages of dying, (V1) 356–357
Physiological stressors, (V1) 239
Physiology of movement, (V1) 841–844, (V1) 842–843f, (V1) 843t
Piaget, Jean, (V1) 147, (V1) 148t, (V1) 154, (V1) 165, (V1) 402
PICOT questions
    acupuncture for neuropathic pain, (V1) 917
    alcohol treatment and family support, (V1) 296
    constipation in pregnancy, (V1) 760
    early treatment of metabolic acidosis, (V1) 1052
    fluid balance, (V1) 682
    formulating searchable questions and, (V1) 110
    health promotion, (V1) 232
    infections, (V1) 517
    medication safety, (V1) 628
    older adults, comorbidity, and risk for surgical site infection, (V1) 1080
    physical activity and well-being of older adults, (V1) 203
    sensory overload in the ICU, (V1) 793
    sexuality, dementia, and competency, (V1) 901
    skin care for pressure injury
        and effect of nutritional support on healing, (V1) 942
        in frail, older woman, (V1) 111
Piercings, (V1) 172, (V1) 944
Pillows, (V1) 869, (V1) 869f
Piloerection, (V1) 447
Pinworms, (V1) 765
Piston syringe, (V1) 964
Pitch in communication, (V1) 377
Placebos for pain relief, (V1) 835
Planning in nursing process, (V1) 47, (V1) 65–67
    cultural competence and, (V1) 324–325
    documentation in, (V1) 420
    health promotion and, (V1) 229–230
    interventions, (V1) 74–75
        using standardized language, (V1) 78–80, (V1) 79b
    patient care, (V1) 67–71, (V1) 68f, (V1) 70f
    patient education, (V1) 409
    patient goals/outcomes, (V1) 71–74, (V1) 73t
    types of, (V1) 66
Plan of care. *See* Care plans
Plantar warts, (V1) 589
Plaque, (V1) 593
Plasma, (V1) 1019, (V1) 1040
    for transfusion, (V1) 1069
Plasma derivatives, for transfusion, (V1) 1069
Plateau, in sexual response cycle, (V1) 894, (V1) 894t
Platelet-derived growth factor, (V1) 949
Platelets, for transfusion, (V1) 1069
Play, infant, (V1) 161
Pleading, (V1) 1169
Pleural membrane, (V1) 978
PLISSIT model, (V1) 907

Pneumonia, (V1) 989, (V1) 990–992
    evidence-based practice on, (V1) 1008
    immunization for, (V1) 1001
    as postoperative complication, (V1) 1098t
    ventilator-assisted, (V1) 532, (V1) 1008–1009
Pneumothorax, (V1) 1009
Poisoning, (V1) 548
    carbon monoxide, (V1) 548, (V1) 564
    food, (V1) 550
    mercury, (V1) 555, (V1) 555t, (V1) 572, (V1) 573b
    in preschoolers, (V1) 166
    prevention of, (V1) 563, (V1) 564
Politics/law and culture, (V1) 316
Pollution, (V1) 550–551, (V1) 570
    physical activity and, (V1) 856
Polypharmacy, (V1) 195, (V1) 198, (V1) 631
Polysaccharides, (V1) 669
Polysomnography, (V1) 932
Polyunsaturated fatty acids, (V1) 672, (V1) 672t
Polyvinyl chloride (PVC) catheters, (V1) 735
Popliteal artery pulse, (V1) 460, (V2) 182p
Population(s)
    age distribution, (V1) 187, (V1) 188f
    aging of, (V1) 24
    biological variations in, (V2) 109
    census data on, (V1) 1110–1111, (V1) 1111f
    diversity of, (V1) 121, (V1) 309–310, (V1) 310b
    life expectancy and, (V1) 186
    migration and distribution of, (V1) 187
    racial diversity of, (V1) 186–187
    vulnerable, (V1) 314, (V1) 1112–1113
Portal of entry, infection, (V1) 519
Portal of exit, infection, (V1) 517
Port wine stains, (V1) 941
Position, body
    for bed-bound patients, (V1) 871–872t
    blood pressure and, (V1) 469
    for bowel elimination, (V1) 767
    devices for, (V1) 868–870, (V1) 869–870f
    dyspnea and, (V1) 994
    for maximum ventilation, (V1) 1002
    for mobility interventions, (V1) 867–873, (V1) 869–870f, (V1) 871–872t
    moving patients in bed, (V1) 873, (V1) 873f
    for physical examination, (V1) 481, (V1) 482–484t
    pulse rate and, (V1) 457
    respiration and, (V1) 464
    for surgery, (V1) 1094
    techniques for, (V1) 870–873, (V1) 871–872t
    for urinary elimination, (V1) 731–732
Positive inotropic agents, (V1) 1023t, (V1) 1033
Positive nitrogen balance, (V1) 671
Positive pressure ventilators, (V1) 1008, (V1) 1008f
Positive self-talk, (V1) 262, (V1) 375
Postanesthesia care unit (PACU), (V1) 1095–1096
    assessment in, (V2) 830
    nursing care in, (V1) 1096–1097, (V1) 1096b
Postconventional, autonomous, or principled stage, in moral development theory, (V1) 149
Posterior chest, (V1) 496
Posterior tibial artery pulse, (V1) 460, (V2) 182p

Postmortem care, (V1) 367, (V2) 130–131
    autopsy in, (V1) 361
Postoperative care
    antiembolism stockings and sequential compression devices, (V1) 1103–1104, (V1) 1104p
    assessment of, (V1) 1097
    gastrointestinal suction, (V1) 1104, (V1) 1105p
    incentive spirometry, (V1) 1103, (V1) 1103f
    interventions in, (V1) 1098–1101t, (V1) 1098–1104
    nursing care in PACU, (V1) 1096–1097, (V1) 1096b
    nursing diagnosis and, (V1) 1097
    pain management in, (V1) 1101–1102, (V1) 1102f
    patient teaching in, (V1) 1102–1103
    potential complications, (V1) 1098, (V1) 1098–1101t
    preparing room for patient's return from surgery, (V2) 826
    recovery from anesthesia, (V1) 1095–1096, (V1) 1096b
    recovery from surgery, (V1) 1096
    recovery rooms, (V1) 1089, (V1) 1095, (V1) 1095f
Postpartum patients, physical activity guidelines for, (V1) 852b
Post-term fetus, (V1) 150
Post-trauma syndrome, (V1) 271
Post-traumatic stress disorder (PTSD), (V1) 254, (V1) 255–256
Postural drainage, (V1) 1003, (V1) 1003f, (V1) 1011p, (V2) 712–713p
Posture, (V1) 379
    body alignment and, (V1) 844, (V1) 844f
Postvoid residual urine volume with portable bladder scanner, (V2) 517–519p
Potable tap water, (V1) 963
Potassium, (V1) 679–680t
    electrolytes, (V1) 1042t, (V1) 1043
Powders, (V1) 612t
Power, sources of, (V1) 1189–1190
PPE. *See* Personal protective equipment (PPE)
Practical boundaries of nursing, (V1) 9
Practical knowledge, (V1) 30
    ethical decision making and, (V1) 140
Practical nursing education, (V1) 10–11
Practices
    definition of, (V1) 314
    health and illness, (V1) 318
Practice theory, (V1) 98
Prayer, (V1) 333, (V1) 344, (V1) 344f
    with clients, (V2) 120
    in holistic healing, (V1) 345
    types of, (V2) 119
Prealbumin, (V1) 698
Preceptors, (V1) 1186–1187
Preconceptual phase, (V1) 162
Preconventional stage, in moral development theory, (V1) 148
Preexisting conditions and surgery, (V1) 1079, (V1) 1079b
Preferred provider organizations (PPOs), (V1) 22

Prefilled unit-dose systems, (V2) 454
Pregnancy
  See also Gestation
  adolescent, (V1) 151, (V1) 176, (V1) 178, (V1) 299
  bowel elimination during, (V1) 760
  cardiovascular function during, (V1) 1021–1022
  constipation in, (V1) 760
  Emergency Medical Treatment and Active Labor Act (EMTALA) and, (V1) 1158
  fetal development during, (V1) 149–150, (V2) 48–49
  maternal age effects on, (V1) 151
  maternal changes during, (V1) 150
  maternal health effects on, (V1) 151
  maternal nutrition effects on, (V1) 151, (V1) 151*f*
  menstrual cycle and, (V1) 883
  nutrition in, (V1) 686
  oral problems with, (V1) 593
  oxygenation and, (V1) 982
  pharmacokinetics and, (V1) 619
  physical activity guidelines for, (V1) 852*b*
  prenatal visits during, (V1) 151–152
  screening during, (V1) 151–152
Preinteraction phase of communication, (V1) 384
Prejudice, (V1) 321
Premature ejaculation, (V1) 902
Premature infants, pulmonary function in, (V1) 980
Premenstrual dysphoric disorder (PMDD), (V1) 897
Premenstrual syndrome (PMS), (V1) 897, (V1) 905–906
Prenatal visits, (V1) 151–152
Preoperational stage, in cognitive development theory, (V1) 148*t*, (V1) 402
Preoperative care
  assessment in, (V1) 1081–1082, (V1) 1093
  guidelines and tools for, (V2) 827–828
  classification of surgeries and, (V1) 1077–1078
  diagnostic testing in, (V2) 830
  interventions in, (V1) 1083–1084, (V1) 1094–1095
    communication with surgical team, (V1) 1088–1089
    confirm that surgical consent has been obtained, (V1) 1084–1085
    measures to prevent wrong patient, wrong site, wrong surgery, (V1) 1088
    preoperative teaching, (V1) 1085–1086, (V2) 825
    preparing the patient physically for surgery, (V1) 1086–1088, (V1) 1087*t*, (V1) 1088*f*
    preparing the postoperative room, (V1) 1089
    transferring patient to operative suite, (V1) 1089, (V1) 1089*f*
  nursing diagnosis in, (V1) 1082–1083, (V1) 1084*t*, (V1) 1093
  perioperative nursing data set (PNDS), (V1) 62, (V1) 1081
  surgical risk factors and, (V1) 1078–1081, (V1) 1079*b*, (V1) 1079*t*, (V1) 1080*b*

Prepackaged bathing products, (V1) 585
Preparing, drawing up, and mixing medications, (V1) 659–660*p*, (V2) 417–425*p*
Preschoolers
  abuse, neglect, and violence involving, (V1) 166
  assessment of, (V1) 166
  cardiovascular function in, (V1) 1020
  common health problems in, (V1) 166
  communicable diseases in, (V1) 166
  communication by, (V1) 380
  development of
    cognitive, (V1) 165
    physical, (V1) 164–165, (V1) 165*b*
    psychosocial, (V1) 165–166, (V1) 165*f*
  development of sexuality in, (V1) 886–887
  enuresis in, (V1) 166
  implementation for, (V1) 166–167
  loss in, (V1) 348
  neurological system examination in, (V1) 505
  nutrition in, (V1) 685
  physical activity guidelines for, (V1) 852*b*
  physical examination of, (V1) 485
  poisoning in, (V1) 166
  pulmonary function in, (V1) 980
  safety of, (V1) 546–547
  sleep requirements and characteristics in, (V1) 918*t*, (V1) 923
  surgical risk in, (V1) 1078
Prescriptions, (V1) 625, (V1) 625*f*
  abbreviations used in, (V1) 625
  communication of, (V1) 626, (V1) 626*b*
  oxygenation and, (V1) 982
  questioning of, (V1) 439
  receiving and documenting verbal and telephone, (V1) 438–439, (V2) 159
  types of, (V1) 625–626
  what to do about incorrect, (V1) 626–627
Presence, as spiritual intervention, (V1) 343
Pressure injuries, (V1) 111, (V1) 582, (V1) 946*t*
  altered level of consciousness and, (V1) 805
  Braden Scale for Predicting Pressure Sore Risk, (V2) 696
  care plan for, (V1) 960–963
  foot, (V1) 589
  Norton Pressure Sore Risk Assessment Scale, (V2) 697
  in patients with morbid obesity, (V1) 588
  PICOT questions on, (V1) 942
  pressure ulcer healing chart, (V2) 699
  PUSH Tool for Evaluation of Pressure Ulcers, (V2) 698
  skin integrity and, (V1) 951–952, (V1) 951–952*f*
Pretrial motions, (V1) 1169
Prevention, levels of, (V1) 220
Previous experience
  with pain, (V1) 816
  with stimuli, (V1) 786
Primary cardiomyopathy, (V1) 1024
Primary defense against infections, (V1) 521
  breaks in, (V1) 525
Primary dressings, (V1) 971, (V1) 971*f*
Primary effects, drug, (V1) 619–621
Primary infections, (V1) 519
Primary (first) intention healing, (V1) 946, (V1) 947*f*

Primary nursing, (V1) 16
Primary prevention, (V1) 220
Primary services, (V1) 18
Primary skin lesions, (V1) 490
Printed materials, for patient teaching, (V1) 411
Prioritization of problems, (V1) 59–60
Prioritizing hypotheses and generating solutions. *See* Planning in nursing process
Privacy and confidentiality, (V1) 129
  bowel elimination and, (V1) 758, (V1) 767
  electronic communications, (V1) 1140
  electronic health records (EHRs), (V1) 1147, (V1) 1149–1150, (V1) 1149*f*
  invasion of privacy law, (V1) 1167
  laws regulating, (V1) 1157–1158
  minimizing malpractice risks, (V1) 1175
  in physical examination, (V1) 480
  social networking, (V1) 1140–1141
  urinary elimination and, (V1) 722, (V1) 731
Private insurance, (V1) 19, (V1) 19*f*
  home healthcare, (V1) 1126
Prn prescription, (V1) 626
Probiotics, (V1) 759
  for pain management, (V1) 823
Problem-intervention-evaluation (PIE) system, (V1) 427
Problem list, (V1) 422, (V1) 422*f*
Problem-oriented record (POR) systems, (V1) 422, (V1) 422*f*
Problem-solving, (V1) 8
  by older adults, (V1) 299
Procedural justice, (V1) 131
Procedures
  abdomen assessment, (V2) 257–263*p*
  adding medications to IV fluids, (V1) 661*p*, (V2) 440–441*p*
  administering feedings through gastric and enteric tubes, (V2) 488–492*p*
  admitting patient to nursing unit, (V1) 236*p*, (V2) 60–62*p*
  airway suctioning, (V1) 1012–1013*p*
  anus and rectum assessment, (V2) 294–295*p*
  apical pulse, (V2) 179–183*p*
  apical-radial pulse deficit, (V1) 452*p*, (V2) 186–187*p*
  applying and removing transparent film dressing, (V2) 676–678*p*
  applying antiembolism stockings, (V2) 815–817*p*
  applying bandages, (V2) 684–687*p*
  applying binders, (V2) 682–684*p*
  applying external (condom) urinary catheter, (V2) 535–537*p*
  applying hydrating dressing, (V2) 678–680*p*
  applying sequential compression devices, (V1) 1104*p*, (V2) 817–819*p*
  assessing for abuse, (V1) 161*p*, (V2) 43–47*p*
  assisting with ambulation, (V2) 625–628*p*
  assisting with percutaneous central venous catheter placement, (V2) 795–797*p*
  bathing, (V1) 602*p*
    providing a complete bed bath using prepacked bathing product, (V2) 346–351*p*
    using a basin and water, (V2) 351–352*p*
  beard and mustache care, (V1) 602*p*, (V2) 369–370*p*

bed and chair monitoring devices, (V1) 573p, (V2) 332–334p
bed making
  occupied, (V1) 603p, (V2) 380–382p
  unoccupied, (V1) 603p, (V2) 377–380p
blood pressure measurement, (V2) 189–193p
body temperature, (V2) 173–179p
bowel elimination, (V1) 779–780
breast and axillae assessment, (V1) 511p, (V2) 240–243p
brief bedside assessment, (V1) 513p, (V2) 295–296p
brushing and flossing, (V1) 602p, (V2) 358–361p
cardiac monitoring, (V1) 1035, (V2) 759–761p
caring for artificial eyes, (V2) 374–375p, (V2) 603p
caring for hearing aids, (V2) 375–377p, (V2) 603p
changing IV dressings, (V2) 783–787p
changing IV solutions and tubing, (V2) 779–782p
checking fingerstick blood glucose levels, (V2) 480–483p
chest and lungs assessment, (V2) 244–250p
chest drainage, (V1) 1014p
colostomy irrigation, (V2) 577–579p
denture care, (V1) 602p, (V2) 361–363p
discharge from healthcare facility, (V1) 237p, (V2) 66–68p
discontinuing peripheral IV, (V2) 790–791p
emptying a closed-wound drainage system, (V2) 691–692p
enema administration, (V2) 565–569p
eye assessment, (V1) 603p, (V2) 220–227p
female genitourinary system, (V2) 290–293p
foot care, (V1) 602p, (V2) 355–358p
general survey, (V1) 510p, (V2) 200–205p
hair assessment, (V2) 215–216p
hand hygiene, (V1) 539p, (V2) 303–304p
head and face assessment, (V2) 218–219p
hearing aid care, (V1) 603p
hearing assessment, (V1) 511p, (V2) 227–231p
heart and vascular system assessment, (V2) 250–257p
host susceptibility to infection and, (V1) 529p
initiating a peripheral intravenous infusion, (V2) 769–774p
inserting indwelling urinary catheter, (V2) 529–535p
inserting intermittent urinary catheter, (V2) 523–528p
intermittent infusion, (V1) 661p, (V2) 446–449p
intradermal injections, (V2) 428–430p
intradermal medication, (V2) 428–430p
intramuscular injections, (V1) 660–661p, (V2) 434–440p
irrigating bladder or catheter, (V2) 540–543p
IV push medications, (V1) 661p, (V2) 441–446p
lipid administration, (V2) 498–500p
male genitourinary system assessment, (V2) 285–289p
measuring postvoid residual urine volume with portable bladder scanner, (V2) 517–519p

mechanical ventilation, (V1) 1014p
medication administration through central venous access device (CVAD), (V2) 450–453p
metered-dose inhaler (MDI) medication, (V1) 659p, (V2) 415–417p
metered-dose inhalers (MDIs), (V1) 659p, (V2) 415–417p
mobility and physical activity, (V1) 879–880p
mouth and oropharynx assessment, (V1) 511p, (V2) 234–238p
moving and turning patients in bed, (V2) 617–621p
nail assessment, (V2) 216–218p
nasal, (V2) 405–407p
nasal medication administration, (V2) 405–407p
nasogastric and nasoenteric tubes
  insertion, (V2) 483–487p
  removal, (V2) 493–494p
nasopharyngeal airway insertion, (V2) 746–747p
neck assessment, (V2) 238–240p
negative pressure wound therapy (NPWT) device, (V2) 671–676p
nose and sinuses assessment, (V1) 511p, (V2) 232–234p
obtaining a urine specimen for testing, (V2) 519–523p
ophthalmic, (V1) 658p, (V2) 400–403p
ophthalmic medication administration, (V1) 658p, (V2) 400–403p
oral, (V2) 396–400p
oral care, (V1) 602–603p
  for unconscious patients, (V1) 602p, (V2) 363–366p
oral medication administration, (V1) 658p, (V2) 396–400p
oral problems with, (V1) 594
oropharyngeal airway insertion, (V2) 744–745p
orotracheal and nasotracheal suctioning, (V2) 730–733p
ostomy appliance changing, (V2) 573–576p
otic, (V1) 658p, (V2) 403–405p
otic irrigation, (V2) 596–598p
otic medication administration, (V1) 658p, (V2) 403–405p
oxygen administration, (V1) 1011p, (V2) 714–718p
parenteral therapy, (V1) 1071–1073p, (V2) 494–498p
percussion, vibration, and postural drainage, (V2) 712–713p
perineal care, (V1) 602p, (V2) 352–355p
peripheral intravenous infusion, (V1) 1071p
peripheral pulse, (V2) 179–183p
personal protective equipment (PPE)
  donning, (V2) 305–307p
  removing, (V2) 307–309p
placing and removing bedpans, (V2) 562–565p
placing fecal drainage devices, (V2) 579–582p
postoperative, (V1) 1104p
preparing, drawing up, and mixing medications, (V1) 659–660p, (V2) 417–425p

providing a complete bed bath using prepacked bathing product, (V2) 346–351p
pulse oximetry, (V1) 1011p, (V2) 709–711p
recapping needles using one-handed technique, (V1) 660p, (V2) 426–428p
recapping of needles, (V1) 426–428p, (V1) 660p
rectal, (V1) 659p, (V2) 409–412p
rectal medication administration, (V1) 659p, (V2) 409–412p
rectal tube insertion, (V2) 571–572p
regulating IV flow rate, (V2) 775–776p
removing and applying dry dressings, (V2) 666–668p
removing and caring for contact lenses, (V2) 372–373p, (V2) 603p
removing indwelling catheter, (V2) 537–539p
removing stool digitally, (V2) 569–571p
removing sutures and staples, (V2) 688–689p
respiration assessment, (V1) 452p, (V2) 187–189p
restraints, (V1) 573p, (V2) 334–337p
selection of peripheral venipuncture site, (V2) 800
sensory-neurological system assessment, (V2) 272–285p
setting up and using volume-control pumps, (V2) 777–779p
setting up disposable chest drainage systems, (V2) 740–744p
shampooing the hair, (V1) 602p, (V2) 366–369p
shaving a patient, (V2) 370–372p, (V2) 602–603p
shortening a wound drain, (V2) 690–691p
skin assessment, (V2) 206–210p
skin closures, (V2) 680–681p
skin medication administration, (V1) 659p, (V2) 412–414p
sputum specimen, (V1) 1011p, (V2) 706–709p
steps for all, (V2) 392–396p
steps to follow for all medications, (V2) 392–396p
sterile fields, (V1) 539p, (V2) 318–320p
sterile gown and gloves, (V1) 539p
  closed method, (V2) 314–3153p
  open method, (V2) 316–317p
subcutaneous injections, (V1) 660p, (V2) 431–434p
surgical hand washing, (V1) 539p
  brushless system, (V2) 311–313p
  traditional method, (V2) 309–311p
teaching patient to deep-breathe, cough, move in bed, and perform leg exercises, (V2) 811–814p
testing stool for occult blood, (V2) 560–562p
topical, (V1) 659p, (V2) 409–412p
tracheostomy, (V1) 1011–1013p
  or endotracheal suctioning (inline closed system), (V2) 729–730p
  or endotracheal suctioning (open system), (V2) 726–728p
transfer of patient to another unit, (V1) 236p, (V2) 63–64p
transfer of patient to long-term care facility, (V1) 237p, (V2) 64–65p

transferring of patients, (V2) 622–625p
upper airway suctioning, (V2) 734–736p
urinary elimination, (V1) 746–747p
vaginal, (V1) 658p, (V2) 407–409p
vaginal medication administration, (V1) 658p, (V2) 407–409p
vital signs, (V1) 452p
wound culture by swab, (V2) 659–661p
Process, communication, (V1) 375–377, (V1) 376f
Process recordings, (V1) 389
Process reviews, (V1) 23
Procurement surgery, (V1) 1078
Prodromal stage, infections, (V1) 519–520
Professional boundaries, (V1) 1176, (V1) 1176b
Professional care, seeking, (V1) 218
Professional composure, (V1) 383
Professional liability insurance, (V1) 1178–1179
Professional values, (V1) 125
Progressive muscle relaxation, (V1) 934
Progressive relaxation, (V1) 260
Progress notes, (V1) 421, (V1) 422, (V1) 426
 "do no use" list for, (V1) 426t
 electronic entry, (V1) 429–430, (V1) 430f
 FACT system, (V1) 429
 Focus Charting, (V1) 428
 narrative format, (V1) 426–427
 problem-intervention-evaluation (PIE) system, (V1) 427
 SOAP format, (V1) 427–428
 use of abbreviations in, (V1) 426
Projection, as defense mechanism, (V1) 247t
Proliferative phase in wound healing, (V1) 948, (V1) 948f
Prolonged immobility, (V1) 860–863
Prone position, (V1) 871t, (V1) 870
Propositions, (V1) 95
Proprietary organizations, (V1) 1124
Proprioception, (V1) 507
Proprioceptors, (V1) 784
Propulsive gait, (V1) 865
Prospective reimbursement system, (V1) 21
Prostaglandins, (V1) 449, (V1) 827
Prostate, (V1) 883, (V1) 884f
 cancer of, (V1) 182
  screening for, (V1) 229
 evaluation of, (V1) 182
 physical examination of, (V1) 509
Prostatectomy, (V1) 891
Prostate gland, (V1) 724
Prostheses removal, preoperative, (V1) 1088
Protective environments (isolation), (V1) 535–536
Protective isolation, (V1) 536
Protein-binding capacity, (V1) 617
Protein-calorie malnutrition, (V1) 693
Protein-controlled diet, (V1) 694
Proteins, (V1) 669–671, (V1) 670t
 cardiovascular function and, (V1) 1022
 functions of, (V1) 671
 metabolism and storage of, (V1) 671
 nitrogen balance, (V1) 671
 skin and, (V1) 942
Protein system, (V1) 1045
Prothrombin time, (V2) 700
Provider's prescriptions, (V1) 421
Proximodistal development, (V1) 144
Proximodistal growth, (V1) 144
Pruritus, (V1) 582, (V1) 943

Psychoanalytic theory, (V1) 145–147, (V1) 147t
Psychogenic pain, (V1) 812
Psychological defense mechanisms, (V1) 147, (V1) 247–248t
Psychological loss, (V1) 348
Psychological needs during active dying, (V1) 365
Psychological responses
 pharmacokinetics and, (V1) 619
 to stress, (V1) 246–251, (V1) 246b, (V1) 247–248t
 stress-induced, (V1) 251–253
Psychological stages of death, (V1) 357
Psychomotor learning, (V1) 398t, (V1) 399
Psychosis, (V1) 892
Psychosocial assessment, (V1) 50
 preschooler, (V1) 165–166, (V1) 165f
Psychosocial development
 adolescent, (V1) 171–172, (V1) 172f
 infant, (V1) 157
 middle adulthood, (V1) 181, (V1) 181f
 neonate, (V1) 155
 in older adults, (V1) 194–195t, (V1) 195f
 school-age children, (V1) 168
 toddler, (V1) 162–163
 young adult, (V1) 179
Psychosocial development theory, (V1) 148, (V1) 191–192
Psychosocial health
 anxiety and, (V1) 277–281, (V1) 278t
 assessment of, (V1) 270–271, (V2) 90–91
  guidelines and tools for, (V2) 93–95
 critical thinking and clinical judgment on, (V2) 96–99
 depression and, (V1) 281–287, (V1) 281t, (V1) 282f, (V1) 287b, (V1) 287f, (V2) 92
 diagnoses in, (V1) 271, (V1) 272t
 full-spectrum nursing model applied to, (V2) 95–96
 interlocking psychosocial influences in, (V1) 266, (V1) 266f
 key concepts in, (V1) 264
 knowledge map on, (V2) 100
 nursing care
  for anxiety, (V1) 279–281
  for depression, (V1) 282–287, (V1) 287b, (V1) 287f
  to promote, (V1) 270–271, (V1) 272t
  for self-concept disturbance and low self-esteem, (V1) 272–277
 planning for, (V1) 271
 psychological and social factors in, (V1) 266, (V1) 266f
 psychosocial theory and, (V1) 266–267
 self-concept in
  components of, (V1) 268–270, (V1) 269f
  defined, (V1) 267
  factors affecting, (V1) 267–268
  formation of, (V1) 267–268
  and low self-esteem and disturbance in, (V1) 272–277
  in preschoolers, (V1) 165
  stress and, (V1) 262
Psychosocial illness, key concepts in, (V1) 264
Psychosocial stressors, (V1) 239
Psychosocial theory, (V1) 266–267
Psychotherapeutic drugs, skin effects of, (V1) 943

Pterygium, (V1) 492
Ptosis, (V1) 492
Puberty, (V1) 167, (V1) 171
 development of sexuality during, (V1) 887
 menstrual cycle and, (V1) 883
Public agencies, (V1) 1124
Public distance, (V1) 381
Public financing of healthcare, (V1) 19–20
Public health nursing, (V1) 1113–1114, (V1) 1114f, (V1) 1117
Public relations, (V1) 1185
Public speaking, (V1) 375
Pulmonary circulation, (V1) 497
 abnormalities of, (V1) 992
Pulmonary embolus, (V1) 992
 as postoperative complication, (V1) 1098t
Pulmonary functions studies, (V2) 753
Pulmonary hypertension, (V1) 992
Pulmonary system
 See also Oxygenation
 abnormalities of, (V1) 989
 components of, (V1) 976–977, (V1) 976–977f
 functions of, (V1) 977–979, (V1) 978–979f
  factors influencing, (V1) 980–984, (V1) 983b
  pathophysiological conditions altering, (V1) 984–993, (V1) 984t, (V1) 985b
 nursing diagnosis of, (V1) 998–999
Pulmonary ventilation, (V1) 462, (V1) 977–978, (V1) 978f
Pulse
 absent or weak, (V1) 461
 apical, (V1) 452p, (V1) 459, (V1) 460, (V1) 460f
  assessment of, (V2) 184–185p
 apical-radial, (V1) 452p, (V1) 460, (V2) 186–187p
 assessment of, (V1) 452p, (V1) 458–461, (V1) 459–460f
 bilateral equality of, (V1) 461
 body production and regulation of, (V1) 457
 data collection on, (V1) 460–461
 equipment for measuring, (V1) 458–459, (V1) 459f
 factors influencing, (V1) 457
 implementation for, (V1) 462
 infections and, (V1) 530
 normal rate of, (V1) 454
 nursing diagnosis and, (V1) 461
 peripheral, (V1) 452p, (V1) 459
  assessment of, (V2) 179–183p
 quality of, (V1) 461
 rhythm of, (V1) 461
 sites for assessing, (V1) 459–460, (V1) 459f
 volume of, (V1) 461
Pulsed irrigations, (V1) 964
Pulse oximetry, (V1) 466, (V1) 996, (V1) 1011p, (V2) 709–711p, (V2) 748
Pulse pressure, (V1) 467
Pump-controlled infusions, (V1) 713
Puncture wounds, (V1) 945t
Pupils, (V1) 492–493
Purified water, (V1) 963–964
Purosanguineous exudate, (V1) 949
Purulent exudate, (V1) 949
PUSH Tool for Evaluation of Pressure Ulcers, (V2) 698
Pustule, (V2) 212p
Pyogenic bacteria, (V1) 949

Pyrexia, (V1) 449–450
Pyridoxine, (V1) 677t
Pyrogens, (V1) 449

Q

Qigong, (V1) 261
QSEN (Quality and Safety Education for Nurses), (V1) 6
Quadriceps, (V1) 876
Quadriplegia, (V1) 864b
Qualitative research, (V1) 108, (V1) 108t
Quality and Safety Education for Nurses (QSEN), (V1) 6, (V1) 105
  on infection prevention, (V1) 516
  on patient safety, (V1) 545
Quality assurance programs, (V1) 91
Quality improvement, documentation of, (V1) 420
Quality of care, (V1) 23
  disparities in, (V1) 310
  evaluation of, (V1) 91
Quantitative research, (V1) 107–108, (V1) 108t
Quasi-intentional torts, (V1) 1166
Questions
  about prescriptions, (V1) 439
  asking too many, (V1) 389
  asking why, (V1) 389–390
  closed, (V1) 50
  open-ended, (V1) 51, (V1) 389

R

Race and ethnicity
  aging and, (V1) 186–187
  biological variations in, (V2) 109
  blood pressure and, (V1) 469
  chronic diseases and, (V1) 195
  definitions of, (V1) 312
  diet and, (V1) 691–692
  health disparities and, (V1) 211, (V1) 310
  life expectancy and, (V1) 186–187
Racism, (V1) 321–322
Radial artery pulse, (V1) 459, (V2) 180p
Radiating pain, (V1) 811
Radiation, (V1) 448
  injury from, (V1) 556–557
Radiation therapy, (V1) 693
Radiofrequency ablation, (V1) 832
Radiography, chest, (V2) 763
Rando, Theresa, (V1) 350t
Range of motion (ROM), (V1) 504, (V1) 845, (V1) 846–851t
  exercises for, (V1) 875–876, (V2) 629
Rape, (V1) 900
Rate of diffusion, (V1) 979
Rationalization, as defense mechanism, (V1) 248t
RDA. See Recommended daily allowance (RDA)
Reaction formation, as defense mechanism, (V1) 248t
Readiness
  for enhanced communication, (V1) 387
  for patient learning, (V1) 400
Real-time location systems (RTLSs), (V1) 1142
Reasoning
  diagnostic, (V1) 56–60, (V1) 58b, (V1) 58f
  inductive and deductive, (V1) 96–97, (V1) 96f
  logical, (V1) 107

Rebound effect, (V1) 640
Recapping of needles, (V1) 426–428p, (V1) 660p
Receiver in communication, (V1) 376–377, (V1) 376f
Reception
  defined, (V1) 784
  key concepts in, (V1) 784
  specialized receptors, (V1) 784
Recommended daily allowance (RDA), (V1) 667, (V1) 673
  calcium and vitamin D, (V1) 1044t, (V1) 1055
Reconstitution of medications, (V1) 646, (V2) 455
Reconstructive surgery, (V1) 1078
Recovery from illness, (V1) 219
Recovery rooms, (V1) 1089, (V1) 1095, (V1) 1095f
Recovery stage of stress, (V1) 244
Recreational therapists, (V1) 18
Rectal body temperature measurement, (V1) 455t, (V2) 175–176p
Rectal medications, (V1) 640
  administration of, (V1) 659p, (V2) 409–412p
  opioid, (V1) 830
Rectal tube insertion, (V2) 571–572p
Rectum, (V1) 509, (V1) 513p, (V1) 756, (V1) 756f
  assessment of, (V2) 294–295p
Rectus femoris injection site, (V1) 652
Recurrent fever, (V1) 450
Red blood cells (RBCs), (V1) 982
  crossmatching, (V1) 1069
  for transfusion, (V1) 1069
Reeve, Christopher, (V1) 333
Referrals to home healthcare, (V1) 1126
Referred pain, (V1) 811
Reflection
  about evaluation, (V1) 90
  in choosing interventions, (V1) 79b
  in critical thinking, (V1) 40b, (V1) 41, (V1) 41f
  during implementation, (V1) 84
Reflective skepticism, (V2) 9
Reflex(es)
  assessing function of, (V1) 506–507
  Babinski, (V1) 154
  crawling, (V1) 153–154, (V1) 154f
  fencing, (V1) 153
  grasp, (V1) 153, (V1) 154f
  Moro, (V1) 153
  rooting, (V1) 153
  startle, (V1) 153
  stepping, (V1) 153, (V1) 154f
  sucking, (V1) 153
  swallowing, (V1) 153
  tonic neck, (V1) 153, (V1) 154f
Reflexology, (V1) 261
Reflex pain response, (V1) 245
Reform, healthcare, (V1) 21–23
Refractory period, in sexual response cycle, (V1) 894
Regeneration, cell, (V1) 245
Regenerative healing, (V1) 946
Regional anesthesia, (V1) 1091–1092, (V1) 1092f
Registered dietitian, (V1) 18–19
Registered nurse first assistant (RNFA), (V1) 1090

Registered nurses (RNs), (V1) 11–12, (V1) 1185
  expanded variety of settings for care by, (V1) 25
  on healthcare team, (V1) 18
  power of, (V1) 1190
Regression, as defense mechanism, (V1) 248t
Regulation, healthcare, (V1) 21
  controlled substances, (V1) 609–610, (V1) 610f
Rehabilitation and therapy notes, (V1) 421
Rehabilitation centers, (V1) 17
Reiki, (V1) 261
Reimbursement, (V1) 421
Reinforcing, (V1) 232
Relapsing fever, (V1) 450
Relationships, loss of, (V1) 348
Relaxation, (V1) 260
  for pain, (V1) 826
Relevance in communication, (V1) 378
Religion(s)
  See also Spirituality
  Buddhism, (V1) 337, (V1) 337f
  Christianity, (V1) 335
  Christian Science, (V1) 336t
  compared to spirituality, (V1) 331t
  culture and, (V1) 312, (V1) 316
  defined, (V1) 330–331
  diet and, (V1) 691–692
  Hinduism, (V1) 336–337
  hygiene and, (V1) 576
  influence on health, (V1) 214
  Islam, (V1) 335–336
  Jehovah's Witness, (V1) 336t
  Judaism, (V1) 334–335
  Mormonism, (V1) 336t
  Native American, (V1) 337, (V1) 338f
  Roman Catholicism, (V1) 336t
  Seventh-Day Adventism, (V1) 336t
  sexuality and, (V1) 890
  support and, (V1) 263
  symbolism associated with, (V1) 332f
Religiosity, impaired, (V1) 341, (V1) 342b
Reminiscence therapy, as spiritual intervention, (V1) 343
Remittent fever, (V1) 450
Remodeling, (V1) 948
REM sleep, (V1) 921, (V1) 921t
  alcohol and, (V1) 924
  disorders of, (V1) 931
Renal calculi, (V1) 724
Renal diet, (V1) 694
Renal failure, as postoperative complication, (V1) 1100t
Renin-angiotensin system, (V1) 1041
Repair, tissue, (V1) 245
Repatterning, (V1) 325
Repetition in patient learning, (V1) 400
Reporting
  defined, (V1) 420
  incident, (V1) 1173–1174
  mandatory reporting laws, (V1) 1160
    minimizing malpractice risks, (V1) 1176–1178, (V1) 1177b
  on sexually transmitted infections (STIs), (V1) 896
  minimizing malpractice risks, (V1) 1172–1174
  oral, (V2) 157–158
    handoff reports in, (V1) 384, (V1) 437–438
    key concepts in, (V1) 420

questioning prescriptions, (V1) 439
receiving and documenting verbal and telephone prescriptions, (V1) 438–439
standardized formats for, (V1) 437–438
transfer reports in, (V1) 438
Reports
evidence, (V1) 75–76
handoff, (V1) 384
occurrence, (V1) 436, (V1) 436b
standardized formats for, (V1) 437–438
transfer, (V1) 438
Repression, as defense mechanism, (V1) 248t
Reproductive system
female, (V1) 882–883, (V1) 883f
male, (V1) 883–885, (V1) 884f
Research, nursing
basing practice on, (V1) 109–114, (V1) 112b, (V1) 112t
defined, (V1) 105
developing priorities for, (V1) 106
educational preparation for, (V1) 106
evidence-based practice and, (V1) 105
history of, (V1) 106
phases of, (V1) 108
practical knowledge on, (V1) 106–114
reasons for learning about, (V1) 105–106
rights of participants, (V1) 109
two approaches to, (V1) 107–108, (V1) 108t
use of nursing theory in, (V1) 98
Research consumer, role and function of, (V1) 7t
Reservoirs, infection, (V1) 517
portal of exit for, (V1) 517
Resident flora, (V1) 516–517
Residual volume, (V2) 753
Resistance stage in stress, (V1) 244
Resistance to change, (V1) 1193–1194
Resistance training, (V1) 852
Resolution, in sexual response cycle, (V1) 894–895, (V1) 894t
Respect
in culturally competent care, (V1) 327
for dignity, (V1) 129
in therapeutic relationship, (V1) 385
Respiration
See also Oxygenation
arterial oxygen saturation and, (V1) 466
assessment of, (V1) 452p, (V1) 464–467, (V1) 465t, (V2) 187–189p
associated clinical signs of, (V1) 466
body regulation of, (V1) 462–463
breath sounds and, (V1) 465–466, (V1) 496, (V1) 499–500f
chest and abdomen movement and, (V1) 466
defined, (V1) 462, (V1) 977, (V1) 978
effort, (V1) 465
external, (V1) 462, (V1) 979, (V1) 979f
factors influencing, (V1) 463–464
internal, (V1) 462, (V1) 979
measuring rate of, (V1) 464–465, (V1) 465t
mechanics of breathing, (V1) 463, (V1) 463f
normal rate of, (V1) 462
nursing diagnosis and, (V1) 467
respiratory depth and, (V1) 465
respiratory rhythm and, (V1) 465
Respiratory acidosis, (V1) 1050t
Respiratory alkalosis, (V1) 1050t
Respiratory anti-inflammatory agents, (V1) 984t

Respiratory arrest, (V1) 1034
Respiratory depth, (V1) 465, (V1) 978
Respiratory disease and sexuality, (V1) 891
Respiratory distress, in neonate, (V1) 155
Respiratory effort, (V1) 465
Respiratory infections
influenza, (V1) 985–989
oxygenation and, (V1) 982, (V1) 985–989
pneumonia, (V1) 989–992
upper
teaching clients how to prevent, (V1) 233
in toddlers, (V1) 980
Respiratory inhalations
metered-dose inhalers and dry powder inhalers, (V1) 641–642, (V1) 641f, (V1) 659p
types of nebulizers for, (V1) 641, (V1) 641f
Respiratory rate, (V1) 464–465, (V1) 465t, (V1) 978
Respiratory rhythm, (V1) 465
Respiratory syncytial virus (RSV), (V1) 985
Respiratory system
See also Oxygenation (gas exchange)
administering medications for, (V1) 1000
age-related changes in, (V1) 193t
evidence-based practice on, (V1) 1008
in neonates, (V1) 152–153
physical activity and, (V1) 860
physical examination of, (V1) 452, (V1) 509
as primary defense against infection, (V1) 521
prior to death, (V1) 357
promoting optimal functioning of, (V1) 1000–1002, (V1) 1001b
responses related to failure of adaptation, (V1) 252t
response to stress, (V1) 244
in toddlers, (V1) 162
unrelieved pain and, (V1) 817
Respiratory therapists (RTs), (V1) 18
Respondeat superior, (V1) 1169
Rest. *See* Sleep and rest
Restating, (V1) 388
Restitution (undoing), as defense mechanism, (V1) 248t
Restless legs syndrome (RLS), (V1) 925–926
Restorative effects, (V1) 621
Restraints, (V1) 554–555, (V1) 571–572, (V1) 573p, (V2) 334–337p, (V2) 339, (V2) 341–342
Restructuring, (V1) 325
Retention enemas, (V1) 771
Reticular activating system (RAS), (V1) 784–785
sleep and, (V1) 920, (V1) 920f
Retirement, (V1) 298–299
Retirement communities, (V1) 189
Retirement homes, (V1) 18
Retractions, (V1) 994
Retrograde ejaculation, (V1) 902
Retrospective system, (V1) 21
Return-flow enemas, (V1) 771
Reversible drug reactions, (V1) 622
Revised Faces Pain Scales, (V2) 611
Rewards, employee, (V1) 1185
Rheumatoid arthritis (RA), (V1) 858
Rh factor, (V1) 1068, (V1) 1068t
Rhizotomy, (V1) 832–833
Rhonchi, (V1) 465
Rhythmic tapping, (V1) 473

Riboflavin, (V1) 676t
RICE (rest, ice, compression, elevation), (V1) 859
Richards, Linda, (V1) 6
Richmond Agitation-Sedation Scale, (V2) 612
Right-sided heart failure, (V1) 1024
Rights of medication, (V1) 630–636, (V1) 635f
Rigor mortis, (V1) 367
Rinne test, (V1) 493–494
Risk-benefit analysis, (V1) 126–127
Rituals
grief, (V1) 353f
marriage, (V1) 315, (V1) 315f
RN-to-BSN programs, (V1) 11
Rodents, (V1) 570
Role conflict, parental, (V1) 271
Role enhancement, (V1) 277
Role modeling, (V1) 231–232
Role-modeling, for patient teaching, (V1) 417
Role performance, (V1) 269
Role strain, (V1) 269
Rolled bandages, (V1) 973
Roller trays, (V1) 873
Roman Catholicism, (V1) 336t
Roman chamomile, (V1) 786
Romberg test, (V1) 494
Room temperature, (V1) 603
Root-cause analysis (RCA), (V1) 552
Rooting reflex, (V1) 153–154, (V1) 154f
Rosemary, (V1) 786
Routes of administration, (V1) 611, (V1) 612–615t, (V1) 619
opioid, (V1) 830–831, (V1) 831f
Rubella, (V1) 151
Rural healthcare, (V1) 1141

S

Saccharide units, (V1) 669
S-Adenosyl methionine (SAMe), (V1) 288
Safe, Effective Nursing Care (SENC), (V1) 5, (V1) 6–7, (V1) 90, (V1) 105–106
application of education and evidence-based practice to client care and sexual health, (V1) 905
assessing and treating pain in patients with cognitive impairment, (V1) 822
chronic illness and self-management through telehealth, (V1) 216
creating a culture of safety, (V1) 546
culturally competent care, (V1) 320–321
detecting and preventing abuse, (V1) 161
effect of authority gradients on teamwork and client safety, (V1) 1198
effects of teamwork and collaboration on activity and exercise outcomes, (V1) 864
handoff reports, (V1) 438
health assessment and cultural adaptation, (V1) 481
impact of nurse self-awareness on client spiritual care, (V1) 331
improving wound care with interprofessional teams, (V1) 957
information technologies living up to their promise, (V1) 1143
limits and boundaries of therapeutic relationships, (V1) 376
managing urinary incontinence, (V1) 730
for patients in palliative care, (V1) 769

perfusion (blood pressure), (V1) 472
preventing ventilator-associated
    pneumonia (VAP) and, (V1) 532
promoting client-centered care in
    community health, (V1) 1119
promoting health and safety through
    self-care management, (V1) 580
providing safe clinical monitoring of
    circulation and perfusion, (V1)
    1027
removing barriers to patient and family
    involvement in care, (V1) 1006
respecting patient and family needs, (V1)
    359
safe use of parenteral nutrition, (V1) 708
surgical team communication, (V1) 1081
teaching clients through collaborative
    partnership, (V1) 401
understanding limitations of technologies
    for medication safety, (V1) 629
use of nursing process to provide legally
    safe nursing care, (V1) 1172
Safe harbor laws, (V1) 1178
Safety
  alarm, (V1) 554
  assessment for, (V1) 557–561, (V1) 562f
  automobile, (V1) 161, (V1) 167, (V1) 177,
    (V1) 179, (V1) 550, (V1) 567, (V1)
    567–568t
  change and psychological, (V1) 1194, (V1)
    1194b
  critical thinking and clinical judgment on,
    (V2) 342–343
  drug quality and, (V1) 608–611, (V1) 610f
  factors affecting
    developmental, (V1) 546–547
    individual, (V1) 547, (V1) 547t
  fighting vector-borne pathogens and, (V1)
    568, (V1) 570
  food, (V1) 568, (V1) 569
  full-spectrum nursing model applied to,
    (V2) 341–342
  home, (V1) 1134–1135
  home healthcare, (V1) 1127, (V2) 839
  hospital bed, (V1) 604, (V1) 604f
  implementation for
    in the healthcare facility, (V1) 571–574,
      (V1) 573b
    in the home, (V1) 563–571
  importance of, (V1) 545, (V1) 545t
  interventions
    choking rescue, (V1) 565, (V1) 566f
    delegation of, (V1) 557
    general, (V1) 563
    home care, (V1) 563–567, (V1) 566f
    preventing drowning, (V1) 565
    preventing firearm injuries, (V1) 564
    preventing home fires, (V1) 549, (V1)
      564–565
    preventing scalds and burns, (V1) 564
    preventing suffocation, (V1) 564–565,
      (V1) 566f
    preventing take-home toxins, (V1) 565
  intraoperative, (V1) 1095
  key concepts on, (V1) 545
  knowledge map on, (V2) 344
  medication, (V1) 628, (V1) 632–633
  medication administration, (V1) 633–636,
    (V1) 635f
  minimizing malpractice risks, (V1) 1175

nonsteroidal anti-inflammatory drugs
    (NSAIDs), (V1) 828
nursing diagnosis and, (V1) 562
oxygen therapy, (V1) 1004, (V2) 749
parenteral medication administration, (V1)
    648
perioperative, (V1) 1076–1077, (V1) 1077b
planning for, (V1) 562
preoperative checklist for, (V1) 1088
reducing pollution and, (V1) 570
Safety Assessment Scale (SAS), (V1) 561,
    (V2) 340–341
school-age child's awareness of, (V1)
    169–170
sleep and, (V1) 934–935
surgical, (V2) 829
teaching for, (V1) 203, (V1) 567–571
transmission-based precautions, (V1) 535,
    (V1) 535t, (V1) 536, (V2) 325–326
using bed and chair monitoring devices,
    (V1) 573p, (V2) 332–334p
using restraints, (V1) 573p, (V2) 334–337p
Safety assessment scale (SAS), (V1) 561, (V2)
    340–341
Safety hazards
  in the community, (V1) 550–551
  in healthcare facilities (See Healthcare
    facilities)
  in the home, (V1) 547–549, (V1) 548b, (V1)
    561
Safety needs, (V1) 100, (V1) 102, (V1) 102f
Safety officers, (V1) 541
Saliva, (V1) 592
Salivary glands and drug excretion, (V1) 618
Salmonella enteritidis, (V1) 517
Sandbags, (V1) 870
Sanders, Cicely, (V1) 358
Sandwich families, (V1) 293, (V1) 297
Sanger, Margaret, (V1) 1114
Sanguineous exudate, (V1) 949
Sanitation, (V1) 550
Saturated fatty acids, (V1) 672, (V1) 672t
  cardiovascular function and, (V1) 1022
  sleep and, (V1) 923
Saturation of oxygen, (V1) 997
Sawtooth waves, (V1) 921t
SBARQ model, (V1) 384, (V2) 143
SBAR (Situation-Background-Assessment-
    Recommendation) report, (V1) 438,
    (V1) 553
Scalds and burns, (V1) 548–549, (V1) 582
  prevention of, (V1) 565
Scales, (V2) 214p
Scalp, (V1) 490
Scalp vein needle, (V1) 1057, (V1) 1057f
Scar, (V2) 214p
Scheduled hygiene, (V1) 578
Scheduling and sequencing, for patient
    teaching, (V1) 410–411
School-age children
  assessment of, (V1) 169
  asthma in, (V1) 168, (V1) 170
  cardiovascular function in, (V1) 1020
  common health problems of, (V1)
    168–169
  communication by, (V1) 380
  development of
    cognitive, (V1) 167–168
    physical, (V1) 167, (V1) 167b
    psychosocial, (V1) 168

development of sexuality in, (V1) 887
diabetes in, (V1) 170
drowning of, (V1) 549
friendships of, (V1) 168, (V1) 168f
hospitalized, (V1) 170–171
hygiene and, (V1) 576
immunizations in, (V1) 169
implementation for, (V1) 169–171
loss in, (V1) 348
nutrition and exercise for weight loss in,
    (V1) 170
nutrition in, (V1) 685–686
obesity in, (V1) 168
physical activity guidelines for, (V1) 852b
physical examination of, (V1) 485
poisoning in, (V1) 548
pulmonary function in, (V1) 980
safety of, (V1) 547
sleep requirements and characteristics in,
    (V1) 918t, (V1) 923
unintentional injury in, (V1) 168–169
violence and risk-taking behaviors in, (V1)
    170
School nursing, (V1) 1116–1117
School readiness of preschoolers, (V1) 166
Schut, Henk, (V1) 352t
Schwartz, Morrie, (V1) 213
Science of Human Caring, (V1) 93–94, (V1) 95,
    (V1) 95b
Scientific/biomedical health system, (V1)
    318
Scientific management, (V1) 1184
Scientific method, (V1) 107, (V1) 107b
Scissors gait, (V1) 865
Sclera, (V1) 492
Scoliosis, (V1) 169, (V1) 857
Scoot sheets, (V1) 873, (V1) 873f
Scope of practice, (V1) 1163–1164
Screener and Opioid Assessment for Patients
    with Pain (SOAPP), (V1) 834–835
Screening
  blood glucose, (V1) 182, (V1) 698
  bowel elimination, (V1) 765
  Braden Scale for Predicting Pressure Sore
    Risk, (V2) 696
  breast, (V1) 180, (V1) 182, (V1) 228–229, (V1)
    495–496, (V1) 906
  cervical cancer, (V1) 229
  cholesterol, (V1) 182, (V1) 1027–1028, (V2)
    763
  circulation, (V2) 763
  colon cancer, (V1) 228
  dental health, (V1) 228
  functional ability assessment, (V2) 17
  health, (V1) 224–226t
  hearing in older adults, (V2) 599
  lipid panel, (V1) 182, (V1) 228, (V1) 1027
  mammogram, (V1) 180, (V1) 182
  mental status, (V2) 283p
  neonatal, (V1) 151, (V1) 155–156
  Norton Pressure Sore Risk Assessment
    Scale, (V2) 697
  nutritional, (V1) 695, (V2) 505–506
  for opioid abuse, (V1) 834–835
  osteoporosis, (V1) 183
  physical examination in, (V1) 479
  during pregnancy, (V1) 151–152
  preoperative, (V2) 830
  PUSH Tool for Evaluation of Pressure
    Ulcers, (V2) 698

scoliosis, (V1) 169
skin cancer, (V1) 229
testicular, (V1) 229, (V1) 906
violence, (V1) 180
vision, (V1) 166
young adults, (V1) 180
Scrotum, (V1) 884f, (V1) 893
Scrub nurse, (V1) 1089
SDOH. *See* Social determinants of health (SDOH)
Sebaceous glands, (V1) 579, (V1) 582
Secondary cardiomyopathy, (V1) 1024
Secondary defense against infections, (V1) 521, (V1) 522t
Secondary effects, drug, (V1) 621–623, (V1) 621b, (V1) 622t, (V1) 623f
Secondary infections, (V1) 519
Secondary intention healing, (V1) 947, (V1) 947f
Secondary prevention, (V1) 220
Secondary services, (V1) 18
Secondary skin lesions, (V1) 490
Secondary sleep disorders, (V1) 931
Secondhand smoke, (V1) 214–215, (V1) 983
Second heart sound, (V1) 501
Second trimester
  fetal development during, (V1) 149–150
  maternal changes during, (V1) 150
Sedation
  conscious, (V1) 1091
  palliative, (V1) 361
Sedatives, (V1) 788
  opioid, (V1) 829
  preoperative, (V1) 1087t
Sedentary lifestyle, (V1) 856
Seizures, (V1) 794, (V1) 797
  caring for patients with, (V1) 805–809
Self
  dynamic, (V1) 267
  loss of aspects of, (V1) 348
Self-actualization needs, (V1) 102, (V1) 102f
Self-administration of medications, (V1) 610
Self-affirmation, (V1) 262, (V1) 375
Self-awareness, (V1) 1182
Self-care
  See also Hygiene; specific body areas
  activities of daily living (ADLs), (V1) 578
  assessment of, (V1) 577
  cough and cold medicines, (V1) 1000
  fatigue and sleep deprivation among healthcare workers, (V1) 919
  food safety, (V1) 569
  grief and loss, (V1) 367–368
  hands-only cardiopulmonary resuscitation, (V1) 1034
  health status and, (V1) 576–577
  on how to prevent upper respiratory infections, (V1) 233
  on how to reduce stress of hospitalization, (V1) 263
  implementation for, (V1) 578
  Internet-based software for aiding, (V1) 1143, (V1) 1143f
  maintaining proper posture, (V1) 845
  nursing diagnosis and, (V1) 577
  planning for, (V1) 578
  postoperative patient teaching topics, (V1) 1103
  smoking cessation, (V1) 1001

taking oral electrolyte supplements, (V1) 1055
teaching clients about sleep hygiene, (V1) 936
teaching clients how to set up a fitness program, (V1) 854
teaching older adults about increasing physical activity and exercise, (V1) 857
teaching parents about medicating children, (V1) 638
teaching patients about incentive spirometry, (V1) 1103
teaching patients how to help prevent surgical site infections, (V1) 1085
teaching patients how to prevent back injury, (V1) 856
teaching patients on limited budget to buy nutritious foods, (V1) 702
teaching patients to prevent fluid and electrolyte imbalances, (V1) 1054
teaching weight-loss tips, (V1) 707
Self-catheterization, (V1) 733
  clean, intermittent, (V1) 739–740
Self-concept
  assessment of, (V2) 90
  components of, (V1) 268–270, (V1) 269f
  defined, (V1) 267
  factors affecting, (V1) 267–268
  formation of, (V1) 267
  nursing care for disturbance and low self-esteem in, (V1) 272–277
  in preschoolers, (V1) 165
  promoting, (V1) 276
  stress and, (V1) 262
Self-efficacy, (V1) 397
Self-esteem, (V1) 269–270, (V1) 269f, (V2) 91
  needs related to, (V1) 102, (V1) 102f
  promoting, (V1) 276
Self-help groups, (V1) 386
Self-knowledge, (V1) 30, (V1) 61
  ethical decision making and, (V1) 139
  sexual health, (V1) 909
Self-management, (V1) 1182
Self-neglect, (V1) 577
Self-payment, home healthcare, (V1) 1126
Self-talk, (V1) 375
  negative, (V1) 375
  positive, (V1) 262, (V1) 375
Semi-Fowler's position, (V1) 870
SENC (Safe, Effective Nursing Care). *See* Safe, Effective Nursing Care (SENC)
Sender in communication, (V1) 375, (V1) 376f
Sensation
  See also Perception
  assessment of, (V2) 599–601
  components of, (V1) 784–786, (V1) 785f
  contrast of, (V1) 785
  critical thinking and clinical judgment on, (V2) 602–603
  full-spectrum nursing model applied to, (V2) 601–602
  knowledge map on, (V2) 604
  responding to, (V1) 785–786, (V1) 785f
  skin and diminished, (V1) 942–943
Sense of self, loss of, (V1) 216
Sensorimotor development in preschoolers, (V1) 165

Sensorimotor stage, in cognitive development theory, (V1) 148t, (V1) 154, (V1) 156–157, (V1) 162
Sensory alterations
  seizures, (V1) 797
  sensory deficits, (V1) 794–801
  sensory deprivation, (V1) 788, (V1) 790–791
  sensory overload, (V1) 788, (V1) 792–793
Sensory deficits, (V1) 794–801
Sensory deprivation, (V1) 788, (V1) 790–791
Sensory overload, (V1) 788, (V1) 792–793
  PICOT questions, (V1) 793
Sensory system
  age-related changes in, (V1) 194t
  alterations in, (V1) 788–802
  assessment of, (V1) 507, (V1) 512p, (V1) 802–803, (V2) 272–285p
  components of sensory experience and, (V1) 784–786, (V1) 785f
  evidence-based practice and, (V1) 806
  factors affecting
    culture, (V1) 788
    illness, (V1) 788
    life-span variations, (V1) 786–787
    medications, (V1) 788, (V1) 789f
    personality and lifestyle, (V1) 788
    stress, (V1) 788
  interventions, (V1) 804–809
  PICOT questions, (V1) 793
  promoting optimal function of, (V1) 804
  seizures, (V1) 794
  self-care ability and, (V1) 577
Septicemia, (V1) 519
  as complication of intravenous therapy, (V1) 1066t
Septic shock, as complication of parenteral nutrition, (V1) 715
Sequential compression devices (SCDs), (V1) 1032, (V1) 1103–1104
  procedure for, (V1) 1104p, (V2) 817–819p
Sequential muscle relaxation (SMR), (V1) 826
Serious Reportable Events (SREs), (V1) 552
Serosanguineous drainage, (V1) 949
Serous exudate, (V1) 949
Serum albumin, (V2) 700
Serum electrolytes, (V2) 830
Serum osmolality, (V1) 1053
Serum prealbumin, (V2) 700
Serum protein levels, (V1) 698–699, (V2) 700
Servant leadership, (V1) 1184
Set point, (V1) 449
Seventh-day Adventism, (V1) 336t
Severe acute respiratory syndrome (SARS), (V1) 300
Severe adverse reactions, (V1) 621
Severe anxiety, (V1) 278t
Severe Mercy, (V1) 234
Sexting, (V1) 175
Sexual arousal, (V1) 893
  disorders of, (V1) 901
Sexual assault, (V1) 897, (V1) 900
  providing care after, (V2) 639
Sexual dysfunction, (V1) 903
Sexual harassment, (V1) 897, (V1) 908, (V1) 1176
Sexual health
  assessment of, (V1) 902
  condom use and, (V2) 641
  contraception method and, (V2) 642–643

critical thinking and clinical judgment on, (V2) 646–648
defined, (V1) 893
full-spectrum nursing model applied to, (V2) 645–646
health history and, (V1) 902, (V2) 640, (V2) 644–645
interventions, teaching, (V1) 904–907
key concepts in, (V1) 882
knowledge map on, (V2) 649
nursing diagnosis, (V1) 903–904, (V1) 904f
sexual and reproductive anatomy and physiology and, (V1) 882–885, (V1) 883–884f
sexual assault and, (V1) 897, (V1) 900, (V2) 639
sexual response cycle and, (V1) 893–895, (V1) 893f, (V1) 894t
disorders of, (V1) 900–902
teaching children about sexual predators and, (V1) 908
Sexual intercourse, (V1) 895
Sexuality
adolescent, (V1) 175–176, (V1) 887–888
dealing with inappropriate behaviors and, (V1) 907–908
defined, (V1) 885, (V1) 885f
development of
in adolescence, (V1) 887–888
from birth through preschool, (V1) 886–887, (V1) 887f
in middle adults, (V1) 888
in older adults, (V1) 888–889, (V1) 889f
from school age through puberty, (V1) 887
in young adults, (V1) 888
evidence-based practice on, (V1) 890
factors affecting
cultural, (V1) 889–890
health and illness, (V1) 891–892, (V1) 892t
lifestyle, (V1) 890–891
religion, (V1) 890
sexual knowledge, (V1) 891
and forms of sexual expression, (V1) 895–896
gender identity and, (V1) 885–886
gender roles and, (V1) 885
multiple partners and, (V1) 528
PICOT questions, (V1) 901
problems affecting
arousal disorders, (V1) 901
counseling for, (V1) 907
dysmenorrhea, (V1) 897
low libido, (V1) 900–901
negative intimate relationships, (V1) 897
orgasmic disorders, (V1) 901–902
premenstrual syndrome, (V1) 897
rape, (V1) 900
sexual harassment and sexual assault, (V1) 897
sexually transmitted infections (STIs), (V1) 896–897
sexual response cycle disorders, (V1) 900–902
sexual orientation and, (V1) 172, (V1) 886, (V1) 888
Sexually transmitted infections (STIs), (V1) 895
in adolescents, (V1) 175–176, (V1) 887–888
common, (V1) 896–897, (V1) 898–899t

detection of, (V1) 897
effects on pregnancy, (V1) 151
incidence of, (V1) 896
mandatory reporting of, (V1) 896
prevention of, (V1) 897, (V1) 906–907
in young adults, (V1) 179–180
Sexual orientation, (V1) 886, (V1) 888
adolescents and emerging, (V1) 172
Sexual pattern alterations, (V1) 903
Sexual response cycle, (V1) 893–895, (V1) 893f, (V1) 894t
disorders of, (V1) 900–902
Shampooing, (V1) 598, (V1) 602p, (V2) 366–369p
Sharing and ethical decision making, (V1) 140
Sharp débridement, (V1) 966–967
sterile technique for, (V1) 972
Sharps disposal, (V1) 536
Shaving, (V1) 599, (V1) 602–603p
Shock phase in stress, (V1) 242
Short-term goals, (V1) 72
Showers, (V1) 586, (V2) 383
Sickle cell anemia, (V1) 464
sensory function and, (V1) 788
Sick role behavior, (V1) 218
Side effects, drug, (V1) 621
opioid, (V1) 829–830, (V1) 829b
systemic, (V1) 640
Siderails, (V1) 555, (V1) 604, (V1) 604f, (V1) 869
Side-stream smoke, (V1) 983
SIDS. *See* Sudden infant death syndrome (SIDS)
Sigma Theta Tau International (STTI), (V1) 14
Sigmoid colon, (V1) 755
Sigmoidoscopy, (V2) 586
Silence, (V1) 389
Silicone catheters, (V1) 735
Silver-alloy catheters, (V1) 735
Simple carbohydrates, (V1) 669
Simple Descriptor Scale (SDS), (V2) 611
Sims' position, (V1) 872, (V1) 872t
Simulations
computer-based, (V1) 1145–1146
high-fidelity mannequins for, (V1) 1146, (V1) 1146f
Single adults, (V1) 292
Single-lumen stethoscopes, (V1) 458
Single parent families, (V1) 292, (V1) 299
Single prescriptions, (V1) 626
Single studies, (V1) 75
Single-use, continuous-flow pump, (V1) 1102, (V1) 1102f
Sinoatrial (SA) node, (V1) 1018
Sinuses, (V1) 511p
assessment of, (V1) 511p, (V2) 232–234p
Situational stressors, (V1) 239
Situational theories, (V1) 1182
Sitz bath, (V1) 587
Skeletal muscles and heat production, (V1) 447
Skeletal system, (V1) 841–843, (V1) 842f
Skilled care, (V1) 17
Skilled nursing services, (V1) 1123, (V1) 1123b
Skills
critical thinking, (V1) 37
development of, (V1) 144
nursing assessment, (V1) 48–49, (V1) 48b

Skin
age-related variations in, (V1) 193t, (V1) 941
anatomy and physiology of, (V1) 579, (V1) 940–941, (V1) 940f
assessment of, (V1) 323–324, (V1) 510p, (V1) 584, (V2) 206–214p
guidelines and tools for, (V2) 694–699
in wound assessment, (V1) 952
Braden Scale for Predicting Pressure Sore Risk, (V2) 696
care for pressure injury to, (V1) 111
characteristics of, (V1) 488
color of, (V1) 488, (V1) 489t
common problems of, (V1) 582–583, (V1) 583t
risk factors for, (V1) 582–583
contamination or infection of, (V1) 943–944
critical thinking and clinical judgment on, (V2) 701–702
cutaneous stimulation of, (V1) 824
diagnostic testing of, (V1) 996
diminished sensation or cognition and, (V1) 942–943
fever and, (V1) 943
fluid loss via, (V1) 1041
foot problems and, (V1) 589
full-spectrum nursing model applied to, (V2) 701
functions of, (V1) 582
impaired circulation and, (V1) 490, (V1) 943
impaired mobility and, (V1) 942
implementation for, (V1) 585–587, (V1) 586b
infections and, (V1) 530
integrity of, (V1) 944
knowledge map on, (V2) 704
lesions of, (V1) 490, (V2) 209–214p
lifestyle and, (V1) 583, (V1) 944
medication application to, (V1) 659p, (V2) 412–414p
medications and, (V1) 943, (V1) 943f
moisture on, (V1) 488, (V1) 943
neonatal, (V1) 153
Norton Pressure Sore Risk Assessment Scale, (V2) 697
nursing diagnosis of, (V1) 584
nutrition and hydration and, (V1) 942
PICOT question for, (V1) 111
planning for problems with, (V1) 585
preparation for surgery, (V1) 1086–1087, (V1) 1094
as primary defense against infection, (V1) 521
procedures
applying and removing transparent film dressing, (V2) 676–678p
applying bandages, (V2) 684–687p
applying binders, (V2) 682–684p
applying hydrating dressing, (V2) 678–680p
applying negative pressure wound therapy (NPWT) device, (V2) 671–676p
closures, (V2) 680–681p
emptying a closed-wound drainage system, (V2) 691–692p
obtaining wound culture by swab, (V2) 659–661p
removing and applying dry dressings, (V2) 666–668p

removing and applying wet-to-damp dressings, (V2) 668–670p
removing sutures and staples, (V2) 688–689p
shortening a wound drain, (V2) 690–691p
sterile wound irrigation, (V2) 662–664p
taping a dressing, (V2) 665–666p
PUSH Tool for Evaluation of Pressure Ulcers, (V2) 698
tags on, (V1) 490
temperature of, (V1) 488
texture of, (V1) 488
tone of, (V1) 488
topical medications for
administration of, (V1) 659p, (V2) 412–414p
lotions, creams, and ointments, (V1) 637
transdermal, (V1) 637, (V1) 639f
turgor of, (V1) 490, (V1) 942
wound healing and (See Wounds)
Skin body temperature measurement, (V1) 456t
Skin cancer screening, (V1) 229
Skinfold measurements, (V1) 696
Skin integrity impairment risk, (V1) 461, (V1) 584
Skull and face, physical examination of, (V1) 491
Slander, (V1) 1166
Slang, (V1) 322
Sleep and rest
in adolescents, (V1) 178
assessment of, (V1) 931–932
guidelines and tools for, (V2) 652–653
circadian rhythms and, (V1) 919
critical thinking and clinical judgment on, (V2) 654–655
cycles of, (V1) 921, (V1) 922f
defined, (V1) 916, (V1) 916f
disorders of
bruxism, (V1) 930
hypersomnia, (V1) 926
insomnia, (V1) 924–925
narcolepsy, (V1) 926
night terrors, (V1) 930–931
nocturnal enuresis, (V1) 721–722, (V1) 931
parasomnias, (V1) 927, (V1) 930–931
REM sleep behavior, (V1) 931
restless legs syndrome (RLS), (V1) 925–926
secondary, (V1) 931
sleep apnea, (V1) 926, (V1) 928–930
sleep deprivation, (V1) 926
sleeptalking, (V1) 930
sleep-wake schedule, (V1) 925
disorders provoked by, (V1) 931
as etiology, (V1) 932–933
evidence-based practice on, (V1) 927
factors affecting, (V1) 922–923
age, (V1) 923
environmental, (V1) 924
illness, (V1) 924
lifestyle, (V1) 923–924
light, (V1) 924
noise, (V1) 924
full-spectrum nursing model applied to, (V2) 653–654
host susceptibility to infection and, (V1) 529, (V1) 531
importance of, (V1) 916–917, (V1) 917f

in infants, (V1) 156
influence on health, (V1) 213
interventions for
bedtime rituals and routines, (V1) 934
creating a restful environment, (V1) 933–934, (V1) 934f
medication, (V1) 935
offering appropriate bedtime snacks or beverages, (V1) 934
promoting comfort, (V1) 934
promoting relaxation, (V1) 934
scheduling nursing care to avoid interrupting sleep, (V1) 933
teaching about sleep hygiene, (V1) 935
key concepts in, (V1) 916
knowledge map on, (V2) 657
NREM, (V1) 920–921, (V1) 920–921t
pain during, (V1) 1032
physical activity and, (V1) 860
in preschoolers, (V1) 166, (V1) 167
as the problem, (V1) 932
quality of, (V1) 922
regulation of, (V1) 920, (V1) 920f
REM, (V1) 921, (V1) 921t, (V1) 924, (V1) 931
requirements and characteristics of, (V1) 918–919, (V1) 918t
in school-age children, (V1) 169
stages of, (V1) 920–921, (V1) 921–922t
stress and, (V1) 259
as symptom, (V1) 933
Sleep apnea, (V1) 926, (V1) 928–930
oxygenation and, (V1) 982
Sleep deprivation, (V1) 926
Sleep history, (V1) 932
Sleep logs, (V1) 932
Sleep-provoked disorders, (V1) 931
Sleep studies, (V1) 932
Sleeptalking, (V1) 930
Sleep-wake schedule disorders, (V1) 925
Sleepwalking, (V1) 927, (V1) 934
Slings, (V1) 972
Slough, wound, (V1) 953, (V1) 957t
Slow-reacting substance of anaphylaxis (SRS-A), (V1) 981
Slow speech, (V1) 487
Slow-wave sleep (SWS), (V1) 920
Sluggish accommodation, (V1) 492
Small-bore NG tubes, (V1) 707
Small intestine, (V1) 755, (V1) 755f
Smart beds, (V1) 1145
Smart pumps, (V1) 628–629
Smell sense
diminished, (V1) 702
neonatal, (V1) 154–155
Smoking, (V1) 213
cardiovascular function and, (V1) 1020, (V1) 1022
chest shape and size and, (V1) 496
exposure to secondhand smoke from, (V1) 214–215
fires and, (V1) 549
host susceptibility to infection and, (V1) 525
nutrition and, (V1) 689–690
osteoporosis and, (V1) 867
oxygenation and, (V1) 982–983
quitting, (V1) 983b, (V1) 1001
respiration and, (V1) 464
skin and, (V1) 944
sleep and, (V1) 923
as vital sign, (V1) 444

Smothering, (V1) 549
SOAP format, (V1) 427–428
SOAR model, (V1) 1185, (V1) 1186t
Social data, (V1) 1111
Social determinants of health (SDOH), (V1) 210–212, (V1) 211f, (V1) 1112, (V1) 1112f
cardiovascular disease and, (V1) 1025
Social distance, (V1) 381
Social functioning and self-concept, (V1) 267
Social isolation, (V1) 218, (V1) 271
homelessness and, (V1) 300–301
Socialization, (V1) 12, (V1) 313
Social justice model, (V1) 138
Social learning theory, (V1) 397
Social media, adolescents and, (V1) 175
Social networking, (V1) 1140–1141
Social organization and culture, (V1) 316, (V1) 327b
Social pressure on adolescents, (V1) 297
Social roles and communication, (V1) 382
Social workers, (V1) 19
Societal trends influencing contemporary nursing practice, (V1) 23–24
Society factors in ethical problems, (V1) 119, (V1) 121
Sociocultural factors
in communication, (V1) 382
in pain, (V1) 816
Socioeconomic status and poverty
dental care and, (V1) 593
hygiene and, (V1) 576
limited income for food and, (V1) 702
physical activity and, (V1) 856
unemployment and, (V1) 299
vulnerable populations and, (V1) 1112–1113
Sodium, (V1) 678, (V1) 680t, (V1) 1041
electrolytes, (V1) 1042t
Sodium-potassium pump, (V1) 1040
Sodium-restricted diets, (V1) 694
Soil contamination, (V1) 551
Solid waste, (V1) 570
Solubility, drug, (V1) 612, (V1) 616
Solutions, (V1) 612t, (V1) 614–615t, (V1) 614t, (V1) 616
bags containing, (V1) 1062
enema, (V1) 771, (V1) 772t
enteral feeding, (V1) 710
hypertonic, (V1) 1057
hypotonic, (V1) 1056–1057
intravenous therapy, (V1) 714, (V1) 1056–1057
changing, (V1) 1064, (V1) 1071–1072p, (V2) 779–782p
isotonic, (V1) 1056
wound irrigation, (V1) 964
Solvent, water as, (V1) 681
Somatic nervous system, (V1) 844
Somatic pain, (V1) 812
Somatization, (V1) 251
Somatoform disorders, (V1) 251
Somatosensory cortex, (V1) 814
Soul, the, (V1) 209
Sounds, breath, (V1) 465–466
Source-oriented record systems, (V1) 421–422
Space and culture, (V1) 315, (V1) 327b
Spastic gait, (V1) 865
Spasticity, (V1) 864b

Special discharge plans, (V1) 69
Special needs persons
 assessments of, (V1) 49–50, (V2) 18
 patient education for, (V1) 402
Specific gravity, urine, (V1) 729–730, (V1) 730f
Speculum examination, (V2) 298–299
Speech
 in general survey, (V1) 487
 impairments in, (V1) 392–393
Speech and language therapists (SLTs), (V1) 18
Spermicides, (V2) 642
Sphygmomanometers, (V1) 470, (V1) 470–471f
 mercury in, (V1) 555
SPICES, (V1) 486
Spinal anesthesia, (V1) 1092, (V1) 1092f
Spindles, sleep, (V1) 920, (V1) 920t
Spine and spinal cord
 injury to, (V1) 859, (V1) 992
  sexuality and, (V1) 891
 oxygenation and, (V1) 992
 posture and, (V1) 844, (V1) 844f
 scoliosis of, (V1) 169, (V1) 857
 and spinal cord stimulator (SCS) for pain, (V1) 824
 transmission of pain to, (V1) 813–814, (V1) 813f
SPIRIT assessment tool, (V1) 341, (V2) 122
Spirits, (V1) 612t
Spiritual care, (V1) 104
 assessment tools for, (V1) 340–341
 barriers to, (V1) 338–340
 of dying patient, (V1) 365–366
 interventions in, (V1) 80, (V1) 343–345
 other nursing activities in, (V1) 345–346
 providers in, (V1) 19
Spiritual development theory, (V1) 149
Spiritual distress, (V1) 341, (V1) 343
Spiritual health assessment, (V1) 50
Spirituality
 See also Religion
 assessment of, (V2) 121–122
 compared to religion, (V1) 331t
 core issues of, (V1) 332–333
 cures, miracles, and spiritual healing and, (V1) 333
 defined, (V1) 331–332
 as etiology, (V1) 341
 evidence-based practice in, (V1) 334
 full-spectrum nursing model applied to, (V2) 123
 history in nursing, (V1) 330
 hygiene and, (V1) 576
 influence on health, (V1) 214, (V1) 333
 key concepts in, (V1) 330
 knowledge map on, (V2) 125
 lack of general awareness of, (V1) 338–339
 nurses' personal biases and, (V1) 338
 prayer and, (V1) 333, (V1) 344, (V1) 344f
  with clients, (V2) 120
  in holistic healing, (V1) 345
  types of, (V2) 119
 responses to stress, (V1) 251
 sources of data on, (V1) 340
Spiritual pain, (V1) 342b, (V1) 342f
Spiritual support, (V1) 343–345, (V1) 344f
Spirometry, (V1) 997
Splinter hemorrhages, (V1) 491
Spokesperson, manager as, (V1) 1185
Sports and stress, (V1) 262
Sprains, (V1) 859

Sprays, (V1) 613t
Sputum, (V1) 995, (V1) 995b
 sampling of, (V1) 996, (V1) 1011p, (V2) 706–709p
Sputum culture, (V2) 753
Stable angina, (V1) 1024
Staffing and workflow management, (V1) 1142
Standard bedside equipment, (V1) 603–604
Standardized communication tools, (V1) 384
Standardized nursing languages, (V1) 61–62, (V1) 1147
 holistic care and, (V1) 80
 for home health and community care, (V1) 79
 home healthcare and, (V1) 1130
 importance of, (V1) 421
 for outcomes, (V1) 74
 in planning interventions, (V1) 78–80, (V1) 79b
 supporting evidence-based practice, (V1) 1147, (V1) 1148b
Standardized plans, (V1) 67–71, (V1) 68f, (V1) 70f
Standardized report formats, (V1) 437–438
Standard precautions, (V1) 534–535, (V1) 535t, (V1) 536, (V2) 323–324
Standards, nutrition, (V1) 666
Standards for Community Health Nursing, (V1) 1119
Standards of practice, (V1) 13, (V1) 420, (V1) 1162
 See also Nurse practice acts
 infection prevention, (V1) 515–516
 minimizing malpractice risks, (V1) 1172
Standing assist devices, (V1) 874, (V1) 875f
Standing prescriptions, (V1) 626
Staphylococcus, (V1) 517
Staples, (V2) 688–689p
Startle reflex, (V1) 153
State laws, (V1) 1160–1161
Statements, (V1) 95
Statins, (V1) 1033
STAT prescriptions, (V1) 625
Statutory law, (V1) 1156, (V1) 1157t
Statutory rape, (V1) 900
Stepfamilies, (V1) 293
Steppage gait, (V1) 865
Stepping reflex, (V1) 153, (V1) 154f
Stereotypes, (V1) 61, (V1) 321
 as barrier to therapeutic communication, (V1) 391
 cultural, (V1) 315
Sterile fields, (V1) 539p, (V2) 318–320p
Sterile gown and gloves
 closed method, (V2) 314–3153p
 open method, (V2) 316–317p
Sterile team, (V1) 1089
Sterile technique, (V1) 537, (V1) 539p
 for artificial airway, (V1) 1006
 home healthcare, (V1) 1132
Sterile urine specimen, (V1) 729
Sterile water, (V1) 963
Sterilization, (V1) 534
 in surgical asepsis, (V1) 536–537
Steroids, skin effects of, (V1) 943
Sterols, (V1) 671
Stertor, (V1) 466
Stethoscopes, (V1) 458–459, (V1) 459f, (V1) 465–466

STI. *See* Sexually transmitted infections (STIs)
Stimuli
 adaptation to, (V1) 784
 brain response to sensations and, (V1) 785–786, (V1) 785f
 chemical, (V1) 813
 defined, (V1) 784
 intensity of, (V1) 785
 mechanical, (V1) 813
 pain, (V1) 813
 perception of, (V1) 784
 previous experience with, (V1) 786
 processing of, (V1) 784
 sensory deficits, (V1) 794–801
 sensory deprivation and, (V1) 788, (V1) 790–791
 sensory overload and, (V1) 788, (V1) 792–793
 thermal, (V1) 813
St. John's wort, (V1) 288, (V1) 823
Stock supply, (V1) 610
Stomach, (V1) 754, (V1) 754f
 nutrition and function of, (V1) 693
 in toddlers, (V1) 162
Stomatitis, (V1) 594
STONES, wound, (V1) 950
Stool
 digital removal of, (V1) 771, (V2) 569–571p
 laboratory studies of, (V1) 765
 normal, (V1) 757
Stork bites, (V1) 941
Strabismus, (V1) 162
Straight catheters, (V1) 735
Strains, (V1) 859
Stranger danger, (V1) 167
Stratum corneum, (V1) 941
Stratum germinativum, (V1) 941
Street talk, (V1) 322
Stress
 See also Adaptation
 adaptation or disease as outcomes of, (V1) 241, (V1) 241f
 and adaptation theory, (V1) 102–103
 alarm stage in, (V1) 242–244, (V1) 243–244f
 assessment of, (V1) 254, (V1) 257b
  guidelines and tools for, (V2) 82–84
 blood pressure and, (V1) 469
 body temperature and, (V1) 449
 bowel elimination and, (V1) 758, (V1) 760
 burnout and, (V1) 253–254, (V1) 254b
 cardiovascular function and, (V1) 1021
 coping and adaptation relation to, (V1) 240–242, (V1) 241f
 crisis intervention and, (V1) 263, (V2) 81
 critical thinking and clinical judgment on, (V2) 85–86
 daily, (V1) 227
 dealing with angry patients and, (V2) 80
 defined, (V1) 239
 exercise for relief from, (V1) 867
 exhaustion or recovery stage of, (V1) 244
 full-spectrum nursing model applied to, (V2) 84–85
 health promotion activities for, (V1) 258–259
 of hospitalization, (V1) 263
 host susceptibility to infection and, (V1) 529, (V1) 533
 implementation for, (V1) 258
 knowledge map on, (V2) 88
 life stress review, (V1) 227

making referrals for, (V1) 264
models of, (V1) 240
nursing diagnosis and, (V1) 257
nutrition and, (V1) 689
planning for, (V1) 257–258
post-traumatic stress disorder (PTSD) and, (V1) 254, (V1) 255–256
pulmonary function and, (V1) 981
pulse rate and, (V1) 457
resistance stage in, (V1) 244
respiration and, (V1) 464
responses to
 general adaptation syndrome (GAS), (V1) 242–245, (V1) 243–244f
 local adaptation syndrome, (V1) 245–246, (V1) 245b
 psychological, (V1) 246–251, (V1) 246b, (V1) 247–248t, (V1) 251–253
 spiritual, (V1) 251
sensory function and, (V1) 788
sleep and, (V1) 917
support systems for, (V1) 262–263
techniques for managing, (V1) 260–262, (V1) 262f
workplace, (V1) 263–264
Stressor(s)
 anticipatory, (V1) 239
 childhood, (V1) 240b
 common approaches to coping with, (V1) 241
 developmental, (V1) 239
 distress/eustress, (V1) 239
 endocrine system response to, (V1) 242–243, (V1) 244f
 external, (V1) 239
 how people respond to, (V1) 242–251
 internal, (V1) 239
 perception of, (V1) 241
 physiological, (V1) 239
 psychosocial, (V1) 239
 situational, (V1) 239
 sympathetic nervous system responses to, (V1) 243
 time, (V1) 239
Stretching injuries, (V1) 859
Striae, (V1) 490
Stridor, (V1) 466, (V1) 994
Stroebe, Margaret, (V1) 352t
Stroke. See Cerebrovascular accident
Stroke volume, (V1) 457
 blood pressure and, (V1) 467–468
Structural abnormalities of pulmonary system, (V1) 989
Structural-functional family theories, (V1) 295
Structure evaluation, (V1) 86
Structure reviews, (V1) 23
STTI. See Sigma Theta Tau International (STTI)
Student care plans, (V1) 69
 mind-mapping, (V1) 71
Student liability, (V1) 1178–1179
Subcultures, (V1) 313–314
 gender, (V1) 314
 nursing and other professional, (V1) 318–319
 old age, (V1) 314
 vulnerable population, (V1) 314
Subcutaneous infusions, (V1) 1060, (V1) 1061f
Subcutaneous injections, (V1) 649–651, (V1) 649f, (V1) 660p, (V2) 431–434p
 opioid, (V1) 830

Subcutaneous tissue, (V1) 941
Subjective data, (V1) 47–48, (V1) 48t
Subjective global assessment (SGA), (V1) 695, (V2) 505
Sublimation, as defense mechanism, (V1) 248t
Sublingual medications, (V1) 636
Substance abuse
 by adolescents, (V1) 172, (V1) 173–174
 cardiovascular function and, (V1) 1021, (V1) 1022
 host susceptibility to infection and, (V1) 525, (V1) 528
 influence on health and illness, (V1) 213
 maternal, (V1) 150
 medications, (V1) 624
 mental illness and, (V1) 287, (V1) 290
 opioids, (V1) 834–835
 oxygenation and, (V1) 982
 treatment for, (V1) 287, (V1) 290
 by young adults, (V1) 180
Substernal retraction, (V1) 466
Substitutive effects, (V1) 620
Subsystems in families, (V1) 295
Sucking reflex, (V1) 153
Suctioning of airways, (V1) 1006–1007, (V1) 1007f, (V1) 1012–1013p, (V2) 726–730p
Sudden infant death syndrome (SIDS), (V1) 150, (V1) 157–158, (V1) 160
Suffocation, (V1) 549
 prevention of, (V1) 564–565, (V1) 566f
Sugars, (V1) 669
Suicide
 by adolescents, (V1) 172
 assisted, (V1) 361
 cues indicating possible risk for, (V1) 287b
 opioids and risk of, (V1) 835
Summarizing conversations, (V1) 389
Sunburn, (V1) 548
Sun exposure, (V1) 944
Superego, (V1) 147
Superficial pain, (V1) 811
Superficial reflexes, (V1) 507
 testing, (V2) 283p
Superficial sensations, testing, (V2) 279p
Superficial wounds, (V1) 946
Supine position, (V1) 872–873, (V1) 872t
Supplemental Nutrition Assistance Program (SNAP), (V1) 701
Supplementation
 oral electrolyte, (V1) 1055
 vitamin and mineral, (V1) 700–701
Supplies. See Equipment and supplies
Supportive effects, (V1) 620
Support systems
 adaptation and, (V1) 241
 assessing, (V1) 256
 assessment of, (V1) 802
 for caregivers, (V1) 205, (V1) 1135
 identifying and using, (V1) 262–263
 physical activity and, (V1) 856
 support groups, for patient teaching, (V1) 411
Suppositories, (V1) 614t
Suppressor cells, (V1) 524
Suppressor T cells, (V1) 524
Suprapubic catheter, (V1) 736, (V1) 736f
Suprasternal retraction, (V1) 466

Suprasystems in families, (V1) 295
Surgery
 bariatric, (V1) 693
 bowel elimination and, (V1) 759–760
 classification of, (V1) 1077–1078
 clean wounds from, (V1) 950
 collaborative wound treatments, (V1) 949
 full-spectrum nursing model applied to, (V2) 831–832
 interruption of pain conduction pathways by, (V1) 832–833
 intraoperative care (See Intraoperative care)
 key concept sin, (V1) 1076
 music used during and after, (V1) 1090
 "never events" in, (V1) 1077
 operative field and, (V2) 826
 perioperative nursing for, (V1) 1076–1077, (V1) 1076b
 positioning for, (V1) 1094
 preexisting conditions and, (V1) 1079, (V1) 1079b
 preoperative care (See Preoperative care)
 preparing a room for patient's return from, (V2) 826
 risk factors in, (V1) 1078–1081, (V1) 1079b, (V1) 1079t, (V1) 1080b
 safety checklist for, (V2) 829
 sexuality and, (V1) 891–892
 skin preparation for, (V1) 1086–1087, (V1) 1094
 urinary diversion, (V1) 740–745, (V1) 744f
 urinary elimination and, (V1) 723–724
 wounds from, (V1) 1079, (V1) 1079t
Surgical asepsis
 avoiding common breaks in sterility and, (V1) 540b
 defined, (V1) 536–537
 donning surgical attire in, (V1) 538
 hand washing method, (V1) 539p
 surgical scrub in, (V1) 537, (V1) 537t
 using sterile technique in nursing care, (V1) 538
Surgical attire, (V1) 538
Surgical consent forms, (V1) 1084–1085
Surgical glue, (V1) 949
Surgical hand washing, (V1) 539p
 brushless system, (V2) 311–313p
 traditional method, (V2) 309–311p
Surgical holding area, (V1) 1089, (V1) 1089f
Surgical patient care
 applying antiembolism stockings, (V2) 815–817p
 applying sequential compression devices, (V1) 1104p, (V2) 817–819p
 critical thinking and clinical judgment on, (V2) 832–833
 knowledge map on, (V2) 834
 managing gastric suction, (V2) 819–824p
 teaching patient to deep-breathe, cough, move in bed, and perform leg exercises, (V2) 811–814p
Surgical scrub, (V1) 537
Surgical site infections, (V1) 1080, (V1) 1085
Surgical staples, (V1) 949, (V1) 949f
Susceptible host for infection, (V1) 519
Suspensions, (V1) 612t
Sutures, (V1) 948–949, (V2) 688–689p
Swabbing, wound, (V1) 958
Swallowing, impaired, (V1) 702–703, (V1) 703f
Swallowing reflex, (V1) 153

Sweat glands, (V1) 579, (V1) 582
    drug excretion and, (V1) 618
    fever and, (V1) 943
Swelling, wound, (V1) 953
SWOT analysis, (V1) 1185, (V1) 1186t
Sympathectomy, (V1) 833
Sympathetic fibers, (V1) 1019–1020
Sympathetic nervous system
    responses to pain, (V1) 817
    responses to stress, (V1) 243
Symptoms of illness, (V1) 218
Synarthroses, (V1) 841
Synchrony, (V1) 919
Syndactylism, (V1) 857
Synergistic drug relationship, (V1) 623
Synovial fluid, (V1) 842
Synovial joints, (V1) 842, (V1) 843t
Syphilis, (V1) 151, (V1) 896, (V1) 899t
Syringes
    irrigation and instillation, (V1) 639, (V1) 639f
    mixing medications in same, (V1) 646
    parenteral medications, (V1) 643–645f, (V1) 644–645
Syrups, (V1) 612t
Systemic circulation, (V1) 497
Systemic diseases and skin, (V1) 583
Systemic effects, drug, (V1) 612
Systemic infections, (V1) 519
    urinary elimination and, (V1) 724
Systemic side effects, (V1) 640
System-specific assessment, (V1) 479
System theory, (V1) 103, (V1) 294
Systole, (V1) 457, (V1) 499
Systolic pressure, (V1) 467, (V1) 473

T

Tablets, (V1) 612t
Tachycardia, (V1) 460
Tachypnea, (V1) 465t, (V1) 994
Take-home toxins, (V1) 549, (V1) 565
Taking action. *See* Implementation
Talk test, (V1) 853b
Tanner model of clinical judgment, (V1) 30–31
Tantrums, (V1) 163
Tape, adhesive, (V1) 971
Taping of dressings, (V2) 665–666p
Target heart rate (THR) method, (V1) 853b
Tartar, (V1) 593
Task groups, (V1) 386
Task versus relationship theories, (V1) 1182
Taste sense
    diminished, (V1) 702
    in neonates, (V1) 786
Tattoos, (V1) 172, (V1) 944
T-binders, (V1) 972
Teaching
    See also Patient education
    five rights of, (V1) 397b
    plans for, (V1) 69, (V1) 409–411, (V1) 410t, (V1) 411f, (V1) 412–414
    strategies for, (V1) 410
Team empowerment, (V1) 553
Team nursing, (V1) 16
    communication with surgical team, (V1) 1081, (V1) 1088–1089
    home healthcare, (V1) 1124
Tearing injuries, (V1) 859
Tea tree, (V1) 786

Technetium scan, (V2) 763
Technologists, (V1) 18
Technology
    barriers to learning with, (V1) 407–408
    for counseling, (V1) 232–233
    culture and, (V1) 316
    ethics and, (V1) 121
    for managing staffing and workflow, (V1) 1142
    in nursing, (V1) 27
    for patient self-care, (V1) 1143–1144, (V1) 1143f
    for patient teaching, (V1) 411
    for reducing error with automation, (V1) 1142–1143
    supporting healthcare professionals, (V1) 1145–1146, (V1) 1146f
    for tracking patients and equipment, (V1) 1142
Teenage pregnancy, (V1) 151, (V1) 176, (V1) 178, (V1) 299
Teeth
    See also Dental hygiene
    care of, (V1) 595–596, (V1) 595f, (V1) 602p, (V2) 358–361p
    decay of, in infants, (V1) 157
    denture care, (V1) 602p, (V2) 361–363p
    developmental variations in, (V1) 592, (V1) 592f, (V1) 593f
    edentulism and, (V1) 191
    eruption of permanent, (V1) 167
    eruption of primary, (V1) 156
    physical examination of, (V1) 494
Telehealth nursing, (V1) 25, (V1) 216, (V1) 1141, (V1) 1141f
Telephone prescriptions, (V1) 438–439, (V1) 626, (V2) 159
Temperature
    See also Body temperature
    cardiovascular function and, (V1) 1021
    equipment for measuring, (V1) 451, (V1) 452–453t, (V1) 454
    measurement scales for, (V1) 450–451, (V1) 451f
    pulmonary function and, (V1) 982
    room, (V1) 603
Temperature therapy, (V1) 824–825
Temporal artery
    body temperature measurement and, (V1) 455t, (V2) 176–177p
    pulse measurement and, (V1) 460, (V2) 183p
Temporary bowel diversions, (V1) 761
Tendons, (V1) 504, (V1) 504f, (V1) 843
Teratogens, (V1) 150
Terminal hair, (V1) 597
Termination phase of communication, (V1) 385
Terminology, medication administration times, (V1) 432
Territoriality, (V1) 381
Tertiary defenses against infection, (V1) 521, (V1) 522–523b, (V1) 524, (V1) 524f, (V1) 525b, (V1) 525f
Tertiary intention healing, (V1) 947, (V1) 947f
Tertiary prevention, (V1) 220
Tertiary services, (V1) 18
Testes, (V1) 883, (V1) 884f, (V1) 893
Testicular cancer screening, (V1) 229, (V1) 906
Testicular self-examination, (V1) 178
    young adults and, (V1) 180

Tetanus immunization, (V1) 958
Theology, (V1) 330
Theoretical definition, (V1) 95
Theoretical knowledge, (V1) 30, (V1) 60
    ethical decision making and, (V1) 139
Theory/theories
    See also Nursing theory
    activity, (V1) 191
    of aging, (V1) 190
    components of, (V1) 94–95
    defined, (V1) 94
    of development, (V1) 103, (V1) 145–148t, (V1) 145–149
    development of, (V1) 96–97, (V1) 96f
    disengagement, (V1) 191
    emotional intelligence, (V1) 1182
    family care and, (V1) 295–296
    of leadership, (V1) 1181–1183, (V1) 1183t
        behavioral, (V1) 1182
        situational, (V1) 1182
        task versus relationship, (V1) 1182
        trait, (V1) 1182
        transactional, (V1) 1183, (V1) 1183t
        transformational, (V1) 1182–1183, (V1) 1183t
    learning, (V1) 397–398
    management, (V1) 1183–1184
    Maslow's hierarchy of human needs, (V1) 100, (V1) 102, (V1) 102f
    from other disciplines used in nursing, (V1) 100–104, (V1) 102f
    paradigms, frameworks, models, and, (V1) 95–96
    psychosocial development, (V1) 148, (V1) 191–192
    sexual health and, (V1) 908
    stress and adaptation, (V1) 102–103
    system, (V1) 103
    validation, (V1) 102
Theory X, (V1) 1184
Theory Y, (V1) 1184
Therapeutic baths, (V1) 586–587
Therapeutic communication, (V1) 363, (V1) 364b
    barriers to, (V1) 389–391
    enhancing, (V1) 387–389, (V1) 388f
    evidence-based practice in, (V1) 392
    key characteristics of, (V1) 385
Therapeutic range of drugs, (V1) 618–619
Therapeutic relationships
    limits and boundaries of, (V1) 376
    phases of, (V1) 384–385
    therapeutic use of self in, (V1) 385
Therapeutic touch (TT), (V1) 261, (V1) 826
Therapists, (V1) 18
Therapy groups, (V1) 386
Thermography, (V1) 495–496
Thermometers, (V1) 451, (V1) 452–453t, (V2) 173–179p
    mercury in, (V1) 555
Thermoreceptors, (V1) 784
Thermoregulation, (V1) 444, (V1) 446
    See also Body temperature
    neonatal, (V1) 153
Theta waves, (V1) 920, (V1) 920f, (V1) 920t
Thiamin, (V1) 675–676t
Third heart sound, (V1) 501
Third spacing, (V1) 1037
Third trimester
    fetal development during, (V1) 150
    maternal changes during, (V1) 150

Thirst, (V1) 1040
Thoracentesis, (V2) 753
Three checks, medication, (V1) 630
Three-dimensional printing, (V1) 1145
Thrill, (V1) 501
Throat, physical examination of, (V1) 509
Throat culture, (V2) 753
Thrombophlebitis
  as complication of intravenous therapy, (V1) 1066t
  as postoperative complication, (V1) 1099t
Thrombus, (V1) 1033
Throughput, in systems theory, (V1) 103
Thyroid gland, (V1) 495
  basal metabolic rate (BMR) and, (V1) 447
Thyroid hormone, (V1) 1041
Thyroid-stimulating hormone (TSH), (V1) 243
Thyroxine, (V1) 447
Ticks, (V1) 570
Tidal volume, (V1) 465, (V2) 752
Timed-release medications, (V1) 616
Timed Up & Go test, (V1) 557
Time management, (V1) 1196–1197
  BOSS tool, (V1) 1198–1199t
  organizing work for, (V1) 1197–1199, (V1) 1199b
  setting goals for, (V1) 1197
  work-life balance and, (V1) 1200, (V1) 1200t
Time orientation, (V1) 315–316, (V1) 327b
Time-released tablets or capsules, (V1) 612t
Time stressors, (V1) 239
  management of, (V1) 259
Timing
  in communication, (V1) 378
  insulin administration, (V1) 650
  of medication administration, (V1) 619
  in patient learning, (V1) 400
Tinctures, (V1) 612t, (V1) 613t
Tinea pedis, (V1) 589
Tissue biopsy, (V1) 958, (V2) 700
Tissue building by proteins, (V1) 671
Tissue perfusion, (V1) 467
  alteration in, (V1) 461
Tobacco use. *See* Smoking
Toddlers
  assessment of, (V1) 164
  common health problems of, (V1) 163–164
  communication by, (V1) 380
  development of
    cognitive, (V1) 162
    physical, (V1) 162, (V1) 162f, (V1) 163b
    psychosocial, (V1) 162–163
    sexuality, (V1) 886
  drowning of, (V1) 549
  immunizations in, (V1) 163
  implementation for, (V1) 164
  infections in, (V1) 163
  loss in, (V1) 348
  neurological system examination in, (V1) 505
  nutrition in, (V1) 685
  physical examination of, (V1) 485
  pulmonary function in, (V1) 980
  safety of, (V1) 546
  sleep requirements and characteristics in, (V1) 918t, (V1) 923
  surgical risk in, (V1) 1078
  unintentional injury in, (V1) 163
  urinary elimination in, (V1) 721–722

To Err Is Human: Building a Safer Health System, (V1) 545
Toilet training, (V1) 162, (V1) 164, (V1) 166, (V1) 721, (V1) 757
Tolerable upper intake level (UL), (V1) 667
Tolerance
  drug, (V1) 624
  pain, (V1) 814
Tongue, (V1) 494, (V1) 494f
Tonic neck reflex, (V1) 153, (V1) 154f
Topical anesthesia, (V1) 832
Topical medications
  administration of, (V1) 659p, (V2) 409–412p
  lotions, creams, and ointments, (V1) 637
  transdermal, (V1) 637, (V1) 639f
Tort law, (V1) 1166
Torts
  intentional, (V1) 1166–1167
  quasi-intentional, (V1) 1166
  unintentional, (V1) 1167–1169
Total care, (V1) 16
Total colectomy with ileoanal reservoir, (V1) 761
Total quality management (TQM), (V1) 23
Touch
  conveying caring through, (V1) 379, (V1) 379f
  in infants, (V1) 787
  mutual masturbation, (V1) 895
  neonatal sense of, (V1) 155, (V1) 786–787
  as spiritual intervention, (V1) 343
  therapeutic (TT), (V1) 261, (V1) 826
Touch therapies, (V1) 261
Toxic reactions to drugs, (V1) 621–622
Toxoplasmosis, (V1) 151
  sensory function and, (V1) 788
Trabeculae, (V1) 841
Trace minerals, (V1) 673, (V1) 680–681t
Trachea, (V1) 977
Tracheostomy, (V1) 1004, (V1) 1011–1013p
  modified sterile technique for, (V2) 719–726p
  or endotracheal suctioning, (V2) 726–730p
Tracheostomy approach to airway suctioning, (V1) 1007
Traditional Chinese medicine (TCM), (V1) 320
Traditional families, (V1) 292
Trait theories, (V1) 1182
Tranquilizers, (V1) 924
Transactional theories, (V1) 1183, (V1) 1183t
Transcellular fluid, (V1) 1037
Transcendence of self, (V1) 102, (V1) 102f
Transcultural assessment model, (V2) 112
Transcutaneous electrical nerve stimulators (TENS), (V1) 824
Transdermal patches, (V1) 613t, (V1) 638, (V1) 639f
  opioid, (V1) 830
Transduction, pain, (V1) 813
Trans-fatty acids, (V1) 672, (V1) 672t
Transfer belts, (V1) 875, (V1) 875f
Transfer boards, (V1) 874, (V1) 875f
Transfer needles, (V1) 654, (V1) 654f
Transfer of patient to another unit, (V1) 236p, (V2) 63–64p
Transfer of patient to long-term care facility, (V1) 237p, (V2) 64–65p
Transfer reports, (V1) 438
Transferrin, (V1) 698
Transferring of patients, (V2) 622–625p

Transfer roller sheets, (V1) 873, (V1) 873f
Transfers, (V1) 235, (V1) 236–237p
Transformational theories, (V1) 1182–1183, (V1) 1183t
Transfusions. *See* Blood infusions
Transgender, (V1) 886
Transient flora, (V1) 516
Transitions, maintaining trust during, (V1) 235–236
Transition to extrauterine life, (V1) 155
Translators, (V1) 326, (V2) 110
Transmission, pain, (V1) 813–814, (V1) 813f
Transmission-based isolation, (V1) 536
Transmission-based precautions, (V1) 535, (V1) 535t, (V1) 536, (V2) 325–326
Transparency, (V1) 553
Transparent film dressing, (V2) 676–678p
Transpersonal caring moments, (V1) 104
Transplant surgery, (V1) 1078
Transport, water and, (V1) 681
Transtheoretical model of change, (V1) 222
Transverse colon, (V1) 755
Trapeze bars, (V1) 869
Trauma
  bone, (V1) 858–859, (V1) 860f
  nutrition and, (V1) 693
  oxygenation and, (V1) 992
  rape, (V1) 900
  vulnerable populations and, (V1) 1113
Treadmill test, (V2) 763
Treatment failure, as health disruption, (V1) 217
Tremor, (V1) 864b
Trial and error, (V1) 107
Trial process, (V1) 1170
Triangular arm binders, (V1) 972
Trichomoniasis, (V1) 898t
Tricyclic antidepressants, (V1) 935
Triglycerides, (V1) 671
Trochanter rolls, (V1) 869, (V1) 870f
Troponin, (V2) 763
Trousseau's sign, (V2) 798
Trust
  communication for establishing, (V1) 388
  established at first patient contact, (V1) 234–235
  home healthcare and, (V1) 1128
  leaders and, (V1) 1191
  versus mistrust, in psychosocial development theory, (V1) 148
Truth, (V1) 130–131
Tubal ligation, (V2) 643
Tub baths, (V1) 586, (V2) 383
Tuberculin skin testing, (V1) 996, (V2) 754
Tuberculosis, (V1) 985
Tubing
  changing IV, (V2) 779–782p
  chest, (V1) 1009–1010, (V1) 1009–1010f, (V1) 1014p, (V2) 750–751p
  parenteral therapy, (V1) 1064
  stethoscope, (V1) 459
Tubular reabsorption, (V1) 718
Tubular secretion, (V1) 718
Tuesdays with Morrie, (V1) 213
Tumors, bone, (V1) 858, (V1) 866
Tunneled central venous catheters, (V1) 1059, (V1) 1060f
Tunneled devices, (V1) 657
Tunneling wounds, (V1) 953
Tunnel wounds, (V1) 945t

Turmeric, (V1) 823
20-hour infusion, (V1) 713
24-hour recall, (V1) 696
24-hour urine collection, (V1) 729
Two-minute briefings, (V1) 1089
Tympanic membrane (TM), (V1) 493
  body temperature measurement using, (V1) 456t, (V2) 177–178p
Tympanites, (V1) 1100t

U

UL. *See* Tolerable upper intake level (UL)
Ulcers, skin, (V1) 945f, (V1) 946t, (V2) 213p
  Braden Scale for Predicting Pressure Sore Risk, (V2) 696
  Norton Pressure Sore Risk Assessment Scale, (V2) 697
  pressure ulcer healing chart, (V2) 699
  PUSH Tool for Evaluation of Pressure Ulcers, (V2) 698
Ultrasonic nebulizers, (V1) 641
Ultrasound, (V2) 587, (V2) 763
Umbilical hernia, (V1) 503
Unauthorized practice, (V1) 1178
Uncomplicated grief, (V1) 354
Unconscious mind, (V1) 147
Unconscious patients
  nose care for, (V1) 601
  oral care for, (V1) 596, (V1) 602p, (V2) 363–366p
Undermining wounds, (V1) 953
Underwater weighing, (V1) 697
Underweight and malnutrition, (V1) 703–706
Unemployment and poverty, (V1) 299
Unexpected/sudden life changes, as health disruption, (V1) 217
Uniform Determination of Death Act, (V1) 356, (V1) 356b
Uniform Law Commission, (V1) 356
Unintentional torts, (V1) 1167–1169
Unit-dose system, (V1) 610, (V1) 610f
Units, insulin, (V1) 624
Unknown situations, as health disruption, (V1) 217
Unlicensed assistive personnel (UAP), (V1) 18, (V1) 26–27
  ear cleaning and hearing aid care by, (V1) 601
  focused nutritional assessment by, (V1) 699
  hygiene care by, (V1) 578–579, (V1) 579f
  pain management by, (V1) 823, (V1) 823b
  power of, (V1) 1190
  unauthorized practice by, (V1) 1178
  wound assessment by, (V1) 958–959
Unoccupied bed making, (V1) 603p, (V2) 377–380p
Unoccupied beds, making, (V2) 377–380p
Unrelieved pain, (V1) 817–818
Unsaturated fatty acids, (V1) 672
Unstable angina, (V1) 1024
Upper airway, (V1) 977
  suctioning of, (V2) 734–736p
Upper respiratory infections (URIs)
  cough with, (V1) 995
  influenza and, (V1) 985–989
  teaching clients how to prevent, (V1) 233
  in toddlers, (V1) 980
Urea, (V1) 698–699

Ureters, (V1) 720
Urethra, (V1) 720–721
Urge incontinence, (V1) 723
Urgent surgery, (V1) 1078
Urinalysis (UA), (V1) 729, (V1) 1053, (V2) 547–548, (V2) 830
  preoperative care, (V1) 1082
Urinary catheterization, (V1) 732–740, (V1) 736f, (V1) 738f
  care plan for, (V1) 748–750
  external (condom), (V2) 535–537p
  insertion of
    indwelling, (V2) 529–535p
    intermittent, (V2) 523–528p
Urinary diversion, (V1) 740–745, (V1) 744f
Urinary elimination
  assessment of
    common diagnostic procedures in, (V1) 727
    guidelines and tools for, (V2) 545–546
    nursing history, (V1) 724
    physical, (V1) 727
    urine tests in, (V1) 727–729, (V1) 728f, (V1) 730f
  critical thinking and clinical judgment on, (V2) 556
  diagnostic testing of, (V2) 547–550
  factors affecting
    developmental, (V1) 721–722
    lifestyle, (V1) 723
    medications, (V1) 723, (V1) 723b
    pathological conditions, (V1) 724
    personal, sociocultural, and environmental, (V1) 722–723
    surgery and anesthesia, (V1) 723–724
  full-spectrum nursing model applied to, (V2) 555
  key concepts on, (V1) 717
  knowledge map on, (V2) 558
  normal patterns in, (V1) 721
  nursing care plan for, (V2) 551–554
  nursing diagnosis and, (V1) 731
  preoperative, (V1) 1087
  procedures
    applying external (condom) urinary catheter, (V2) 535–537p
    inserting an intermittent urinary catheter, (V2) 523–528p
    irrigating bladder or catheter, (V2) 540–543p
    measuring postvoid residual urine volume with portable bladder scanner, (V2) 517–519p
    obtaining a urine specimen for testing, (V2) 519–523p
    removing indwelling catheter, (V2) 537–539p
  promoting normal, (V1) 731–732, (V1) 732b
  steps in, (V1) 721
  teaching clients about clean, intermittent self-catheterization, (V2) 544
  urinary catheterization and, (V1) 732–740, (V1) 736f, (V1) 738f
    care plan for, (V1) 748–750
  urinary diversion and, (V1) 740–745, (V1) 744f
Urinary incontinence, (V1) 201, (V1) 741–744
  management of, (V1) 730
Urinary retention, (V1) 733–735
  as postoperative complication, (V1) 1100t

Urinary system
  disorders of, (V1) 724
  kidneys filtering and regulating in, (V1) 717
  nephrons forming urine in, (V1) 717–718, (V1) 719–720f
  organs of, (V1) 717f, (V1) 718f
  response to stress, (V1) 244
  terms associated with, (V1) 729b
  ureters transporting urine in, (V1) 720
  urethra transporting urine, (V1) 720–721
  urinary bladder storing urine in, (V1) 720
Urinary tract infection (UTI), (V1) 725–726
  indwelling catheters and, (V1) 737–738, (V1) 738f
  as postoperative complication, (V1) 1100t
Urine
  assessment of, (V1) 727–729, (V1) 728f, (V1) 730f
  characteristics of normal, (V1) 721
  fluid loss via, (V1) 1041
  formation of, (V1) 717–718, (V1) 720f
  obtaining a urine specimen for testing, (V2) 519–523p
  osmolality, (V1) 1053
  storage in the urinary bladder, (V1) 720
  transported by ureters, (V1) 720
  transported by urethra, (V1) 720–721
U.S. Bureau of the Census, (V1) 1110–1111
U.S. Constitution, (V1) 1156, (V1) 1157t
USDA *Dietary Guidelines for Americans 2020-2025*, (V1) 667, (V1) 667lb
U.S. Public Health Service (USPHS), (V1) 1113–1114
Uterus, (V1) 882, (V1) 893
Utilitarianism, (V1) 126–127
Utilization review, (V1) 421

V

Vaccinations. *See* Immunizations
Vagina, (V1) 882
Vaginal medications, (V1) 640, (V1) 658–659p
  administration of, (V1) 658p, (V2) 407–409p
Vaginal ring, (V2) 642
Vaginismus, (V1) 901
Valerian root, (V1) 937
Validation
  of data, (V1) 51–52
  of messages, (V1) 388
Validation theory, (V1) 102
Valsalva maneuver, (V1) 757
Values
  See also Ethics
  attitudes, beliefs, and, (V1) 124–126
  clarification of, (V1) 133, (V1) 134t
  conflicts in, (V1) 123
  critical thinking and clinical judgment applied to, (V2) 34–36
  defined, (V1) 124
  knowledge map for, (V2) 38
  neutrality in, (V1) 125–126
  nursing, (V1) 318–319
  professional versus personal, (V1) 125
  related to ethics, (V1) 125
  transmission of, (V1) 125, (V1) 126t
Valve incompetence, (V1) 1025
Valves, heart, (V1) 1017, (V1) 1017f, (V1) 1024–1025
Valve stenosis, (V1) 1024–1025
Vanauken, Sheldon, (V1) 234

Vancomycin-resistant enterococci (VRE), (V1) 164
Vascular response to stress, (V1) 245
Vascular system, (V1) 502, (V1) 511–512p, (V1) 1019–1020
 altitude and, (V1) 982
 assessment of, (V2) 250–257p
Vasectomy, (V2) 643
Vasocongestion, (V1) 893
Vasoconstriction, (V1) 447
Vasodilation, (V1) 447
Vasodilators, (V1) 1023t, (V1) 1033
Vasomotor center, (V1) 1020
Vastus lateralis injection site, (V1) 652, (V1) 652f
Vector, (V1) 519
Vector-borne pathogens, (V1) 550
 fighting, (V1) 568, (V1) 570
Vegetarian/vegan diets, (V1) 667–668, (V1) 690
Veins, (V1) 502, (V1) 1018
 abnormalities of, (V1) 1025
 jugular, (V1) 502
Vellus hair, (V1) 597
Venipuncture, (V1) 1062–1063
 site selection for, (V2) 800
Vernix caseosa, (V1) 153
Venography, (V2) 763
Venous access devices, parenteral nutrition, (V1) 714
Venous return, (V1) 1032
Venous stasis ulcers, (V1) 946t, (V1) 959–960
Venous system, (V1) 497
Ventilation
 altitude and, (V1) 982
 defined, (V1) 977
 factors affecting, (V1) 978
 mechanical, (V1) 1008–1009, (V1) 1008f, (V1) 1014p
 medications promoting, (V1) 984t
 positioning for maximum, (V1) 1002
 problems of, (V1) 999
 pulmonary, (V1) 462, (V1) 977–978, (V1) 978f
Ventilation-perfusion scan, (V2) 753
Ventilator-associated pneumonia (VAP), (V1) 532, (V1) 1008–1009
 oral care and, (V1) 596
Ventricles, (V1) 1017, (V1) 1017f
Ventrogluteal muscle injection site, (V1) 651–652, (V1) 651f
Venules, (V1) 1018
Veracity, (V1) 130–131
Verbal communication, (V1) 377–378
Verbal prescriptions, (V1) 438–439, (V1) 626, (V2) 159
Vesicle, (V2) 211p
Vials, (V1) 645–646, (V1) 646f, (V1) 659p
Vibration, chest, (V1) 1003, (V1) 1011p, (V2) 712–713p
Vicarious liability, (V1) 1169
Video recordings, (V1) 389
Violence
 See also Child abuse and neglect
 assessing risk for, (V1) 561
 against healthcare workers, (V1) 557, (V1) 574
 and neglect as family health challenge, (V1) 301–302
 and risk-taking behaviors in school-age children, (V1) 170

screening for, (V1) 180
 sexual, (V1) 897, (V1) 900
 workplace, (V1) 382–383
 young adults and, (V1) 180
Viruses, emerging, (V1) 520
Visceral pain, (V1) 811, (V1) 812
Vision
 annual eye examination for, (V1) 182
 communicating with clients having impaired, (V2) 598
 contact lenses and, (V1) 600, (V2) 372–373p, (V2) 603p
 in infants, (V1) 787
 in neonates, (V1) 154, (V1) 786
 in preschoolers, (V1) 166
 prior to death, (V1) 357
 in school-age children, (V1) 167, (V1) 169
 in toddlers, (V1) 162
Visual acuity, (V1) 491–492
Visual Analog Scale (VAS), (V2) 610
Visual field, (V1) 492
Visualization studies, (V1) 260–261
 bowel elimination, (V1) 765, (V2) 586–588
 urinary system, (V1) 727, (V2) 549–550
Vital capacity, (V2) 753
Vital signs (VS)
 blood pressure (See Blood pressure)
 body temperature (See Body temperature)
 critical thinking and clinical judgment on, (V2) 195–196
 defined, (V1) 444
 delegating, (V1) 476
 documentation of, (V1) 445
 evaluating, (V1) 476
 full-spectrum nursing model applied to, (V2) 194
 in general survey, (V1) 487
 key concepts in, (V1) 444
 knowledge map on, (V2) 197
 normal findings for adults, (V1) 445, (V1) 445t
 pain as fifth, (V1) 444, (V1) 819
 pulse (See Pulse)
 respiration (See Respiration)
 when to measure, (V1) 445, (V1) 445t
Vitamin A, (V1) 673, (V1) 674t
Vitamin B complex, (V1) 673, (V1) 675–678t
Vitamin C, (V1) 673, (V1) 678t
 bowel elimination and, (V1) 758
 skin and, (V1) 942
Vitamin D, (V1) 673, (V1) 674t
 bone formation and, (V1) 857
 osteoporosis and, (V1) 866
 recommended daily allowance for, (V1) 1044t
 skin and formation of, (V1) 582
 supplementation of, (V1) 700
Vitamin E, (V1) 673, (V1) 674–675t
Vitamin K, (V1) 673, (V1) 674–675t
 supplementation of, (V1) 700
Vitamins, (V1) 673, (V1) 674–678t
 bowel elimination and, (V1) 758
 cardiovascular function and, (V1) 1022
 teaching clients about supplementation with, (V1) 700–701
Vocabulary, (V1) 377, (V1) 487
Vocational nursing education, (V1) 10–11
Voided urine, (V1) 728
Volkmann canals, (V1) 841

Volume-control infusion sets, (V1) 656, (V1) 656f, (V1) 1063, (V1) 1071p, (V2) 777–779p
Volume in communication, (V1) 377
Voluntary agencies, (V1) 1124
Vomiting. See Nausea and vomiting
VQ scan, (V2) 763
VS. See Vital signs (VS)
Vulnerable populations, (V1) 314, (V1) 1112–1113
Vulva, (V1) 882

W

Waddling gait, (V1) 865
Waist-to-hip ratio (WHR), (V1) 696
Wald, Lillian, (V1) 6, (V1) 1114
Walkers, (V1) 877–878, (V1) 878f
Walking aids, (V1) 877–878, (V1) 877–878f, (V2) 630–631
Water
 See also Hydration
 as essential nutrient, (V1) 681
 PICOT questions on, (V1) 682
 for wound care, (V1) 963–964
Water-borne pathogens, (V1) 550
Water contamination, (V1) 551
Water-soluble drugs, (V1) 616
Water-soluble vitamins, (V1) 673, (V1) 675–676t
Watson, Jean, (V1) 93–94, (V1) 208
Watson's 10 caring processes, (V1) 93–94, (V1) 95, (V1) 95b, (V2) 27–28
Wearable devices, (V1) 1143–1145
Wear-and-tear theory, (V1) 190
Weather hazards, (V1) 551, (V1) 570–571
 physical activity and, (V1) 856
Web conferencing, (V1) 1141
Weber test, (V1) 493–494
Webinars, (V1) 1141
Weight
 See also Obesity and overweight
 body mass index (BMI) and, (V1) 487–488
 in school-age children, (V1) 169
 diets for losing, (V1) 691, (V1) 694
 gain of
  infant, (V1) 156
  during pregnancy, (V1) 151, (V1) 151f
  preschooler, (V1) 164–165
  school-age children, (V1) 167
  toddle, (V1) 162
 in general survey, (V1) 487
 ideal, (V1) 683
 loss of
  teaching school-age children about, (V1) 170
  tips for, (V1) 707
 pharmacokinetics and, (V1) 619
 standards of, (V1) 683
 underwater, (V1) 697
 underweight and malnutrition, (V1) 703–706
Wellness, (V1) 208
 See also Health
 assessment of, (V1) 50, (V1) 223, (V1) 226–229
 as balancing act, (V1) 234
 defined, (V1) 208–209
 environmental factors and, (V1) 214
 envisioning, (V1) 234

goals for, (V1) 74
how people experience, (V1) 212–215, (V1) 214t
how to honor each client's unique experience with, (V1) 233–235
as individual experience, (V1) 209
influence of lifestyle on, (V1) 213
influence of personal relationships on, (V1) 213–214, (V1) 214t
interventions for, (V1) 80
key concepts of, (V1) 208–209
PICOT question for, (V1) 203
using conceptual models to understand, (V1) 209–210, (V1) 210f
Western medicine, (V1) 317
Wet-to-damp dressings, (V2) 668–670p
Wet-to-dry dressings, (V1) 967
Wheal, (V2) 212p
Wheel of wellness, (V1) 221–222, (V1) 222f
Wheezing, (V1) 465, (V1) 994
Whirlpool treatments, (V1) 967
Whistleblowing, (V1) 119, (V1) 121, (V1) 122
White blood cells (WBCs), (V1) 521, (V1) 522t, (V1) 524, (V2) 700, (V2) 753
hyperbaric oxygen therapy (HBOT) and, (V1) 949
for transfusion, (V1) 1069
White willow bark, (V1) 823
WHO. *See* World Health Organization (WHO)
Whole blood, (V1) 1069
Whooping cough, (V1) 466
Will to live, (V1) 219–220, (V1) 220f
Windshield survey, (V1) 1119
Wing-tipped catheter, (V1) 1057, (V1) 1057f
Wisdom, in nursing informatics, (V1) 1139
Wisdom teeth, (V1) 592
Withdrawal (coitus interruptus), (V2) 642
Women, Infants, and Children (WIC), (V1) 701
Wong-Baker FACES pain rating scale, (V2) 611
Worden, William, (V1) 351t
Work, meaningful, (V1) 213, (V1) 260
Working phase of communication, (V1) 385
Work-life balance, (V1) 1200, (V1) 1200t
Workplace stress, (V1) 263–264
Workplace violence, (V1) 382–383
Work redesign, (V1) 22
Work-related social support groups, (V1) 386
Workstation privacy filters, (V1) 1150
World Health Organization (WHO), (V1) 208, (V1) 516
on trans-fats, (V1) 672–673
Wound culture, (V2) 700
Wounds
acute, (V1) 944
assessment
delegation of, (V1) 958–959
focused nursing history in, (V1) 952
focused physical examination in, (V1) 952–953, (V1) 954–956t, (V1) 956–958, (V1) 957t

guidelines and tools for, (V2) 694–699
laboratory data for, (V1) 958
care plan for, (V1) 959–974
asepsis measures, (V1) 972
cleansing, (V1) 960, (V1) 963–964
débridement, (V1) 966–967
with drainage devices, (V1) 965, (V1) 965f
dressings for, (V1) 967, (V1) 968–970t, (V1) 971–972, (V1) 971–972f
irrigation, (V1) 964–965
providing moist wound healing, (V1) 967
supporting and immobilizing, (V1) 972–973
using heat and cold therapy, (V1) 973–974, (V1) 973–974f
chronic, (V1) 945, (V1) 945f, (V1) 946t, (V1) 951–952, (V1) 951–952f
cleansing of, (V1) 960
closed, (V1) 944
closures for, (V1) 948–949, (V1) 949f, (V2) 680–681p
cold therapy for, (V2) 694
collaborative treatments for, (V1) 949
contamination or infection of, (V1) 943–944, (V1) 950
critical thinking and clinical judgment on, (V2) 701–702
defined, (V1) 944
dehiscence of, (V1) 950, (V1) 950f
depth and location of, (V1) 945–946
diagnostic testing of, (V2) 700
drainage from, (V1) 949, (V1) 956–957, (V1) 965, (V1) 965f, (V2) 690–691p
evidence-based practice on, (V1) 966
evisceration of, (V1) 950–951, (V1) 951f
extent and type of tissue in base of, (V1) 953, (V1) 956, (V1) 957t
fistula, (V1) 951, (V1) 951f
full-spectrum nursing model applied to, (V2) 701
healing of
complications of, (V1) 949–951, (V1) 950–951f
length of time for, (V1) 944–945
phases in, (V1) 947–948, (V1) 948f
types of, (V1) 946–947
heat therapy for, (V2) 693
hemorrhage from, (V1) 949–950
infected, (V1) 943–944, (V1) 945, (V1) 950
as postoperative complication, (V1) 1101t
irrigations of, (V1) 964
knowledge map on, (V2) 704
level of contamination of, (V1) 945
location of, (V1) 953
nursing diagnosis and, (V1) 959
obtaining culture by swab from, (V2) 659–661p
open, (V1) 944
size of, (V1) 953
skin integrity and, (V1) 944, (V1) 952

sterile irrigation of, (V2) 662–664p
surgical, (V1) 1079, (V1) 1079t
and tissue pain, (V1) 958
types of, (V1) 944–946, (V1) 945f, (V1) 945t, (V1) 946t, (V1) 953
full-thickness, (V1) 946
partial-thickness, (V1) 946
superficial, (V1) 946
untreated, (V1) 958
Writing, expressive, (V1) 826
Written discharge plans, (V1) 66
Written prescriptions, (V1) 625, (V1) 626

X

Xerosis, (V1) 941
X-ray, chest, (V2) 753, (V2) 763, (V2) 830

Y

Ylang-ylang, (V1) 786
Yoga, (V1) 260
Young adults
assessment of, (V1) 180
cardiovascular function in, (V1) 1021
development of
cognitive, (V1) 179
physical, (V1) 179
psychosocial, (V1) 179
exercise by, (V1) 180
health risk factors in families with, (V1) 297–298, (V1) 298f
implementation for, (V1) 180
loss in, (V1) 348
nutrition in, (V1) 686
obesity in, (V1) 180
physical examination of, (V1) 485–486
pulmonary function in, (V1) 981
returning to the next, (V1) 298
sexuality in, (V1) 888
sexually transmitted infections (STIs) in, (V1) 179–180
sleep requirements and characteristics in, (V1) 918t, (V1) 923
stressors in, (V1) 240b
substance abuse and violence among, (V1) 180
surgical risk in, (V1) 1078
Young-old adults, (V1) 190
assessment of, (V1) 200–201
implementation for, (V1) 201–202
Youth Risk Behavior Surveillance System (YRBSS), (V1) 887

Z

Zinc, (V1) 680t, (V1) 681t
skin and, (V1) 942
Zolpidem tartrate, (V1) 924
Z-track technique, (V1) 653